Fundamentals of Surgery for Physician Assistants

Sam Atallah • Jelena Dragoljevic
Editors

Fundamentals of Surgery for Physician Assistants

Springer

Editors
Sam Atallah
Department of Surgery, Piedmont Hospital
Mercer University School of Medicine
Macon, GA, USA

Jelena Dragoljevic
Telemed2U
Roseville, CA, USA

ISBN 978-3-032-21068-5 ISBN 978-3-032-21069-2 (eBook)
https://doi.org/10.1007/978-3-032-21069-2

This Springer imprint is published by the registered company Springer Nature Switzerland AG
The registered company address is: Gewerbestrasse 11, 6330 Cham, Switzerland

Foreword

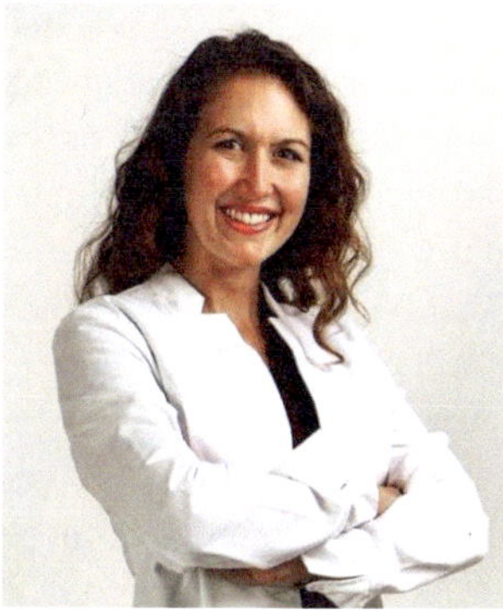

As a brand new second year PA Student, I clasped my freshly scrubbed hands together at the center of my chest sweating underneath my gown and gloves. My breath fogged up my face shield as I had not yet mastered the art of crimping my mask over my nose. My heart raced with excitement and an equal level of nervousness as I was in the operating room for the first time on my colorectal surgery rotation with Dr. Atallah. This was the moment I had been waiting for.

This was the moment of truth.

I would soon find out if I could handle the guts and glory of an exploratory laparotomy. The circulator pulled up a step, and I stepped up into my greatness as I stood shoulder to shoulder with surgeons, fellows, residents, and PA students around the patient. I intently listened to every detail during the timeout and attempted to calm my nervous system by deepening my breath. The incision was made and the smoke from electrocautery started to make me feel sick. I could feel the gaze of the surgeons and surgical technicians on me as I focused on the acute abdomen before me.

At that very moment I almost called it quits. Dr. Atallah asked me to give him my hands. He placed them inside of the abdomen and allowed me to run the bowel. He showed me what was normal and what was abnormal. He pointed out the multiple abscesses and how these distorted the once healthy anatomy.

In that very moment my entire life changed.

My love for surgery was born and the unshakable desires to learn, best serve our patients, and one day teach the medical community simultaneously were created.

This textbook will serve as a valuable resource throughout your career as a surgical PA. Give yourself permission to dive deep into studying the details of the anatomy illustrations. Immerse yourself in developing the skill set of fine-tuning your history and physical exam through the examples provided over these pages. But most importantly apply what you learned here within these chapters to the life-saving real experiences you will practice on the floor, in the clinic, and in the OR.

What you bring to the table as a surgical PA influences the entire surgical team. The role of the surgical PA has evolved into a vital cog in the wheel of modern surgical care, bridging the gap between patients, surgeons, and the healthcare team.

Often, surgical PAs are known as the common provider to the patient. From their first consultation, to rolling back to the OR to post-op follow-up evaluations, surgical PAs create continuity of care that alleviates the anxiety of the perioperative experience. As medicine continues to advance, so too must the knowledge and skills of those who assist in surgical procedures, manage perioperative care, and contribute to positive patient outcomes. Consider this textbook as your comprehensive resource, equipping you with the essential clinical, technical, and decision-making expertise necessary to excel in this dynamic field.

Written by experienced surgical professionals, this text covers fundamental principles as well as advanced concepts, ensuring that readers—from students to seasoned practitioners—can refine their proficiency in surgical techniques, patient management, and interdisciplinary collaboration. Each chapter is designed to provide not only foundational knowledge but also real-world application, preparing surgical PAs for the complexities of modern surgical practice while maintaining their own mental well-being.

As the demand for skilled surgical PAs grows, so does the need for high-quality educational materials tailored to this profession. Dr. Atallah genuinely prepared me well for my entrance into the surgical PA profession as my first, and honestly most influential preceptor. I know his meticulous involvement in this publication will prepare you equally as well. This textbook stands as a testament to the dedication and expertise of those who have contributed to its creation, offering a valuable guide for anyone pursuing excellence in surgical patient care.

It is with great enthusiasm that I introduce this resource. Confident that it will serve as an indispensable tool for surgical PAs committed to enhancing their knowledge, skills, and impact within the surgical team.

No matter what, never give up on being the best surgical PA you can be. The world needs your intelligent and wholehearted care.

President of The American Association of Surgical PAs

Michelle Dellene
Lombard, IL USA

Preface

There has been tremendous growth in the number of PAs in the healthcare, with more than 125,000 active PAs in the United States as of 2021. This has quadrupled since 1980. In addition, there are currently 11,000 PAs in training in the United States in 277 accredited programs.

With such considerable growth, projected to continue well into the future, it is important to tailor and curate information *for the PA*. Approximately 25% of PAs pursue a surgical specialty upon graduation, so it's imperative to have educational content geared toward the physician assistant, and other advanced practice providers (APPs) as well.

The growth in this provider market has outpaced our ability to provide appropriate didactic content, including textbooks that are made to educate PAs commensurate with *their* level of training and background. That has been the impetus behind *Fundamentals of Surgery for Physician Assistants.*

Fifty years ago, outside of the classroom, education was found in books and only books. Today, education has been highly enriched by electronic media, generative AI (Chat GPT, Open Evidence), video education, and a multitude of student-friendly aides. While all of this has improved one's ability to learn, it doesn't replace the value of books—which help teach principles and—when done properly—direct students and practicing PAs to *what's important.* While generative AI can be very useful and has proven itself increasingly accurate, student learners need *direction* and *guidance.* In other words, AI and new modes of education enhance formal education and texts, but don't replace them. For this reason, even 50 years from now, books will *still* have a role in education and PA training!

Fundamentals of Surgery for Physician Assistants carries several advantages. First, it is written with expert perspectives from 42 institutions, and 70 contributing authors, many of whom are PAs/APPs themselves… an aspect that ensures the APP's *point of view* is taken into consideration. Second, as editors, our main objective was to assure that the content was expressed in a manner suitable for the PA level of training, and that the content covers the critical information needed to be learned—especially for PAs during their clinical year who are preparing for the surgery End of Rotation (EOR) exam and, afterwards, for the PANCE. Finally, it was important to present this material in a way that could be more easily grasped. To this end, hundreds of tables, figures, and clinical images have been used throughout.

Although *Fundamentals of Surgery for Physician Assistants* was designed specifically with the PA in mind, there is obviously crossover information suitable for all APPs. Indeed, several of the contributing authors are PAs and NPs, which strengthens this resource, and broadens its applicability. Ultimately, we hope that this becomes a valuable learning aide for all student learners and that it becomes integral to formal education programs.

Macon, GA, USA
Raleigh, NC, USA

Sam Atallah
Jelena Dragoljevic

Acknowledgments

The Editors are grateful for the invaluable contributions of the following:

Kiruthika Andappan
Casey Arlotta
Olivia Atallah
Brooke Bailey
Mandy Lane
Sergio W. Larach
Jenna Hendler
Darlene Buehrer
Noemi Cabrera
Anna Flint
Alex Garcia
Hannah Gordon
Patricia Gutierrez
Brittyn Hamer
Brianne Kimura
Annamarie Kondek
Ayleen Martinez
Earl Mullis
Katerina 'Kat' Nelson
Harold Neyra
Chelsea Ramos
Sophie Ruiz
Natasia Schaefer
Emily Smithies
Kristopher Spring
Yami Sousa
Tatiana Villante
Tom Woodyard

Whether large or small, your contributions helped to make this book a better product!

Sam Atallah
Jelena Dragoljevic

Contents

Editors and Contributors

About the Editors

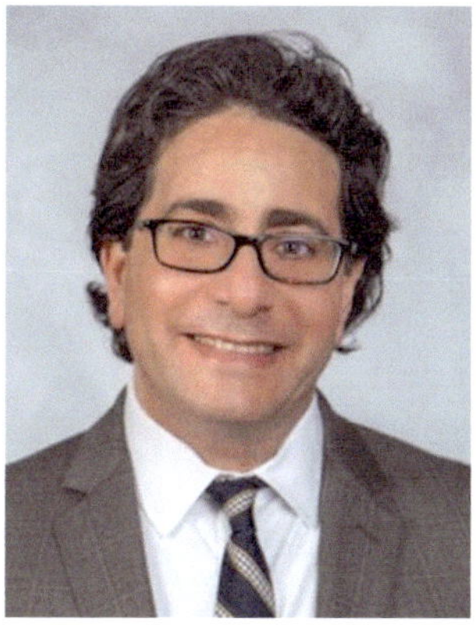

Sam Atallah, MD earned his medical degree from UT-Southwestern Medical School (Dallas, TX) with residency and fellowship training in general and colorectal surgery completed at Texas Medical Center (Houston, TX). Since 2011, he has been a preceptor for PAs during their core general surgery rotations year-round. He has precepted over 200 PA students from Nova Southeastern University (Orlando), South College (Atlanta), and Mercer University (Atlanta).

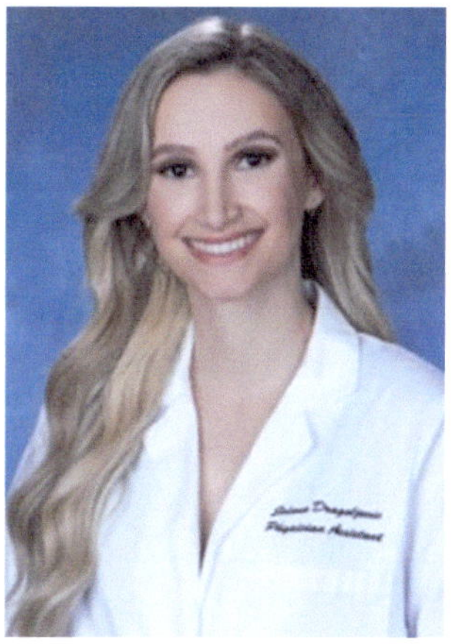

Jelena Dragoljevic, PA-C earned her Bachelor of Science in Health Sciences from the University of Central Florida and her Master of Science in Physician Assistant Studies from Nova Southeastern University in Orlando. She has experience in both urology and endocrinology. Her contributions to the text aim to reinforce the clinical relevance of the material for PA students and practicing PAs.

Contributors

Oladapo O. Akinmoladun Madigan Army Medical Center, Tacoma, WA, USA

Amber Amick Atrium Health/Sanger Heart & Vascular Institute, Charlotte, NC, USA

Ali Amirkhosravi Medical Laboratory Sciences, Department of Biomedical Sciences and Technology, AdventHealth University, Orlando, FL, USA

Cynthia Araradian Department of Surgery, Oregon Health and Science University, Portland, OR, USA

Frank R. Arko III Vascular and Endovascular Surgery, Atrium Health/Sanger Heart & Vascular Institute, Charlotte, NC, USA

Sam Atallah Department of Surgery, Piedmont Hospital, Mercer University School of Medicine, Macon, GA, USA

Goran Augustin University Hospital Centre Zagreb, Zagreb, Croatia
School of Medicine University of Zagreb, Zagreb, Croatia

Ali Azizzadeh Cedars-Sinai Medical Center, Los Angeles, CA, USA

Donna Bahroloomi Cedars-Sinai Medical Center, Los Angeles, CA, USA

Jessica Barbosa Department of Trauma and General Surgery, Legacy Health, Legacy Medical Group, Portland, OR, USA
Department of Emergency Medicine, OHSU - Hillsboro Medical Center, Portland, United States

Ronald Barbosa Department of Trauma and General Surgery, Legacy Health, Legacy Medical Group, Portland, OR, USA

Rishi Batra Division of Colorectal Surgery, Department of Surgery, University of Nebraska Medical Center, Omaha, NE, USA

Holly Bonnette, NP Department of General and Gastrointestinal Surgery, Massachusetts General Hospital, Boston, MA, USA

Liliana Bordeianou, MD Department of General and Gastrointestinal Surgery, Massachusetts General Hospital, Boston, MA, USA

Colette Brottman, PA-C Department of Surgery, University of Chicago—Medicine, Chicago, IL, USA

Richard F. Burgess Department of Physician Assistant Program, South College, Orlando, FL, USA

Melissa Camp Division of Surgical Oncology, Breast Surgery Section, Johns Hopkins University School of Medicine, Baltimore, MD, USA

Steven Capece Department of Colon and Rectal Surgery, Kelsey Sebold Medical Clinic, Pearland, TX, USA

Mark Chaet Florida State University, Medical School, Orlando Regional Campus, Tallahassee, FL, USA

Hannah Chelliah Reproductive Endocrinology, Brown Fertility, Orlando, FL, USA

B. Bobby Chiong SBH Health System, Department of Interventional Radiology, Bronx, NY, USA

William Cobb Department of General Surgery, AdventHealth Orlando, Orlando, FL, USA

Jennifer S. Davids Department of Surgery, Boston Medical Center, Boston University Chobanian and Avedisian School of Medicine, Boston, MA, USA

Rafaela de Araújo Molteni Moretti Pontifícia Universidade Católica do Paraná (PUCPR), Health Sciences Postgraduate Program, IBD outpatient clinics, Curitiba, PR, Brazil

Kathleen Donais Vanderbilt University Medical Center, Nashville, TN, USA

Bozana Dragoljevic Department of Pharmacy, Veterans Affairs Hospital, Daytona, FL, USA

Jelena Dragoljevic Telemed2U, Roseville, CA, USA

Elizabeth Dunham Department of Neurosurgery, Mayo Clinic, Jacksonville, FL, USA

Craig P. Eberson Department of Orthopaedic Surgery, Brown University, Warren Alpert Medical School, Providence, RI, USA

Mohamed El Khourassani AdventHealth – Orlando, Department of Medical Oncology, Orlando, FL, USA

Anthony L. Estrera Department of Cardiothoracic and Vascular Surgery, McGovern Medical School at UTHealth Houston, Houston, TX, USA

Paula Ferrada, MD, FACS, FCCM, MAMSE Inova Health System, Fairfax, VA, USA

Landon Fike Vanderbilt University Medical Center, Nashville, TN, USA

Caitlin A. Fitzgerald Department of Surgery, Division of Trauma, Bariatrics, and Acute Care Surgery, Baylor College of Medicine, Houston, TX, USA

Neil Floch Department of Surgery, Yale School of Medicine, New Haven, CT, USA

Greenwich Hospital, Greenwich, CT, USA

Susana Fortich Department of Surgery, University of Texas Medical Branch, Galveston, TX, USA

W. Christopher Fox Department of Neurosurgery, Mayo Clinic, Jacksonville, FL, USA

Katherine Frederick-Dyer Vanderbilt University Medical Center, Nashville, TN, USA

Matthew Fuglestad Division of Colorectal Surgery, Department of Surgery, University of Nebraska Medical Center, Omaha, NE, USA

Trent Gabriel Atrium Health/Sanger Heart & Vascular Institute, Charlotte, NC, USA

Mariem Galuia AdventHealth – Orlando, Department of Medical Oncology, Orlando, FL, USA

John R. Gerke Department of Physician Assistant Program, South College, Orlando, FL, USA

Julia Gillette Department of Orthopaedic Surgery, Brown University, Warren Alpert Medical School, Providence, RI, USA

Bhuwan Giri Digestive Disease Institute, Cleveland Clinic Foundation, Cleveland, OH, USA

Martha Grajewski Department of Surgery, University of Connecticut, University of Connecticut Health Center, Farmington, CT, USA

Renee Walker Green Department of General Surgery, McGovern Medical School, Houston, TX, USA

Haley Harris Department of Surgery, NewYork-Presbyterian Hospital, Weill Cornell Medicine, New York, NY, USA

Shelby Harris Department of General Surgery, AdventHealth Orlando, Orlando, FL, USA

Heitham T. Hassoun Cedars-Sinai Medical Center, Los Angeles, CA, USA

Michaiah Nichole Hughes Shock Trauma Center, University of Maryland Medical Center, Baltimore, MD, USA

Tam T. T. Huynh Department Cardiovascular Surgery, Houston Methodist Hospital Houston, Houston, TX, USA

Sandra A. Hyder Department of Graduate Studies, Cizik School of Nursing at UTHealth Houston, Houston, TX, USA

Lillian S. Kao Department of General Surgery, McGovern Medical School, Houston, TX, USA

Danielle Kohler Department of General Surgery, Cleveland Clinic, Cleveland, OH, USA

Christopher Kolokythas Shock Trauma Center, University of Maryland Medical Center, Baltimore, MD, USA

Callan Kosnik Multicare Health Network, Tacoma, WA, USA

Paulo Gustavo Kotze Pontifícia Universidade Católica do Paraná (PUCPR), Health Sciences Postgraduate Program, IBD outpatient clinics, Curitiba, PR, Brazil

Rosemary Kozar Shock Trauma Center, University of Marylnd School of Medicine, Baltimore, MD, USA

Sean J. Langenfeld Division of Colorectal Surgery, Department of Surgery, University of Nebraska Medical Center, Omaha, NE, USA

Michelle Le Florida State University, Medical School, Orlando Regional Campus, Tallahassee, FL, USA

Chelsea Liles Department of Physician Assistant Program, South College, Orlando, FL, USA

Mary Lou Department of Orthopaedic Surgery, Brown University, Warren Alpert Medical School, Providence, RI, USA

Carlina A. Maria, DHA MassGeneral Brigham, Boston, MA, USA

Stephanie Martinez-Ugarte Department of General Surgery, McGovern Medical School, Houston, TX, USA

Jeffrey Matthews, MD, FACS Department of Surgery, University of Chicago—Medicine, Chicago, IL, USA

David W. McFadden Department of Surgery, University of Connecticut, University of Connecticut Health Center, Farmington, CT, USA

Jonathan Messing, DNP, MBA, ACNP-BC Inova Health System, Fairfax, VA, USA

Kimberly Miles Department of General Surgery, Cleveland Clinic, Cleveland, OH, USA

Steven D. Miller Department of Thoracic Surgery, Oklahoma Heart Hospital, Oklahoma City, OK, USA

Sarah L. Mims Division of Pediatric Surgery, Department of Surgery, University of Texas Medical Branch, Galveston, TX, USA

Abdul Mohammed Advanced Endoscopy Fellow, Center for Interventional Endoscopy, Advent Health Orlando, Orlando, FL, USA

Joseph Moschella Department of Orthopaedic Surgery, Brown University, Warren Alpert Medical School, Providence, RI, USA

Sara Myers Department of Surgery, Boston Medical Center, Boston University Chobanian and Avedisian School of Medicine, Boston, MA, USA

Mariam Naveed Gastroenterology and Hepatology Fellowship, AdventHealth Medical Group Gastroenterology Altamonte Springs, Altamonte Springs, FL, USA

Melina Norberto, PA-C Lakeland, FL, USA

Annabella Olson Department Cardiovascular Surgery, Houston Methodist Hospital Houston, Houston, TX, USA

Marcus Oosenbrug Department of Colorectal Surgery, Medstar Georgetown University Hospital, Washington, DC, USA

Roy Phitayakorn UIC College of Medicine, Chicago, IL, USA

Division of Surgical Oncology, Department of Surgery, UI Health, Chicago, IL, USA

Sunshine Pille Multicare Health Network, Tacoma, WA, USA

Joseph Portoghese Department of General Surgery, AdventHealth Orlando, Orlando, FL, USA

Vincent Pretorius Department of ENT, University of Cape Town, Cape Town, South Africa

Ravi S. Radhakrishnan Division of Pediatric Surgery, Department of Surgery, University of Texas Medical Branch, Galveston, TX, USA

Laila Rashidi Multicare Health Network, Tacoma, WA, USA

Sreelakshmi Reddivari Department of Surgery, University of Connecticut, University of Connecticut Health Center, Farmington, CT, USA

Samantha J. Rivard Department of Surgery, Boston Medical Center, Boston University Chobanian and Avedisian School of Medicine, Boston, MA, USA

Brittney J. Roberts Department of Thoracic Surgery, Oklahoma Heart Hospital, Oklahoma City, OK, USA

Michael J. Rosen Department of General Surgery, Cleveland Clinic, Cleveland, OH, USA

Hunter Ruokonen College of Health Professions and Sciences, University of Central Florida, Orlando, FL, USA

Shaghayegh Sabbaghan Kermani Department of Surgery, Massachusetts General Hospital, Harvard Medical School, Boston, MA, USA

Heather Sales Physician Assistant Department, Nova Southeastern University, Orlando, FL, USA

Michael J. Snyder Section of Colon and Rectal Surgery, McGovern School of Medicine, Houston, TX, USA

Scott R. Steele Digestive Disease Institute, Cleveland Clinic Foundation, Cleveland, OH, USA

Marco Swanson Dermatology and Plastic Surgery of Arizona, Tucson, AZ, USA

Pooja Thyvalappil Department of Orthopaedic Surgery, Brown University, Warren Alpert Medical School, Providence, RI, USA

Tracy Totten Atrium Health/Sanger Heart & Vascular Institute, Charlotte, NC, USA

Tammie Trinh Shock Trauma Center, University of Maryland Medical Center, Baltimore, MD, USA

Lisa M. Truett Vanderbilt University Medical Center, Nashville, TN, USA

V. Liana Tsikitis Department of Surgery, Oregon Health and Science University, Portland, OR, USA

Brian Untch Department of Surgery, Memorial Sloan Kettering Cancer Center, New York, NY, USA

Stacy Laack Valentine, DMSc, PA-C Physician Assistant Department, Nova Southeastern University, Orlando, FL, USA

Maura Walsh Department of Surgery, Oregon Health and Science University, Portland, OR, USA

Steven D. Wexner Department of Colorectal Surgery, Medstar Georgetown University Hospital, Washington, DC, USA

Miranda Wood Department of General Surgery, McGovern Medical School, Houston, TX, USA

Heather Yeo Department of Surgery, NewYork-Presbyterian Hospital, Weill Cornell Medicine, New York, NY, USA

Ahmed Zakari AdventHealth – Orlando, Department of Medical Oncology, Orlando, FL, USA

Jana Zeineddine, MD Department of General and Gastrointestinal Surgery, Massachusetts General Hospital, Boston, MA, USA

The Clinical Rotation Experience for Physician Assistant Students

1

Stacy Laack Valentine and Heather Sales

This chapter will discuss the clinical rotation experience during Physician Assistant/Associate (PA) training, including an overview of the clinical year, professionalism on rotations, and strategies for success on the surgical rotation.

Overview of the Clinical Year

The clinical year represents a pivotal stage in the education of PA students. It marks the transition from the didactic, classroom environment to hands-on patient care in real-world clinical settings. In the clinical year, the technical skills learned will merge with medical knowledge and create growth. Initially, navigating the world outside the classroom may seem challenging, but with time, this environment will become more familiar.

PA students develop competence in the following categories developed by the American Academy of Physician Associates (AAPA): knowledge for practice, interpersonal and communication skills, person-centered care, interprofessional collaboration, professionalism and ethics, practice-based learning and quality improvement, and society and population health [1]. These competencies are learned during PA training and continually practiced throughout a PA's career.

Among the most vital competencies emphasized in the clinical year is professionalism, a cornerstone of effective health care practice. Professional behavior not only shapes the patient-provider relationship but also determines how PA students are perceived by preceptors, patients, and future employers. This is imperative to success in all rotations; however, professionalism is particularly critical in surgical rotations, where teamwork, precision, and high-pressure decision-making are constant.

S. L. Valentine (✉) · H. Sales
Physician Assistant Department, Nova Southeastern University, Orlando, FL, USA
e-mail: SLaack@nova.edu; heather.sales@noval.edu

According to the Accreditation Review Commission on Education for the Physician Assistant (ARC-PA), there are required rotation settings that each PA student must gain experience in during the clinical year [2]. These core rotations include Internal Medicine, Family Medicine, Pediatric Medicine, Women's Health (prenatal care and gynecology), Surgery, Behavioral Health, and Emergency Medicine. PA programs may also offer selective or elective rotations, in which the student can choose additional specialties, including but not limited to Cardiology, Pulmonology, Endocrinology, Dermatology, Orthopedics, etc.

Each rotation must have a preceptor, or someone who is an expert in that medical setting, who will educate and guide the PA student. Preceptors take on this role to share knowledge. They want students to learn as much as possible about their field of practice. They will help piece together book knowledge with real-world medicine and how to navigate between the two. Tips and tricks will be shared during each rotation. Preceptors are expected to provide real-time feedback and facilitate learning through supervised patient care, case discussions, and procedural instruction. The goals of each rotation include improving diagnostic acumen, enhancing patient communication, and demonstrating increasing autonomy as clinical experience accumulates. Students will practice these skills and develop competency upon completion of their clinical year.

Professionalism on Rotations

Professionalism in PA education encompasses ethical conduct, accountability, communication skills, and respect for patients and colleagues. The AAPA defines professionalism through a code of conduct that emphasizes integrity, compassion, excellence, and respect for the dignity of others [1]. These principles must be evident in every aspect of clinical training, from patient interactions to interprofessional collaboration.

S. Atallah, J. Dragoljevic (eds.), *Fundamentals of Surgery for Physician Assistants*,
https://doi.org/10.1007/978-3-032-21069-2_1

On the rotation, professionalism is practiced and evaluated. The preceptor has an obligation to ensure that PA students are held to a high professionalism standard. Students must become proficient in this skill upon completion of their clinical year. Assessment tools, such as the preceptor evaluation, play a critical role in evaluating professionalism. The student should know the learning outcomes regarding professionalism for each rotation and seek opportunities to demonstrate professional behavior. The rotation setting is also an excellent time to ask questions about behaviors and what is expected in that setting. Although the student is expected to demonstrate professional behaviors during the clinical year, this is also a time to learn and grow. Making mistakes is a part of the learning process and can be seen as a positive opportunity, as long as the student remembers to humbly accept criticism and aim to demonstrate improvement in areas where they are lacking, especially professionalism. Early intervention and remediation of unprofessional behaviors are ideal. This will ensure successful proficiency in the competency.

Professionalism in the clinical year can be more challenging as it is not fully encapsulated in the didactic year. Some professionalism skills carried over from the didactic year include professional dress and respect. This is practiced and perfected during the first year of PA education, but is much different in the clinical year. On rotations, professional dress is defined by the setting in which it takes place. Different attire is often seen in a surgical ward versus an outpatient clinic, and it is essential for the PA student to be aware of what is expected. Business casual and a white coat are accepted in most clinical settings, whereas scrubs are accepted in the surgical setting. Asking the preceptor before the rotation begins is the best way to ensure the proper professional attire is worn.

Respecting all health care team members is a significant part of professionalism on rotations. This is achieved through actions and words. Using proper etiquette, such as saying please and thank you, and addressing others on the health care team with appropriate titles (doctor, nurse, etc.) is professional behavior. Asking others how they wished to be addressed is key to being professional. In the surgical suite, understanding the roles of the health care team is imperative. Communicating to ensure a clear understanding of everyone's role during the procedure is essential to prevent a break in the sterile field and detrimental mistakes.

Although professionalism is critical in all rotations, surgical rotations often rank among the most demanding and formative experiences during the PA clinical year. These rotations expose students to the operating room (OR), perioperative patient care, and surgical pathology. Given the intensity of surgical training environments, professionalism takes on heightened importance.

In the surgical setting, PA students must navigate unique responsibilities, such as assisting in the OR, managing postoperative patients, and participating in surgical rounds [3]. These duties demand technical competence, emotional intelligence, and interprofessional collaboration, requiring the PA student to maintain professionalism. In this environment, PA students encounter ethical challenges, including informed consent, end-of-life care, and intraoperative decision-making. Professionalism in surgery involves not only adhering to rules and showing respect but also advocating for patient-centered care under challenging circumstances. Clear communication and collaboration with the entire health care team are imperative while maintaining respect and being effective during the high-stress environment of surgery.

Strategies for Success on the Surgical Rotation

The transition to full-time clinical care on rotations can be overwhelming. PA students often face long hours, emotionally charged situations, and steep learning curves. These stressors can challenge even the most resilient students. Maintaining a positive mindset is an excellent strategy for success during the clinical year. PA students should approach each rotation without judgment and with an open mind. Students should understand that each classmate has a different experience on rotations. Different personalities will meld or clash, so a rotation that many love may be disliked by others and vice versa. PA students should begin rotations as if they are guests in a new home. Proper introductions, including learning the names of the health care team and treating everyone with respect, are key to a successful rotation experience.

PA students must understand that, like all experiences, not all rotations will be well-liked or enjoyed. Different people have different preferences when it comes to specialties. However, during the rotation, students should treat it as though it is their primary interest. Remember that the professionals in that field have chosen it and enjoy their work.

All rotations will offer different experiences for each PA student. Settings also differ, such as inpatient versus outpatient care. Although each rotation has its own way of functioning, the surgical setting operates like a well-oiled machine. Each member of the health care team plays a vital role within the OR, and they work alongside one another almost as if choreographed. Understand the PA student's role by discussing expectations with the preceptor before entering the OR.

Preparation for surgical rotations requires mastery of basic surgical principles, including sterile technique, anatomy, and documentation. The ARC-PA emphasizes that students must be adequately prepared to contribute meaningfully to patient care in the surgical setting [2]. Punctuality, preparedness, and a proactive attitude are essential for success in the OR.

There are key strategies and professional expectations for a PA student on a surgery rotation (see Table 1.1). PA students are expected to know what needs to be completed before reporting the following day. Does the rounding of admitted patients need to be completed first? What is the expected arrival time of the PA student if the first surgery is at 7:00 am? Is there any charting or paperwork that needs to be completed prior to the start of the day? The PA student needs to be fully aware of the expectations before surgery. During the surgery is not the time to discuss the preceptor's expectations of the student.

This table outlines key professional expectations for PA students during surgical rotations. It serves as a practical guide to promote effective learning, patient safety, and interprofessional collaboration in the surgical setting.

Table 1.1 Dos and don'ts for PA students on surgical rotation [4–6]

Category	Do	Don't
Professionalism	Do introduce oneself to all team members; maintain a respectful tone and demeanor	Do not be passive or disengaged; do not gossip or use informal language
In the operating room	Do arrive early, review the case, and maintain sterile technique	Do not touch sterile fields if not scrubbed; do not speak unnecessarily
Preparation	Do study anatomy and procedures prior to surgeries	Do not show up unprepared or guess when uncertain
Patient care	Do assist with exams, documentation, and rounds under supervision	Do not overstep the student role; do not violate patient confidentiality
Communication	Do speak clearly; confirm instructions when needed	Do not interrupt or assume; do not speak beyond the student scope
Learning attitude	Do ask thoughtful questions and seek regular feedback	Do not take feedback personally; do not display disinterest
Teamwork	Do offer assistance to the surgical team; express appreciation to all roles	Do not act entitled or ignore the instructions of any team member
Documentation	Do follow charting guidelines and supervisor instructions closely	Do not chart independently unless explicitly directed
Appearance	Do wear clean scrubs, closed-toe shoes, and display a visible ID badge	Do not wear fragrances or bring food/drinks into the OR
Body language	Do maintain professional posture and attentiveness	Do not slouch, cross arms, or look at phone during clinical hours

The student should obtain a list of the surgeries scheduled for the next day. They should use their time at home to prepare and review the surgeries planned for the following day. This includes understanding the potential complications that could arise from the patient's underlying conditions. The student should practice the necessary skills for the procedure, focusing on the suturing techniques that may be used for wound closure.

The surgical rotation will involve long hours and continuous standing for the PA student. Now is not the time to complain about the demanding hours or physical fatigue. The health care team in the room understands the intensity of the surgical setting. The PA student can best prepare for these stressors in the surgical environment by having a pair of compression socks, comfortable closed-toed shoes, a good night's rest, and adequate nourishment at the start of each day.

Every rotation, whether enjoyable or not, serves as a learning experience and an opportunity for growth. The medical knowledge and skills gained during any clinical rotation are often transferable and applicable to other areas of practice. For example, assessing and treating a patient in a behavioral health setting can enhance a PA student's ability to care for a behavioral health patient during an emergency medicine rotation. Suturing a patient in the surgical rotation can help a student become more proficient in suturing, thereby providing better care in the urgent care setting. The goal is to absorb as much knowledge as possible from each rotation experience. The preceptors will share invaluable tips and insights to help shape PAs into competent practicing providers.

Reflection and self-evaluation are key components of rotation success. Students are encouraged to set personal goals, seek feedback regularly, and engage in reflective writing or discussions to process their clinical experiences. These practices not only enhance learning but also reinforce professional growth.

Conclusion

The clinical year of PA education is a transformative period that demands the integration of knowledge, technical skills, and professional behaviors. Professionalism, rooted in ethical conduct and patient-centered care, is fundamental to the success of PA students and the quality of care they deliver. Surgical rotations, although challenging, offer rich opportunities for growth in these areas. By successfully completing the clinical year, PA students will develop the professionalism necessary for lifelong success in medicine.

References

1. American Academy of Physician Associates. Competencies for the physician associate profession. AAPA. 2025. https://www.aapa.org/career-central/employer-resources/employing-a-pa/competencies-physician-associate-profession/. Accessed 28 Apr 2025.
2. Accreditation Review Commission on Education for the Physician Assistant. Accreditation Standards for Physician Assistant Education, 5th ed. ARC-PA; 2024. https://www.arc-pa.org/wp-content/uploads/2024/07/Standards-5th-Ed-July-2024.pdf. Accessed 20 Apr 2025.
3. Davis CH, DiLalla GA, Perati SR, Lee JS, Oropallo AR, Reyna CR, Cannada LK, Association of Women Surgeons Publications Committee. A review of professionalism in surgery. Proc (Bayl Univ Med Cent). 2024;37(6):993–7. https://doi.org/10.1080/08998280.2024.2403375.
4. Murphy B. Ready for the OR? 5 tips for your surgical clerkship rotation. American Medical Association. November 29, 2023. https://www.ama-assn.org. Accessed 1 May 2025.
5. American Academy of Physician Associates. Tackling Clinical Rotations. https://www.aapa.org. Accessed 1 May 2025.
6. Springer Publishing. Preparing for your surgical rotation. https://connect.springerpub.com. Accessed 1 May 2025.

Basics of Anesthesia and Surgery

2

Sam Atallah

Introduction

This chapter is divided into two parts. *Part 1* provides a review of the fundamentals and theory of anesthesia, including important applied principles of physiology. It contains ideas that a surgical physician assistant (PA) should master to excel in this field. In *Part 2,* practical aspects of surgery are detailed, geared for the PA in training and in surgical practice.

Part 1: Theory and Principles

The Air We Breathe

It is important to know the concentration of oxygen (O_2) in the atmosphere that we are breathing. This is fundamental to *everything* in anesthesia care, ventilator management, and for understanding many aspects in medicine. **The concentration of O_2 is 21%** (technically 20.9% at sea level). *This is essential to know, so commit it to memory!* In the medical arena, we refer to atmospheric O_2 as **"room air"** and you will often see this abbreviated as **RA**.

Well, if our atmosphere is only 21% O_2, then what is the composition of the remaining 79%? The answer is *mainly* **nitrogen.** Yes, there are other trace gases, but for our purposes we do not need to worry about them, but the ratio and composition of atmospheric oxygen and nitrogen is **fundamental**.

S. Atallah (✉)
Department of Surgery, Piedmont Hospital, Mercer University School of Medicine, Macon, GA, USA
e-mail: atallah@post.harvard.edu

Measuring Oxygen

Pulse oximetry measures **oxygen saturation,** often abbreviated as **SpO_2** or **"O_2-sats."** Note that SpO_2 is *not* the same as oxygen concentration in the air we are breathing at all. Typical SpO_2 for most healthy adults range from 94% to 100% on RA (21%). For patients who are on supplemental oxygen and for whom we are measuring and recording their O_2 sats, it is important to note what percent of oxygen the patient is breathing, as it will be greater than 21% and may be as high as 100% for ventilated patients. We term the amount of O_2 a person is breathing the *fraction of inspired oxygen*, often abbreviated **FiO_2**.

Arterial blood gas **(ABG)**, measured in millimeters of mercury (mmHg), is yet another way to assess oxygenation. Whether we measure a person's arterial blood *gas* (i.e., the *partial pressure* of oxygen, **pO_2**) or their oxygen saturations via pulse oximetry (SpO_2), we have to *also know the FiO_2 at the time the measurement was taken.* Note that pO_2 *differs* from O_2-sats and can even exceed 100 in certain conditions. The normal range for arterial O_2 ranges from 75 to 100 mmHg. A good rule of thumb is that a **pO_2 of 60 correlates with an O_2 sat of 90%**. This information is summarized in Table 2.1.

Table 2.1 Important terms related to oxygenation

Core term	Normal value	Common abbreviation	Special notes
Atmospheric oxygen (O_2)	21%	RA, "room air"	Value approximate, at sea level
Atmospheric nitrogen (N)	79%	n/a	Value approximate, at sea level
Oxygen saturation	94–100%	SpO_2, "O2-sats," "sats"	Obtained by pulse oximetry
Arterial blood gas oxygen	75–100 mmHG	Arterial O_2, pO_2	Represents the partial pressure of oxygen in the blood
Fraction of inspired oxygen	21–100%	FiO_2	Fundamental value to know for interpreting oxygenation

S. Atallah, J. Dragoljevic (eds.), *Fundamentals of Surgery for Physician Assistants*,
https://doi.org/10.1007/978-3-032-21069-2_2

Why Do We Breathe?

This seems like such a silly question. But is it? We have to take some time to *really* understand the answer. Of course, we need O_2 to live, and this is the typical answer given by most PA students when asked. But is the need for O_2 what controls our *urge* to breathe? Is it what makes us exhale and take in a breath?

Let us think about this for a second. Imagine you are breathing in a room, as you are now. We just learned that RA = 21% FiO_2. Now suppose we remove all the oxygen in that room so now we are breathing an FiO_2 of 0%. How would you react to this? Would you breathing become erratic and would your respiratory rate increase? Would you feel like you were drowning? Would you feel like you could not breathe and that you were "suffocating"?

The answer is *you would not feel or experience these things.* Instead, you would continue to breathe normally *almost* as if nothing has changed. Slowly you would become confused and unable to focus, and eventually you would succumb to anoxia. Why is this the case?

Let us try and understand why you do not feel as if you are "suffocating" when there is no oxygen in the room. The reason is that respiratory drive is dependent on **blood CO_2 concentration (not blood O_2 concentration)**. As long as you are able to clear CO_2 out of your body, you do not feel any sort of respiratory distress, at least not initially. Even though there was no oxygen in the room in this example, you were still able to clear the CO_2 out through normal exhalation. *The act of clearing out CO_2 from our body is called* ***ventilation*** *and bringing in O_2 is called* ***oxygenation.*** These are the most important functions of the pulmonary system, and we have to understand that they are *completely separate* from one another.

To summarize, as long as we are able to ventilate (breathe off CO_2) we will not feel like we are "starving for oxygen," even if we become dangerously hypoxic. **Simply put, we do not "notice" if our O_2 levels drop, <u>we only notice when our CO2 level builds up</u>**. Real world scenarios that exemplify this principle, include carbon monoxide (CO) poisoning (were CO competitively binds to hemoglobin; with a binding affinity 200X that of O_2) leading to hypoxia, but *not* difficulty ventilating. Patients who experience CO poisoning do not feel short of breath and are essentially "unaware" of the condition. As another example, perhaps everyone who has traveled on a plane has heard the flight attendants say: *in case of sudden cabin depressurization … don the oxygen mask.* This universal aviation safety instruction is emphasized because there is *no sensation of, or awareness for a hypoxic environment* during the unlikely event that [the partial pressure of] oxygen falls due to sudden cabin depressurization or similar emergency.

While the main effects of hypoxia manifest as confusion, restlessness, dizziness, and headache, there can be noticeable alterations in ventilation—namely, the respiratory rate (**RR**) would increase and/or the tidal volume, $\mathbf{T_v}$ (i.e., the amount of air inhaled with each breath). This happens not because your body senses it needs more oxygen, but rather because when oxygen is not available, aerobic cellular respiration is not possible, and we resort to *anerobic* respiration, which is much less efficient (generates few ATP) and also generates **lactic acid**, dropping blood pH, which as we shall see is corrected by breathing off more CO_2—clinically evident as *tachypnea.*

Acid-Base and pH Regulation

The regulation of blood pH is more tightly controlled than anything else. Our body strives to maintain control over pH, and it is done primarily through respiratory *ventilation.* Blood pH is often given as a narrow range of normal, but we can just use the number **7.45 as normal.** At this pH, the **acid dissociation constant**, or **pKa**, is optimal for most enzymes. In plain terms, this is the pH at which most cellular enzymes are working at their best.

Although a pH of 7.0 is technically "neutral," our body would *not* tolerate this low pH relative to *our* normal, and in medicine, this would be considered *extremely acidic.* A pH level of 6.99, for example, is rarely survivable.

This is quite interesting, because there are parts within the human body that can tolerate high acidity (e.g., low pH), such as the stomach which has a pH of ~2. Furthermore, many beverages we consume are actually acidic (pH 2.52–5.0). Despite this, **our blood pH is very tightly regulated and is kept at ~7.45**. There are many conditions that can lead to pH derangements. The most relevant of which are *hemorrhagic shock and sepsis.*

pH Buffering

Recall that the most important pH buffering system in our body is the **bicarbonate buffering system**. Bicarbonate (HCO_3^-), or *bicarb* for short, is an anion that acts as a *weak base.* By definition, a **base** is a molecule that can *accept* a proton (hydrogen, H^+) and the definition of an **acid** is any molecule that can *donate* a proton (H^+). When blood pH drops, bicarb springs into action, "mopping up" excess H^+ and thereby preventing acidosis. When the blood pH is high (alkalotic), the weak acid carbonic acid (H_2CO_3) donates hydrogen, in a reversible fashion, as shown:

$$H_2CO_3 \leftrightharpoons H^+ + HCO_3^-$$

This is the metabolic side of the **acid-base equation**. In instances of lactic acidosis, bicarb is our body's way of "mopping up acid" so that pH can be normalized. While this equation is fundamental in medicine and in the medical management of the surgical patient, it is not complete. What about the respiratory side of the acid-base equation?

You have probably learned that in respiratory acidosis, the pCO_2 is elevated. But how exactly does an elevated carbon dioxide lead to a drop in blood pH? The answer is that carbon dioxide combines with water to form carbonic acid, as follows:

$$H_2O + CO_2 \leftrightharpoons H_2CO_3$$

Thus, the higher the consideration of CO_2, the more the reaction shifts towards the right. Remember that carbonic acid is a weak acid, and the more carbonic acid that forms, the more likely it is to donate a hydrogen proton. Thus, we get something that looks like this:

$$H_2O + CO_2 \leftrightharpoons H_2CO_3 \leftrightharpoons H^+$$

Do you now understand why an increase in CO_2 leads to an increase in acidity? We can now combine the respiratory side of the equation and the metabolic side of the equation into one, as follows:

$$\text{[Respiratory] } H_2O + CO_2 \leftrightharpoons H_2CO_3 \leftrightharpoons H^+ + HCO_3^- \text{ [Metabolic]}$$

This is probably one of the most important general chemistry equations in applied medicine and physiology, and it is fundamental understanding acid-base. It is important to understand that the metabolic and respiratory sides of the equation are **connected.** You may have also learned about, for example, *compensated* states; in reality *it is all connected through a single equation.*

Examine the above acid-base equation closely. How do you think we can *control pH?* It turns out we really have **only one way to control pH,** and it is through *ventilation.* Let us run through examples so that this makes more sense. Let us suppose a patient has a metabolic acidosis and the pH is 7.27. What would our body's reaction be to this? Certainly, bicarb would work to mop up as much hydrogen (acid) as possible, but there would be a limit to this and eventually we would run out of buffer, leading to what is often referred to as a **base deficit.** So now what? Well, we need to drive the equation towards the left, which is done by *lowering carbon dioxide,* which is done by **breathing faster and/or deeper**. This will thus *compensate* for the acidity caused by the metabolic side of the equation. *This is why patients who are acidotic present with tachypnea and often dyspnea.* So, ***ventilation is our way of controlling blood pH.***

Did you know that when patients are ventilated in the ICU, one of the most important uses of the ventilator is to help *control* blood pH? Indeed, for infirm patients who are septic or acidotic for other reasons, **normalizing blood pH is one of the most important goals for the critical care team.**

Safe Induction of Anesthesia and Denitrogenation

If you were to take in a deep breath and hold it, how long could you hold your breath for? A minute? Longer? What will your O_2 sats read on pulse oximetry at the beginning of the breath holding, and just before you have to take in a breath again because you cannot hold it anymore? The answer is that your O_2 sats would not drop significantly and may remain the same, because *our blood CO_2 rises well before our O_2 begins to fall* triggering our brain to have the sensation of having to take in a breath.

Now imagine holding your breath again, only this time it is after giving you an oxygen tank to breath from, so that you breathe in not RA (21%), but rather 100% FiO_2 for 10 minutes prior to holding your breath. Doing this would clear out the lungs of the 80% nitrogen they would normally contain and fill them with "pure oxygen." The process of doing this to "get rid of" the nitrogen in the lungs is called **denitrogenation** (Fig. 2.1). You can think of denitrogenation as a way of "washing out" the nitrogen and thus increasing the alveolar concentration of oxygen, effectively providing the lungs with a much larger reservoir of O_2.

Let us ask a hypothetical question. With your lungs now denitrogenated, how much longer do you think you will be able to hold your breath for? The answer is not any longer—because respirator drive and the urge to breath is dependent on CO_2 build up, which still continues to build up at the same rate, *regardless* of what percent O_2 is in the lungs.

The first step performed during the induction of anesthesia is denitrogenation, which fills the lungs with pure oxygen. But, if we cannot hold our breath any longer due to CO_2 build up, what exactly is the advantage of denitrogenation? It is that it substantially increases the time before O_2 saturations will fall creating an important safety buffer in case there is a problem securing the airway. Problems securing the airway are infrequent, but quite possible due to a variety of factors including bronchospasm, laryngospasm, vocal cord edema, and difficult anatomy making intubation challenging, which could result in inadvertent esophageal intubation. *Thus, loss of an airway, or the inability to secure a proper airway, is a challenging aspect of anesthesia.* If securing an airway takes too much time (4–6 minutes), the

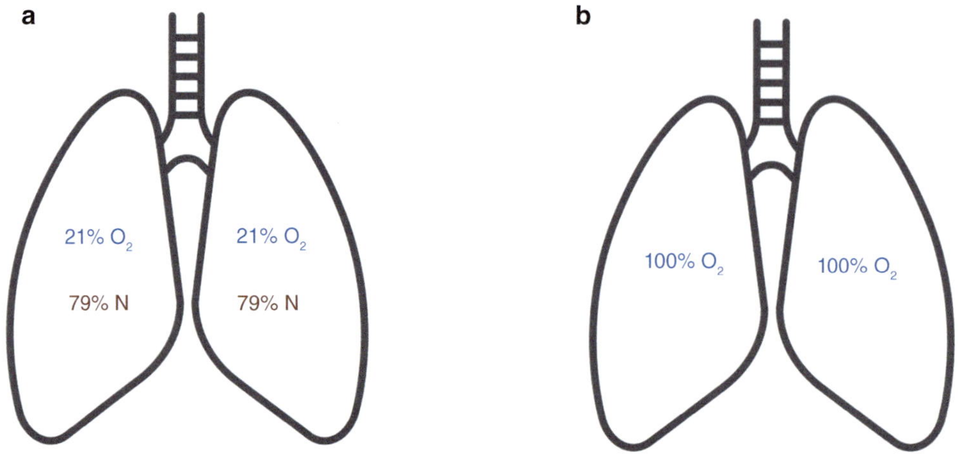

Fig. 2.1 Denitrogenation. (**a**) The composition of gas within lung alveoli is 21% oxygen and 79% nitrogen. (**b**) The process of denitrogenation removes the nitrogen, filling the lungs with pure oxygen. This increases the oxygen reserve, resulting in a longer time before oxygen desaturation

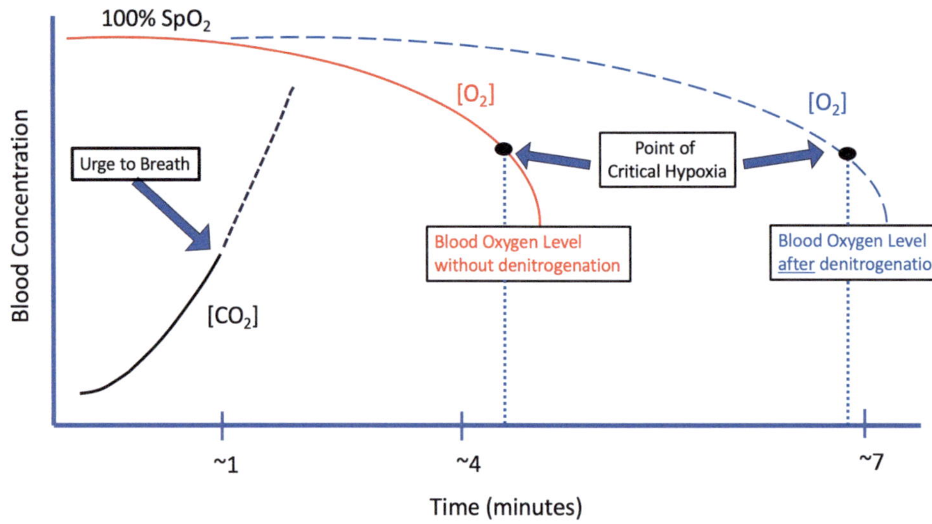

Fig. 2.2 Illustrated are the changes that occur in terms of blood carbon dioxide and oxygen levels. When ventilation ceases, CO_2 rises much more rapidly than O_2 levels fall. If you were to stop ventilating by holding your breath, CO_2 would accumulate, triggering a mounting urge to breathe that cannot be overcome. For most healthy adults, this is around 1 min (black curve), at which point oxygen saturations remain normal. Any disruption in ventilation will lead to a continued and rapid rise in CO_2, but as long as oxygenation is maintained, critical organs (especially kidneys and brain) can recover without permanent injury. The predicted fall in SpO_2 is shown with (blue curve) and without (red curve) denitrogenation. Denitrogenation has no effect on carbon dioxide build up, but increases the time before critical anoxic injury occurs, which is the reason it is routinely performed prior to intubation

outcome could be devastating with an unrecoverable anoxic brain injury being the most dreaded outcome. *Denitrogenation buys time, lengthening the time before SpO_2 falls, at which point irreversible brain injury would result due to prolonged hypoxia* (Fig. 2.2).

Anesthetic Monitoring

The anesthetist is at the helm of patient safety during operation. Maintaining homeostasis requires vigilant attention to vital signs and other parameters. Let us address each of these.

1. *Temperature:* Patients under anesthesia are prone to a drop in their core body temperature, which is carefully monitored. Human enzymes work best at normal body temperature (37 °C/98.6 °F). At this temperature, the *kinetic energy of molecules is optimal for enzyme-substrate interaction.* Methods to keep patients warm include delivery of warmed crystalloid fluids, and the application of an external warming blanket (e.g., Bair Hugger™). While in very specific circumstances it may be desirable to cool body core temperature below normal, in general, body temperature should be maintained at or close to 37 °C. Should body temperature rise unexpectedly during surgery (or in the immediate post-operative period), one must consider

malignant hyperthermia as a possible etiology; failure to recognize this condition with prompt treatment could result in patient morbidity and/or mortality.

2. *Blood Pressure and Heart Rate:* A multitude of factors can affect blood pressure (BP), which is prone to erratic variances upon the induction of and emergence from anesthesia and potentially at other times during the course of the operation. During surgery, blood pressure is checked at routine intervals (3–5 minutes) noninvasively using a sphygmomanometer. In circumstances in which beat-to-beat monitoring is required, an arterial line can be placed from continuous waveform monitoring of BP. In addition to diastolic and systolic pressures, the **mean arterial pressure** (MAP) is also monitored, which is mathematically defined as follows:

$$\text{MAP} = \frac{(2 \times \text{Diastolic BP}) + \text{Systolic BP}}{3}$$

MAP is a quite useful metric, because *it more accurately reflects organ and tissue perfusion, better than systolic and diastolic blood pressures do.* Maintaining MAPs >70 mmHg is considered ideal, particularly for organs sensitive to poor perfusion pressures (e.g., brain, kidney). Importantly, anesthetics can decrease MAP, and thus monitoring these values is an important aspect of anesthetic titration, which is one reason that it is carefully monitored and *balanced with respect to the level of stimulus* resultant from surgery. Some patients may require a vasopressor (such as norepinephrine) to improve MAP, particularly when the patient has labile blood pressure due to cardiovascular disease or due to an underlying condition (such as sepsis).

Blood pressure and heart rate can be raised, mostly by decreasing the level of anesthesia, but they can also be lowered (if they are too high) pharmacologically. This can be done with Labetalol (an alpha-1 adrenergic blocker), or in some instances, an Esmolol drip for tighter control. Mostly, however, heart rate is used as a good indicator of depth of anesthesia. *If patients become light under anesthesia, one of the most important and first indications is that the heart rate will begin to rise.* The blood pressure will also rise, but recall that BP is only measured at periodic intervals, unless an arterial line is in place.

It is worth noting that certain instances during surgery can result in *bradycardia.* Let us consider this vignette. A stable fit patient is undergoing routine laparoscopic appendectomy, a few minutes after insufflating the abdominal cavity with CO_2, the patient's heart rate drops from 75 to 23 bpm. What can explain this? What are the next steps? This is actually not an infrequent occurrence and can be best understood as a *vagal overstimulation* caused by gas distention of the abdomen. This can happen during colonoscopy as well as the colon is distended with air resulting in a vagal "overload." Because it is caused by the gas distention, **the most important first step is to stop the procedure** (immediately desufflate the abdomen). What if this does not work, and the patient remains profoundly bradycardic? Remember that the heart is innervated by the autonomic nervous system which includes the parasympathetic and the sympathetic systems. The sympathetic system increases heart rate (e.g., *fight or flight* response) while the parasympathetic lowers heart rate (e.g., *rest and digest* response). In this situation, the parasympathetic system has been "over stimulated" so the best treatment would be a parasympatho*lytic* agent, such as **atropine** sulfate, which can be administered intravenously.

3. *Electrocardiogram (EKG):* Usually patients are monitored with a three-lead EKG thus producing a so-called rhythm "strip." In addition to heart rate, rhythm strips provide clinical data regarding *P* waves (arterial depolarization), *QRS* complex (ventricular depolarization), and *T* waves (ventricular repolarization) and can thus be **used to assess for cardiac changes,** possible *ST*-segment depression (indicative of myocardial ischemia), or *ST*-segment elevation (suggestive of acute myocardial injury/infarction). An entire spectrum of arrhythmias can occur during surgery and range from sporadic ectopy (quite common during central line placement), to atrial fibrillation, to ventricular fibrillation, and even asystole. Fortunately, through the delivery of safe anesthesia and via appropriate risk-stratification, the risk of a serious cardiac events for non-cardiac surgery, particularly in the operative/perioperative period, is uncommon.

4. *Capnography:* **Capnography** is the noninvasive, real-time monitoring of exhaled, or **end-tidal CO_2—** abbreviated **$EtCO_2$**. It measures the partial pressure of exhaled CO_2. *Capnography represents one of the most important developments in anesthetic care and is a standard in the monitoring of all sedated/anesthetized patients.* Note, $EtCO_2$ is the gold standard when assessing proper tube placement after endotracheal (ET) intubation. It is the best way to assure the ET tube is in the airway, as opposed to the esophagus. **The most dreaded complication of intubation is esophageal intubation,** *not* right main-stem bronchus intubation. *Failure to immediately recognize that an advanced airway, specifically an endotracheal tube, has been placed in the esophagus can have devastating outcomes leading to anoxic brain injury and potentially death.* While auscultation of the lungs and listening to breath sounds, looking for the chest rising and falling, and even chest X-ray are all good techniques to assure proper ET tube placement, they are *not* the gold standard and are not a substitute for capnography, even when intubations are carried out in the field.

In addition to assuring that the patient is being ventilated, the anesthetist is able to interpret the quantitated $EtCO_2$ reading, which can alert the surgical team about potential decompensation, including (cardiac) pump failure and CO_2 embolus. These are special circumstances that are beyond the scope of this chapter.

5. *Pulse Oximetry:* Patients under sedation of any type are monitored with continuous waveform pulse oximetry, SpO_2. This provides the anesthetist with constant information about arterial oxygenation, which can be affected by a variety of factors, including bronchospasm and aspiration. It not only provides information about peripheral blood oxygen saturation, but it also provides a continuous waveform reading corresponding to heart rate. Additionally, pulse oximetry provides an *audible tone.* The *pitch* of the tone varies with the degree of oxygenation. Patients with an SpO_2 of 100% will have a very *high* pitched tone, while patients with SpO_2 of 60%, for example, will have a *low* pitched tone alerting the surgeon and anesthetist audibly, without having to directly observe the monitor (Fig. 2.3).
6. *Quantitative Twitch Monitoring:* Patients under anesthesia, particularly when undergoing abdominal surgery, are pharmacologically "relaxed"—or technically, *paralyzed.* This can be done with a variety of agents, including succinylcholine (depolarizing) and rocuronium (non-depolarizing) neuromuscular blockers. Anesthesiologists utilize a twitch monitor (Fig. 2.4) that helps titrate the right amount of muscle relaxation/paralysis and re-dose when and if required. Essentially, a probe is placed over a nerve (such as the facial nerve) and an electrical stimulus is discharged assessing the response to the corresponding muscle or group of muscles. The most common of these methods is called **train of four (TOF)**. Here 2 Hz (pulse per second) is delivered as four electrical stimuli to the nerve. If the muscle contracts all four times, the paralysis is minimal and the paralytic agent may require redosing. If there are no twitches, then the patient's paralysis is considered "too deep," which can make reversal more challenging. The ideal number of twitches for a patient for which paralysis is required during surgery is **one twitch.** Many aspects of surgery are simplified by having paralysis and this greatly improves the delivery of surgical care. Importantly, in order to emerge from anesthesia and transition the patient back to breathing on their own, the paralysis must be *off.* This has to be delicately balanced and timed with the closure of surgery, and can be somewhat difficult to perfectly time.

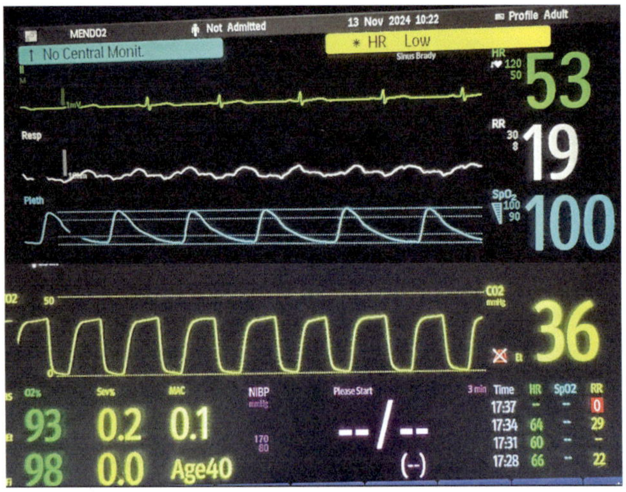

Fig. 2.3 A typical anesthesia monitor displays continuous pulse oximetry or SpO2 (blue), EKG strip (green), respirations (white) in this patient who is spontaneously breathing, and waveform capnography showing end-tidal CO_2 ($EtCO_2$, yellow). Capnography is an essential part of modern anesthetic monitoring and it is mandatory on all anesthetized or sedated patients. It provides information about whether or not the patient is breathing (in sedated patients) and whether or not they are being appropriately ventilated. In this graph, the $EtCO_2$ waveform that correlates with exhaled breaths demonstrates consistent and good gas exchange, suggesting the patient is being adequately ventilated. Anesthesiologists also monitor other parameters (not shown) including temperature and blood pressure

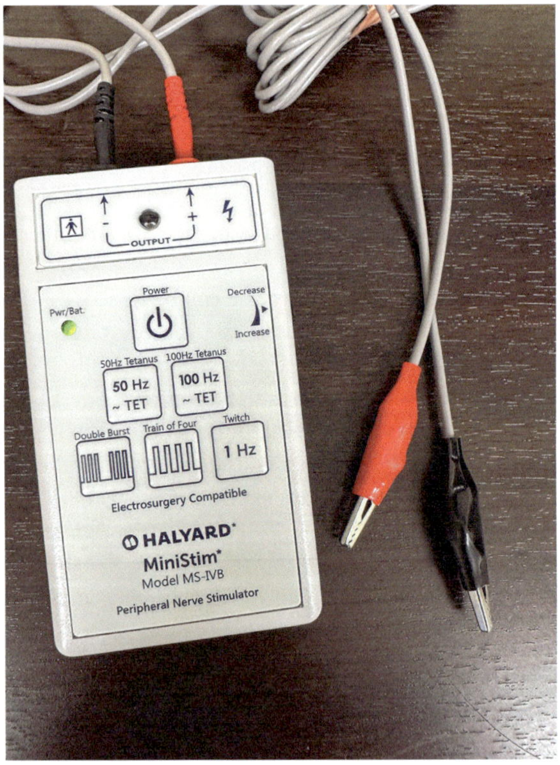

Fig. 2.4 A peripheral nerve stimulator, typical of the type used by anesthetists is shown. The red and black leads are affixed to EKG style pads and attached to the patient's skin overlying specific nerves. When activated, the motor (muscle) response, which correlates with level of pharmacologic paralysis, can be monitored. Redosing of paralytics such as rocuronium is based on interpretation of the stimulator reading

Part 2: Practical Aspects and Applied Surgery

The Operating Theater Team

Surgery is complex and is performed by not one person, but rather a team. The team size may vary, but at a minimum includes an attending (primary) surgeon, an anesthetist, a surgical technician, and a nurse circulator (Fig. 2.5). Other personnel can include first assists (FAs), secondary surgeons, student learners, surgical residents/fellows, and, of course, PAs. Physician assistants are often given autonomy during some portions of the operation (such as closing). More importantly, they provide crucial assistance during key portions of operation and it is important to understand the roles of a PA and the importance of those roles—and how they can be implemented safely.

Patient Safety and Your Personal Safety

One of the most important principles in medicine and surgery is maintaining safety, not only of the patient *but also for yourself as a PA, and other personnel and healthcare staff.* Whether you are a practicing PA or PA in training, you are considered part of the surgical team, and each person in that team plays an important role in delivering safe surgical care. Your safety is paramount, and it is important to always wear personal protective equipment (PPE) while scrubbed into surgery. PPE includes a gown, mask, preferably double-gloves, shoe covers, and eye protection (Fig. 2.6).

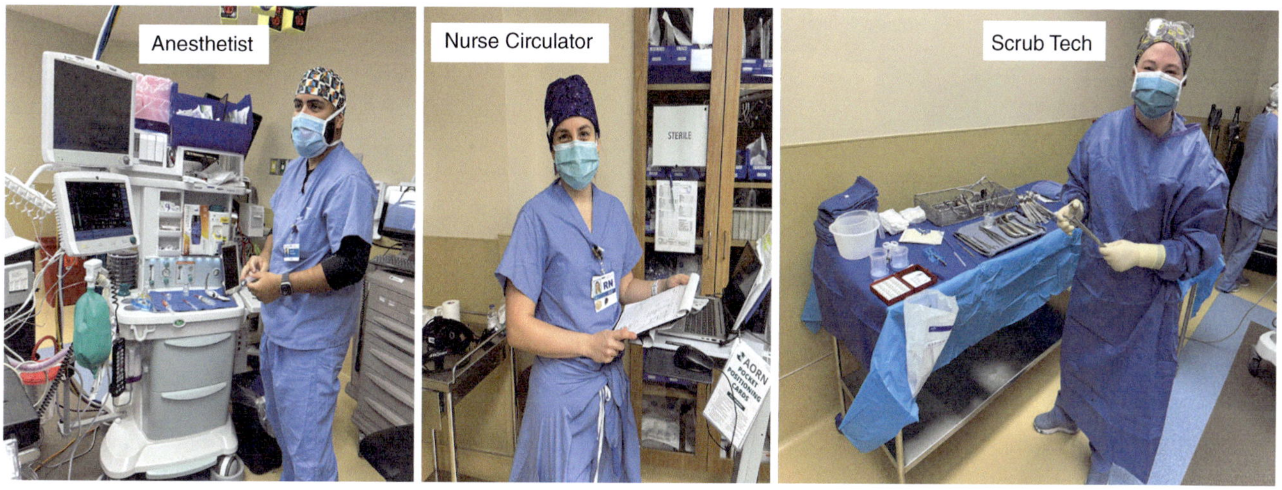

Fig. 2.5 Surgery is performed by a team of specially trained personnel. In addition to the surgeon and/or physician assistant(s), the team consists of at least three other individuals—an anesthetist, a circulator, and a scrub technician. These individuals are always present in the operating room from before the operation begins to after it is completed. The scrub tech has many responsibilities, including maintaining the sterile field, assuring instrument and sponge counts are correct, and organizing the sterile instruments in a manner that is in sync with the steps of the operation. The scrub tech usually has a strong knowledge of the operation being formed and can anticipate which instruments are needed and when. The nurse circulator is not scrubbed into the sterile field and is available to obtain items needed and bring them into the field. The circulator is often the person overseeing the operation globally and keeps track of start and stop times, for example, and completes very detailed charting during each case. In the United States, anesthetist can be a mid-level provider, such as a **certified registered nurse anesthetist (CRNA)** or **anesthesiologist assistant (AA)**, or an **anesthesiologist**, who is a physician (MD/DO) specialized in anesthesia, and who often overseas CRNAs or AAs

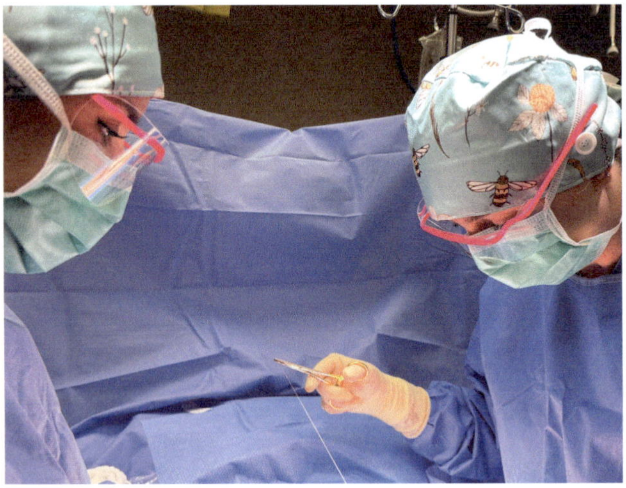

Fig. 2.6 Two PAs close skin at the completion of abdominal laparoscopic surgery. Note their eye protection. Eye protection is mandatory in most operating rooms. Wearing corrective lens (eye-glasses) is somewhat protective from direct splashes, but wrap-around style eye shields offers more robust protection. Single use eye protection (as shown) is usually made available to all operating room personnel

Pre-operative Safety

Patient safety in surgery begins prior to entry into the OR. It is important to confirm the patient's identifier information, confirm the operation and planned operative approach (laparoscopic, robotic, or open), and verify sidedness when applicable. *The PA who is assisting in surgery should carefully review the patient's clinical history, medications, allergies, and other relevant clinical data including recent imaging and blood laboratory results.* Surgeons want their PAs (in practice or in training) to **take ownership of knowing their patients.**

For patients requiring medical clearance, this should be verified as well. Importantly, concerns about the patient's preparedness to undergo surgery should be brought up to the attending surgeon and anesthesiologist prior to transferring the patient to the operating theater. Every member of a surgical team has a role in assuring that proper patient safety is delivered. *The goal is to assure that the correct operation is performed on the correct patient on the correct side and/or level (when applicable) 100% of the time.* Having a robust **safety culture** is crucial in the surgical arena.

Operating Room Safety and Protocols

1. *Time Out:* Medical errors are an important source of morbidity in the US healthcare system, and the operating room and surgical care delivery (in particular) are heavily scrutinized, due to the high stakes, high risk nature of surgery. One of the most important safety regulations to be implemented is that <u>no surgery can commence without a</u> <u>**"Time Out."**</u>

   This hard-stop provides a verbal review of the name of the operation and anatomic side (left versus right when applicable), the patient name, the surgeon name, as well as other important aspects, such as whether or not the patient has received intravenous antibiotics 30 min prior to surgery.

   At the completion of the operation, every surgical team member participate in what is termed a **debrief.** Here, the operation performed is reviewed, and the specimen(s), if applicable, are labeled and verified. Other parameters, including wound classification, estimated blood loss (EBL), the patient's overall condition and stability, are also discussed, as are the final instrument and sponge counts. Note that surgical sponges and other devices which are not radio-opaque have been purposely made so that they *do* show up on X-rays (Fig. 2.7).

   Remember, <u>you</u> are part of the surgical team and should always speak up during time out if something said is opposed to what you believe to be the case. For example, if you read that the patient is having a right carpal tunnel release, but during time out it is stated the patient is having a left carpal tunnel release, *voice your concern immediately, you will <u>not</u> be faulted even if you were wrong.*
2. *Maintain a Sterile Field:* During scrub training, PAs are taught and trained about how to maintain a sterile field. There are important rules to follow, such as always keeping your hands above the level of the elbows (Fig. 2.8). Once scrubbed in, you should never touch your shoulders, neck, or face as this would break the sterile field (Fig. 2.9). At times you may inadvertently break the sterile field by touching something outside of the field. Do not worry if this happens, all OR personnel including surgeons have done this from time to time. The important thing is to recognize that you have contaminated yourself and simply inform the scrub tech you have contaminated yourself. The scrub tech will direct you to next steps, which may include changing a glove, applying a sterile "sleeve" to the contaminated portion of the gown, or simply re-scrubbing. *Do not feel ashamed or embarrassed, swiftly report the contamination and understand that this is not uncommon and no one will "blame" you for it.*
3. *Protective Attire:* As stated previously, your safety during surgery is crucial. It is important to protect yourself from bodily fluids and splashes and so-called "sharps" (needles, blades). While all operating room attire includes hair covering (e.g., hairnet), a sterile gown, and sterile gloves, it is highly recommended that you also wear shoe covers and eye protection to maximize your level of protection (Fig. 2.10). Some patients may have known blood-

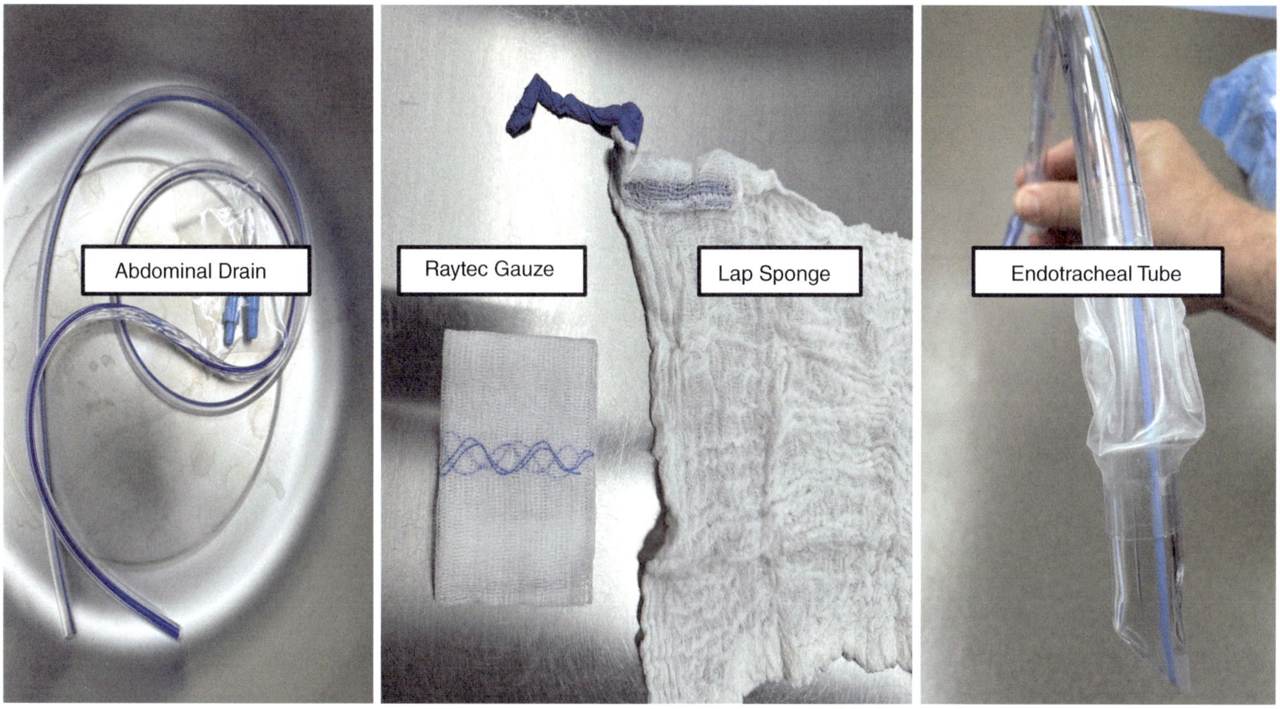

Fig. 2.7 What do these seemingly unrelated items have in common? The answer is they all contain a special, radio opaque marker which is in a universal blue color. Thus, surgical sponges are modified with the blue, radio opaque marker so that they can be located if lost in the abdomen by X-ray. Abdominal drain position can also be determined by this, as can the depth of an endotracheal tube, which is how right mainstem intubation, for example, can be deduced radiographically

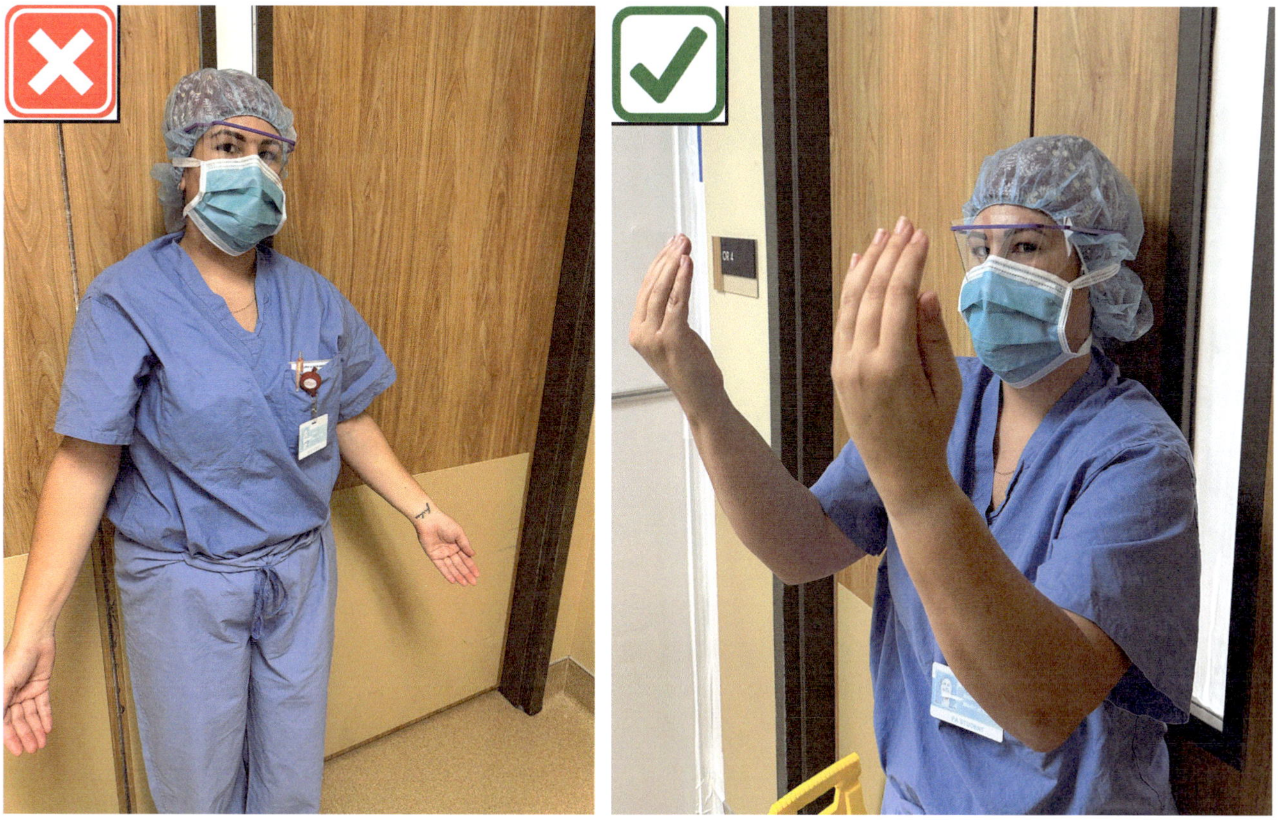

Fig. 2.8 After scrubbing (usually done at sinks situated outside of the operating room), a PA enters through the doorway to the OR by pushing the door open with her back. Shown is the incorrect and correct method, emphasizing that your hands should not drop below elbow level

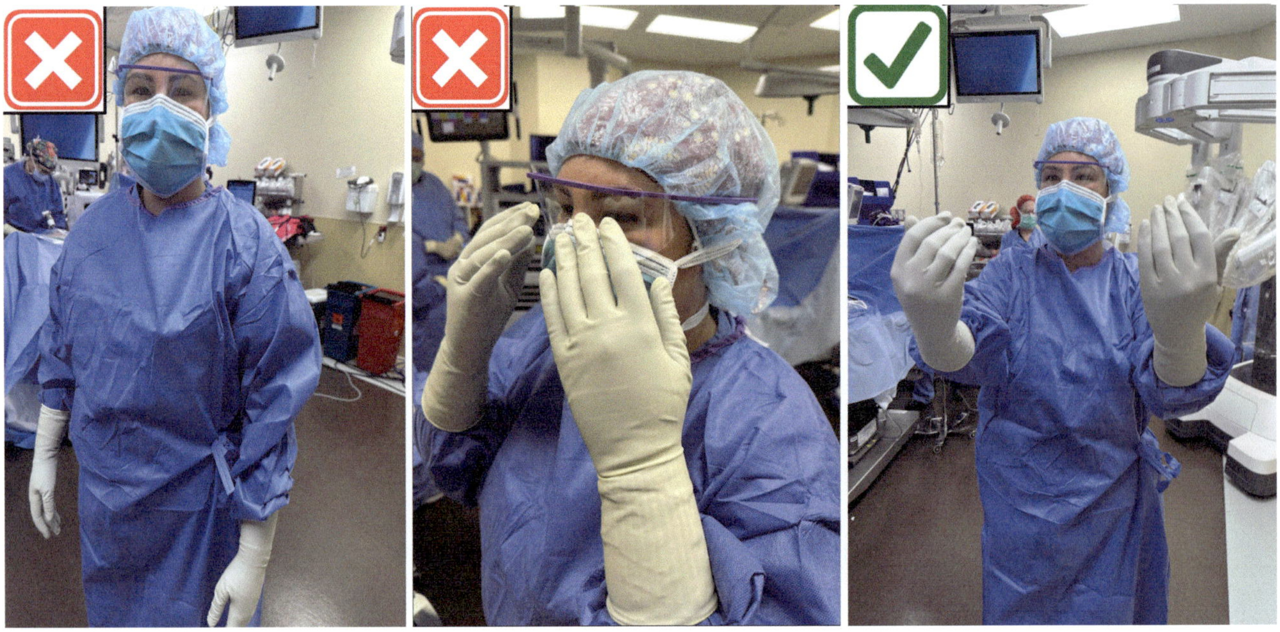

Fig. 2.9 Dos and Don'ts when scrubbed in for surgery. Even after scrubbing in, do not drop your hands below elbow level, and do not raise hands above chest level and never touch your face, head, or neck, as these are not parts of the sterile field. The only exception to raising your hand above head level is to adjust the overhead light (which contains a sterile light handle) and this is certainly permissible. Note this PA's personal protection includes a facemask for eye protection

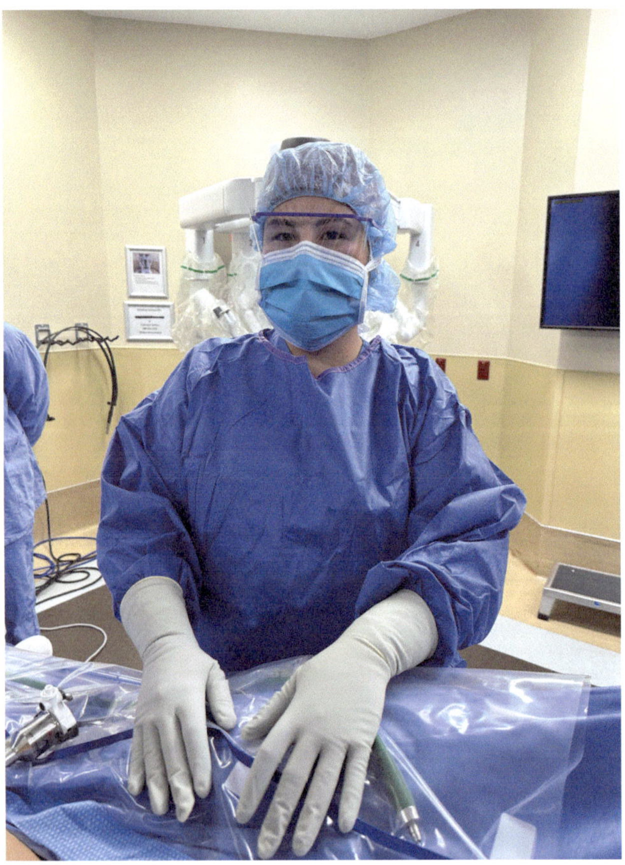

Fig. 2.10 Scrubbed and ready for surgery. Here, a PA student is scrubbed in and ready to go. Note the protective attire, including sterile gown, gloves, mask, hairnet, and eye protection. Note that she has her hands on the patient drape approximately at elbow level. This is a good place to position your hands

borne pathogens, such as hepatitis C, and HIV; but the policy used is that *every patient should be treated with the same high level of protection.* That is, we do not "do anything differently" if a patient has a known disease that could be spread via accidental needle stick (i.e., via the hematogenous route). There are special protocols in place, however, for *specific* types of communicable *airborne* pathogens, such as COVID-19, tuberculosis, as well as certain other infections, such as *Clostridium difficile* colitis, the details of which are beyond the scope of this introductory chapter.

4. *Personal Health and Wellness:* There are occasions when a PA, especially those in training, may feel suddenly ill and/or dizzy. Pre-syncope and syncope are not rare among persons experiencing the operating room environment for the first time. *If you feel unwell or faint for any reason and you are scrubbed into surgery, immediately scrub out and immediately notify the team and the nurse circulator.* This is completely understandable. You will never be reprimanded. You may also feel unwell for other reasons; *always understand that your health and wellbeing come first.*
5. *Radiation Safety:* Some operations may require the administration of intra-operative radiation—for example, fluoroscopy and portable X-ray. All OR personnel should wear protective lead, including a thyroid shield. Radiation exposure varies in accordance to the **inverse square law.** This law states that radiation exposure is as follows:

$$R \propto \frac{1}{d^2}$$

Where R represents the radiation exposure, and d represents distance from the radiation beam. Thus, if you are standing 2 feet from the radiation beam, your exposure would be $\frac{1}{2^2}$ or 25%, but if you were standing 6 feet away, the exposure falls exponentially to $\frac{1}{6^2}$ or 2.78%. Thus, at the 6-feet mark, most of the radiation exposure has diminished, which is why **6 feet is considered a safe distance away from (most) radiation fields.** With appropriate precautions, there is minimal risk to OR personnel during operations that employ even substantial and/or repeated use of fluoroscopy (such as orthopedics). Notwithstanding, if you are pregnant or think you may be pregnant, notify the attending surgeon and avoid radiation exposure if at all possible.

6. *Laparoscopic Basics and Safety:* Minimally invasive surgery includes robotic and laparoscopic surgery. Such approaches require "keyhole" access to the abdominal cavity via trocars and insufflation of the abdominal cavity with a gas, namely CO_2. The gas insufflation acts like an invisible retractor that distends the abdominal cavity allowing a field of view. CO_2 is used because it can be both (a) monitored by the anesthetist via $EtCO_2$ and, more importantly, (b) controlled through respiratory rate and tidal volume, as we have learned, to vent off the CO_2 when it begins to build up.

   You may wonder why O_2 is not as a gas for insufflation, after all, "oxygen is good," right? Well, oxygen may be good, *but it is also highly flammable.* Surgeons frequently use heat energy devices in the operating room, and during laparoscopic surgery including electrocautery (see later), harmonic scalpel, and/or vessel sealing devices that, due to the thermal energy they release, would make the *combustion a very high risk in the presence of high concentrations of oxygen.*

   Fire safety in the operating room is more important than you would think. In the United States alone, there are an estimated 600–800 operating room fires annually. Operation in some anatomic sites, such as the trachea, are challenging due to the requirement to oxygenate the patient that can be potentially hazardous depending on the specifics of the case. Other factors include the type of skin prep used, as some are alcohol-based, making them potentially flammable in certain circumstances, for example, *if they are not given the proper dry time.* It is important to know that the camera lens of the robotic scope and laparoscope becomes quite hot, and this could lead to a fire if it comes into contact with the paper drapes for a long enough period of time. As a general rule, *never leave the scope tip on the drapes while the light is in the ON position* (Fig. 2.11).

7. *Trocar Basics and Safety:* A trocar is a hollow cylindrical device used to gain minimally invasive access to the

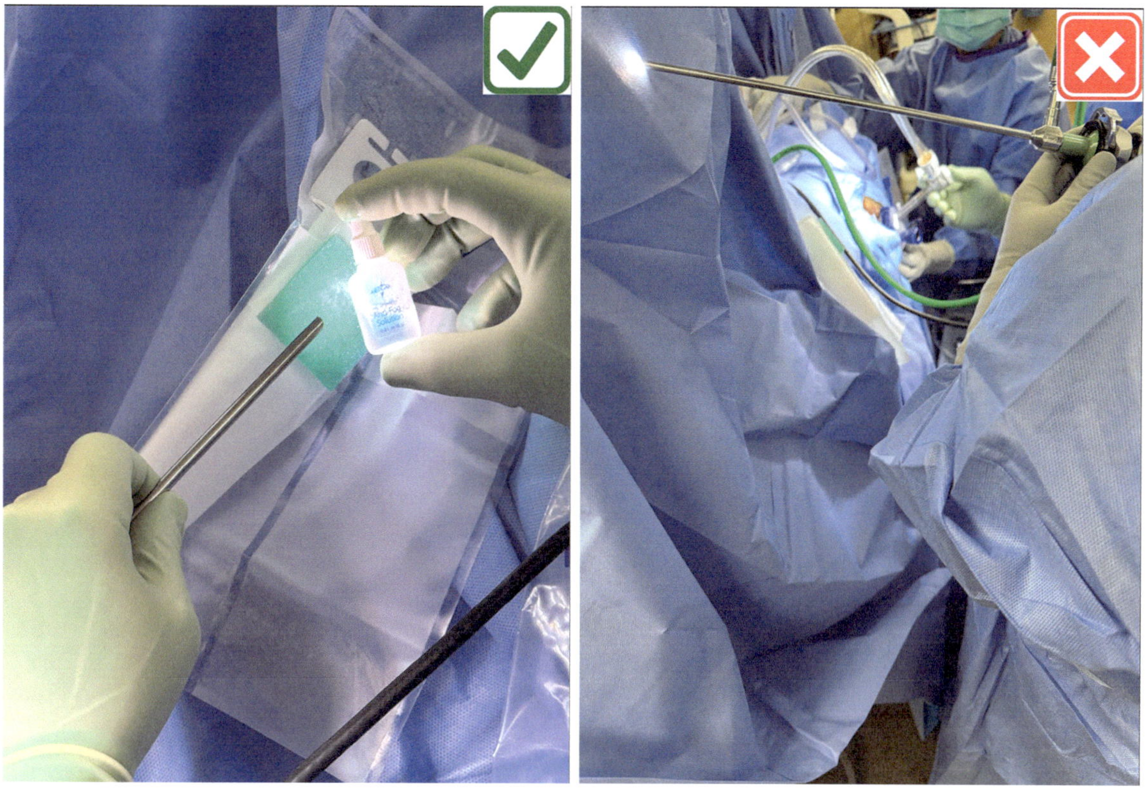

Fig. 2.11 Shown is the permissible point of contact of the scope tip outside of the abdominal cavity while the scope light is on. Here, it is a defogging solution (Fred™, Medtronic, Inc.) being applied to help keep the optics clear. Antifog agents are surfactants that minimize the surface tension of H_2O. The scope tip (lens) can often require frequent defogging and cleaning since they tend to smudge easily. The scope tip, however, should never be left against the drape as it can burn the drape or even the patient. As an added safety precaution, it is recommended that the scope light be placed in the STANDBY or OFF position when not in use

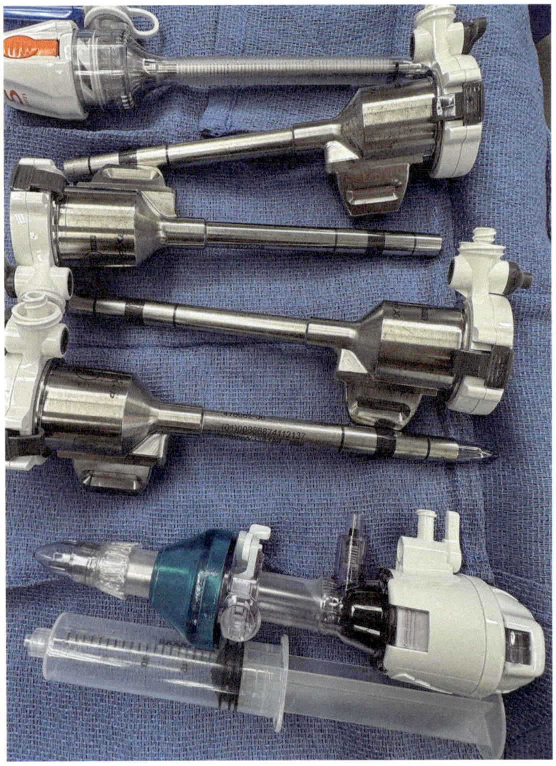

Fig. 2.12 An assortment of trocars of variable types are shown. A 5 mm disposable trocar (top, orange-white) and a 12 mm Hassan-Type trocar (bottom) are shown with their obturators in place. Pictured between them are metal, reusable 8 mm da Vinci Robotic trocars. Robotic trocars are sometimes also referred to as *ports* or *cannulas*. All trocars are delivered and positioned into the abdominal cavity using obturators that can be sharp or dull. When the obturator is removed, the trocar serves as a cylindrical access channel into the abdominal cavity

abdominal cavity for laparoscopy and/or robotic-assisted surgery. Trocars may be re-usable (metal) or disposable (plastic) (Fig. 2.12). Trocar placement is necessary to access the abdominal cavity and there are different techniques for this. Trocar placement, which involves placing a 5–12 mm blunt or sharp-ended instrument through the abdominal wall, is a safe procedure but must be performed under direct vision (Fig. 2.13) and requires special training as there is a potential for organ injury (such as the bladder, small bowel, or stomach), or even vascular injury.

The dome of the bladder is at risk for injury when low midline trocars are placed and it can be "hard to see." This is one reason laparoscopy and robotics approaches *usually include urinary catheter placement to decompress the bladder; nasogastric or orogastric tubes are used to decompress the stomach as well.*

Small bowel, in particular, can be densely adherent to the anterior abdominal wall and is at risk for injury. Trocar injury to small bowel can be repaired without difficulty, as long as it is recognized. A *missed* small bowel injury, however, is a **serious condition that can lead to sepsis** and other morbidity including the need for re-operation. *The most serious immediate complication from trocar placement is* ***vascular injury****,* which can lead to rapid and life-threatening blood loss if not swiftly controlled.

At the completion of surgery, trocars are ideally removed under direct vision. Trocar sites that are >8 mm in diameter require fascial closure, while trocars of a smaller diameter require only skin closure—but there are exceptions, such as at the umbilicus. Skin is typically closed with a subcuticular absorbable monofilament suture; alternatively, skin clips can be used.

The PA's Role Assisting During Surgery

Even for PA students on surgery rotation, many attending surgeons (preceptors) will encourage active participation during surgery. Teamwork is essential. But what exactly are PAs expected to do? The following section outlines the typical role of a PA in the operating room, although this may vary widely depending on surgeon comfort and PA experience and preparedness.

1. *Retraction:* One of the most important tasks relegated to PAs in training and in practice is retraction. Retraction provides exposure to the operative field, which is a cornerstone of all surgery, regardless of specialty. Proper retraction takes skill and sometimes considerable manual force. Although student learners often feel that retracting is a menial task, when performed properly, *it provides an immense aid to the surgeon.* Retraction can be laparoscopic or open and can involve both abdominal wall musculature or more delicate anatomic structures. *It is imperative that the retraction* ***force****, together with* ***direction*** *(defined as a* ***vector****) is* <u>*constant*</u>*,* and this is often one of the most challenging aspects of manual retraction, especially for beginners (Fig. 2.14). This requires the PA retracting to **pay close attention**.

   A person retracting should be cognizant of *what* they are retracting as *different forces are required depending on the anatomy.* For example, abdominal wall and fascial retraction often requires moderate amounts of manual retraction force, while small bowel mandates gentle

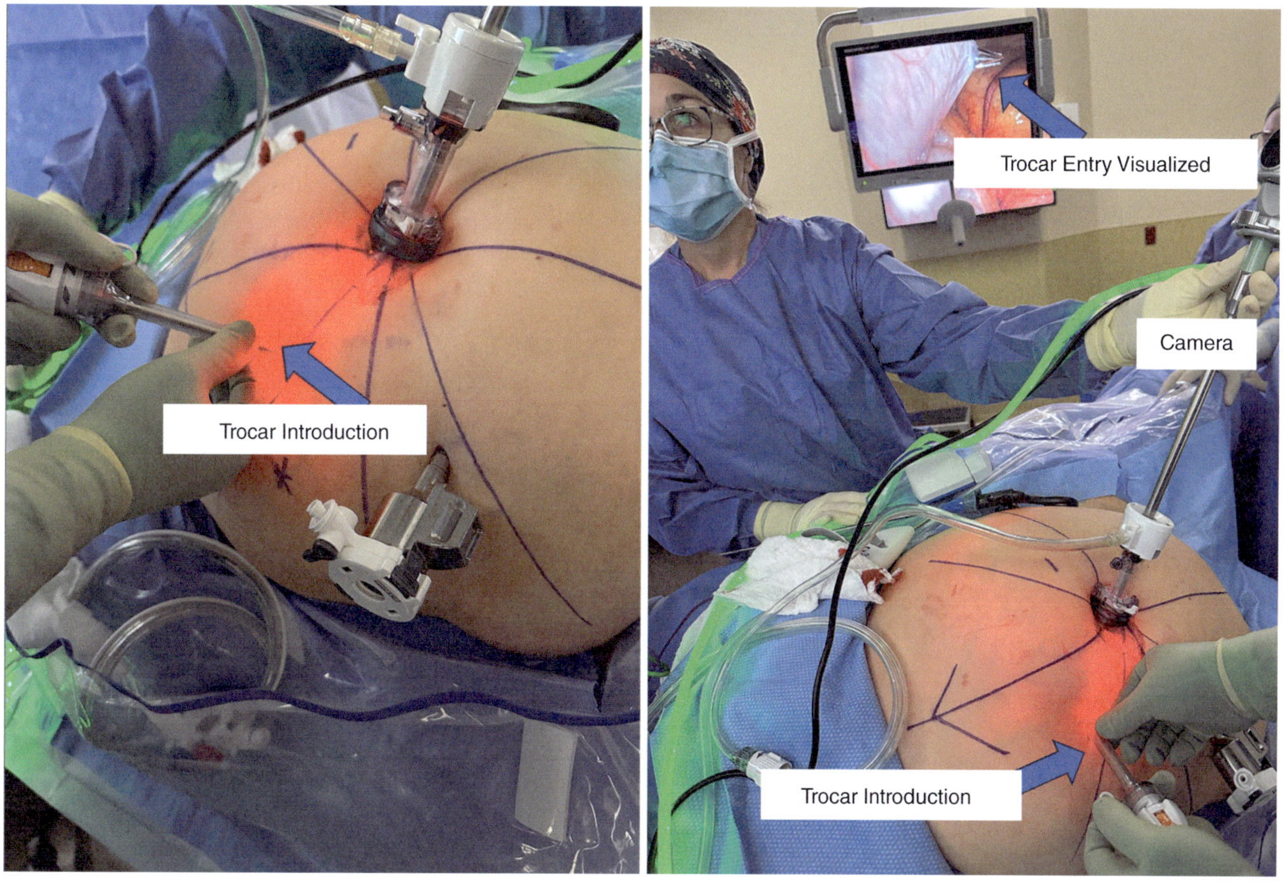

Fig. 2.13 Trocar placement is an advanced skill that PAs can perform after proper education and training. Here, the trocar is introduced in the desired trajectory with both hands on the trocar, one at the base, and one further along the trocar's shaft. A camera is aimed at the trocar to directly observe the tip as it enters the abdominal cavity. The person placing the trocar and the laparoscopic camera operator *always have their eyes on the monitor* during this phase

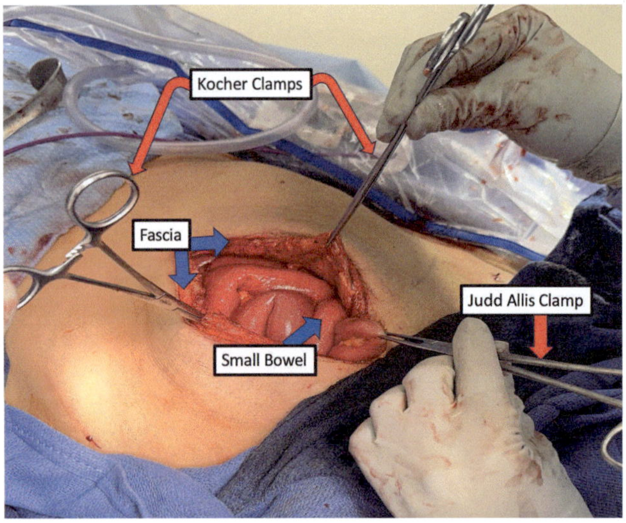

Fig. 2.14 Manual retraction of different anatomy is illustrated. The instrument names are not what is important, but rather an understanding of the forces used. Retractors may be placed on different types of targets to help expose the surgical field and anatomic targets. They can be placed on the fascia, *the toughest and strongest layer of the abdominal wall.* Here, two Kocher clamps on fascia are being retracted in an *upward and outward* direction, which is common. *Fascia is a strong layer, and therefore the retraction on this part of the anatomy is often very strong and a lot of force is used.* In counter distinction, *the force applied to the much more delicate small bowel requires very gentle and delicate retraction.* Certain graspers are designed for delicate tissue (like bowel), while others are designed for tougher and thicker tissue (like fascia). Here, a Judd Allis is used to delicately grasp the small bowel. This fine instrument is not suitable for fascia, just as the Kocher clamp is not suitable for small bowel

retraction to avoid a crush injury or serosal tear. In some open operations, self-retaining retractors can be employed providing circumferential retraction and obviating the need for manual retraction. Such retractor systems can be metal, ratcheting systems (e.g., Thompson Retractor System, BookWalter Retractor System) *or* disposable (Alexis, Applied Medical, Inc.). Disposable self-retraining retractor systems also serve as a wound protector (Fig. 2.15a, b).

2. *Suturing:* In counter-distinction to retraction, suturing is usually the skill most PA students are excited to do. Depending on surgeon comfort level and PA experience, it is common for a PA to suture skin during the closing portion of the operation. This is where PAs can hone their skills, as the patient is anesthetized, and the operative environment has a rich supply of personnel to help with closing skin. There are many types of skin suturing techniques that can be learned, and they are covered elsewhere. *PA Students are encouraged to have practiced suturing in a dry lab model, including instrument and hand knot-tying so that they can focus on making the most of their time in the OR during closing.*
3. *Cutting:* Cutting suture is an important aid to the surgical team, and PAs both in training and in practice routinely perform this task. Every surgeon has a specific style of how they want their suture cut and you will find surgeons can be quite particular about the length of the tail. Surgeons want the tail of a knotted stitch to be *not*

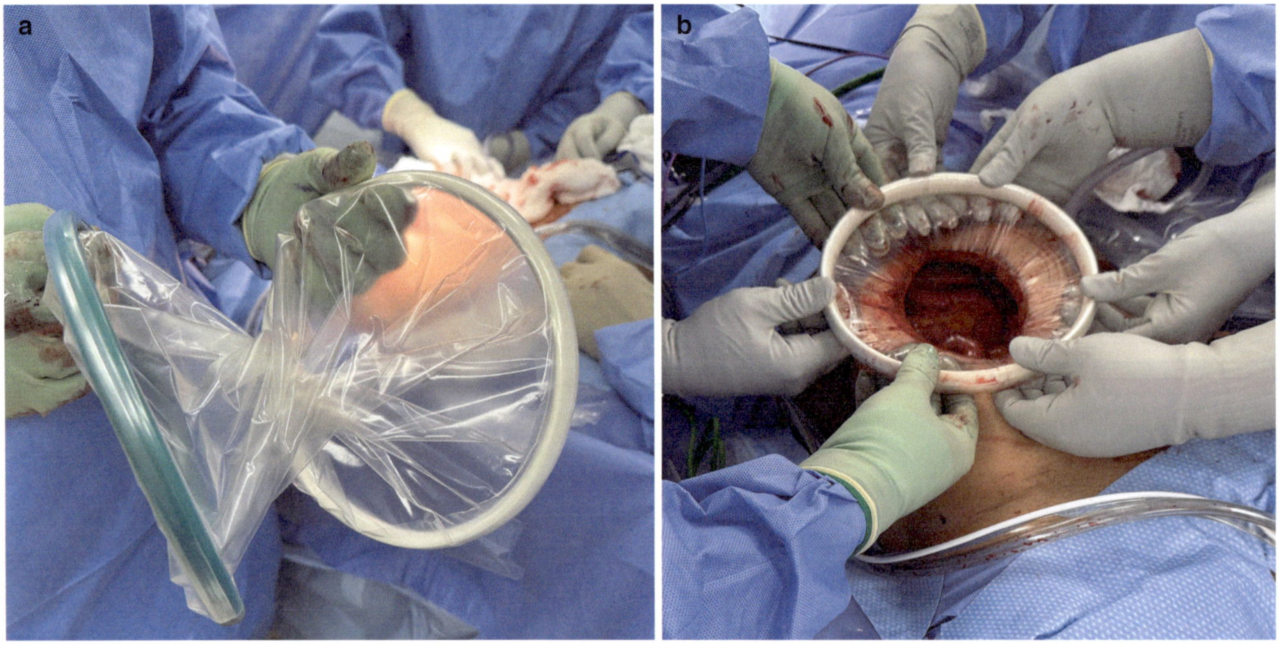

Fig. 2.15 (**a**) A self-retaining disposable retractor for use with open abdominal surgery. The device consists of an inner (green) and an outer (white) ring; the rings are connected by a tough plastic material. The green ring is placed against the peritoneum and the white ring is placed outside of the body cavity. (**b**) The retractor is positioned with a manual inward twisting of the outer ring. Note that the plastic serves as a wound protector

too long and *not too short.* At first, you may feel that you are always disappointing the team when you are starting out, but it just takes practice!

As a general rule, monofilament suture knots should be cut longer than braded suture—usually the tail should be 1 cm or so; braided suture can be cut shorter, usually 5 mm. The reason is that monofilament (for example, PDS) tends to slip, and a short tail is less secure in this case. The technique of cutting with surgical scissors is important. Precision and stability are paramount, and cutting with the tip of the scissor rather than the base is best practice (Fig. 2.16). Not only should sutures be cut to the proper length, but the tail length should also be consistent—such that all tails are the *same length.*

4. *Knot-tying:* While PAs often have exposure to knot-tying using instruments as this is the common technique for laceration management, in the operating room, emphasis is given to tying knots *manually*, via the one and two hand techniques. Instrument tying is still used to close skin, as this does conserve suture material. However, for more critical knots, *surgeons like there to be more force in the knot construction to assure it is sturdy, especially when it is being placed on a critical artery, for example.*

   Other types of advanced knots can be made that are typically only performed by surgeons and not PAs—these would include laparoscopic and robotic suturing and knot-tying. Robotic and laparoscopic knot-tying, although still performed, is much less common due to the advent of self-locking or "barbed" suture (e.g., V-Loc™ Wound Closure Device) that cinches tissue together without the need for knots.

5. *Suctioning and Maintaining a Dry Surgical Field:* Perhaps equally as important as retraction is maintaining a clear field by suctioning and/or dabbing the surgical field with a sterile gauze sponge. *Even minor bleeding can obscure the surgical field*, and a good assistant is hyper-alert to this, meticulously dabbing and suctioning fluid and blood from the field to maintain a dry field.

   Suctioning is also important to clearing plumes of smoke that can result from heat-generating dissectors (e.g., electrocautery). Keeping the field free of smoke not only helps clear the field of view for improved exposure, but it also removes the hazardous material so it is not inhaled by the surgical team members (Fig. 2.17).

6. *Irrigation:* There is an old proverb in surgery—*"The Solution to Pollution Is Dilution."* In other words, if you

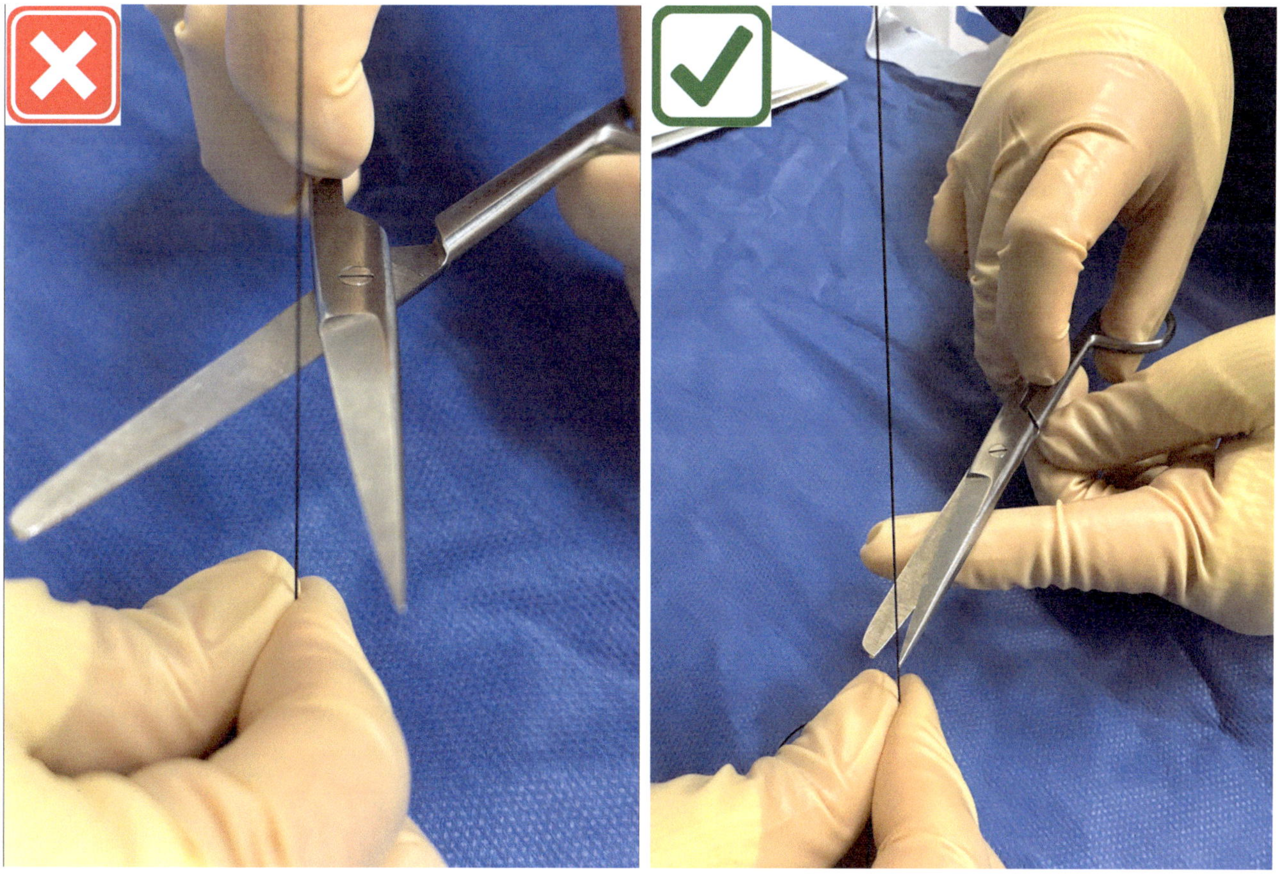

Fig. 2.16 The technique of cutting is important. Being cautious and precise is a key tenet of cutting. As shown, the base of the scissor should not be used to cut, only the tip

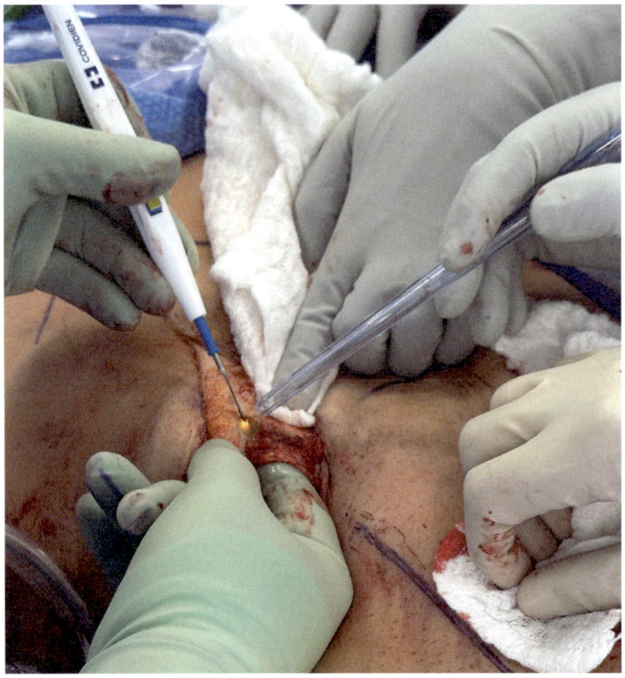

Fig. 2.17 A suction tip is used to reduce the smoke generated by the electrocautery device. Suctioning keeps the operative field clean and is an extremely important part of modern surgery. It is not as simple as it looks, and it takes experience to become adept at suctioning

want to clean up a surgical site from bacteria and debris, particularly in contaminated fields, copious irrigation with a **sterile saline** solution is good practice. In instances when the spillage is tumor cells, the irrigation of choice is **sterile water**, as this is more likely to *lyse free-floating cancer cells due to an osmotic pressure gradient.* While some surgeons will add dilute betadine or antibiotics (e.g., gentamycin) to the irrigation fluid, there is no data to support this practice regardless of wound classification and level of contamination.

7. *Incision:* PAs in practice and in training may be permitted to make skin incision, depending on surgeon's comfort level and PA aptitude. This is usually accomplished with a #10, 11, or 15 blade (cold knife). Cold knife blades are single-use disposable instruments that are extremely sharp.

   Safe handling of the knife blade and calling out loud, "knife back" when returning the knife to the scrub tech is standard procedure and must be followed (Fig. 2.18). Cutting should be performed orthogonal to the dermis; the *belly* of the blade should be used to cut the skin in a slow steady motion (Fig. 2.19).

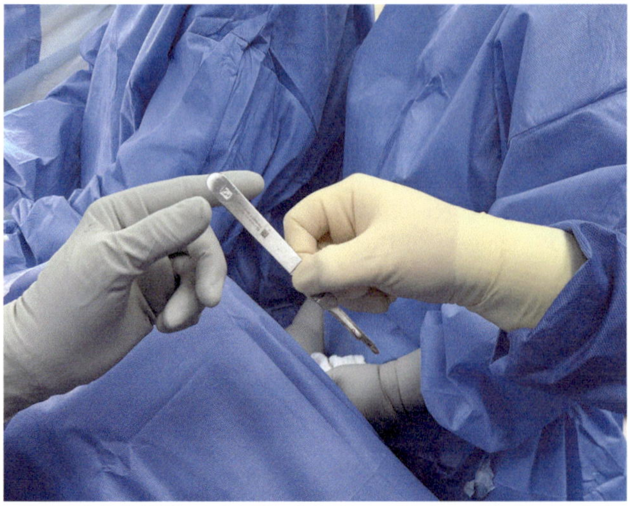

Fig. 2.18 A #15 blade cold knife is passed from a scrub tech to a PA during surgery. This demonstrates a safe and standard technique of passing the knife with the blade side down

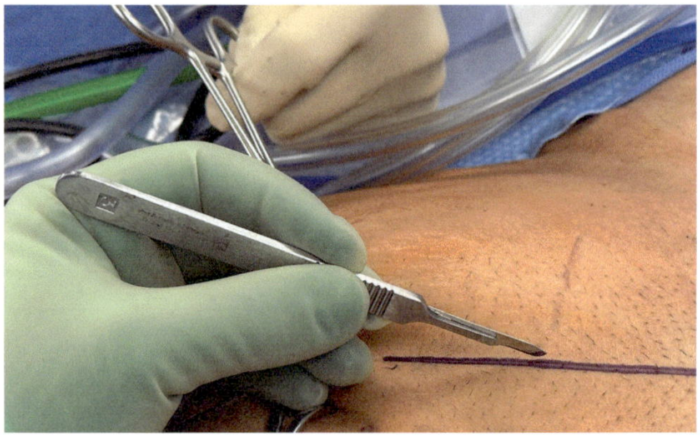

Fig. 2.19 Proper technique of using a cold knife here just prior to opening incision. Cutting is best with the "belly" of the blade, not the tip. Note that the tip is orthogonal (perpendicular) to the skin. When cutting, a slow, steady motion is made along the planned direction of incision, which can be marked as shown using a sterile skin marker

8. *Driving the Laparoscopic Camera:* Perhaps one of the most frustrating parts of assisting in surgery is driving the laparoscopic camera (Fig. 2.20). This is because it is hard for PAs in training and new PAs in practice to understand fully what view the surgeon wants to see. Moreover, the view desired is constantly changing for many types of more complex surgery. Until you become familiar with specific operations, you will not be able to easily follow the steps and it may seem confusing.

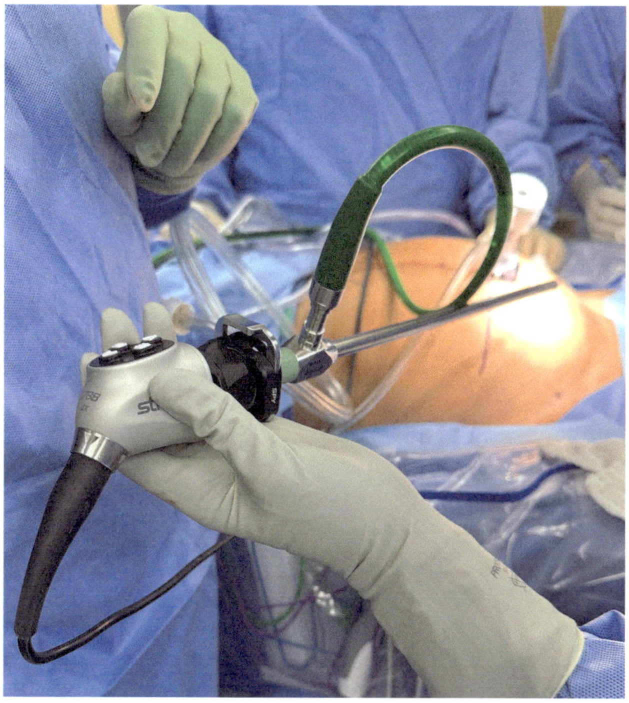

Fig. 2.20 A typical laparoscopic camera is shown. Laparoscopes consist of (**a**) a camera cord (black) connected to the camera head with controls, (**b**) a long metal shaft that contains the scope lens at the tip, and (**c**) a light cord, here shown in green. As demonstrated, the operator cradles the camera such that the control panel on it (black with white icons) faces *upward, toward the OR ceiling. This is essential to maintain the horizon level.* The image is transmitted to usually at least two LCD monitors for viewing (not shown)

Students are often told multiple commands very quickly, such as "come in, look left, back out, come out and clean, etc.," and this can be anxiety provoking, especially for the novice assistant. Still, there are important principles that should be consistently followed during all laparoscopic camera driving. They are as follows: (a) never take your eyes off the monitor as long as the camera is in the body cavity, (b) always keep the surgeon's main operating instrument in the center of the field of view, (c) always keep the horizon level, and finally (d) always hold the camera steady (Fig. 2.21).

One special aspect of minimally invasive scopes (robotic and laparoscopic) is that the camera lens can be flat-ended *or* angled. Flat-ended lens are called ZERO DEGREE scopes (0°) and angled scopes can be either 45 DEGREE (45°) or 30 DEGREE (30°) scopes. Angled lenses are preferred by some but not all surgeons to gain a better viewpoint of the surgical field, by "looking in a specific direction."

Think of it in terms of how we see things. Look out in front of you. You probably can see the ground, the ceiling, and walls, but if you look up at the ceiling (without moving your head), you will see the ceiling much better; but now you may not see the ground, or barely so, as it has shifted to the limit of your peripheral field of view. This is essentially how moving the scope tip of an angled scope operates. It is like moving your eyes to look at something without moving your head and thus without shifting your *frame of reference.*

Robotic scopes are not driven by assistants like the laparoscope, but are instead controlled by the surgeon. In robotics, there are two main ways the angled scope can be set to—either the lens looking up or down, often expressed as 30 UP or 30 DOWN (Fig. 2.22). In laparoscopy, when a 30° or 45° scope lens is used, the angle can be adjusted to optimize the viewpoint, and this is one of the more challenging aspects of advanced camera driving during laparoscopy (Fig. 2.23).

9. *Application of Cautery:* PAs in practice and in training usually become quite familiar with cautery and its various applications. Rather than using a "cold knife" or scalpel to cut through skin and tissue, an instrument that uses thermal energy can be used. *Such devices do not dull with repeated use like scalpels do*, and do not contain an actual sharp cutting blade. One of the most commonly used surgical devices is electrocautery, often referred to simply as **Bovie** (named after its creator, William T. Bovie, Harvard University) (Fig. 2.24).

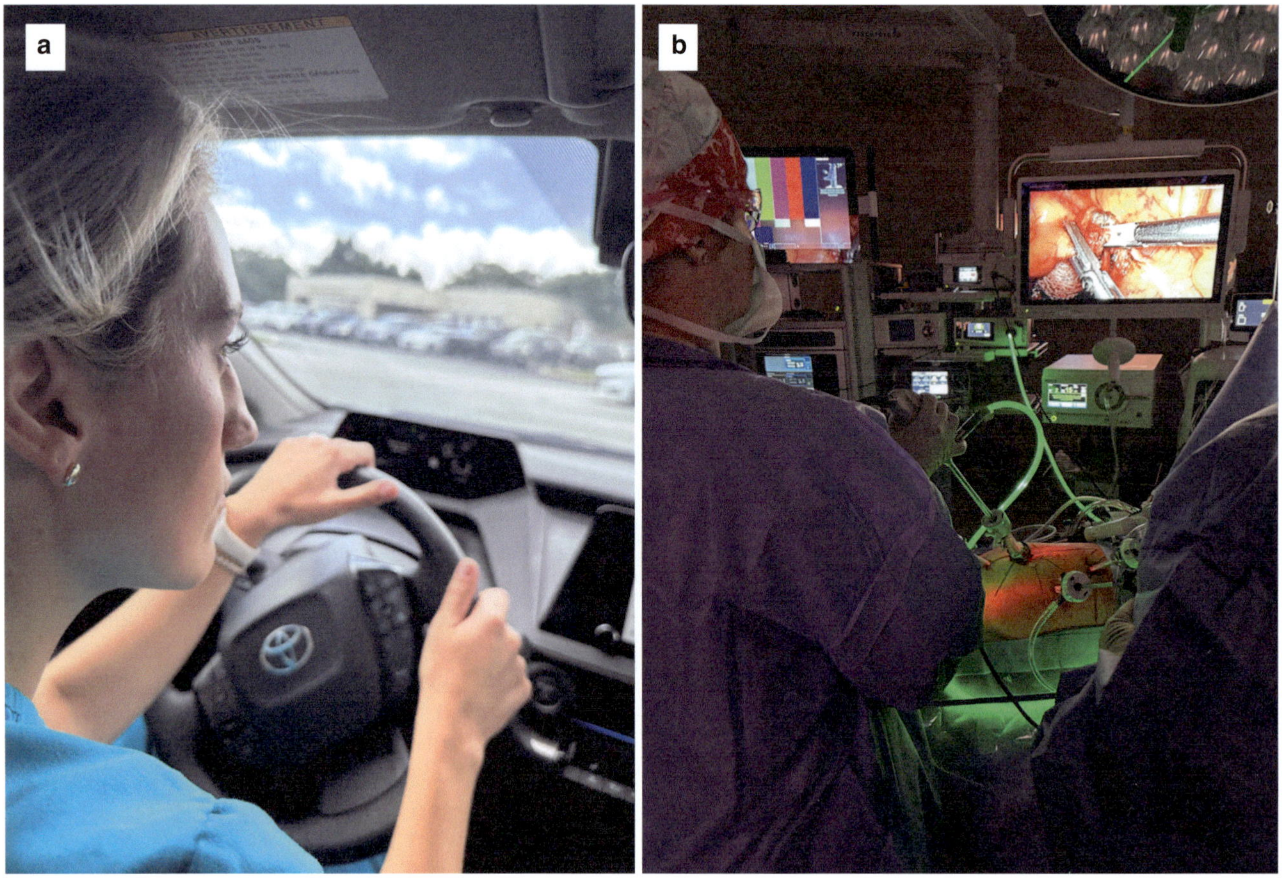

Fig. 2.21 (**a**) A driver keeps her eyes on the road, never needing to look down at the steering wheel even when executing a turn. This same principle applies to PAs who are "driving" the laparoscope, who must always focus on the operative field and not their hands operating the scope device. (**b**) PAs often assist in laparoscopic surgery by driving the camera (laparoscope). The principles of maintaining the *horizon*, surgeon instrument in the *center* of the LCD monitor, while holding the scope *steadily*. Note that the PA has her *eyes on monitor* and is not looking at her hands or the scope itself

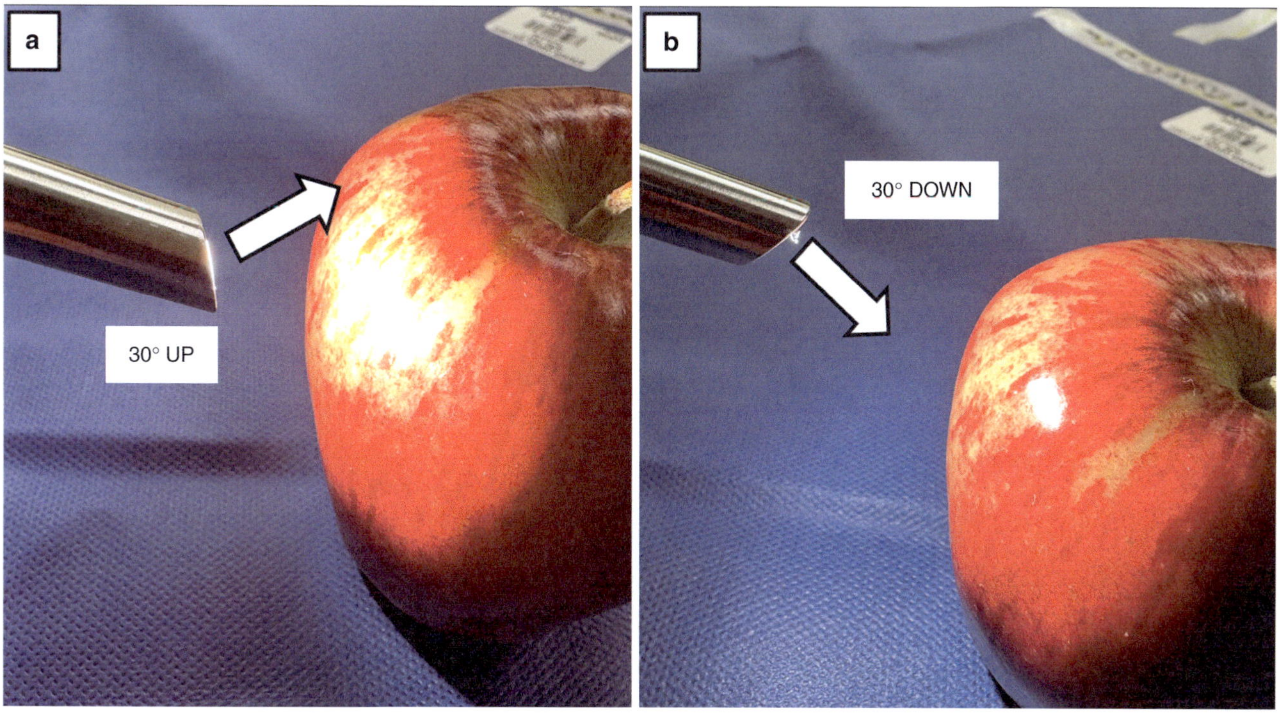

Fig. 2.22 A 30° angled scope lens is shown in the 30 UP and 30 DOWN configuration which are common base-setting for robotic cameras. Robotic cameras, unlike laparoscopic cameras, can be completely controlled by the surgeon. While 0° lens are used by some surgeons, many prefer the angled lens because it allows the surgeon to see the target anatomy from a better vantage point, particularly in more complex cases

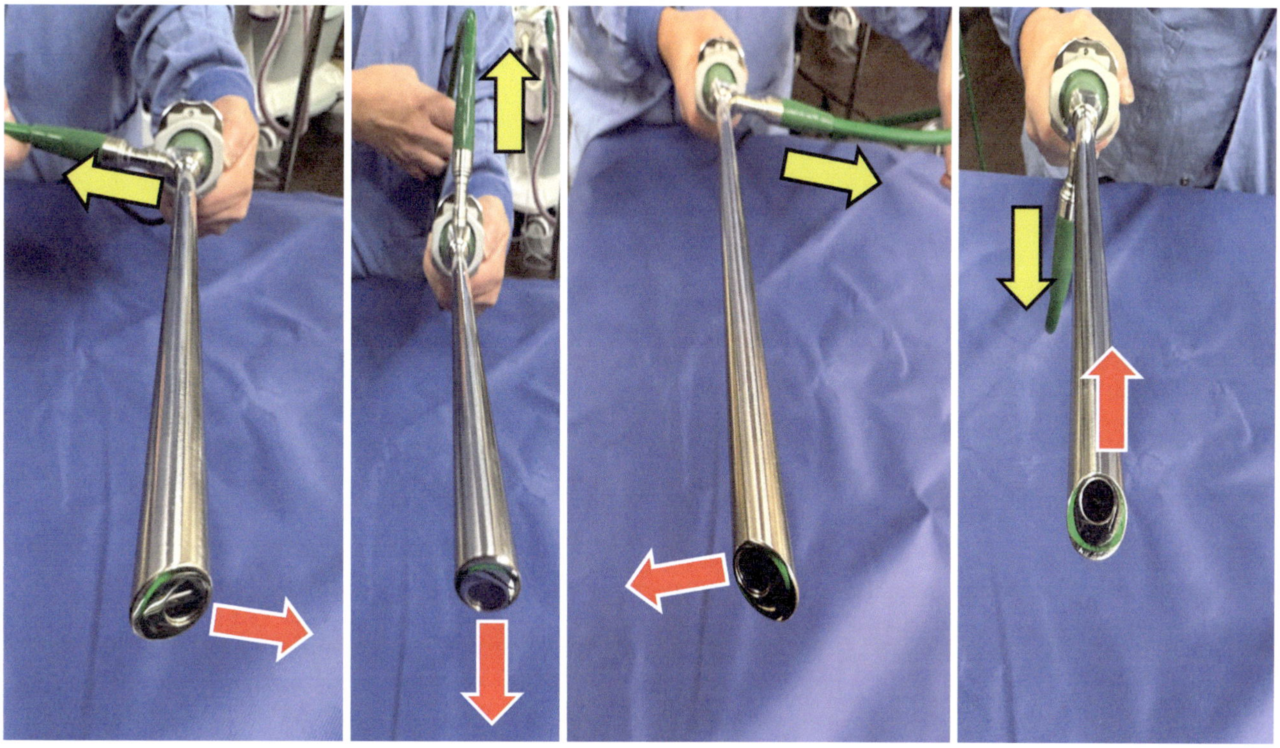

Fig. 2.23 In laparoscopic surgery, *the position of the light cord dictates the direction of the lens*. Thus, if the operator moves the light cord *downward*, the lens will be looking *upward*, and if the light cord is directed *leftward*, the lens will be looking *rightward*, and so on. The light cord is able to rotate along the scope access in 360° allowing for the lens direction to be perfectly optimized

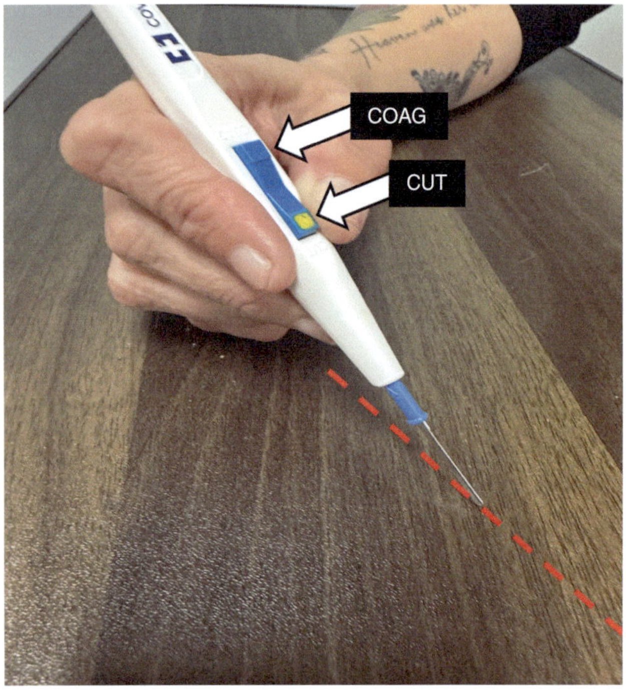

Fig. 2.24 The proper technique for holding the Bovie pencil is just like holding an ordinary pencil. The tip is often Teflon coated metal, and there are many different types and styles that can be easily exchanged into the Bovie. The device is connected to a generator through a cord (not shown) and a separate cord connects to a grounding pad, usually affixed to the patient overlying a large muscle group, such as the quadriceps. The Bovie has two controls, a yellow button, which delivers cutting current, and a blue button that delivers coagulation current. The purity of cutting current can be adjusted on the generator as well as the energy settings, but a main rule of thumb is that for operation of the Bovie on skin, *cutting* current is used (yellow button), and for everything else, coagulation is used (blue button). Note the general angle of the tip to the table and how the tip is perpendicular to the table (not slanting to one side or the other). It is important to realize that anything the blade tip contacts on a patient will be cauterized. *Therefore, only use the tip, and be cognizant that the other portions of the active blade are not in contact with the patient*

The advantage of electrocautery is that, unlike a cold knife, it coagulates tissue as it cuts through them resulting in greatly improved hemostasis. Electrocautery is excellent for cutting through vein-rich subcutaneous tissue (that otherwise tends to bleed easily) but can also be used on most soft tissues, muscle, fascia, peritoneum, stomach, etc.

Without getting into too much detail, electrocautery requires the patient to be *a part of a circuit*. This is done by placing a **grounding pad** adherent to the patient. In such a circuit design, only the patient can be effected by cautery. Thus, as long as the circuit is intact, you cannot be burned by the cautery device even if you were to touch it onto your bare skin. *The surgeon and PA are safe from thermal injury during electrocautery.*

There are some instances when this rule is broken, and that is when the surgeon, PA, or other personnel inadvertently becomes a part of the circuit, at which time the risk of burn/injury from the cautery device is possible. The other point to make about cautery is that it works by *direct contact*, and the energy does not pass through the air for any significant distance (perhaps just a few millimeters depending on the cautery setting).

There are many applications of electrocautery, including dissecting, cutting, cauterizing blood vessels, fulgurating lesions (e.g., condyloma acuminata), and more. The Bovie device can be used both laparoscopically and in open procedures. One of the most important uses is its application for tissue dissection, whereby it is important that a PA assistant *does not advance the tip beyond the dissection plane*, which is often referred to as "**pass-point**"—in reference to *passing beyond the intended point of dissection* (Fig. 2.25).

10. *Light Adjustment:* For laparoscopic and robotic surgery, there is no need for light adjustment (except for adjusting brightness). However, during open surgery, and during open phases of laparoscopic and robotic surgery, external light beam adjustment is absolutely crucial. Adjustments to the main overhead lights are often required multiple times during operation, as the lights tend to "drift" and can get bumped as well, sending the beam of maximum light intensity off of the area of interest. In addition, the surgical field is not constant and the beam can only focus on one small area at a time, so it has to often be redirected. *A good assistant is aware of the external overhead light beam and constantly strives to optimize its position.* Even when a surgeon is using a headlight, it is still important to optimize the external overhead lighting such that it is always focused on the operative field.
11. *Other:* Clamping tissue and picking up tissue to prove counter-tension is an essential aspect of surgery. Being able to control and handle clamps and retractors requires practice as it is not as easy as it looks for beginners (Fig. 2.26). Being able to slowly release a hemostat (with either the left or right hand), for example, is a very important task. This slow release of a clamp usually takes place as a vessel is being simultaneously tied off by the surgeon with suture. Due to the high stakes involved if the control of the vessel is lost, most surgeons will not entrust novice PAs to handle this critical task until they have demonstrated competency.

Other skills that should be mastered by surgical PAs include the proper method of surgical skin stapling (Fig. 2.27), which altogether differs from the surgical staplers commonly used for bowel surgery (Fig. 2.28).

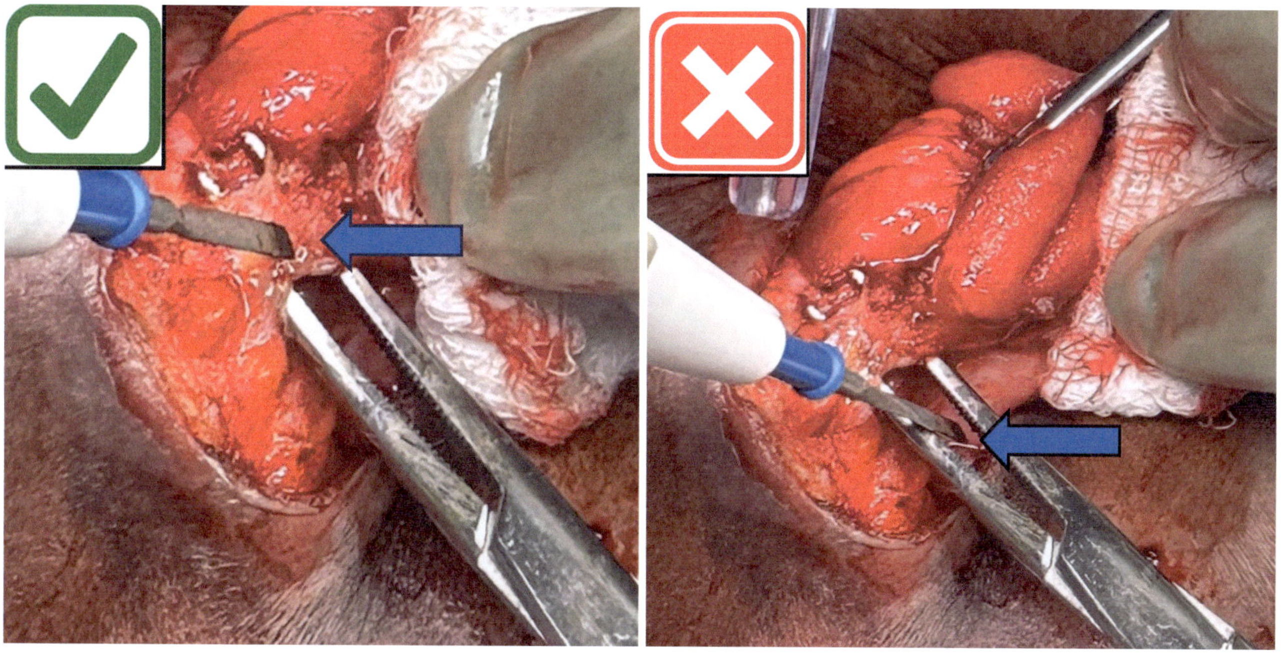

Fig. 2.25 One important role for a PA in surgery is to assist in tissue dissection and exposure by operating the Bovie to divide through certain tissue along the plane of dissection. Usually the surgeon will expose the tissue to be divided, as is shown here with a hemostat or similar dissection tool. The exposed tissue is the *only thing* that should be divided and the tissue beneath this should never be cut or divided, as this can result in serious injury and damage to surrounding organs and/or vessels. If the Bovie tip falls below this plane, it is called **"pass point."** So if you hear a surgeon say to you, *"don't pass point"* it is in reference to this

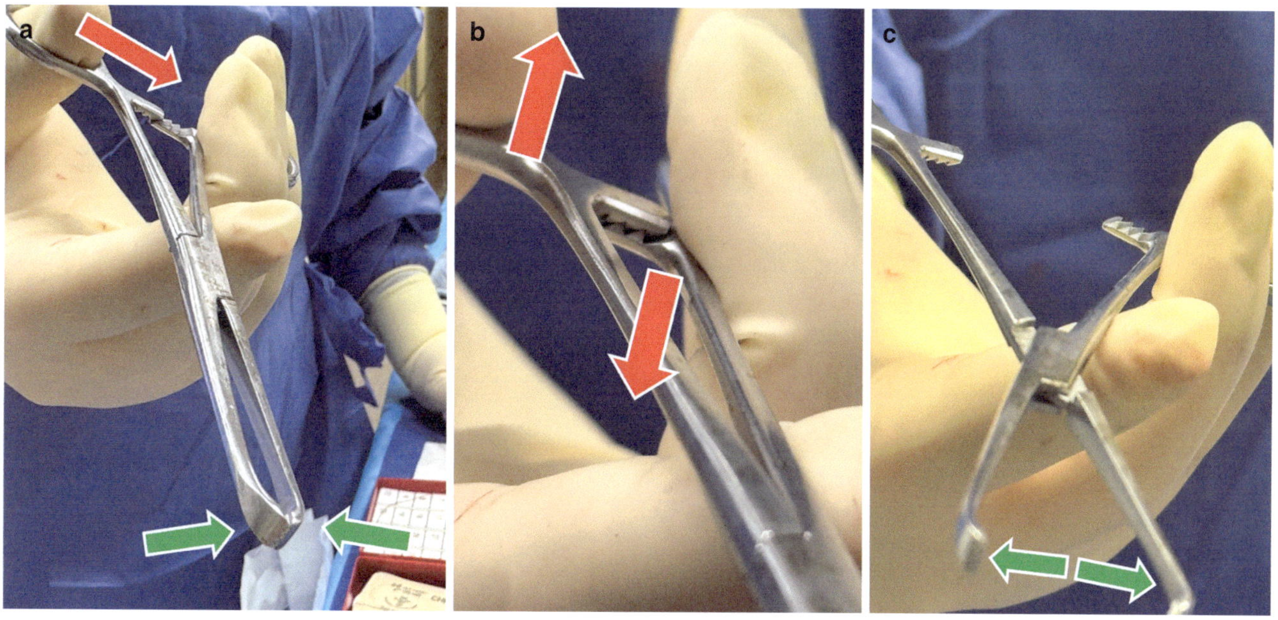

Fig. 2.26 The correct operation of surgical instruments, especially graspers, is important—and this is a skill that novice PAs and PAs in training should strive to master. Graspers and hemostats have a universal clamping mechanisms that ratchets near the finger loops. (**a**) The operation to close the device is simple, and it is just like closing a pair of scissors, only once closed the rachets lock it into place so it cannot open. Closing is not difficult to learn as it is intuitive and easy. What is not easy is understanding how to open the device. (**b**) To release the self-locking ratchet, one must apply counter pressure to the handle in opposite directions (red arrows), which will release the lock and allows the grasper to open (green arrows), as shown in (**c**). This is a simple skill that PAs should practice until they master it completely *and* can do it with either their left or right hand. Note: due to the way handles and ratchets are designed, it will be more difficult to do this with your left hand, so be sure to practice!

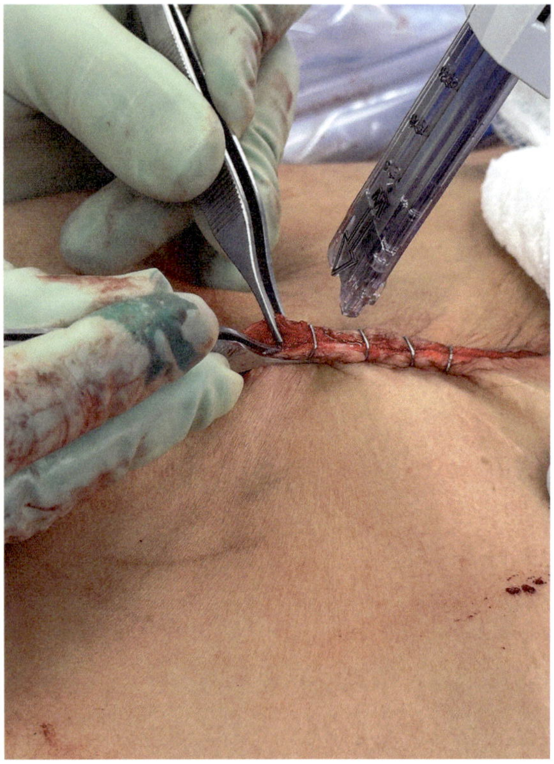

Fig. 2.27 Closure of skin can be performed using suture or by using skin staples (clips) as shown. The staples are delivered through a single-use stapling gun that delivers one staple at a time when the handle is depressed. An arrow on the tip shows where the center of the staple will be when fired, and the person operating the stapler lines this up precisely to the center of the wound edges. As shown, stapling skin requires an assistant to bring the skin edges together using toothed forceps (such as Adson forceps) to reapproximate the tissue in preparation for stapling. Note that the skin edges are purposely everted, which is proper technique for stapling skin

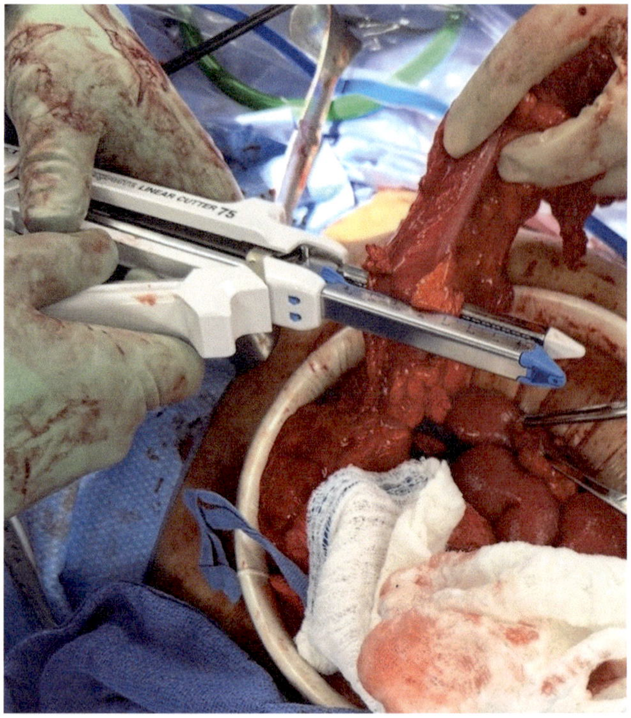

Fig. 2.28 Bowel and other organs including the liver and lung can be divided using surgical staplers. There are a multitude of different types, shapes, and sizes suitable for open, laparoscopic, and robotic platforms. For bowel, staplers can be used to transect and simultaneously seal the two ends of bowel, as is shown here. In other instances, using specialized surgical (circular) staplers, the bowel can be reconnected, a process termed anastomosis. Surgical staplers use high-grade titanium staples, which are a nonferrous metal and do not activate metal detectors at airports, for example

Laser Operation and Safety

Lasers in surgery are quite different in method and operation than electrocautery. Common operative lasers include the argon beam laser and the CO_2 laser (Fig. 2.29a, b). Like electrocautery, *lasers do not dull like scalpels do.* Lasers use thermal energy to cut and coagulate tissue, similar to cautery, but there are key differences that have to be understood in comparison to electrocautery. First, laser energy *does* travel through the air, thus it *does not* require direct contact to cauterize tissue. Second, it *does not* require the patient to be part of the circuit. **This means that anything the laser is pointed towards can potentially be cauterized and/or burned.** This includes the patient drapes (fire risk), OR personnel and or their gowns, your hands, or other inadvertent targets. *Special protective eyewear is mandatory and special laser safety education is strongly recommended and mandatory in some institutions.*

Understanding Surgical Anatomy

Surgeons are anatomists. They study anatomy to become surgeons, and review and relearn anatomy to become better surgeons. Without a strong foundation in anatomy, a surgeon is not likely to be competent. As PAs, very detailed knowledge about human anatomy is not necessary, but it is important to know how a surgeon thinks anatomically when approaching a surgical procedure.

In school, you probably learned about anatomy, particularly **gross human anatomy**, but this differs from **surgical anatomy**. **Surgical anatomy** can best be defined as understanding the *relationship of one structure to another*, as well as understanding *points of left-right asymmetry*. Finally, surgical anatomy also includes a strong understanding of *where critical structures are found*, which should be avoided when they are not the anatomic target of operation. Let us look at each of these points closer.

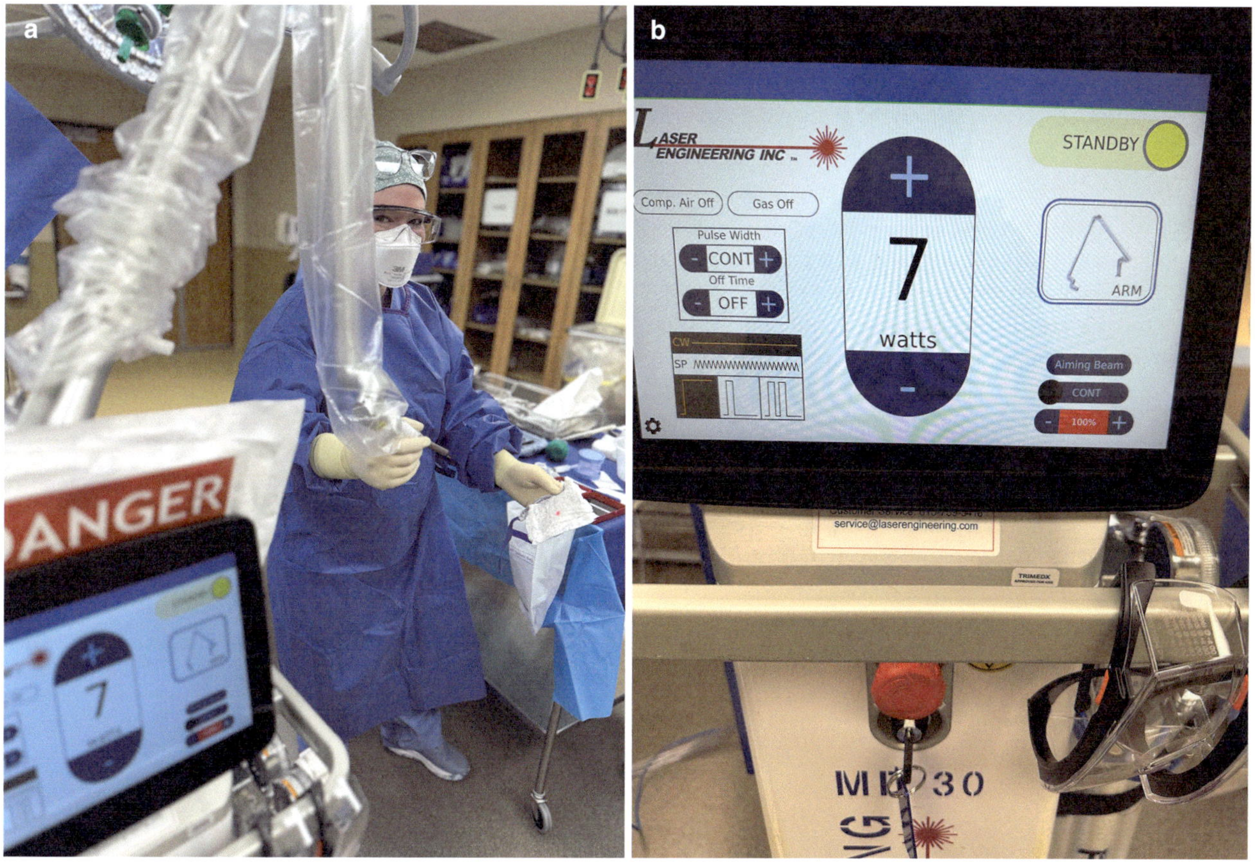

Fig. 2.29 (**a**) A surgical technician hold the hand piece to a CO_2 laser (in standby mode) at a scrub sponge for demonstration purposes. Note that a laser "red dot" beam is projected onto the sponge. This is exactly the same as the laser pointers you are familiar with, and it is not the actual CO_2 laser beam itself. Since the CO_2 laser beam is invisible, a red light, secondary pointer laser is used to let the surgeon know where the CO_2 is targeting, as the laser pointer mirrors the CO_2 laser beam. The device is connected to a generator (**b**) that requires a key to activate and is usually set to 5–10 Watts. For safety reasons, the laser is usually switched to standby mode (as shown) unless it is actively being used

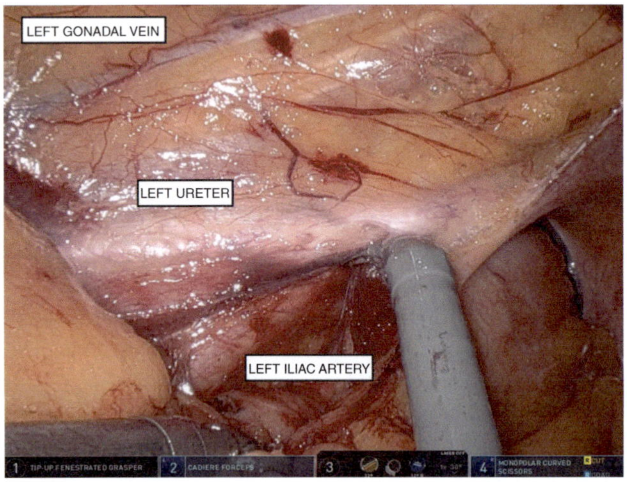

Fig. 2.30 A robotic console view of the left pelvis and retroperitoneal structures is shown. This image exemplifies what is meant by *surgical* anatomy. Understanding the relationship between the ureter and the iliac vessel, and understanding that the ureter courses *over/above* and not beneath the iliac vessel, is an important distinction. At this level, the gonadal vessels lie *lateral to* the ureter. The relationship of one organ structure to another defines *surgical* anatomy. Surgeons rely on a strong understanding of surgical anatomy in order to perform operations safely and effectively.

1. *Relationship of One Structure to Another:* Surgeons want to know very important details about how structures are "arranged." As an example, in gross human anatomy you probably learned that the ureter is a tiny tube that connects the kidney (where urine is formed) to the bladder (where urine is stored), but in *surgical anatomy* we learn that the ureter courses above (rather than deep to) the common iliac vessels, and is medial to, not lateral to, the gonadal vein below the level of the sacral promontory (Fig. 2.30). There are multiple other examples like this. Surgeons spend a lot of time understanding these relationships so they always "know where they are" and so they minimize complications as they dissect near or at an organ or structure(s) of interest.
2. *Points of Left-Right Asymmetry:* It turns out our body is not a perfect mirror image and there are important anatomic differences with clinical relevance. Examples include well-known unilateral structures—e.g., the appendix exists on the right side only, as does the gallbladder. It also includes several other subtle differences. Some examples are: (a) the *thoracic duct* drains into the *left* subclavian vein; (b) the recurrent laryngeal nerve courses around the *aortic arch* on the *left*, but loops around the *subclavian vein* on the *right*; and (c) the *left* gonadal vein drains into the renal vein, but the *right* gonadal vein drains directly into the inferior vena cava.

   Another example includes the difference in angulation of the right and left main stem bronchus, where the right is not very angulated, and the left is quite angulated. As a clinical correlate, this is the reason that when intubation is performed and the ET tube is advanced beyond the carina, it is much more likely to slide into the right mainstem bronchus and almost never the left.

   From a PA standpoint, it is not so important to memorize all these differences, just know that they exist and that they can be quite important to surgeons especially.
3. *Where critical structures are found:* Remember that the goal of any operation is to (a) reach the target anatomy via dissection, (b) excise the target anatomy (for example, appendix or gallbladder) *or* repair the target anatomy (for example, mesh repair of an inguinal hernia), and this has to be executed (c) without causing collateral damage to surrounding and potentially very critical structures.

   As a good example, let us consider one of the most common general surgical procedures performed—the laparoscopic cholecystectomy (Lap Chole). Here, a surgeon must remove the gallbladder without causing injury to the common bile duct (CBD). This is because CBD injury is very serious and repair can be complex and problematic. General surgeons who perform this operation are keenly aware of identifying the relevant anatomy so that the gallbladder can be removed without injury to surrounding critical structures such as the CBD which lies in very close proximity to the gallbladder.

Selected Readings and Additional Resources

1. Donaldson MS, Corrigan JM, Kohn LT, editors. To err is human: building a safer health system. Institute of Medicine, Committee on Quality of Health Care in America; 2000.
2. Guideline for hand hygiene in healthcare settings. J Am Coll Surg. 2004;198:121–7.
3. Gupta V, Jain G. Safe laparoscopic cholecystectomy: adoption of universal culture of safety in cholecystectomy. World J Gastrointest Surg. 2019;11(2):62.
4. Hopkins E, Sanvictores T, Sharma S. Physiology, acid base balance. 2018.
5. Macdonald AG. A brief historical review of non-anaesthetic causes of fires and explosions in the operating room. Br J Anaesth. 1994;73:847–56.
6. Pocock G, Richards CD, Richards DA. Human physiology. Oxford University Press; 2018.
7. Popowicz P, Leonard K. Noninvasive ventilation and oxygenation strategies. Surg Clin North Am. 2021;102(1):149.
8. Townsend CM, et al. Sabiston textbook of surgery: the biological basis of modern surgical practice. Elsevier Health Sciences; 2016.
9. Wolf GL, Sidebotham GW, Lazard JL, Charchaflieh JG. Laser ignition of surgical drape materials in air, 50% oxygen, and 95% oxygen. Anesthesiology. 2004;100:1167–71.

Medical Treatment and Management Protocols for the Surgical Patient

3

Sam Atallah

Introduction

Perhaps the most important idea to understand for PAs being introduced to surgery is that most of what has to be learned and mastered in surgery has almost nothing to do with the operation itself. Instead, the focus of surgery as a rotation or even as a career is centered on the *medical management of the surgical patient.*

There are a multitude of scenarios, principles, and core information related to this topic, many of which are delineated in this chapter. The role of the PA in surgery and the nuts and bolts of surgery protocols and standards are discussed.

Part 1: General Guidelines for PAs on the Surgical Service

Expectations for PAs on Surgery

PAs must have meticulous attention to detail and a strong work ethic. They should be extremely knowledgeable about their patients. Surgeons expect you to ***know your patients*** and to be a **fully engaged team member**. Even as a student, you want to *take ownership* of patients on the surgical service. Do not think of patients as "someone else's" but as <u>your</u> patient as well! Thus, if you asked to assess a patient preoperatively (a.k.a., "*pre-op*"), attending surgeons expect the PA to know all of the patient's medical and surgical history, their medications, allergies, and other relevant information (e.g., findings on pertinent radiographic imaging, if applicable).

Most importantly, a PA should know the <u>indication for surgery</u> and <u>diagnosis</u> of the patient when pre-oping them. If you find yourself asking the attending surgeon in the middle of an operation *"why are we doing this surgery?", "does the patient have a cancer?", "what operation are we doing?",* then you demonstrate to your attending surgeon a lack of preparedness, and these are examples of questions you should know the answers to prior to the commencement of operation. *Always be prepared. Always know your patients!*

As PAs gain clinical experience, they also gain a more solid foundation in managing patients, and understanding what is important to pay attention to when evaluating patients. *The emphasis should always be on the medical management of the surgical patient, with patient safety as the top priority care.* By nature, surgery is a high risk and high stakes endeavor, which demands meticulous attention to every detail. Managing a surgical patient requires a solid foundation in medicine.

PA Communication on the Surgical Service

Communication is one of the most important roles you will have as a PA on the surgical service. Communication is with three groups: **(a)** the surgical and medical team (attending surgeon and/or surgical residents/fellows; consulting physicians, radiologists, practitioners, and hospitalists), **(b)** the nursing care team and ancillary services (such as respiratory and physical therapists), and **(c)** the patient and the patient's family and loved ones. Examples of each of these are provided in Table 3.1.

You may be asked to present patients to your attending surgeon on rounds, or even in clinic. Many patients on the surgical ward are post-ops recovering from their surgery. An important role of the PA is to stay informed about patient progress and communicating this to the attending surgeon or surgical team (e.g., interns, residents, fellows). When discussing patients, surgeons always want to know where a patient is, *at a <u>point in time</u>, relative to the time of an index event.*

S. Atallah (✉)
Department of Surgery, Piedmont Hospital, Mercer University School of Medicine, Macon, GA, USA
e-mail: atallah@post.harvard.edu

S. Atallah, J. Dragoljevic (eds.), *Fundamentals of Surgery for Physician Assistants*,
https://doi.org/10.1007/978-3-032-21069-2_3

Table 3.1 The role of communication for the PA

A. **Communication with the surgical and medical team**
a. Discuss the status of post-operative patients b. Review the care plan and review the medical history, address any concerns preoperatively (for example, medical clearance) c. Review with the internists and hospitalists the plan of care
B. **Communication with the nursing team/ancillary services**
a. Talk to the nursing staff. Discuss concerns they may have. Discuss and learn about the patient's progress in the hospital b. When applicable, discuss with the physical therapist, respiratory therapist and other ancillary support staff the progress of the patient. This may include evaluation from speech and swallow specialists c. For patients who are hospitalized and require additional care afterwords, such as a rehabilitation facility, discuss patient placement with the patient care coordinator
C. **Communication with patient and patient family/loved ones**
a. Explain the operation to the patient and address questions they may have. In general, you should be able to explain the risks and benefits of the operation, and answer questions such as, "what happens if I don't have the surgery?", "what are the risks of this operation?", "how long is the operation?", "can you explain this surgery to me in simple terms?" b. Relay information about the patient, for example after surgery inform the family that the surgery has been, for example, successfully completed and that the patient is in recovery c. Set expectations about the operation and the recovery pathway. Patients often have very practical questions that they want to have answered. For example, "how long will I be in the hospital after my operation?", "when can I start driving again?", "when can I start working out after my surgery?", "will I have any restrictions and for how long?", "will I be able to eat regular food?" d. Express compassion and empathy when speaking to patients and family. Surgery is not only high stakes, it is also anxiety provoking and perhaps more in this field than in any other, surgeons want their PAs to be a calming and caring member of the care team. This is an aspect of medicine in which a PA can shine and truly fill their role as a physician extender

For example, on the trauma surgical service, an important point of time is knowing the time of a car accident (motor vehicle accident/MVA) which in this case is an important *index event.* Thus, a key question to ask in obtaining a history from a MVA patient is knowing *how long ago* was the accident? This is relevant in almost all fields of medicine as it can determine approach and treatment. For example, knowing the *weeks of gestation* in a female with contractions on the obstetrical service or knowing the time of onset of focal neurologic deficits in a patient with suspected cerebrovascular accident (CVA). This gives clinicians an important **frame of reference**, and the same applies to the surgical patient.

Surgeons think of their post-op patients in terms of ***time since an index event,*** which is usually **the day they had their surgery**. This day is abbreviated **POD** which stands for "**P**ost-**O**perative **D**ay," and **POD 0** denotes the day *of* surgery, and **POD 1** denotes the first day after surgery, and so on. *It is very important for PAs to be very well tuned into this.*

Table 3.2 Communicating to physicians—examples of how to communicate in various scenarios

DON'T: "You did a colectomy a few days ago and he has a fever today"
DO: "Mr. Jones is POD 4 from a laparoscopic right hemicolectomy and is febrile to 38.2 °C this am"
DON'T: "This patient fell from a ladder and passed out and so they brought him here"
DO: "This trauma patient sustained a fall from an approximately 12-foot ladder 3 h ago and was found unresponsive at the scene"
DON'T: "I have a young guy here who developed pain in his testicle"
DO: "A 17 yo male presented to the ED with sudden onset left testicular pain that began 45 min prior to arrival"
DON'T: "This is a lady you removed her pancreas cancer awhile back and she's here for follow up"
DO: "Mrs. Jones is a 78 yo female status-post Whipple operation for pT1 adenocarcinoma at the head of the pancreas who is now 7-months post-op here for follow-up today"
DON'T: "Hey this patient is just here for his scan results"
DO: "Mr. Jones is a 56 yo male who was recently diagnosed with a low-lying rectal cancer, biopsy proven invasive adenocarcinoma and is undergoing a staging workup. His CT-scans show no evidence of metastasis. You sent him for a dedicated MRI of the rectum, and he is here to review the results. The MRI report shows the lesion to be T3N1 with the lower border at 4 cm from the anal verge

For example, if you are rounding on a 67 yo patient, Mr. Jones, who had a left colectomy Monday and it is now Thursday, the first thing a PA student or PA-C would relay is this information, usually conveyed as follows: "Mr. Jones is a 67 yo **POD 3** from left colectomy." *This frames in the mind of the surgeon an understanding of the expected progress, potential problems encountered, anticipated exam findings one would expect at* <u>*that*</u> *point in time.*

The same frame of reference is also kept when evaluating surgical patients in the clinic. For example, you may say, "Mr. Jones is a 67 yo 2 **years** status post left colectomy for cancer" which is drastically different than if the patient was 2 **days** or 2 **weeks** post-op.

Communication should be informative, succinct, and should capture the details of the encounter in a way that *makes sense.* Be specific when sharing information. For patients who have had CT-scans or other imaging completed, be sure to know *what* the results were and <u>take time to read through the radiology report</u>. PAs are <u>expected to be knowledgeable</u> about their patients, and not just someone who is "passing information along" to the attending physician.

Table 3.2 provides examples of what to say, and what not to say while communicating to other members of the healthcare team. Indeed, this is a skill that improves with experience and time in clinical practice; but start honing your communication skills as a student!

Part 2: Managing Surgical Patients Pre-operatively

General Protocols: Getting Your Patient Ready for Surgery

This section will cover various aspects related to the preparation of the surgical patient. It is meant to provide an introduction to the *general* approach and is not intended to be comprehensive. This is intended as a *pre-op-101* for PA students and newcomers to the surgical field. If you are just starting out caring for surgical patients, you will want to get familiar with the process. While hospitals and surgical centers have different protocols and styles, in the United States, there are general guidelines and approaches regarding the delivery of surgical care that are fairly universal across the country and they are outlined herein.

1. **Written Consent:** All patients who are undergoing surgery must have a consent form signed by the patient and signed by the surgeon that delineates, at a minimum, the planned operation. **No patient will enter an operating room without a signed consent**. Of course, there are permissible exceptions under very specific circumstances—such as emergent cases in patients who are not able to provide consent (for example, secondary to altered level of consciousness, or trauma). Another caveat is that if the patient is unable to sign, but has a power of attorney (POA), or a next of kin who can sign of the patient's behalf. *As a PA, when pre-oping patients, you should check the consent, and confirm that it is filled out properly (correct procedure) with the patient's/surgeon's signature.*
2. **History and Physical Examination:** One of the most important documents that is required to be either physically available, or available electronically, is the *History and Physical Examination Form,* you will hear this often abbreviated as **H and P**. This is a crucial part of documentation, and surgeons and surgical ancillary staff look to this as a source that not only is informative regarding the patient's past medical history, medications, allergies, etc., but, importantly, the H and P spells out the diagnosis of the patient and the indication for surgery; in cases where the operation is "sided" (left versus right), the proper side to be operated on is expressly stated. In the United States, most hospitals and surgical centers require the form be available and up-to-date (usually within 30-days prior to the date of operation).
3. **Orders:** Both outpatient and inpatients require a completed **order set**, which is nowadays standardized in most healthcare systems. An example order set is shown in Fig. 3.1. It provides a menu of items that can be chosen for a specific procedure. Orders delineate exactly what the planned operation is going to be, on whom it is going to be, and when it is going to be. It also covers essential preoperative orders which vary depending on the case specifics. Commonly, an order for **venous thromboembolic prophylaxis** (VTE), *also known as* **deep vein thrombosis** (DVT) **prophylaxis**, is provided, as well as orders for pre-operative antibiotics which are routinely given for prophylaxis for select operations, delivered systemically and ideally **30 min prior to incision**. You may be surprised to learn that not all operations require antibiotics for prophylaxis (discussed later).
4. **Medical or Cardiac Clearance Documentation:** Some patients may have a significant pre-existing condition that requires medical or cardiac clearance, as deemed necessary by the attending surgeon and/or anesthetist. Examples include history of coronary artery disease, heart failure, and chronic pulmonary disease. *Critical aortic stenosis* places patients at very high risk for a cardiac event, as the coronary arteries are the first branch off of the aorta (Fig. 3.2), and flow through these vital arteries can plummet due to the effects of anesthesia. A PA's role in surgery is to assure that, if a medical/cardiac clearance was required, it is physically available "on the chart" (or electronically) and that the patient's operative risk stratification has been reviewed; and, importantly, *any recommendations made by the clearing physician have been followed prior to proceeding with surgery.*
5. **Marking the Patient (Sided Operations):** Some patients undergo operations that are non-sided and thus do not require side (left versus right) skin marking on the patient. For example, laparoscopic appendectomy does not require marking the patient because there is only one appendix. However, operations such as inguinal hernia repair do require marking as part of the **safety culture** of insuring correct side surgery. Thus, if a patient is undergoing a left inguinal hernia repair, the standard is to mark that side with a skin marker, using the word "Yes" and then both the attending surgeon and the patient (when able) sign the side to be operated on with the skin marker (Fig. 3.3a, b). *This is not performed by the PA but rather the operating surgeon(s);* still, it is important to know about skin marking. This is one important step to assuring that wrong-side surgery remains a "never event." ***Other Special Markings:*** Sometimes other markings are made on the patient, and this depends on the case and procedure. Plastic surgeons typically will make several skin markings with a marker to maintain a visual perspective and understanding of the operation, particularly for cosmetic procedures. In general surgery and colorectal surgery, patients are often marked at the best site for a stoma, if a stoma (ileostomy, colostomy) is planned. Usually this is done when the patient is sitting up, because there can

Fig. 3.1 An example of a pre-operative order set is shown. Order sets like this do not just make putting orders easier for clinicians, they help standardize the delivery of healthcare and helps reduce errors of omission. Overall, order sets improve care quality

Patient: ____________________

Surgeon: ___________________

1. Diagnosis: ___________________________________
2. Allergy:__________________Height:_____ Weight:_____
3. Date of Procedure: _____________________________
4. Post-Operative Care: O Admit In Patient O Admit Observation O Outpatient
5. Obtain Surgical Consent for: ________________________
6. Diet: O NPO after MN on __________ (date) O clear liquids until _____(time)
7. Labs: O In Pre-op day of surgery O Within 30 days prior to surgery
   Check All that apply:
   O CBC O aPTT/PT/INR O Type and Screen O Urinalysis
   O CMP O Urine ßHCG O Type and Cross
8. Diagnostics: O EKG O Chest-Xray O CT-scan (of)_______ reason: ______
9. Request Pre-op Clearance: O Cardiology O Pulmonology O Medical
10. Pre-op VTE prophylaxis: O Sequential Compression Device O Enoxaperin (Lovenox) 40 mg subcutaneous one does in pre-op within one hour prior to incision
11. Pre-operative Intravenous (IV) Antibiotics (to be given 30 min prior to incision)
    O Cefazolin (Ancef) 1gm 2gm
    O Ertapenem (Invanz) 1gm
    O Vancomycin Dose: ___________
    O Ciprofloxacin 400mg
    O Metronidazole (Flagyl) 500mg
    O Other: ____________________
12. Other Medications: Indocyanine Green (ICG) on-call to OR, one vial
13. IV: O Establish Intravenous Access in Pre-Op Holding O Other: _______________
14. IV-Fluids: O Normal Saline (NS 0.9%) O Lactated Ringers (LR) O Other ___________
    IV Fluid Rate ____________ ml/hr
15. Other: ____

Provider Signature: ____________________ **Date:** ____________ **Time:** __________

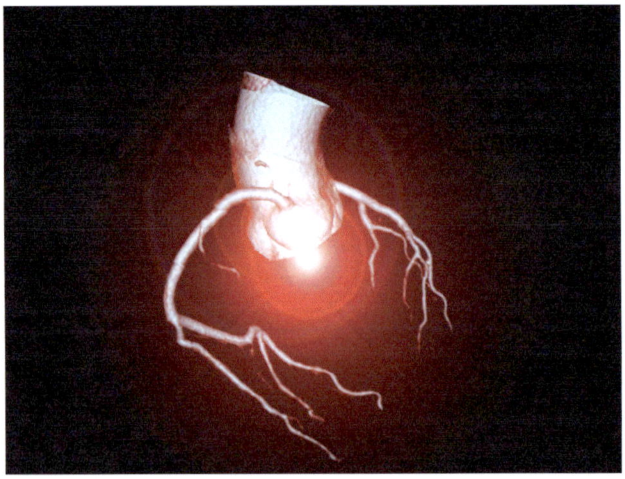

Fig. 3.2 A 3-D rendering of the proximal aorta, including the aortic valve is shown. Notice that the first branches from the aorta are actually the left and right main coronary arteries, and they are immediately distal to the aortic valve, as shown. In patients with critical aortic stenosis, their heart is already working harder to push blood through the narrowed valve. A drop in blood pressure during anesthesia can worsen this, causing a further decline in perfusion to the coronary arteries, which could lead to myocardial ischemia and/or arrythmia

be natural skin creases that are not suitable for stoma maturation and should be avoided. Where available, a stoma nurse will mark the patient and provide appropriate teaching to the patient.

6. **Relevant Additional Consent Forms and Non-consent Forms:** In many hospitals, "major cases" require the patient have been informed about the possibility of a *blood transfusion*, in case of emergency, but in some very complex operations, blood transfusion may even be planned. Blood consent is important to have *prior* to surgery. Patients should be explained the risks of blood transfusion verbally. Importantly, *not all patients consent to receiving blood products due to religious reasons—for example,* ***Jehovah's Witness***. Religious beliefs must be respected. Additionally, it is important to understand which blood products specifically a patient will or will not accept. Some will accept certain blood products such as cell saver and albumin, but not others—such as packed red blood cells (PRBCs), and/or fresh frozen plasma (FFP). It is important to check and document this in the chart.

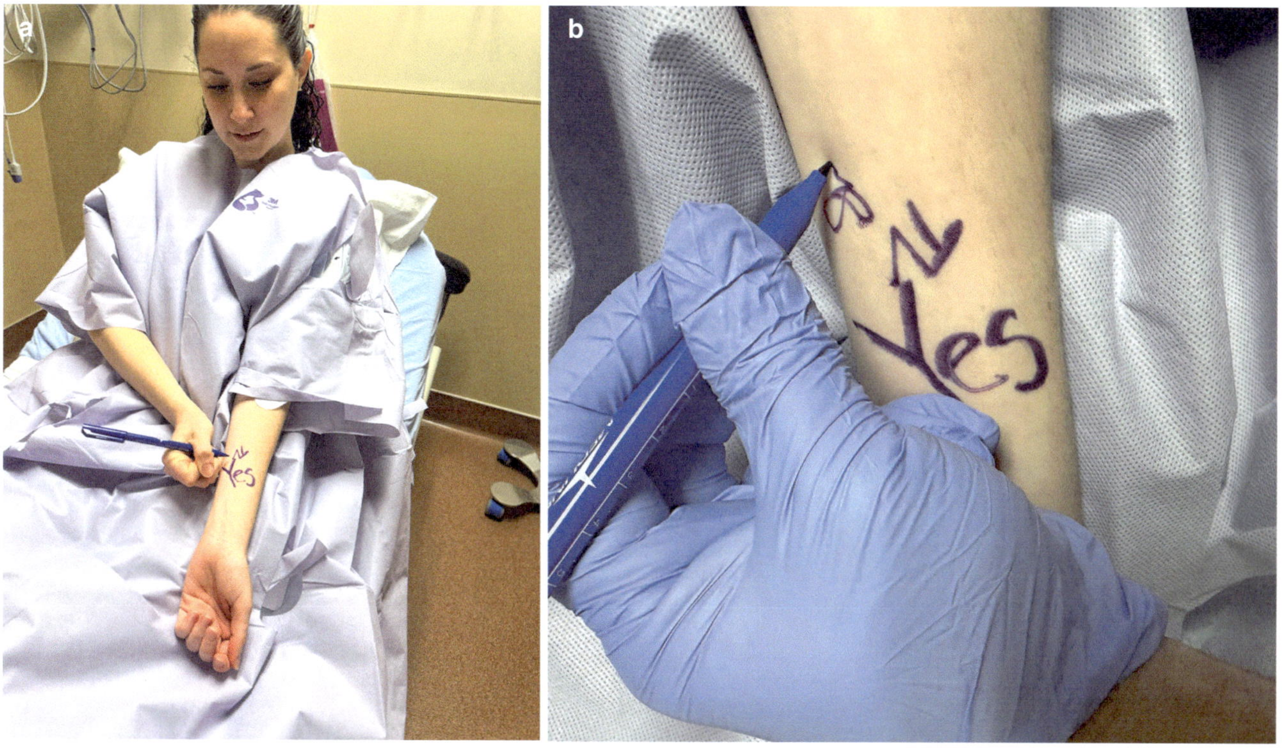

Fig. 3.3 (**a**) A patient is being prepared for a left upper extremity operation. A skin marker is used to clearly mark "YES" indicating this is the correct side of surgery. It is best practice to have the patient sign or initial the correct extremity and (**b**) have the surgeon also sign or initial the correct side. These are important steps in modern surgical safety culture that help insure that wrong side surgery is a *never event*

7. **Educating Your Patient About the Operation:** Patients are often not knowledgeable about the details of the operation. Most only have a basic understanding of anatomy and it is difficult to understand the operation the same way that persons with a clinical background understand it. *Be patient!* They may have many valid questions. Spend time explaining the operation, and what to expect after surgery. Focus on using terms that are simple to understand and process. For example, rather than saying "the surgeon is going to do an oncologic partial colectomy," say "the surgeon is going to remove a portion of your bowel that contains the cancer." The latter is easier for laypersons to process and comprehend. Setting expectations helps patients with the process and improves the overall care delivery; PAs play an important role in facilitating this. *On the one hand, PAs have to learn how to talk in highly specific medical terms when discussing patient care with other healthcare providers, while on the other hand, they have to be able to conversate with patients in a totally different and basic manner so that they understand more clearly. It is almost like you have to learn to speak in two different languages!*

Risk Stratification

Patients may have pre-existing conditions that increase their risk of undergoing surgery and may place them at high risk for complications post-operatively. Table 3.3 provides a general appreciation for the types of conditions that are important to consider. As a PA, you want to have an idea of what pre-existing conditions pose challenges. For example, a history of prior high-dose pelvic external beam radiotherapy makes operating on the pelvis *very challenging* because the tissue is likely to exhibit post-radiation changes, and it is *difficult for radiated tissue to heal after surgery.* Chronic steroid use also impedes healing. Pre-existing conditions such as severe (Child-Pugh *C*) liver cirrhosis, critical aortic stenosis, and pulmonary fibrosis also pose risks for surgery and significantly increase the odds of post-operative morbidity. As a PA on surgery, you do not have to risk stratify patients, but be *knowledgeable about the types of conditions that pose risk.*

Table 3.3 Pre-existing conditions and the relative risk for complications post-op

Condition	Relative risk
Critical aortic stenosis	+++++++
Liver cirrhosis (child's C)	++++++
Hyperkalemia, > 6.0	++++++
Myocardial infarction <6 months	+++++
Pulmonary fibrosis	+++++
Pulmonary hypertension	+++++
Severe COPD/emphysema	++++
Immune compromised status	++++
Chronic corticosteroid use	++++
CHF	+++
Prior radiation exposure	++++
Sepsis	+++++
Acidosis	+++
History of smoking	+++
Drug abuse/esp. cocaine	+++
Diabetes	++
HTN	++
Prior coronary artery stents	++
Prior coronary artery bypass grafting	++
Asthma	+

Diet Management Prior to Surgery

Rule number 1: Patients must be fasting prior to elective surgery to decrease the risk of **aspiration** during the induction of anesthesia. The medical term for fasting is *nothing* per os, or simply ***NPO***.

Rule number 2: *How long* a patient is required to be fasting prior to elective surgery *depends on the diet.*

Practice guidelines are available that meticulously detail the standard of care in pre-op fasting protocols [1–3], and they are briefly reviewed here.

Clear liquids can be consumed up to **2 h** before a planned procedure where sedation or a general anesthetic is required. Note: regional anesthetics (such as spinal anesthesia) follow the same guidelines. *A word of caution:* for patients with known or suspected **gastroparesis**, many experts believe 2 h is *insufficient.*

Clear liquids are defined as "*any liquid you can see through*" with the exception of alcohol which is impermissible. A clear liquid by definition thus cannot be hazy and cannot contain pulp or fat ingredients, such as milk. Specific examples of clear and non-clears are delineated in Table 3.4.

Preoperative Fasting of Light Solid Food So-called **Solid Food** is not a homogenous category and can be subdivided into *Regular* Solid Foods and *Light* Solid Food. **Light solid food (including a small amount of milk)** may be consumed up to **6 h** before a planned procedure where sedation or a general anesthesia are required. Examples of light solid foods include toast, cereal (with a small amount of milk), coffee with milk, crackers, and fruit juices that contain pulp.

Table 3.4 Examples of clear liquid and non-clear liquid diets

Clear liquid diet
Water
Apple juice
Black coffee (without milk or creamers)
Clear tea
Sports drinks (e.g., Powerade®, Gatorade®)
Clear carbonated drinks (Sprite®, 7-Up®)
Clear protein drinks like Ensure Clear®,
Non-clear liquid diet
Milk
Coconut water
Jello™
Hot chocolate
Coffee or tea that contains any additive—e.g., milk, cream,
Orange juice (with or without pulp)
Smoothies
Most gastric tube feeds (if applicable)

These guidelines assume the patient has normal gastric emptying (beware that many diabetic patients have delayed gastric emptying and it is better to err on the side of safety).

Preoperative Fasting of Regular Solid Food For regular solid foods, which may include fatty foods, fried foods, and/or meats such as chicken or steak, fasting requires **8 h** prior to planned operation for elective cases. Patients who require emergent surgery and who have not fasted have an increased risk of aspiration. Protocols such as ***rapid sequence intubation*** **(RSI)** are important in mitigating the risk of aspiration in these settings.

To summarize, these are the fasting/NPO recommendations for patients prior to elective surgery:

- Regular solid food diet: permissible, up to **8 h** prior to operation
- Light solid food diet: permissible, up to **6 h** prior to operation
- Clear liquid diet: permissible, up to **2 h** prior to operation
- Strict NPO: no diet is permissible **<2 h** prior to operation

Important Genetic Mutations and the Pre-surgical Patient

G6PD Mutation Glucose-6-phosphate dehydrogenase (G6PD) deficiency *is the most prevalent enzyme deficiency, with an estimated 400 million people affected worldwide* [4, 5]. It is an inborn error of metabolism and occurs due to a mutation in the gene that results in a lack of the G6PD enzyme production. The gene lies near the telomeric end of the long (q) arm of the X chromosome, Xq28 (Fig. 3.4), making it a condition that far more frequently affects males (since males only possess *one* X chromosome). In Mendelian

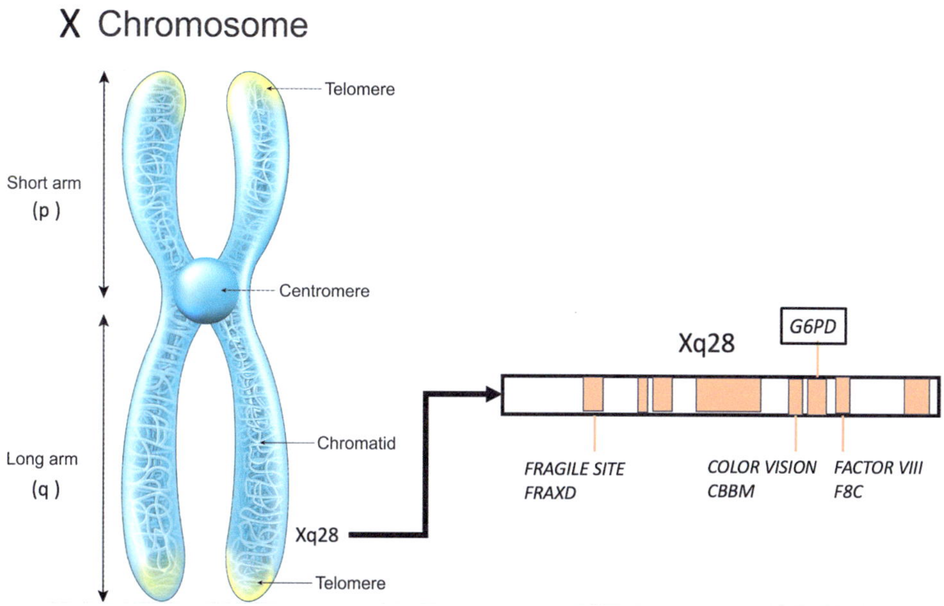

Fig. 3.4 The glucose-6-phosphate dehydrogenase (G6PD) gene is on the long or *q* arm of the X-chromosome and lies near the telomeric end (Xq28). A mutation in this X-linked trait primarily affects males. G6PD is a gene that codes for an enzyme critical for protecting red blood cells from oxidative damage. G6PD is important for the pentose phosphate pathway, which helps generate molecules that protect cells from oxidative stress. Individuals with this mutation may experience hemolytic anemia (destruction of red blood cells) in response to certain triggers, like infections, and certain medications (e.g., sulfa drugs, aspirin)

genetics, this disease inheritance pattern is described as **X-linked recessive**.

Importantly, patients with G6PD deficiency can exhibit oxidative stress resulting in *hemolysis.* Certain anesthetics can cause this, while others tend to be protective. For example, propofol and remifentanil are considered safe for G6PD deficient patients, and perhaps sevoflurane, an inhalational general anesthetic.

As a PA, who may be administering *local anesthetics* in the operating room and while doing minor procedures, it is important to know that *some local anesthetics can cause methemoglobinemia and should be avoided in G6PD deficient patients.* This is especially true for *lidocaine* (an amide) and *tetracaine* (an ester). In addition, *prilocaine* and *benzocaine* (known to induce methemoglobinemia) should be avoided. Some studies have shown the long-acting local anesthetic *bupivacaine* to be safe in the setting of G6PD deficiency.

Other important medications used in surgery include SILVADENE Cream 1% (silver sulfadiazine), which is commonly used as a topical therapy for burns. However, in G6PD-deficient individuals, this may result in hemolysis.

Malignant Hyperthermia Unlike G6PD deficiency which is relatively common, malignant hyperthermia (MH) is quite *rare* with approximately 800,000 individuals affected worldwide (an approximate incidence of ~1 in 10,000). The inheritance pattern is autosomal dominant (AD), which means the offspring of a person with MH has a 50% probability of carrying the disease (Fig. 3.5). MH is caused by a genetic mutation in the *RYR1* gene on chromosome 19q13 which codes for the ryanodine receptor that affects calcium homeostasis [6]. MH results in an abnormal release of calcium from the sarcoplasmic reticulum in muscle cells causing severe metabolic derangements with resultant rise in core body temperature (often quite high: > 104 °F/40 °C).

With MH, there is also notable muscle rigidity, tachypnea, tachycardia, and acidosis. Importantly, ***these symptoms can occur during surgery or in the immediate post-operative period*** (e.g., in the recovery room, or post anesthesia care unit, PACU). Certain anesthetic agents are triggers for MH. This especially includes halothane, sevoflurane, and depolarizing paralytics/muscle relaxants—namely *succinylcholine.* MH is an emergent, life-threatening condition. The main treatment is **Dantrolene** [7, 8]. When preoping your patient, it is important to ask about a family history of MH. Patients with a family history are best treated as though they have the genetic mutation with care to avoid triggering agents.

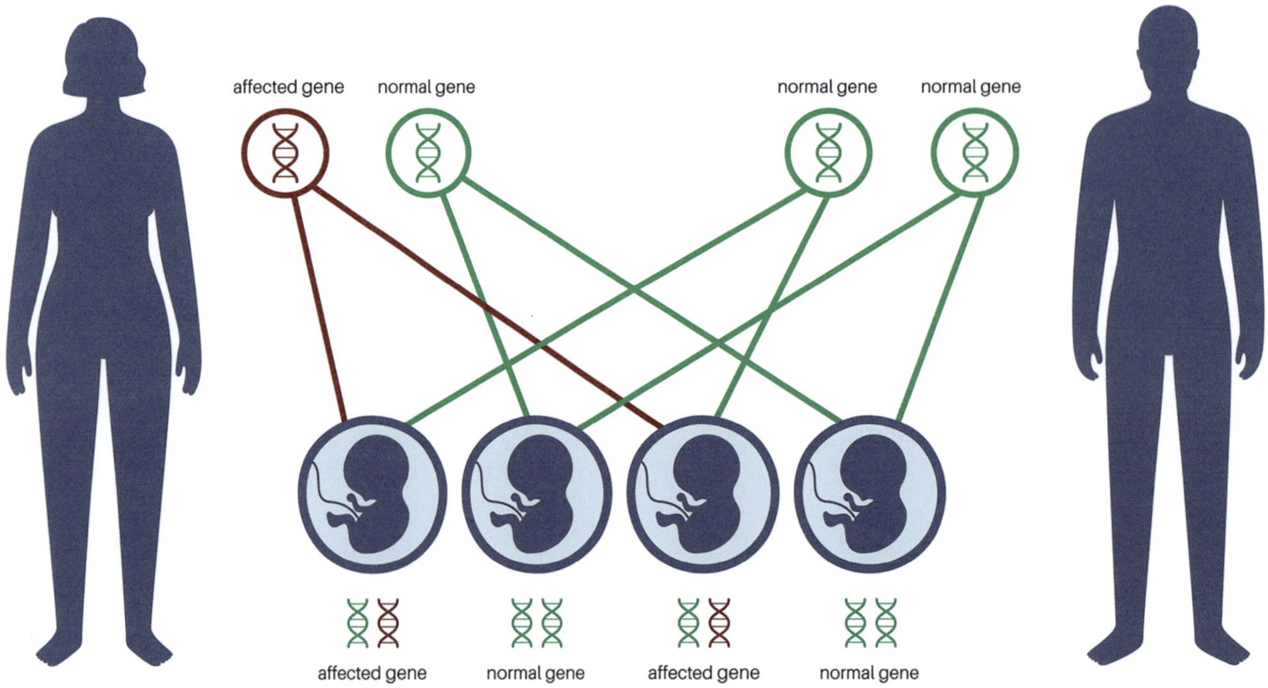

Fig. 3.5 The autosomal dominant (AD) inheritance pattern means there is a 50% chance or probability of inheriting the affected gene. Thus, if the mother has the disease, there is a 50–50 chance her children will be affected, regardless of whether they are born male or female. AD is a common inheritance pattern for several clinically relevant conditions, including malignant hyperthermia, protein C and S deficiency, and factor V Leiden mutation. Familial adenomatous polyposis syndrome (FAP), hereditary non-polyposis colorectal carcinoma (HNPCC), Lynch syndrome, BRCA1, and BRCA2 are all inherited as AD

Antibiotic Prophylaxis Prior to Operation

To minimize the risk of infection, antibiotics are often administered prophylactically, most often **30 min prior to incision** [9–11]. Importantly, some types of operation do not require the routine use of antibiotics for prophylaxis. If there is no proven risk-reduction in **surgical site infection (SSI)** for the type of operation being performed, then antibiotics are not recommended and should not be administered. The reason is not only that the antibiotic is unnecessary, but it can actually cause harm to the patient. For example, the patient could have an adverse reaction to the antibiotic, or the patient could develop *Clostridium difficile* (aka, antibiotic-associated) colitis [12, 13]. Therefore, clinicians must be judicious and exercise stewardship with the administration of antibiotics pre-operatively. Always check the patient's allergy profile prior to ordering an antibiotic, and chose an appropriate alternative if needed. Table 3.5 provides the typical antibiotics used for common operations in general surgery and their doses; operations that do not typically require antibiotics are also shown. Note, this assumes the host is immune competent; for immune compromised patients, special considerations for antibiotic prophylaxis are given.

There are a few points to consider for specific types of operations:

- **Appendectomy**: In case of perforated appendicitis, more broad-spectrum antibiotics (like Piperacillin-Tazobactam or Ceftriaxone + Metronidazole) are used.
- **Cholecystectomy**: Routine use of antibiotics for clean procedures, but in cases of infected gallbladder (e.g., cholecystitis), broader coverage is preferred.
- **Hernia repair**: Antibiotics are not needed unless there is contamination, infection, or specific high-risk factors.
- **Anorectal operations:** Antibiotics are not indicated for most of the common procedures, including hemorrhoidectomy, fistulotomy, sphincterotomy, anal skin tag excision.
- **Colorectal resection**: Preoperative antibiotics are critical to prevent infections due to gut flora; broad-spectrum coverage (such as Ertapenem) is typically used sometimes in combination with a mechanical bowel preparation (see later).
- **Mastectomy**: Antibiotics are used to reduce the risk of post-operative wound infection.
- **Thyroidectomy**: Generally, antibiotics are not required unless there is a high risk of contamination, or an immune compromised state.

Allergic Reactions While you should verify the patient's allergy history prior to prescribing any medication, it is particularly true for patients undergoing surgery who are being

Table 3.5 Common general surgical procedures and pre-operative antibiotics

Surgical procedure	Preoperative antibiotics	Antibiotic(s) used	Recommended dose
1. Appendectomy	Yes	Cefazolin (or Clindamycin + Gentamicin if allergic to beta-lactams)	**Cefazolin**: 2 g IV 30 min before incision (or **Clindamycin** 600 mg + **Gentamicin** 5 mg/kg)
2. Cholecystectomy	Yes	Cefazolin (or Metronidazole + Ceftriaxone if allergic to beta-lactams)	**Cefazolin**: 2 g IV 30 min before incision (or **Metronidazole** 500 mg + **Ceftriaxone** 1 g)
3. Hernia repair (inguinal)	Not usually	None	No antibiotics needed unless infection risk is high (e.g., contaminated cases)
4. Colorectal resection	Yes	Ceftriaxone + Metronidazole *Or* Ertapenem	**Ceftriaxone** 1 g IV + **Metronidazole** 500 mg IV, 30 min prior to incision; or **Ertapenem** 1 gm IV, 30 min prior to incision
5. Mastectomy (breast)	Yes	Cefazolin	**Cefazolin**: 2 g IV 30 min before incision
6. Gastrostomy tube placement	Not usually	None	Antibiotics not routinely given unless high infection risk (e.g., immunocompromised patients)
7. Thyroidectomy	Not usually	None	No antibiotics needed unless infection risk is high (e.g., contaminated surgery)
8. Bariatric surgery (gastric bypass)	Yes	Cefazolin + metronidazole	**Cefazolin**: 2 g IV + **Metronidazole** 500 mg IV, 1 h before incision
9. Laparotomy (exploratory)	Yes	Cefazolin (or piperacillin-tazobactam for contaminated cases)	**Cefazolin**: 2 g IV, or **Piperacillin-Tazobactam** 3.375 g IV if risk of contamination
10. Hemorrhoid-ectomy	No	None	Antibiotics are not indicated for the majority of anorectal procedures

prescribed/ordered an antibiotic. One of the most common allergies you will encounter is to **Penicillin** (PCN), which can include allergic reactions as serious as anaphylaxis. Another common allergy is to *sulfonamides* ("sulfa" drugs), which include trimethoprim-sulfamethoxazole (TMP/SMZ) (e.g., Bactrim, Septra) as well as sulfasalazine (e.g., Sulfazine).

In surgery, *PCN is the more significant allergy, and some of the antibiotics given for prophylaxis may have cross over reactivity with PCN*. This is true for the *cephalosporins* in particular. *Clindamycin, vancomycin*, and *aztreonam* are good alternatives for patient with a PCN allergy, but it is important that the appropriate bacterial flora is covered. Other alternatives include the fluoroquinolones (e.g., moxifloxacin, levofloxacin).

Note that each surgeon may have a specific preference for the antibiotic regimen they would like to administer. Some types of surgery may require additional antibiotics preoperatively. For example, some surgeons prefer to prescribe a Nichols Prep prior to colon resection.

Because each surgeon may have specific preferences and because institutions may also have set-protocols regarding preoperative antibiotics, *always check* and follow the guidelines and recommendations set forth by the surgeon and hospital.

Special Circumstances For patients with pre-existing heart conditions who are at risk for ***infective endocarditis***, prophylactic antibiotic treatment is sometimes recommended before certain medical (or dental procedures). The American Heart Association (AHA) guidelines for endocarditis prophylaxis have evolved over the years, and the indications for antibiotics have become more specific. Conditions that may require prophylaxis include prosthetic heart valves (including bioprosthetic and mechanical valves), a personal history of infective endocarditis, a personal history of congenital heart disease, and cardiac transplant recipients.

The choice of antibiotics depends on the procedure being performed and the patient's risk factors. The most common regimen includes amoxicillin (oral) 2 grams orally 30–60 min before the procedure. Usually this is managed by the treating cardiologist. The decision to administer antibiotics should be based on the individual patient's health history and risk profile [14, 15].

Bowel Preparation

For patients undergoing colonic surgery, a bowel preparation, or **"bowel PREP,"** is often prescribed prior to surgery. Bowel PREPs are cathartic agents that help clear out the colon of residual stool. Bowel PREPs are usually polyethylene glycol (PEG) based (e.g., MiraLAX®, GoLYTELY®). A bowel PREP can include other agents, as well as water-based enemas and other laxative agents. Some surgeons prefer to add oral antibiotics to the Bowel PREP as well, such as the **Nichol Condon Prep**, administered the day prior to planned operation, as follows:

- 1 g oral neomycin given at 2 pm, 3 pm, and 10 pm
- 1 g erythromycin base given at 2 pm, 3 pm, and 10 pm

Management Anticoagulants Prior to Surgery

You will encounter many patients who are on *blood thinning agents* (anticoagulants) for a variety of reasons in the preoperative setting, among the most common are **aspirin** (acetylsalicylic acid) and **coumadin** in the out-patient setting, and **heparin** in the in-patient setting (Fig. 3.6).

Other blood thinners include **clopidogrel** (Plavix®), which is a prodrug whose metabolites interfere with platelet aggregation [17, 18]. Additionally, **rivaroxaban** (XARELTO®), **fondaparinux** (Arixtra®), as well as **apixaban** (Eliquis®) are relatively newer anticoagulants that act as reversible inhibitors of factor Xa and are referred to as *direct oral anticoagulants* (DOACs) [19].

There are different reasons patients may be on anticoagulation, and they can be classified as either **(a)** preventative or **(b)** therapeutic. In the case of aspirin, it can be *non-prescribed* as it is available over the counter (OTC). Specific, common reasons for prescribed blood thinners include, but are not limited to, history of chronic atrial fibrillation, treatment of DVT/PE, coronary artery stents, peripheral vascular disease, genetic predisposition to clotting—*especially,* **Factor V Leiden gene mutation—**and **protein C and S deficiency** (both conditions inherited as autosomal dominant and result in a *hypercoagulable state*).

PAs in surgical practice need to have a strong understanding of blood thinners, their effect on the coagulation cascade and/or clotting (Fig. 3.7). It is important to have in your mind general guidelines about when and if a blood thinner can be held prior to surgery. Importantly, there are tradeoffs that have to be considered. On the one hand, performing surgery on patients who are taking blood thinners increase the risk of untoward bleeding, but on the other hand, discontinuing blood thinners prior to surgery can result in even more significant morbidity—such as coronary stent occlusion.

There are three questions to ask yourself in the management of blood thinners when considering the surgical patient [16]. They are as follows:

1. **What is the thromboembolic risk of the patient?**
2. **What is the risk of bleeding with the planned operation/procedure?**
3. **Most importantly,** ***is it safe to interrupt anticoagulation or antithrombotic therapy?***

Aspirin (Acetylsalicylic Acid) Aspirin is a non-steroidal anti-inflammatory drug (NSAID). Its mechanism of action is that it is a permanent inhibitor of cyclooxygenase (COX-1), preventing thromboxane synthesis within platelets, and thus affecting the *platelet plug* (platelet aggregation), which is the *first step in normal coagulation.* Thus, you can think of aspirin as a **permanent inhibitor of platelets**. For patients taking aspirin, the platelet *count is normal, but the platelet function is not.* Since the half-life of platelets is approxi-

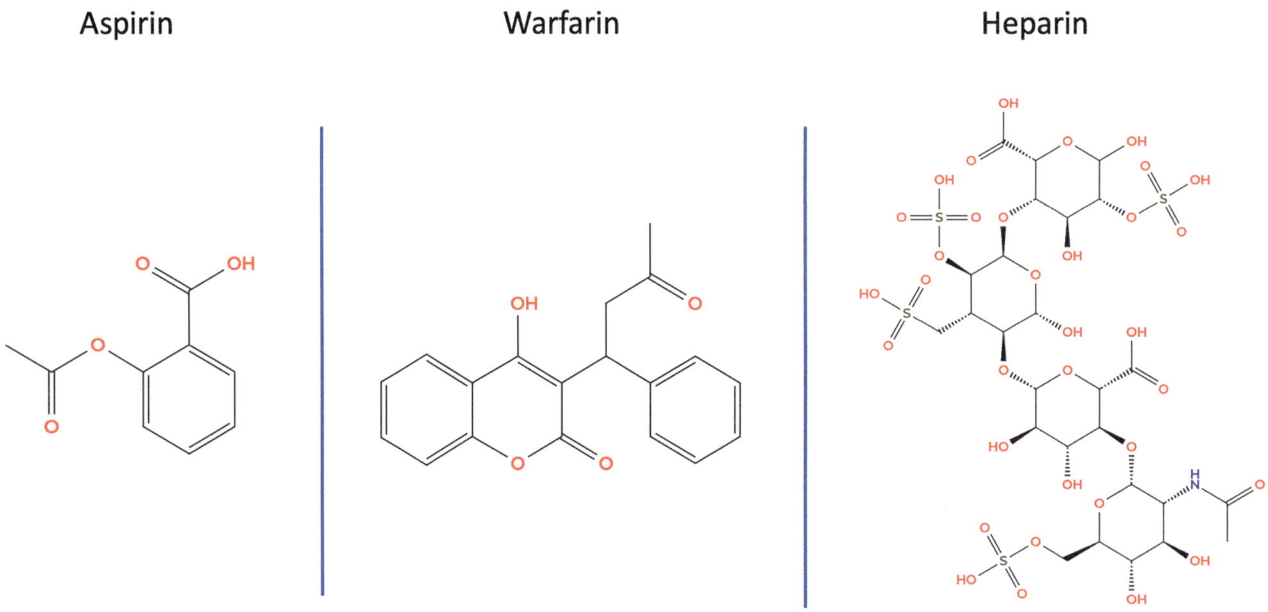

Fig. 3.6 The chemical structures of aspirin (acetylsalicylic acid), warfarin (coumadin), and heparin are shown. These are important anticoagulants that act on different points of the clotting cascade

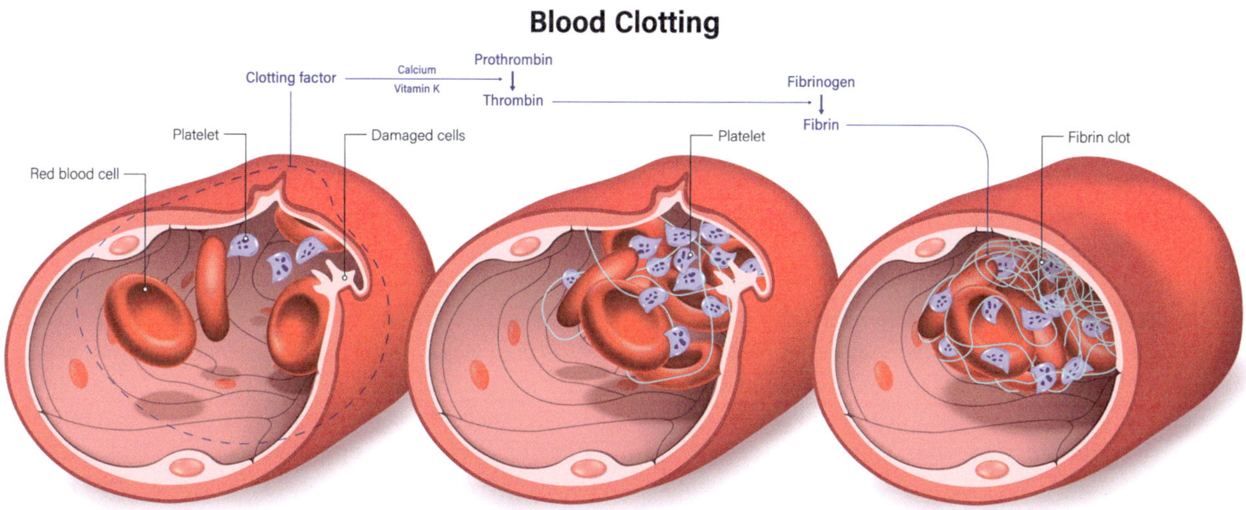

Fig. 3.7 Blood clotting (coagulation) is a complex process that helps stop bleeding when blood vessels are injured. Platelets play a crucial role in clot formation. When a blood vessel is injured, platelets are activated creating the "platelet plug." Prothrombin is a protein present in blood plasma and is essential for the formation of thrombin during clotting. When the clotting process begins, prothrombin is converted into thrombin with the help of other clotting factors. Thrombin is an enzyme that plays a central role in clot formation, as it activates fibrinogen, a soluble plasma protein, converting it into insoluble fibrin strands. These fibrin strands form a mesh-like structure that strengthens the platelet plug

mately *7 days,* it is recommended that *if* a decision to hold this blood thinner prior to surgery is made, it should be held 1 week prior to planned surgery. *Note well:* patients on aspirin do not have abnormal coagulation labs. That is, the PT, INR, aPTT, and platelet (PLT) count are not affected.

For patients who take "preventative aspirin" that is not prescribed by a physician, then aspirin should be discontinued 1 week prior to planned surgery, regardless if the patient is taking a "baby aspirin" (81 mg) or standard adult dose (325 mg).

For patients who have been prescribed aspirin, it is best to have the treating physician (e.g., cardiologist) make the recommendation of whether or not aspirin should be discontinued. This is especially important in patients with *cardiac stents* and those with *carotid artery atherosclerotic disease*, as well as patients with pre-existing vascular (arterial) *grafts.* For *some* minor operations, it is considered safe to proceed with the operation without discontinuing aspirin, but this is surgeon dependent. *As a PA on surgery, always check with the surgeon to see whether or not it is safe to proceed with a planned operation without discontinuing aspirin.*

Coumadin (Warfarin) Coumadin inhibits the synthesis of vitamin K-dependent clotting factors, which are *Factors II, VII, IX, and X* as well as the anticoagulant *proteins C and S.* The coumadin level can be monitored with a routine coagulation profile to check the **PT and INR**. Patients on coumadin are monitored and their dose is titrated to a specific INR.

A classic indication for coumadin therapy is *atrial fibrillation.* While typically it is considered "safe" to discontinue coumadin 3 days prior to operation, newer data suggests more scrutiny is required. As a general rule, always check with the patient's treating medical practitioner to determine when and if it is safe to discontinue coumadin prior to operation.

Coumadin, unlike heparin, *takes time* to achieve therapeutic levels, on the order of days, not hours. Therefore, it is considered a slow onset drug. This also means that it takes a substantial time for the effect of the drug to dissipate once it has been discontinued. In patients who require emergent surgery on therapeutic doses of coumadin, **vitamin K** (10 mg, slow IV push) and/or **fresh frozen plasma (FFP)** can be administered as reversal agents.

Heparin Unlike coumadin, IV heparin is a rapid "on/off" that allows for quick titration to a therapeutic level (as determined by the **PTT**). Its anticoagulation properties also quickly diminish after the discontinuation of the infusion. You may encounter patients who are on a *heparin drip* in the in-patient setting. Typically, the drip can be discontinued 4 h prior to surgery, and a PTT drawn prior to operation to ensure it is in normal range. Specifics of when a heparin drip should be discontinued prior to surgery should be discussed with the medical team as well as the attending surgeon.

Bridging Sometimes patients who are on long-acting anticoagulation (*esp.* coumadin) will be "bridged" with heparin. That is, their oral coumadin will be discontinued and as the PT/INR normalize. Simultaneously, they will be started on heparin leading up to the day of surgery. Then, the heparin will be stopped *approximately* 4 h prior to surgery. This allows for better "control" of the anticoagulation, which capitalizes on the heparin's rapid on/off characteristics.

Anticoagulant bridging can be performed with *low molecular weight heparin*, LMWH (Lovenox), or *unfractionated heparin* (UFH). This is especially useful for patients who are outpatients *and* where the time off of anticoagulation (prior to surgery) *needs to be minimized* [20].

After the operation, the reverse is done and the patient is bridged back to coumadin. Bridging is a strategy that is used for particularly high-risk patients. Examples include patients who have undergone coronary artery stent placement within the last 3 months as well as patients with mechanical heart valves. While there are different approaches to bridging, the following is a general "how to" approach:

Prior to Operation:
- The patient discontinues warfarin 5 days prior to surgery.
- Three days before surgery, the patient starts on subcutaneous LMWH at therapeutic doses (this depends on renal function).
- Two days before surgery, assess INR (goal INR < 1.5).
- Discontinue LMWH 24 h prior to planned surgery.

After Operation:
- Once the patient restarted a diet, and the patient is stable (not bleeding or dropping their hemoglobin), it is generally safe to restart warfarin by the second post-operative day.
- Always assess the post-surgical bleeding risk and adequacy of homeostasis before the resumption of any anticoagulant. *As operations have variable levels of complexity and bleeding risk, always discuss the decision to resume anticoagulation with the surgeon.*

Special Considerations Consider postponing elective surgery in patients with coronary artery disease who have had recent stent placement. The *type* of coronary artery stent placed is relevant for this. There are two types of cardiac stents, **bare metal** and **drug eluting**.

- Postpone elective surgery for **6 weeks** after the placement of **bare metal stents.**
- Postpone elective surgery for **6 month**s after the placement for **drug-eluting stents**.

Managing Antihypertensive Medications

Hypertension (HTN) is extremely prevalent among adults, and there is an increased incidence with age. It has been reported that 60% of patients >60 years have HTN, defined as a blood pressure that is consistently measured at or above 140/90. It is recommended that patients who are taking **angiotensin receptor antagonists** (e.g., Losartan, Valsartan) and/or **angiotensin-converting enzyme (ACE) inhibitors** (e.g., Lisinopril, Enalapril) should *withhold these medications 24 h prior to surgery.* This does not apply to patients undergoing cardiac surgery, whereby holding ACE inhibitors and/or angiotensin receptor blockers can increase mortality.

Beta blockers (e.g., propranolol, metoprolol, atenolol) are no longer considered first line treatment for HTN, but this class of medication is still commonly prescribed. If your patient is taking a beta blocker, it is generally recommended that the he/she *continues the medication and it should not be discontinued prior to a planned surgery.*

Data on discontinuing loop diuretics, thiazide diuretics, and calcium channel blockers is lacking, and these medications thus do not need to be discontinued prior to planned operation, unless recommended by the treating physician [21].

Managing Diabetic Medications

Diabetes mellitus (DM) is a chronic disease that affects an estimated 1 in 10, or 537 million persons worldwide. Patients with diabetes are often prescribed either insulin or oral hypoglycemics (such as metformin). Managing diabetic patients in the perioperative period can be quite challenging. DM patients often have gastroparesis, so they require a longer fasting period prior to surgery. When DM patients are fasting, they cannot receive their normal dose, for example, of insulin as this can cause their blood sugar level to drop dangerously low. In addition, however, the stress of surgery will tend to raise blood sugar levels substantially, making glycemic control challenging.

Some experts recommend dose reduction of insulin on the day prior to surgery. Treatment is often individualized. The goal is to maintain glycemic control. Be aware that ***hypo*****glycemia is far worse than *hyper*glycemia**.

Since managing diabetic medications can be nuanced and because it depends on multiple factors, it is best to defer to the treating internist for guidance. Nowadays, hospitalists and treating internists and endocrinologists manage most diabetic medications in the perioperative period and it is best to consult them for their expertise. Protocols may vary according to region and institution [22].

Special Medications

Glucagon-like peptide-1 (GLP-1) receptor agonists [23, 24] include medications such as **Semaglutide** (Ozempic®) and **Tirzepatide** (Mounjaro®) and are approved in the United States to treat diabetes (Type II). Ozempic has been popularized by many clinicians as a weight loss drug, although not approved for this. More recently (2023), a formulation of Tirzepatide was approved for weight loss by the FDA under the brand name Zepbound®.

These medications are now in widespread use. According to a 2024 KFF health poll, one in eight adult Americans have taken a GLP-1 receptor agonist. This means as PAs, it is important to be familiar with this class of medications, which have specific guidelines when it comes to fasting, and they can be summarized as follows:

- For patients on daily dosing: hold GLP-1 agonists on the day of the procedure/surgery.
- For patients on weekly dosing: hold GLP-1 agonists 1 week prior to the procedure/surgery.

Minor Procedures and the Injection of Local Anesthetics

Local anesthetic agents provide *preemptive* analgesia. There are two main classes of local anesthetics, **esters** and **amides**. Amides are more frequently used as a choice of local anesthetic for surgery—this includes *lidocaine* and *bupivacaine,* with the latter being more long-acting and thus preferred in most settings.

Note that there are *limits on the amount of local anesthetic that can be safely administered, and this amount is weight-based.* The maximum safe dose also depends on whether or not the local anesthetic contains epinephrine "epi" (either 1:100,000 or 1:200,000). For example, the safe maximum does of lidocaine (plain) is 4.5 mg/kg (not to exceed 300 mg). For lidocaine (*with* epi, 1:100,000), the dose is *higher* at 7 mg/kg in adults. For a 1% solution of lidocaine, there are 10 mg per 1 ml. To calculate the safe dose, you will need to be able to convert milligrams (mg) to a volume amount in milliliters (ml).

Let us work through an example. Suppose you have 67 kg female patient that requires skin suturing. You plan to inject a local anesthetic, 1% lidocaine (plain). We can calculate the maximum safe dose that can be injected as follows:

$$\text{max Dose for 1\%Lidocaine}\left(\text{plain}\right): 4.5\,\text{mg} / \text{kg}$$

$$\text{For this Patient}: 4.5\,\text{mg} \times 67\text{kg} = 301.5\,\text{mg}$$

$$\text{1\%Lidociane solution} = 10\,\text{mg} / \text{ml}$$

$$\frac{301.5\,\text{mg}}{10\,\text{mg} / \text{ml}} = 30.15\,\text{ml}$$

Thus, the maximum amount (volume) of a 1% lidocaine solution that can be safely administered is ~30 ml. As a PA, you should be familiar with the safe doses of injections. You should be able to perform simple calculations like this. Do not just "inject local" without knowing the safe dose and limits.

A Case Problem for Surgical PAs

Consider a real-world example. Suppose your attending asks you to pre-op the next patient for surgery, a planned elective excision of a lipoma. You review the patient's history. He is a 67 yo male with no prior medical history and no prior surgeries. He is currently asymptomatic, but review of systems reveals he has been under "a lot of stress lately" due to his mother dying unexpectedly 2 weeks prior. Exam is remarkable for a resting heart rate of 115 and blood pressure of 175/89. Based on this, you decide you check a rhythm strip which is shown in Fig. 3.8. What would you do?

Although the patient does not report symptoms, the findings on cardiac exam (tachycardia, hypertension) and the findings on EKG should alert the PA pre-oping the patient that this *patient needs a cardiac workup immediately and that the planned surgery should be canceled.* The EKG strip shows inverted T-waves and ST-segment depression (both indicative of myocardial ischemia). If the patient's procedure was being performed at an ambulatory surgical center, the patient should be transported to the nearest emergency department without delay.

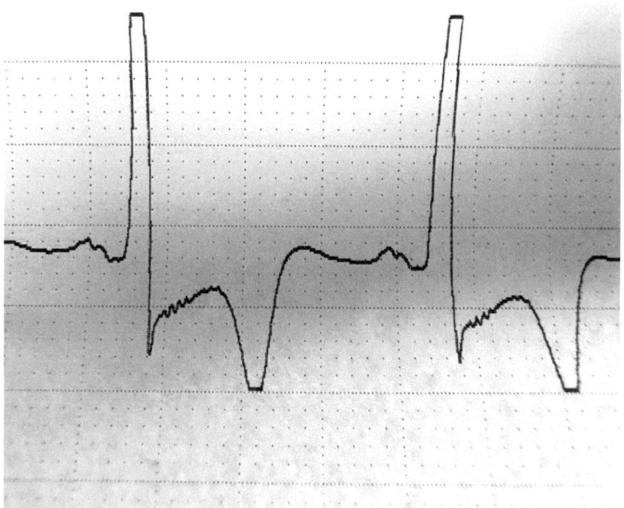

Fig. 3.8 An EKG rhythm strip obtained from a patient in pre-op holding prior to a planned elective operation. The EKG is abnormal with inverted T-waves and ST-segment depression that could indicate myocardial ischemia

This example is prototypical of the type of problem you will need to be able to solve and reason through, *not* only for didactic examinations but also for managing patients on any surgical service line. As a PA student, be prepared to answer *these* types of questions, and be less concerned with questions related to the practice of surgery itself. For example, you will not be expected to name all the steps involved in performing a robotic ileocolic resection, Ivor Lewis esophagectomy, or other operation. As a PA, *focus on the medical management of the surgical patient.*

Part 3: General Protocols for the Post-operative Patient

One of the first steps to be performed after surgery is to enter orders for the patient. Nowadays this is done electronically using the electronic medical record (EMR) system. There are usually pre-selected **post-op order sets**. An example is shown in Fig. 3.9. Order sets spell out what care the patient will receive. Specifically, they assign a level of care, provide a menu of nursing care options, assign diet, activity, fluids, blood draws, and medications. As a practicing PA, you will often be the one entering these orders, so you want to become familiar with them.

The most important value of order sets is that they *standardize the delivery of healthcare for the surgical patient* and likely diminish the chance of errors. Order sets for the surgical patient, especially for those admitted after elective surgery, are usually geared towards a "fast-track" discharge pathway and follow the guidelines known as enhanced recovery after surgery, or *ERAS*.

Enhanced Recovery After Surgery (ERAS)

One of the most important advancements in the care of the surgical patient is a bundled approach that is designed *to minimize narcotic pain medication use, accelerating the return of gut function, and decreasing hospital length of stay (LOS) post-operatively*. This approach is termed **enhanced recovery after surgery (ERAS)** [25–28]. ERAS is not "any *one* thing" but a *spectrum of interventions* that also varies from center to center and can be thus thought of as "a menu to choose from." ERAS protocols should be used *consistently*.

ERAS Protocols: Key Elements and General Guidelines

(A) **Minimally Invasive Surgery:** Minimally invasive (robotic/laparoscopic) surgery is termed **MIS**. This approach minimizes post-operative pain and narcotic usage, accelerating time to discharge from the hospital and thus decreasing LOS.
(B) **Long-Acting Local Anesthetics:** Where available, Exparel is an important part of ERAS (Fig. 3.10). Exparel is *liposomal bupivacaine*, and in this formulation the anesthetic effect can last up to 96 h—although more typically 12–36 h. Exparel is commonly administered in combination with 0.25% or 0.50% bupivacaine in a 1:1 ratio, so that both immediate and long-acting analgesia is achieved.
(C) **Intravenous (IV) Non-Narcotic Analgesics:** IV acetaminophen (Ofirmev®; 1000 mg IV Q6 hours, *weight dependent*) and, in select patients who do not have a contraindication, IV ketorolac (15 mg IV Q6 hours) can be considered and are generally preferred over IV narcotics—such as IV morphine and IV hydromorphone (Dilaudid) which are typically reserved for *breakthrough* pain.
(D) **Neuromodulators:** Although typically used as an anticonvulsant medication, oral **gabapentin** 100–300 mg can be effective as an analgesic for the surgical patient and is often used in ERAS protocols.
(E) **Diet:** Early resumption of oral intake and avoiding nasogastric (NG) tubes in most instances are important in assuring the prompt return of gut function.
(F) **Activity:** Early and frequent ambulation and encouragement of mobility post-operatively improves the return of gut function. "Bed rest" is highly discouraged in most instances. For patients who have difficulty with mobility, the aid of **physical therapy** (PT) and/or **occupational therapy** (OT) is an important ancillary service that should be used liberally.
(G) **Early Discontinuation of Urinary Catheter:** Where applicable, removing a catheter can help improve the patient's mobility and should be encouraged, *if and only if* appropriate.
(H) **Patient Education:** Expectations for a fast-track recovery should be established during preoperative consultation. It should also be encouraged during rounds on patients post-operatively.

ADMISSION
- o ADMIT TO IN-PATIENT STATUS
- o ADMIT TO OBSERVATION STATUS

LEVEL OF CARE
- o ICU
- o SURGICAL WARD

NURSING CARE
- o PULSE OXIMETERY Q 4 HOURS
- o VITAL SIGNS Q 4 HOURS
- o NOTIFY DOCTOR FOR CHANGE IS STATUS
- o DRESSING CHANGES DAILY
- o SITZ BATHS DAILY
- o STOMA CARE
- o FLUSH DRAINS Q 12 HOURS
- o ENCOURAGE INSENTIVE SPIROMETER USE 4 TIMES PER HOUR

ACTIVITY
- o BED REST
- o AD LIB/ AMBULATE
- o PHYSICAL THERAPY
- o PATIENT MAY SHOWER

DIET
- o RENAL DIET
- o CARDIAC DIET
- o REGULAR DIET
- o CLEAR LIQUID DIET
- o FULL LIQUID DIET
- o NOTHING PER OS (NPO)

IV FLUIDS
- o TO KEEP OPEN (TKO)
- o NS AT 125 ML/HR
- o LR AT 125 ML/HR
- o $D_5$1/2 NS c 20KCl @ 125 ML/HR
- o OTHER

ANTIBIOTICS
- o INVANZ 1GM IV Q 24 HRS
- o CIPRO 400 MG IV Q 12 HRS
- o FLAGYL 500 MG IV Q 8 HRS
- o CEFAZOLIN (ANCEF) 1GM IV Q 8 HRS
- o NONE

ANALGESIC MEDICATIONS
- o KETOROLAC (TORADOL) 15 MG IV Q 6 HRS
- o OXYCODONE/ACETOMENEPHEN (PERCOCET) 5/325, ONE P.O. Q 4 HRS
- o DILUDID 0.2MG IV PUSH, Q 6 HRS, PRN SEVERE PAIN
- o OTHER

ANTI-EMETIC MEDICATIONS
- o ONDANSETRON (ZOFRAN) 4MG IV Q 4 HRS, PRN NAUSEA/VOMITING
- o PROCHLORPERAZINE (COMPAZINE) 5MG IV Q 4 HRS, PRN NAUSEA/VOMITING

DVT PROPHALAXIS
- o SPONTANEOUS COMPRESSION DEVICES (SCD), WHILE IN BED
- o LOW MOLECULAR WEIGHT HEPARIN (ENOXAPARIN) 40 MG SUBQ DAILY
- o FUNDAPARINUX (ARIXTRA) 2.5 MG SUBQ DAILY

LABORATORY
- o CBC WITH DIFFERENTIAL IN AM
- o COMPLETE METABOLIC PANNEL (CMP) IN AM
- o LIVER FUNCTION TESTS (LFTS) IN AM
- o OTHER

RADIOLOGY
- o CHEST X-RAY IN AM
- o CT ABDOMEN/PELVIS WITH AND WITHOUT CONTRAST IN AM
- o OTHER

CONSULTS
- o CONSULT HOSPITALIST FOR MEDICAL MANAGEMENT
- o CONSULT CARDIOLOGY

Fig. 3.9 A typical order set for post-operative care is shown. Like pre-operative order sets, it too contains a menu of options to choose from, depending on the case specifics. Nowadays, many aspects of surgical post-op care are standardized, including deep vein thrombosis (DVT) prophylaxis, pain-control regimens, diet, and nursing care

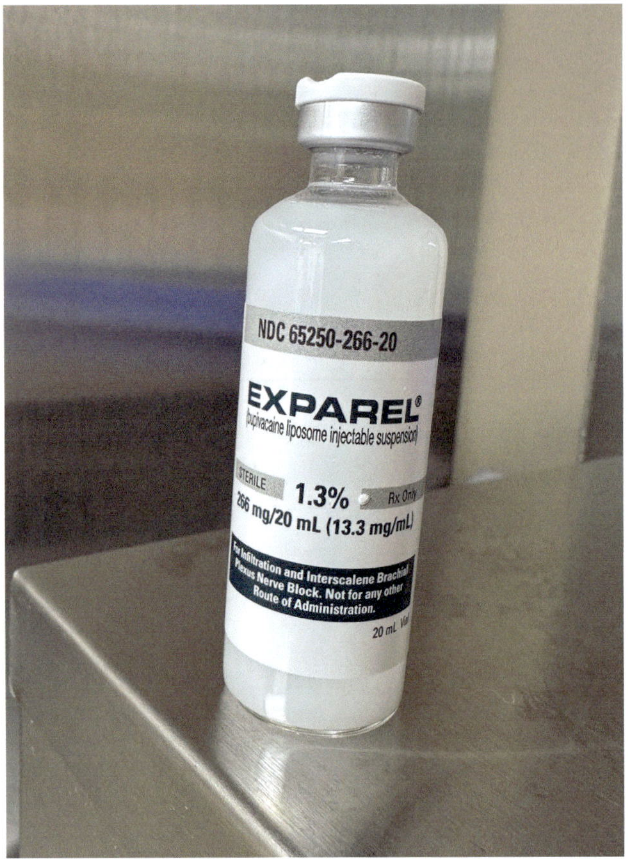

Fig. 3.10 Exparel is a milky-colored local anesthetic, as shown here. Exparel is liposomal bupivacaine. This formulation allows its anesthetic properties to last substantially longer, on the order of 72–96 h. Exparel can be mixed with bupivacaine (plain) which provides both short *and* long-term analgesia. Medications like this are important in ERAS protocols, because they decrease patient-narcotic requirements and enhance the return of gut function, especially after GI surgery

Patient Mobility, Stability, and Fall Risk Post-operatively

Realize that for some patients, even if physically able, they may lack *coordination and balance* after surgery. This can be multifactorial and can be secondary to post-surgical pain, the effect(s) of medications, and even psychologic factors. Recognize when patients may be a **fall risk**. *Falls are an important cause of preventable hospital morbidity.*

Patients who are bedridden and immobile are at risk for developing other morbidity, including *sacral decubitus ulcers* (that are very difficult to heal) and DVT. Surgeons believe in the teaching that *"the bed is the enemy,"* meaning that the more mobile and out of bed (OOB) the patient is, the *quicker they will recover.* Thus, patients are routinely counseled to spend as much time OOB as possible during their recovery.

Of course, there are exceptions to this rule, and there are instances when bedrest is required, but this is not the norm. In orthopedics and neurological surgery, special circumstances dictate post-op mobility. *Always check with your attending surgeon if you have questions, it is better to ask than not to!*

The Recovery Pathway

Post-op patients are expected to follow a so-called *recovery pathway.* This means they are meeting milestones at an expected timeframe, and it is important to monitor these patients to assure that they are progressing *on track*, and not falling off track or faltering.

There are *specific points in time* during a patient's recovery process where clinicians can anticipate certain issues and/or events that require immediate attention. Let us examine some of the more common and important ones. A list of important morbidity (complications) which may affect post-operative patients is shown in Table 3.6.

While all of these are important, it is good to have *some* idea of the level of importance and level of concern you should have for the various types of post-operative events. For example, a *common bile duct (CBD) injury* is an

Table 3.6 Types of complications encountered after abdominal surgery

Complication	Level of concern	Incidence
Bleeding, minor	++	+++
Bleeding, major	+++++	+
Return to O.R. (all causes)	+++++	+
Fever	++	++++
Intra-abdominal infection	++++	+++
Anastomotic leak	+++++	++
Bile duct injury	+++++	+
Ischemic bowel	+++++	+
Bladder perforation	++++	+
SSI (surgical site infection)	++	+++
Fascial dehiscence	+++	+
DVT	+++	+++
Pneumonia	+++	++
Arrythmia	+++	+++
Myocardial infarction	+++++	+
Renal failure	++++	++
Sepsis	+++++	++
Special problems, Nec Fasc	+++++	+
Bowel ischemia	+++++	+
Bowel obstruction	++++	++
Ileus	+	++++
Atelectasis	+	+++++
Seroma	+	++

extremely serious complication after surgery, while fortunately *very* rare; whereas ileus is a more common occurrence but is not considered to be a serious post-op complication. Table 3.6 provides you with a *general* appreciation for the types of complications you may see, their *relative* incidence, and *level of significance.*

Discharge Planning

As patients progress along their recovery pathway, an important question becomes, is the *patient ready for discharge?* The *general* criteria for discharge of the post-operative patient are:

1. Resumption of oral intake without nausea or vomiting
2. Return of gastrointestinal function (bowel movements/flatus)
3. Pain controlled with oral analgesics alone
4. Return to their baseline (pre-op) mobility and physical activity
5. Have clinical exam findings that are normal

Assuming the patient meets these criteria, it is important to consider the next question, which is *where* will the patient be discharged? For most patients they will simply be discharged to home. However, this may not always be the case, and some patients (e.g., the elderly, those involved in major vehicular accident) may need extra time to recuperate, but do not meet the criteria to stay hospitalized. These patients are often transitioned to a *rehabilitation center* or a *skilled nursing facility* that provides supportive care outside of the hospital environment. In these situations, a case or patient *coordinator* will usually assist with finding placement.

Table 3.7 Key reasons why fluid management is important for the surgical patient

Post-op patients exhibit **third-spacing**, which moves fluid outside of the vascular tree
Fluid shifts and other fluid losses (for example, from NG tube suction, drains, high output ostomies, burns) can result in **pre-renal renal failure** (pre-renal azotemia) which can have *significant downstream effects on overall recovery*
Fluid that shifts outside of the vascular tree can limit perfusion to critical structures that need maximum perfusion (oxygenated blood flow) **necessary to ensure proper healing** (for example, a colonic anastomosis after colectomy)

Part 4: The Medical Management of the Surgical Patient

Post-operative Patient Fluid Balance

Fluid management is an important aspect of care for the surgical patient, especially post-operatively and for certain conditions—for example, in *burn patients* who have a disruption of normal control from fluid loss provided by the skin barrier.

Surgeons have a keen interest in their patient's fluid balance and *hydration status* for multiple reasons (Table 3.7). It is important that the surgical PA is aware of the *total fluid intake,* or **"ins,"** often shortened to ***I's***, and the *total fluid output,* **"outs,"** often shortened to ***O's,*** and referred to combined as ***"I's and O's."***

Overall Fluid Balance In *general medicine,* practitioners focus on the *overall* fluid balance as referenced to a patient's *baseline* weight or "dry" weight. Recall that a substantial portion of our body weight is actually water, although this does vary by age (Fig. 3.11). We know that day-to-day variations in weight are mostly due to changes in fluid balance; thus, *tracking a patient's weight allows us to track overall fluid balance.* Since 1 L of water is equivalent to 1 kg, changes like this can be tracked daily by *weighing the patient*—either by directly weighing the patient on a scale or, for ICU patients, weighing the bed itself (since most are equipped with a built-in scale).

Overall fluid balance is important to monitor. For example, suppose there is a patient in the ICU who is receiving multiple boluses of IVF, and their weight has trended up by 7 kg over 48 h. This would imply an overall "positive fluid

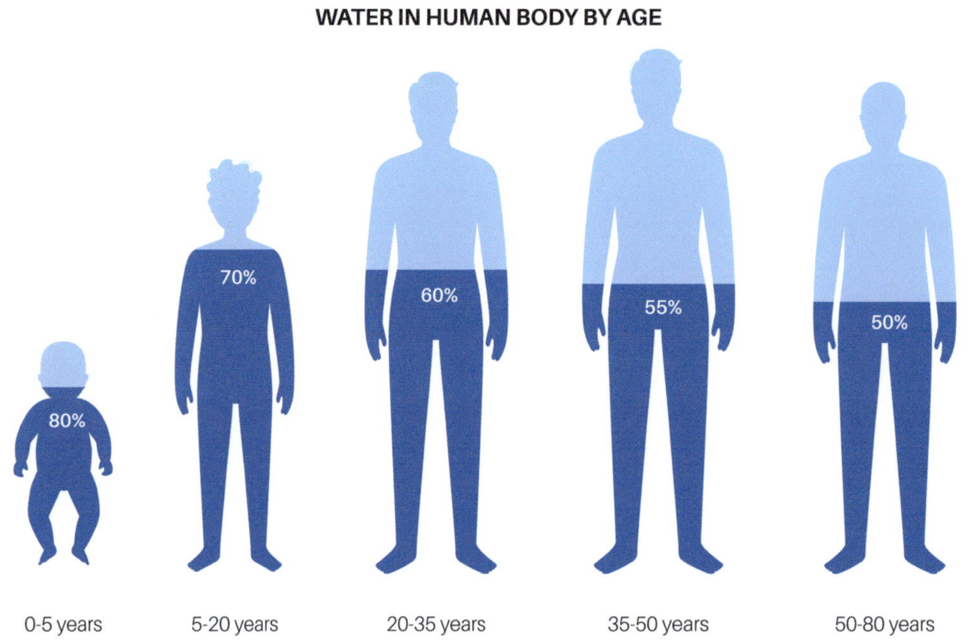

Fig. 3.11 Water is a very significant part of the human body, especially for infants and young children. While the percent of our body weight attributable to water declines with age, it is still an important fraction of our overall body composition and is closely tied to changes in our weight from day to day. For hospitalized patients, it is the water-weight that is changing and thus *body weight changes from day to day* are a proxy for *overall fluid balance*

balance" and the patient would be considered 7 kg over their dry weight. Patients with too much fluid onboard can develop important complications, including pulmonary edema, that may require drug-directed therapy (see later).

Intravascular Fluid Balance While overall fluid balance should be considered, there is a way to think about fluid balance in a more granular way: namely to focus attention on the portion of volume that is *within the vascular tree*. Note that post-surgery, *patients may be overall fluid overloaded, but at the same time be intravascularly depleted.*

In surgery, we always focus on intravascular volume status, as we want to *ensure maximal perfusion to end-organs,* which is critical at all times, but *especially* for the post-operative patient. There are different ways to assess this. Patients may be intravascularly depleted if they are *tachycardic* and have an *elevated BUN:Cr ratio,* with *diminished* and/or *amber colored* UOP. In the ICU setting, in patients with central lines, a low *central venous pressure* (CVP) would be found. This topic will be covered later (see ***the problem of hypovolemia***).

Maintenance Fluid and the 4-2-1 Rule

It is imperative that the post-operative patient be well hydrated, and this is assured by providing intravenous (IV) fluids. IV fluids are either **colloid** or **crystalloid**. The latter can be further subdivided into *maintenance* and *resuscitation* fluids (Fig. 3.12). Maintenance fluids are designed to provide hydration to patients who have *no* oral intake, or who have *low* amounts of intake (due to a variety of reasons, including nausea and/or poor appetite). A common maintenance fluid is **$D_5$1/2NS with 20 mEq KCL**, which is designed to be isotonic while providing a small amount of potassium repletion as well as 5% dextrose. Maintenance fluids are so named because they *maintain normovolemia* in patients who have poor or no oral intake as it repletes the volume of fluid lost through *urination* (estimated to be 900 ml/24 hr for a 75 kg person) as well as *insensible fluid losses* (estimated to be 400–800 ml daily).

Maintenance fluid administration rates can be calculated, and the calculation varies *according to patient weight* using the **4-2-1 rule**, as follows:

4 ml/kg/h for the first 10 kg
2 ml/kg/h for the second 10 kg
1 ml/kg/h for each kg over 20 kg

Let us work though an example for a patient who weighs 77 kg.

$$4\,\text{ml} \times \text{first}\,10\,\text{kg} = 40\,\text{ml}\,/\,\text{h}$$
$$2\,\text{ml} \times \text{second}\,10\,\text{kg} = 20\,\text{ml}\,/\,\text{h}$$

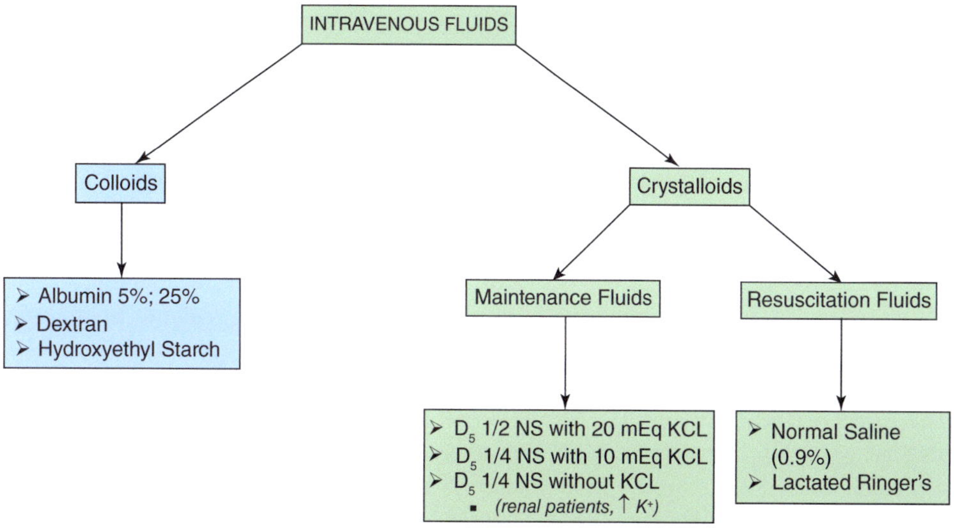

Fig. 3.12 A diagram illustrating the different types of intravenous fluids is shown. PAs on surgery should be familiar with the different categories

So, for the first 20 kg of the patient's weight, 60 ml/h are required to provide maintenance fluid. But of course, we need to account for his entire weight. We have accounted for the first 20 kg, so what remains is: 77 kg *minus* 20 kg or 57 kg. For this remaining weight we only multiply by 1 ml/kg

$$1\text{ml} \times 57\text{kg} = 57\text{ml} / \text{h}$$

Now adding all these values up according to the 4-2-1 rule, we have:

$$40\text{ml} / \text{h} + 20\text{ml} / \text{h} + 57\text{ml} / \text{h} = 117\text{ml} / \text{h}$$

Thus, maintenance IVF rate for this patient would be **117 ml/h**. In most post-op order sets, you will find preselected rates and these typically vary but are usually on the order of 110–125 ml/h, which are common maintenance rates selected for routine adult patients who have been admitted to a hospital after operation.

The maintenance fluid can be tapered and eventually discontinued once the patient is tolerating a diet. Note that the IV itself usually will stay positioned and "heparin locked," or hep-locked, in case it is needed and for the delivery of some IV medications. IV lines are an important point of access and thus usually are kept in place until discharge.

Monitoring Urine Output

On surgery, you need to have a strong understanding of how to calculate normal urine output (UOP). For adults, expected urine output for patients with normal urine function varies **according to weight**, and can be calculated as **½ ml per kg per hour**.

$$\text{Normal Adult } UOP = \frac{1}{2}\ \text{ml} / \text{kg} / \text{hr}$$

In pediatric patients <1 year of age, this is **1** ml/kg/hr. As an example, for a 40 kg adult patient, urine output would be predicted to be 20 ml/hr, while for a patient who weighs 80 kg, one would expect urine output to be 40 ml/hr. This is best monitored in patients who have an indwelling catheter connected to graduated urinary meter bag (e.g., Foley bag).

Knowledge about UOP is *very important to surgeons,* who are interested in knowing the ***hourly*** UOP. Be aware that nurses and hospital staff do not usually keep track of UOP "by the hour." Typically, they chart urine output "per shift" which can be per 8 h or 12 h.

To work through a practical example, let us suppose a 67.5 kg adult patient with normal renal function has reported to have a urine output of 355 ml recorded by a surgical nurse during her 12-h shift. What is the patient's UOP per hour? Is this normal or below normal?

Since the output is recorded over 12 h, we first need to determine how much urine the patient made *per hour.* This can simply be determined by dividing the total volume of urine made by 12, as follows:

$$355\,\text{ml} \div 12\,\text{h} = 29.58\,\text{ml} / \text{hr}$$

Now we need to calculate the patient's *expected* urine output for *his* weight, according to the formula:

$$\text{Predicted } UOP = 1/2\,\text{ml} \times \text{kg} \times \text{hr}$$

$$\text{Predicted } UOP = 1/2\,\text{ml} \times 67\,\text{kg} \times \text{hr} = 33.5\,\text{ml} / \text{hr}$$

Thus, in this example, the patient's *actual* UOP (29.58 ml/hr) is slightly lower than what is *predicted* (33.5 ml/hr). Since the discrepancy is minimal, this would typically be monitored only. PAs on the surgical service should always be tuned in to UOP. *Be able to calculate UOP on all your patients. Patients with low urine output may have intrinsic renal failure or may have pre-renal azotemia due to low intravascular volume and require increase perfusion though increased fluid resuscitation.*

Key Pearl UOP may be low due to *third spacing* (see next), sepsis, or other reason. Always look for and treat the underlying condition. Diuretics should not be administered simply to improve UOP. *Surgeons (especially) do not approach the problem of low UOP by "forcing it" with medication.*

The Problem of Hypovolemia

The Effect of Third Spacing Due to fluid losses related to surgery, post-op patients may exhibit intravascular volume depletion, even if their overall fluid balance is the same, which is related to **third spacing**. This is a transient condition whereby fluid shifts from the bloodstream into the interstitial spaces. Third spacing is typical after abdominal surgery. Third space fluids mobilize (return back to the vascular tree) at *48–72 h after operation.* It is important to keep patients well hydrated during this period of time. This is compensated for by maintaining the patient on IV fluids. The objective is to keep the patient intravascularly optimized and the "pressure head" normal. Caution is advised in the IV fluid *rate and volume* for patients with a known cardiac history (particularly CHF) or chronic pulmonary disease, as too much volume can result in a CHF exacerbation and/or pulmonary edema.

How to Determine Hypovolemia An important clue that a patient may be under resuscitated is if the urine is dark or amber colored and the heart rate is elevated. Importantly, blood chemistry analysis is also very useful in this setting, in two ways. *First,* the hemoglobin and hematocrit (**Hb/HCT**) values, and particularly the trend, can indicate under-resuscitation if, for example, the Hb and HCT *increase. Second,* the blood urea nitrogen (BUN) and creatine (Cr) **ratio** is very useful in this setting. As a PA, it is important to understand that BUN and Cr are not just "kidney numbers." Instead, the BUN and Cr must always be interpreted together; it is the ***ratio*** of BUN:Cr that is *fundamental to understanding certain conditions including fluid management and hypovolemia.* Normally, the **ratio of BUN:Cr is 10:1**.

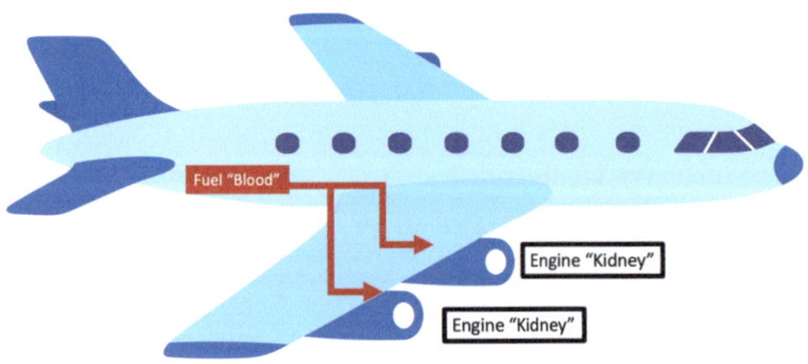

Fig. 3.13 To understand the relationship between blood flow and the kidneys, it is helpful to consider the analogy of a jet plane. Jet engines require fuel to work, and if they are not fed fuel, they stop working. The same is true for kidneys, which rely on a robust pressure head (arterial blood perfusion) to function. Patients who are "dehydrated" or more accurately *intravascularly deplete,* lack adequate perfusion to all organs, but the kidneys are particularly sensitive to these changes. If the blood urea nitrogen (BUN) is elevated to >20 and the creatinine (Cr) is normal at 1.0, this would indicate there is *nothing wrong with the kidneys themselves,* they just need more blood flow. In our analogy, the engines are working just fine, they just need more fuel. Medically, a BUN:Cr ratio of 20:1 or greater suggests *pre-renal* renal failure, which would indicate the patient needs *fluid resuscitation,* typically with normal saline (NS) or lactated ringer's (LR) solution

Understanding the BUN:Cr Ratio To help us understand BUN and Cr and their relationship to one another, let us use an airplane as an analogy (Fig. 3.13). Think of a plane flying through the sky, when suddenly the engines are not generating enough thrust, or the engines stops working altogether, and the aircraft starts losing altitude. There are two main possibilities here. First, there could be an actual mechanical problem with the engines themselves, and there is plenty of good fuel running to them. The second possibility is that the engines could be totally fine, but the problem is that they are not receiving fuel or *enough* fuel for them to function.

We can think of "fuel" as being analogous to *blood flow* or simply intravascular volume. Thus, *fuel* going to the *engines* is like *blood* going to the *kidneys.* **Blood urea nitrogen** (BUN) is a good proxy of blood flow going to the kidneys. If the blood flow to the kidneys is poor, the BUN is elevated. If the blood flow is adequate, then the BUN is normal, usually around 10.

Actual kidney function is indicated by Cr, whereby a Cr ≤ 1.0 is considered normal, and represents "good, working kidneys." Remember, the normal ratio of BUN:Cr is 10:1. If the ratio is higher than 20:1, the kidneys are *under*-perfused and the patient has *pre-renal azotemia* (low intravascular volume) [29]. This is sometimes referred to as *pre-renal, renal failure.*

Let us work through an example. Suppose a 56 yo female patient has undergone a robotic assisted liver resection. As a PA, you order blood chemistries on POD 4 and discover the BUN:Cr measures 37:0.9. You compare this to the patient's previous lab values and observe that the BUN:Cr measured 10:0.9 on POD 1. How would be interpret this change, and what intervention would you undertake?

In this example, the BUN:Cr ratio has risen from normal on POD 1, to high, at a ratio well over 30:1. This would indicate the kidneys are functioning perfectly well, since the Cr is normal (like the engines on our jet plane example) *but* the BUN being elevated tells us there is not enough blood flow to the kidneys, which is analogous to the working engines on a jet plane not being delivered enough fuel to operate properly.

Stated another way, there is nothing intrinsically wrong with the kidneys themselves—the normal Cr tells us they are working perfectly well—they just need more "fuel" or *blood flow*. The treatment is *fluid resuscitation* which can be delivered by IV bolus of NS or LR, depending on preference, and typically 1–2 L is given and the patient reassessed for response to therapy.

Intrinsic Renal Failure Sometimes intrinsic renal failure is seen post-operatively, such as from acute tubular necrosis (ATN) [30–32]. Here, the problem is not a lack of perfusion to the kidneys, it is that they are not functioning properly. In our airplane analogy, this would be as though the engines are receiving enough fuel, but there is something mechanically wrong with the engines themselves. In this instance, the Cr would rise (for example, from a baseline of 1 to 2 or 3 and sometimes higher). *Doubling of the Cr is very significant* and a workup should be performed to rule out post-renal obstruction and acute renal failure. A renal ultrasound is usually indicated and a nephrologist should be consulted.

Deep Vein Thrombosis (DVT) Prevention and Management

Perioperative risk factors for DVT include emergency surgery, BMI >35 kg/m^2, corticosteroid use, ileus, immobility, underlying malignancy, and a pre-existing hypercoagulable state. Prolonged, extensive open operations also increase the risk of developing a DVT, whereas the risk with MIS is less. Patients with inflammatory bowel disease (IBD) have a 2–3X increased risk of DVT and pulmonary embolism (PE) compared with the general population.

Mechanical DVT Prophylaxis **Sequential compression devices (SCDs)**, also referred to as intermittent pneumatic compression (IPC) devices, decrease venous stasis and promote fibrinolysis, essentially by decreasing the activation of coagulation pathways through stimulation of the vascular endothelium.

DVT Chemoprophylaxis Low molecular weight heparin (LMWH) and low-dose unfractionated heparin (LDUH) are anticoagulants used to prevent DVT in post-operative patients. Low molecular weight heparin (LMWH) **enoxaparin** (**Lovenox**®) is most commonly used and is typically administered subcutaneously, once daily (40 mg). Alternatively, **dalteparin** (Fragmin®) can be given.

IVC Filter For patients with a known lower extremity DVT and who require surgery, an **inferior vena cava** (IVC) **filter** should be considered. An IVC filter is placed in the inferior vena cava by an *interventional radiologist (IR)*. It acts as an umbrella to "catch" any clot that breaks off and threatens forming a pulmonary embolus, a potentially life-threatening condition.

There is limited data supporting IVC filter placement for patients who have a contraindication to chemoprophylaxis.

DVT Diagnosis and Treatment Lower extremity DVT is diagnosed through clinical evaluation, supported by **duplex ultrasound**, which is the *gold standard for detecting blood clots* in the deep veins of the lower extremity. Patients may complain of calf pain and have a positive Homan's sign (although this is unreliable). D-dimer testing is also unreliable in the post-surgical patient. Treatment typically involves anticoagulation therapy with medications, such as heparin, to prevent clot growth and reduce the risk of embolism. Compression stockings are often recommended to reduce swelling and prevent post-thrombotic syndrome. Early diagnosis and appropriate treatment are crucial for preventing complications. An IVC filter can be considered in select patients.

As an important pearl for PAs, know that a bilateral lower extremity ultrasound to rule out a DVT is **NOT a test that evaluates the *arterial* system**. If you suspect arterial occlusion, this requires a different mode of radiographic imaging, such as a *CT-angiogram*.

Post-operative Hemorrhage

For the vast majority of routine, elective operations, post-op bleeding requiring reoperation is *rare*. When such bleeding occurs, it is most likely to occur within the **first 24 h**, and up to 48 h (POD 0–2).

Such bleeding, requiring a return to the OR, is related to what surgeons term **mechanical bleeding**, which means it is brisk and usually attributable to a *pulsatile arterial vessel* which *is* amenable to surgical intervention for control. Mechanical bleeding differs from other, more smoldering types of bleeding, such as venous oozing, which is often compounded by coagulopathy, and for which re-operation is of little or no benefit. The general approach to the management of a patient who is bleeding post-operatively is shown below, and as a surgical PA, you should become familiar with this.

Post-operative Hemorrhage Management

- **Examine Patient Vitals:** Tachycardia together with hypotension may indicate *hemorrhagic shock*; heart rate trends and blood pressure trends with close monitoring are imperative. Tachycardia can be difficult to interpret due to post-operative pain, which should also be taken into consideration; however, *hypotension is not an expected finding in a post-operative patient,* as they will typically be *hyper*tensive due to pain.

- **Examine Patient Abdomen:** A physical exam should be performed. Check for abdominal distension which could be an indication of hemoperitoneum, or blood accumulating in the abdominal cavity. Check the surgical wounds as well for bleeding. Remove existing dressings for closer inspection of the surgical wounds. If the patient has drain in place, check the color and quantity of the drain output. For example, a high output of 150 ml/h that is *sanguinous* should alert you to active bleeding that requires a return to the OR, and the surgeon should be notified immediately.
- **Assess Coagulation Profile:** In any patient with a bleeding diathesis, assess derangements in blood coagulation by checking "COAGS" which is a standard blood panel that includes: **PT (Prothrombin Time)**, **PTT (Partial Thromboplastin Time)**, and **INR (International Normalized Ratio)**.
- **Assess Complete Blood Count:** The complete blood count (**CBC**) provides not only information on hemoglobin and hematocrit (**Hb/HCT**, or **H/H**) but also provides information about the platelet (**PLT**) count. Platelet counts under 20 K with active bleeding would strongly benefit from a PLT transfusion and can also be given at a healthcare provider's discretion at higher levels. Recall that patients who are on amino-salicylates (aspirin) have *NORMAL* platelet counts, but because the platelets are permanently inhibited, they are *NON-FUNCTIONAL* due to aspirin products permanently inhibiting PLTs via the cyclooxygenase pathway.
- **Track and Trend H/H:** All patients who are bleeding require the H/H be carefully monitored for stability or instability. The period of time for which an H/H is drawn depends on the suspected severity of bleeding. For example, if only minor bleeding is suspected, monitoring H/H every 12 h or 24 h could be considered reasonable; while patients who you are concerned are bleeding at a faster rate, it should be checked much more frequently—with an H/H drawn every 6 or even 4 h. There is no specific "rule" about how frequently to track and trend H/H, and this is often left to the healthcare provider's discretion. If the H/H is stable over a 24–48 h period, then generally the H/H monitoring can be spaced out and possibly discontinued. COAGs and PLTs can also be monitored in a similar fashion, when and if needed.
- **Prepare for Possible Transfusion:** Type and **Cross** the patient's blood for transfusion. When you give this order, the blood bank will match the patient's blood to actual banked blood and set aside those units for transfusion, should the patient require transfusion. This is important to do for all active bleeding patients, even if you think it is minor at the time of initial evaluation. Review the patient and/or family desires regarding transfusion and obtain informed consent.
- **Discontinue or HOLD Coagulopathic Medications:** Patients are often placed routinely on blood thinners for DVT prophylaxis, such as Lovenox®, or Heparin. They may be on other medications as well, including warfarin. In actively bleeding patients, these medications should be immediately held.
- **Consider REVERSAL of Specific Anticoagulants:** If the patient is on a high dose of heparin and is actively bleeding, consider administering protamine sulfate. For patients on high dose of warfarin, consider treatment with vitamin K and/or fresh frozen plasma (FFP).
- **Change Diet to NPO:** As bleeding may require a return to the operating room, making the patient NPO is prudent, until you determine that the bleeding can be managed medically. The important thing here is that if you think a patient *may* be returning to the OR to control bleeding, make him/her NPO **immediately**.
- **Strongly Consider Re-assigning the Patient to Higher Acuity Unit:** All patients who are admitted after surgery are assigned a level of care in a designated unit. Patients after routine surgery only require basic level care and are often assigned to the medical or surgical ward post-op. When patients develop an acute problem, such as active post-surgical bleeding, their care is no longer considered routine. Depending on the severity of the bleeding, strong consideration should be given to transferring the patient to a higher acuity level of care, such as the intensive care unit (ICU). It is important to move the patient to the ICU *before* they become hemodynamically unstable. A greater level of care is available to patients in the ICU with highly trained and experienced nursing personnel, with *a much improved nurse to patient ratio.*
- **Notify the Surgeon:** The attending surgeon should always be notified as soon as bleeding in a patient post-operatively is suspected. Ultimately, the surgeon is the team leader who will decide whether or not the patient can be managed medically (for example, by correcting an underlying coagulopathy), or if local treatment is required (e.g., silver nitrate for minor wound bleeding), or if an urgent return to the operating theater is required.

Table 3.8 Important causes of elevated WBC *other than* infection

Stress from surgery and anesthesia
Hematologic malignancy—Leukemia
Physiologic stress
Steroids
Acute myocardial infarction (AMI)

Post-operative Fever

General Aspects. Many patients who undergo surgery may require hospital admission post-operatively for medical management, careful monitoring, assistance with mobility, and pain management. An important role of the PA on a surgical service is to "round" on these post-operative patients and assess their progress until discharge. This includes daily physical examinations including assessment of logged vital signs that are obtained at regular intervals.

Because *fever* may be a sign of an important problem that requires intervention, it is important to not only be familiar with these common causes but also to understand at which point in time (i.e., *which* post-operative day) one would anticipate their occurrence.

Medical students and PA students are often taught the **"5 W's"** as an acronym to help remember the potential causes of fever (temp >99.5 °F) in post-op patients. The 5 W's are as follows:

- **I**. **W**ind—pneumonia (*formerly* atelectasis)
- **II**. **W**ound—wound infection
- **III**. **W**alk—deep vein thrombosis (DVT)
- **IV**. **W**ater—urinary tract infection (UTI)
- **V**. **W**onder drugs—patients on medication(s) for a long period of time, "drug fever"

The "5 W's" are not just something to commit to rote memorization. PAs should have a good understanding of when the events tend to occur and related management. It is important to realize that the **cause of fever may *not* be related to an underlying infection**. Interestingly, an elevated WBC *also* does *not* always indicate infection (Table 3.8).

Core Principle: Not all fevers and not all elevations in WBC are secondary to infection

An important idea in surgery is that different causes of fever carry different levels of importance. For example, an anastomotic leak (a type of deep space/body cavity infection) is far more serious than, for example, a wound infection (which is usually superficial and which can be treated with local therapy. While they are both technically "infections" and they both cause fever, they are treated *much differently.* Nonetheless, understanding basic causes of fever in the surgical patient is a good *starting point.* It at least gives you some context as to what to look for on patients who are febrile. Let us take a closer look at the five W's ***(I.–V.):***

I. ***Wind***—This represents *pneumonia.* Historically, atelectasis was considered a cause of early post-operative fever, but *recent data and a systematic review of the literature do not support a causal relationship between atelectasis and post-operative fever* (although atelectasis *is* common after surgery). Thus, the long-standing dogma that atelectasis causes fever in the early post-operative period is invalid, and instead most attribute early post-op fever to the *release of cytokines,* such as **interleukin-6**, as part of the inflammatory response to surgical trauma.

Notwithstanding, it is important to be knowledgeable about atelectasis—which represents alveolar collapse, is common in the first 24–48 h after operation, and is typically self-limited. Treatment recommendations include deep breathing exercises and use of an incentive spirometer (IS) to help re-expand alveoli is probably useful, as atelectasis is associated with hypoxemia (Fig. 3.14). Patients are set a target inspiratory goal of 1000–1500 ml and are asked to use IS several times a day.

Atelectasis is a benign condition that **does not cause fever** and does not require pharmacologic treatment. In counter-distinction, pneumonia *dose* require intervention—often treated with systemic, broad-spectrum antibiotics.

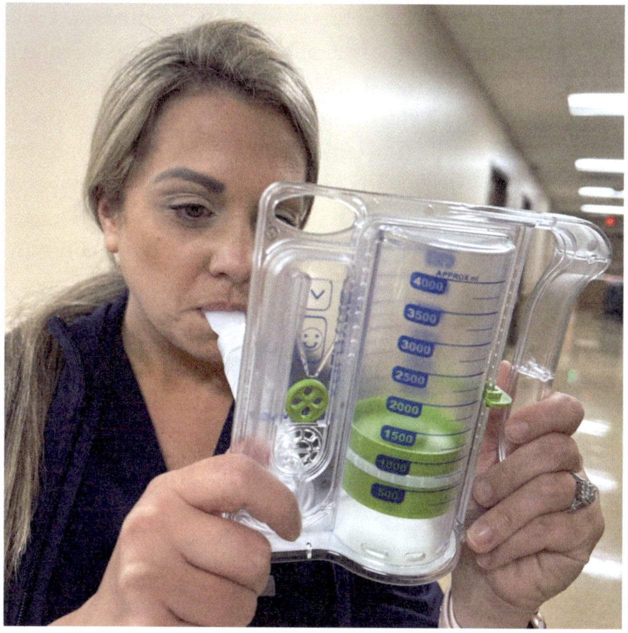

Fig. 3.14 Standard post-operative protocols for hospitalized patients include **incentive spirometry (IS)**, as shown. Patients who undergo anesthesia are prone to developing *atelectasis,* whereby the alveoli are not expanding fully. Atelectasis is not the same as "a collapsed lung" and usually is a self-limited condition. It was historically believed to be associated with fever in the first 24–48 h post-op, *but this is no longer the case.* Incentive spirometry is a useful way to help re-expand the lungs, and patients are given an incentive spirometer with instructions for use at regular intervals (e.g., hourly). Rather than blowing air out, patients *suck air in,* causing the disk (green) to rise. The goal is to have the bottom of the disk rise to 1500–2000

There are two important kinds of pneumonia. First, during intubation, especially for patients who undergo surgery with a full stomach, *aspiration* of acidic gastric contents is possible leading, potentially, to severe pneumonitis. **Aspiration pneumonia** is a serious condition and it manifests early (POD 0–1). The second type of pneumonia manifests at a later time and is often bacterial and often associated with prolonged ventilation, for example, in patients who require vent-support post-operatively. The time frame for this type of pneumonia is variable but typically would be observed POD 5–10 post-op.

II. ***Wound***—*Wound infections* are bacterial in origin and are more likely to be observed in patients who have had an operation that is considered "contaminated." That is, ones in which there was risk of bacterial infection—such as from bowel resection, which is bacteria-rich. Wound infections are termed ***surgical site infections,*** or **SSI**s, as they are often abbreviated. SSIs are superficial in nature, as opposed to a deep space or body cavity infections, which tend to be more serious.

Wound infections are typical around POD 7–10. Patients present with fever and the wound that is draining yellowish purulent fluid with or without erythematous borders. There may be cellulitis (blanching erythema) along the periphery.

The main treatment of a wound infection is to *open the wound;* it is *not* antibiotics, although antibiotics can be given adjunctively, especially if there is associated cellulitis. A wound culture can be helpful in some cases, but is not mandatory. The wound can be opened by removing the skin clips and/or sutures. The wound should be opened down to the level of the fascial closure. Packing the wound can be done with dry gauze or saline soaked gauze that is repacked twice or three times daily.

One of the most important principles to understand is that antibiotics are not the first line treatment for certain types of infections, *even though* the infection is bacterial in nature. Examples are provided in Table 3.9.

Core Principle: Not all bacterial infections are treated primarily with antibiotics

Necrotizing Fasciitis. There is an important type of wound infection that is not treated by opening the wound and is very much worth mentioning. That is *necrotizing fasciitis* [33, 34]. Necrotizing fasciitis is sometimes referred to as "gas gangrene" because the bacteria are gas forming; thus *crepitus* is an important clinical feature of this life-threatening condition. In the lay press, you may hear necrotizing fasciitis be described as "flesh eating bacteria" as well. Regardless of the terminology, *this is an extremely important clinical entity to be able to diagnose and manage swiftly.*

Necrotizing fasciitis may present *earlier* than typical wound infections (POD 1–3), and the wound may exhibit *blistering, bullae, and crepitus.* Opening the wound reveals what is typically described as *dish-water brown*

Table 3.9 Different types of infection and their respective primary mode of treatment

Type of infection	Bacterial infection?	Primary treatment	Remarks
Necrotizing fasciitis	Yes	Surgical debridement (emergent)	Life-threatening emergency; antibiotics are an important adjunct; hyperbaric oxygen therapy also be considered, only adjunctively
Wound infection/surgical site infection (SSI)	Yes	Open the wound/local wound care	Wound infections are characterized by a purulent exudate. Opening the wound and packing it with gauze is the treatment of choice
Soft tissue abscess	Yes	Incision and drainage (I and D)	Soft tissue, abscesses require I and D. The abscess cavity can be packed or left open, and heals by secondary intention
Abdominal/pelvic abscess	Yes	Interventional radiology (IR) drainage	Often done via placement of a pigtail catheter under CT-guidance
Appendicitis	Yes	Appendectomy	Some studies suggest antibiotics can be used for uncomplicated appendicitis, but this is still controversial and has not been accepted as a standard of care
Cellulitis	Yes	Antibiotics	Classic findings include warm skin, pain, swelling and especially blanching erythema

fluid with a *devitalized* appearance; the wound can also be extremely malodorous. A Gram stain may reveal *gram* ***positive*** *rods* (classic for *Clostridium perfringens*) although other bacteria and a mixed flora are quite possible.

Necrotizing fasciitis is a surgical emergency. While antibiotics and even hyperbaric oxygen can be utilized adjunctively, the standard of care is *emergent surgical debridement.* This means a surgeon "cuts out the dead tissue" until healthy, viable (bleeding) borders are encountered. This may leave large tissue defects, increasing fluid losses. Patients may also require more than one operation, sometimes with scheduled "second look" operations to re-evaluate the surgical site to assure (infection) *source control.*

Central line sepsis. Patients in the hospital environment may have a central venous access catheter (central line) for the management of multiple infusion medications and/or blood products, for monitoring of the central venous pressure, for hemodialysis access, and for a multitude of other reasons. Central lines are prone to infection leading to bacteremia and sepsis. This is especially true for *femoral* lines. Patients with line sepsis may have fever spikes (102 °F or higher) in an *undulant* fashion and may develop leukocytosis as well as systemic signs of infection. While IV antibiotic therapy is an important aspect of treatment, **central line removal** (ideally with culture of the catheter tip) is required. Skin flora (*esp. Staphylococcus epidermidis*) are the most common bacteria to seed the catheter and result in line sepsis.

III. ***Walk***—for *deep vein thrombosis* (DVT). What is probably more important than recognizing that a DVT can be associated with fever is to *make sure that patient who are admitted on the surgical ward have DVT prophylaxis,* this is especially pertinent for patient at high risk of forming a DVT due to a hypercoagulable state (Table 3.10).

IV. ***Water***—*Urinary Tract Infection:* UTIs are not infrequent among female patients due to a short urethra, but in the hospital environment, where post-operative patients may have indwelling foley catheters, males can also be afflicted. The goal is to minimize the time for which the catheter is required for two reasons. First, it improves patient mobility, which is important in the recovery process and is part of the ERAS protocol discussed earlier. Second, early removal of urinary catheters is an important intervention that has been proven to diminish the rate of UTIs among hospitalized post-operative patients. Patients with UTI may present with fever most commonly POD 3–5. Symptoms include dysuria, and/or burning with urination. Findings on urine analysis (UA) may be positive

Table 3.10 Common causes of a hypercoagulable state

Cause	Category	Details
Genetic mutations	Hereditary	**Factor V Leiden mutation**: A mutation that makes factor V resistant to inactivation **Prothrombin gene mutation**: A mutation leading to elevated prothrombin levels **Antithrombin III deficiency**: Decreased levels of an important anticoagulant **Protein C or S deficiency**: Deficiency of proteins that inhibit clotting
Antiphospholipid syndrome (APS)	Autoimmune	Characterized by the presence of antiphospholipid antibodies (e.g., lupus anticoagulant)
Cancer	Acquired	Certain cancers, especially solid tumors, increase procoagulant activity through tumor markers and cytokines
Estrogen use	Hormonal	Oral contraceptives or hormone replacement therapy increase clotting risk due to elevated estrogen levels
Pregnancy	Physiological	Increased clotting factors, decreased fibrinolysis, and venous stasis contribute to a higher risk of thrombosis
Immobilization	Environmental/behavioral	Prolonged immobility (e.g., long-term bed rest, travel) leads to venous stasis and increased clot risk
Obesity	Metabolic	Increased fat tissue can lead to chronic inflammation and increased clotting factor production
Chronic inflammation	Inflammatory	Conditions like rheumatoid arthritis and inflammatory bowel disease increase clotting risk through inflammatory cytokines
Heparin-induced thrombocytopenia (HIT)	Drug-induced	A paradoxical increase in clotting risk due to antibodies forming against heparin-platelet factor 4 complexes
Hyperhomocysteinemia	Metabolic	Elevated homocysteine levels, often due to genetic mutations or vitamin deficiencies, can damage blood vessels and promote clotting

for **leukocyte esterase**, **nitrites**. **Urine culture** is the gold standard and **quantitative colony count**: of $\geq 10^5$ CFU/mL in a midstream clean-catch sample is generally considered diagnostic for a UTI. Common treatment options include oral trimethoprim-sulfamethoxazole (TMP-SMZ), nitrofurantoin (Macrobid, Macrodantin), and ciprofloxacin (Cipro).

V. ***Wonder Drugs****—chronic medications.* Some patients develop so-called drug fever. Importantly, these patients are NOT the patients who just had surgery a few days ago. Drug fever is an uncommon cause of fever in the post-op patient. It is most typically seen in patients with a *complex and protracted medical stay.* These patients may be on a *multitude of infusion medications* (including antibiotics) who have typically been hospitalized for weeks and who develop temperature spikes in the background of a normal WBC and no other signs of infection and no other discernable cause of fever. If everything else is excluded, then medications (*esp.* antibiotics) can be considered the cause and sometimes a "drug holiday" is recommended whereby the medications are held or altogether discontinued.

Interpreting the White Blood Cell Count

For most patients after surgery, it is quite common to observe an elevated white blood cell count (WBC), especially on POD 1. On this day, the reason is almost never due to "infection" and is more likely due to the physiologic stress resultant from the physical "assault" of surgery. This is a normal physiologic response, and an elevated WBC after surgery is actually expected and is predictable. It is usually used as a *baseline,* and if followed (track and trend), the WBC would gradually decrease in the coming days post-op, assuming the recovery is proceeding as expected.

The WBC *Sink—an important pitfall.* We are trained to think that an elevated, up-trending WBC is concerning, and that a down-trending WBC is "reassuring." Interestingly, this is *not* always the case.

Core Principle: In certain instances, a down-trending WBC is more concerning than an up-trending WBC.

This is an idea that deserves your attention and understanding. This is of particular importance in monitoring patients post-op, who may develop potentially life-threatening infections, and who will often exhibit an acute drop in their white blood cell count—referred by clinicians as a **WBC *sink***. A WBC sink occurs when the overall (absolute) WBC drops due to the *white blood cells leaving the blood stream to fight an (often severe) infection outside of the blood stream.*

Table 3.11 Interpreting WBC + *differential* in post-op patients

	A	B	C
WBC	10→7	8→12	7→3
PMN	82→67	75→80	68→94
BANDS	N/A	0→1	0→40
Concern	None	Moderate	High

But how do you know if a patient has a WBC sink, or if there WBC is just normalizing? This can usually be determined by the CBC *differential.* When a CBC is obtained in post-op patients, it should always be obtained *with* a differential. This provides *much* greater information than the absolute WBC alone.

One important aspect of the differential is that it provides the percent polymorphonuclear leukocytes (PMNs) and BANDS (young neutrophils). A rise in PMNs is known as a **LEFT SHIFT**, and a rise, or even presence of bands, is known as a **BANDEMIA**. *Importantly, even if the absolute WBC is normal or down-trending, if a left shift and/or bandemia is present, the patient likely has a serious and potentially life-threatening infection.* Always correlate with physical exam findings and notify the attending surgeon immediately to determine next steps, which may include CT body imaging or return to the OR, depending on the overall clinical picture.

To help explain this important principle, let us consider a *MOC* example, as shown in Table 3.11. Here, three WBC trends are shown for post-surgical patients. ***(A)*** represents the WBC absolute number is normalizing, and *so is the differential* which initially demonstrated a slight left shift. This is an expected pattern after surgery. Bands are usually not present and therefore not reported on a differential unless they are present. For ***(B)***, there is a slight rise in the absolute WBC and an associated mild left shift. The slight rise in bands is not regarded as a bandemia. This pattern is typical of common types of infections, for example, SSIs or wound infections. It needs to be addressed and the source for elevated WBC identified and promptly treated; it is of moderate clinical concern. In the final column, ***(C)***, a *WBC sink is shown.* Here, the absolute WBC is *decreased,* however, analysis of the differential clearly shows a left shift and bandemia. *This is suggestive of a very serious infection and requires immediate attention. As a PA, you should always notify the attending surgeon if you observe a WBC sink on lab evaluation.*

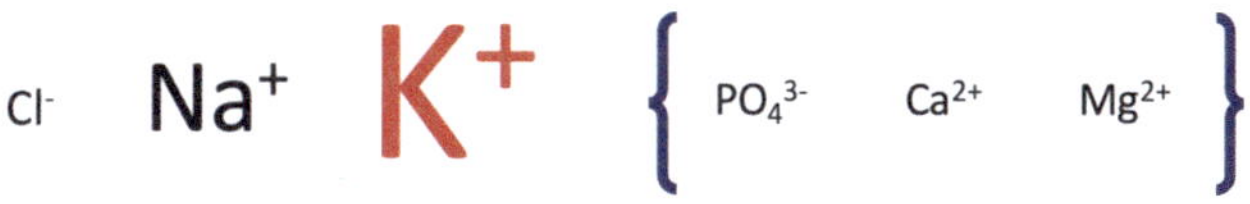

Fig. 3.15 The relevant electrolytes in the human body Cl^-, Na^+, K^+, Ca^{2+}, Mg^{2+}, and PO_4^{3-} are shown according to their relative importance, with K^+ being the most important electrolyte clinically. While all electrolytes carry some level of importance, in clinical medicine they are not all equal. In most routine lab draws, for example, Ca^{2+}, Mg^{2+}, and PO_4^{3-} are not even assessed, and thus are shown here in brackets

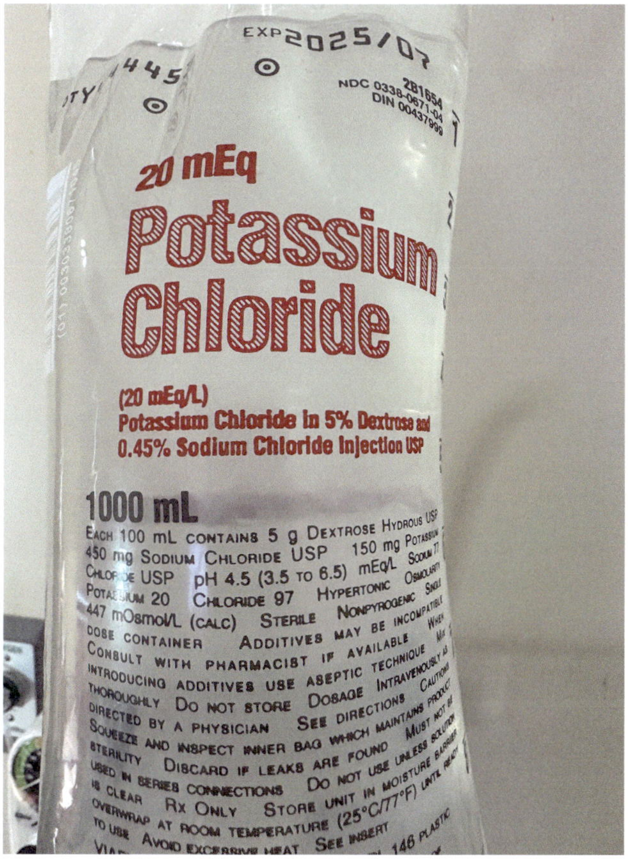

Fig. 3.16 Crystalloid intravenous fluid bags for normal saline are printed with black ink. However, if even a small amount of potassium (K^+) is added to the solution, then the writing is switched to red, as a type of "warning." This underscores how serious of an electrolyte potassium can be. Hyperkalemia, in particular, can be deadly

Blood Chemistry and the Importance of Potassium (K^+)

Surgical patients can have electrolyte derangements, which can have downstream effects on end organs, and which can impede the healing process during the recovery phase. The common electrolytes monitored are sodium (Na^+), chloride (Cl^-), and potassium (K^+). These electrolytes are often reported on a routine *complete metabolic panel* or **CMP**, sometimes referred to as a CHEM7. Additionally, calcium (Ca^{2+}), magnesium (Mg^{2+}), and phosphate (PO_4^{3-}) are electrolytes that can be assessed but are not (in most hospitals) part of a routine CMP.

Rather than thinking about these as just "electrolytes in your body" and assessing if they are "high or low" try and understand that a *weighted level of importance* is placed on them, and these electrolytes are not all the same level of importance (Fig. 3.15).

The electrolytes with the <u>most importance</u> overall is **potassium (K^+)**. This electrolyte is so important, that even if a small amount (e.g., 10 mEq/L) is mixed with a normal saline solution, *the writing on the bag is changed from black ink to red ink* (Fig. 3.16). This is done for patient safety **as a high potassium can result in life threatening arrythmias and even death**.

The normal range for potassium is 3.5–5.0 mEq/L. Most potassium is concentrated *intracellularly* (ranging from 140 to 150 millimoles per liter. For K^+, which is an ion with a plus-one charge, millimoles, and milliequivalent are the *same*). Thus, outside the cells, $[K^+_{\text{serum}}]$ is 3.5–5.0 mEq/L, but inside the cells, $[K^+_{\text{intracellular}}]$ is 140–150 mEq/L. *That is a huge difference and a very large gradient!*

This gradient is crucial for maintaining proper cellular function, including resting membrane potential, electrical excitability, and various cellular processes. The gradient is maintained by the *sodium-potassium pump* (Na+/K+ ATPase), which actively transports potassium ions into the cell while pumping sodium ions out, helping to keep this concentration gradient intact (Fig. 3.17).

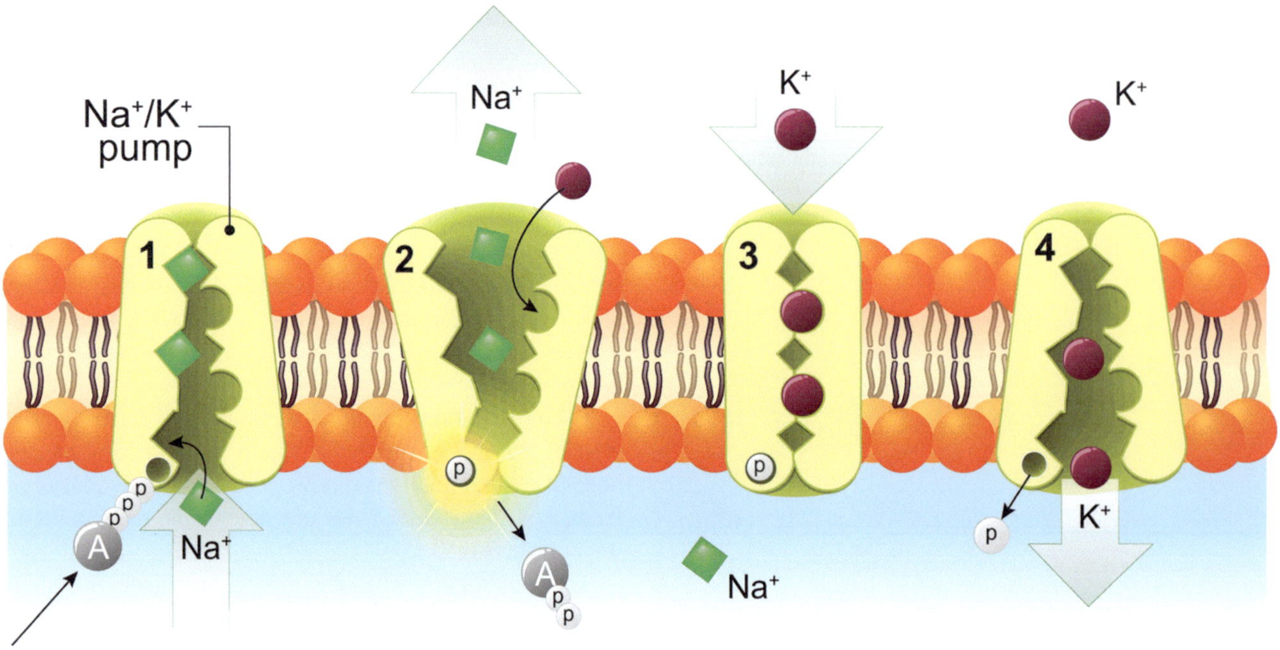

Fig. 3.17 The primary mechanism responsible for maintaining the potassium gradient is the sodium-potassium pump (Na^+/K^+ ATPase). This pump actively transports three sodium ions (Na^+) out of the cell and two potassium ions (K^+) into the cell, against their concentration gradients, using energy from adenosine triphosphate (ATP). As a result, the intracellular concentration of K^+ is kept high, and the extracellular concentration is kept low, maintaining the potassium gradient (high K^+ inside, low K^+ outside)

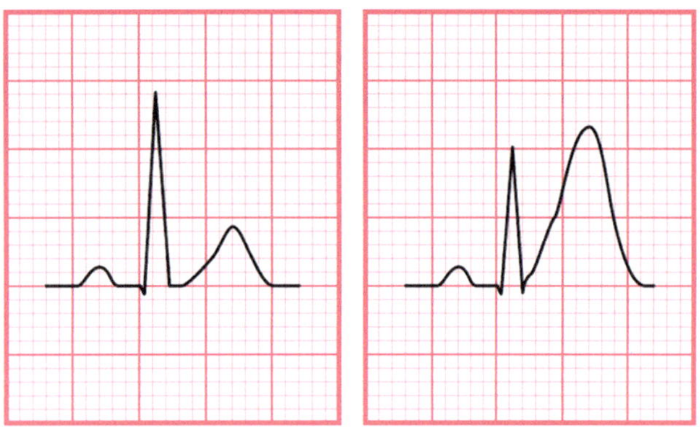

Fig. 3.18 Patients with hyperkalemia can develop a hyperacute, or *peaked* T-waves (as shown on the EKG—*right*). Hyperkalemia can be deadly due to its effects on the heart, which is why recognizing and normalizing this critical electrolyte derangement is very important. Patients with peaked T-waves are at risk for developing *torsades de pointes,* a potentially life-threatening ventricular arrythmia

Some methods of treating hyperkalemia take advantage of this large gradient, whereby medications act to move K^+ into cells. Clinically, we do not care about what the intracellular potassium concentration $[K^+_{\text{intracellular}}]$ is, only the concentration in the blood stream $[K^+_{\text{serum}}]$ which is what is measured and analyzed.

Aberrant Hyperkalemia If blood is drawn on a patient and there is a delay in processing, sometimes the sample drawn can hemolyze, resulting in the red blood cells "spilling out their contents" which includes that high concentration of potassium $[K^+_{\text{intracellular}}]$. Now, when the blood sample is analyzed, an aberrantly high potassium value is measured. This is not uncommon in clinical medicine. Thus, if your blood sample comes back with a very high potassium (for example 7.2 mEq/L), check to see that the specimen is not **hemolyzed**. This may be reported as a LAB ERROR as well. The sample should be repeated with a new blood draw.

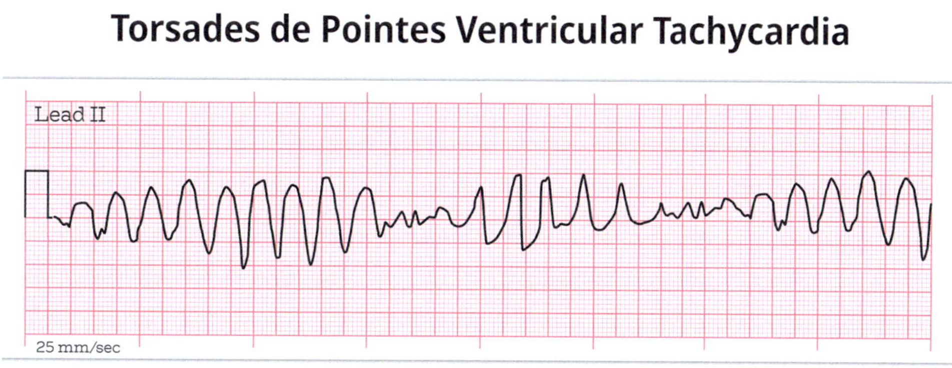

Fig. 3.19 This EKG shows *torsades de pointes,* a ventricular arrythmia that can be fatal and is associated with hyperkalemia. Calcium gluconate is the best choice to treat severe hyperkalemia because it stabilizes the cardiac membrane. *The most significant danger of hyperkalemia is on the heart*

Table 3.12 Methods to lower potassium (K+) and correct hyperkalemia

Treatment	Description	Indication
Calcium gluconate/ calcium chloride	Stabilizes the cardiac cell membrane and reduces the risk of arrhythmias	Used for severe hyperkalemia (especially if there are ECG changes)
Sodium bicarbonate	Helps shift potassium from extracellular to intracellular space by alkalinizing the blood	Effective in metabolic acidosis or in acute situations like kidney failure
Insulin and glucose	Insulin drives potassium into cells; glucose is given to prevent hypoglycemia	Common treatment for moderate to severe hyperkalemia
Beta-2 agonists (e.g., albuterol)	Stimulate beta-2 receptors, which promotes the shift of potassium into cells	Often used in combination with insulin for faster effect
Sodium polystyrene sulfonate (Kayexalate)	Binds potassium in the intestines and removes it via the stool	Used for chronic hyperkalemia or in cases where other treatments are not effective
Diuretics (e.g., furosemide)	Increases potassium excretion via the kidneys	Often used in patients with kidney function intact or mild hyperkalemia
Dialysis	Removes potassium directly from the blood in cases of severe hyperkalemia, especially in kidney failure	Reserved for severe cases or patients with end-stage renal disease
Dietary modifications	Reducing potassium-rich foods (bananas, tomatoes, potatoes) can help manage mild hyperkalemia	Used for mild or chronic hyperkalemia, especially with kidney disease

For patients with confirmed hyperkalemia, it is important that the [K^+] be lowered to normal range as quickly as possible. Hyperkalemia can lead to EKG changes, classically **peaked T-waves** (Fig. 3.18). These are nicknamed "tombstone T waves" not only because of their shape but also because they can lead to a potentially fatal ventricular arrythmia, **torsades de pointes** (French, "twisting points") (Fig. 3.19).

Table 3.13 Optimizing perfusion

Improve Hb-carrying capacity (PRBC for anemia <7.0 gm/dL)
Improve blood pressure and especially *mean arterial pressure*
Treat underlying cause (pulmonary edema, heart failure, sepsis)
Optimize FiO_2
Optimize lung function via nebulized breathing treatments and respiratory therapy

To stabilize the cardiac membrane, in patients with critically high potassium levels, the best treatment is **calcium gluconate (1–2 grams IV)**. Other options include **insulin and glucose** which draws K^+ intracellularly. A multitude of other tactics can be used [35], as shown in Table 3.12. If all else fails, **hemodialysis** is an option and is, indeed, an *absolute indication for treating refractory hyperkalemia.*

Hypokalemia *Hypo*kalemia ($K^+ < 2.4$ mEq/L) is not as concerning as *hyper*kalemia, and the condition can usually be easily corrected through potassium repletion (intravenous or oral). Clinically, hypokalemia is important in the post-surgical patient as it can contribute to a **prolonged *adynamic ileus*** in patients who have undergone intestinal surgery.

Oxygen Saturation Optimization Post-op

Obviously, patients who have undergone a surgical procedure need to *heal.* This requires *good tissue profusion* and is contingent on the delivery of *well-oxygenated blood,* among other things (such as protein and other nutrients). While blood SpO_2 (pulse oximeter readings) can be easily monitored and supplemental oxygen given if and when needed, in certain situations the optimization of oxygen delivery may *not always* be as simple as increasing FiO_2. Patients may exhibit a physiologic *shunt* and would thus *remain hypoxemic despite attempts to increase* FiO_2. One must sometimes

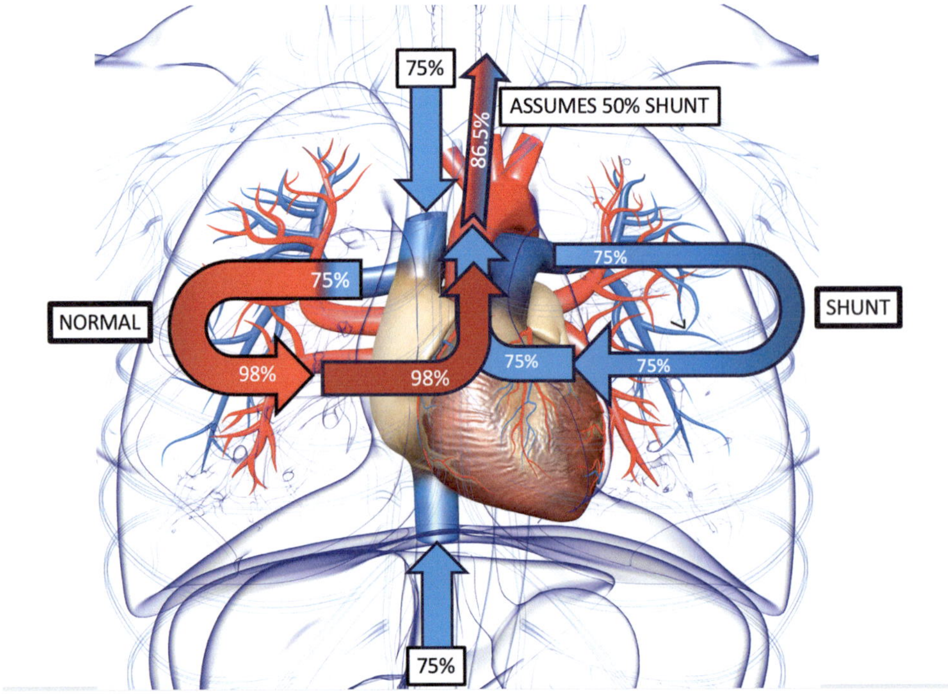

Fig. 3.20 This schematic illustrates the effect of a 50% pulmonary shunt. For simplicity, the diagram shows what normally happens on the *patient* right, marked "normal." On the *patient* left, the shunt effect is depicted. Normally, the 75% saturated blood undergoes oxygenation to, in this example 98% (range 95–100%), which is then driven out to the systemic circulation via the left ventricle. In the shunted side, the venous blood that is 75% saturated does not pick up any oxygen, so it returns to the systemic circulation the same way it came back to the heart (75% saturated). Mathematically, for a 50% shunt, this is mixed together with blood that is oxygenated in equal halves. Thus: (98% + 75%) ÷ 2 = 86.5%. Patients who shunt like this tend remain hypoxemic despite supplemental oxygen

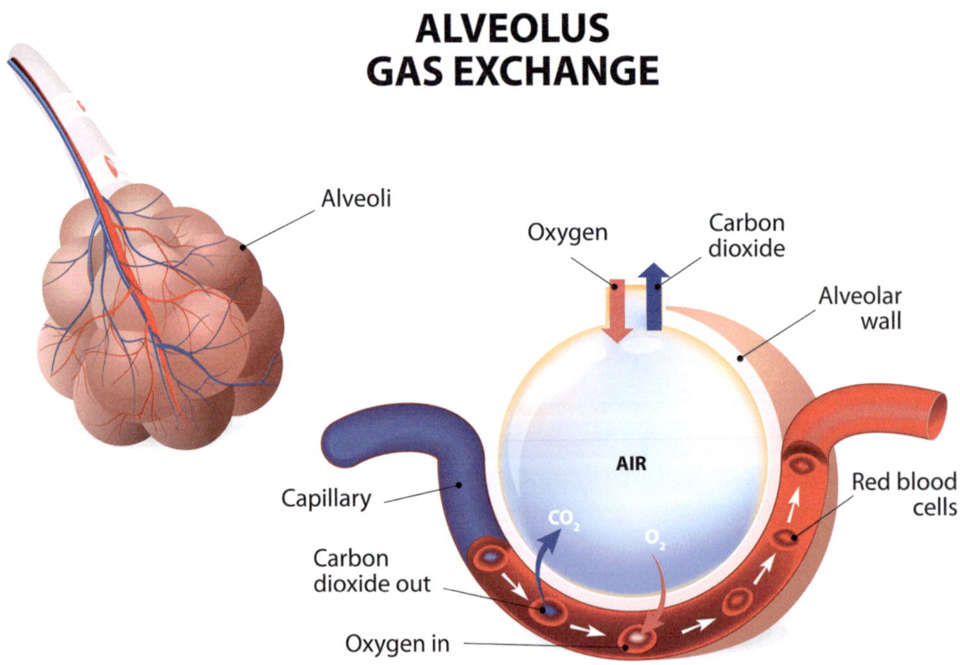

Fig. 3.21 Gas exchange occurs in the alveoli of the lungs, where CO_2 is released and O_2 is absorbed into the blood stream via capillary networks. Collectively, alveoli have a very high surface area which is important in maintaining efficient gas exchange. Disease processes that affect the lung parenchyma can impede gas exchange. This is especially true for intrinsic disease, such as acute respiratory distress syndrome (ARDS) and COVID-19 pneumonia

consider alternate methods to improve end-organ perfusion and oxygenation (Table 3.13).

Understanding Shunts and the Effect on End Organ Oxygenation There are important factors that can impede the delivery of oxygen to the periphery and to tissue in the process of healing, especially **shunts**. There are specific conditions in which a patient can develop a shunt—including sepsis, ARDS, and pulmonary edema. It is important to understand what this means for clinical management.

To help us understand this, let us look at an example, as shown in Fig. 3.20. Here, the effect of a 50% pulmonary shunt is demonstrated. Venous blood that returns to the heart is *de*oxygenated, but not totally deoxygenated. In fact, hemoglobin is still 70–75% saturated with oxygen as it returns to the right heart.

This blood then travels through the pulmonary artery to the lungs where gas exchange occurs and the blood is oxygenated as it passes through capillaries within the alveoli (Fig. 3.21). Under normal conditions, a level of 95–100% Hb-O_2 saturation is achieved. This blood is then driven to the systemic circulation providing well oxygenated blood.

When a pulmonary shunt is present, however, the gas exchange that normally occurs in the alveoli is restricted. Some alveoli may function perfectly well, while others may not be function at all. In this example, we have supposed that one-half of the alveoli are working normally, and the other one-half are not allowing for gas exchange at all. This would represent a 50% shunt.

In this setting we can calculate the effect on arterial blood. If we assume that there is a 50% shunt, and that deoxygenated blood is normally oxygenated to 98%, one-half of the blood returning would not get oxygenated (the shunt side) and would return to the systemic circulation with 75% Hb-O_2 saturation. The other half (the normal side), would be oxygenated at 98%. Finding the mean will provide the predicted saturation of arterial blood in the circulation as follows:

$$(98\% + 75\%)/2 = 86.5\%$$

Thus, in our example of a 50% shunt, the patient would be quite hypoxic, with saturations in the mid-80 s. Importantly, even if you add supplemental oxygen to this patient, they would *remain* hypoxemic because the most you can improve the oxygenation is on the non-shunted side, which would improve the value from 98% to 100% potentially. However, this would not improve systemic arterial oxygenation by much, as shown:

$$(100\% + 75\%)/2 = 87.5\%$$

More generally, this can be expressed as a weighted mean, where the percent of the shunt, ***n***, expressed as a decimal, can be calculated as:

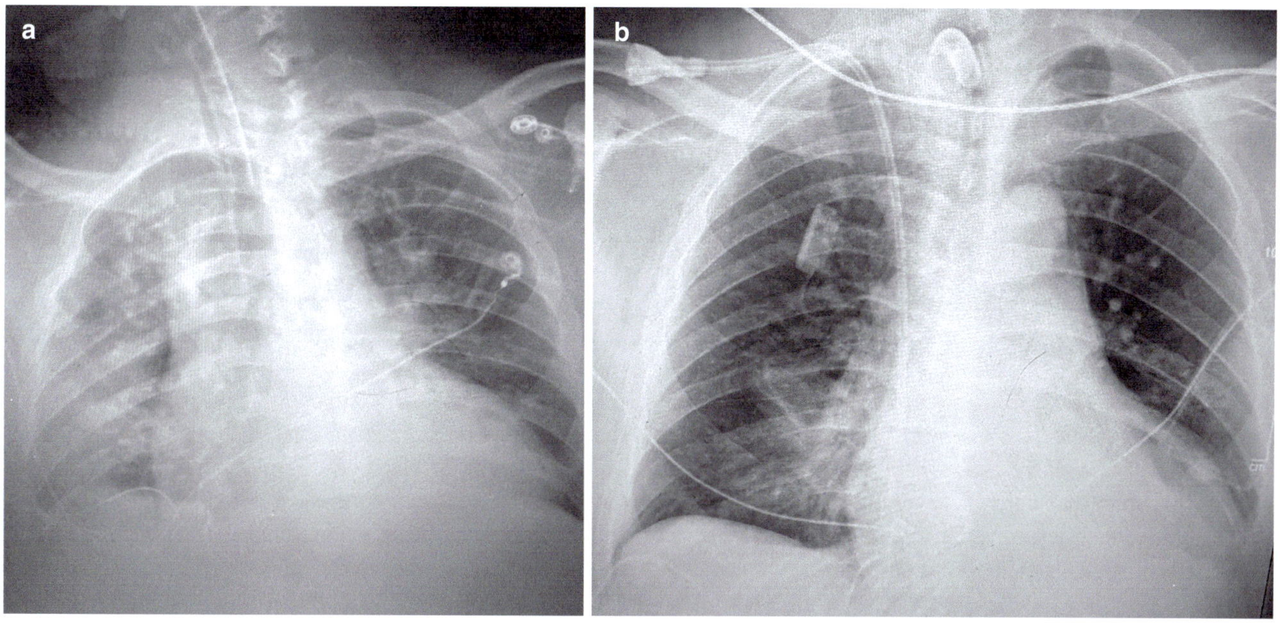

Fig. 3.22 (**a**) A chest x-ray (CXR) of a patient with pulmonary edema is shown prior to treatment. Normally, the lung fields should appear black (appearance of air on x-ray) not white (appearance of fluid on x-ray). These "wet lungs" result in hypoxia, which leads to downstream effects on tissue and end-organ perfusion. (**b**) After treatment with albumin 5% solution (500 ml) to osmotically draw the fluid out of the lung parenchyma and back into the vascular tree, *and* subsequent diuretic to clear the excess volume; the so-called *Albumin-Lasix Sandwich.* Note the marked improvement in aeration; clinically, the patient's oxygenation was dramatically improved as well

$$\Sigma[\left(B_o \times (1-n)\right)] + [B_d \times n]$$

Where ***B**o* represents the oxygenated blood *not* affected by the shunt, and ***B**d* represents the blood affected by the shunt (both expressed as a percent). For example, if the venous return to the heart is 70% rather than 75%, and the oxygenated blood is oxygenated to 95% from the normal, non-shunted side, with a 65% shunt (expressed as a decimal), we can predict the systemic oxygenation to be as follows

$$\Sigma[\left(95\% \times (1-.65)\right)] + [70\% \times .65]$$

$$\Sigma[33.25\%] + [45.5\%] = 78.25\%$$

The take away points are as follows. (1) Patients who shunt may be profoundly hypoxic, and they remain hypoxemic despite supplemental oxygen. (2) The degree of hypoxia is proportional to the fraction of blood being shunted. (3) The larger the shunt, the more hypoxic the patient. If you encounter this type of supplemental oxygen-resistant hypoxia, consider the possibility that the patient may be shunting. Look for potential causes. *For post-surgical patients, always consider* ***sepsis***, although intrinsic lung disease (e.g., ARDS, COVID-19, pneumonia) should also be considered, and chest imaging (two-view chest x-ray, CXR) is useful in this setting.

Challenges in Medical Management To test our understanding, consider a patient who has undergone abdominal surgery for resection of a gastric tumor. Suppose the surgery was successful, however, the patient has developed CHF and now has secondary pulmonary edema, as shown in the CXR (Fig. 3.22a). You attempt to increase FiO_2 by placing the patient on high flow NC, 6 L O_2, but there is no improvement, due to shunting.

How could you improve oxygenation in another way? You know the problem is that the lungs are "wet" (thus interfering with normal gas exchange) and you want to "dry them out" but *how?* One approach would be to administer albumin, usually as a 5% solution with vol. 250 ml, or alternatively as a 25% drip. This would shift fluid out of the interstitium and lung parenchyma, moving the fluid back into the vascular tree. However, this would increase the vascular volume and further challenge the patient's heart, which is currently in failure. To solve this problem, Lasix®/furosemide can be administered, which would eliminate the excess volume by increasing urine output. This is known as an *Albumin-Lasix Sandwich.* This is one way to dry out the lungs, improve aeration, and thus gas exchange, and ultimate end-organ perfusion *without "overloading" the heart* (Fig. 3.22b). Ultimately, this acts to *optimize organ perfusion, which is vital after surgery.* This example ties many principles together and is representative of how a strong foundation in medicine is necessary for the management of the surgical patient.

Part 5: Select Problems in General Surgery

Septic Shock

Sepsis is one of the most serious conditions that can affect patients post-operatively. This is especially true for patients who have undergone GI surgery, who are at increased risk for gram-negative bacteremia and potentially septicemia. There is a significant concentration of bacteria within stool in the GI tract—on the order of 10^{10} to 10^{12} bacteria per gram of stool. Bacteria have a symbiotic relationship within our GI tract, and inside the tract, high concentrations of bacteria is normal and does not (usually) cause problems. *However,* when bacteria spills into the abdominal or peritoneal cavity (which is normally sterile) during or after surgery, the bacteria can cause serious infection and sepsis.

Sepsis may be heralded by fever, tachycardia, an elevated WBC, and other signs of systemic inflammatory response. But in addition to these findings, *septic patients tend to shunt,* and thus will be *hypoxemic,* despite increasing supplemental oxygen, as discussed in the previous section. Septic shock, like all forms of shock, results in a labile blood pressure, and maintaining normotension is challenging.

Patients with septic shock have a very low *peripheral vascular resistance* (↓ ↓ ↓ PVR)—because bacteria interfere with the ability of the arterial capillary bed to clamp down. Because the vessels cannot clamp down in the periphery, the extremities feel warm to the touch, which is why septic shock is sometimes referred to *"warm shock."* This is in counter-distinction to *hemorrhagic* shock, where the peripheral vessels are able to clamp down (↑ ↑ ↑ PVR), resulting in "cold and clammy" extremities. Keep this in mind, as it is a very important point of distinction between the two types of shock (septic and hemorrhagic).

Patients with septic shock should immediately be transferred to the intensive care unit for a higher level of care, which generally includes aggressive IVF resuscitation (first and foremost), broad-systemic antibiotics, and vasopressors when indicated. Advanced monitoring, including arterial lines and/or central lines, are often placed as well.

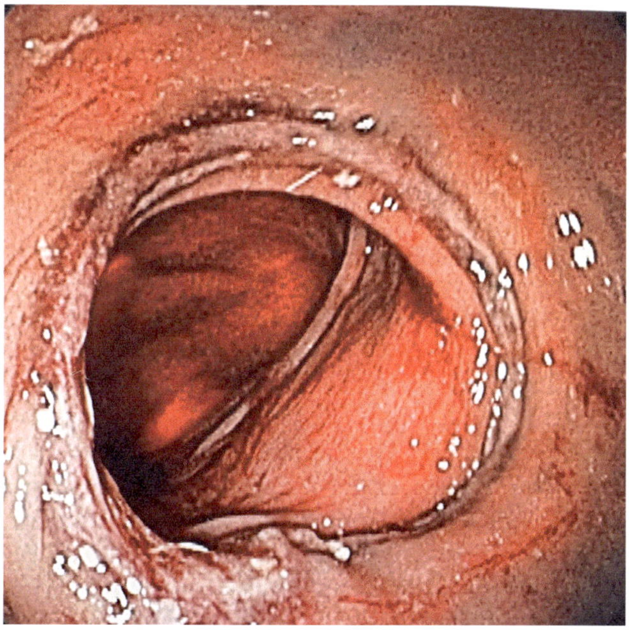

Fig. 3.23 After a segment of intestine has been removed, surgeons reconnect the remaining bowel by either suturing methods or by using mechanical, specialized stapling devices. Here, an endoluminal view of a mechanical, circular stapling is shown. Connections between two segments of bowel like this are termed an **anastomosis**. Such connections are designed to be airtight and watertight, but they can leak afterwards, as a disruption between the two joined ends can sometimes happen. **Anastomotic leaks** are a serious type of complication after intestinal surgery

If you suspect a patient may be septic and/or has unexplained hypotension or hypoxia post-op, notify the surgeon immediately and transfer the patient to the ICU. As a PA, taking care of in-patients, you want to develop a strong **safety culture**—always think to yourself—*what is the safest thing to do for the patient?*

Anastomotic Leak

When surgeons remove or *resect* a segment of intestine, they reconnect the bowel using either specialized mechanical stapling devices or by sewing the bowel back together. Either way, this connection is termed an **anastomosis** (Fig. 3.23). In most cases, the connection is made airtight and watertight and does not cause a problem. However, in some instances the connection can leak, usually days after the patient's surgery.

An **anastomotic leak** is an important and serious type of complication, **which represents a failed** healing of the bowel at its point of connection [36, 37]. This results in stool contents leaking into the abdominal cavity. Typically, this happens *between POD 3–10.* Such leaks are uncommon beyond 14 days post-op, although small chronic and "walled off" leaks can manifest later.

Table 3.14 Clinical findings that suggest an anastomotic leak

Elevated C-reactive protein (↑ ↑ ↑ CRP)
Clinical deterioration
Increasing abdominal pain and pain med requirements
Peritonitis
CT-scan that shows *contrast extravasation* and *free air*
High index of suspicion
Left shift, WBC sink
Hypoxia
Acidosis

This can be very useful information when evaluating a post-operative patient as it allows you to focus on what *is probable* and what is *not probable* for a specific point in time. For example, a patient who is *6-weeks* post-op from laparoscopic colectomy who present to the emergency room with abdominal pain is *not likely* to have an anastomotic leak, but a patient who is *6-days* post-op *is* in the "window for a leak." Leaks are one of the *most important things to rule out* in a patient who has had intestinal surgery with anastomosis during the appropriate time frame.

Clinical Findings Patients may present with nausea, vomiting, worsening abdominal pain and **peritonitis**. Patients with peritonitis require surgery. Indeed, another name for peritonitis is a "**surgical abdomen**." Signs of peritonitis includes *guarding,* a *rigid abdomen,* and *rebound tenderness.* Patients with peritonitis prefer to *lie motionless,* which is quite different than other causes of abdominal pain, such as ureteral stones, which tends to result in the patient *writhing* in constant motion.

Anastomotic leaks may not only result in fever, but generally a *very* ***high*** *fever* (e.g., 102–103 °F). However, patients with serious conditions, such as sepsis and anastomotic leak may or *may not* mount a febrile response. Notwithstanding, *when a high fever is observed in adults post-op, one should carefully rule out serious conditions, that include but are not limited to sepsis, intra-abdominal infection, or anastomotic leak.* Table 3.14 outlines findings that could suggest anastomotic leak. As a general rule, colonic anastomotic leaks are *more serious* than small bowel anastomotic leaks.

Tips for PAs Adults generally do not mount febrile responses to the same degree as observed in the pediatric patient population. In pediatrics, patients can *easily* mount a *very* high febrile response (104–105 °F) even if due to a *minor* viral URI; while for the most part, adults *cannot* mount such high fevers. This is an inherent distinction

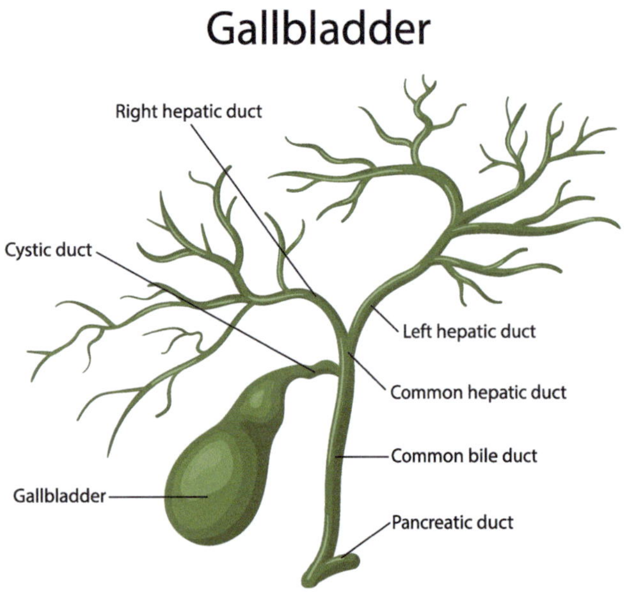

Fig. 3.24 The gallbladder is an outpouching from the biliary tree, and its relation to the biliary tree is shown. Of particular importance is the close proximity of the **cystic duct** (which has to be divided to remove the gallbladder) and the **common bile duct**, or CBD. If the CBD is inadvertently transected, it can result in very serious morbidity, and repair is difficult and highly complex. *CBD injury is the most dreaded complication from cholecystectomy.* Fortunately, CBD injury is extremely rare

between the pediatric and adult patient population, and one reason why it is commonly taught that "pediatric patients are <u>not</u> small adults."

Select Operative Injuries

Surgeons operate by focusing on target anatomy with care to avoid critical structures that may lie in close proximity. Some types of injury may not be evident at the time of surgery, and you need to be aware of them if you are a PA on the surgical service. Among the more important general surgical injuries are outlined in this section.

I. ***Common Bile Duct Injury:*** Among the most important structures that general surgeons try and avoid is the common bile duct (CBD). A substantial fraction of general surgery involved the elective or urgent removal of a gallbladder, which is most often done with minimally invasive techniques (laparoscopic/robotic) but can sometimes be performed open. The operation requires ligation of the cystic duct, which is a branch from the CBD. When surgeons operate in this area, they go to great lengths to visualize and confirm this duct so that the CBD is not inadvertently injured [38–40], and ICG can be useful for delineating the structures of the biliary tree (Fig. 3.24). The CBD drains bile into the digestive system via the *ampulla of Vader.*

   Clinical Findings: Signs of CBD injury include *jaundice,* caused by bile leakage or obstruction, leading to an accumulation of bilirubin in the bloodstream. This may appear within hours or days after surgery. Abdominal pain, especially in the right upper quadrant can occur due to bile leakage, inflammation, or bile duct obstruction. The pain may be continuous or intermittent. Fever is often present, and may indicate infection or bile peritonitis resulting from bile leakage. Other signs and symptoms may include nausea, vomiting, and dark urine. The latter secondary to increased levels of conjugated bilirubin, which gets excreted in the urine. This happens due to the obstruction of bile flow.

   Laboratory tests may show elevated levels of liver enzymes (such as AST, ALT, alkaline phosphatase, and bilirubin) due to bile duct obstruction or bile leakage into the peritoneum.

   Treatment requires reoperation. Repairing the CBD is highly complex and is often referred to an expert liver surgeon. This results in substantial morbidity to patients and thus is one of the most important structures surgeons seek to avoid injuring during cholecystectomy.

II. ***Ureteral Injury and Transection:*** Excluding special procedures performed by urologists, such as removal of the bladder (cystectomy) and creation of an ileal conduit (a surgical method to re-route urine after cystectomy), the ureters are structures *carefully identified and preserved during certain operations.* This is particularly the case during sigmoid or *low anterior resection* (LAR) of the rectosigmoid colon, and during some *gynecologic procedures* where the ureter(s) may be prone to injury due to their close proximity.

   Diagnosis of Ureteral Injury. Injury to the ureter requires reoperation and/or placement of percutaneous nephrostomy tubes to drain the affected kidney.

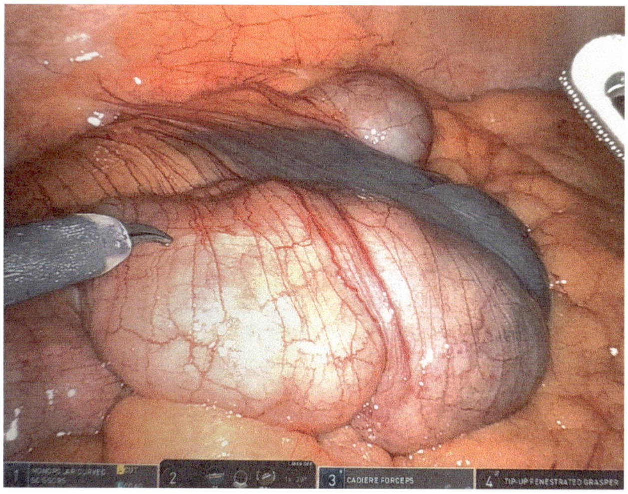

Fig. 3.25 A video still frame during robotic colectomy is shown. On the left is an 8 mm, sharp ended robotic instrument. Here, the tip is visible, but it had to be delivered to this point, and during delivery, it may not have been visualized, and there exists a small risk that the scissor tip shown *could* have caused injury to a structure, such as a loop of small bowel, *"off camera."* Although rare, such off camera inadvertent injuries are believed to be one potential mechanism whereby a small bowel injury, for example, could be missed at the time of surgery

Diagnosis can be made by *CT-urogram,* and a *renal ultrasound* may demonstrate hydro-ureter (a dilated ureter) if the ureter has been ligated (tied off). Patients may complain of increased or unusual levels of pain on the affected side, and the Cr may be elevated over baseline. For patients who have an intra-abdominal drain, the output may be clear, and the volume may increase as it may contain urine spilling into the abdominal cavity. Checking the drain fluid for Cr levels is of value to confirm a urine leak. If an injury to the urinary system is confirmed, a *urologist should be consulted for evaluation and next-steps in treatment.*

III. ***Small Bowel Injury:*** An injury to small bowel at the time of surgery, which can occur during lysis of adhesions (LOA), and which is promptly repaired (usually by primary suture repair), is not regarded as a complication, and there is usually no untoward sequelae from such injuries if immediately recognized and fixed. However, if a small bowel injury is not recognized at the time of surgery, it can have catastrophic consequences and is considered a major complication.

Small bowel injuries can be missed if they are small and/or overlooked, and in some instances, they occur in an area that is "off camera" during minimally invasive surgery. In this case, the injury occurs outside of the field of view, so it can be missed. This can happen, for example, if a robotic (sharp) scissor tip instrument is being introduced from a port site that is out of the field of view, and as it is delivered to the target site, it inadvertently injures a bowel (Fig. 3.25).

Special Considerations and Challenges

Post-op patients who have undergone abdominal surgery are going to have abdominal pain, and often abdominal distention as well. They will also have tenderness on palpation during physical examination. In other circumstances, these signs and symptoms would be concerning for an acute intra-abdominal process, but these findings are *expected* for post-op patients.

Sometimes it is difficult to tell if the symptoms are normal findings or if there is, in fact, an acute intra-abdominal process (such as infection, abscess, small bowel injury, or anastomotic leak). You may think a CT scan would be helpful, but it is too difficult to interpret, especially in the *early* post-op period. For example, the scan may show some "free air" and fluid throughout the abdominal cavity, but these findings are not atypical for patient who have had recent surgery. Thus, it may not be clear if what is seen on CT scan represents "post-op changes" or whether there is an acute or developing intra-abdominal process.

One must rely on clinical judgement and the overall clinical picture. One good rule of thumb is that patients should improve (have less pain, for example) *each day.* If you are a PA rounding on surgical patients, keep track of how patients are on exam compared to previous days.

References

1. Force AT. Practice guidelines for preoperative fasting and the use of pharmacologic agents to reduce the risk of pulmonary aspiration: application to healthy patients undergoing elective procedures: a report by the American Society of Anesthesiologists Task Force on Preoperative Fasting. Anesthesiology. 1999;90:896–905.
2. Brady MC, Kinn S, Stuart P, Ness V, Cochrane Wounds Group. Preoperative fasting for adults to prevent perioperative complications. Cochrane Database Syst Rev. 1996;4(5)
3. Joshi GP, Abdelmalak BB, Weigel WA, Harbell MW, Kuo CI, Soriano SG, Stricker PA, Tipton T, Grant MD, Marbella AM, Agarkar M. 2023 American Society of Anesthesiologists Practice Guidelines for preoperative fasting: carbohydrate-containing clear liquids with or without protein, chewing gum, and pediatric fasting duration-a modular update of the 2017 American Society of

Anesthesiologists Practice Guidelines for preoperative fasting. Anesthesiology. 2023;138(2):132–51.
4. Cappellini MD, Fiorelli GE. Glucose-6-phosphate dehydrogenase deficiency. Lancet. 2008;371(9606):64–74.
5. Luzzatto L, Nannelli C, Notaro R. Glucose-6-phosphate dehydrogenase deficiency. Hematol Oncol Clin. 2016;30(2):373–93.
6. Rosenberg H, Pollock N, Schiemann A, Bulger T, Stowell K. Malignant hyperthermia: a review. Orphanet J Rare Dis. 2015;10:1–9.
7. Hopkins PM. Malignant hyperthermia: advances in clinical management and diagnosis. Br J Anaesth. 2000;85(1):118–28.
8. Schneiderbanger D, Johannsen S, Roewer N, Schuster F. Management of malignant hyperthermia: diagnosis and treatment. Ther Clin Risk Manag. 2014;10:355–62.
9. Woods RK, Dellinger EP. Current guidelines for antibiotic prophylaxis of surgical wounds. Am Fam Physician. 1998;57(11):2731–40.
10. Dale WB, Peter MH, Surgical Infection Prevention Guidelines Writers Workgroup. Antimicrobial prophylaxis for surgery: an advisory statement from the National Surgical Infection Prevention Project. Clin Infect Dis. 2004;38(12):1706–15.
11. Stevens DL, Bisno AL, Chambers HF, Dellinger EP, Goldstein EJ, Gorbach SL, Hirschmann JV, Kaplan SL, Montoya JG, Wade JC. Practice guidelines for the diagnosis and management of skin and soft tissue infections: 2014 update by the Infectious Diseases Society of America. Clin Infect Dis. 2014;59(2):e10–52.
12. Wren SM, Ahmed N, Jamal A, Safadi BY. Preoperative oral antibiotics in colorectal surgery increase the rate of Clostridium difficile colitis. Arch Surg. 2005;140(8):752–6.
13. Carignan A, Allard C, Pepin J, Cossette B, Nault V, Valiquette L. Risk of Clostridium difficile infection after perioperative antibacterial prophylaxis before and during an outbreak of infection due to a hypervirulent strain. Clin Infect Dis. 2008;46(12):1838–43. PMID:18462108.
14. Cahill TJ, Baddour LM, Habib G, Hoen B, Salaun E, Pettersson GB, Schäfers HJ, Prendergast BD. Challenges in infective endocarditis. J Am Coll Cardiol. 2017;69(3):325–44.
15. Hubers SA, DeSimone DC, Gersh BJ, Anavekar NS. Infective endocarditis: a contemporary review. Mayo Clin Proc. 2020;95(5):982–97. Elsevier.
16. Gutierrez JJ, Rocuts KR. Perioperative anticoagulation management. In: StatPearls [Internet]. Treasure Island (FL): StatPearls Publishing; 2023.
17. Ageno W, Gallus AS, Wittkowsky A, Crowther M, Hylek EM, Palareti G. Antithrombotic therapy and prevention of thrombosis: American College of Chest Physicians evidence-based clinical practice guidelines. Chest. 2012; https://doi.org/10.1378/chest.11-2292.
18. Lucà F, Oliva F, Abrignani MG, Di Fusco SA, Parrini I, Canale ML, Giubilato S, Cornara S, Nesti M, Rao CM, Pozzi A. Management of patients treated with direct oral anticoagulants in clinical practice and challenging scenarios. J Clin Med. 2023;12(18):5955.
19. Ferri N, Colombo E, Tenconi M, Baldessin L, Corsini A. Drug-drug interactions of direct oral anticoagulants (DOACs): from pharmacological to clinical practice. Pharmaceutics. 2022;14(6):1120.
20. Cools F, Johnson D, Camm AJ, Bassand JP, Verheugt FW, Yang S, Tsiatis A, Fitzmaurice DA, Goldhaber SZ, Kayani G, Goto S. Risks associated with discontinuation of oral anticoagulation in newly diagnosed patients with atrial fibrillation: results from the GARFIELD-AF Registry. J Thromb Haemost. 2021;19(9):2322–34.
21. Rismiati H, Lee HY. Perioperative Management of Hypertensive Patients. Cardiovasc Prev Pharmacother. 2021;3(3):54–63.
22. Crowley K, Scanaill PÓ, Hermanides J, Buggy DJ. Current practice in the perioperative management of patients with diabetes mellitus: a narrative review. Br J Anaesth. 2023;131(2):242–52.
23. Levin PA, Nguyen H, Wittbrodt ET, Kim SC. Glucagon-like peptide-1 receptor agonists: a systematic review of comparative effectiveness research. Diabetes Metab Syndr Obes. 2017;10:123–39.
24. Madsbad S. Review of head-to-head comparisons of glucagon-like peptide-1 receptor agonists. Diabetes Obes Metab. 2016;18(4):317–32.
25. Gustafsson UO, Scott MJ, Schwenk W, Demartines N, Roulin D, Francis N, McNaught CE, Macfie J, Liberman AS, Soop M, Hill A. Guidelines for perioperative care in elective colonic surgery: enhanced recovery after surgery (ERAS®) society recommendations. World J Surg. 2013;37:259–84.
26. Moningi S, Patki A, Padhy N, Ramachandran G. Enhanced recovery after surgery: an anesthesiologist's perspective. J Anaesthesiol Clin Pharmacol. 2019;35(Suppl 1):S5–S13.
27. Thorell A, MacCormick AD, Awad S, Reynolds N, Roulin D, Demartines N, Vignaud M, Alvarez A, Singh PM, Lobo DN. Guidelines for perioperative care in bariatric surgery: enhanced recovery after surgery (ERAS) society recommendations. World J Surg. 2016;40:2065–83.
28. Ljungqvist O, Scott M, Fearon KC. Enhanced recovery after surgery: a review. JAMA Surg. 2017;152(3):292–8.
29. Blantz RC. Pathophysiology of pre-renal azotemia. Kidney Int. 1998;53(2):512–23.
30. Esson ML, Schrier RW. Diagnosis and treatment of acute tubular necrosis. Ann Intern Med. 2002;137(9):744–52.
31. Gill N, Nally JV Jr, Fatica RA. Renal failure secondary to acute tubular necrosis: epidemiology, diagnosis, and management. Chest. 2005;128(4):2847–63.
32. Abuelo JG. Normotensive ischemic acute renal failure. N Engl J Med. 2007;357(8):797–805.
33. Misiakos EP, Bagias G, Patapis P, Sotiropoulos D, Kanavidis P, Machairas A. Current concepts in the management of necrotizing fasciitis. Front Surg. 2014;1:36.
34. Allaw F, Wehbe S, Kanj SS. Necrotizing fasciitis: an update on epidemiology, diagnostic methods, and treatment. Curr Opin Infect Dis. 2024;37(2):105–11.
35. Larivée NL, Michaud JB, More KM, Wilson JA, Tennankore KK. Hyperkalemia: prevalence, predictors and emerging treatments. Cardiol Ther. 2023;12(1):35–63.
36. Litchinko A, Buchs N, Balaphas A, Toso C, Liot E, Meurette G, Ris F, Meyer J. Score prediction of anastomotic leak in colorectal surgery: a systematic review. Surg Endosc. 2024;38(4):1723–30.
37. Bruce J, Krukowski ZH, Al-Khairy G, Russell EM, Park KG. Systematic review of the definition and measurement of anastomotic leak after gastrointestinal surgery. Br J Surg. 2001;88(9):1157–68.
38. Martin RF, Rossi RL. Bile duct injuries: spectrum, mechanisms of injury, and their prevention. Surg Clin N Am. 1994;74(4):781–803.
39. Manguso N, Zuckerman R. Identification and management of bile duct injuries. Surg Clin. 2024;104(6):1229–36.
40. Dickens EO. Common bile duct injury in cholecystectomy. JAMA Surg. 2024;159(5):591–2.

Hemostasis and Disseminated Intravascular Coagulation

4

Ali Amirkhosravi and Hunter Ruokonen

Overview of Hemostasis

Hemostasis is a process by which blood is maintained in a fluid state and confined to the circulatory system. This system is also primed to rapidly react to vascular injury to prevent blood loss by sealing the injured segment of the blood vessel wall. In accomplishing this, the body relies on four major components including the vascular endothelium, platelets, the coagulation system, and the fibrinolytic system. The balance between coagulation and fibrinolysis is imperative and excessive or reduced activity in either system can potentially lead to thrombotic or bleeding complications.

The Vascular Endothelium

Vascular endothelial cells participate in hemostasis by maintaining blood fluidity through exhibiting anticoagulant characteristics [1] and by separating blood's hemostatic components from reactive subendothelial structures. In normal hemostasis, the endothelial cells secrete bioactive molecules such as prostacyclin and nitric oxide which inhibit clot formation and stimulate vasodilation [2]. Furthermore, the endothelial cells suppress coagulation factors by releasing heparan sulfate and thrombomodulin [3]. Following vascular damage, endothelial cells regulate vascular tone by producing endothelins that cause local vasoconstriction, ultimately minimizing blood loss [4].

Platelets

Platelets participate in hemostasis by adhering to the damaged area of the blood vessel wall. They then spread on the exposed subendothelial matrix, become activated and release internal constituents involved in both hemostasis and wound healing. Next, additional platelets delivered to the site adhere to the initial layer of platelets as well as to one another thus forming large aggregates. This is widely known as the platelet plug. The activated platelets become degranulated and begin to release their alpha and dense granule contents, including coagulation factors V, VIII, and fibrinogen, that participate in the coagulation system. Furthermore, the released factors, by both alpha and dense granules, can act as platelet agonists, thus amplifying further platelet activation and aggregation. Platelet contribution to hemostasis can be assessed in the laboratory by measuring the platelet count and platelet aggregation ability.

The Coagulation Mechanism

The coagulation mechanism is composed of a series of reactions that function as a biological amplifier and culminate in the conversion of soluble circulating fibrinogen into a fibrin meshwork at the site of vascular injury. The fibrin clot acts as a "glue" holding the platelets together providing stability to what is known as the hemostatic plug. The coagulation

A. Amirkhosravi (✉)
Medical Laboratory Sciences, Department of Biomedical Sciences and Technology, AdventHealth University, Orlando, FL, USA
e-mail: Ali.Amirkhosravi@ahu.edu

H. Ruokonen
College of Health Professions and Sciences, University of Central Florida, Orlando, FL, USA

S. Atallah, J. Dragoljevic (eds.), *Fundamentals of Surgery for Physician Assistants*,
https://doi.org/10.1007/978-3-032-21069-2_4

reactions involve inactive circulating precursor proteins (e.g., factor X) that are converted into their active forms (designated with an "a" after the coagulation factor [e.g., factor Xa]) with each activated factor catalyzing the next coagulation reaction ultimately resulting in the formation of fibrin.

In vivo, the coagulation cascade is initiated by the glycoprotein tissue factor (TF), which, under normal physiological conditions, is limited to extravascular sites and is not in contact with flowing blood. However, following vascular injury, TF is exposed to flowing blood. The exposed TF rapidly binds to and causes the activation of coagulation factor VII to VIIa. The resulting TF/VIIa complex then acts in concert with activated platelet membrane phospholipid to activate factor IX into IXa and X to Xa. Factor Xa, again in concert with activated platelets, calcium ions, and factor Va, goes on to convert prothrombin (factor II) into thrombin (IIa). Thrombin, the pivotal enzyme of the coagulation system, drives fibrin formation and stabilization as well as continuous platelet and further coagulation precursor protein activation. Specifically, thrombin cleaves fibrinogen (factor I) to generate fibrin while converting factor XIII to factor XIIIa which causes the crosslinking of fibrin molecules thereby stabilizing the blood clot. The cleaved fibrinogen forms insoluble fibrin clots that act as a woven mesh, further stabilizing the thrombus [5]. Importantly, thrombin also causes direct activation of platelets.

To prevent excessive blood clotting after vascular injuries, TF-dependent coagulation reactions are regulated by natural anticoagulant inhibitors. Tissue factor pathway inhibitor (TFPI) can inhibit factor Xa as well as TF/VIIa complex. Other natural coagulation inhibitors include antithrombin (AT) which blocks factors IXa, Xa, and thrombin, and activated protein C which regulates thrombin generation by inhibiting factors Va and VIIIa. In the clinical laboratory, blood coagulation is most commonly assessed by measuring the clotting times: prothrombin time (PT) and partial thromboplastin time (PTT).

The Fibrinolytic System

As quickly as fibrin clot is formed, it begins to be degraded in the bodies effort to return to a pre-injury state. The purpose of the fibrinolytic system is to prevent excessive clotting which could lead to serious complications such as restricting blood flow or organ damage. Like the inactive factors in the coagulation cascade, the fibrinolytic system also has circulating inactive precursors. Plasminogen activators convert the proenzyme plasminogen to the active fibrinolytic enzyme plasmin whose job is to degrade fibrin. Thrombus degradation results in the formation of soluble fibrin degradation products (FDPs) including the D-Dimer fragment. Any plasmin released into the blood is neutralized by α_2-antiplasmin, thus preventing non-specific degradation of plasma proteins. In the clinical laboratory, fibrinolytic activity could be assessed by measuring FDP concentration in blood.

Introduction to DIC

Disseminated intravascular coagulation (DIC) was first described in the nineteenth century in experimental animals following the injection of fresh organ extracts or the infusion of hemolyzed erythrocytes [6, 7]. The recognition of a hemorrhagic state being associated with DIC came several decades later in humans with blood transfusion reactions [8]. Since then, DIC syndrome has been recognized to be a potentially life-threatening disease affecting the hemostatic system. The syndrome is characterized by systemic intravascular activation of coagulation resulting in widespread deposition of fibrin in the circulation [9]. The continuous activation of coagulation may result in depletion of coagulation factors and platelets (consumption coagulopathy), which may result in bleeding. Thus, DIC could be divided into two stages: (1) overactive clotting and (2) bleeding.

According to the Scientific and Standardization Committee of the International Society on Thrombosis and Hemostasis (ISTH), DIC is defined as "an acquired syndrome characterized by the intravascular activation of coagulation with a loss of localization arising from different causes" [10]. A substantial body of experimental and clinical evidence indicate that the initiation of coagulation in DIC is caused by tissue factor (TF) expression. Consequently, the excessive TF procoagulant activity in combination with downregulated physiological anticoagulant pathways and impaired fibrinolysis lead to systemic fibrin deposition. The clot formation occurs primarily in the microvasculature and could result in organ dysfunction and damage. Furthermore, the bidirectional interaction between coagulation activation and inflammation may further contribute to the pathogenesis of DIC [9].

DIC is an acquired consumptive thrombohemorrhagic syndrome, and its clinical presentation can be thrombosis and/or hemorrhage [11]. There is a high degree of complexity and variability in the clinical presentation of DIC which is dependent on the balance between fibrin clot formation in the microvasculature, the consumption of platelets, coagulation factors, and the physiological coagulation inhibitors. Therefore, the intensity of symptoms in DIC varies from mild to life-threatening according to etiology. It can be subclinical, present acutely or chronically, and based on severity and stage, can be classified as early (non-overt) and decompensated (overt) [12]. It is important to emphasize that DIC is always secondary to various underlying clinical conditions and remains a significant clinical challenge to clinicians in many medical specialties.

Pathophysiology of DIC

Initiation of Coagulation in DIC by Tissue Factor

Whereas normal hemostasis involves the intricately regulated and localized process of thrombus formation in response to endothelial damage in which clotting and fibrinolysis are limited to the site of injury, DIC represents a pathological, uncontrolled, and systemic activation of coagulation.

The manifestations of this thrombohemorrhagic syndrome are the result of excess formation of the pivotal coagulation enzyme, thrombin (Fig. 4.1). Thrombin can directly activate platelets and catalyze the activation and subsequent consumption of certain coagulation factors. On the other hand, thrombin induces the release of tissue plasminogen activator (t-PA) from the vascular endothelial cells which is converted to the fibrinolytic enzyme plasmin in the presence of fibrin.

Coagulation activation in DIC can be triggered by several different underlying conditions. However, the driving pathophysiological mechanisms of DIC appear to be inflammatory cytokine-initiated activation of tissue factor (TF)-dependent thrombin generation and fibrin clot formation, insufficient control of physiological anticoagulant pathways and dysregulated fibrinolysis [13]. The emergence of TF can be caused by several mechanisms such as monocyte activation (e.g., during septic infection), endothelial injury, placental abruption, or malignancy [14–16]. Upon exposure to circulating blood, the aberrantly expressed TF forms a complex with coagulation factor VII (FVII). This TF/VIIa complex then directly activates factors IX and X. Factor Xa converts prothrombin (factor II) to thrombin (IIa) which then converts fibrinogen to fibrin.

Role of Thrombin in Consumption Coagulopathy

Thrombin plays a central role in the pathogenesis of DIC. First, it proteolytically converts fibrinogen to fibrin to form fibrin thrombi in the microvessels. Continuous fibrin formation leads to a decrease in plasma fibrinogen concentration. Thrombin also potentiates clot formation by increasing the activity of factors V (FV) and VIII (FVIII) and renders the fibrin clot more resistant to fibrinolysis through its ability to activate FXIII [17]. Thrombin binds to specific platelet receptors and causes activation, aggregation, and secretion leading to a decrease in circulating platelets. Overall, excessive thrombin generation accounts for the rapid consumption of fibrinogen, platelets, and factors II, V, VIII, and XIII [18], whereas the depletion of coagulation factors IX and X is due to rapid clearance [19].

Role of Activated Platelets

Platelet activation in DIC could occur directly by thrombin as well as through interaction with disrupted (activated) endothelium [20]. Platelet aggregates contribute significantly to clotting activation in DIC. For example, activated platelets enhance prothrombin activation by offering their surface (increased anionic phospholipid availability) for FV binding which serves as a receptor for factor Xa [21, 22]. In addition, thrombin stimulates the release of FV from platelets which then binds to the platelet surface to accelerate coagulation [23].

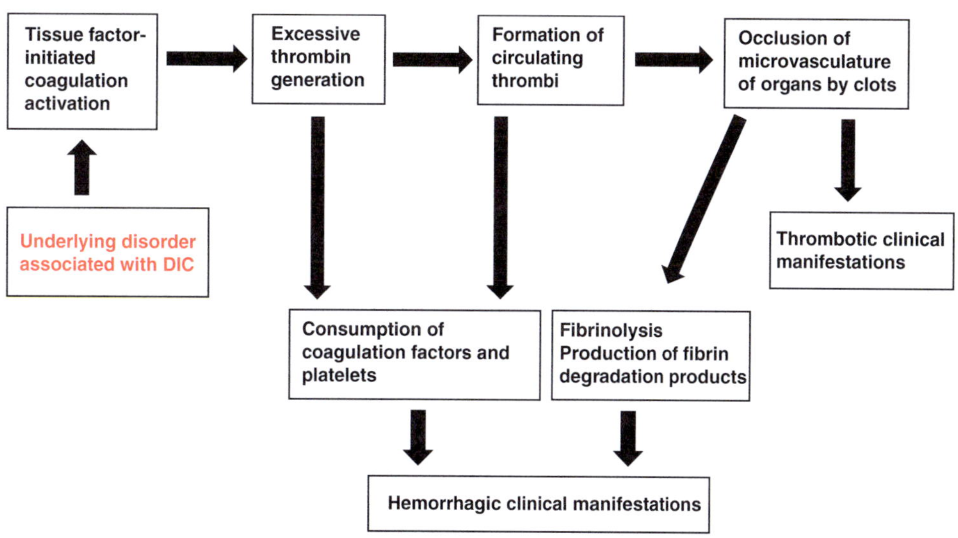

Fig. 4.1 Events during disseminated intravascular coagulation leading to thrombotic and hemorrhagic clinical manifestations

Endothelial Disruption and Insufficient Physiological Anticoagulant Activity

The normal vascular endothelium is central to the natural anticoagulant mechanisms involved in maintaining hemostasis. These include protein C, protein S, and antithrombin. During inflammation, the endothelium tends to lose its anticoagulant properties. Following endothelial damage, vascular subendothelial procoagulants such as TF and collagen are exposed to circulating blood. In addition, vascular permeability is increased resulting in the extravasation of anticoagulant proteins [13]. Furthermore, protein C and S are lost due to consumption, under production (in the liver), and degradation [24]. In patients with DIC, protein C level is decreased because of PC biding to its inhibitor forming a PC/plasma PC inhibitor complex during the consumptive process [25]. Finally, inflammation causes glycocalyx and surface anticoagulant proteins to be cleaved off into the circulation resulting in a decrease in anticoagulant properties of the endothelium.

Dysregulated Fibrinolysis

The balance between the procoagulant enzyme thrombin and the fibrinolytic enzyme plasmin determines the clinical manifestation of DIC. If there is a thrombin predominance and a decreased plasmin formation (hypofibrinolysis), the clinical picture is characterized by thrombosis in the microvasculature, organ ischemia, and bleeding due to consumption of coagulation factors. However, it is also possible for fibrinolysis to be enhanced in DIC (hyperfibrinolysis). The pathophysiology of the underlying disease determines whether fibrinolysis is impaired or enhanced in DIC [26].

In the microcirculation, plasmin degrades fibrin whereas in other (larger) vessels, plasmin activates and degrades fibrinogen. If enough plasmin is available in circulation, fibrinogen degradation products (X, Y, D, and E) are produced which can inhibit the formation of polymerized fibrin clots [27]. In DIC, when fibrinogen and platelet concentrations are low, these degradation products contribute to the bleeding manifestation.

In sepsis-associated DIC, both plasminogen activator inhibitor-1 (PAI-1) and tissue plasminogen activator (tPA) are released from activated endothelial cells [28]. In addition, PAI-1 released from activated platelets is a contributory factor to hypofibrinolysis in DIC. Other factors that could contribute to hypofibrinolysis include overconsumption and underproduction of plasminogen and increased thrombin-activatable fibrinolysis inhibitor (TAFI) [12].

Cancer-related DIC is more commonly associated with hyperfibrinolysis [29]. In this situation, secondary fibrinolysis as a compensatory mechanism to degrade fibrin clots in the microcirculation is likely the contributing factor to the hyperfibrinolytic activity.

Clinical Disorders Associated with the Pathogenesis of DIC

DIC is always secondary to one or more underlying clinical conditions which share the ability to cause systemic coagulation activation by exposure of TF procoagulant activity and the release of inflammatory mediators. Therefore, the recognition of clinical disorders which may lead to the development of DIC is most important to appropriate management of patients.

The pathogenesis of DIC is associated with a wide range of disorders including severe infection, trauma, malignancy, pregnancy complications, liver disease and others (Table 4.1). Some of the more common conditions associated with acute or chronic DIC are described.

Table 4.1 Clinical conditions associated with DIC

Conditions associated with acute DIC	Conditions associated with chronic or subacute DIC
Infections	Malignancy Solid tumors Leukemia
Acute obstetric complications Placental abruption Preeclampsia and "HELLP" syndrome Amniotic fluid embolism	Retained dead fetus syndrome
Severe liver disease	Liver disease
Trauma or massive tissue necrosis	Vascular abnormalities Hemangioma Vascular aneurysm
Heat stroke	Recreational drugs
Snakebite	
Acute hemolysis	
ABO transfusion incompatibility	
Purpura fulminans	
Transplant rejection	
Severe toxic and immunological insults	

Conditions Associated with Acute, Severe DIC

Infections

Many gram-negative organisms can cause severe DIC with histopathologic evidence usually seen in patients with gram-negative shock who die quickly after presentation [30, 31]. Gram-positive bacterial infections are a less common cause of DIC and viral diseases such as influenza A, cytomegalovirus could be associated with consumptive coagulopathy [32, 33]. The pathophysiologic mechanism causing DIC during infection could be endothelial damage or disturbance resulting in TF expression, down regulation of the anticoagulant features of endothelial cells (e.g., thrombomodulin), and increased secretion of PAI-1 [34]. In addition, monocytes can become activated by bacterial endotoxins to express TF and promote a prothrombotic state [35].

Acute Obstetric Complications

A wide range of obstetric disorders can present with DIC as a complication, including placental abruption [36], postpartum hemorrhage, retained dead fetus [37], amniotic fluid embolism, preeclampsia (or eclampsia), and hemolysis, elevated liver enzyme, and low platelets (HELLP) syndrome [38]. The clinical manifestation of DIC in obstetric complications is varied, and the site of coagulation consumption may be limited to a single extravascular location, be disseminated in blood, or both. In placental abruption, coagulation consumption results from a combination of localized intrauterine hemorrhage and systemic fibrin formation caused by the release of TF from the placental tissue and/or the amniotic fluid components [39, 40].

Obstetrical (especially post-partum) hemorrhage is a major cause of DIC in pregnancy [41, 42] although there is debate as to whether the consumption coagulopathy seen in such patients is truly DIC or is simply the large blood loss that results in a depletion of coagulation factors [43]. However, evidence suggest that maternal coagulopathy associated with post-partum bleeding is more likely due to a procoagulant state and thrombin generation caused by TF release into the maternal circulation following the separation of membranes and the placenta [44].

In preeclampsia and HELLP syndrome, although sensitive markers of thrombin generation are increased, the levels of fibrinogen and other clotting factors are not significantly different from those in normal pregnancy [45] and overt intravascular consumption is only seen in those with complicating abruptions.

Liver Disease

Patients with acute or chronic liver disease could develop episodes of DIC including those with peritoneovenous shunts and fatty liver of pregnancy [46, 47]. The cause of DIC in cirrhosis and fatty liver disease is likely to be associated with impaired synthesis of coagulation factors. With peritoneovenous shunts, DIC could develop due to the TF activity of monocytes and macrophages of ascitic fluid.

Trauma

DIC could present as a complication of trauma in various situations such as head injury, soft-tissue trauma, burns, fractures, fat embolism, and gunshot wounds [48]. In these scenarios, the exposure of TF to blood (e.g., from necrotic brain tissue) is probably the initiator of the DIC process. Furthermore, in cases of severe trauma, DIC-associated fibrin clots in the lung microvasculature can lead to pulmonary dysfunction [49].

Conditions Associated with Subacute or Chronic DIC

In contrast to acutely ill patients who present with acute severe DIC, other patients such as those with malignancy may have relatively mild or protracted clinical manifestations of consumptive coagulopathy. Subacute or chronic DIC can occur especially in patients with mucin-producing adenocarcinomas and acute promyelocytic leukemia (APL). Retained dead fetus syndrome can also be a cause of subacute or chronic DIC which could present as a slow-developing and a compensated form of DIC [50].

Solid Tumors

Patients with solid tumors or hematological malignancies could present with DIC. The clinical association between solid tumors and thrombohemorrhagic disorders was first described by Trousseau in 1865 [51]. With solid tumors, the consumptive coagulopathy can have various clinical manifestations including venous thromboembolism, thrombocytopenia secondary to decreased bone marrow production, nonbacterial endocarditis, and microangiopathic hemolytic anemia. The pathophysiologic mechanism of DIC in patients with solid tumors is complex, but TF expressed on the surface of tumor cells, monocytes or tumor cell-associated microparticles appears to be the major trigger [52, 53].

Hematologic Malignancies

DIC could also be a complication of APL. In APL, although hemorrhagic effects of DIC are more common, evidence of thrombosis have been observed in up to 25% of patients [54]. Promyelocytic cells can express both TF and fibrinolytic activity with procoagulants being the predominant clinical presentation [54, 55].

Diagnosis of DIC

Since DIC is secondary to a wide variety of underlying disorders, both the clinical and the laboratory manifestations are variable and depend on the features of the DIC as well as the features of the underlying condition(s). Therefore, timely diagnosis of DIC, although challenging, could be achieved by assessing the entire clinical picture and considering the patient's clinical condition and all laboratory results. It is also important to know that DIC is a dynamic process and laboratory tests used must reflect the rapid changes in hemostatic function and keep pace with the clinical nature of the syndrome [43]. The laboratory tests include platelet count, partial thromboplastin time (PTT), prothrombin time (PT), fibrinogen, fibrin degradation products (FDP), and antithrombin activity assay. Screening tests such as platelet count, PT, and PTT provide information regarding the degree of coagulation activation and consumption.

Platelet Count

Serial measurement of platelets and observing a downward trend in platelet count is a sensitive sign of DIC. Thrombocytopenia is present in almost all DIC patients [56] and the reduction in platelets correlates with markers of thrombin generation. However, since some of DIC's underlying conditions themselves are associated with a drop in platelets, the specificity of platelet count for DIC is relatively low [57].

Fibrinogen, PT, and PTT

Although fibrinogen is consumed in DIC, its plasma levels can remain within the normal range since fibrinogen is also an acute-phase reactant. For this reason, isolated measurement of fibrinogen level is not a sensitive test for the diagnosis of DIC, but sequential measurements can provide more useful diagnostic information. PT and PTT are prolonged in about half the cases of DIC [58] for multiple reasons including rapid consumption of coagulation factors, loss of coagulation factors due to bleeding, or deficient liver function. However, in almost half of DIC cases, due to the presence of activated clotting factors (e.g., thrombin and FXa), PT and PTT are normal or shortened. So, for PT and PTT, repeated measurements are necessary to provide useful diagnostic information.

Fibrin Degradation Products

In DIC, fibrin D-Dimer and other fibrin degradation products (FDP) are elevated. This reflects increased fibrin formation and degradation. However, the specificity of FDP for DIC is limited since many conditions other than DIC are associated with elevated levels. Examples include venous thromboembolism, recent surgery, trauma, and liver and kidney dysfunction [59]. Elevated D-Dimer and FDP, in combination with changes in PT and PTT and falls in platelet count, rather than FDP alone, can be useful for the diagnosis of DIC.

Antithrombin and Protein C as Markers of DIC

Both antithrombin and protein C are reduced during DIC. The measurement of these natural anticoagulants has been shown to provide useful prognostic information [60, 61]. However, the availability of chromogenic and enzyme-linked immunoassays for antithrombin and protein C may be limited in some laboratories. Furthermore, due to low sensitivity and specificity, single measurements of both antithrombin and protein C are not very useful for the diagnosis of DIC.

Point-of-Care Tests

Thromboelastography (TEG) and thromboelastometry (ROTEM) are viscoelastic point-of care tests that can be used for the diagnosis of DIC. By measuring clot formation velocity, clot firmness, and clot lysis index in addition to clotting time, these methods provide a global hemostatic profile. For example, prolonged clot times and decreased clot firmness has been associated with overt DIC in patient with sepsis [62, 63]. In addition, TEG and ROTEM are sensitive to hyperfibrinolysis and may provide useful information to physicians toward using anti-fibrinolytic agents in DIC patients with bleeding [12].

Scoring System for DIC

The diagnostic criteria of overt DIC were established by the International Society on Thrombosis and Hemostasis (ISTH) in 2001 [10]. Based on the criteria, the ISTH recommended a 5-step diagnostic algorithm (Table 4.2) to calculate a DIC

Table 4.2 ISTH scoring system for the diagnosis of overt DIC [64]

Presence of underlying conditions known to be associated with DIC	
Does the patient have a condition associated with DIC? Y/N	
If yes, proceed to tests	
If no, do not use the scoring system	
Ordering of laboratory tests	
Platelet count	
Fibrinogen	
Prothrombin time (PT)	
D-Dimer and FDP	
Scoring of test results	
Test result	*Score*
Platelet count > 100 × 10^9/L	0
Platelet count < 100 × 10^9/L	1
Platelet count < 50 × 10^9/L	2
Fibrinogen >1 g/L	0
Fibrinogen <1 g/L	1
PT < 3 seconds	0
PT >3 but < 6 seconds	1
PT > 6 seconds	2
D-Dimer and FDP	0
No increase	1
Moderate increase	2
Large increase	
Cumulative score:	
≥ 5 Overt DIC	
< 5 Non overt DIC: [repeat testing the following days recommended]	

score using simple and widely available laboratory tests including platelet count, fibrinogen, PT, and fibrin markers (D-Dimer or FDP) [64]. This scoring system requires the presence of an underlying disorder and pertains to conditions that could cause both acute and chronic DIC and has a sensitivity and specificity of 91% and 97%, respectively [65], with an increasing cumulative DIC score correlating strongly with mortality.

Since detecting DIC in its earlier stages would be useful for therapeutic considerations, the ISTH introduced the sepsis-induced coagulopathy scoring system in 2019 [66]. This scoring system was specifically designed to detect the compensated stage of DIC in sepsis, which can lead to overt DIC.

Management of DIC

The cornerstone to the management of DIC is the treatment of the underlying condition such as vigorous antibiotic treatment of patients with sepsis. In addition, supportive care must be provided to manage the coagulation abnormalities in DIC as well as correction of conditions such as hypovolemia and hypoxemia. In many cases, following specific and prompt treatment of the underlying condition and other supportive therapy, DIC will resolve spontaneously.

Transfusion of platelets is done in thrombocytopenic patients who bleed and have a count of <50 × 10^9/L and in non-bleeding patients with counts of 10–20 × 10^9/L [64]. Fresh frozen plasma transfusion may be given to correct the coagulation defect.

Anticoagulant therapy is used in DIC patients to restore organ perfusion and prevent organ failure caused by microvascular thrombosis. These include unfractionated and low molecular weight heparins. Experimental evidence suggest that direct thrombin inhibitors may reduce hypercoagulability in endotoxin-induced coagulation activation [67]. There is also evidence to support a beneficial effect of antithrombin substitution in DIC patients with sepsis [60, 61].

Hyperfibrinolysis secondary to DIC can occur in cancer patients such as those with adenocarcinoma or APL. The treatment of such patients with antifibrinolytic agents (e.g., tranexamic acid) may be beneficial [68].

Concluding Remarks

DIC is always a result of one or more underlying conditions and is manifested by a wide range of thrombotic and hemorrhagic pathology. Clinical presentation of DIC is also complex and its course is variable and unpredictable. Because of these complexities, the diagnosis of patients with early DIC prior to overt microvascular thrombosis, organ dysfunction, and bleeding is challenging. Finally, since DIC complicates many different clinical disorders and has different clinical manifestations, its treatment remains to be extremely complex, and despite the use of numerous therapeutics, prognosis of DIC patients remains poor. Studies involving clinical and laboratory observations of patient groups with the same underlying condition are needed for better understanding of the history and evolution of DIC as well as for identifying appropriate therapeutic interventions and proper individualized clinical management.

References

1. Félétou M. Chapter 2, Multiple functions of the endothelial cells. In: The endothelium: part 1: multiple functions of the endothelial cells—focus on endothelium-derived vasoactive mediators. San Rafael: Morgan & Claypool Life Sciences; 2011. Available from: https://www.ncbi.nlm.nih.gov/books/NBK57148/.
2. Mitchell JA, Ali F, Bailey L, Moreno L, Harrington LS. Role of nitric oxide and prostacyclin as vasoactive hormones released by the endothelium. Exp Physiol. 2008;93(1):141–7. https://doi.org/10.1113/expphysiol.2007.038588. Epub 2007 Oct 26. PMID: 17965142.
3. Esmon CT. The interactions between inflammation and coagulation. Br J Haematol. 2005;131(4):417–30. https://doi.org/10.1111/j.1365-2141.2005.05753.x. PMID: 16281932.
4. Haynes WG, Webb DJ. Endothelin as a regulator of cardiovascular function in health and disease. J Hypertens. 1998;16(8):1081–98. https://doi.org/10.1097/00004872-199816080-00001. PMID: 9794709.

5. Depasse F, Binder NB, Mueller J, Wissel T, Schwers S, Germer M, Hermes B, Turecek PL. Thrombin generation assays are versatile tools in blood coagulation analysis: a review of technical features, and applications from research to laboratory routine. J Thromb Haemost. 2021;19(12):2907–17. https://doi.org/10.1111/jth.15529. Epub 2021 Sep 26. PMID: 34525255; PMCID: PMC9291770.
6. Nauyen B. Unterschungen Ober Blutgerinnung I.M. Lebeden Tiere und Ihre Folgen. Arch Exp Pathol Pharmak. 1873;1:1.
7. Foa P, Pellacani P. Sulfermento fibrinogeno: Sulleazioni tossiche, escercitate da alcuni organi Freschi. Arch Sci Med (Torino). 1884;7:113.
8. Krevans J, Jackson DP, Conley CL, Hartmann RC. The nature of the hemorrhagic disorder accompanying hemolytic transfusion reactions in man. Blood. 1957;12(9):834–43. PMID: 13459931.
9. Levi M, van der Poll T. A short contemporary history of disseminated intravascular coagulation. Semin Thromb Hemost. 2014;40(8):874–80. https://doi.org/10.1055/s-0034-1395155. Epub 2014 Nov 6. PMID: 25377321.
10. Taylor FB Jr, Toh CH, Hoots WK, Wada H, Levi M. Scientific subcommittee on Disseminated Intravascular Coagulation (DIC) of the International Society on Thrombosis and Haemostasis (ISTH). Towards definition, clinical and laboratory criteria, and a scoring system for disseminated intravascular coagulation. Thromb Haemost. 2001;86(5):1327–30. PMID: 11816725.
11. Thachil J, Toh CH. Current concepts in the management of disseminated intravascular coagulation. Thromb Res. 2012;129(Suppl 1):S54–9. https://doi.org/10.1016/S0049-3848(12)70017-8. PMID: 22682134.
12. Adelborg K, Larsen JB, Hvas AM. Disseminated intravascular coagulation: epidemiology, biomarkers, and management. Br J Haematol. 2021;192(5):803–18. https://doi.org/10.1111/bjh.17172. Epub 2021 Feb 8. PMID: 33555051.
13. Gando S, Levi M, Toh CH. Disseminated intravascular coagulation. Nat Rev Dis Primers. 2016;2:16037. https://doi.org/10.1038/nrdp.2016.37. PMID: 27250996.
14. Osterud B, Flaegstad T. Increased tissue thromboplastin activity in monocytes of patients with meningococcal infection: related to an unfavourable prognosis. Thromb Haemost. 1983;49(1):5–7. PMID: 6845273.
15. Dicke C, Amirkhosravi A, Spath B, Jiménez-Alcázar M, Fuchs T, Davila M, Francis JL, Bokemeyer C, Langer F. Tissue factor-dependent and -independent pathways of systemic coagulation activation in acute myeloid leukemia: a single-center cohort study. Exp Hematol Oncol. 2015;4:22. https://doi.org/10.1186/s40164-015-0018-x. PMID: 26251762; PMCID: PMC4527228.
16. Thaler J, Koder S, Kornek G, Pabinger I, Ay C. Microparticle-associated tissue factor activity in patients with metastatic pancreatic cancer and its effect on fibrin clot formation. Transl Res. 2014;163(2):145–50. https://doi.org/10.1016/j.trsl.2013.06.009. Epub 2013 Aug 21. PMID: 23973167.
17. Gormsen J, Fletcher AP, Alkjaersig M, Sherry S. Enzymatic lysis of plasma clots: the influence of fibrin stabilization on lysis rates. Biochem Biophys Res Commun. 1967;120:654.
18. Minna JD, Robboy SJ, Coleman RW. DIC in man. Springfield: Charles C Thomas; 1974.
19. Wesseler S. Studies in intravascular coagulation. III. The pathogenesis of serum-induced venous thrombosis. J Clin Invest. 1955;34(4):647–51. https://doi.org/10.1172/JCI103114. PMID: 14367519; PMCID: PMC438671.
20. Page MJ, Pretorius E. A champion of host defense: a generic large-scale cause for platelet dysfunction and depletion in infection. Semin Thromb Hemost. 2020;46(3):302–19. https://doi.org/10.1055/s--0040-1708827. Epub 2020 Apr 12. PMID: 32279287; PMCID: PMC7339151.
21. Weiss HJ, Vicic WJ, Lages BA, Rogers J. Isolated deficiency of platelet procoagulant activity. Am J Med. 1979;67(2):206–13. https://doi.org/10.1016/0002-9343(79)90392-9. PMID: 572637.
22. Miletich JP, Kane WH, Hofmann SL, Stanford N, Majerus PW. Deficiency of factor Xa-factor Va binding sites on the platelets of a patient with a bleeding disorder. Blood. 1979;54(5):1015–22. PMID: 497393.
23. Ittyerah TR, Rawala R, Colman RW. Immunochemical studies of factor V of bovine platelets. Eur J Biochem. 1981;120(2):235–41. https://doi.org/10.1111/j.1432-1033.1981.tb05694.x. PMID: 7032911.
24. Massberg S, Grahl L, von Bruehl ML, Manukyan D, Pfeiler S, Goosmann C, Brinkmann V, Lorenz M, Bidzhekov K, Khandagale AB, Konrad I, Kennerknecht E, Reges K, Holdenrieder S, Braun S, Reinhardt C, Spannagl M, Preissner KT, Engelmann B. Reciprocal coupling of coagulation and innate immunity via neutrophil serine proteases. Nat Med. 2010;16(8):887–96. https://doi.org/10.1038/nm.2184. Epub 2010 Aug 1. PMID: 20676107.
25. Marlar RA, Endres-Brooks J, Miller C. Serial studies of protein C and its plasma inhibitor in patients with disseminated intravascular coagulation. Blood. 1985;66(1):59–63. PMID: 3924142.
26. Asakura H. Classifying types of disseminated intravascular coagulation: clinical and animal models. J Intensive Care. 2014;2(1):20. https://doi.org/10.1186/2052-0492-2-20. PMID: 25520834; PMCID: PMC4267600.
27. Marder VJ, Shulman NR. High molecular weight derivatives of human fibrinogen produced by plasmin. II. Mechanism of their anticoagulant activity. J Biol Chem. 1969;244(8):2120–4. PMID: 4238528.
28. van Deventer SJ, Büller HR, ten Cate JW, Aarden LA, Hack CE, Sturk A. Experimental endotoxemia in humans: analysis of cytokine release and coagulation, fibrinolytic, and complement pathways. Blood. 1990;76(12):2520–6. PMID: 2124934.
29. Levi M. Disseminated intravascular coagulation in cancer: an update. Semin Thromb Hemost. 2019;45(4):342–7. https://doi.org/10.1055/s-0039-1687890. Epub 2019 Apr 30. PMID: 31041800.
30. Rapaport SI, Tatter D, Coeur-Barron N, Hjort PF. Pseudomonas septicemia with intravascular clotting leading to the generalized Shwartzman reaction. N Engl J Med. 1964;271:80–4. https://doi.org/10.1056/NEJM196407092710206. PMID: 14149259.
31. Preston EF, Malia RG, Sworn MJ, et al. Intravascular coagulation and E. coli septaecemia. J Clin Pathol. 1973;26:120.
32. McKay DG, Margaretten W. Disseminated intravascular coagulation in virus diseases. Arch Intern Med. 1967;120(2):129–52. PMID: 4952942.
33. Talley NA, Assumpcao CA. Disseminated intravascular clotting complicating viral pneumonia due to influenza. Med J Aust. 1971;2(15):763–6. https://doi.org/10.5694/j.1326-5377.1971.tb92529.x. PMID: 5117272.
34. Schuster HP. Epilogue: disseminated intravascular coagulation and antithrombin III in intensive care medicine: pathophysiological insights and therapeutic hopes. Semin Thromb Hemost. 1998;24(1):81–3. https://doi.org/10.1055/s-2007-995826. PMID: 9515783.
35. ATA S, Mackman N. Monocyte tissue factor expression: lipopolysaccharide induction and roles in pathological activation of coagulation. Thromb Haemost. 2023;123(11):1017–33. https://doi.org/10.1055/a-2091-7006. Epub 2023 May 11. PMID: 37168007; PMCID: PMC10615589.
36. Onishi K, Tsuda H, Fuma K, Kuribayashi M, Tezuka A, Ando T, Mizuno K. The impact of the abruption severity and the onset-to-delivery time on the maternal and neonatal outcomes of placental abruption. J Matern Fetal Neonatal Med. 2020;33(22):3775–83.

https://doi.org/10.1080/14767058.2019.1585424. Epub 2019 Mar 8.
37. Romero R, Copel JA, Hobbins JC. Intrauterine fetal demise and hemostatic failure: the fetal death syndrome. Clin Obstet Gynecol. 1985;28(1):24–31. https://doi.org/10.1097/00003081-198528010-00004. PMID: 3987131.
38. Thachil J, Toh CH. Disseminated intravascular coagulation in obstetric disorders and its acute haematological management. Blood Rev. 2009;23(4):167–76. https://doi.org/10.1016/j.blre.2009.04.002. Epub 2009 May 12. PMID: 19442424.
39. Page EW, Fulton LD, Glendening MB. The cause of the blood coagulation defect following abruptio placentae. Am J Obstet Gynecol. 1951;61(5):1116–22. https://doi.org/10.1016/0002-9378(51)90313-4. PMID: 14838003.
40. Beller FK, Epstein MD. Traumatic placental abruption. Report of a case with hemorrhagic diathesis due to fibrinogen consumption. Obstet Gynecol. 1966;27(4):484–8. PMID: 5907369.
41. Rattray DD, O'Connell CM, Baskett TF. Acute disseminated intravascular coagulation in obstetrics: a tertiary centre population review (1980 to 2009). J Obstet Gynaecol Can. 2012;34(4):341–7. https://doi.org/10.1016/S1701-2163(16)35214-8. PMID: 22472333.
42. Erez O, Novack L, Beer-Weisel R, Dukler D, Press F, Zlotnik A, Than NG, Tomer A, Mazor M. DIC score in pregnant women--a population based modification of the International Society on Thrombosis and Hemostasis score. PLoS One. 2014;9(4):e93240. https://doi.org/10.1371/journal.pone.0093240. PMID: 24728139; PMCID: PMC3984105.
43. Levi M. Disseminated intravascular coagulation (DIC) in pregnancy and the peri-partum period. Thromb Res. 2009;123(Suppl 2):S63–4. https://doi.org/10.1016/S0049-3848(09)70013-1. PMID: 19217479.
44. de Boer K, ten Cate JW, Sturk A, Borm JJ, Treffers PE. Enhanced thrombin generation in normal and hypertensive pregnancy. Am J Obstet Gynecol. 1989;160(1):95–100. https://doi.org/10.1016/0002-9378(89)90096-3. PMID: 2521425.
45. Kobayashi T, Terao T. Preeclampsia as chronic disseminated intravascular coagulation. Study of two parameters: thrombin-antithrombin III complex and D-dimers. Gynecol Obstet Investig. 1987;24(3):170–8. https://doi.org/10.1159/000298799. PMID: 3319818.
46. Ragni MV, Lewis JH, Spero JA. Ascites-induced LeVeen shunt coagulopathy. Ann Surg. 1983;198(1):91–5. https://doi.org/10.1097/00000658-198307000-00018. PMID: 6859998; PMCID: PMC1352939.
47. Pockros PJ, Peters RL, Reynolds TB. Idiopathic fatty liver of pregnancy: findings in ten cases. Medicine (Baltimore). 1984;63(1):1–11. https://doi.org/10.1097/00005792-198401000-00001. PMID: 6690883.
48. Ordog GJ, Wasserberger J, Balasubramanium S. Coagulation abnormalities in traumatic shock. Ann Emerg Med. 1985;14(7):650–5. https://doi.org/10.1016/s0196-0644(85)80881-7. PMID: 4014813.
49. Watkins J, Wild G. The early diagnosis of impending coagulopathies following surgery and multiple trauma. Klin Wochenschr. 1985;63(19):1019–27. https://doi.org/10.1007/BF01737639. PMID: 3851975.
50. Graeff H, Kuhn W. Coagulation disorders in obstetrics. Major Probl Obstet Gynecol. 1980;13:1–157. PMID: 7453244.
51. Trousseau A. Phlegmasia alba dolens: Clinique Medicale de l'Hotel Dieu de Paris, vol. 3. London: The New Sydenham Society; 1865. p. 94.
52. Gonmori H, Maekawa T, Kobayashi N, Tanaka H, Tsukada H, Takada M, Andou K. The role of tissue thromboplastin in the development of DIC accompanying neoplastic diseases. Bibl Haematol. 1983;49:23–39. https://doi.org/10.1159/000408444. PMID: 6667248.
53. Callander NS, Varki N, Rao LV. Immunohistochemical identification of tissue factor in solid tumors. Cancer. 1992;70(5):1194–201. https://doi.org/10.1002/1097-0142(19920901)70:5<1194:aid-cncr2820700528>3.0.co;2-e. PMID: 1381270.
54. Gralnick HR, Sultan C. Acute promyelocytic leukaemia: haemorrhagic manifestation and morphologic criteria. Br J Haematol. 1975;29(3):373–6. https://doi.org/10.1111/j.1365-2141.1975.tb01834.x. PMID: 1059471.
55. Daly PA, Schiffer CA, Wiernik PH. Acute promyelocytic leukemia--clinical management of 15 patients. Am J Hematol. 1980;8(4):347–59. https://doi.org/10.1002/ajh.2830080403. PMID: 6932177.
56. Spero JA, Lewis JH, Hasiba U. Disseminated intravascular coagulation. Findings in 346 patients. Thromb Haemost. 1980;43(1):28–33. PMID: 6773170.
57. Akca S, Haji-Michael P, de Mendonça A, Suter P, Levi M, Vincent JL. Time course of platelet counts in critically ill patients. Crit Care Med. 2002;30(4):753–6. https://doi.org/10.1097/00003246-200204000-00005. PMID: 11940740.
58. Bick RL. Disseminated intravascular coagulation: objective clinical and laboratory diagnosis, treatment, and assessment of therapeutic response. Semin Thromb Hemost. 1996;22(1):69–88. https://doi.org/10.1055/s-2007-998993. PMID: 8711492.
59. Nakamura Y, Tomura S, Tachibana K, Chida Y, Marumo F. Enhanced fibrinolytic activity during the course of hemodialysis. Clin Nephrol. 1992;38(2):90–6. PMID: 1387598.
60. Mesters RM, Mannucci PM, Coppola R, Keller T, Ostermann H, Kienast J. Factor VIIa and antithrombin III activity during severe sepsis and septic shock in neutropenic patients. Blood. 1996;88(3):881–6. PMID: 8704245.
61. Fourrier F, Chopin C, Goudemand J, Hendrycx S, Caron C, Rime A, Marey A, Lestavel P. Septic shock, multiple organ failure, and disseminated intravascular coagulation. Compared patterns of antithrombin III, protein C, and protein S deficiencies. Chest. 1992;101(3):816–23. https://doi.org/10.1378/chest.101.3.816. PMID: 1531791.
62. Adamzik M, Eggmann M, Frey UH, Görlinger K, Bröcker-Preuss M, Marggraf G, Saner F, Eggebrecht H, Peters J, Hartmann M. Comparison of thromboelastometry with procalcitonin, interleukin 6, and C-reactive protein as diagnostic tests for severe sepsis in critically ill adults. Crit Care. 2010;14(5):R178. https://doi.org/10.1186/cc9284. Epub 2010 Oct 7. PMID: 20929576; PMCID: PMC3219282.
63. Haase N, Ostrowski SR, Wetterslev J, Lange T, Møller MH, Tousi H, Steensen M, Pott F, Søe-Jensen P, Nielsen J, Hjortrup PB, Johansson PI, Perner A. Thromboelastography in patients with severe sepsis: a prospective cohort study. Intensive Care Med. 2015;41(1):77–85. https://doi.org/10.1007/s00134-014-3552-9. Epub 2014 Nov 21. PMID: 25413378.
64. Levi M, Toh CH, Thachil J, Watson HG. Guidelines for the diagnosis and management of disseminated intravascular coagulation. British Committee for Standards in Haematology. Br J Haematol. 2009;145(1):24–33. https://doi.org/10.1111/j.1365-2141.2009.07600.x. Epub 2009 Feb 12. PMID: 19222477.
65. Bakhtiari K, Meijers JC, de Jonge E, Levi M. Prospective validation of the International Society of Thrombosis and Haemostasis scoring system for disseminated intravascular coagulation. Crit Care Med. 2004;32(12):2416–21. https://doi.org/10.1097/01.ccm.0000147769.07699.e3. PMID: 15599145.
66. Iba T, Levi M, Thachil J, Helms J, Scarlatescu E, Levy JH. Communication from the Scientific and Standardization Committee of the International Society on Thrombosis and Haemostasis on sepsis-induced coagulopathy in the management of sepsis. J Thromb Haemost. 2023;21(1):145–53. https://

doi.org/10.1016/j.jtha.2022.10.022. Epub 2022 Dec 22. PMID: 36695377.

67. Pernerstorfer T, Hollenstein U, Hansen JB, Stohlawetz P, Eichler HG, Handler S, Speiser W, Jilma B. Lepirudin blunts endotoxin-induced coagulation activation. Blood. 2000;95(5):1729–34. PMID: 10688831.

68. Thachil J, Falanga A, Levi M, Liebman H, Di Nisio M, Scientific and Standardization Committee of the International Society on Thrombosis and Hemostasis. Management of cancer-associated disseminated intravascular coagulation: guidance from the SSC of the ISTH. J Thromb Haemost. 2015;13(4):671–5. https://doi.org/10.1111/jth.12838. Epub 2015 Jan 28. PMID: 25556711.

Pharmacology for the Surgical Patient

5

Bozana Dragoljevic

Introduction

Pharmacological concepts involved in the care of a surgical patient can be categorized into preoperative, intraoperative, and postoperative considerations. In the preoperative period, a comprehensive medication reconciliation must be performed to evaluate for the need to interrupt chronic medication therapy when applicable. Other considerations include pre-anesthetics, antimicrobial prophylaxis, and perioperative anticoagulation management prior to the procedure. Intraoperatively, antimicrobial prophylaxis may be considered again in addition to anesthesia and pain management. After surgery, the concepts of antimicrobial selection and pain management are re-evaluated as the patient is prepared for the recovery period. Anti-emetics and chronic disease state management may be considered in this period as well. Caring for the surgical patient in the perioperative period involves overlapping concepts which must be evaluated after transitioning from each step in the process.

Preoperative

Medication Reconciliation

In the preoperative setting, comprehensive clinical evaluation of the surgical patient, among other components, includes a complete *medication reconciliation.* Documentation of the use of prescription medications, over-the-counter medications, and herbal supplements is necessary in order to prevent potential complications during and post-surgery and to reduce perioperative morbidity and mortality. As many patients may not disclose herbal supplement use, it is important to directly seek this information from patients during the preoperative assessment in order to avoid interactions with anesthetic medications and prevent unexpected intraoperative complications resulting from hemodynamic changes or increased bleeding risk. For example, use of *Ginkgo biloba*, ginseng, ginger, or garlic may predispose a patient to higher bleeding tendency during or after surgery. Other herbal supplements which may interact with anesthetics (through a prolonged or inadequate effect) or result in unexpected adverse effects include echinacea, St. John's wort, kava, and valerian (Table 5.1) [1, 2].

Aside from medication reconciliation, collection of the patient's history of allergies to medications or adverse reactions to anesthetics during prior procedures is useful during preoperative evaluation when determining the treatment plan. In addition to medication history, a patient's *social history* which includes possible use of nicotine, alcohol, and illicit substances should also be documented.

Premedications

Premedications or pre-anesthetics are drugs administered prior to procedures which are used to ensure optimal conditions for the patient which include reduction in pain, anxiety, and risks associated with uncontrolled comorbid conditions.

Opioids and other analgesics can be used to relieve preoperative pain and prepare the patient for surgery/recovery. Multimodal pain management relies on the synergistic effects of multiple analgesics which have effects on different pain pathways to improve clinical outcomes and reduce use of opioids. **Nonsteroidal anti-inflammatory drugs (NSAIDs)** have *analgesic* and *anti-inflammatory* effects through the ***inhibition of cyclooxygenase (COX)-1 and COX-2*** and by decreasing prostaglandin synthesis. Side effects associated with this drug class include ***gastric adverse effects*** (dyspepsia, peptic ulcer disease, bleeding), ***renal effects*** (acute kidney failure, worsening hypertension, electrolyte and fluid abnormalities), and ***cardiovascu-***

B. Dragoljevic (✉)
Department of Pharmacy, Veterans Affairs Hospital, Daytona, FL, USA

S. Atallah, J. Dragoljevic (eds.), *Fundamentals of Surgery for Physician Assistants*, https://doi.org/10.1007/978-3-032-21069-2_5

Table 5.1 Commonly used herbal supplements and associated adverse reactions [1, 2]

Herbal supplement	Adverse effects	Perioperative considerations
Ginkgo biloba	Anti-platelet effects	Increased bleeding risk
Garlic	Anti-platelet effects Hypoglycemic potential May lower blood pressure	Increased bleeding risk Hemodynamic instability Altered blood glucose control
Ginseng	Anti-platelet effects Hypoglycemic potential	Increased bleeding risk Altered blood glucose control
Ginger	Anti-platelet effects Hypoglycemic potential	Increased bleeding risk Altered blood glucose control
Echinacea	Altered taste Allergic reactions Immunosuppressive or immunostimulatory effects Hepatotoxicity	May increase the metabolism of IV midazolam
St. John's wort	Nausea, vomiting, constipation Neurologic/CNS effects (e.g., dizziness, lethargy, headache) Serotonergic effects	Increases metabolism of many drugs (e.g., midazolam, lidocaine) Adrenergic desensitization, cardiovascular effects, decreased response to vasopressors
Kava	Anxiolytic and sedative effects	Increases sedative effects of anesthetics
Valerian	Sedation Hypnosis	Increases sedative effects of anesthetics and midazolam

lar effects (exacerbation of heart failure, increased risk of adverse cardiovascular outcomes) among others. **Acetaminophen** acts in the central nervous system to provide *analgesic* and *antipyretic* effects; however, the exact mechanism is unknown. As *it is metabolized primarily through the liver,* it is important to consider a patient's *hepatic function* prior to use of this medication and to adjust the dose accordingly [3].

Benzodiazepines may be used to help patients with preoperative anxiety with midazolam, lorazepam, and diazepam commonly used via intravenous route. *Midazolam has the fastest onset of action* and is typically used at a dose of 1–2 mg in the preoperative setting. In those with significant concern for anxiety, an oral benzodiazepine dose may be used the night before or the morning of the procedure. Consideration of adverse effects, paradoxical reactions, sedation, and cognitive effects should be considered prior to the use of these mediations. Other drugs that may have a role in reducing anxiety include clonidine and dexmedetomidine (Precedex™) which could also have anesthesia sparing effects [4].

Postoperative nausea and vomiting (PONV) occurs during the first 24 h after a procedure. Risk factors for PONV include female sex, history of PONV or motion sickness, postoperative opioid use, younger age, nonsmoking, type of surgery, duration of anesthesia, among others. As antiemetic medications are associated with many adverse effects, it is important to assess the patient's risk for developing PONV to determine the number and type of antiemetics to use to limit these adverse effects while preventing nausea and vomiting. Several classes of antiemetic drugs can be used which include 5-hydroxytryptamine (5-HT3) receptor antagonists (e.g., ondansetron, palonosetron), dopamine (D2) receptor antagonists (e.g., metoclopramide, prochlorperazine), neurokinin-1 (NK1) receptor antagonists (e.g., aprepitant, fosaprepitant), corticosteroids (e.g., dexamethasone, methylprednisolone), and antihistamines (e.g., meclizine, promethazine). ***Ondansetron is the most commonly utilized 5-HT3 receptor antagonist and is considered the "gold standard" antiemetic.*** It has stronger anti-vomiting effects when compared to anti-nausea effects and *is recommended at a dose of 4 mg IV* which is as effective as an 8 mg *orally disintegrating tablet* for nausea prevention. Combination therapy with antiemetics from multiple categories as mentioned above is more effective than using a single agent alone due to additive effects at different receptors that target nausea and vomiting pathways. For example, ondansetron is commonly used with droperidol or dexamethasone for additional anti-nausea benefits [5]. Other antiemetic combinations recommended by the Consensus Guidelines for the Management of Postoperative Nausea and Vomiting by the American Society of Anesthesiologists task force on postoperative care are summarized in Table 5.2.

Antimicrobial Prophylaxis

Preoperative antibiotic prophylaxis is used to decrease the incidence of ***surgical site infections (SSIs)***. The Centers for Disease Control and Prevention (CDC) released guidelines in 2017 related to the prevention of surgical site infections due to the financial and human burden these infections cause. The guidelines recommend administration of antimicrobial agents when indicated by clinical practice guidelines with a goal of achieving bactericidal concentrations in both serum and tissues when the incision is made. (https://jamanetwork.com/journals/jamasurgery/fullarticle/2623725).

The CDC guidelines mentioned provide general recommendations regarding prophylaxis and defer details related to timing and antimicrobial selection to other organizations such as the American Society of Health-System pharmacists, the Infectious Disease Society of America (IDSA), the

Table 5.2 Antiemetic combination therapy for adults [5]

Droperidol and dexamethasone
5-HT3 receptor antagonist and dexamethasone
5-HT3 receptor antagonist and droperidol
5-HT3 receptor antagonist, dexamethasone, and droperidol
Ondansetron and casopitant or transdermal scopolamine

Source: Adapted from Gan et al. [5]

Table 5.3 Preoperative cefazolin dosing recommendations

Antimicrobial	Adult dose	Half-life	Time to peak (serum)	Redosing interval
Cefazolin	2 g (or 3 g if weight ≥120 kg)	1.2–2.2 h	IV: within 5 min	4 h from time of pre-op dose initiation

Surgical Infection Society (SIS), and the Society of Healthcare Epidemiology of America (SHEA). These organizations collaborated to publish guidance in 2013 to create a standardized approach to appropriate and safe use of antimicrobial medications [6].

The ideal antimicrobial agent should target the most common pathogens associated with contamination of the surgical site at an appropriate and effective dose for the shortest duration of time. Patient-specific factors such as allergies and renal/hepatic function should also be considered when choosing the appropriate agent to ensure safe medication use.

These guidelines recommend administering antimicrobial agents ***within 60 minutes prior to an incision*** with consideration for administration duration of specific agents that may require an infusion time which is longer than 60 min (i.e., fluoroquinolones or vancomycin). Recommendations for surgical antimicrobial prophylaxis ***are based on the type of procedure*** and most frequently include use of **beta lactams** such as **cefazolin** and **cefuroxime.** Alternative agents may be used in those with beta lactam allergies, which include clindamycin, vancomycin, fluoroquinolones, aminoglycosides, metronidazole plus clindamycin, and others, depending on the procedure type [6]. As ***cefazolin*** *is the most commonly utilized antimicrobial* and has been most extensively studied in the surgical setting, details regarding initial dosing, pharmacokinetic properties, and redosing are provided Table 5.3.

Perioperative Anticoagulation Management

The general approach for perioperative anticoagulation management involves **four steps:**

- **assessing thromboembolic risk**
- **assessing bleeding risk related to the procedure**
- **deciding whether to interrupt anticoagulation therapy**
- **deciding whether to bridge anticoagulation**

The American College of Chest Physicians clinical practice guidelines for Perioperative Management of Antithrombotic Therapy outline the key principles of risk stratification as it relates to a patient's thromboembolic risk vs. procedure-related bleeding risk. The risk of developing an arterial thromboembolism (ATE) in patients with atrial fibrillation, a mechanical heart valve, or a history of venous thromboembolism (VTE) can be categorized into high-, moderate-, or low-risk categories. In those with atrial fibrillation, the **CHA_2DS_2-VASc score** is used to determine thromboembolic risk while the type of valve and presence of major risk factors for stroke are used to stratify ATE risk in those with a mechanical heart valve. Patients with a history of VTE are stratified into one of the three thromboembolic risk categories based on whether the VTE was provoked or unprovoked, the time after the episode, and other patient-specific factors.

Assessing procedure-related bleeding risk can be classified into "high," "low-to-moderate," or "minimal" bleed risk categories. *Procedures with minimal bleed risk typically do not require interruption of anticoagulation or may require minimal interruption such as holding therapy on the day of the procedure only.* Low-to-moderate bleed risk procedures require short periods of anticoagulation interruption. High bleed risk procedures typically require longer periods of anticoagulation interruption and resuming therapy typically is delayed when compared to low-to-moderate bleed risk procedures.

The American College of Chest Physicians provides three antithrombotic patient care pathways which describe management of specific antithrombotic therapies. *In patients who are taking warfarin, the guidelines recommend interruption of warfarin therapy at varying intervals based on bleeding risk.* In minimal bleeding risk, warfarin therapy is not interrupted. In *low-to-moderate bleeding risk*, ***warfarin*** *is discontinued* ***5 days prior*** to the procedure and is resumed on the evening of the procedure or the day after the procedure typically. In both low-to-moderate and high bleed risk, if the decision to **bridge** is made, subcutaneous low-molecular-weight heparin (LMWH) is used (e.g., **enoxaparin** or **dalteparin**) starting *3 days prior to the procedure* with the last dose being given on the morning or the day prior to the procedure. Resuming LMWH after the procedure is recommended at full dose on day 1 after the procedure in low-to-moderate bleed risk and on day 3 in high bleed risk procedures (with low dose LMWH used in the first 24–72 h after the procedure). Most **direct oral anticoagulants (DOACs)** are interrupted ***1–2 days prior*** to the procedure based on bleeding risk with the exception of dabigatran which requires interruption 4 days prior to the high bleeding risk procedures and 2 days prior to low/moderate bleeding risk procedures. DOACs can be resumed approximately 24 h after low/moderate bleeding risk procedures and 48–72 h after high bleeding risk procedures. Finally, recommendations are also provided for patients receiving antiplatelet therapies such as **aspirin** or **$P2Y_{12}$ inhibitors** (*ticagrelor, clopidogrel, prasugrel*). Aspirin may be continued depending on the surgery and procedural bleeding risk. ***Clopidogrel*** *typically requires a* ***5-day*** *interruption,* while ***ticagrelor*** *requires* ***3–5 days*** *of interruption* and ***prasugrel*** *requires* ***7–10 days*** *of interruption.* All three can be resumed within 24 h after the procedure.

Managing anticoagulation therapy in surgical patients *requires an interdisciplinary approach* with the healthcare team which involves the surgeon, nurse, anesthesiologist, pharmacist, and other disciplines. Each member plays a role from the preoperative setting to the time the patient is discharged to reduce morbidity and mortality related to anticoagulation management [7, 8].

Management of Chronic Medications

Certain chronic medications, aside from anticoagulants and antiplatelets as discussed previously, may require interruption prior to certain procedures. **Glucagon-like peptide-1** receptor agonists (GLP-1Ras, e.g., **Ozempic®**) are commonly prescribed for type 2 diabetes and weight loss treatment and widespread clinical use has resulted in safety concerns among providers caring for patients in the perioperative setting. *As these medications result in delayed gastric emptying, patients may be at an increased risk of* ***pulmonary aspiration*** *due to residual gastric contents despite fasting prior to the procedure.* Additionally, GLP-1RAs *are commonly associated with nausea, vomiting, constipation, and abdominal pain which are symptoms that may be seen in those with preoperative and postoperative complications.* This potentially leads to *difficulty in distinguishing between the cause of symptoms and may delay treatment of complications.* While several organizations have provided guidance regarding management of GLP-1RAs, the decision to hold therapy is based on shared decision-making to assess a patient's individual risk. *The American Society of Anesthesiologists recommends holding* ***daily dosed GLP-1RAs on the day of surgery*** *and* ***weekly dosed GLP-1RAs for 1 week*** *prior to surgery* in patients for whom the decision to hold therapy has been made [9].

Another medication class with widespread use for the management of type 2 diabetes, chronic kidney disease, and congestive heart failure are **sodium-glucose cotransporter-2** (SGLT2) **inhibitors.** Due to a potentially increased risk of euglycemic diabetic ketoacidosis with the use of these medications, current guidance recommends ***holding SGLT2 inhibitors 3 days before surgery*** *to avoid risk of ketoacidosis.* However, a retrospective cohort study published in the *Journal of the American Medical Association* (JAMA) Surgery in February 2025 suggests preoperative use of SGLT2 inhibitors is not associated with an increased risk of diabetic ketoacidosis in patients with type 2 diabetes. The authors suggest that current guidance may be revised in the future to allow for preoperative use; however, additional research is needed. As with GLP-1RAs, shared decision-making may be used to determine whether holding SGLT2 inhibitors prior to procedures is appropriate based on patient-specific risk factors [10].

Intraoperative

Anesthesia

Anesthesia protocols are dependent on the type of procedure and may involve conscious sedation through the use of IV medications and local anesthetics for minor procedure. Other procedures requiring general anesthesia involve the use of induction agents, inhaled anesthetics, IV anesthetics, opioids, and neuromuscular blockers.

Local anesthetics are ***sodium channel blockers*** and can be classified into **esters** or **amides** (Fig. 5.1). They have a localized effect if administered into a specific area via injection or topically but can also be given intravenously. Esters include procaine, tetracaine, and benzocaine while amides include lidocaine, bupivacaine, and ropivacaine. Table 5.4 summarizes the differences between ester and amides.

IV anesthetics are used in general anesthesia for induction to produce rapid unconsciousness. ***Propofol*** (Fig. 5.2) can be used for both *induction and maintenance* of anesthesia. ***Etomidate, dexmedetomidine,*** *and* ***ketamine*** (a *dissociative* anesthetic) may also be used for *induction.* ***Inhaled anesthetics*** are used for *anesthesia maintenance* and are rapidly absorbed in the alveoli. These include ***sevoflurane*** and ***desflurane*** (Fig. 5.3a, b), as well as ***isoflurane*** and (historically) halothane (Fig. 5.4a, b). Synthetic opioids such as ***fentanyl*** and ***remifentanil*** or semi-synthetic opioids such as ***hydromorphone, hydrocodone,*** *and* ***oxycodone*** can provide a rapid onset of *analgesia* when administered intravenously. ***Neuromuscular blockers*** are categorized into depolarizing and non-depolarizing agents which include ***succinylcholine*** (**non-depolarizing**) and other depolarizing agents such as ***cisatracurium, pancuronium, rocuronium,*** and ***vecuronium*** [11].

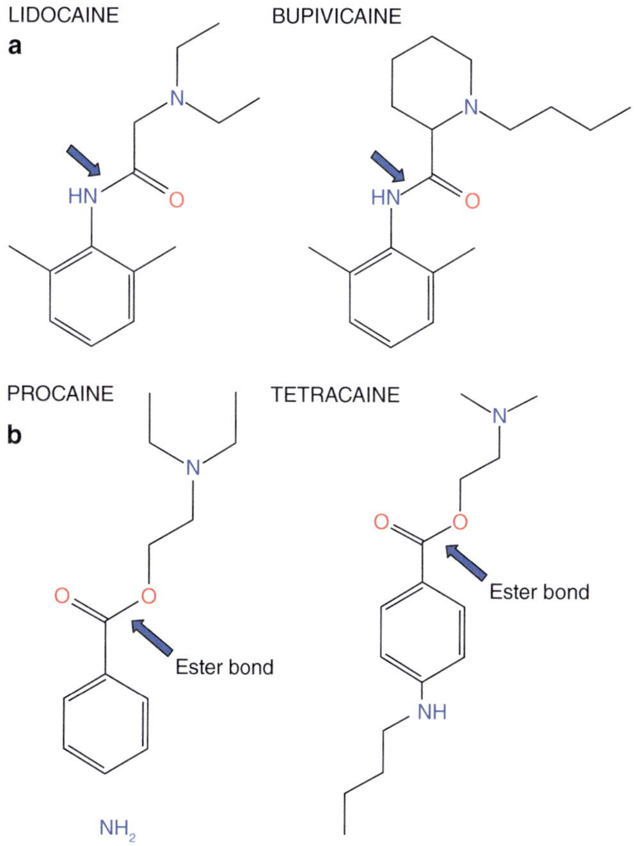

Fig. 5.1 Ester anesthetics and amide anesthetics have important differences at a molecular level. (**a**) The molecular structure of two of the most common amide anesthetics, *lidocaine* and *bupivacaine,* are illustrated. *Amides* are named so because they contain an *amide bond (arrows)* which represents a covalent bond between a carboxylic acid group (—COOH) and an amine group (—NH_2). Amide bonds are common in our body, especially *in proteins*, where they are typically referred to as "*peptide bonds*." In addition to being a local anesthetic, lidocaine is also a *class IB antiarrhythmic.* (**b**) In contrast to amides, esters are so named, not surprisingly, because they contain an *ester bond*, which happens when carboxylic acid (—COOH) reacts with an alcohol group (—OH) to form a bond (—CO—O—), as shown in (**b**), *arrows*. *Procaine* and *tetracaine*, depicted here, are examples of ester anesthetics. Did you know that *cocaine* (available as 4% or 10% topical solution) can *also* be used as a local anesthetic? It, too is an *ester anesthetic,* and is used for topical anesthesia of mucous membranes, most commonly in otolaryngologic procedures (such as nasal surgery)

Table 5.4 Comparison of amide vs. ester local anesthetics

Feature	Amide anesthetics	Ester anesthetics
Chemical bond	–NH–CO– (amide bond)	–CO–O– (ester bond)
Stability to hydrolysis	Stable	Easily hydrolyzed
Primary site of metabolism	Liver (CYP450 enzymes)	Plasma (cholinesterases)
Duration of action	Longer (slow breakdown)	Shorter (rapid breakdown)
Allergy risk	Low (no PABA production)	Higher (PABA byproducts)
Examples	Lidocaine, bupivacaine, ropivacaine	Procaine, tetracaine, benzocaine

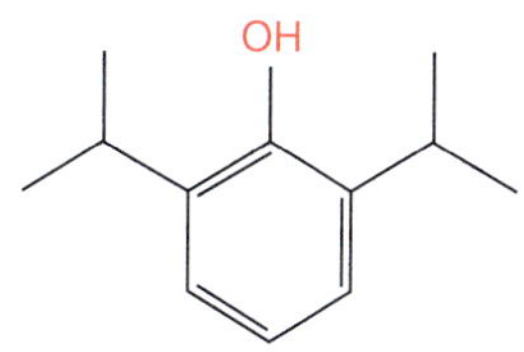

Fig. 5.2 The molecular structure of propofol, which contains an aromatic (phenol) ring, is shown. Propofol is a *short-acting* intravenous sedative-hypnotic and is among the *most frequently used in procedural sedation, including monitored anesthesia care (MAC).* Outside of the operating room, it is commonly used to sedate patients undergoing endoscopic procedures, and in the intensive care unit, especially for mechanically ventilated patients. Marketed under the brand name *Diprivan* in the United States, it has a rapid onset of action and it dissipates quickly, due to *rapid redistribution* and *hepatic metabolism*

Pain Management

Intraoperative pain management involves the use of opioids as described briefly above. The **Enhanced Recovery After Surgery (ERAS)** guidelines recommend the use of short and ultra-short acting opioids such as fentanyl and remifentanil intraoperatively if needed *rather than* morphine due to a lower risk of adverse effects such as respiratory depression and nausea in the postoperative period. Some opioids may also be used together with local anesthetics intraoperatively.

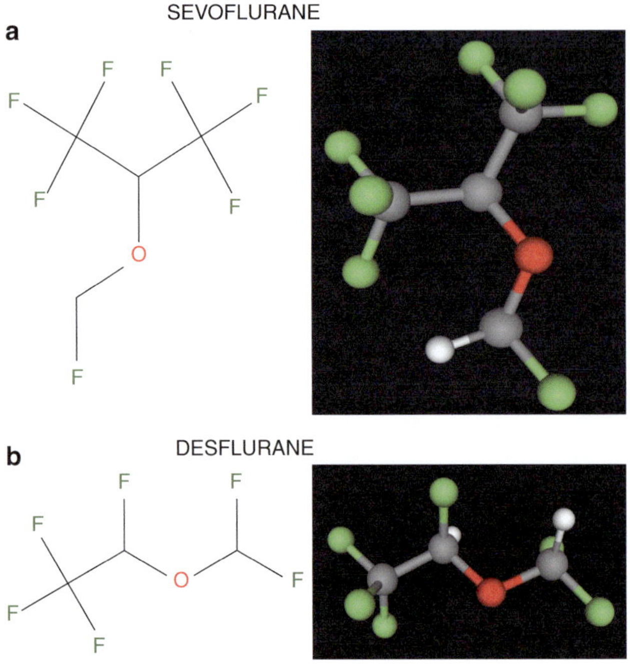

Fig. 5.3 Inhalational (general) anesthetics contain the suffix ***flurane***, with *sevoflurane* and *desflurane* being among the ones most typically used and collectively these are termed *halogenated ether anesthetics*. The chemical structure and molecular models for (**a**) sevoflurane and (**b**) desflurane are depicted. Note the similarities between the two molecules and that they are rich in **Fluorine** (F), which is one of the ***halogen atoms*** (Group VIIA from the Periodic Table). Inhalational anesthetics *inhibit excitatory neurotransmission* by blocking presynaptic voltage-gated sodium channels, which reduces glutamate release. Although somewhat complex, the overall effect is profound depression of cortical and subcortical neuronal activity

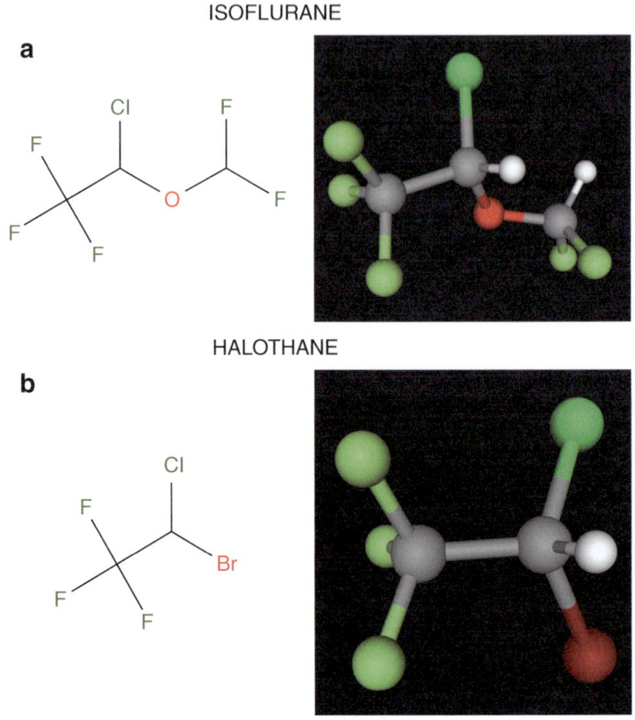

Fig. 5.4 The molecular structure for (**a**) *isoflurane* and (**b**) *halothane* is depicted. Halothane is no longer used due to hepatoxicity and potential cardiac effects, and is thus of historical interest only. Inhalational anesthetics are *volatile* anesthetics, meaning they are readily vaporized. By definition, they are all *general* anesthetics, and their common denominator is that *they contain one or more halogens,* which include Fluorine (F), Chlorine (Cl), Bromine (Br). You can see that isoflurane contains two halogens (F and Cl), while Halothane contains three (Br, F, and Cl)

In some cases, ketamine may be administered intraoperatively for major surgeries and may be appropriate in patients with significant opioid tolerance or for those who are unable to tolerate opioids. However, the ERAS Society guidelines do not recommend the routine use of ketamine in elective surgery based on limited evidence [12–14]. Specific dosing recommendations and notes on intraoperative analgesics are described in Table 5.5.

Table 5.5 Intraoperative analgesic dosing [12]

Drug	Dosing	Renal/hepatic dose adjustment	Notes
Fentanyl	0.5–2 mcg/kg IV in incremental boluses	No renal dose adjustment for single or infrequent boluses for short interventional procedures Hepatic dose adjustment required in patients with liver impairment (child-Turcotte-Pugh class C)	Short-acting synthetic opioid One thousand times more potent than morphine Can cause respiratory depression, bradycardia, constipation, meiosis, urinary retention
Remifentanil	Single IV dose (if used alone): 1 mcg/kg over 30–60 s Continuous infusion (if used alone): 0.1 mcg/kg/min beginning 5 min prior to local anesthetic or 0.05 mcg/kg/min if administered after local anesthetic	No renal dose adjustment No hepatic dose adjustment	Expensive, ultra-short acting synthetic opioid Causes minimal "drug hangover" No residual analgesia Adjusted body weight for initial dosing in obese patients
Ketamine	Bolus: 0.25–0.5 mg/kg Infusion: 0.2–0.3 mg kg^{-1} h^{-1} or 2.5–10 mcg kg^{-1} min^{-1}	No renal dose adjustment, however, prolonged use should be avoided in those with altered kidney function No hepatic dose adjustment	Increased secretions, risk of laryngospasm, hallucinations
Lidocaine	Induction IV dose of 1.5 mg/kg followed by 2 mg/kg/h intraoperatively for open and laparoscopic abdominal surgery; less commonly used in clinical practice	In both renal and hepatic impairment, a lower maintenance infusion rate should be used with close monitoring	Can cause dizziness, seizures, bradycardia

Postoperative

Pain Management

The ERAS Society recommends **avoidance of opioids in the postoperative setting** if possible and reliance on multimodal analgesia instead. When opioids are used, the oral route is preferred in patients who are able to take medications by mouth. Other medications previously discussed in the preoperative setting can be used again postoperatively and include acetaminophen, NSAIDs, gabapentinoids (e.g., **gabapentin**), and others as part of a multimodal approach to analgesia. Normal adult dosing is provided for each medication; however, reviewing the product labeling is recommended for potential renal and hepatic dose adjustments for each analgesic mentioned. **Acetaminophen** can be given at doses of 500–1000 mg every 6 h postoperatively, and **celecoxib** can be given at a dose of 200 mg twice daily postoperatively. Gabapentin is typically given as a 600-mg dose postoperatively (single or multiple doses) [12].

Antiemetics

If patients experience nausea and vomiting postoperatively, an antiemetic from a different drug class should be administered than what was given prior to surgery. If antiemetics were not administered prophylactically, then a 5-HT3 receptor antagonist is recommended for postoperative nausea and vomiting. The recommended postoperative dose is lower than the prophylactic dose. For example, the recommended post-op dose of ondandestron (**Zofran**®) is 4 mg. It is important to note that palonosetron has not been studied for use in postoperative nausea and vomiting treatment. Other antiemetics that may be used dexamethasone IV, droperidol IV, or promethazine IV [5].

Antibiotics

Postoperative antibiotic use is not needed for most surgical procedures. The Centers for Disease Control and Prevention recommends against administering additional prophylactic antibiotic doses in clean and clean-contaminated procedures after the incision is closed and the operation has been completed [15].

References

1. Lucenteforte E, et al. J Clin Anesth. 2000;12(6):468–71.
2. Ang-Lee MK, Moss J, Yuan CS. JAMA. 2001;286(2):208–16. https://doi.org/10.1001/jama.286.2.208.
3. Riley CL. Anesthesiol Clin. 2017;35(2):e115–43.
4. Sharp D. Premedication. In: Freeman BS, Berger JS, editors. Anesthesiology core review: part one basic exam. McGraw-Hill Education; 2014.
5. Gan TJ. Anesth Analg. 2014;118(1):85–113. https://doi.org/10.1213/ANE.0000000000000002.
6. Bratzler DW, et al. Am J Health-System Pharm. 2013;70:195–283.
7. https://www.ncbi.nlm.nih.gov/books/NBK557590/.
8. Douketis JD, et al. Chest. 2022;162(5):e207–43. https://doi.org/10.1016/j.chest.2022.07.025. Epub 2022 Aug 11.
9. Kindel TL, et al. Surg Obes Relat Dis. 2024;20(12):1183–6.
10. Dixit AA, et al. JAMA Surg. 2025;160(4):423–30. https://doi.org/10.1001/jamasurg.2024.7082.
11. https://www.ncbi.nlm.nih.gov/books/NBK493199/#:~:text=Benzodiazepines%20are%20often%20used%20as,duration%20of%20action%20than%20lorazepam.
12. Beverly A, et al. Anesthesiol Clin. 2017;35(2):e115–43.
13. Chou R, et al. J Pain. 2016;17(2):131–57.
14. Kaye AD, et al. Anaesthesiol Intensive Ther. 2020;52(2):154–64. https://doi.org/10.5114/ait.2020.95020.
15. Berríos-Torres SI, et al. JAMA Surg. 2017;152(8):784–91. https://doi.org/10.1001/jamasurg.2017.0904.

Wound Healing

6

John R. Gerke, Chelsea Liles, and Richard F. Burgess

Introduction

Wound healing is a complex and dynamic process essential for restoring tissue integrity following surgical interventions. For physician associates (PAs), understanding wound healing mechanisms is crucial to optimizing patient outcomes and minimizing complications. This chapter provides a comprehensive overview of the wound healing process, emphasizing the stages of healing, factors influencing this process, and practical implications for surgical practice.

The wound healing process is traditionally divided into four overlapping stages: hemostasis, inflammation, proliferation, and remodeling [1]. Each stage involves a carefully orchestrated sequence of cellular and molecular events essential for successful tissue repair. This chapter will delve into the biological mechanisms underpinning each stage, discuss advances in surgical techniques and wound care, and address common complications and management strategies. By the end of this chapter, readers will gain a thorough understanding of wound healing and practical insights for improving surgical outcomes through effective wound management.

Hemostasis

Hemostasis is the initial and critical phase of the wound healing process, essential for preventing blood loss and forming a foundation for subsequent healing stages. This phase involves vascular constriction, platelet plug formation, and activation of the coagulation cascade, culminating in a stable clot.

J. R. Gerke (✉) · C. Liles · R. F. Burgess
Department of Physician Assistant Program, South College, Orlando, FL, USA
e-mail: jgerke@south.edu

Vascular Constriction

The body's immediate response to tissue injury is vasoconstriction of the damaged blood vessels. This reaction, mediated by smooth muscle contraction, reduces blood flow to the injured area. This rapid constriction, though brief, is vital for minimizing blood loss and facilitating platelet adhesion [1].

Platelet Plug Formation

After vascular injury, platelets quickly adhere to the exposed subendothelial matrix, particularly binding to collagen fibers and von Willebrand factor (vWF). This adhesion is mediated by glycoprotein receptors on platelet surfaces, such as glycoprotein Ib (GpIb), which binds to vWF, and integrin $\alpha 2\beta 1$, which binds to collagen. Upon adhesion, platelets become activated, morphing from smooth discs to spiky structures and releasing contents from their granules.

Activated platelets release adenosine diphosphate (ADP), serotonin, and calcium, which intensify platelet aggregation and recruit additional platelets to the site of injury. The release of thromboxane A2 (TXA2), a vasoconstrictor and platelet aggregator, further amplifies platelet activity, forming a primary platelet plug that temporarily stabilizes the wound site.

Coagulation Cascade

While the platelet plug provides an initial seal, it is insufficient to withstand mechanical forces without reinforcement. Therefore, the coagulation cascade is activated to create a fibrin mesh that stabilizes the plug. The coagulation cascade includes two pathways—intrinsic and extrinsic—that converge into a common pathway, leading to fibrin formation.

Extrinsic Pathway: Triggered by external trauma and the exposure of tissue factor (TF), the extrinsic pathway activates

S. Atallah, J. Dragoljevic (eds.), *Fundamentals of Surgery for Physician Assistants*,
https://doi.org/10.1007/978-3-032-21069-2_6

factor VII, forming a TF-VIIa complex that activates factor X.

Intrinsic Pathway: Activated by trauma within blood vessels, the intrinsic pathway begins with the activation of factor XII and involves a sequence of activations that culminates in the activation of factor X.

Common Pathway: Factor Xa, in complex with factor V and calcium ions, converts prothrombin to thrombin. Thrombin then cleaves fibrinogen to fibrin, creating an insoluble fibrin network that reinforces the platelet plug.

Regulation of Hemostasis

Hemostasis is finely regulated to prevent excessive clotting (thrombosis) and bleeding (hemorrhage). Key regulatory mechanisms include:

- **Antithrombin**: Inactivates thrombin and coagulation factors (Xa, IXa).
- **Protein C and Protein S**: Degrade factors Va and VIIIa, reducing thrombin generation.
- **Tissue Factor Pathway Inhibitor (TFPI)**: Inhibits the TF-VIIa complex and factor Xa.
- **Fibrinolysis**: The breakdown of fibrin clots via plasmin, facilitated by tissue plasminogen activator (tPA) and urokinase.

Clinical Implications and Surgical Considerations

Effective hemostasis is critical during surgery to prevent blood loss and stabilize the wound environment. Surgeons employ various methods to control bleeding:

- **Mechanical Methods**: Sutures, staples, and compression techniques.
- **Thermal Methods**: Electrocautery and laser coagulation for localized hemostasis.
- **Chemical Agents**: Fibrin sealants and thrombin can enhance clot stability.

Knowledge of hemostasis mechanisms enables PAs to anticipate bleeding risks and optimize surgical outcomes, particularly for patients with coagulopathies who require careful management.

Inflammation

Inflammation is the second essential phase of wound healing, characterized by a coordinated immune response to remove pathogens, debris, and damaged tissue from the wound site. This phase typically lasts a few days and includes vascular changes, cellular infiltration, and the release of chemical mediators, all of which prepare the wound for tissue repair.

Vascular Changes

After hemostasis, local blood vessels undergo several key changes:

- **Vasodilation**: Mediated by histamine, nitric oxide, and prostaglandins, vasodilation increases blood flow to the injury, resulting in redness (erythema) and warmth.
- **Increased Vascular Permeability**: Histamine and bradykinin enhance blood vessel permeability, allowing plasma proteins and immune cells to move into the tissue. This vascular permeability results in swelling (edema) and delivers immune cells and proteins essential for wound healing.

Cellular Infiltration

Leukocytes, primarily neutrophils and macrophages, play a critical role in wound healing through a multi-step process of recruitment:

- **Margination and Rolling**: Leukocytes slow down and roll along the endothelium via selectins and integrins.
- **Adhesion**: Integrins on leukocytes firmly attach to endothelial adhesion molecules (ICAM-1, VCAM-1).
- **Transmigration (Diapedesis)**: Leukocytes move through endothelial gaps to the wound site, guided by chemotactic signals.

Neutrophils, the first responders, arrive within hours to phagocytize pathogens and debris, releasing proteolytic enzymes and reactive oxygen species (ROS) to further degrade damaged tissue. They are soon followed by monocytes, which differentiate into macrophages upon reaching the wound.

Mediators of Inflammation

Several chemical mediators orchestrate inflammation, including:

- **Cytokines**: Produced by immune cells, cytokines like interleukin-1 (IL-1), interleukin-6 (IL-6), and tumor necrosis factor-alpha (TNF-α) amplify the inflammatory response and recruit more leukocytes.
- **Chemokines**: Molecules such as IL-8 and MCP-1 attract leukocytes to the wound through chemotaxis.
- **Histamine and Serotonin**: Released by mast cells and platelets, these mediators increase vascular permeability and vasodilation.
- **Prostaglandins and Leukotrienes**: Derived from arachidonic acid, these lipids modulate vasodilation, permeability, and leukocyte chemotaxis.

Functions of Inflammatory Cells

- **Neutrophils**: These cells phagocytize pathogens and debris, releasing ROS and proteases that degrade tissue and kill microbes.
- **Macrophages**: Macrophages continue phagocytosis and release cytokines and growth factors, including transforming growth factor-beta (TGF-β) and vascular endothelial growth factor (VEGF), which promote the transition from inflammation to the proliferative phase.

Resolution of Inflammation

To prevent excessive tissue damage, inflammation must be resolved in a timely manner. Regulatory mechanisms include:

- **Anti-inflammatory Cytokines**: Cytokines such as IL-10 and TGF-β suppress pro-inflammatory signals.
- **Apoptosis of Neutrophils**: Programmed cell death of neutrophils prevents prolonged inflammation, facilitating clearance by macrophages.
- **Lipoxins and Resolvins**: Derived from fatty acids, these specialized pro-resolving mediators actively promote the resolution of inflammation.

Clinical Implications and Surgical Considerations

While inflammation is necessary for clearing pathogens and initiating repair, excessive inflammation can impede healing and lead to chronic wounds or fibrosis. Surgical site infections are a major cause of prolonged inflammation; sterile techniques and prophylactic antibiotics (where appropriate) are therefore critical. Foreign material, such as sutures (in particular braided, non-absorbable) or implanted devices and vascular access catheters, can also prolong inflammation, so biocompatible materials and proper technique are essential.

Surgeons can enhance patient outcomes by managing inflammation with anti-inflammatory medications and minimizing tissue trauma. Preoperative management, including **glycemic control** and optimization of immune health, can further reduce the risk of complications related to excessive inflammation [2].

Proliferation

The proliferation phase is a critical stage in wound healing, occurring approximately 3–5 days after injury and lasting several weeks. This phase focuses on tissue restoration and includes four key processes: epithelialization, angiogenesis, fibroplasia (collagen deposition), and wound contraction.

Epithelialization

Epithelialization involves the migration of new epithelial cells across the wound bed to reestablish the skin barrier. Epithelialization is an important step in healing and has important clinical implications. Initial epithelialization begins rapidly over the course of the first 24–48 h. This underlies the common practice of removing surgical dressings within the first 24–48 hours postoperatively. While the incisions can be re-dressed, in most instances, they are left open to air as the epithelialization process is well under way. The skin, however, is not completely airtight and watertight until about 7–10 days post operatively, which is one reason why surgeons often recommend patients avoid submersion in bodies of water for the first 2 weeks after surgery.

Epithelialization is a process with the following phases:

- **Keratinocyte Activation and Migration**: Keratinocytes, the primary cells of the epidermis, become activated at the wound edges and begin migrating across the wound bed, producing enzymes to degrade the provisional matrix.
- **Proliferation**: Growth factors like epidermal growth factor (EGF) and transforming growth factor-alpha (TGF-α)

stimulate keratinocyte proliferation to cover the wound surface.

- **Basement Membrane Reestablishment**: After keratinocytes cover the wound, the basement membrane is restored, crucial for returning the skin to its protective function.

Angiogenesis

Angiogenesis, or the formation of new blood vessels, is essential for delivering oxygen and nutrients to the regenerating tissue.

- **Endothelial Cell Activation**: Endothelial cells in existing blood vessels are activated by hypoxia and angiogenic factors such as vascular endothelial growth factor (VEGF) and fibroblast growth factor (FGF).
- **Capillary Sprouting**: Activated endothelial cells form capillary sprouts that extend into the wound bed, gradually forming new capillary loops to support tissue regeneration.
- **Vessel Maturation**: New capillaries stabilize through interactions with pericytes and the extracellular matrix, forming a functional blood supply.

Fibroplasia (Collagen Deposition)

Fibroplasia involves the synthesis of new extracellular matrix (ECM) by fibroblasts, providing structural integrity to the wound.

- **Fibroblast Activation**: Fibroblasts, drawn to the wound by chemotactic signals, proliferate and become activated to produce ECM components.
- **Collagen Synthesis**: Initially, fibroblasts produce type III collagen, forming a loose, provisional matrix. Over time, type III collagen is replaced by the stronger type I collagen.
- **ECM Formation**: Fibroblasts also secrete glycosaminoglycans and proteoglycans, contributing to a scaffold that promotes cell attachment and organization.

Wound Contraction

Wound contraction, driven by myofibroblasts, significantly reduces wound size.

- **Myofibroblast Differentiation**: Fibroblasts differentiate into myofibroblasts in response to growth factors like TGF-β and mechanical tension.
- **Contraction Mechanism**: Myofibroblasts express alpha-smooth muscle actin (α-SMA), allowing them to contract and generate tensile forces that pull the wound edges inward.

Regulation of the Proliferative Phase

The proliferative phase is regulated by a complex network of growth factors, cytokines, and cell interactions.

- **Growth Factors**: Key growth factors like VEGF, FGF, EGF, and TGF-β stimulate cellular proliferation, migration, and ECM production.
- **Cytokines**: Cytokines, including IL-1 and TNF-α, modulate cellular activities and support healing by maintaining a balanced inflammatory response.
- **Cell–Cell and Cell–Matrix Interactions**: Integrins and other adhesion molecules support cell migration, attachment, and signal transmission, essential for wound stabilization.

Clinical Implications and Surgical Considerations

Understanding the proliferative phase allows surgical practitioners to optimize wound healing. Several strategies can enhance this phase:

- **Infection Control**: Maintaining sterility is crucial, as infection prolongs inflammation and disrupts cell activities.
- **Nutritional Support**: Nutrients, especially proteins, vitamin C, and vitamin A, support collagen synthesis and cellular function. **Vitamin A** is particularly important to reverse the deleterious effects of corticosteroids on wound healing.
- **Comorbidity Management**: Managing conditions like diabetes and vascular insufficiency can improve outcomes.

Advanced techniques, such as debridement, tissue engineering, and hyperbaric oxygen therapy, can also enhance the proliferative phase by creating a favorable environment for cell migration and growth.

Remodeling

Remodeling is the final and longest phase of wound healing, beginning around 3 weeks after injury and lasting for months to years. During this phase, the provisional extracellular matrix formed in the proliferative phase is replaced with a mature, organized matrix, restoring tensile strength and tissue functionality.

Collagen Maturation and Reorganization

The remodeling phase is primarily characterized by the reorganization and maturation of collagen fibers to strengthen the tissue.

- **Collagen Cross-Linking**: Type III collagen is gradually replaced by type I collagen, which undergoes extensive cross-linking through enzymes such as lysyl oxidase, enhancing tensile strength.
- **Collagen Realignment**: Fibroblasts and myofibroblasts reorganize collagen fibers along the lines of mechanical stress, a process influenced by physical activity and cellular contraction.

Extracellular Matrix Remodeling

The extracellular matrix (ECM) undergoes degradation and reformation to replace the initial matrix with a more durable structure.

- **Matrix Metalloproteinases (MMPs)**: MMPs degrade the temporary ECM components, allowing for the deposition of a stable matrix.
- **Balance of MMPs and TIMPs**: Tissue inhibitors of metalloproteinases (TIMPs) regulate MMP activity, maintaining a balance between ECM degradation and synthesis.

Cellular Activities

Cellular remodeling is coordinated by fibroblasts and myofibroblasts, which produce ECM components and contract the wound.

- **Myofibroblasts**: These cells express smooth muscle actin and facilitate wound contraction. After contraction, they undergo apoptosis to prevent excessive scarring.
- **Apoptosis**: Apoptosis of fibroblasts, endothelial cells, and other cells reduces cellular density, allowing the tissue to return to its pre-injury state.

Restoration of Vascularity and Innervation

The vasculature and nerves are remodeled to support the healed tissue's metabolic needs.

- **Vascular Remodeling**: Newly formed capillaries stabilize as mature blood vessels, while excess vessels regress, maintaining necessary but not excessive blood supply.
- **Nerve Regeneration**: Damaged nerve fibers regenerate, restoring sensation and functionality to the affected area. Nerve regeneration occurs slowly, at a rate of 1 mm per day. Nerves that are not severed but damaged can also heal over a period of 6–12 months. Age can affect the rate of regeneration.

Functional Recovery and Tensile Strength

The ultimate goal of remodeling is to restore functional capability and tensile strength to the tissue.

- **Tensile Strength**: Healed wounds typically regain about 70–80% of the tensile strength of uninjured tissue over time. The most important layer (fascia) reaches 90% of its tensile strength by 3 months after abdominal surgery. While variable, by 6 weeks from abdominal surgery, the fascia has regained 50–70% of its tensile strength. As an important clinical correlate, patients are recommended to avoid strenuous activity and heavy lifting until they reached the 6 weeks post op mark; however, there is an important risk of wound-related problems including hernia formation and even fascial dehiscence.
- **Mechanical Loading**: Controlled mechanical loading, such as early mobilization and physical therapy, supports collagen alignment and improves strength.
- **Scarring**: The extent of scarring depends on the balance between collagen deposition and degradation; excessive scarring may result in hypertrophic scars or keloids. Keloids are pronounced hypertrophic scars that develop in patients with a genetic predisposition for their formation. Keloid formation has been linked to genetic factors involved in collagen production and remodeling and is more common in persons of African, Asian, and Hispanic origin.

Clinical Implications and Surgical Considerations

Understanding remodeling helps clinicians manage long-term healing and minimize complications. Key considerations include:

- **Scar Management**: Techniques such as silicone gel sheets, pressure therapy, and laser treatments can reduce scarring and improve cosmetic outcomes. While Vitamin E use is often advocated for scar reduction, the scientific evidence is mixed and inconclusive.
- **Rehabilitation**: Early mobilization and physical therapy enhance collagen alignment and strength by applying mechanical stress.
- **Monitoring and Intervention**: Chronic wounds or abnormal scarring may require interventions such as surgical revision or the application of growth factors to promote proper remodeling.

Patient-specific factors, such as age, nutrition, and comorbidities, significantly influence remodeling. Older patients and those with conditions like diabetes often experience delayed or impaired remodeling, requiring tailored management to support healing.

Factors Influencing Wound Healing

Wound healing is influenced by numerous factors beyond age, nutritional status, and pre-existing medical conditions. These factors can be grouped into local and systemic influences, each affecting the body's capacity to repair tissue effectively. Recognizing and addressing these factors can significantly improve outcomes, particularly in complex cases where healing is delayed.

Infection

Infection is a primary barrier to effective wound healing, as bacterial contamination triggers prolonged inflammation, disrupting collagen synthesis and reducing tissue strength. Early control through sterile techniques, wound hygiene, and, when needed, antibiotics, is critical for preventing infection and optimizing healing [1, 3].

Wound Oxygenation and Blood Supply

Oxygen is essential for collagen synthesis, immune function, and overall cellular activity in wound repair. Conditions such as vascular disease or localized pressure on the wound can impair blood flow, reducing oxygen availability and slowing healing. Interventions like hyperbaric oxygen therapy can enhance oxygen delivery and improve outcomes, especially in hypoxic wounds [4].

Moisture Balance

A balanced moisture level in the wound environment promotes cell migration and autolytic debridement. Excessive dryness leads to scab formation, which can impede healing, while too much moisture causes maceration. Hydrocolloid and hydrogel dressings are effective tools for maintaining optimal moisture and supporting a faster healing process [3, 5].

Tissue Perfusion and Edema

Adequate blood flow is essential not only for oxygenation but also for nutrient delivery and immune cell transport. Reduced perfusion, common in diabetes, and peripheral artery disease delay healing. Edema raises interstitial pressure, reducing capillary flow and further compromising healing. Compression therapy and elevation can help manage edema and improve perfusion [1, 6].

Mechanical Stress and Wound Tension

Mechanical stress on the wound, such as from movement or tension, disrupts new tissue formation, increasing inflammation and slowing healing. High-tension areas, like over joints, are particularly susceptible. Immobilization techniques, bandaging, and careful suturing help minimize stress, especially during early healing [7].

Chronic Inflammation

Chronic inflammation prevents wounds from progressing to subsequent healing stages. Conditions like venous ulcers often remain inflamed due to a persistent immune response that breaks down new tissue. Addressing underlying inflammatory causes and removing necrotic tissue are essential for treating chronic wounds [2].

Foreign Bodies and Necrotic Tissue

Foreign bodies and necrotic tissue provide a growth medium for bacteria and act as barriers to healing. Removing debris and non-viable tissue through debridement is crucial for establishing a clean wound bed conducive to repair [1].

Environmental Temperature and Humidity

Temperature and humidity affect cellular activity and blood flow at the wound site. Warm, humid conditions accelerate healing, while cold, dry environments slow cellular processes. In clinical settings, maintaining wound temperature and humidity through controlled environments or appropriate dressings can support healing [3, 8].

Psychological Stress and Hormonal Influences

Psychological stress triggers cortisol release, which suppresses immune responses and impairs healing. Elevated cortisol levels reduce angiogenesis and collagen deposition, both vital for wound repair. Techniques that reduce stress and provide patient support can positively influence outcomes [9].

Medication Use

Certain medications, like corticosteroids and NSAIDs, may impair certain aspects of healing, particularly in high-risk or prolonged use by suppressing inflammation or immune function. Immunosuppressive drugs also weaken the immune response, prolonging healing. Awareness of medication effects allows clinicians to adjust wound care plans as needed [3].

Smoking and Substance Use

Nicotine's vasoconstrictive properties reduce blood flow to the wound, while carbon monoxide in cigarette smoke limits oxygen transport. Additionally, excessive alcohol use impairs immune function, prolonging inflammation. Smoking cessation programs are often essential for patients with surgical wounds [1, 4].

Wound Size, Type, and Depth

Larger or deeper wounds require extensive tissue repair, prolonging healing time. Jagged or irregular wounds, in contrast to clean surgical incisions, can complicate the repair process, increasing healing time [5].

Radiation Therapy

Patients may have had prior external beam radiotherapy for treatment of a malignancy. For patients who require surgery and who have had antecedent radiotherapy, wound healing (within the prior radiation field) is **dramatically reduced and often problematic.** Radiation therapy damages blood vessels and connective tissues, reducing oxygen and nutrient delivery to the wound. Tissue fibrosis in irradiated areas often creates a rigid wound bed with limited perfusion. Special dressings and careful management are necessary for wounds in irradiated regions to address these challenges [1].

Complications of Wound Healing

Wound healing can be complex and, despite optimal techniques, may lead to complications. Recognizing and addressing these complications promptly is essential to prevent worsening outcomes, especially in surgical settings. The most common complications include dehiscence, infection, and abnormal tissue responses, each requiring a tailored approach to management.

Dehiscence

Dehiscence, or the separation of the fascia, may be partial or complete and can involve superficial or deep tissue layers (Fig. 6.1). Complete dehiscence poses a significant risk, potentially leading to evisceration of underlying organs [10].

To surgeons, the word "dehiscence" carries a very specific meaning. It is used in reference to **fascia only.** Some non-surgeon clinicians refer to skin separation as "dehiscence," but this is distinct from true fascial dehiscence and should not be used interchangeably. **Fascial dehiscence is a surgical problem that mandates a swift return to the operating room.** To avoid confusion, **only use the term dehiscence when referring to fascia.**

Dehiscence usually occurs within the first 1–2 weeks post-surgery, often due to infection, poor surgical technique, or excessive mechanical stress. Abdominal wound dehiscence, for example, can result in mortality rates up to 44% [11]. Proper closure techniques, choosing appropriate suture material, and spacing sutures effectively are crucial for preventing dehiscence. Strenuous activity, trauma, or direct pressure on the wound should be minimized postoperatively to allow proper tissue healing.

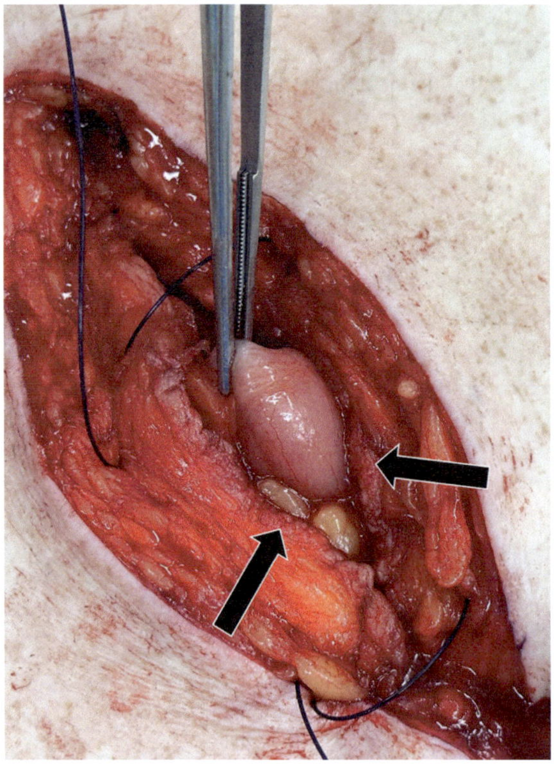

Fig. 6.1 Fascial dehiscence and small bowel evisceration are depicted. In addition to skin separation, the strength layer of the anterior abdominal wall, the fascia (black arrows), has also separated and the strong monofilament suture (#1 PDS) used to close the fascia has somehow unraveled, which may be due to a technical failure or other reasons. Fascial closure is the "main layer" and most important layer to be closed when the abdominal or pelvic cavity is entered. As a consequence of fascial dehiscence, a loop of small bowel, being grasped with forceps, has started to eviscerate and is clearly visible. Fascial dehiscence and small bowel evisceration both mandate a prompt return to the operating room

Infection

Infection is one of the most common and serious complications in wound healing, as it can prevent the wound from progressing through the normal healing phases, leading to dehiscence and other complications. Surgical site infections can occur in contaminated wounds or those with inadequate postoperative care, particularly if a patient has comorbidities that increase infection risk, such as diabetes or immunosuppression [12].

For infected or at-risk wounds, prophylactic antibiotics may be indicated, particularly for grossly contaminated wounds. Postoperative infection management includes regular assessment for signs of infection (redness, warmth, pus), wound cultures, and antibiotic therapy as needed. Optimizing glycemic control, nutritional support, and patient compliance with wound care instructions are also critical to reducing infection risk [13].

Abnormal Tissue Response (Keloid/Contracture/Hypertrophic Scarring)

Abnormal scarring, such as keloids, hypertrophic scars, or contractures, can occur when wound healing produces excessive or disorganized collagen deposition. Keloids extend beyond the wound margin and generally do not regress, whereas hypertrophic scars remain within the wound boundary and may diminish over time [14]. Scar contractures often develop over joint surfaces, affecting function and appearance.

Risk factors for abnormal scarring include genetics, darker skin pigmentation, younger age, and areas with tension. Preventative measures, including silicone gel sheets, pressure therapy, and early range-of-motion exercises, may reduce scar formation. Corticosteroids are commonly used for treating both hypertrophic scars and keloids, though keloids often require more aggressive, multimodal treatment, including surgery or radiation [15].

Foreign Body Response and Necrosis

Foreign bodies, such as sutures or remnants of dressings, can lead to prolonged inflammation and tissue necrosis, increasing infection risk and delaying healing. Necrotic tissue must be promptly removed through debridement, as it provides a breeding ground for bacteria and inhibits wound closure. When necrosis occurs, particularly in contaminated or high-tension wounds, specialized management may be needed to salvage the tissue and promote healing.

Delayed Healing and Chronic Wounds

Certain factors, such as poor circulation, diabetes, and chronic inflammation, can convert acute wounds into chronic wounds that do not progress through the normal stages of healing. Chronic wounds, including venous or diabetic ulcers, remain in a prolonged inflammatory state that degrades new tissue.

Chronic wounds require a tailored approach, often involving debridement, advanced dressings, or topical growth factors. Regular monitoring and intervention, including addressing underlying health conditions, are crucial for chronic wound management.

Clinical Implications and Surgical Considerations

Surgeons and wound care professionals play a critical role in preventing and managing wound complications. Proactive measures, such as preoperative patient optimization (e.g., smoking cessation, glycemic control) and selecting appropriate closure techniques, reduce complication risks. In the postoperative phase, regular wound assessment and prompt intervention for early signs of complications are essential for optimal outcomes.

Understanding these common complications and implementing preventive and therapeutic strategies enable clinicians to minimize morbidity, enhance healing, and improve patient satisfaction.

Wound Care

Effective wound care is critical in surgical settings to prevent complications, promote healing, and ensure optimal outcomes. Proper wound care involves assessment, cleaning, dressing, and monitoring, each adapted to the surgical patient's unique needs. By understanding and applying these fundamentals, PAs can play a significant role in enhancing wound healing.

Wound Assessment

A thorough wound assessment is the first step in wound care, as it informs care decisions and helps identify potential complications. Key factors include wound size, depth, type, and location, as well as signs of infection, inflammation, and exudate levels. PAs should regularly evaluate wounds for erythema, warmth, swelling, and purulent discharge—early indicators of infection or delayed healing [1, 3].

Wound Cleaning

Cleaning is essential to reduce bacterial load and prevent infection. In surgical settings, sterile saline or mild antiseptic solutions are often used to clean wounds, as harsher solutions like hydrogen peroxide or iodine may damage healthy tissue [5]. Gentle cleansing helps avoid disruption of healing tissue, especially in wounds healing by primary intention. For open or contaminated wounds, irrigation under moderate pressure can reduce bacterial contamination and promote a cleaner wound bed [7].

Surgical Debridement

Surgical debridement, or removal of necrotic tissue and foreign material, is often necessary for wounds healing by secondary intention, when devitalized tissue is present. Surgical debridement is frequently performed in the operating room and is the most efficient method for managing specific types of wound infections. **Surgical debridement is the gold standard for the treatment of necrotizing fasciitis.** Alternates to surgical debridement can be considered in select settings, via autolytic, enzymatic, and mechanical debridement. These options may also be appropriate depending on the wound type and patient condition. Maintaining a moist environment with appropriate dressings can facilitate autolytic debridement by leveraging the body's own enzymes [6]. For wounds that are not contaminated, and which are open and being managed with bedside dressing changes, as the dry gauze is removed from the bed of the wound it naturally pulls off dead cells and effectively the dressing change itself is a form of debridement for this reason. Of note, when wet-to-dry gauze dressing changes are applied, they should not be soaked in saline prior to removal, as they are best removed dry to help with the debridement process (since the dried gauze helps "pull off" the dead cells more effectively).

Moisture Management and Dressing Selection

Maintaining a balanced moisture level is key for wound healing. A moist environment supports cell migration and reduces scab formation, while excessive moisture leads to maceration of surrounding skin. Dressing selection is guided by wound characteristics, such as exudate levels and depth:

- **Standard "Wet to Dry" Gauze Dressings**: This is the most basic and probably most cost-effective method to use. Ordinary gauze can be placed into the base of the wound after applying a small amount of saline to the gauze. It is important to pack the wound at its base, as the wound heals from inside out. The average wound takes 4–6 weeks to heal by secondary intention, and assessment of the wound edges for granulation tissue (which appears as "beefy red") color is an important aspect of wound assessment. The simplicity of the dressing change allows non-medical persons, such as family or friends, to assist patients with their dressing changes after only minimal instruction.
- **Hydrocolloid and Hydrogel Dressings**: Suitable for wounds with minimal to moderate exudate, helping to maintain a moist environment conducive to healing [4].
- **Foam Dressings**: Absorb excess exudate in wounds with moderate to heavy drainage, providing cushioning to reduce pressure and friction [7].
- **Alginate Dressings**: Derived from seaweed, alginate dressings are effective for heavily exudative wounds, absorbing significant moisture while supporting healing [1].

Regular dressing changes, based on the wound's exudate levels and healing progress, are essential for preventing complications and promoting recovery. As a rule of thumb, wound dressings should be changed in accordance to how often they become saturated. If a dressing becomes saturated with once-daily dressing changes, for example, then increasing the frequency to twice or three times a day will remedy the problem.

Infection Prevention and Management

Infection control is paramount in surgical wound care. To minimize bacterial contamination, sterile or aseptic techniques should be used when handling wounds and changing dressings. Prophylactic antibiotics may be warranted in high-risk wounds, especially those involving implants or contaminated sites. Prompt treatment of infected wounds—via wound cultures, antibiotic therapy, or additional interventions—is critical to prevent further complications [5, 8] (Fig. 6.2).

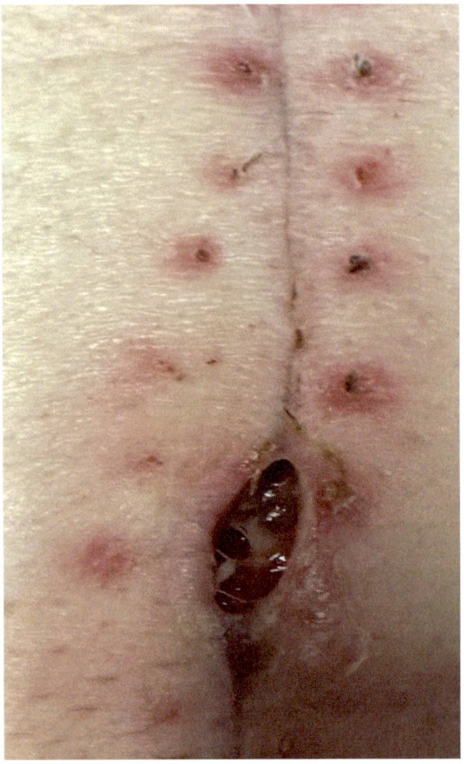

Fig. 6.2 A surgical wound demonstrating minor skin disruption after staple removal. This skin separation is not dehiscence and should not be referred to as such. Minor skin separation like the one shown requires local wound care only and generally heals by secondary intention over a period of 2–4 weeks

Wound Closure Techniques

The closure method affects both the healing trajectory and care requirements. Surgical wounds can be closed by primary, secondary, or tertiary intention:

- **Primary Intention**: Direct closure of wound edges with sutures or staples, typically requiring minimal care beyond regular dressing changes and infection monitoring.
- **Secondary Intention**: Left open to heal naturally, often used in contaminated or infected wounds, requiring frequent cleaning, moisture management, and debridement.
- **Tertiary Intention**: A hybrid approach where wounds are left open initially and then closed surgically once infection risk subsides [1].

Understanding closure methods enables PAs to tailor wound care practices to specific needs and anticipate potential complications, for example, the development of a stitch granuloma (Fig. 6.3).

Patient Education

Patient education is an essential part of wound care, especially for outpatient management. Educating patients on wound hygiene, recognizing infection signs, and adhering to follow-up care improves compliance and reduces complications. Patients should be encouraged to keep wounds clean and dry, minimize stress on healing areas, and report any signs of infection [9].

Advanced Wound Care Techniques

For complex or chronic wounds, advanced techniques may be necessary. Negative pressure wound therapy (NPWT) is a valuable tool, using controlled suction to promote wound closure by reducing edema and enhancing perfusion. Hyperbaric oxygen therapy also aids in wound healing by increasing tissue oxygenation and stimulating angiogenesis [4, 8]. Familiarity with these techniques enables PAs to make appropriate referrals and collaborate with specialists for optimal healing outcomes.

Clinical Implications and Surgical Considerations

Effective wound care in surgical settings requires a comprehensive approach. Accurate assessment, appropriate cleaning, debridement, moisture control, infection prevention, and

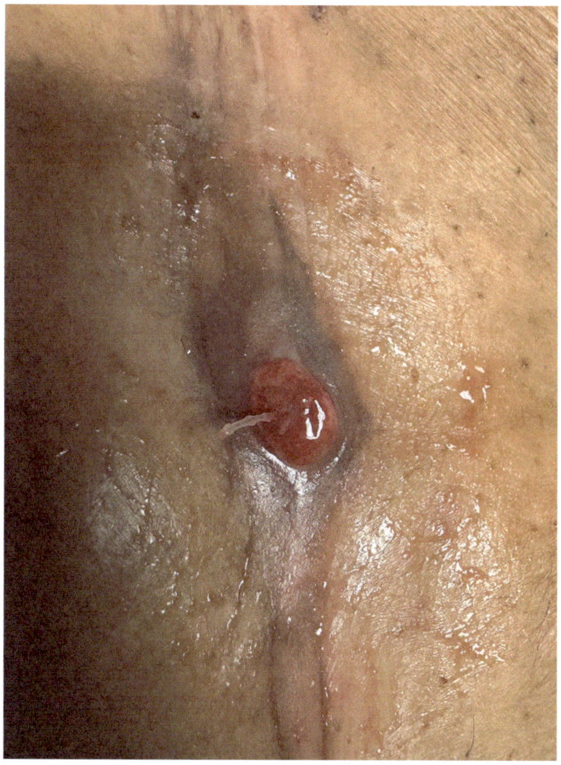

Fig. 6.3 A patient represented to the clinic 6 weeks post-op complaining of drainage from the surgical wound and was presumed by the primary care doctor treating her that this was an infection. However, this would not be in the typical time frame for a wound infection. The differential diagnosis would include possible enterocutaneous fistula or foreign body reaction, which classically occurs secondary to suture. Careful inspection of the wound reveals healthy granulation tissue surrounding a visible stitch. Treatment includes removing the stitch with or without application of a topical chemical cautery agent, such as silver nitrate

understanding closure techniques are all essential components. By remaining informed about advanced techniques and adapting to patient-specific needs, PAs can provide high-quality care that supports healing and minimizes complications.

Conclusion

Wound healing is a complex, multi-stage process influenced by numerous biological and external factors. For surgical patients, understanding the phases of hemostasis, inflammation, proliferation, and remodeling is essential to effective wound management and improved patient outcomes. Physician associates (PAs) play a critical role in preventing complications, promoting optimal healing, and managing wounds, both in the immediate postoperative setting and beyond.

Effective wound care involves not only technical skill but also an in-depth understanding of factors that impact healing, such as infection, oxygenation, and wound tension. By recognizing potential complications like dehiscence, infection, and abnormal scarring early**, PAs can implement timely interventions** to support tissue repair. Advanced wound care techniques, including negative pressure wound therapy and hyperbaric oxygen therapy, further equip practitioners to handle complex or chronic wounds.

Through comprehensive assessment, tailored wound care strategies, and ongoing patient education, **PAs can optimize surgical outcomes and contribute to overall patient health.** As wound care evolves with new research and techniques, staying informed and adaptable ensures that clinicians continue to provide high-quality, evidence-based care.

References

1. Guo S, DiPietro LA. Factors affecting wound healing. J Dent Res. 2010;89(3):219–29.
2. Lindley LE, Stojadinovic O, Pavlovic S, Brem H. The role of inflammation in wound healing. Adv Wound Care. 2016;5(3):119–36.
3. Ousey K, Cook L. Understanding wound bed preparation and wound debridement. Nurs Stand. 2011;25(36):48–56.
4. Sen CK. Wound healing essentials: let there be oxygen. Wound Repair Regen. 2009;17(1):1–18.
5. Martin P. Wound healing—aiming for perfect skin regeneration. Science. 2013;276(5309):75–81.
6. Percival SL, Cutting KF. Microbiology of wounds. In: Microbiology of wounds. CRC Press; 2012. p. 1–13.
7. Chadwick P, McCardle J, Mohamudally A. Mechanisms of wound healing and their clinical applications. J Wound Care. 2009;18(8):346–50.
8. Thackham JA, McElwain DL, Long RJ. The use of hyperbaric oxygen therapy to treat chronic wounds: a review. Wound Repair Regen. 2008;16(3):321–30.
9. Walburn J, Vedhara K, Hankins M, Rixon L, Weinman J. Psychological stress and wound healing in humans: a systematic review and meta-analysis. J Psychosom Res. 2009;67(3):253–71.
10. Rosen RD, Manna B. Wound Dehiscence. In: StatPearls [Internet]. Treasure Island (FL): StatPearls Publishing; 2023. 2026 Jan–. PMID: 31869176.
11. Chun JJ, Yoon SM, Song WJ, et al. Causes of surgical wound dehiscence: a multicenter study. J Wound Manag Res. 2018;14(2):74-79. https://doi.org/10.22467/jwmr.2018.00374.
12. Zabaglo M, Leslie SW, Sharman T. Postoperative Wound Infections. [Updated 2024 Mar 5]. In: StatPearls [Internet]. Treasure Island (FL): StatPearls Publishing; 2026 Jan-. Available from: https://www.ncbi.nlm.nih.gov/books/NBK560533/
13. World Union of Wound Healing Societies (WUWHS). Wound exudate: effective assessment and management. London, UK: Wounds International; 2019. Available at: https://woundsinternational.com/wpcontent/uploads/2023/02/836aed9753c3d8e3d8694bcaee336395.pdf.
14. Limandjaja GC, Niessen FB, Scheper RJ, Gibbs S. Hypertrophic scars and keloids: Overview of the evidence and practical guide for differentiating between these abnormal scars. Exp Dermatol. 2021;30(1):146-161. https://doi.org/10.1111/exd.14121.
15. Xia G, Dohi T, Abdelhakim M, Tosa M, Ogawa R. The effects of systemic diseases, genetic disorders and lifestyle on keloids. Int Wound J. 2024;21(4):e14865. https://doi.org/10.1111/iwj.14865.

Suturing

7

Sam Atallah

Introduction

Surgical suturing is a fundamental skill in operative medicine, essential for closing wounds, promoting healing, minimizing infection, and achieving optimal cosmetic outcomes. One of the most important practical roles in surgery for PAs is suturing. While the tools and techniques have evolved over time, the core principles of effective suturing remain consistent: (**a**) proper needle handling, (**b**) tension control, (**c**) tissue approximation *without strangulation*, and, of course, (**d**) sterile technique. Knot-tying is an important aspect of suturing and will be covered separately in the next chapter.

Objectives of Suturing: Dermis

Suturing is the basis for a varied number of operations that span from vascular and cardiac surgery to gastrointestinal surgery. Suturing underpins the critical phases of many operations, and the details of such applications are beyond the scope of this introductory chapter. Here, we focus on dermal and/or subcuticular suturing as this is the most common type PAs perform in the real world. Many PAs become quite adept at closing skin and in many instances are as good if not better than attending surgeons at this!

It is important to understand the main goal of surgical suturing which are to:

- Approximate wound edges
- Promote healing by primary intention
- Restore function and appearance of the tissue
- Minimize scarring and improve cosmesis

Closing skin is not a must. Many erroneously believe that if you do not close a surgical wound, it will become infected. However, recall that the treatment for a wound infection is to *open* the wound (and pack the wound). Thus, it is *not true* that a closed wound prevents infection, and, if anything, it increases the risk of surgical site infection. For this reason, in abdominal cases where there is severe fecal contamination, the fascia is close, but the skin is left open and the wound is packed with surgical gauze. In some cases, a vacuum-sealed specialized foam apparatus is used (e.g., Wound VAC®). The point is, closure of the dermis in these instances would almost certainly lead to a wound infection, while leaving the wound open is protective. Although this may seem counterintuitive, it is an important principle to understand!

Types of Sutures

A diagram illustrating the various categories of sture is shown in Fig. 7.1. While there are a multitude of different sutures available (Table 7.1), you do not have to memorize each and every one. However, PAs are expected to be very familiar with the different *categories*. Sutures come in sealed, sterile packaging, in most cases, there is one suture per package (Fig. 7.2).

A. **Absorbable vs. Nonabsorbable**
   - *Absorbable sutures* (e.g., Vicryl, Chromic Gut, PDS): Degraded by the body over time, at variable rates. This type of suture is the ***go-to* for most applications**. This type of suture is especially used to **close skin as a subcuticular stitch.** *As a* **surgical** *PA, this is the type of suture you will work with the most.*
   - *Nonabsorbable sutures* (e.g., Nylon, Prolene, Silk): Must be removed or are used for long-term strength, *often in vascular and cardiothoracic surgery.* Can be used for interrupted sutures (especially laceration

S. Atallah (✉)
Department of Surgery, Piedmont Hospital, Mercer University School of Medicine, Macon, GA, USA
e-mail: atallah@post.harvard.edu

S. Atallah, J. Dragoljevic (eds.), *Fundamentals of Surgery for Physician Assistants*,
https://doi.org/10.1007/978-3-032-21069-2_7

repair in the ER). *As an emergency department PA, this is the suture you will work with the most.*

B. **Monofilament vs. Braided (Multifilament)**

- ***Monofilament*** (e.g., nylon, Prolene): Single strand, lower infection risk, but harder to handle. Monofilament is excellent for running a stitch as it *slides through the tissue better*. So, if you are closing skin in a running subcuticular stitch, you'll want to use a monofilament, absorbable suture (Fig. 7.3). If you are closing skin in an interrupted manner, a *non-absorbable monofilament* (Prolene or nylon) is commonly selected.
- ***Braided*** *or Multifilament* (e.g., Silk, Vicryl): Braided suture exhibits *better handling* and *knot security*, but can harbor bacteria more easily. **It is often taught that the bacteria can** *seed the interstices of the braided suture*. While this is true, in practice we do not tend to see infected braided suture to any measurable degree.

C. **Suture Thickness**

Sutures also come in various thickness (Fig. 7.4). The scale is counterintuitive, in that a 10-0 (pronounced "TEN O") is extremely small (Fig. 7.5), while a 2-0 is quite strong. Very thick and strong suture has a "number" designation, the larger the number the greater the strength. Thus, a #2 (pronounced, "number two") PDS is stronger than a #1 PDS suture, and both are much stronger than a 3-0 PDS. For closing skin, *3-0 and 4-0 are the most common sizes used.*

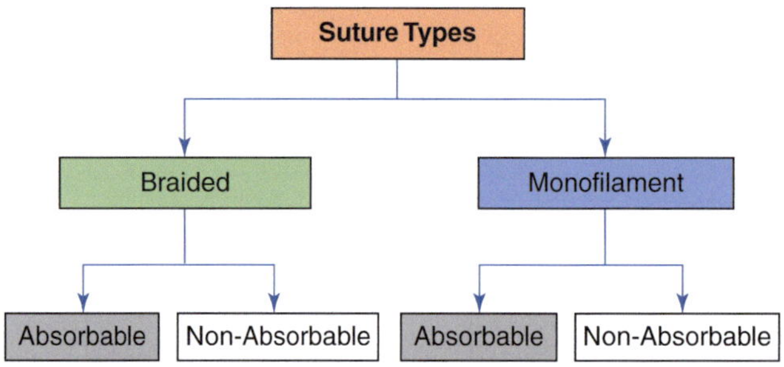

Fig. 7.1 Suture can be either **braided** or **monofilament**. Both monofilament and braided sutures can be either absorbable or nonabsorbable. Braided suture has excellent knotting characteristics, meaning the knots, when formed, are quite secure and do not tend to slip. Monofilament, which is smooth, like fishing line, has poorer knotting characteristics when compared to braided suture. However, monofilament suture is excellent for running, such as with a subcuticular skin closure. PAs should be familiar with the different classifications of suture, as illustrated in this diagram

Table 7.1 Comparison of common suture materials

Suture type	Absorbability	Filament type	Duration	Tissue reaction	Common uses	Notes
Chromic gut	Absorbable	Monofilament	~10–14 days	Moderate	Mucosa, oral cavity, GI, OB/GYN	Natural origin (bovine); enzymatic absorption
Vicryl (Polyglactin 910)	Absorbable	Braided	~3 weeks	Mild	General soft tissue, ligatures	Coated version (Vicryl plus) has antibacterial properties
Monocryl (Poliglecaprone 25)	Absorbable	Monofilament	~1–2 weeks	Very low	Subcuticular skin closure, cosmetic use	Excellent for low tissue reactivity
PDS II (Polydioxanone)	Absorbable	Monofilament	Up to 6 weeks	Low	Fascia, abdominal wall, pediatric cases	Long-lasting absorbable, less pliable
Nylon (Ethilon)	Nonabsorbable	Monofilament	Long-term/ permanent	Minimal	Skin closure, scalp, extremities	Poor knot security; often removed after healing
Prolene (Polypropylene)	Nonabsorbable	Monofilament	Long-term/ permanent	Minimal	Vascular, hernia mesh, skin closure	High memory; slippery, requires extra throws
Silk	Nonabsorbable	Braided (natural)	Gradual loss over months	Moderate to high	Ties, drains, some GI surgeries	Excellent handling; incites higher inflammation
Ethibond (Polyester)	Nonabsorbable	Braided	Long-term/ permanent	Mild to moderate	Cardiac, tendon, ligament repair	Strong, but prone to form stitch granulomas, and can harbor bacteria

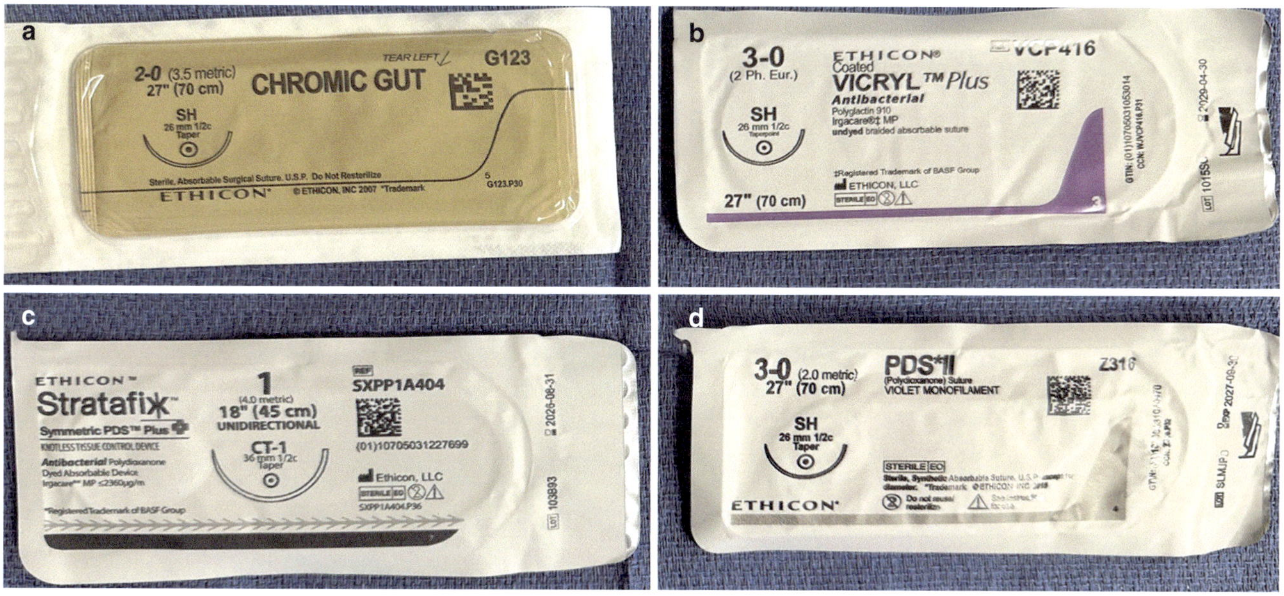

Fig. 7.2 An assortment of commonly used sutures are shown: (**a**) 2-0 Chromic, (**b**) 3-0 Vicryl, (**c**) #1 Stratafix, and (**d**) 3-0 PDS. While some sutures come in packs of eight, most are single (one suture with needle per package). Each package not only includes information about the suture size, length, and type, but it also provides information about the needle shape and tip type (cutting or tapered). In all of these examples, a tapered need is attached and its arch size *depicted to scale* is shown on the package itself

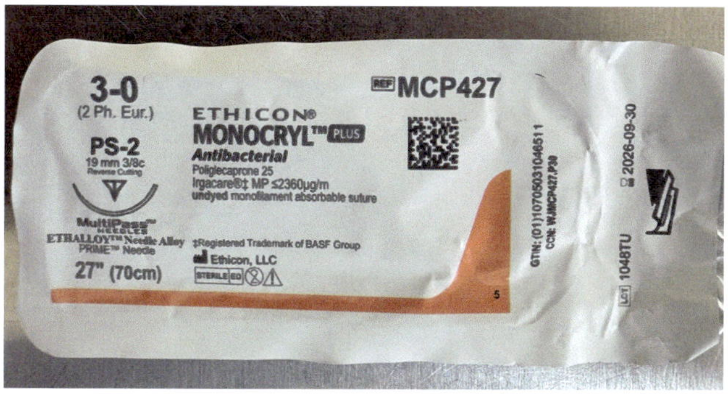

Fig. 7.3 One of the most common sutures used to close skin is shown. In either 3-0 or 4-0, this absorbable monofilament polymer consisting of 75% glycolide and 25% ε-caprolactone, in the United States, it is almost universally referred to by its brand name, **Monocryl™**. This has very good characteristics for subcuticular skin closures and does not cause a significant inflammatory response in most patients. Note that the needle tip has a triangular shape (as shown on the package just above the needle arc illustration). This is known as a *cutting* **needle,** which actually has three sharp blades near the needle's tip. A cutting needle is almost *always preferred when closing and/or suturing skin,* and *almost never* used when suturing anywhere else. The reason is that the dermis is quite tough, and so it is best to use a needle that has blades at the end. Note: although the package says "*reverse*" cutting, this is never referred to as that in the real world, and it is simply known as a *cutting needle*

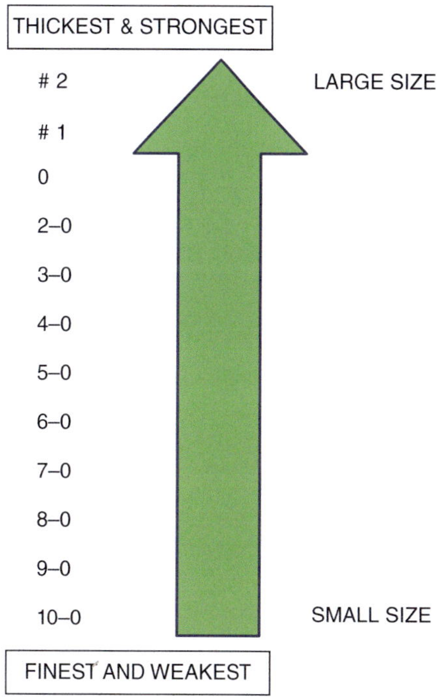

Fig. 7.4 The universal system used for suture thickness and strength is shown. Each suture is suitable for specific applications. Sutures are often matched based upon the strength needed for a specific tissue. For example, when closing the strongest and most important layer of the anterior abdominal wall (fascia), a thick and strong suture is selected, such as **#1** (verbalized as "*number-one*") PDS. Very fine suture is reserved for special applications. For example, **10-0** (verbalized as "*ten-O*") may be used in ophthalmologic surgery but never in general surgery. In general surgery, you will *most commonly use #1, 0, 2-0, 3-0, and 4-0*. Note that there is no 1-0

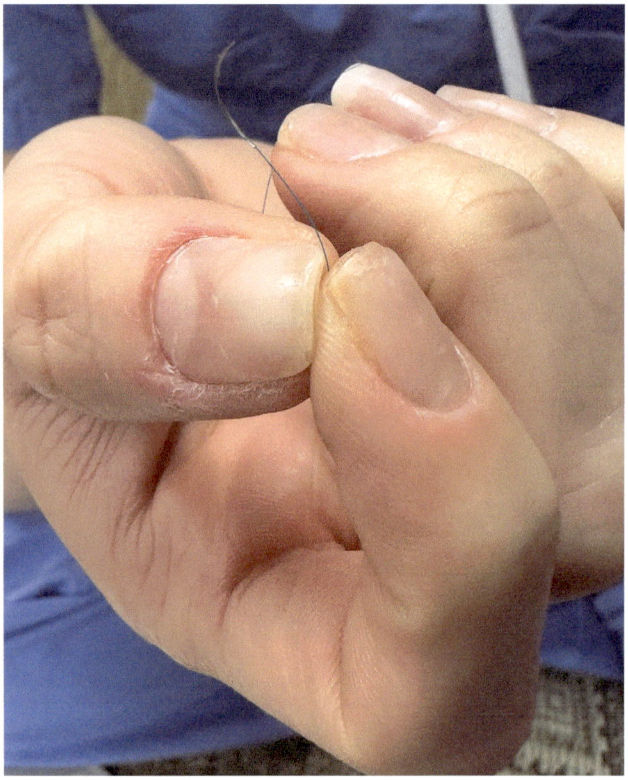

Fig. 7.5 A 10-0 monofilament suture is shown. Although this has important applications in some fields, such as microsurgical procedures in ophthalmic or nerve surgery, it is too small and weak to be used in the field of general surgery. The 10-0 suture diameter is roughly 20–30 microns. Comparatively, human hair diameter typically ranges from 17 to 180 microns, but is usually around 70 microns. Thus, a 10-0 suture is roughly the same diameter as human hair

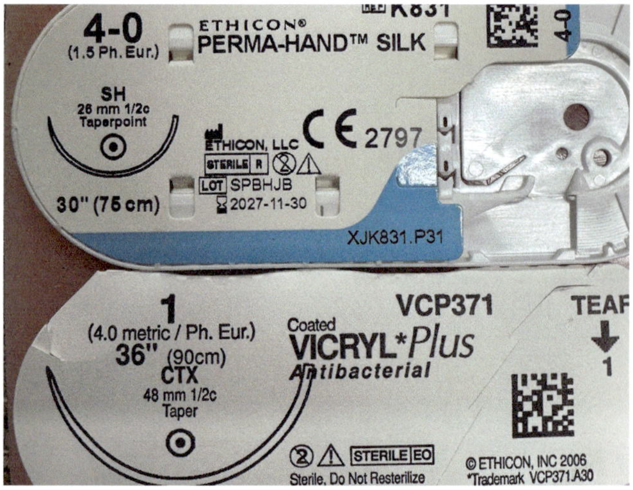

Fig. 7.6 Two single-paged sutures are shown, a 4-0 Silk on an SH needle (top) and a coated #1 Vicryl on CTX needle (bottom). The larger CTX needle is paired with a stronger and thicker suture. Illustrated on the packages is the size of the needle (drawn to scale) to make choosing the proper needle easier as it provides a visual reference

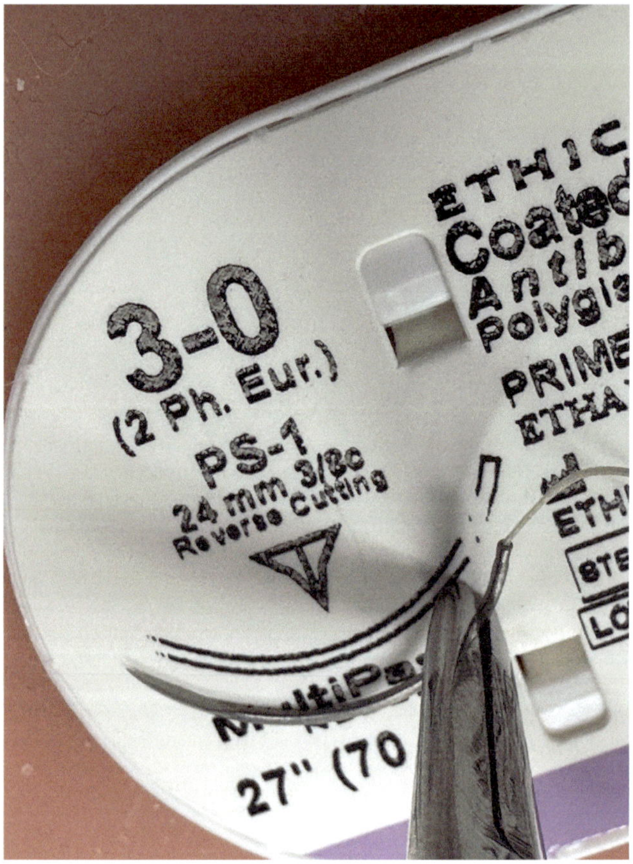

Fig. 7.7 The package of a cutting 3-0 Vicryl on a PS-1 cutting needle is shown, with the suture removed and the needle placed to overlie the needle illustration that is drawn to scale. It is important to choose the right needle for the right surgical task. The needle is a cutting type that is actually bladed near the tip. Such a (cutting) needle is appropriate for use on the dermis only

Suture Needle Types

Surgical needles are classified by:

- **Shape**:
  - **Curved:** This is by far the *most common* shape/design you will use in surgery. Curved needles come in different sizes and each application has a desired size. For example, if you are closing fascia on an obese patient, you will want to select a needle with a large arc. Large arc needles are also constructed stronger so they can handle more force without bending and are easier to use in these situations. Curve needles are given designated abbreviated names, such as **SH** (thin, small) and **CTX** (large, thick) (Fig. 7.6**)**. The names (SH, CTX, etc.) do not need to be committed to memory. The best way to gage the needle size is by the appearance on the package which shows an illustration of the needle size (Fig. 7.7)**.**
  - **Straight:** Used nowadays for very special applications such as to suspend the uterus during pelvic sur-

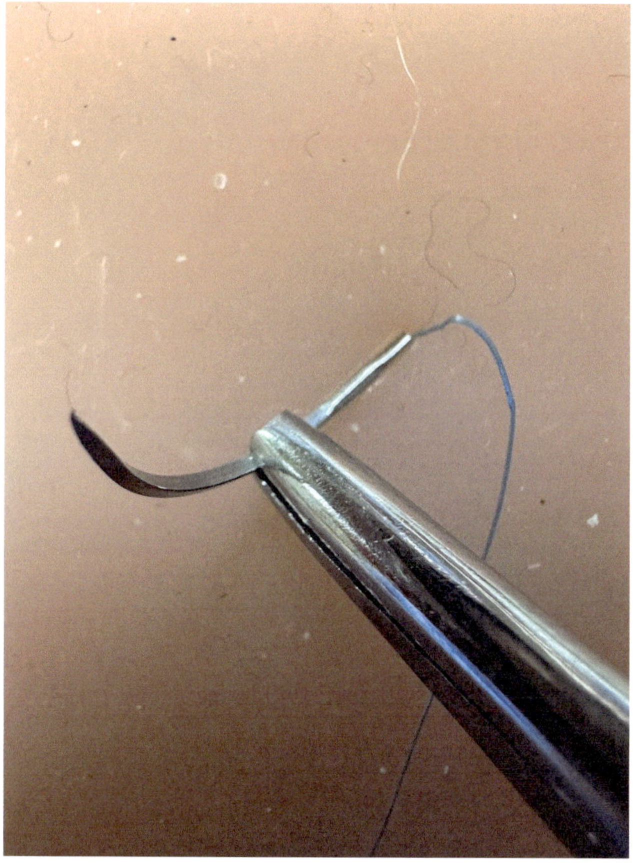

Fig. 7.8 A cutting needle, suitable for skin suturing, is shown. Notice the triangular end near the tip which is bladed and ideal for tough tissues, such as dermis. Generally, cutting needles are not used except on dermis

gery during minimally invasive surgery; it can also be used to sew dermis by hand without a needle driver in a more "old school" fashion, and this is *rarely* performed today).

- **Tip**:
  - *Tapered*: For soft, most *if not all* internal tissue (e.g., muscle, bowel, biliary).
  - *Cutting [Reverse Cutting]*: For tougher tissues like **skin.** As a general rule, *always use a cutting needle when operating* ***on skin*** and *do not* use a cutting needle on other anatomy (Fig. 7.8).

Needles are typically **swaged** (pre-attached) to the suture to minimize tissue trauma. They can also be designed **to "pop-off"** the needle when a tugging motion is applied. The so-called pop-offs come in packs of eight typically. They are ideal when many stitches need to be placed in rapid succession.

Common Suturing Techniques—Skin

A. **Simple Interrupted Suture**
- Most basic and versatile technique.
- Each stitch is individually tied, offering strong wound closure, and allows removal of individual sutures if infection develops.
- *Commonest technique used for laceration repair* (Fig. 7.9)
- *Most common in ER setting.*

B. **Continuous (Running) Suture**
- Faster to apply and distributes tension evenly.
- Less control over individual stitches; a break in the suture line can compromise the entire closure.

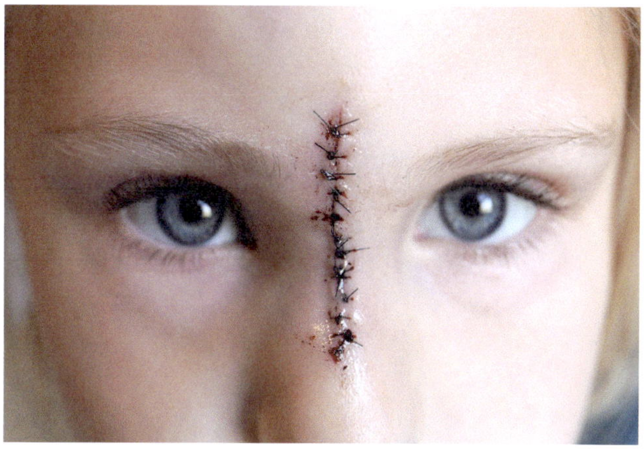

Fig. 7.9 A pediatric patient underwent repair of a 5-cm vertical facial laceration in the emergency department (ED), using the common technique of simple, *interrupted* sutures. This is the most come method to repair lacerations in the ED. In the OR, however, surgical skin incisions are closed most often with a *subcuticular* suture. The primary goals of facial laceration repair are hemostasis, infection prevention, and achieving optimal cosmetic outcomes. In children, minimizing pain and anxiety is essential and should be integrated into all aspects of care, including the use of topical anesthetics and child-friendly techniques. Wound assessment is critical in determining the appropriate closure method. Simple, clean, linear, low-tension lacerations with well-approximated edges are suitable for closure with tissue adhesives or adhesive strips. These methods are particularly advantageous in pediatric patients due to reduced pain, faster application, and avoidance of suture removal. Sutures are indicated for deeper, gaping, or high-tension wounds, or when layered closure is required. Wounds with significant contamination, devitalized tissue, mammalian bites, or those crossing mucocutaneous junctions should not be closed primarily with adhesives or strips. Absorbable sutures (e.g., 5-0 fast-absorbing gut) are also effective, with cosmetic results similar to adhesives and strips, and are appropriate for wounds requiring deeper closure or in children where suture removal would be problematic. Adhesive strips are equivalent to other methods for simple, low-tension wounds. Combining adhesives with strips does not improve cosmetic outcomes but may assist in wound approximation when manual alignment is challenging. Routine prophylactic antibiotics are not indicated for simple facial lacerations

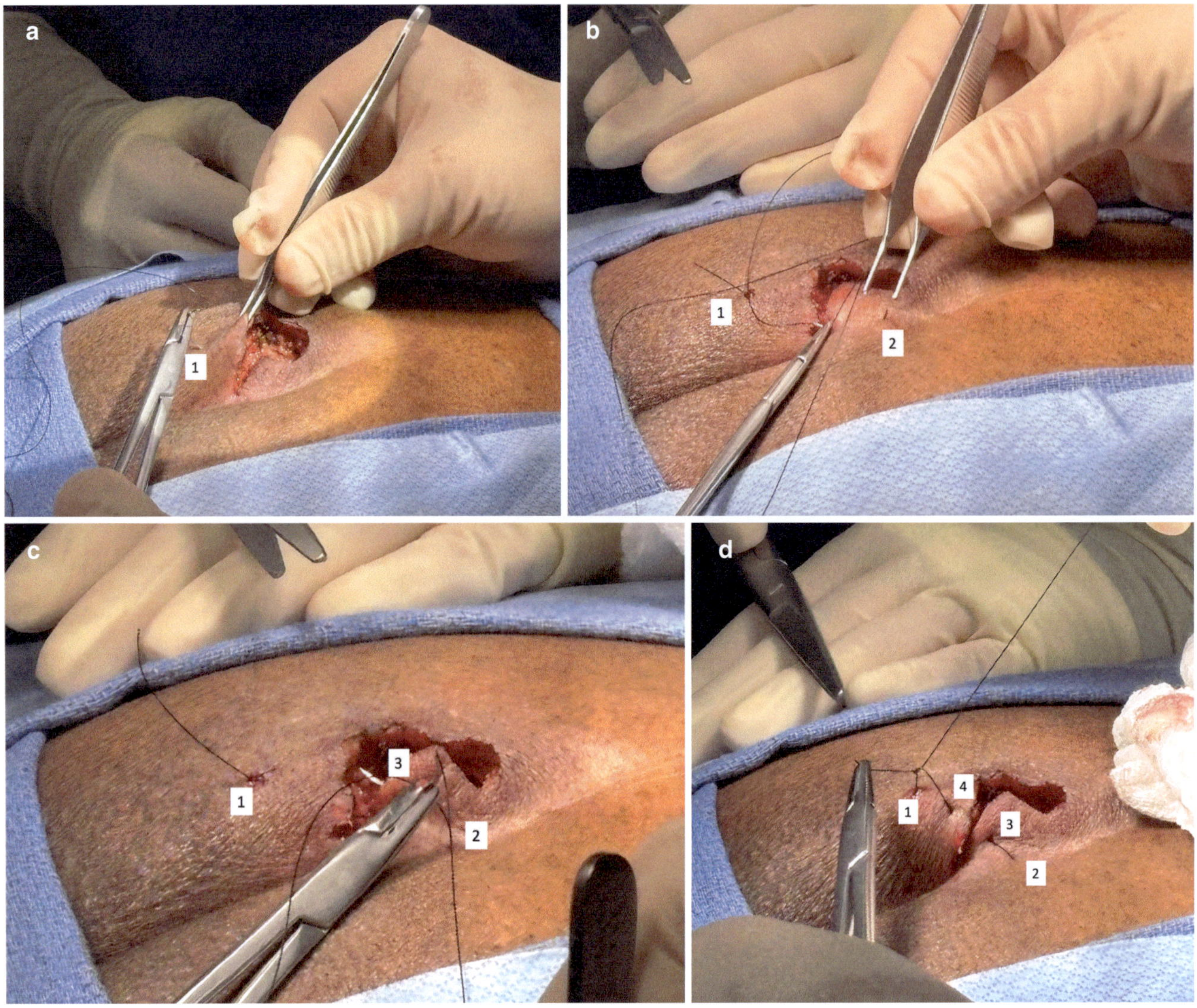

Fig. 7.10 The technique for the vertical mattress is shown to reapproximate the dermis after cyst excision, here using a 2-0 nylon suture on a cutting needle. The general approach is often remembered as "*far-far/near-near*" which refers to the distance the suture bites are taken relative to the wound edge. (**a**) The first bite is taken "far" from the wound edge. (**b**) The suture needle and thread has been driven to the opposite side (going through the wound itself) for another "far" bite. (**c**) The needle direction is now reversed "backhanded" and a near side bite is obtained on the ipsilateral side. (**d**) A final bite is taken near the wound edge, back on the same side that the stitch sequence was started, placing the knot on the starting point. Vertical mattress closures are ideal for high-tension areas and are an alternative to simple interrupted stitches

- This suture is among the *most popular for closing small to mid-size surgical wounds* and is usually done in a subcuticular fashion (see below).

C. **Mattress Sutures**
- *Vertical mattress*: Good for eversion of skin edges and deeper tissue approximation; very robust suture design especially for areas with high skin tension (Fig. 7.10a–d).
- *Horizontal mattress*: Good for skin or where tension is high; robust and secure stitch.

D. **Subcuticular Suture**
- A buried, continuous stitch just under the skin, excellent for many skin closures in surgery, but is not used in the ER setting.
- Excellent cosmetic result, commonly used in plastic surgery, pediatric procedures, and for closure of laparoscopic and robotic port sites, as well as many other applications in general surgery. *If you are a PA, you will want to gain experience with this type of stitch in the operating room!*

Technique Tips

- Use minimal tension—**tight stitches can cause ischemia and necrosis.**
- **Approximate, don't strangulate**—the edges should just meet.

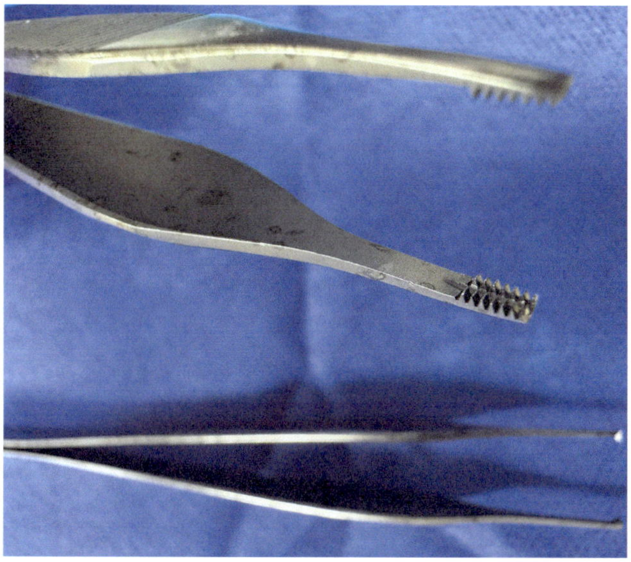

Fig. 7.11 One of the most difficult things for new PA students to grasp is that suturing is a ***two*-handed task.** Much focus is given to the hand that is managing the needle with the needle driver. While this is important, so too is the *grasper* used to provide *counter-traction.* Since many PAs close skin, it is important to know that skin retraction is best carried out using pickups *with teeth*, as shown. Common forceps used are **Adson forceps** (background) or **Adson-Brown** forceps (foreground). Other forceps can also be used, *as long as they have teeth.* This not only provides a better grasp on the dermis, but it is also less traumatizing than using smooth forceps (pickups). As a general rule, *do not use smooth forceps to grasp/retract the dermis!*

- Maintain sterility throughout the procedure.
- Handle tissue gently with forceps, not fingers, to reduce trauma.
- Forceps (usually held in non-dominant hand) provide **counter-tension** (Figs. 7.11 and 7.12).
- Knot security is critical; typically, 3–5 throws are standard for braided suture, more for more slippery monofilament suture materials (e.g., Prolene, PDS).

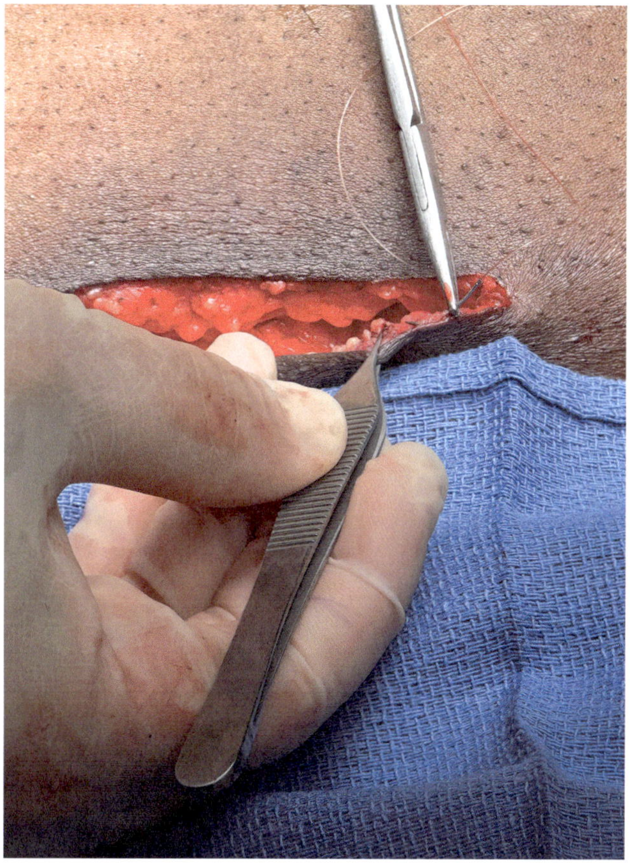

Fig. 7.12 Subcuticular closure of a Pfannenstiel skin incision is shown, here using a running 3-0 Monocryl® (absorbable) suture. Note that the needle is placed at the nose of the needle driver. Most importantly, note that the surgeon's other hand is used to provide *upward and outward counter tension,* using a pair of toothed (Adson) forceps. Providing proper counter-tension, and learning to "operate with both hands" in this manner, is one of the most important skills to learn in surgery

Table 7.2 Typical timing for skin suture removal based on the body location[a]

Location	Suture removal time
Face	3–5 days
Scalp	7–10 days
Neck	5–7 days
Chest or abdomen	7–10 days
Back	10–14 days
Arms and hands	7–10 days
Legs and feet	10–14 days
Joints (e.g., knees, elbows)	10–14 days

[a]These are *general* guidelines *only*. Consider steri-strips when removing suture earlier than ideal target dates. Note: Subcuticular sutures and/or absorbable sutures do not require removal. Patients with poor nutritional status and steroid require a longer duration prior to stitch removal

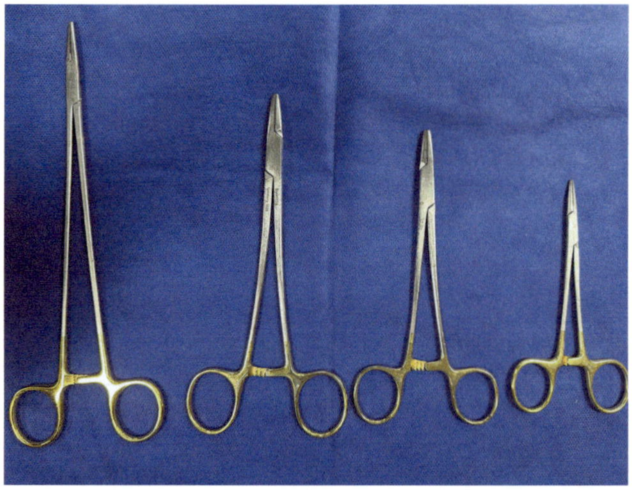

Fig. 7.13 Different-sized *needle drivers,* which are used for suturing, are shown. While long-handled needle drivers are ideal to reach difficult to access areas "deep" in the body, short-handled needle drivers are much better suited for closing skin, where reach and access are generally not a problem. As a PA, always chose the shortest-handled needle driver for closing skin, because it is easier to handle as there is less distance between your hand and the driver tip. This results in better control and dexterity. The smaller drivers are also lighter which is another reason they are easier to handle

Suture Removal and Follow-Up (Table 7.2)

- Sutures are typically removed in 5–14 days depending on location and healing status.
- Facial sutures: ~5 days.
- Trunk and limbs: 7–10 days.
- Joints or high-tension areas: up to 14 days.
- Educate patients on wound care, signs of infection, and when to follow up.
- Suture can cause a local inflammatory reaction, and this is classically observed as erythema at the suture entry and exit points through the dermis.

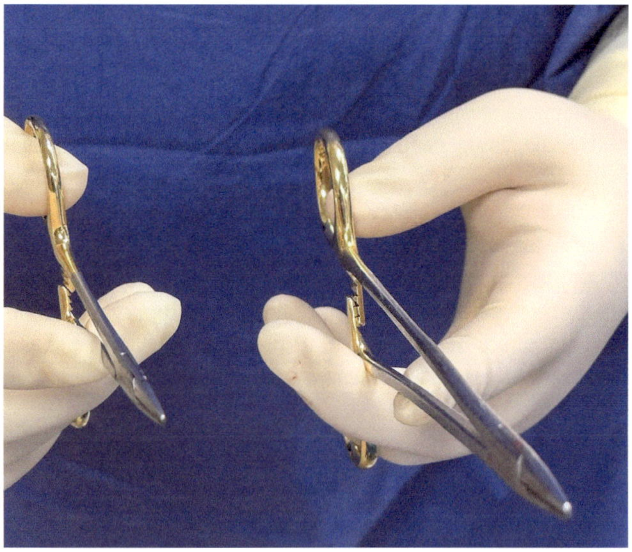

Fig. 7.14 Two needle drivers are shown demonstrating the difference in shaft length. Which of these would you select to close dermis? The shorter needle driver is always easier to handle and is more stable. If given a choice, select the smaller needle driver when closing skin!

Needle Driver Technique

The **needle drivers**, also known as a needle holder, are what is used to carry out the task of suturing and are available in differing sizes (Figs. 7.13 and 7.14). It is an essential surgical instrument used to grasp and manipulate suturing needles with precision and control. Mastery of the needle driver is critical for safe and effective suturing, and there are slight differences for right- and left-hand dominant use (Figs. 7.15 and 7.16). These instruments are all designed for right-hand use, but left-handed surgeons and PAs can still use them in their left hand quite effectively despite this handicap minimizing tissue trauma and ensuring secure wound closure. Proper technique enhances accuracy, knot security, and efficiency during surgical procedures.

- ✔ Needle at tip of driver
- ✔ Driver at needle arc half-way point, or slightly toward back end
- ✔ Needle tip points outwardly, about 10–15 degrees
- ✔ Needle is perpendicular to the driver
- ✔ Sewing direction is *RIGHT TO LEFT* or toward yourself

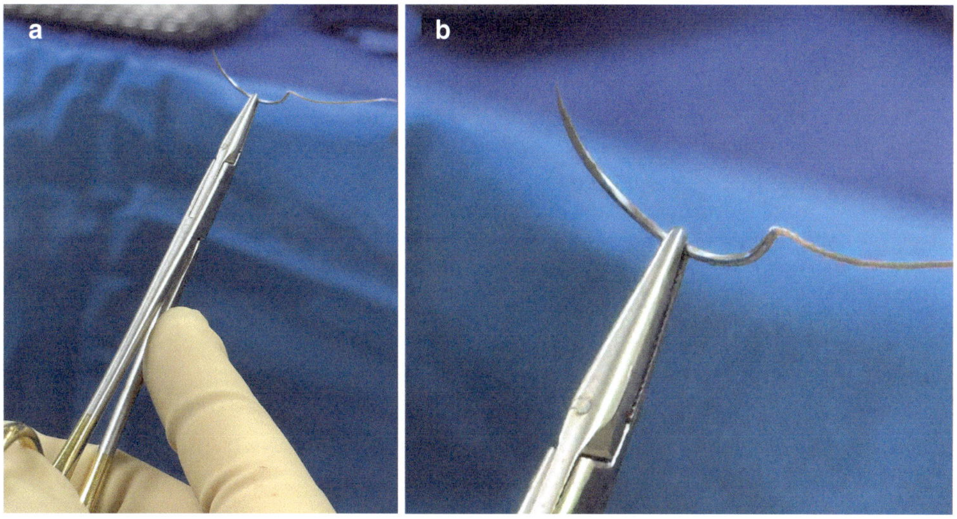

RIGHT-HANDED TECHNIQUE

Fig. 7.15 (**a**) Shown is the correct suture needle placement on the needle driver for a right-handed (forehand) throw; alternatively, this is a left-handed *back hand* configuration (**b**) close-up showing needle tip detail. Placement of the needle on the needle driver correctly will set you up for success, and you will struggle less if you properly configure the needle on the driver. Ideally, the needle should be grasped at the tip of the driver, and directed at a slightly outward angle. Grasping the needle at the center of the arc or slightly toward the back (away from the pointed tip) is good technique. Right-hand dominant persons should sew *right to left or* toward themselves

- ✔ Needle at tip of driver
- ✔ Driver at needle arc half-way point, or slightly toward back end
- ✔ Needle tip points outwardly, about 10–15 degrees
- ✔ Needle is perpendicular to the driver
- ✔ Sewing direction is *LEFT TO RIGHT* or toward yourself

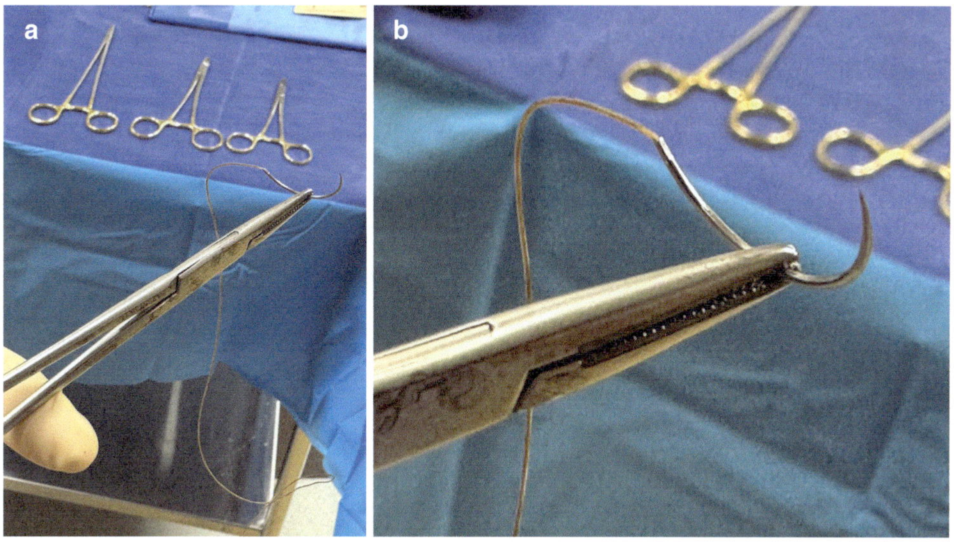

LEFT-HANDED TECHNIQUE

Fig. 7.16 (**a**) Shown is the correct suture needle placement on the needle driver for a left-handed (forehand) throw; alternatively, this is a right-handed *back hand* configuration (**b**) close-up showing needle tip detail. The setup is the mirror image of the right-handed needle setup. Left-hand dominant persons should sew *left to right or* toward themselves

Anatomy of the Needle Driver

A *standard* needle driver includes the following components:

- **Jaws:** Serrated or smooth tips that hold the needle.
- **Box Lock:** The hinge joint allowing controlled movement.
- **Ratchet:** Interlocking teeth that lock the instrument closed.
- **Shanks:** The arms that connect the jaws to the finger rings.
- **Finger Rings:** Loops for the thumb and ring finger, used to control the instrument.

It is important to become familiar with the operation of a needle driver. It should become second nature to you if you want to excel as a PA in a surgical field. If you are using a needle driver for the first time, spend time practicing opening and closing the instrument outside of the operating room. Practice sets are available and are encouraged to use. Many operative instruments use the same basic design as a needle driver, so if you become good at opening and closing a needle driver, you can use the same skill to open and close a hemostat, right angle, Allis clamp, and more. While standard needle drivers are what you will use almost exclusively, there are other specialized needle drivers that have a different design, such as Castroviejo needle holders.

Proper Grip and Handling

Finger Placement: Thumb and ring finger are placed in the rings. The index finger rests along the shank for stability and guidance. Avoid inserting fingers too deeply into the rings; fingertip control allows finer movement and faster release.

Tripod Technique: A tripod configuration, with the index finger supporting and guiding the shaft, provides the best balance of precision and strength. Some prefer a palm grip in certain situations.

Needle Placement on Needle Driver

Grasp Location: The needle should be held at the center of the needle arc or toward the back, although this is not written in stone. Some teach that the needle drive should grasp the needle "one-third" the distance from the needle's swaged end, but surgeons have varied opinions about this. In general, avoid grasping near the needle tip.

Needle Angle: Orient the needle at a 90° angle to the jaws of the driver. The curve of the needle should follow the natural arc of wrist rotation to facilitate smooth passage through tissue. Aiming the needle tip slightly outward at 5–15° can be helpful, especially when closing skin with a running subcuticular layer.

Jaw Position: Close the jaws only to the second or third ratchet click—this secures the needle so that it is in snug a position and is less likely to torque as it is driven though tissue.

Driving the Needle Through Tissue

Wrist Rotation: Rotate the wrist, not the entire arm, to drive the needle along its natural curve.

Avoid pushing or forcing the needle; allow the curve to guide motion.

Entry and Exit: Enter the tissue *at a 90° angle* to minimize trauma and maximize precision.

Drive the needle in a smooth arc, emerging perpendicular on the opposing edge.

Controlled Passage: Use only the amount of needle needed to pass through the tissue. Do not "pull through" aggressively; gently draw the needle out with forceps or hand-over-hand technique if needed.

Suture Cutting

The cutting of suture should be carried out using surgical scissors that are designed for cutting suture specifically. They are called **suture scissors**. Cutting suture should *not* be performed using more specialized scissors used for fine dissection, for example, such as Metzenbaum scissors ("Metz"), as this can damage them.

Suture cutting is an important step after the suture knot has been secured and must be done precisely and meticulously. Best practice of suture cutting is to (a) be prepared to cut even before the knot-tying has been completed; (b) hold the scissor in your dominant hand, with the scissor screw facing upward; (d) cut using the scissor tip; (e) use your non-dominant hand to provide support during the cutting process as this improves stability and precision (Fig. 7.17a, b).

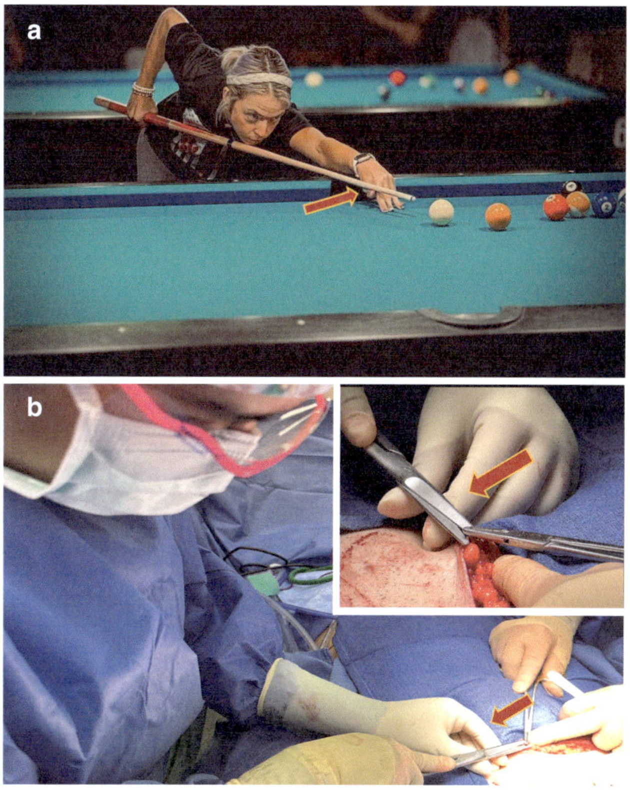

Fig. 7.17 What does playing a game of pool (billiards) have to do with surgery? (**a**) A player lines up her pool cue to strike the ball at a precise point. Although the force and strike will come from her dominant hand, she uses her non-dominant (left) hand to steady the cue near its tip (arrow). This use of the non-dominant hand to steady an instrument, particularly in open surgery, also applies. (**b**) A surgical PA steadies her hand (arrows) in preparation for cutting sutures. Note the use of the non-dominant hand to steady the tip (inset). [*photo (a) courtesy of Mandy Lane, with permission*]

Knot-Tying

8

Ronald Barbosa and Jessica Barbosa

Introduction

Knot-tying is a foundational skill in surgery and is performed on a regular basis in almost all surgical and even in many nonsurgical specialties and procedures. Proper knot-tying technique is critical to achieving good tissue approximation, and in general, it is worthwhile to become comfortable enough with the different techniques that the act of tying knots does not add to the overall cognitive burden of performing the procedure. Many years of observation of trainees at different stages has shown that discomfort with tying knots leads to considerable discomfort in performing a procedure overall.

Many different knots have been described in the surgical literature, but the square knot remains by far the most commonly taught and used knot (Fig. 8.1). Though some have argued that other types of knots may have increased strength or decreased tendency to unravel, the square knot remains the most popular, in part because it easy to conceptualize and teach.

The various techniques described here are basically different ways to create square knots. Each technique has its own advantages and disadvantages, and selection of one technique is often a matter of preference. In practice, surgeons often switch back and forth between techniques frequently.

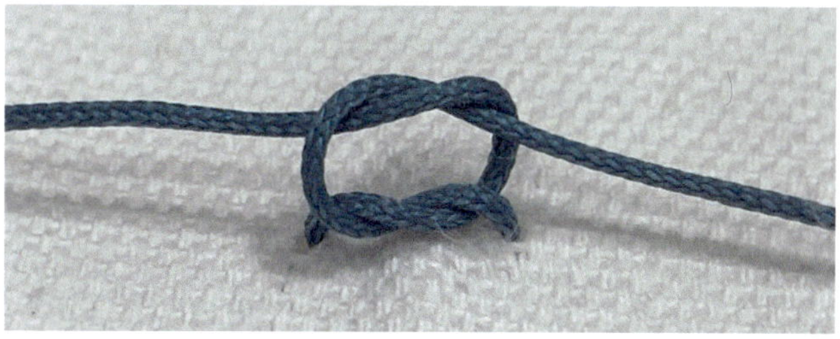

Fig. 8.1 Square knot

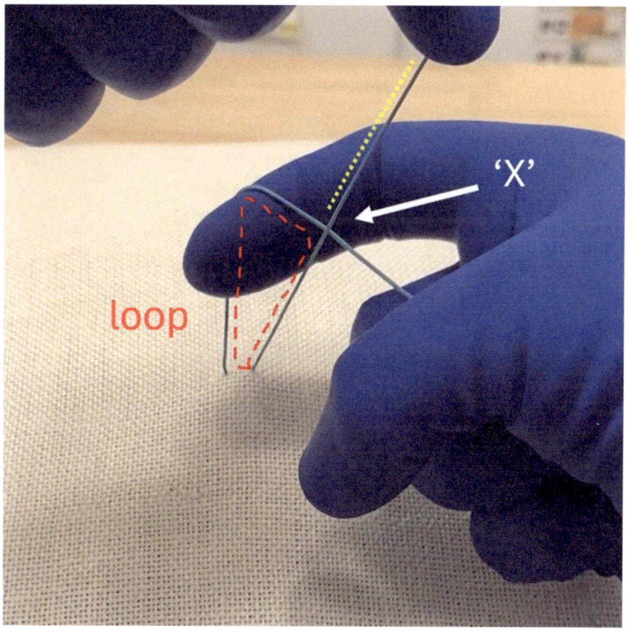

Fig. 8.2 The general theme of square knot-tying involves creating a loop (red dashes) though which the strand in the nondominant hand (yellow dashes) will be passed

The Concept of the Loop

Regardless of the technique used, the process of tying a square knot involves creating a loop that one of the strands will be passed through. In the case of hand-tying (one- or two-handed), the loop is created by bringing the two strands together to form an "X" (Fig. 8.2). The second part

R. Barbosa (✉)
Department of Trauma and General Surgery, Legacy Health, Legacy Medical Group, Portland, OR, USA

J. Barbosa
Department of Trauma and General Surgery, Legacy Health, Legacy Medical Group, Portland, OR, USA

Department of Emergency Medicine, OHSU - Hillsboro Medical Center, Portland, United States

S. Atallah, J. Dragoljevic (eds.), *Fundamentals of Surgery for Physician Assistants*,
https://doi.org/10.1007/978-3-032-21069-2_8

of the knot will also be a variation of this. For instrument tying, the "X" is not created, but the concept is the same: a loop is created, and the other strand is passed through it. Each of the techniques is simply a different method for accomplishing the same thing. These will now each be examined in detail.

Two-Handed Knot-Tying

The two-handed knot-tying technique is often the first technique taught to trainees. It has a number of advantages, including increased ability to control tension across the knot, and the ability to avoid "pulling up" on the tissues excessively (Fig. 8.3), as compared to the one-handed technique. In addition, when the suture strands are short, it is much easier to tie using the two-handed method.

Starting Position

When creating the square knot, it is generally better to have the strands start in a "crossed" position. This allows for the setting down of the first throw to be done with one's hands in a more natural position (Fig. 8.4). If one starts with the strands in an uncrossed position, then the hands will have to be crossed when the first throw is set down, which is considerably more awkward (Fig. 8.5). The strand that is "on top" will dictate which of the two types of throws that will be done first. Here we will start with the left strand on top (Fig. 8.6).

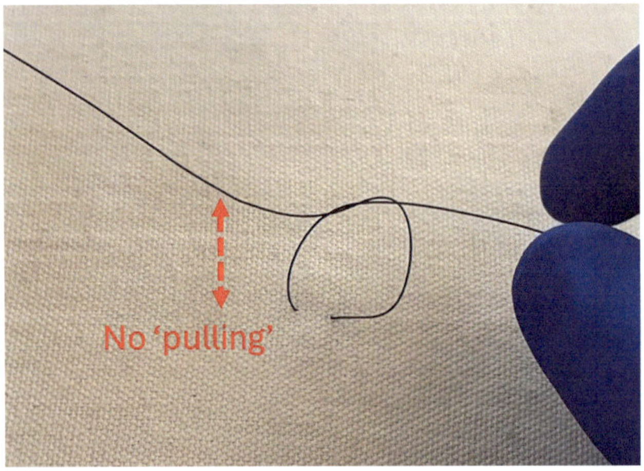

Fig. 8.3 It is important to minimize "pulling up" on tissues when tying knots

First Throw

Step 1: Each of the strands is grasped by one hand as though you were "shaking hands" with the strands (Fig. 8.7).

Step 2: The R strand is tented upward, using the index finger (Fig. 8.8).

Step 3: The L strand is brought over to the other strand. This forms both the "loop" and the "X" (Fig. 8.9).

Step 4: The index finger and thumb are now pinched together (Fig. 8.10).

Step 5: The pinched thumb and finger are now passed through the loop, so that they are now on the other side of the loop (Fig. 8.11).

Step 6: The strand being held by the L hand is now grasped using the finger and thumb of the R hand (Fig. 8.12). The "pinching" of the R thumb and index finger will need to be briefly relaxed to accomplish this.

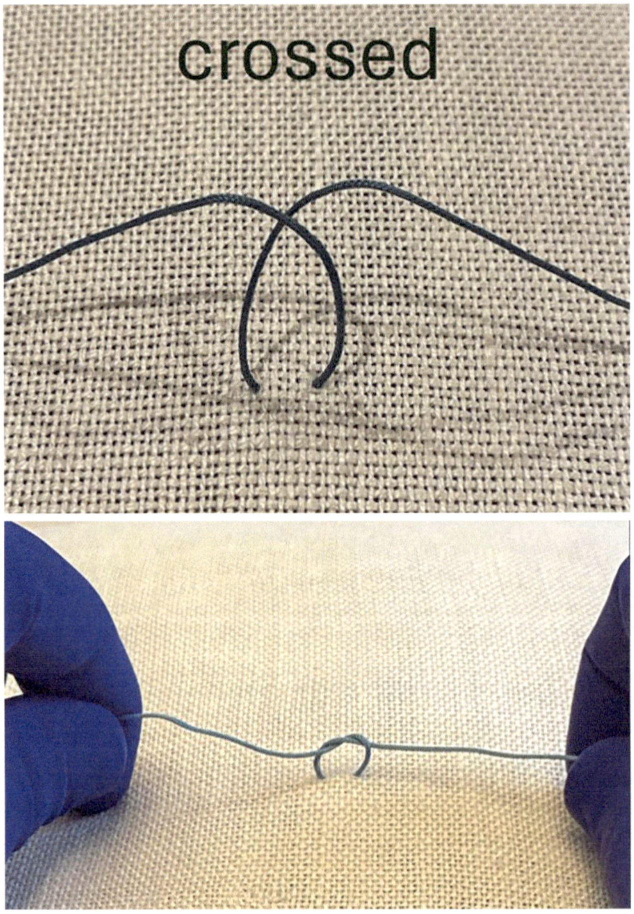

Fig. 8.4 Starting the first throw with crossed strands means that the hands do not need to be crossed when the throw is set down. This tends to be much easier and more precise

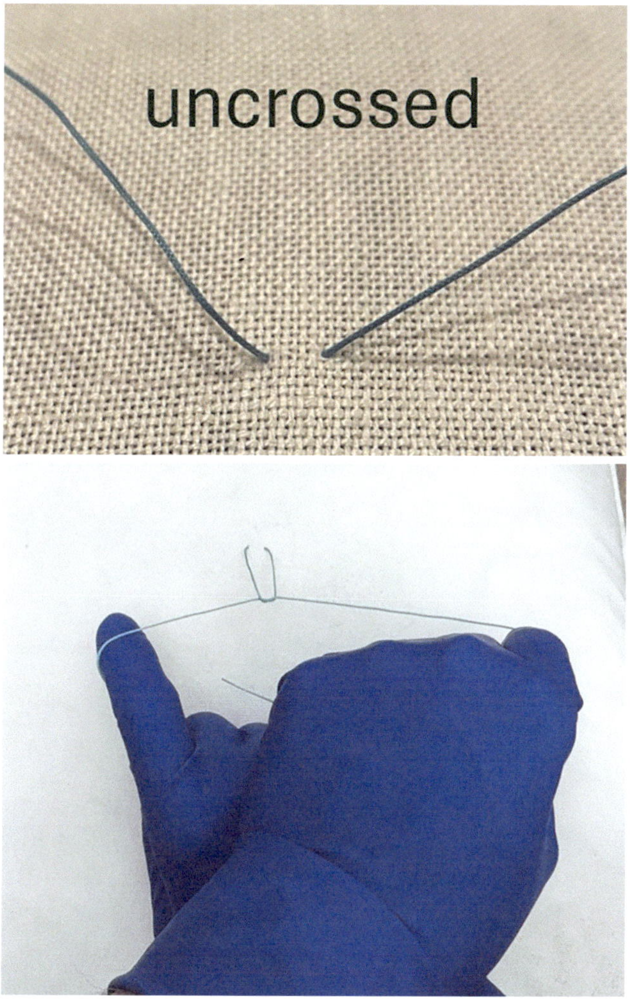

Fig. 8.5 If the first throw is started with the strands in an uncrossed position, the hands must be crossed as the throw is set down, which is awkward

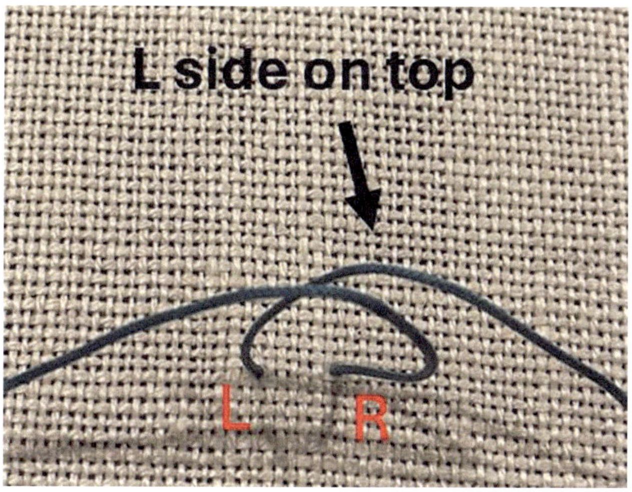

Fig. 8.6 The strand that starts off "on top" will dictate which of the two types of throws will be done first. It is easier to consistently start with either the left or right strands on top. In this example, we have chosen the L strand

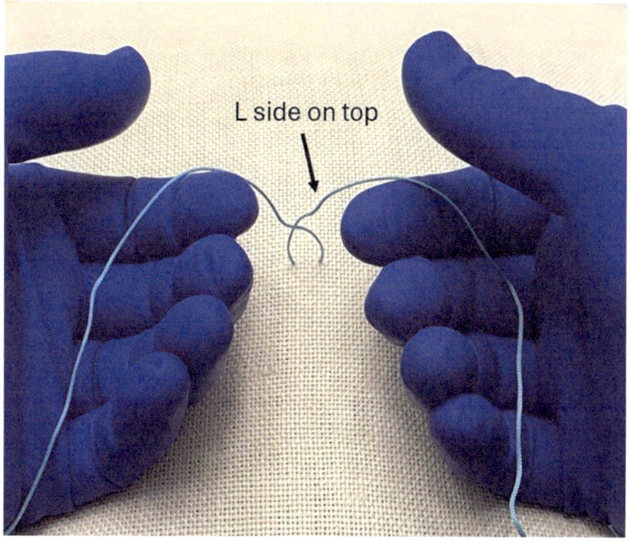

Fig. 8.7 One strand is grasped in each hand, similar to a handshaking position

Step 7: Keeping the thumb and finger pinched, the strand is brought through the loop in the opposite direction (Fig. 8.13). It should be noted that in order to be able to pass the L strand through the loop, it needs to be briefly released by the L hand, and then picked back up again once it is through the loop (Fig. 8.14).

Step 8: The two strands are pulled in opposite directions to complete the first throw (Fig. 8.15). It is often advantageous to use the L hand to "set down" the throw for additional security, especially when tying in deeper cavities.

Second Throw

Step 1: The R strand is tented up again, this time with the thumb (Fig. 8.16).

Step 2: The L strand is brought over to the R, forming the X and the loop (Fig. 8.17).

Steps 3–6: These steps are essentially the same as in the first throw. The index finger and thumb are pinched, and then brought through the loop. The strand in the L hand is grabbed, and then brought back through the loop in the other direction (Fig. 8.18). Once again, the strand must be released briefly to do this.

Step 7: One thing that does differ in the second throw is that after the strand has been brought through the loop, the strands will be crossed, and that will need to be corrected by crossing your hands, so that the knot becomes square (Fig. 8.19).

Error: In the final step, if the hands are not crossed, then the knot will not become square and will be considerably less stable (Fig. 8.20).

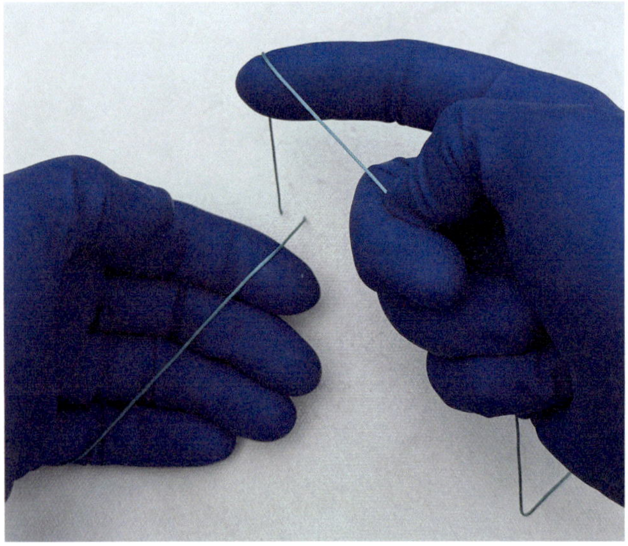

Fig. 8.8 The R strand is tented up using the index finger

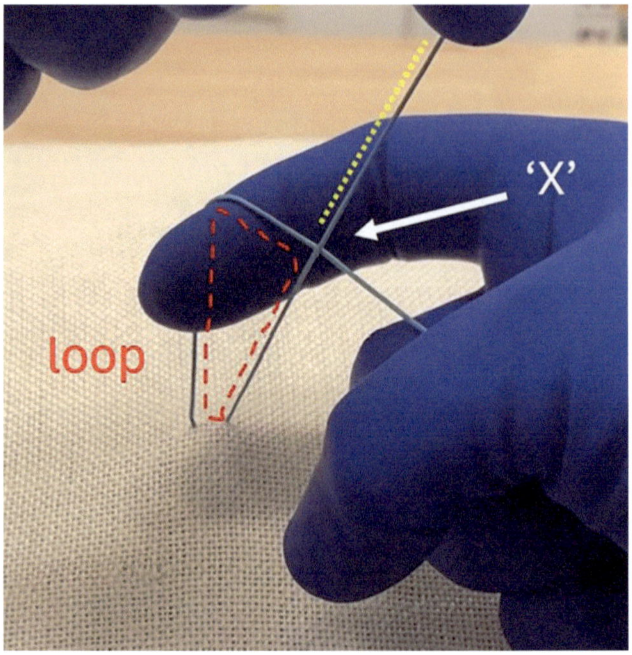

Fig. 8.9 The strand in the L hand (yellow dashed line) is brought over to form the "loop" and the X

Fig. 8.10 Having made the loop, the next step is to pinch the index finger and thumb together

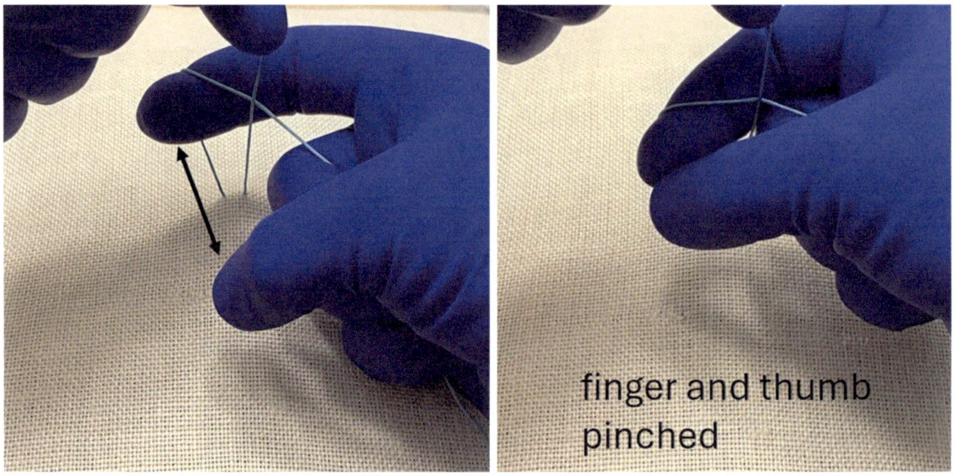

Fig. 8.11 The pinched finger and thumb are passed through the loop, so that the thumb is now on the other side of the loop

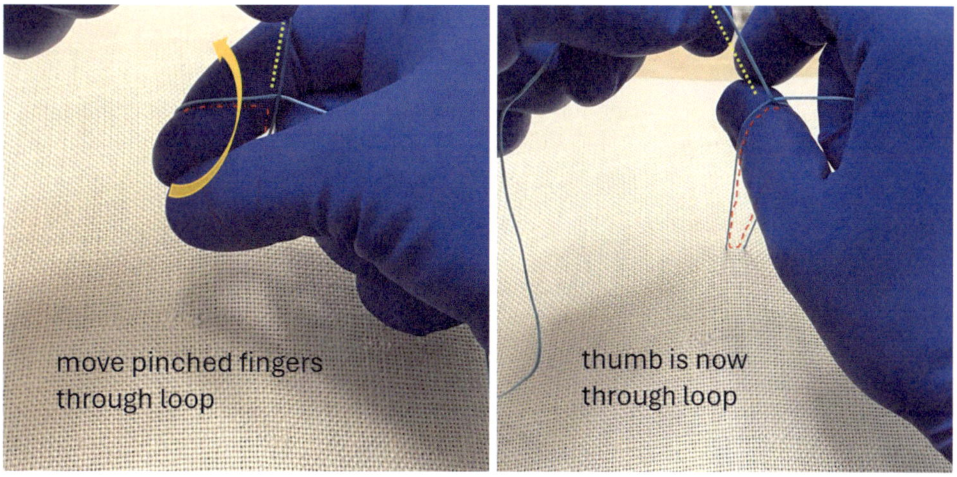

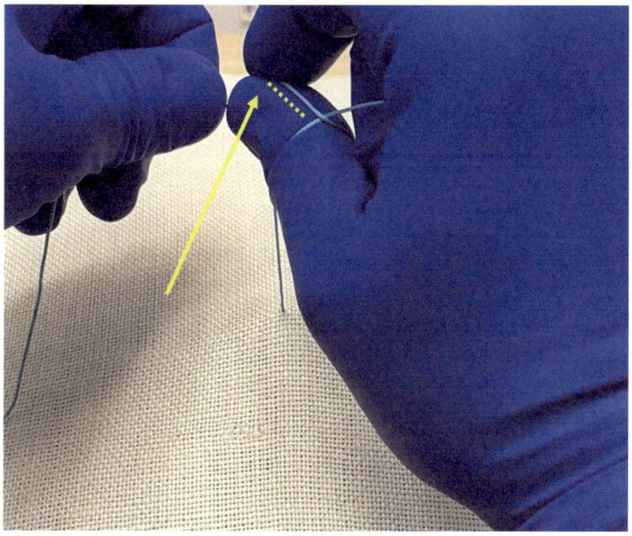

Fig. 8.12 The strand in the L hand is grabbed by the R finger and thumb, which must be briefly unpinched and then pinched again

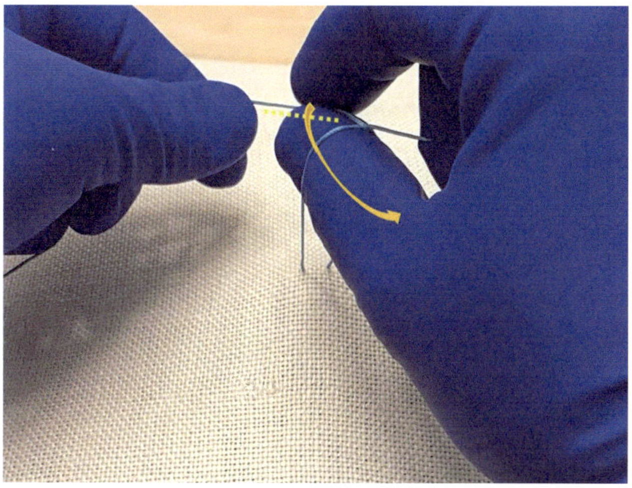

Fig. 8.13 The L strand is brought through the loop in the opposite direction

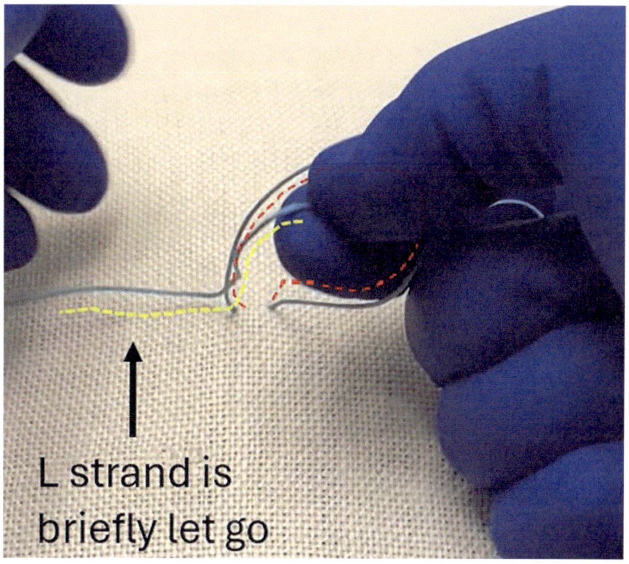

Fig. 8.14 To pass the L strand through the loop, it will be necessary to briefly let off of the strand. The strand is picked up again after it is through the loop

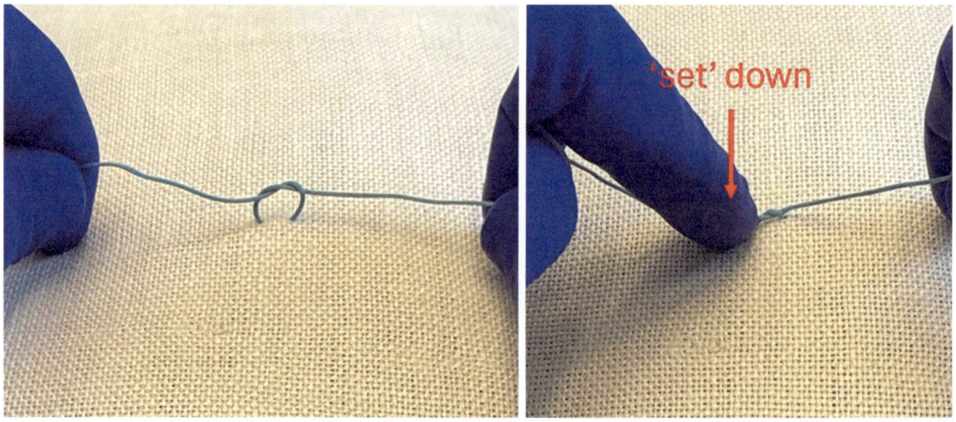

Fig. 8.15 Each strand is then pulled in opposite directions to complete the first throw. When tying in deep cavities, it is usually necessary to "set down" the throw using the L index finger

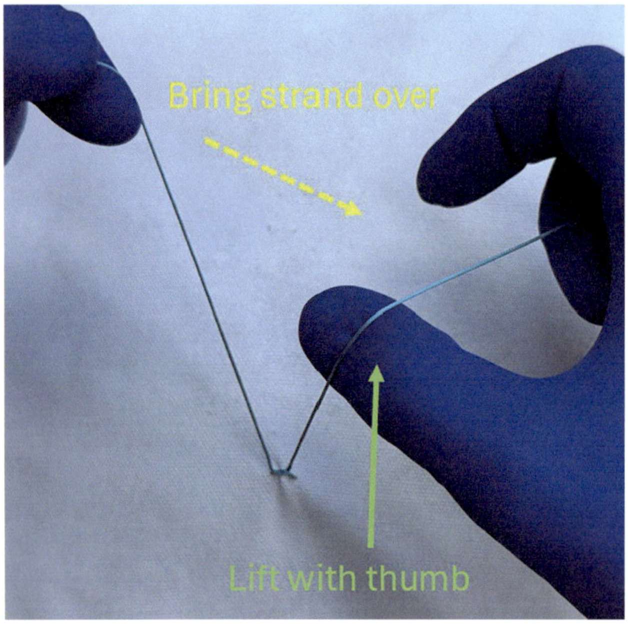

Fig. 8.16 The R strand is tented up with the thumb, and the L strand is brought over

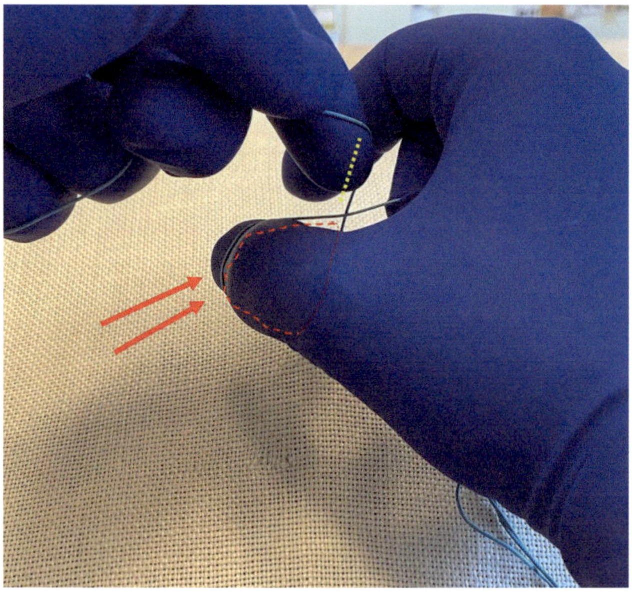

Fig. 8.17 The X and the loop have been formed

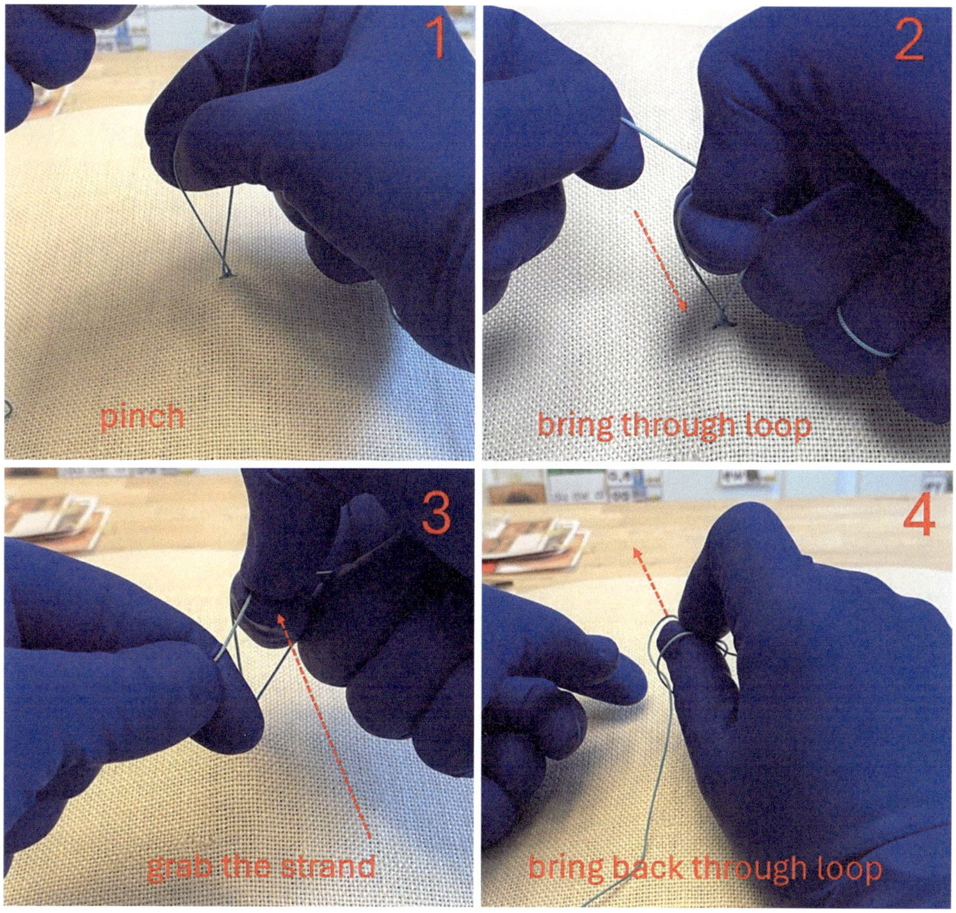

Fig. 8.18 Steps of the second throw of the two-handed knot. These are analogous to the same steps that were executed on the first throw

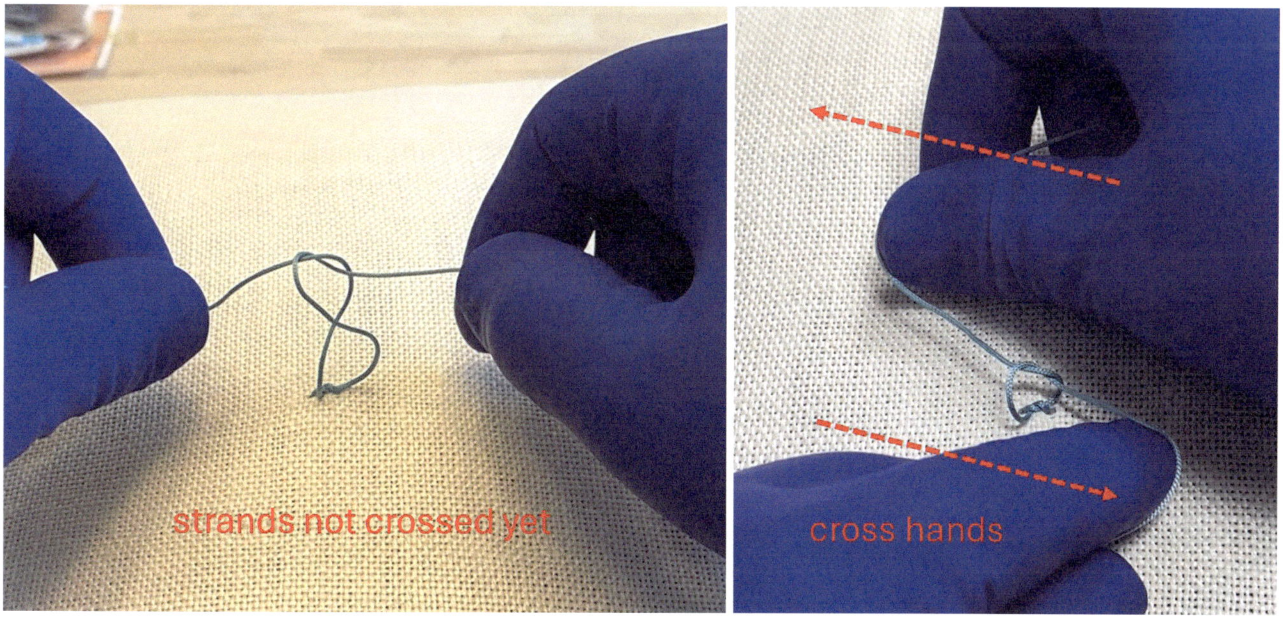

Fig. 8.19 The strands will be crossed at this point, and this needs to be corrected by crossing your hands, which creates the proper orientation for the square knot

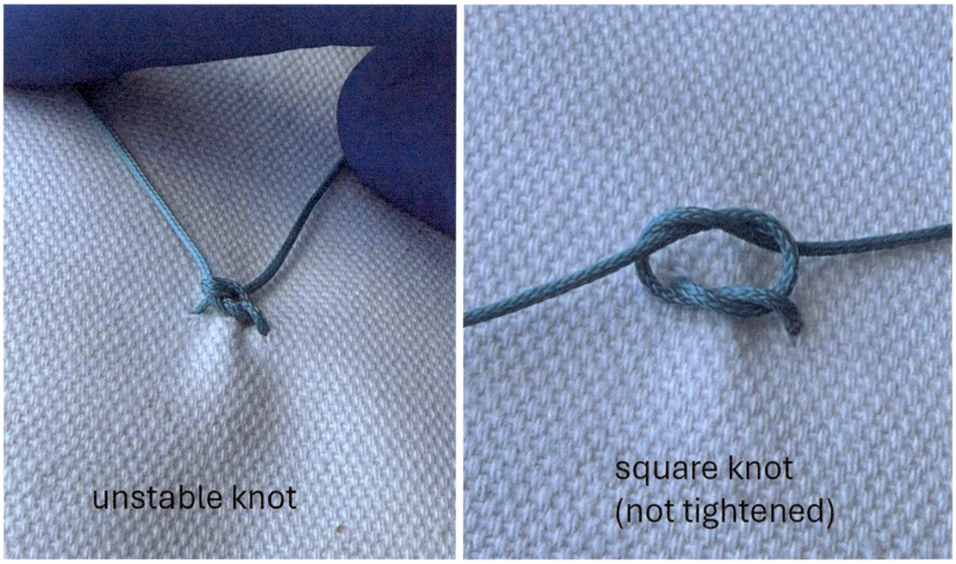

Fig. 8.20 Failure to cross the hands in the final step leads to an unstable knot instead of a true square knot

One-Handed Knot-Tying

In recent years, one-handed knot-tying has become possibly the most popular technique for tying knots. It is often favored by trainees because it tends to be faster than the two-handed knot and because it can be performed without setting the needle holder down.

The main disadvantage of one-handed tying is that there is almost always a tendency to "pull up" on the tissues much harder than when a two-handed knot is used (Fig. 8.21). If the tissues are sturdy, this may not matter. However, when the tissue is friable, there will be a tendency for the suture to tear through if it is pulled too hard. This is much more commonly observed with one-handed knots. The other disadvantage is that the one-handed technique is much harder to perform when the suture strands are relatively short (Fig. 8.22). This is difficult to show in picture form, but in general, it is much easier to tie short strands using a two-handed or an instrument tie technique.

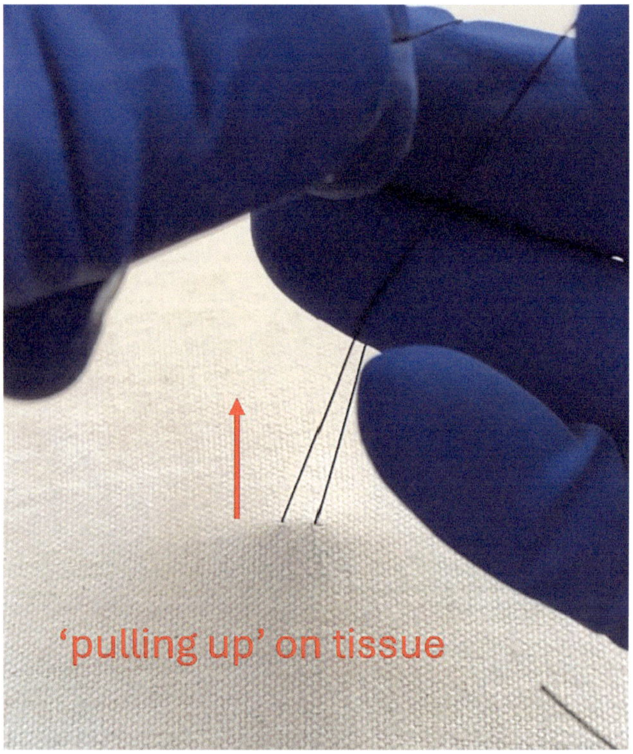

Fig. 8.21 Excessive "pulling up" on tissues is more common with one-handed knots

Starting Position

Most people prefer to tie one of the specific halves of the ONE-handed knot first, and to do this, a right-handed person will have to have the R strand start off on top (Fig. 8.23).

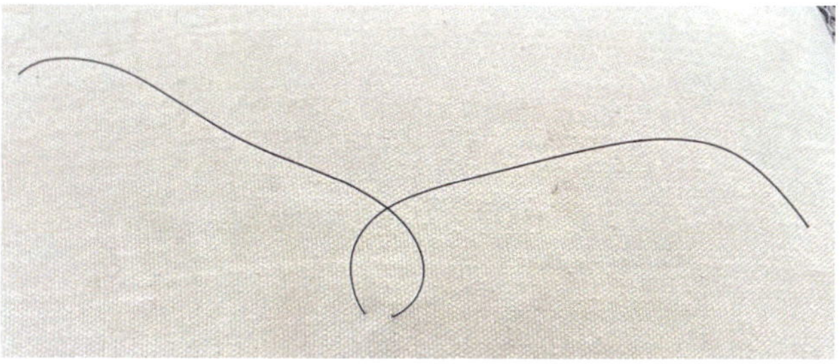

Fig. 8.22 When suture strands are short, they are much harder to tie using a one-handed technique. Two-handed tying or instrument tying is easier

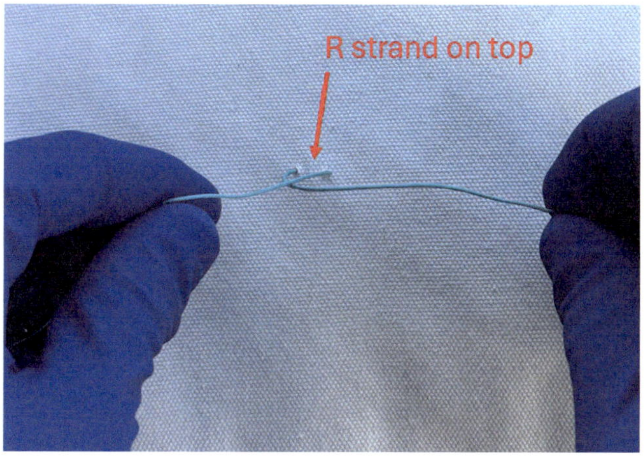

Fig. 8.23 Initial position of the one-handed knot. The R strand is on top

First Throw

Step 1: Use the R hand to grab the strand that it is holding between the thumb and index finger. Simultaneously, use the opposite edge of the R hand to apply tension to the strand (Fig. 8.24).

Step 2: Bring the strand in the L hand over to the lateral edge of the third finger of the R hand (Fig. 8.25). This action forms the X and the loop.

Step 3: Use the third finger to grab the strand being held in the R hand (Fig. 8.26).

Step 4: Pinch the strand between the third and fourth fingers (Fig. 8.27).

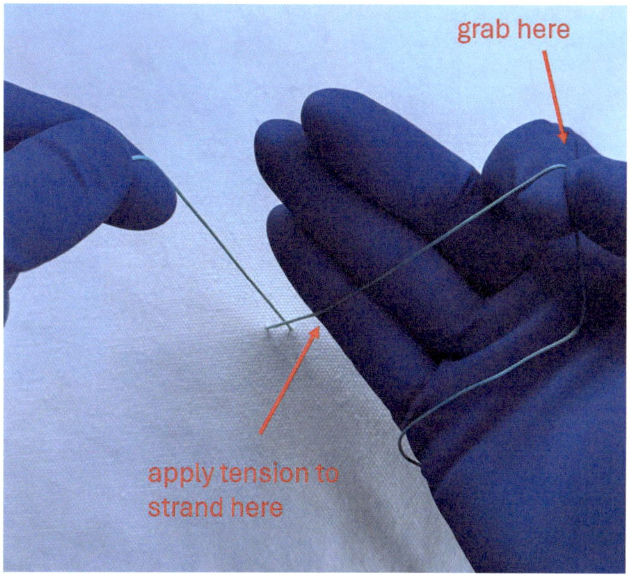

Fig. 8.24 The R strand is grabbed with the thumb and index finger, and the opposite edge of the hand is used to apply tension to the strand

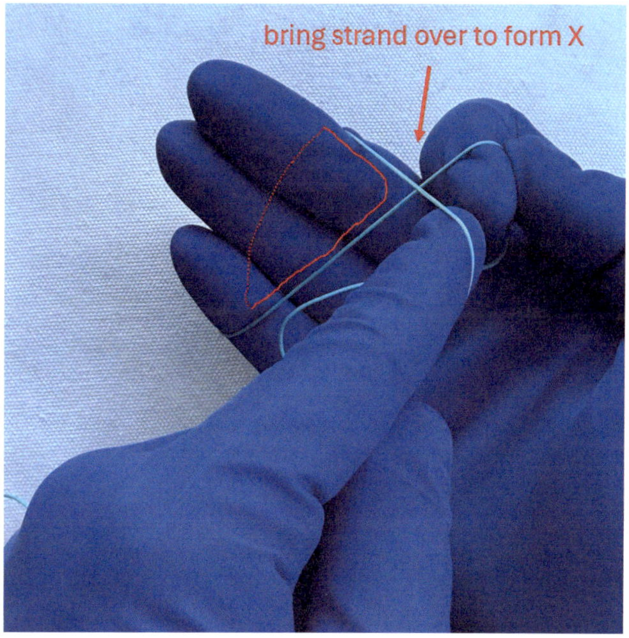

Fig. 8.25 The L strand is brought over the lateral edge of the R third finger. This creates the X and the loop

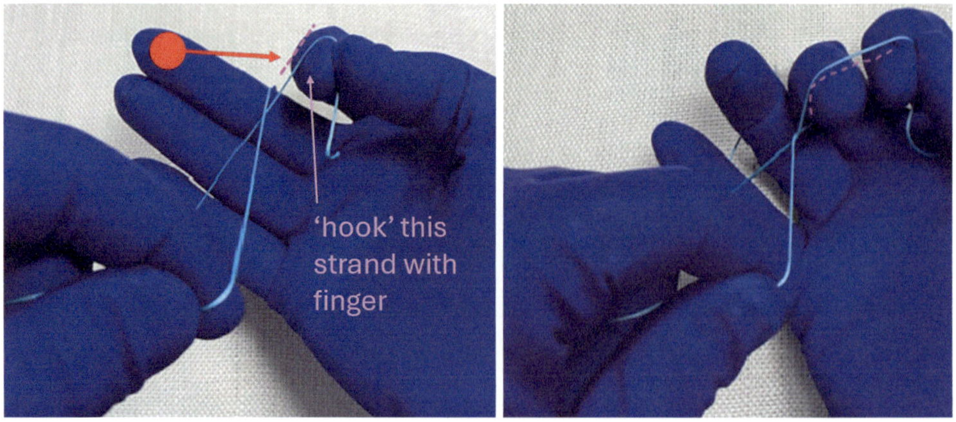

Fig. 8.26 The R third finger is used to grab the section of strand held by the thumb and index finger (pink line)

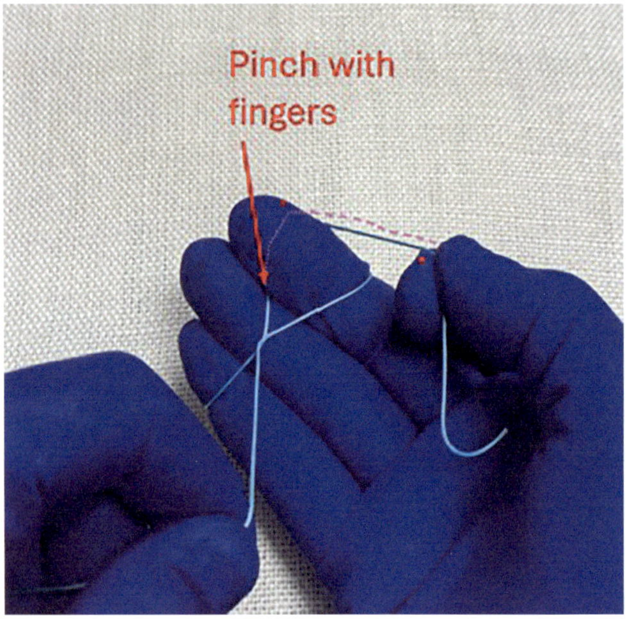

Fig. 8.27 This section of strand is pinched between the third and fourth fingers

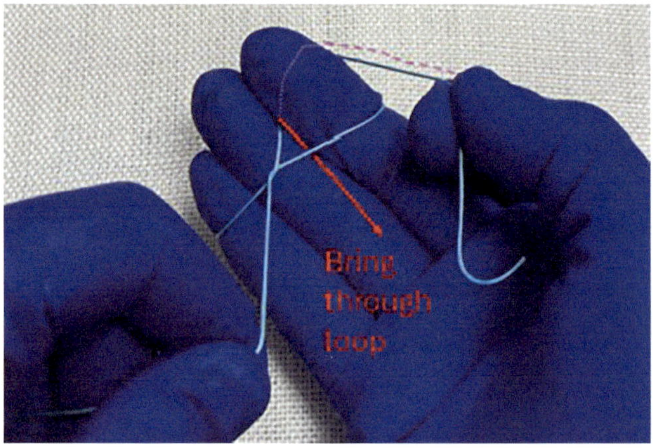

Fig. 8.28 The strand is brought through the loop using the pinched third and fourth fingers

Step 5: Bring this strand though the loop using your pinched fingers (Fig. 8.28).

Step 6: Each strand can now be pulled outward, setting down the first throw (Fig. 8.29).

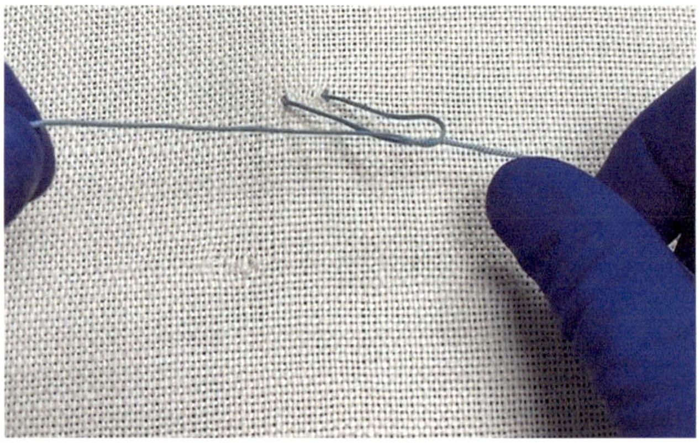

Fig. 8.29 Both strands are pulled outward, setting down the first throw

Second Throw

Step 1: Hold the R strand using the index finger and thumb. There should be a short gap in between the finger and thumb (Fig. 8.30). Keep the strand under a little tension.

Step 2: Bring the L strand over to create the loop and the X (Fig. 8.31).

Step 3: Bring the R index finger around the L strand and use the back of the index finger to grab the section of strand shown by the yellow dashed line (Fig. 8.32).

Step 4: Use the R index finger to bring the strand through the loop in a "flicking" motion (Fig. 8.33). This is often considered the most difficult part of the one-handed knot.

Step 5: The hands must now be crossed in order to set down the second throw as a square knot (Fig. 8.34). Failure to cross the hands will result in an unstable knot.

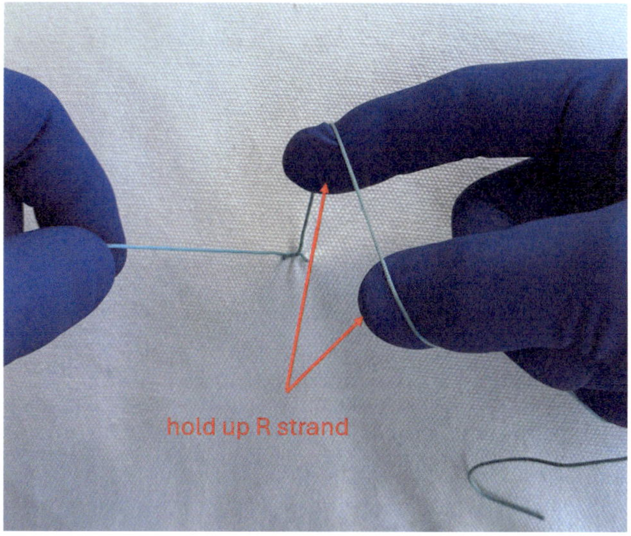

Fig. 8.30 Starting position of the second throw. The R strand is held up under tension using the index finger and thumb

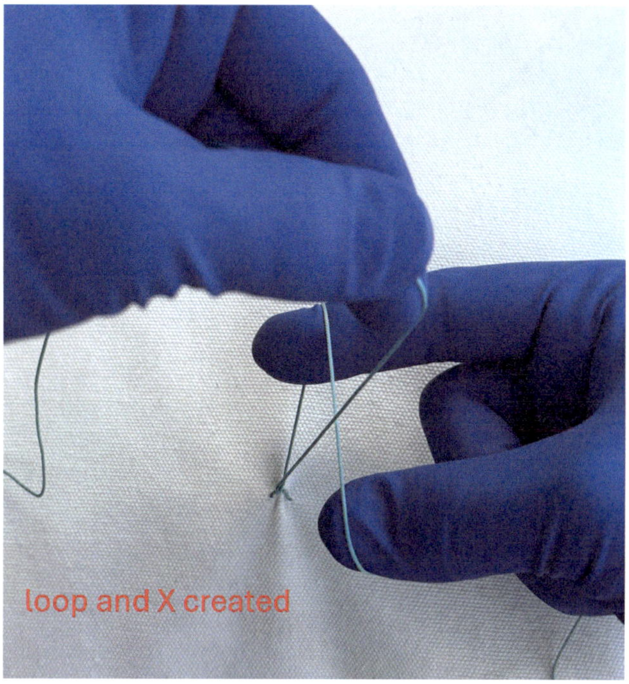

Fig. 8.31 The L strand is brought over to create the X and loop

Fig. 8.32 The R index finger is brought around the L strand and the back of the finger is used to grab the section of strand shown by the pink line

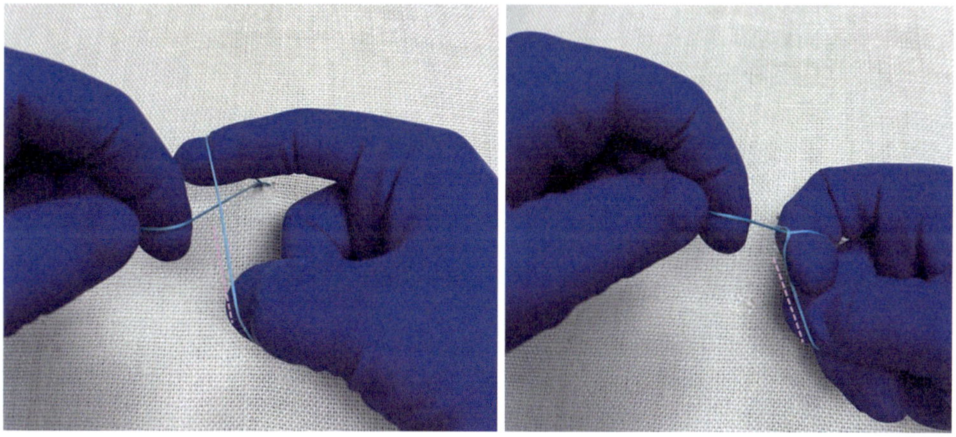

Fig. 8.33 The strand is brought through the loop in a flicking motion

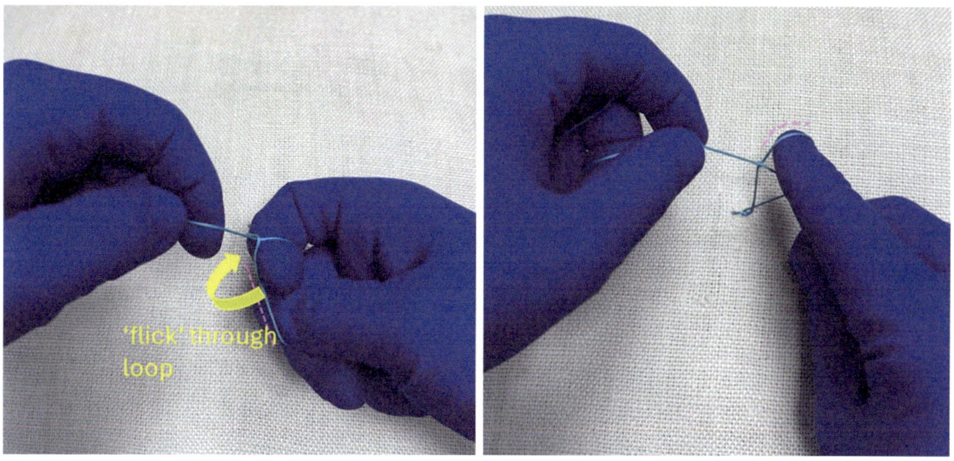

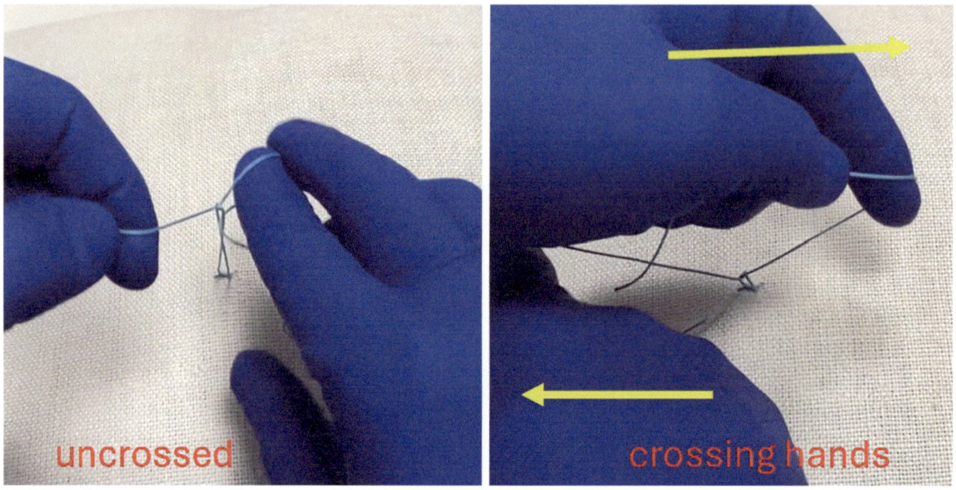

Fig. 8.34 The hands must be crossed to complete the square knot

Instrument Tying

Square knots may also be performed using an instrument-tying technique. In this technique, the needle holder is used to manipulate one of the strands instead of the hand.

One of the advantages of instrument tying is that is conserves suture material to a much greater extent than hand tying does, and typically, a single suture can be used to perform several knots, instead of needing a new suture for each knot (Fig. 8.35). The main disadvantage is that it is considerably more difficult to tie an instrument knot in a confined area, such as deep in a body cavity (Fig. 8.36). For this reason, instrument tying is typically only performed when the knot is on a well-exposed area on the surface of the body. In general, the technique of instrument tying is perhaps the easiest one to learn and remember, and many practitioners, particularly those who are not primarily in surgical specialties, tend to use this as their primary method of knot-tying.

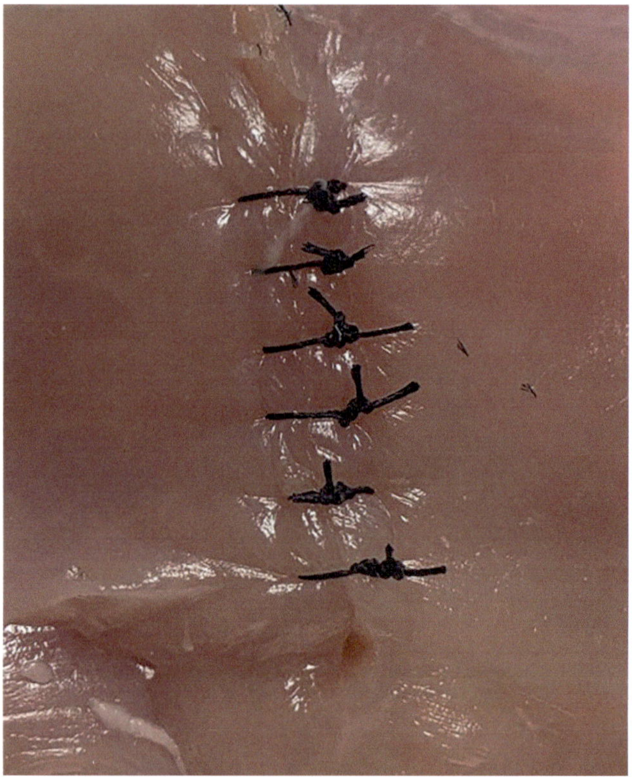

Fig. 8.35 Instrument tying is useful when suture material needs to be conserved. These knots were all tied using a single silk suture

Technique

Step 1: The suture is pulled though the tissue enough that the section of strand to be grabbed is relatively short (Fig. 8.37). Tying will be considerably more awkward if this is left too long.

Step 2: The suture is wrapped around the needle holder (Fig. 8.38).

Step 3: The short strand is grabbed with the needle holder (Fig. 8.39). It should be grabbed close to the end of the strand, but does not need to be at the very end.

Step 4: The strands are crossed and pulled outward to set down the first throw (Fig. 8.40).

Step 5: The suture is looped around the needle holder again (Fig. 8.41).

Step 6: The end of the strand is grabbed and pulled through the loop (Fig. 8.42).

Step 7: The strands are each pulled outward, setting down the second throw (Fig. 8.43).

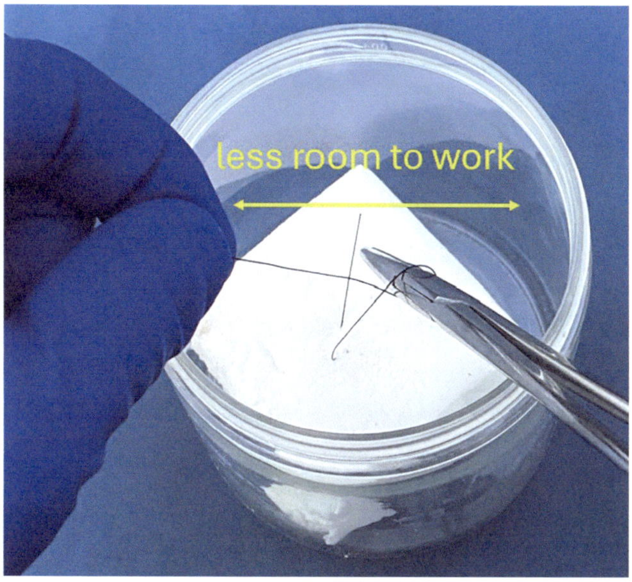

Fig. 8.36 Instrument tying is more difficult when tying deep in a body cavity or any time where there is limited space

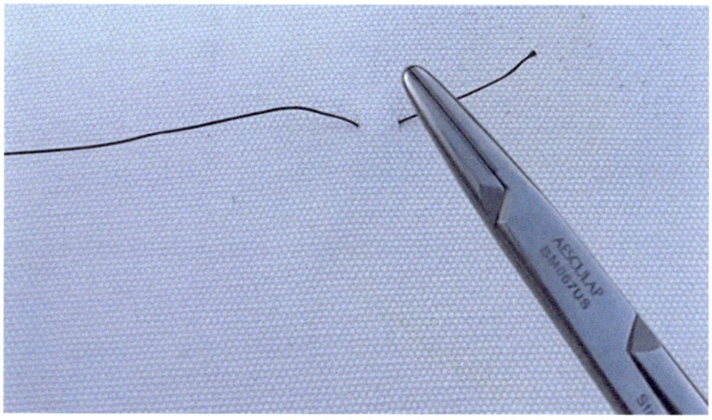

Fig. 8.37 Starting position for instrument tying. One strand should be left short

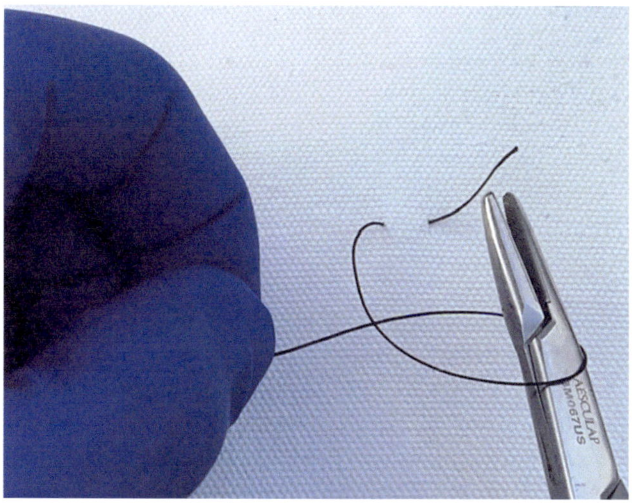

Fig. 8.38 The suture is wrapped around the needle holder, which forms the loop

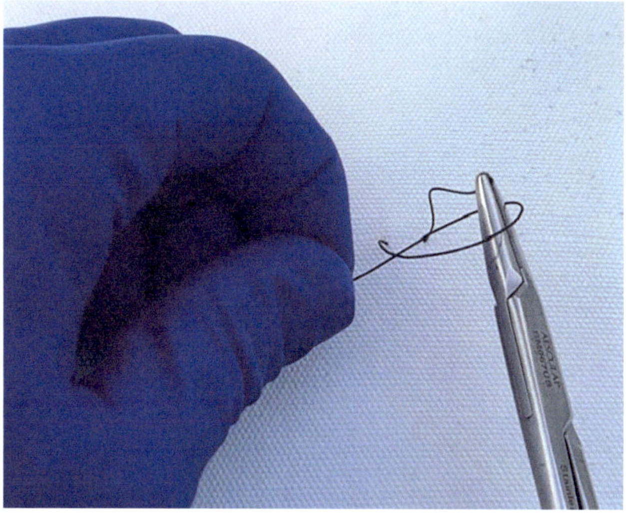

Fig. 8.39 The short strand is grabbed with the needle holder

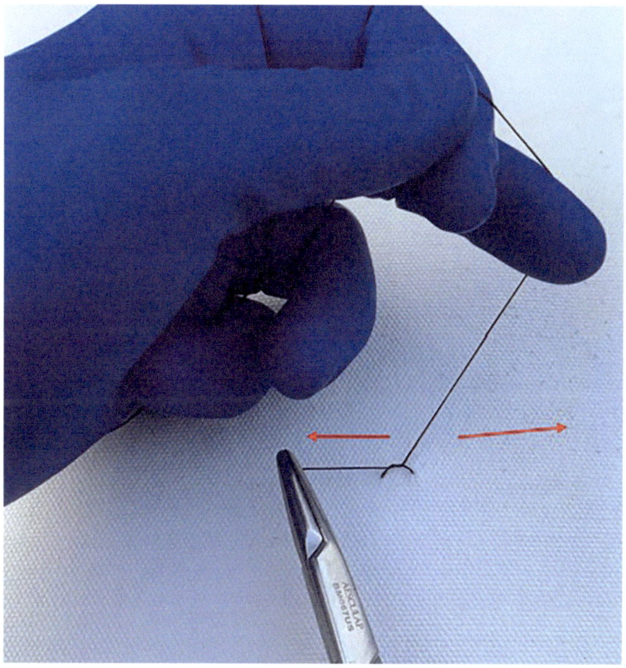

Fig. 8.40 The strands are crossed and pulled outward. This sets down the throw

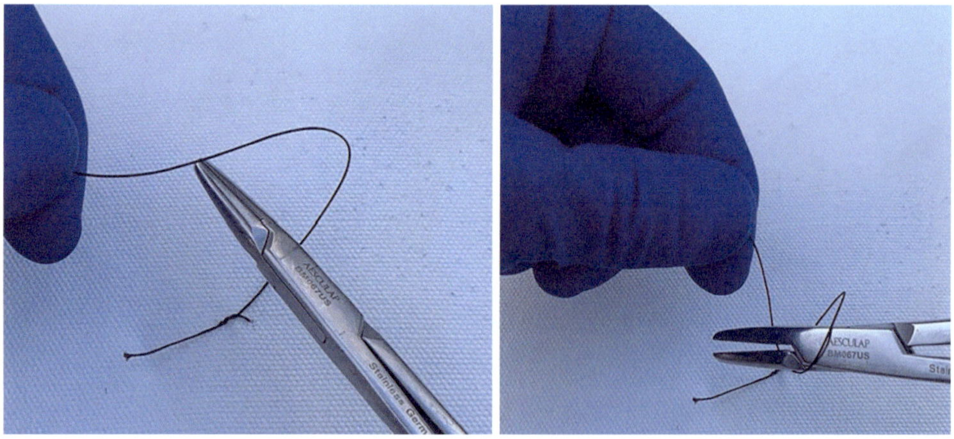

Fig. 8.41 The suture is wrapped around the needle holder again, forming a loop

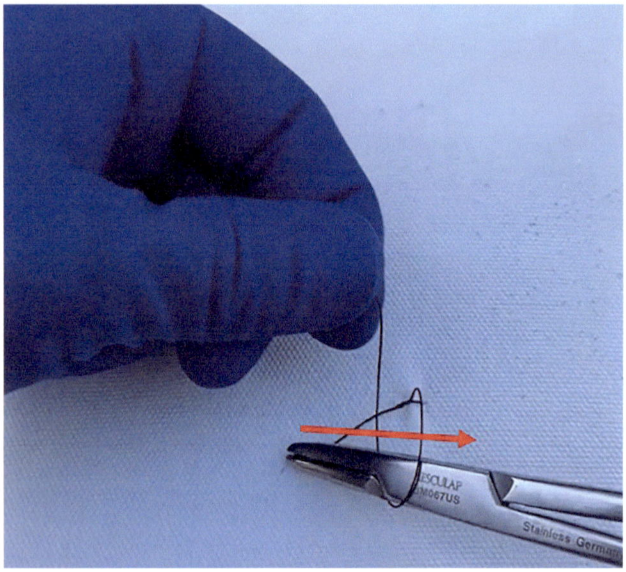

Fig. 8.42 The end of the strand is grabbed and pulled through the loop

Common Errors

Errors are often made at the beginning of an instrument tie when the strand is left too long. The surgeon is unable to reach the end of the suture and tends to grab the midportion of the strand instead (Fig. 8.44). When the strand is pulled through, it often becomes caught, leading to an improper knot (Fig. 8.45). In contrast, if the suture strand is left too short at the beginning, it will tend to pull out of the tissue when the suture is wrapped around the needle holder (Fig. 8.46).

Repeated use of the same suture to perform instrument-tied knots will eventually cause fraying of the end of the suture (Fig. 8.47). Care must be taken to limit the frayed portion of the strand to the section that will be cut off later.

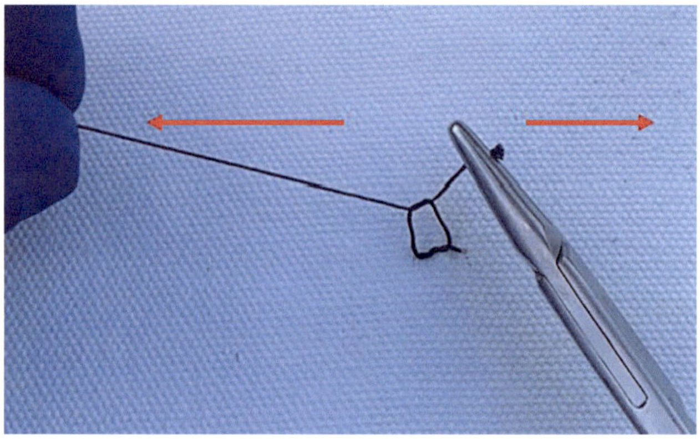

Fig. 8.43 Pulling the strands outward completes the second throw

Loosening of the First Throw

One extremely common issue in knot-tying is that when tissues are approximated, there is a tendency for the edges to retract and cause loosening of the first throw of a square knot. If subsequent throws of a square knot are placed on top of a loose first throw (as often happens), then the suture will be too loose and will need to be redone (Fig. 8.48). This problem is more common in monofilament sutures and sutures made of stiffer materials. Softer, braided sutures like silk or polyglactin 910 (Vicryl) are less prone to this, which is much of the reason for why they are popular. Two of the most common methods for correcting or preventing a loose first throw are the surgeon's knot and the slip knot.

Surgeon's Knot

The "surgeon's knot" involves performing the first throw of the knot twice, instead of once, as in a typical square knot. The additional throw increases the friction in the knot and

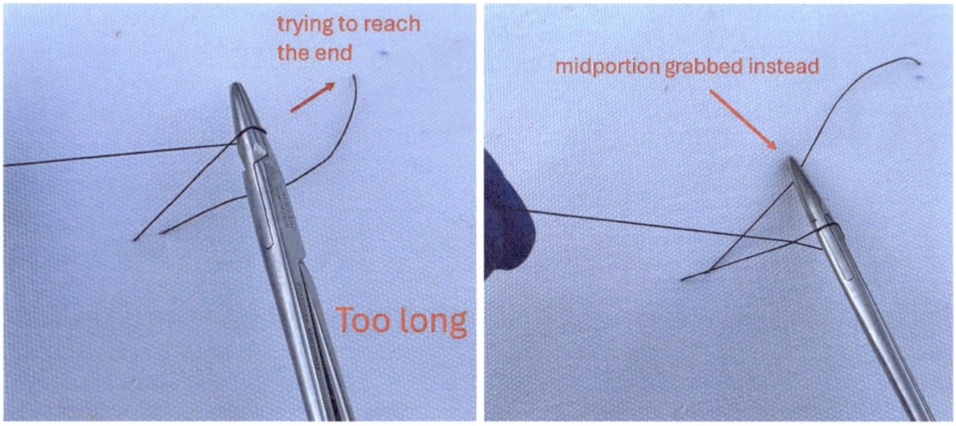

Fig. 8.44 Starting with a strand that is too long often leads to the midportion of the strand being grabbed instead

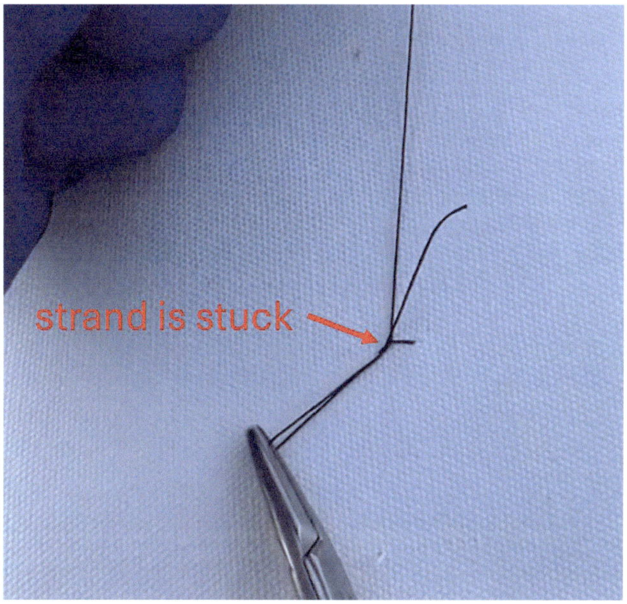

Fig. 8.45 Trying to pull through a strand that is too long has resulted in the strand becoming stuck

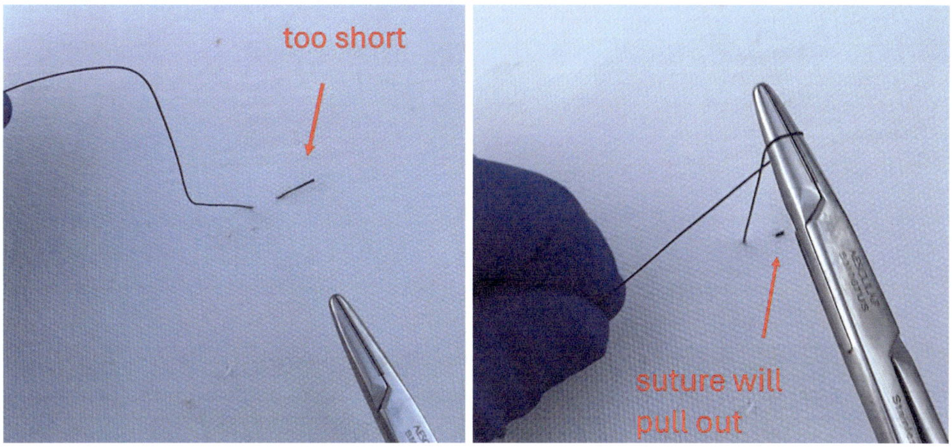

Fig. 8.46 Starting with a strand that is too short tends to cause the suture to pull out of the tissue

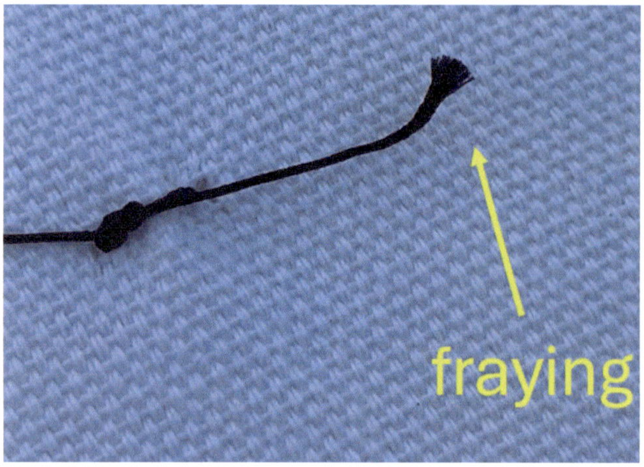

Fig. 8.47 Fraying from repeated use of the same suture for instrument tying

tends to keep the first throw in place while the second throw is performed (Fig. 8.49). Figure 8.50 shows the appearance of the suture after the first "throw" has been done twice. The throw is then set down, and the second throw may then be performed.

A surgeon's knot may also be done while instrument tying and is even more straightforward. On the first throw, the strand is wrapped around the needle holder twice, instead of just once (Fig. 8.51). The throw is set down, and the remainder of the knot is done in the usual manner.

It should be emphasized that performing the throw in the same direction twice should only be done on the first throw. All of the subsequent throws are done in the regular manner with single throws being executed in an alternating fashion. Stacking "surgeon's" throws on top of each other would lead to a bulky and less secure knot.

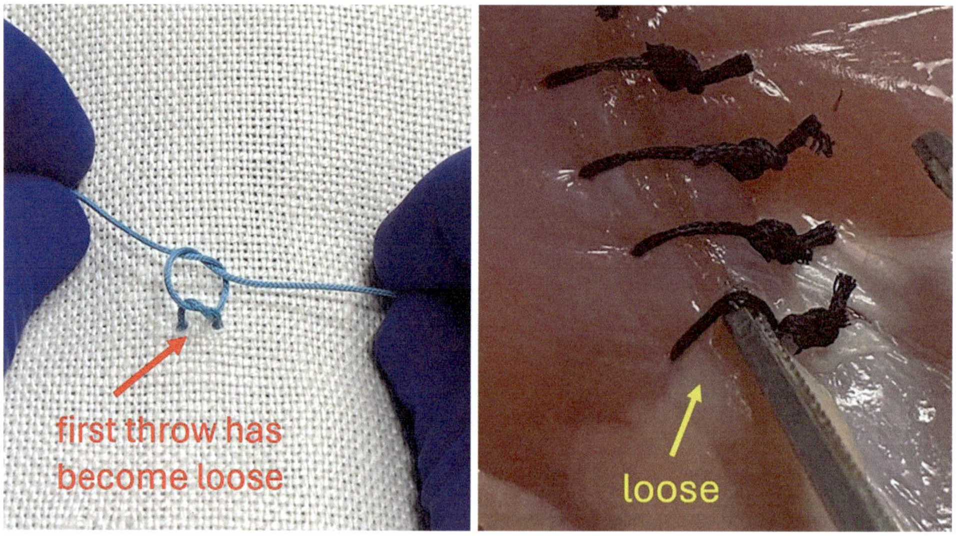

Fig. 8.48 If the second throw is tied on top of a loose first throw, then the entire knot will end up being loose

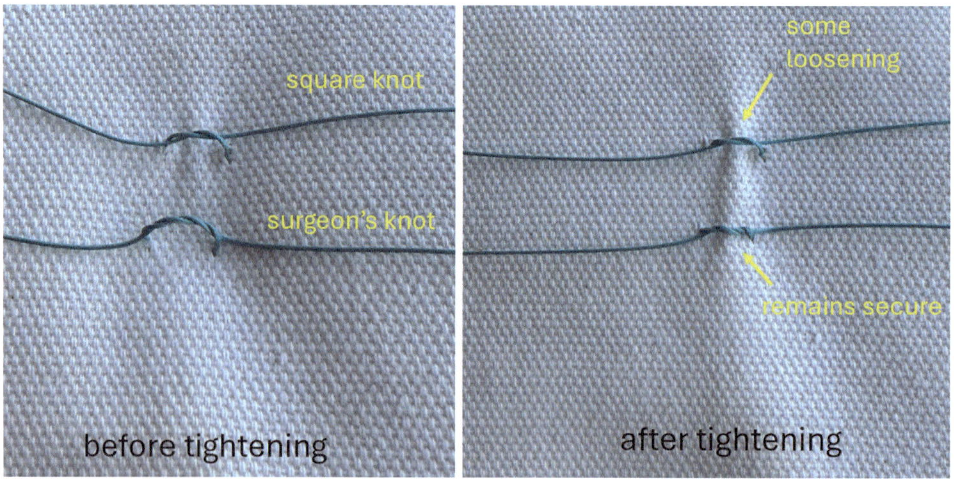

Fig. 8.49 The increased friction created in the first throw of the "surgeon's knot" tends to keep it in place

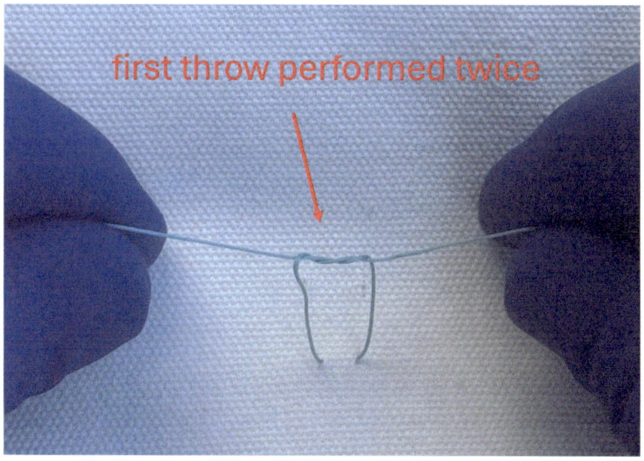

Fig. 8.50 The first throw of a surgeon's knot before it is set down

Slip Knot

The slip knot is perhaps an even more common method for preventing loosening of the first throw. To perform a slip knot, the first throw of a square knot is done in the usual manner and is set down. It will then usually loosen a bit. The second throw is then done in the same direction (the first "half" is performed again) instead of alternating to the opposite direction, as one would normally do. One of the strands is held almost straight up in the air, while the other one is set down (Fig. 8.52). Once this throw is set down, it will tend to stay in place without loosening (Fig. 8.53). The second throw can then be performed in the other direction, as would be normally done for a square knot. Only the first throw should be "slipped" in a slip knot; slip knots are not done on top of each other. Subsequent throws should all be done by alternating the first and second halves of the usual square knot. Slip knots are used very commonly in many surgical specialties, with some surgeons using them for a high percentage of knots overall.

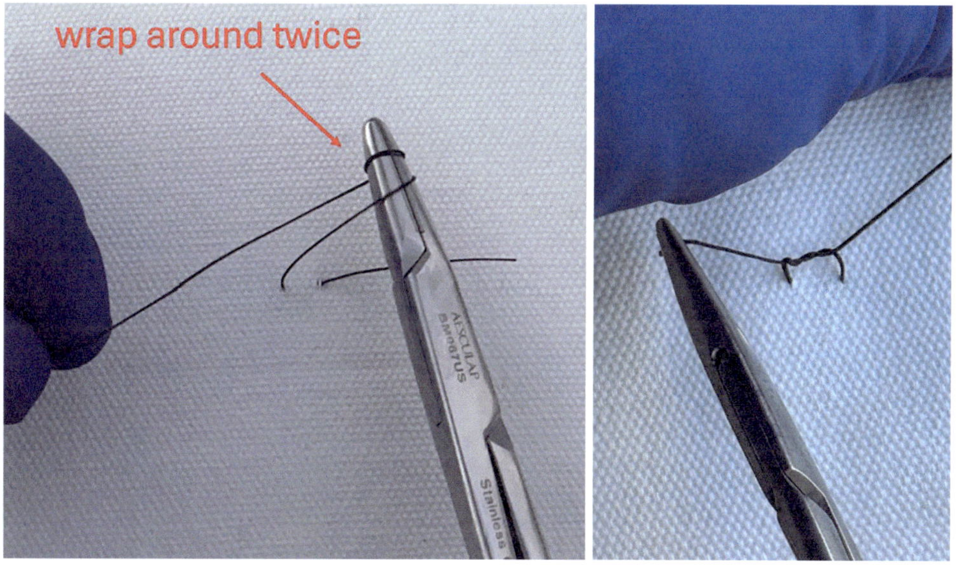

Fig. 8.51 To perform a surgeon's knot while instrument tying, the strand is passed around the needle holder twice

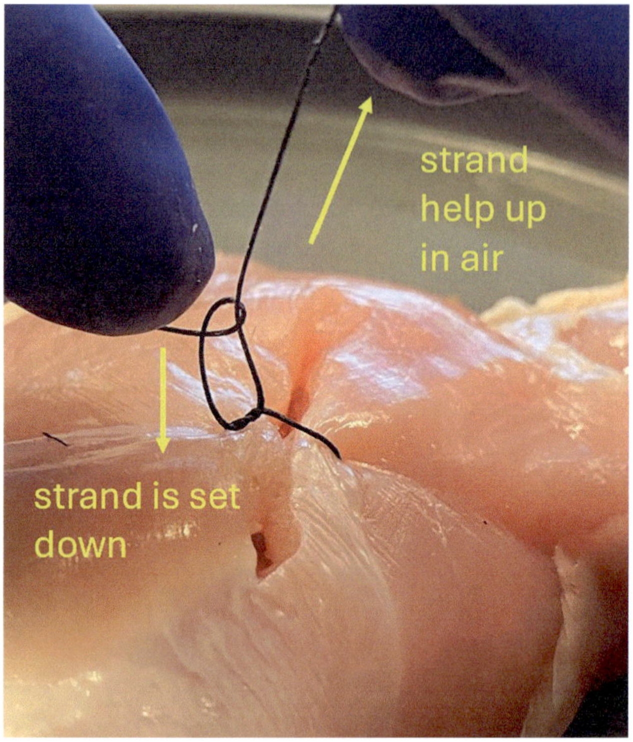

Fig. 8.52 While performing a slip knot, one hand is held nearly straight up in the air while the other strand is set down

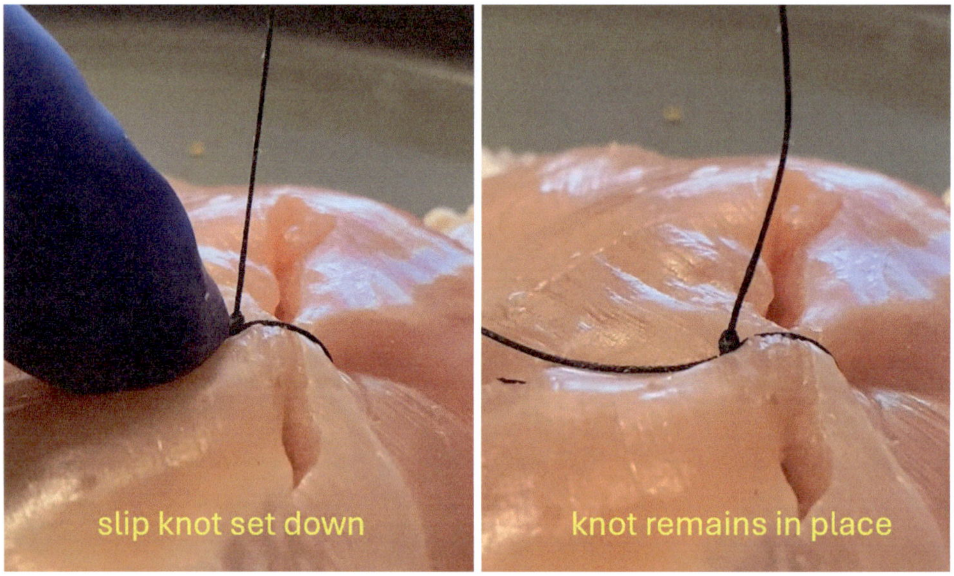

Fig. 8.53 The slip knot tends to stay in place, keeping the tissues approximated until the second throw is done

Gallbladder and Biliary Disease

9

Miranda Wood, Stephanie Martinez-Ugarte,
Renee Walker Green, and Lillian S. Kao

Anatomy and Physiology of the Gallbladder and Biliary System

- *Gallbladder:*
  The **gallbladder** is located in the right upper quadrant (RUQ) of the abdomen, on the inferior surface of the liver. Its primary function is to store and concentrate **bile acids** produced by the liver. When a fatty meal enters the duodenum, it activates *enteroendocrine cells* (I-cells), which release *cholecystokinin* (CCK) into the bloodstream [1]. CCK causes contraction of the gallbladder wall and relaxation of the **sphincter of Oddi**, leading to the release of stored bile from the gallbladder via the cystic duct. This drains via the **common bile duct** and eventually into the duodenum to aid in fat digestion.
- *Biliary Tree*
  The biliary tree is a system of tracts whose primary role is transporting bile acids produced in the liver to the duodenum. *Bile acids help break down and absorb fats, fat-soluble vitamins* (A, D, E, and K), *and other nutrients*. After a meal, partially digested proteins and fats enter the duodenum from the stomach and stimulate the release of **secretin** from the duodenum, which increases bile production and release. The biliary tree is commonly divided into ***intra*hepatic** (inside the liver) and ***extra*hepatic** (outside the liver) bile ducts. The extrahepatic biliary tree is formed by hepatic ducts (right and left), the common hepatic duct, the cystic duct, and the common bile duct (Fig. 9.1). After exiting the liver, the right and left hepatic ducts form the common hepatic duct. The cystic duct (from the gallbladder) joins the common hepatic duct and forms the common bile duct. The common bile duct passes through the pancreas, where the pancreatic duct joins, ultimately draining into the duodenum via the **ampulla of Vater**. *Most of the bile acid is reabsorbed in the terminal ileum* (80%) and colon (~15%), with only 5% of bile excreted into the stool. Bacteria in the intestine digest this bile and convert it to **stercobilinogen**, a brown pigment that gives a distinct brown color to stool [2].

M. Wood · S. Martinez-Ugarte · R. W. Green · L. S. Kao (✉)
Department of General Surgery, McGovern Medical School,
Houston, TX, USA
e-mail: Lillian.s.kao@uth.tmc.edu

S. Atallah, J. Dragoljevic (eds.), *Fundamentals of Surgery for Physician Assistants*,
https://doi.org/10.1007/978-3-032-21069-2_9

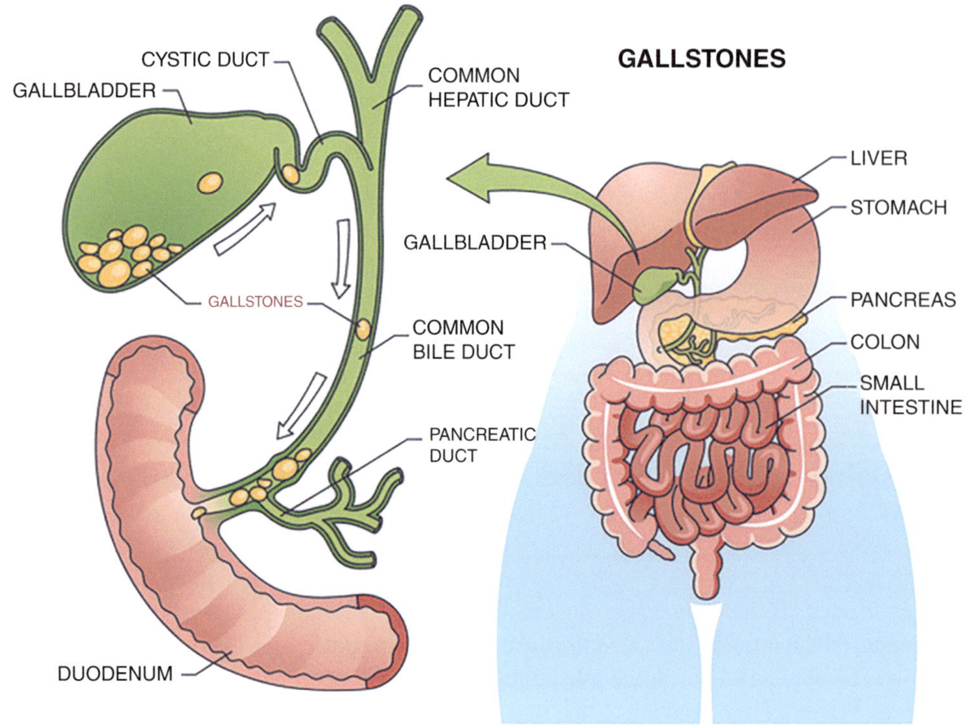

Fig. 9.1 The relevant biliary anatomy is depicted, which is extremely important to understand in relation to the disease states discussed in this chapter. Within the gallbladder, gallstones can exist without symptoms (*asymptomatic* cholelithiasis), or they can lead to conditions—most important of which are (**a**) *biliary colic* (*symptomatic* cholelithiasis) and (**b**) *acute cholecystitis*. Note that gallstones can also leave the gallbladder (arrows) where they can enter the common bile duct (CBD) and get stuck there causing pressure buildup and interfering with normal bile drainage into the duodenum. When gallstones get trapped in the CBD, or anywhere in the biliary tree, it is termed chole*docho*lithiasis (as opposed to cholelithiasis). Choledocholithiasis can then lead to more serious conditions, such as (**a**) *gallstone pancreatitis* and (**b**) *ascending cholangitis*. As a general rule, choledocholithiasis (CBD stones) are treated *primarily with ERCP*, while gallbladder disease (biliary colic, acute cholecystitis) *is treated surgically* (i.e., cholecystectomy)

Common Gallbladder and Biliary Disorders

- *Cholelithiasis (Gallstones)*
  Gallstones are pebble-like structures present in 10–15% of adults [3]. *The most common type of gallstones are* ***cholesterol stones,*** but there are also **pigmented stones** (black and brown). Cholesterol gallstones form due to an imbalance of the content of bile acids or due to the concentration of the bile acids within the gallbladder. Risk factors for cholesterol stones include *obesity, high-fat diet, older age, family history of gallstones, female gender, rapid weight loss, pregnancy, diabetes, and patients of Native American or Latin American descent* [4]. **Black pigmented stones** are common in hemolytic disorders due to excess levels of conjugated bilirubin excretion, such as in *sickle cell disease.* **Brown pigment stones** are usually tiny (<1 cm) and form due to *bacterial infection and bile stasis.* In the United States, brown-pigmented stones most often occur as primary bile duct stones due to biliary strictures [5]. However, in Asia, brown-pigmented stones are associated with stasis caused by parasite infections such as roundworms and liver flukes [5].

  Gallbladder disease related to gallstones is quite prevalent, and **750,000 cholecystectomies are performed annually in the United States alone**. Even though gallstones are common, *most patients remain* ***asymptomatic*** *from their gallstones throughout life and do not experience any symptoms.* Most gallstones are diagnosed incidentally in these patients due to imaging for other reasons. Studies report that about 80% of these patients will remain asymptomatic [6]; therefore, prophylactic cholecystectomy (removal of the gallbladder) is *not* recommended [6]. However, cholecystectomy should be considered in asymptomatic patients with *sickle cell disease and immunosuppressed patients (such as transplant patients) to prevent complications.*
- *Biliary Colic*
  Of all the patients with gallstones, about 3% of patients end up developing symptoms per year [7]. This happens because gallstones can cause *obstruction of the cystic*

duct. As the gallbladder contracts to release bile, the bile cannot be expelled due to the obstruction, causing distention of the gallbladder and abdominal pain. Patients will describe recurrent attacks with intervals of feeling well once the stone dislodges and stops obstructing the cystic duct.

Symptoms: The typical symptoms are RUQ pain or epigastric pain radiating to the back, nausea, and sometimes vomiting *after* a fatty meal. These episodes can last from 30 min up to 4 h. Pain after a meal is referred to as **post-prandial pain**, which is classic in patients with biliary colic. **Laboratories**, including white blood cell (WBC) count, alanine aminotransferase (ALT), aspartate aminotransferase (AST), and bilirubin, are normal in this patient population. **Imaging:** an abdominal ultrasound is the standard of care for diagnosis, which will demonstrate stones inside the gallbladder. **Treatment:** if the abdominal ultrasound is positive for stones and the patient has the classic symptoms of biliary colic, *elective* cholecystectomy is recommended (Fig. 9.2). While patients are waiting for surgery, it is recommended that they follow a low-fat diet and eat small meals to prevent attacks.

- *Acute Cholecystitis*

Acute cholecystitis *is associated with gallstones* in up to 95% of cases, with 5% occurring as acalculous cholecystitis (usually in critically ill patients). Acute cholecystitis often begins as an episode of biliary colic. However, the pain in acute cholecystitis **does not go away** and may persist for days. This process occurs due to an inflammatory process caused by a stone that obstructs the cystic duct and leads to gallbladder wall thickening (gallbladder wall >4 mm). **Symptoms:** The patient often presents with fever, anorexia, **unremitting RUQ pain**, nausea, and vomiting. **Murphy's sign**, an inspiratory pause with deep palpation in the RUQ, is characteristic of acute cholecystitis. On **laboratory** evaluation, patients may have an increased WBC count and a normal to mild increase in AST and ALT levels. Bilirubin levels should be normal. If bilirubin levels are elevated, specifically direct bilirubin, concerns about a stone obstructing the biliary tree should be raised. **Imaging**: on ultrasound, the gallbladder wall will be inflamed with **gallbladder wall thickening**, and often, **pericholecystic fluid** will be present. Focal tenderness over the gallbladder when compressed by the sono-

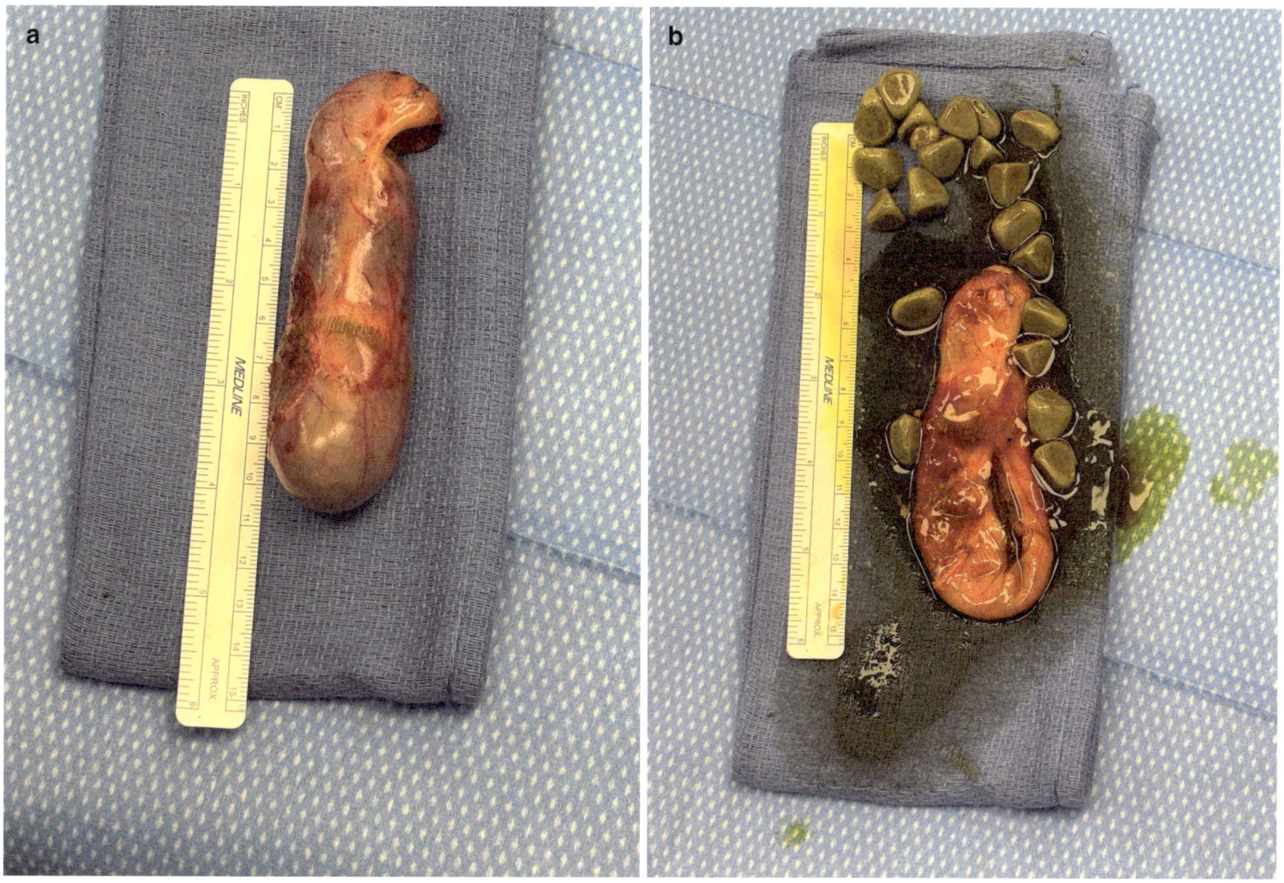

Fig. 9.2 (**a**) The gallbladder is a somewhat oval-shaped organ located beneath the right liver, and is connected via the cystic duct to the common bile duct. Its primary function is to store and concentrate bile produced by the liver, releasing it into the duodenum in response to cholecystokinin during digestion, particularly after fatty meals. The gallbladder wall is composed of mucosa, a muscular layer, and serosa, and its blood supply is via the cystic artery. Shown here is the resected, 10cm gallbladder in a patient who underwent cholecystectomy for biliary colic. (**b**) When opened, the specimen contains multiple gallstones, as shown. (photographs courtesy Harold Neyra, MD, with permission)

Table 9.1 Comparison between biliary colic and acute cholecystitis

Feature	Biliary colic	Acute cholecystitis
Definition	Transient obstruction of the cystic duct by a gallstone	Inflammation of the gallbladder, usually due to persistent cystic duct obstruction
Etiology	Gallstone temporarily lodged in the cystic duct	Gallstone impacted in cystic duct causing inflammation and infection of the gallbladder
Pain characteristics	Recurrent RUQ pain, often postprandial	**Persistent**, severe RUQ pain, shoulder or back
Pain duration	Transient (1–5 h typically)	>6 h, often lasting >12–24 h; pain does not go away
Associated symptoms	Possible nausea, vomiting, but not typical	Nausea, vomiting, fever, anorexia
Fever	Absent	Present (low-grade to moderate)
Murphy's sign	Usually negative	Positive (inspiratory arrest during RUQ palpation)
Leukocytosis	Usually normal	Elevated WBC count
Liver function tests (LFTs)	Typically normal	May be mildly elevated
Ultrasound findings	Gallstones, no wall thickening or pericholecystic fluid	Gallstones, gallbladder wall thickening, pericholecystic fluid, sonographic murphy's sign
HIDA scan (if performed)	Normal gallbladder filling	Non-visualization of gallbladder (due to cystic duct obstruction)
Treatment	Pain management, elective cholecystectomy	Hospitalization, IV fluids, antibiotics, urgent, or early cholecystectomy
Complications if untreated	Recurrent episodes; 10–20% risk of progression to acute cholecystitis	Empyema, gangrene, perforation, sepsis

graphic probe, or a *sonographic Murphy's sign,* also supports the diagnosis of acute cholecystitis. While ultrasound is the gold-standard imaging for gallbladder evaluation, it is not the most sensitive test. A **hepatobiliary iminodiacetic acid (HIDA)** test is approximately 94–96% sensitive, while the sensitivity of ultrasound is 80–81%. An HIDA scan is a nuclear medicine scan. Although it is more sensitive than ultrasound, its use is reserved for situations in which acute cholecystitis is suspected, but the ultrasound evaluation is limited, equivocal, or nondiagnostic. **Treatment:** Patients should receive fluid resuscitation, broad-spectrum antibiotics, a multimodal pain regimen, and *early* (within 72 h) cholecystectomy [8]. When inflammation is severe, bailout procedures have been proposed for the intraoperative management of acute cholecystitis. Examples of bailout strategies include placement of a surgical cholecystostomy tube or performance of a subtotal cholecystectomy, where only a small remnant of gallbladder is left behind, which may or may not be sutured closed.

The subtotal cholecystectomy is referred to as a fenestrating or reconstituting subtotal cholecystectomy if the remnant is left open or closed, respectively. While subtotal cholecystectomies are performed to reduce the risk of a bile duct injury, they are associated with a higher rate of postoperative bile leaks. If patients are too sick to undergo surgery, *they may be treated with antibiotics and biliary decompression* via *a cholecystectomy tube that can be placed by interventional radiology. Decompressing the gallbladder provides time for the patient to stabilize before surgery* [9]. Once the patient has recovered from the acute illness, cholangiography should be performed to evaluate the cystic duct's patency. If the cystic duct is patent, the cholecystostomy tube can be removed within 4 weeks (once the tract is mature). Elective cholecystectomy surgery can be scheduled within 6–8 weeks unless the patient is not medically clear or no stones are seen in the gallbladder. The differences between biliary colic and acute cholecystitis are delineated in Table 9.1.

- *Choledocholithiasis*

  It is estimated that approximately 10–20% of patients undergoing cholecystectomy also have common bile duct (CBD) stones. The medical term for stones within the CBD is **choledocholithiasis** (as illustrated in Fig. 9.1). The incidence of CBD stones increases with age, with 25% of patients >60 years who undergo cholecystectomy having CBD stones. Conversely, 5% of CBD stones are associated with no stones in the gallbladder. The most common mechanism of choledocholithiasis is the passage of stones from the gallbladder through the cystic duct and into the CBD [10–12]. However, gallstone formation can occur even after a patient has had a cholecystectomy. These are referred to as *primary duct stones*. They are generally composed of **pigmented calcium bilirubinate** and are usually the result of *biliary stasis.* Patients who have had a prior cholecystectomy can also have retained stones in the CBD, causing choledocholithiasis. **Symptoms**: Presentation is usually similar to cholelithiasis with RUQ pain, nausea, and vomiting. On **laboratory** evaluation, bilirubin, alkaline phosphatase, AST, and ALT are generally elevated. WBC counts can be elevated, *but the lack of this finding does not exclude choledocholithiasis.* It is also possible for lipase to be elevated, though this does not happen in every case. **Imaging:** Choledocholithiasis can occur with or without acute cholecystitis. *A dilated CBD on transabdominal ultrasound is suggestive of, but not specific for, choledocholithiasis.* A cutoff of 6 mm is often used to classify a duct as being dilated. However, this may change with advancing age or with a history of cholecystectomy. Patients >60 years old can have a CBD diameter of 6–8 mm. After cholecystectomy, the CBD diameter can be as large as 10 mm [13, 14]. In patients with a normal CBD diameter and with laboratory values concerning for choledocholithiasis, a **magnetic resonance cholangiopancreatogram (MRCP)** can be performed depending on availability. **Treatment:** If there is concern for cholangitis, the patient should be started immediately on broad-spectrum antibiotics and undergo emergent **endoscopic retrograde cholangiopancreatography (ERCP)** for biliary decompression. If ERCP is not possible (due to the patient being too sick or unstable), then percutaneous decompression of the gallbladder can be performed. If the patient is hemodynamically stable without concern for cholangitis, there are a few options for treatment depending on available expertise and patient preference. Patients may undergo ERCP followed by cholecystectomy, a cholecystectomy with intraoperative cholangiogram ± postoperative ERCP, or a cholecystectomy with a laparoscopic common bile duct exploration. For patients with primary or retained CBD stones who have previously had a cholecystectomy, ERCP is generally performed for stone removal. Bilirubin, AST/ALT, alkaline phosphatase, and lipase should be trended.

- *Cholangitis*
  Cholangitis is one of the *main complications of choledocholithiasis.* **Acute cholangitis** is an *ascending bacterial infection associated with partial or complete obstruction of the bile ducts.* Mechanical obstruction of the biliary flow allows ascending bacterial contamination from the gastrointestinal tract. Significant bacterial contamination and biliary obstruction are requisite for the development of cholangitis.

  Gallstones that enter into the CBD are the most common cause of obstruction in cholangitis. Other causes include primary sclerosing cholangitis, strictures, parasites, instrumentation of the ducts, indwelling stents, and partially obstructed biliary-enteric anastomosis. The most common causative organisms include *Escherichia coli*, *Klebsiella pneumoniae*, *Streptococcus faecalis*, *Enterobacter*, and *Bacteroides fragilis*. **Symptoms:** Classic symptoms of **"Charcot's Triad"** include *fever, epigastric and/or RUQ pain, and jaundice.* The addition of *shock* and *altered mental status* is known as "**Reynolds' Pentad**." **Laboratory evaluation**: elevated WBC and liver function tests support the diagnosis. **Imaging:** Abdominal imaging can be helpful; however, the initial diagnosis is made clinically. Ultrasound is beneficial to identify gallstones and dilated ducts. CT/MRCP can show pancreatic and periampullary masses and dilated ducts. **Treatment:** The initial treatment for cholangitis includes broad-spectrum IV antibiotics, fluid resuscitation, and rapid biliary decompression. Drainage of the biliary tree can be accomplished by *ERCP (first choice) or percutaneous drainage of the biliary system by interventional radiology.* If these services are not available, stabilized patients may need to be transferred to another hospital. Of note, *patients with cholangitis can deteriorate rapidly and may require intensive care unit monitoring and vasopressor (blood pressure) support.*
- *Gallstone Pancreatitis*
  Gallstones are associated with approximately 40–50% of all cases of pancreatitis in the United States. Gallstones in the *common bile duct* (not in the gallbladder) can provoke attacks of acute pancreatitis through *transient or persistent obstruction of the pancreatic duct by a stone passing through or impacting the ampulla* (refer to Fig. 9.1). The exact mechanism by which obstruction of the pancreatic duct leads to pancreatitis is unclear. However, it may be related to increased ductal pressures causing leakage of pancreatic enzymes into the glandular tissue. **Symptoms:** Patients presenting with pancreatitis have abdominal pain (most commonly in the RUQ or epigastrium) or back pain with or without nausea and vomiting. **Laboratory evaluation:** This will reveal *lipase elevation* with and sometimes elevated amylase. If gallstones obstruct the biliary tree during diagnosis, liver transaminases and bilirubin may also be elevated. **Imaging:** Evaluation of the biliary tree with ultrasound is essential to confirm the presence of gallstones, as there may be other etiologies for the acute pancreatitis. Computed tomography (CT) may be used to diagnose more severe forms of pancreatitis, and *MRCP can assist in the identification of a retained CBD stone* (because MRCP is much better at imaging the biliary tree than ultrasound). **Treatment:** The initial management of gallstone pancreatitis is *supportive (i.e., non-operative)*, including admission for *bowel rest, IV hydration, and pain control.* Antibiotics are not indicated in the absence of signs of infected pancreatic necrosis. When gallstones or sludge are present in the gallbladder, and the pancreatitis is mild and self-limited, a cholecystectomy with intraoperative cholangiogram is indicated as soon as the pancreatitis has clinically resolved. *It is strongly recommended that cholecystectomy be performed during the same admission whenever possible due to the high rate of recurrence and increased morbidity of subsequent attacks of pancreatitis.* If obstructing CBD gallstones are present, *ERCP with sphincterotomy and stone extraction may be necessary.* The long-term outcome of patients with gallstone pancreatitis is related to its severity with localized morbidity, including pancreatic necrosis, splenic vein thrombosis with gastric varices, hemorrhagic pancreatitis, and pancreatic abscess formation. Systemic morbidity can result in multisystem organ failure or even death.

- *Bile Duct Injuries*
  The majority of **bile duct injuries** are due to *surgical trauma* (transection, thermal, traction, and ischemic injuries caused during surgery), with a small proportion due to external abdominal trauma. Bile duct injuries can result in bile leaks and strictures. Understanding the anatomy and anatomical variations of the liver and biliary tract can help prevent these injuries. The identification of the "**critical view of safety**" during a cholecystectomy (clearance of fat and fibrous tissue from the *hepatocystic triangle*, the lower one-third of the gallbladder is separated from the liver to expose the *cystic plate*, and only two structures are seen entering the gallbladder) and intraoperative cholangiography have been shown to reduce bile duct injuries [15, 16]. **Symptoms:** Patients with bile duct injuries resulting in strictures or those with retained gallstones may present within days or weeks from their index operation with recurrent RUQ pain, resulting in *obstructive jaundice* and even cholangitis, depending on the location of the obstruction and/or retained stone. However, patients with **bile leaks** usually present with *abdominal distention, bloating, pain, and mild jaundice from the biliary ascites.* **Laboratories**: Elevated bilirubin and serum alkaline phosphatase will reflect biliary obstruction and cholestasis. Patients with biliary ascites may also present with leukocytosis. **Imaging:** Ultrasounds and CT scans can identify fluid collections caused by bile leaks (termed **bilomas**). However, ERCP can help in the diagnosis and **treatment** of bile leaks, biliary strictures, and noncircumferential bile duct injuries amenable to endoscopic treatment by placement of a common bile duct stent or sphincterotomy for the treatment of retained gallstones. Nonetheless, circumferential transection of the common bile duct requires surgical repair with a *Roux-en-Y hepaticojejunostomy* reconstruction (a connection is made between the hepatic duct and jejunum). Management of a bile duct injury may benefit from consultation with a hepatobiliary surgeon and/or transfer to a higher level of care.
- *Cholangiocarcinoma (Biliary Cancer)*
  Cholangiocarcinomas have a prevalence of 0.01–0.46%, accounting for approximately 3% of all gastrointestinal malignancies. They can be located intrahepatic (10% of cases), perihilar (40% of cases), or extrahepatic biliary tree (50% of cases) [17]. **Symptoms** are usually due to *biliary obstruction* by the tumor and include jaundice, clay colored stools, dark urine, and pruritus. Other symptoms that can be seen include fever, weight loss, and abdominal pain. *Intrahepatic* cholangiocarcinomas instead usually have a history of dull RUQ pain, weight loss, and elevated alkaline phosphatase. Some patients with intrahepatic cholangiocarcinomas can be asymptomatic. **Laboratory evaluation:** Patients with extrahepatic cholangiocarcinoma generally have labs consistent with biliary obstruction including elevated bilirubin and alkaline phosphatase, with a mild to moderate increase in AST and ALT. Patients with intrahepatic cholangiocarcinoma often exhibit elevated alkaline phosphatase levels; however, in most cases, their bilirubin remains within the normal range or is only mildly elevated. All patients suspected of cholangiocarcinoma should have *tumor markers* (**CA 19-9**, **CEA**, and **AFP**) checked. **Imaging:** Often, patients with cholangiocarcinoma have undergone a RUQ ultrasound for the jaundice workup. However, in a patient suspected of cholangiocarcinoma who has not undergone imaging, an *MRCP is often the initial test of choice.* ERCP and endoscopic ultrasound are essential for diagnosis and management. **Treatment:** If a patient presents with a distal biliary tree obstruction, an ERCP may be performed to relieve the obstruction. Otherwise, the patient will require an oncologic workup to determine resectability and treatment strategy.

Special Populations

- *Pregnant Patients*
  Gallstones are one of the leading non-obstetric indications for surgery in pregnant patients. *They are more common in pregnant patients compared to nonpregnant patients* [18]. Gallstones occur in approximately 6–8% of pregnant individuals. However, only around 1% have reported incidence of gallstone-related disease. As in nonpregnant patients, gallstone disease is split into *biliary colic*, *acute cholecystitis*, and *choledocholithiasis.* Risk factors for gallstone formation during pregnancy include prior history of gallstones, obesity, and multiparity. **Symptoms, laboratories and imaging studies** are generally similar to those of nonpregnant patients (see previous sections above). **Treatment:** Treatment of gallstone disease in pregnant patients varies depending on the severity of the disease, center availability, and patient preference. For patients with uncomplicated biliary colic, diet modification and pain control are appropriate treatments. Patients can opt for elective cholecystectomy after the initial postpartum period. For patients with complicated disease as well as uncontrollable or recurrent pain, a cholecystectomy may be performed. **This is safe during the entirety of pregnancy**. For patients with *choledocholithiasis,* decompression may be performed with **ERCP**. If the patient is unstable or there is concern for cholangitis, the patient *should undergo emergent decompression with ERCP, and broad-spectrum antibiotics should be started immediately. Obstetricians should be consulted* regarding perioperative fetal heart rate monitoring and in case of a need for an emergent cesarean section.

- *Patients Post Bariatric Procedures*
  Rapid weight loss after bariatric surgery *increases the risk of developing gallstones. Therefore, patients with gallstones or a prior history of biliary colic may benefit from prophylactic cholecystectomy at the time of* ***bariatric surgery***. For those patients who did not have a cholecystectomy and developed acute cholecystitis after bariatric surgery, their symptoms, workup, and treatment are similar to those without bariatric surgery. However, patients who underwent a Roux-en-Y gastric bypass for weight loss and develop choledocholithiasis may require special procedures (such as a laparoscopic-assisted trans-gastric rendezvous procedure or an endoscopic ultrasound-directed transgastric ERCP) to access and clear their pancreaticobiliary system. The standard ERCP scope cannot reach the ampulla due to the extended distance between the gastric pouch and biliary system created by the Roux-en-Y gastric bypass.
- *Post-cholecystectomy Syndrome (PCS):*
  The term **post-cholecystectomy syndrome** refers to the persistence or new development of gastrointestinal symptoms after cholecystectomy, which can be due to biliary disease or a misdiagnosis. **Symptoms:** The presenting symptoms are usually abdominal pain, dyspepsia, nausea, and diarrhea. *For many patients, the symptoms improve with dietary modifications and symptom control.* In this instance, they are thought to be caused by changes to the biliary anatomy after cholecystectomy, such as increased CBD pressure. **Laboratories**: Patients with abnormal liver functions, jaundice, and/or cholangitis should undergo **imaging** with transabdominal ultrasounds, **HIDA scans**, or MRCP to explain the symptoms. Choledocholithiasis, biliary stricture, and chronic pancreatitis are the most common causes of biliary PCS. *Sphincter of Oddi dysmotility* (which may be treated with endoscopic sphincterotomy), long cystic duct remnant, and neuromas have also been identified as a cause of PCS but are rare. Patients with no source of biliary pathology to explain their symptoms may benefit from further workup with an esophagogastroduodenoscopy to rule out acid reflux and hiatal hernias, which may cause similar symptoms. The **treatment** of PCS depends on the underlying cause.

Cholecystectomy and Postoperative Care

Minimally invasive laparoscopic cholecystectomy is the standard-of-care operation to treat gallbladder disease with conversion rates of less than 5% [19]. **Robotic cholecystectomy** has become more prevalent in recent years; however, it has been shown to have a longer operative time without any significant decrease in intraoperative complications or length of hospital stay [20]. Outcomes might change over time as surgeons become more comfortable using the robotic platform. This operation is usually done via four small incisions, which are sutured closed at the end, and often, a dermal adhesive (or skin glue) is applied. Rarely is a drain left in place in the gallbladder fossa to assess for postoperative bleeding or bile leak. The drain should be evaluated daily and removed once these concerns are ruled out.

Postoperative care: Patients can shower 24 h after surgery with soap and water but avoid scrubbing the incision, removing the skin glue (which will fall off on its own), and submerging in water. The patient should be sent home on a multimodal pain regimen, *minimizing opioid medications as much as possible.* Patients should be advised to keep their incisions *clean and dry.* In addition, patients should maintain a low-fat diet after surgery since they might experience mild diarrhea as their bodies try to adjust. They should also avoid strenuous activity for at least 6 weeks to prevent incisional hernias. For follow-up, patients should be seen in the clinic within 2 weeks of their surgery to review their gallbladder pathology report and assess postoperative recovery or sooner if any concerning signs arise.
Concerning Signs:

- Severe abdominal pain not controlled with oral medications (right shoulder pain is common after laparoscopic cholecystectomy due to pneumatic insufflation)
- Fever, chills
- Jaundice
- Vomiting, inability to tolerate any food or liquids
- Hypotension
- Tachycardia

If a patient exhibits any of these symptoms, *refer them to the nearest emergency room for immediate evaluation.*

References

1. Geoghegan J, Pappas TN. Clinical uses of gut peptides. Ann Surg. 1997;225:145–54. [PubMed: 9065291].
2. Haisley KR, Hunter JG. Gallbladder and the extrahepatic biliary system. In: Brunicardi F, Andersen DK, Billiar TR, Dunn DL, Kao LS, Hunter JG, Matthews JB, Pollock RE. eds. Schwartz's principles of surgery, 11e. McGraw-Hill Education; 2019. https://accesssurgery.mhmedical.com/content.aspx?bookid=2576&sectionid=216215815. Accessed 11 Mar 2025.
3. Stinton LM, Shaffer EA. Epidemiology of gallbladder disease: cholelithiasis and cancer. Gut Liver. 2012;6(2):172–87. [PubMed: 22570746].
4. Nakeeb A, Comuzzie AG, Martin L, et al. Gallstones: genetics versus environment. Ann Surg. 2002;235:842–9. [PubMed: 12035041].

5. Stewart L, Oesterle AL, Erdan I, et al. Pathogenesis of pigment gallstones in Western societies: the central role of bacteria. J Gastrointest Surg. 2002;6:891–903. [PubMed: 12504229].
6. Sakorafas GH, Milingos D, Peros G. Asymptomatic cholelithiasis: is cholecystectomy really needed? A critical reappraisal 15 years after the introduction of laparoscopic cholecystectomy. Dig Dis Sci. 2007;52:1313–25. [PubMed: 17390223].
7. Attili AF, De Santis A, Capri R, et al. The natural history of gallstones: the GREPCO experience. The GREPCO Group. Hepatology. 1995;21:655–60. [PubMed: 7875663].
8. Kao LS, Ball CG, Chaudhury PK, for Members of the Evidence Based Reviews in Surgery Group. Evidence-based reviews in surgery: early cholecystectomy for Cholecystitis. Ann Surg. 2018;268(6):940–2. https://doi.org/10.1097/SLA.0000000000002867.
9. Cherng N, Witkowski E, Sneider EB, et al. Use of cholecystostomy tubes in the management of patients with primary diagnosis of acute cholecystitis. J Am Chem Soc. 2012;214:196–201.
10. Aleknaite A, Simutis G, Stanaitis J, Valantinas J, Strupas K. Risk assessment of choledocholithiasis prior to laparoscopic cholecystectomy and its management options. United European Gastroenterol J. 2018;6:428–38.
11. Collins C, Maguire D, Ireland A, Fitzgerald E, O'Sullivan GC. A prospective study of common bile duct calculi in patients undergoing laparoscopic cholecystectomy: natural history of choledocholithiasis revisited. Ann Surg. 2004;239(1):28–33.
12. Harmon LA, Shah PK, McIntyre RC, Schulick RD. Choledocholithiasis. In: surgical decision making. 6th ed; 2020. p. 146–7. https://doi.org/10.1016/B978-0-323-52524-4.00154-9.
13. Prat F, Meduri B, Ducot B, Chiche R, Salimbeni-Bartolini R, Pelletier G. Prediction of common bile duct stones by noninvasive tests. Ann Surg. 1999;229(3):362–8. https://doi.org/10.1097/00000658-199903000-00009. PMID: 10077048; PMCID: PMC1191701.
14. Abboud PA, Malet PF, Berlin JA, Staroscik R, Cabana MD, Clarke JR, Shea JA, Schwartz JS, Williams SV. Predictors of common bile duct stones prior to cholecystectomy: a meta-analysis. Gastrointest Endosc. 1996;44(4):450–5. https://doi.org/10.1016/s0016-5107(96)70098-6.
15. Strasberg SM, Brunt LM. Rationale and use of the critical view of safety in laparoscopic cholecystectomy. J Am Coll Surg. 2010;211(1):132–8.
16. Traverso LW. Intraoperative cholangiography reduces bile duct injury during cholecystectomy. Surg Endosc. 2006;20(10):1659–61.
17. De Oliveira ML, Cunningham SC, Cameron JL, Kamangar F, Winter JM, Lillemoe KD, Choti MA, Yeo CJ, Schulick RD. Cholangiocarcinoma: thirty-one-year experience with 564 patients at a single institution. Ann Surg. 2007;245(5):755–62. https://doi.org/10.1097/01.sla.0000251366.62632.d3. PMID: 17457168; PMCID: PMC1877058.
18. Balinskaite V, Bottle A, Sodhi V, Rivers A, Bennett PR, Brett SJ, Aylin P. The risk of adverse pregnancy outcomes following nonobstetric surgery during pregnancy: estimates from a retrospective cohort study of 6.5 million pregnancies. Ann Surg. 2017;266(2):260–6. https://doi.org/10.1097/SLA.0000000000001976.
19. Sakpal SV, Bindra SS, Chamberlain RS. Laparoscopic cholecystectomy conversion rates two decades later. JSLS. 2010;14(4):476–83. [PubMed: 21605512].
20. Delgado LM, Pompeu BF, Pasqualotto E, et al. Robotic-assisted cholecystectomy versus conventional laparoscopic cholecystectomy for benign gallbladder disease: a systematic review and meta-analysis. J Robot Surg. 2024;18(1):242. https://doi.org/10.1007/s11701-024-01989-5.

Pancreatic Disease

10

Sreelakshmi Reddivari, David W. McFadden,
and Martha Grajewski

Introduction

The pancreas has been a feared and avoided organ for surgeons for centuries. We were once taught that the pancreas was "put in the back of the abdomen to keep us [surgeons] from disturbing it." One textbook from the early 1980s compared the pancreas to a skunk, in that one should either "kill it or leave it alone." On the surgical service, one the most popular expressions of surgeons you will hear to this day is: *"don't mess with the pancreas!"* Fortunately, pancreatic diseases today are approached surgically with safety and efficacy, despite its unique challenges for surgical intervention.

The **pancreas** (Fig. 10.1) is an essential digestive organ responsible for both *endocrine and exocrine function*. Pancreatic disorders, including acute and chronic pancreatitis, pancreatic cysts, and pancreatic cancer, are challenging to manage and associated with a large burden on healthcare resources. Acute pancreatitis is one of the most common reasons for emergency hospitalizations. Chronic pancreatitis is associated with poor quality of life, largely related to abdominal pain, and associated exocrine insufficiency. Pancreatic cysts are increasingly detected on cross-sectional abdominal imaging examinations. Although only small numbers and specific types of pancreatic cysts can progress to pancreatic cancer, diagnostic uncertainty can elicit undesirable anxiety from patients and treating physicians. Finally, the incidence of pancreatic adenocarcinoma is increasing, and it is the seventh leading cause of cancer-related death in the industrialized world and the third most common in the United States. This chapter will guide Physician Assistants (PAs) in understanding the principles of pancreatic disease and surgery, including indications, procedures, complications, and postoperative management.

PAs play a critical role in pancreatic surgery, contributing to:

- Preoperative patient assessment and education: Conducting comprehensive patient evaluations, explaining surgical procedures, and addressing patient concerns.
- Surgical preparation: Assisting with patient positioning, prepping the surgical field, and ensuring necessary supplies are available.
- Intraoperative assistance: Holding retractors, handling instruments, and providing suction as needed.
- Postoperative care: Monitoring vital signs, managing pain, and assessing for complications.
- Patient education and discharge planning: Educating patients about postoperative recovery, medication management, and follow-up care.

S. Reddivari · D. W. McFadden (✉) · M. Grajewski
Department of Surgery, University of Connecticut, University of Connecticut Health Center, Farmington, CT, USA
e-mail: reddivari@uchc.edu; dmcfadden@uchc.edu; grajewski@uchc.edu

S. Atallah, J. Dragoljevic (eds.), *Fundamentals of Surgery for Physician Assistants*,
https://doi.org/10.1007/978-3-032-21069-2_10

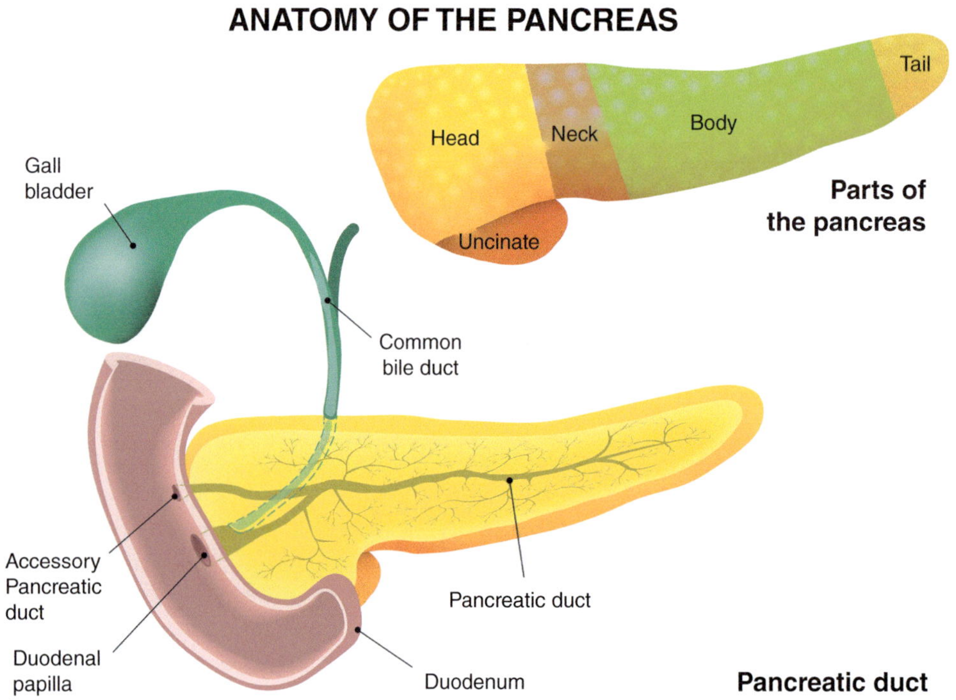

Fig. 10.1 The pancreas is a *retroperitoneal organ* located in the upper abdomen, extending transversely from the duodenum on the right to the spleen on the left. It is divided into the head, neck, body, uncinate process, and tail. The head lies within the curve of the duodenum, while the tail approaches the splenic hilum; the tail of the pancreas is often described as "tickling the spleen" due to its close proximity. The pancreas is closely related to the *posterior* abdominal wall, with the body and tail lying anterior to the first and second lumbar vertebrae. This anatomic relationship explains why inflammation of the pancreas *often causes pain that radiates to the back,* as the retroperitoneal location allows inflammatory processes to irritate the celiac plexus and adjacent somatic nerves, resulting in referred pain patterns. The pancreas has both exocrine (acinar and ductal cells producing digestive enzymes) and endocrine (islets of Langerhans producing hormones) functions. In pancreatitis, premature activation of digestive enzymes within the acinar cells leads to autodigestion, local inflammation, and peripancreatic fat necrosis. The resulting inflammatory response and tissue injury stimulate visceral afferent fibers, producing severe epigastric pain that may radiate to the back, chest, or flanks

Pancreas Anatomy and Physiology

The pancreas is a digestive organ that measures about 6 inches in length while weighing approximately 3.5 ounces. It lies retroperitoneally, crossing the bodies of the L1 and L2 vertebrae on the posterior abdominal wall. The head lies upon the inferior vena cava and right renal vein and is surrounded by the C loop of the duodenum. The tail of the pancreas extends up into the splenic hilum (Fig. 10.2). A small tongue of tissue named the uncinate process lies behind the superior mesenteric vessels as they rise from the retroperitoneum. The body of the pancreas continues from the neck and passes over the aorta. The anterior surface of the pancreatic body is covered with peritoneum while the posterior surface is retroperitoneal. Posteriorly, the pancreatic body is in contact with the aorta, the superior mesenteric artery (SMA), the left adrenal gland, the left kidney, and renal vessels**. This close proximity to critical structures is the reason the pancreas must be handled with extreme care**.

The pancreas has a rich vascular supply from both the celiac and the superior mesenteric arteries. The venous drainage is into the portal vein via the splenic vein. The common bile duct passes through a posterior groove in the head of the pancreas adjacent to the duodenum. This anatomy makes the common bile duct susceptible to obstruction by a pancreatic head mass, resulting in jaundice. The main pancreatic duct (duct of Wirsung) courses along the gland from the tail to the head and joins the common bile duct before entering the duodenum at the ampulla of Vater. The accessory pancreatic duct (duct of Santorini) enters the duodenum 2–2.5 cm proximal to the ampulla of Vater (Fig. 10.3).

The pancreas functionally and anatomically consists of two main parts: The exocrine component is the larger, approximately 80%, and produces pancreatic enzymes that are secreted into the main pancreatic duct. The main pancreatic duct carrying the pancreatic secretions joins the bile duct to form the hepatopancreatic ampulla, or ampulla of Vater,

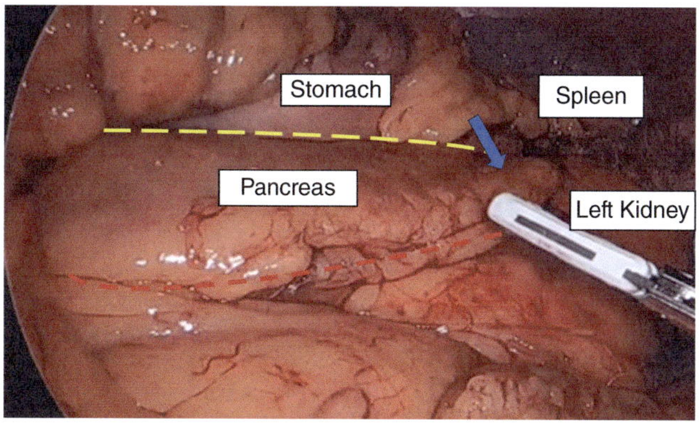

Fig. 10.2 Intraoperative view during a laparoscopic procedure in which the transverse colon and splenic flexure [of the colon] have been moved out of the way to expose the retroperitoneum. The body and tail of the pancreas are shown, with the inferior (red dashed line) and superior border (yellow dashed line) denoted. Note the close proximity to other organs, including the greater curvature of the stomach, the left kidney (which is surrounded by *Gerota's fascia*); also note the proximity of the tail of the pancreas (blue arrow) to the splenic hilum. As you start out in surgery, many things look the same and while at first the pancreas may seem just like "yellow fat" that blends in with other tissue, with experience you will learn to tell the difference

which opens into the descending portion of the duodenum. The sphincter of Oddi around the ampulla controls bile and pancreatic juice flows through the ampulla and inhibits reflux of duodenal substances into the ducts.

Digestive enzymes include amylase that breaks down carbohydrates, lipase that processes fats, and proteases that cleave proteins into amino acids. The smaller endocrine portion of the pancreas consists of tiny clusters of cells called islets of Langerhans. The islets of Langerhans contain beta cells, which produce insulin. The islets also contain alpha cells, which produce glucagon, delta cells (somatostatin), and F cells (pancreatic polypeptide). Daily pancreatic output consists of a clear, alkaline solution of 1–2 liters containing digestive enzymes. Secretion is hormonally stimulated by secretin and cholecystokinin (CCK) and by parasympathetic vagal discharge.

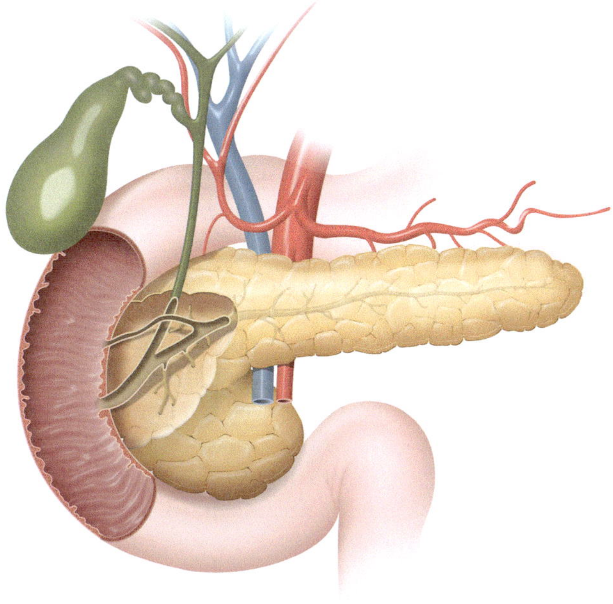

Fig. 10.3 The pancreas is a retroperitoneal organ that lies posterior to the stomach and is *closely related and attached to the duodenum* on its right side. The head of the pancreas is nestled within the C-loop of the duodenum, while the body and tail extend toward the spleen. The **common bile duct (CBD)** descends posterior to the first part of the duodenum and then courses *through or behind the head of the pancreas*, where it joins the main pancreatic duct (**duct of Wirsung**). These two ducts typically unite to form a short common channel before draining into the second portion of the duodenum at the **ampulla of Vater**, regulated by the **sphincter of Oddi.** The gallbladder is located under the liver and stores bile, which is delivered via the **cystic duct** to the CBD. The anatomical proximity of the CBD, pancreatic duct, and duodenum means that obstruction (e.g., by **gallstones**) at or near the ampulla of Vater can block both bile and pancreatic juice outflow, leading to ***biliary (gallstone) pancreatitis***. *This shared drainage explains why gallstones or tumors can cause both jaundice and pancreatitis, and why pain may radiate to the back due to retroperitoneal inflammation and neural irritation*

Pancreatic Diseases

Acute Pancreatitis

Acute pancreatitis is a pancreatic inflammatory condition of variable severity. Fortunately, 80–90% of patients develop mild or moderately severe disease without associated organ failure, while the remaining patients develop severe disease, which carries an approximate 20% mortality rate. Acute pancreatitis is responsible for over 250,000 hospitalizations per year in the United States and is the most common inpatient primary gastrointestinal diagnosis. The median length of stay is 4 days and an overall low mortality of 1–2%. The estimated cost annually approaches $3 billion. Hospitalization rates increase with age and are higher among blacks and males. Acute pancreatitis management comprises supportive care, attending to the underlying causes, and averting complications. Depending on local culture, patients with acute pancreatitis may be admitted to internal medicine or hospitalist services, with surgery frequently playing a consulting role.

There are many causes of acute pancreatitis; ***gallstones and alcohol account for 80–90% of cases in the United States***. Gallstones continue to be the leading cause, with alcohol second. Acute pancreatitis also occurs in 5–10% of patients following endoscopic retrograde cholangiopancreatography (ERCP). Hypertriglyceridemia is the cause of acute pancreatitis in 1–4% of cases with serum triglyceride levels usually greater than 1000 mg/dL. Although often mentioned, less than 2% of cases of acute pancreatitis are drug-related.

Symptoms and Signs

In acute pancreatitis, patients exhibit sudden epigastric or upper abdominal pain, with nausea and vomiting. The revised Atlanta criteria state that the diagnosis can be made if two of the following three criteria are met:

- **Upper abdominal pain, *frequently radiating to the back.***
- **Threefold increase in amylase or lipase.**
- **Radiographic evidence of acute pancreatitis.**

Physical examination findings are variable depending on the severity of the disease, but may include tachycardia, fever, hypotension, severe abdominal tenderness with guarding, and abdominal distention. If an abdominal mass is found, it usually represents a swollen pancreas (phlegmon) or, later in the process, a pseudocyst or abscess. Rarely, **bluish discoloration is present in the flank (*Grey Turner sign*)** or **periumbilical area (*Cullen sign*)**, indicating hemorrhagic pancreatitis with retroperitoneal bleeding. Other acute upper abdominal conditions including acute cholecystitis, penetrating or perforated duodenal ulcer, proximal small bowel obstruction, acute appendicitis, and mesenteric infarction must always be seriously considered in the differential diagnosis.

Laboratory and Imaging

The combination of clinical assessment and laboratory tests will aid in diagnosis of acute pancreatitis and assess the severity of the disease. Patients usually have a moderate leukocytosis, and the hematocrit may be elevated from dehydration or low from retroperitoneal blood loss in hemorrhagic pancreatitis.

Liver function tests will usually show increased transaminases (3× normal) if gallstones are the cause. The serum amylase concentration elevates to greater than three times normal within 8 hours after onset and remains elevated for several days. The magnitude of hyperamylasemia is not correlative with disease severity. Elevated amylase levels may occur in other acute abdominal conditions, such as gangrenous cholecystitis, small bowel obstruction, mesenteric infarction, and perforated ulcer. *Elevated serum lipase* is detectable early and for several days after the acute attack and *is more specific for pancreatitis*. Acute pancreatitis with normal serum amylase may occur in hyperlipidemia or chronic ("burned out") pancreatitis.

On initial presentation a comprehensive metabolic panel is obtained. Magnesium and phosphorous should be assessed as well. Additional biomarkers that are valuable are c-reactive protein level, procalcitonin, and interleukins (IL). However, their lack of rapid availability limits their use (Table 10.1).

Imaging Studies

Plain abdominal films, although frequently bypassed for cross-sectional imaging, are abnormal in two-thirds of cases, but relatively nonspecific. One common finding is isolated

Table 10.1 Indications for laboratory and radiologic testing in pancreatitis

Indication	Test
General	Complete blood count,
Etiology (if suspected *gallstone pancreatitis*)	Comprehensive metabolic panel, *Lipase and amylase level.*
Etiology (if suspected hypertriglyceridemia)	Ultrasonography (*Right upper quadrant ultrasound*)
	Contrast-enhanced computed tomography (CT scan)
	Alkaline phosphatase level,
	Bilirubin level,
	Magnetic resonance cholangiography (MRCP); ERCP (may be therapeutic to clear stones out of the bile duct)
	Triglyceride level,
	Arterial blood gas,
	Calcium level,
	C-reactive protein level, LDH urinalysis

dilation of a segment of bowel ("sentinel loop") consisting of jejunum, transverse colon, or duodenum adjacent to the pancreas. Gas distending the right colon that abruptly stops in the mid or left transverse colon (colon cutoff sign) is due to colonic spasm adjacent to the pancreatic inflammation. Glandular calcifications may be evident, signifying chronic pancreatitis. Chest films may reveal pleural effusion, often on the left side. Radiopaque gallstones will be apparent on plain x-rays; however, only 15% of gallstones are radioopaque.

Ultrasound may be precluded by the inclination to perform computed tomography (CT) scanning study early on but in the presence of hyperamylasemia is usually the first radiologic imaging ordered. In a patient with mild pancreatitis, an ultrasound that confirms gallstones is all that may be needed initially, diagnostically. Many authors recommend initial CT scanning only if the patient is severely ill. However, a ***CT scan is the "gold" standard for diagnostic imaging***; it is often performed with a special pancreas protocol that is designed to image the pancreas. It plays a major role to establish disease severity by assessing the inflammatory process and complications, such as *pancreatic abscess and pancreatic necrosis*. Therefore, a CT scan should be **strongly considered**, especially in patients with severe abdominal pain and clinical suspicion, for complications of pancreatitis. The accuracy of contrast-enhanced CT for the diagnosis of pancreatic complications is 95%. A CT scan must be performed in patients with severe diseases with little to no improvement after 3–4 days of conservative therapy. CT findings may show normal appearing pancreas, pancreatic phlegmon, pancreatic phlegmon with extension to adjacent extrapancreatic spaces, pancreatic necrosis, pancreatic pseudocyst, or abscess.

An MRI (magnetic resonance imaging) is comparable to a CT scan in providing information about the severity of acute pancreatitis. The MRI study is capable of diagnosing with 92% specificity in severe pancreatitis. An MRI can be advantageous over a CT for evaluation of pancreatic duct and pancreatitis associated fluid collection, along with a more accurate detection of stones in the common bile duct (CBD). Using an MRI is particularly beneficial for patients where IV contrast is contraindicated and with renal insufficiency. The only significant disadvantage of the MRI is seen in patients with claustrophobia. Its cost and availability preclude MRI currently as a first-line imaging.

The severity of pancreatitis is classified into mild, moderate severe, and severe, based upon the involvement of organ failure on the revised 2012 Atlanta classification system. Organ failure is defined as shock (SBP <90 mm Hg), renal failure, pulmonary insufficiency, or gastrointestinal bleeding. Similarly, acute pancreatitis is classified morphologically into two subtypes: interstitial edematous pancreatitis (80–85% of cases) and necrotizing pancreatitis (20% of cases). Acute inflammation, edema of the pancreatic parenchyma, and peripancreatic tissues in the CT scan are defined as interstitial edematous pancreatitis. Progression of the interstitial edematous pancreatitis leads to pancreatic or peripancreatic tissue death, also known as **necrotizing pancreatitis**.

Prognostic scores to assess the patient with acute pancreatitis include **APACHE II score** (acute physiology and chronic health evaluation II). This score is based on the age and the pre-existing organ insufficiencies and uses 12 variables to reflect the severity of the disease. The **BISAP** (bedside index of severity of acute pancreatitis) provides a quick and reliable score. It is used during the first 24 hours of admission. A score > 3 indicates increased risk of death (Tables 10.2 and 10.3).

Fluid Collections in Severe Pancreatitis

Historically, all peripancreatic fluid collections were referred to as pancreatic pseudocysts. The discrepancy in the nomenclature along with the high-quality diagnostic imaging and

Table 10.2 Clinical use of BISAP vs. APACHE II in acute pancreatitis

Feature	BISAP score	APACHE II score
Initial risk stratification	Used within 24 hours to identify patients at risk for severe disease or death	Used on ICU admission to stratify overall severity of illness
Score thresholds for action	Score ≥ 3 suggests severe pancreatitisScore 0–1: low risk	Score ≥ 8 indicates high risk for complications and mortality
Guides level of care	High BISAP (≥3): Consider ICU monitoring or step-up in care	Higher scores justify ICU admission or aggressive monitoring
Imaging decisions	High score may prompt early CT to assess for necrosis or complications	Not used directly for imaging, but supports clinical decision for it
Fluid resuscitation	Guides early aggressive IV fluid management in high-risk patients	Reinforces need for hemodynamic monitoring and volume optimization
Antibiotics/ intervention	Suggests close monitoring for infected necrosis or organ failure	High score increases suspicion for infection; may prompt early consults
Surgical consultation	Consider early consult in BISAP ≥3 with clinical deterioration	Consult often warranted in high APACHE II + necrosis or sepsis
Prognosis communication	Helps communicate mortality risk (e.g., 15–20% with score ≥ 3)	Useful for prognostic discussions and goals of care planning
Resource allocation	Assists triage in ED or resource-limited settings	Useful for ICU triage and prioritization
Follow-up planning	Lower scores may support early discharge planning	High scores may prompt closer follow-up and transitional care

Table 10.3 Severity scoring systems for acute pancreatitis

Feature	BISAP score	APACHE II score
Purpose	Early prediction of severity and mortality (within 24 hours)	Comprehensive ICU severity scoring; used for prognosis
Scoring range	0–5	0–71
Timing of use	Within first 24 hours of admission	Typically at admission and updated every 24 hrs
Variables included	BUN >25 mg/dLImpaired mental status (GCS <15)SIRS ≥2Age > 60Pleural effusion	12 physiologic variables + age & chronic health points: Temperature, MAP, HR, RR PaO_2, A-a gradient pH, Na, K, Cr, Hct, WBC GCS Chronic health status
Ease of use	Simple, bedside tool	Complex, requires calculator/software
Prognostic use	Mortality risk stratification	ICU mortality risk prediction
Interpretation	Score ≥ 3 suggests high risk	Higher score = greater severity/mortality risk
Advantages	Quick and easy; good early triage tool	Detailed and comprehensive
Limitations	Less sensitive for gradation of severity	Time-consuming; may overestimate severity

improved pathophysiology understanding led to the 2012 revised Atlanta criteria. Herein, the pancreatic fluid collections are classified into **acute peripancreatic fluid collection (APFC), acute necrotic collection (ANC), pancreatic pseudocyst**, and **walled-off pancreatic necrosis (WOPN)** (Table 10.4).

APFC is an extra-pancreatic fluid collection seen within 4 weeks after the onset of interstitial edematous pancreatitis without necrosis. These collections appear homogeneous, without encapsulation and confined to normal retroperitoneal fascial planes. Pancreatic pseudocysts are homogeneous fluid collections with amylase-rich fluid without solid debris. They are located outside the pancreas and take >4 weeks to mature. ANC collections contain both fluid and necrotic material. They occur in the setting of acute necrotizing pancreatitis and develop within 4 weeks with heterogeneous, variable amount of fluid and necrotic tissue. ANCs incur a 30% risk of infection. Image findings appear as multiloculated heterogeneous fluid and debris. WOPN is an encapsulated collection of peripancreatic necrosis that develops around 4 weeks after necrotizing pancreatitis. Imaging shows a heterogeneous collection with fluid and varying

Table 10.4 Comparison of pancreatic fluid collections (per revised Atlanta Classification)

Feature	APFC(acute peripancreatic fluid collection)	ANC(acute necrotic collection)	Pseudocyst	WON(walled-off necrosis)
Timing of onset	<4 weeks	<4 weeks	≥4 weeks	≥4 weeks
Underlying pancreatitis	Interstitial (mild/moderate)	Necrotizing pancreatitis	Interstitial pancreatitis	Necrotizing pancreatitis
Contents	Fluid only	Fluid + necrotic material	Encapsulated fluid	Encapsulated fluid + necrotic debris
Wall formation	None	None initially	Well-defined wall	Well-defined wall
Imaging (CT/MRI)	Homogeneous fluid; no wall	Heterogeneous, no defined wall	Round/oval with capsule	Heterogeneous with capsule and debris
Clinical relevance	Often asymptomatic; may resolve	Systemic symptoms; organ failure possible	Pain, infection, obstruction possible	High risk of infection/sepsis/ organ failure
Initial management	Supportive care	Supportive; monitor closely	Observation if asymptomatic	Supportive; monitor for complications
Indications for intervention	Rarely needed	If infected or complications	Infection, pain, obstruction	Infection, sepsis, persistent symptoms
Preferred treatment	None	Antibiotics ± drainage if infected	Drainage (endoscopic preferred)	Step-up: antibiotics → drainage → necrosectomy
Prognosis	Excellent	Variable; depends on necrosis extent	Good with treatment	Variable; high morbidity if infected

degrees of loculations with no fluid densities. Detection of debris within the fluid collections is the distinction between pseudocyst and WOPN.

Management

In all, 85–90% of acute pancreatitis cases are self-limited and subside spontaneously, usually within 3–7 days after onset, and do not manifest organ failure or local complications. The medical treatment is guided by the severity of the disease. Fundamentally, management is fluid resuscitation to restore the tissue perfusion, nutrition support, pain management, remove the predisposing causes such as gallstones or alcohol, and managing the local complications. Attention to *hydration, pain control, and bowel rest* will generally suffice. If gallstones are the presumptive cause, laparoscopic cholecystectomy is recommended on that same admission. If alcohol was the cause, alcohol counseling and follow-up are mandatory on the index admission.

Early, aggressive intravenous fluid resuscitation to mitigate systemic complications from a secondary systemic inflammatory response is required. The patient is initially made NPO (nil per os) to decrease pancreatic stimulation and administered intravenous analgesics and supplemental oxygen. Lactated Ringer's or normal saline is initially given or "bolused" at 15–20 mL/kg, followed by 2–3 mL/kg per hour to maintain urine output over 0.5 mL/kg per hour. Serial bedside evaluations are used every 6–8 hours to assess vital signs, oxygen saturation, and change in physical examination to optimize fluid resuscitation. The bedside aspect of these evaluations cannot be overemphasized. Decreasing hematocrit and BUN during the first 24 hours is evidence that sufficient fluids are being administered. Serial measurements and bedside assessment for fluid overload are continued, and fluid rates are maintained at the current rate. Adjustments in fluid resuscitation may be required in patients with cardiac, pulmonary, or renal disease. Hypoxemia should be suspected in every patient, and oxygen saturation should be monitored for the initial hospital stay. Severely ill patients may require endotracheal intubation and mechanical ventilation.

Nasogastric tubes are to be used only if symptomatically required. Therefore, in patients without nausea, vomiting, or evidence of intestinal obstruction or ileus, early oral nutrition is beneficial and provides better outcomes. For patients unable to tolerate oral intake, early nutritional support should be initiated within the first 24–72 hours. Enteral feeding should be used during the acute episode. Total parenteral nutrition (TPN) avoids pancreatic stimulation and should be used for nutritional support only if enteral feeding is not practical for 5 or more days. Nasogastric or naso-jejunal route is preferred enteral nutrition feeding over TPN.

Surgery is generally contraindicated in uncomplicated acute pancreatitis. However, if the diagnosis is uncertain in a patient with severe abdominal pain, diagnostic laparoscopy or laparotomy will not aggravate pancreatitis. If mild to moderate pancreatitis is found when an operative evaluation has been performed for diagnosis, cholecystectomy should be performed if gallstones are present, but the pancreas should be left undisturbed. Biliary pancreatitis can be diagnosed by ultrasound. Cholecystectomy should be performed on these patients during the same hospitalization soon after the attack resolves. A longer delay is associated with a high incidence of recurrent pancreatitis, estimated at 30% within 6 weeks.

In patients with severe necrotizing pancreatitis, current tenets hold that ***debridement*** *of dead peripancreatic tissue, often (40%) colonized by bacteria, reduces the mortality rate of acute severe necrotizing pancreatitis*. Contrast-enhanced CT scans are evaluated for the presence of non-enhancing areas that indicate lack of vascular perfusion and/or the presence of necrotic peripancreatic fat or pancreatic parenchyma. Percutaneous needle aspiration detects the presence of bacterial colonization. Endoscopic and/or surgical debridement is performed, often using a "Step-Up" technique. The mortality associated with acute pancreatitis is 1–2%. **The mortality associated with severe necrotizing pancreatitis is 50% or more, but appropriate surgical therapy lowers the figure to about 20%**.

Chronic Pancreatitis

Chronic pancreatitis (CP) is an inflammatory disorder characterized by progressive pancreatic parenchymal destruction with subsequent fibrosis. Chronic pancreatitis causes chronic abdominal pain and endocrine and/or exocrine pancreatic insufficiency. Chronic pancreatitis is usually caused by ***alcoholism***, but a minority of cases are due to an inherited predisposition (familial pancreatitis), hyperlipidemia, hypercalcemia, or duct obstruction. Pancreatic ductal hypertension results, caused by an increased viscosity of pancreatic juice, partial obstruction by calculi, diminished distensibility of the fibrotic pancreas. The increased pressure leads to ductal dilation, impaired blood flow, and additional functional damage. Frequent signs and symptoms include persistent or recurrent abdominal pain, pancreatic calcification on x-ray in 50%, pancreatic insufficiency in 30%, malabsorption, and diabetes mellitus.

The pain is ***deep in the upper abdomen*** and ***radiates through to the back***. **Clinical pearl**: for any patient who *reports having back pain* with associated abdominal symptoms *always consider pancreatic disease*. **Patients classically lean forward in a sitting position to ease the pain.** Attacks of acute pancreatitis may occur, layered over the pattern of chronic pain. Many patients become addicted to the narcotics prescribed for pain or continue using alcohol to mitigate symptoms.

Laboratory evaluations reveal that serum amylase levels may be elevated, but often not, presumably as the pancreatic fibrosis has damaged much of the enzyme-forming capacity of the parenchyma. About 75% of patients with calcific pancreatitis and 30% of those with noncalcific pancreatitis have insulin-dependent diabetes. Elevated bilirubin and/or alkaline phosphatase levels result from fibrotic constriction of the lower end bile duct. Nutrition labs should be assayed.

Magnetic resonance cholangiopancreatography (MRCP) and/or endoscopic retrograde cholangiopancreatography (ERCP) are useful in securing the diagnosis of chronic pancreatitis (ERCP is a procedure, MRCP is a specific kind of imaging and not a procedure). Pancreatic pseudocyst and neoplasm may be ruled out and preoperative planning for those thought to be surgical candidates. Representative findings include ductal stones and irregularity, with dilation and stenoses. Retrograde cholangiography may be performed to determine if the common bile duct is narrowed, to determine whether ductal stones are present, and to help the surgeon avoid operative injury to the bile duct.

Major complications of chronic pancreatitis include pancreatic pseudocyst, biliary obstruction, duodenal obstruction, malnutrition, and diabetes mellitus. *Adenocarcinoma of the pancreas occurs with greater frequency in patients with chronic pancreatitis*, seen in about 7% of patients. Malabsorption and steatorrhea are managed with medical support. Alcohol abstinence is crucial.

Surgical therapy is uncommon and may be of value to relieve chronic intractable pain. The best surgical candidates are those whose pain persists after cessation of alcohol.

Surgery in most cases facilitates drainage of the pancreatic duct or resects diseased pancreas or that serves both purposes. The choice of operation can usually be made preoperatively based on the findings of a retrograde pancreatogram and CT scans. Concomitant bile duct obstruction should be treated by choledochoduodenostomy.

A dilated pancreatic duct reflects obstruction, and procedures to improve ductal drainage usually relieve pain. The usual finding in calcific chronic alcohol pancreatitis is an **irregular dilated duct (1–2 cm in diameter) with points of stenosis (*"chain of lakes"*) appearance and ductal calculi**. A longitudinal pancreaticojejunostomy (Puestow procedure) is applicable in these patients. The duct is anteriorly incised from the tail into the head of the gland and anastomosed side-to-side to a Roux-en-Y segment of proximal jejunum. Pain improves postoperatively in about 80% of patients, but improvement of pancreatic insufficiency is unusual. This procedure, however, has a low rate of success when the pancreatic duct is narrow (<6 mm). In the absence of a dilated duct, pancreatectomy is the best procedure, and the extent of resection can often be determined from a CT scan and pancreatogram. In patients with small ducts, the most severe disease is usually located in the head of the gland, and pancreaticoduodenectomy (Whipple procedure) is the operation of choice. Pain relief is satisfactory in about 80% of patients treated by these operations. Total pancreatectomy is indicated when a previous pancreaticoduodenectomy or distal pancreatectomy has failed to give satisfactory pain relief. Difficulties in controlling diabetes mellitus occur in 30–40% of patients who have had total pancreatectomy with some mortality. Hence, total pancreatectomy is contraindicated in unreformed alcoholics.

Celiac plexus block may be used to obtain pain relief before proceeding with a major pancreatic resection in small duct pancreatitis. Table 10.5 compares the management of chronic and acute pancreatitis.

Pseudocyst

Pseudocysts in CP are encapsulated collections of fluid with a high amylase content. They likely result from disruption of a pancreatic duct after an episode of acute pancreatitis or direct trauma. The walls of a pseudocyst consist of inflammatory fibrosis of the peritoneal, serosal, and mesenteric membranes. Pseudocysts develop in about 2% of cases of acute pancreatitis and are single in 85%. The term pseudocyst, or false cyst, denotes an absence of an epithelial lining, whereas true cysts are lined by epithelium. This is important as *true cysts can be malignant or premalignant*, and *the presence of epithelium on a biopsy proscribes simple drainage as treatment*. Complications of pancreatic pseudocysts include infection, rupture, and hemorrhage.

Findings on CT that predict cysts are unlikely to resolve spontaneously include *size > 4 cm, wall calcifications, and thick walls*. The indications for treating pancreatic pseudocysts are to lessen symptoms and prevent complications. Their natural history is more nonthreatening than previously believed, so initial expectant management is reasonable. Expectant management is imperative in the first 6–12 weeks as 40% will spontaneously resolve. Thereafter, for cysts greater than 6 cm, treatment is usually recommended over expectant management because most cysts can be promptly eliminated by percutaneous catheter drainage or surgical/endoscopic drainage into the stomach or intestine. This avoids the need for prolonged follow-up with repeated imaging and avoids the risks of complications.

Complications of pancreatic pseudocysts include infection, which is present in 5–20% of pseudocysts and managed with drainage. Hemorrhage is the most feared and secondary to erosion into surrounding vessels. Treatment is prompt angiographic embolization.

Operative management of pseudocysts requires external or internal drainage, excision, or pancreatic resection. Percutaneous drainage is indicated for patients whose cyst does not communicate with the duct and has no appropriate window for endoscopic drainage. It can be used for nonma-

Table 10.5 Clinical comparison of acute vs. chronic pancreatitis

Feature	Acute pancreatitis	Chronic pancreatitis
Definition	Sudden inflammation of the pancreas, typically reversible	Long-standing, irreversible inflammation with progressive destruction of pancreatic tissue
Etiology (common causes)	Gallstones Alcohol Hypertriglyceridemia Medications ERCP TraumaIdiopathic	Chronic alcohol use (most common) Genetic (CFTR, SPINK1) Autoimmune Obstructive (stricture/tumor) Recurrent acute pancreatitis
Onset	Sudden onset of abdominal pain	Gradual or insidious; may follow repeated acute episodes
Pain	Severe, acute epigastric pain radiating to the back; worsens with eating	Chronic epigastric pain; may be intermittent or persistent; may decrease over time
Systemic involvement	Often present (fever, tachycardia, SIRS, shock)	Less common unless complicated
Pancreatic enzymes	Markedly elevated amylase and lipase	May be normal or mildly elevated
Imaging findings	Enlarged pancreas Edema/inflammation Fluid collections Necrosis (in severe cases)	Calcifications Ductal dilatation or strictures Atrophy Pseudocysts
Pathology	Inflammatory edema, fat necrosis, hemorrhage	Fibrosis, glandular atrophy, calcifications, ductal changes
Complications	Pancreatic necrosis Pseudocysts ARDS Renal failure Shock	Diabetes mellitus (type 3c) Exocrine insufficiency Chronic pain Pseudocyst Pancreatic cancer (↑ risk)
Exocrine function	Usually preserved	Often impaired (malabsorption, steatorrhea, weight loss)
Endocrine function	Usually preserved	Often impaired → pancreatic diabetes (Type 3c)
Management: Acute phase	IV fluids Pain control NPO initially Treat underlying cause	Not applicable
Management: Chronic phase	Not applicable	Pain management Pancreatic enzyme replacement Nutritional support Treat diabetes Endoscopic/surgical interventions if obstruction present; Peustow procedure
Prognosis	Usually good with full recovery; prognosis depends on severity	Progressive disease; variable prognosis; increased risk of pancreatic cancer

ture (<6 weeks old) cysts that are infected. The initial treatment of choice for mature cysts is endoscopic drainage via cystoenteric drainage (cyst-gastrostomy or cyst-duodenostomy). Surgical internal drainage is reserved for patients who cannot have endoscopic drainage or fail endoscopic drainage via Roux-en-Y cyst-jejunostomy, cyst-gastrostomy, or rarely cyst-duodenostomy. The surgeon must obtain a biopsy of the cyst wall at time of drainage to rule out malignancy. The presence of epithelium means a true cyst with malignant potential.

Pancreatic Cancer

An estimated 66,000 patients will develop pancreatic cancer in the United States in 2024, and 52,000 will die of the disease. Tumors of the pancreas can be categorized as being of endocrine or exocrine origin and are discussed herein (Table 10.6). Pancreatic carcinoma is the fourth leading cause of death due to cancer in men and women, with a median age of diagnosis of 65. Risk factors of pancreatic cancer include *cigarette smoking, dietary consumption of meat and fat, previous gastrectomy (>20 years earlier), family history, chronic pancreatitis, and race.* Familial or genetic causes are less than 10% at present but are expected to grow based upon improving technology. In two-thirds of cases, the tumor is in the head of the gland; the remainder occurs in the body or tail. Pancreatic cancer includes both the exocrine and endocrine tumors depending on type of cells. ***Ductal adenocarcinoma accounts for 90% of the cancers***. Pancreatic adenocarcinoma is characterized by early local extension to contiguous structures and metastases to regional lymph nodes and the liver. Pulmonary, peritoneal, and distant nodal metastases occur later.

Most affected patients (75%) will have adenocarcinoma of the head of the pancreas and over 50% will have metastatic disease at time of diagnosis. Symptoms are nonspecific and vague therefore the diagnosis is often delayed until the disease in advanced stage.

Table 10.6 Pancreatic tumors

Exocrine	Endocrine
Ductal adenocarcinoma (> 90%)	Insulinoma
Acinar cell carcinoma	Gastrinoma
Pancreatoblastoma	Glucagonoma
Solid pseudopapillary tumor	Vasoactive intestinal peptide –releasing tumor (Vipoma)
Serous cystadenocarcinoma	Somatostatinoma
Mucinous cystadenocarcinoma	Non-functioning neuro-endocrine tumors

Advanced cases may present with symptoms of obstructive jaundice, diabetes, or pancreatic exocrine insufficiency. Back pain occurs in 25% of patients and is associated with an even more dismal prognosis. Jaundice is constant in most patients but may fluctuate. Cholangitis occurs in only 10% of patients with malignant bile duct obstruction. *A palpable nontender gallbladder in a jaundiced patient suggests neoplastic obstruction of the common duct (**Courvoisier sign**), most often due to pancreatic cancer.* Jaundice is often accompanied by pruritus, especially of the hands and feet. Dark, malodorous urine may be the initial perceived symptom.

Carcinomas of the body and tail of the pancreas are distal to the bile duct, so jaundice is uncommon. In fact, *more than half (52%) of patients with resectable pancreatic cancer present with **painless jaundice***. They may also report *antecedent weight loss*. In patients with hepatomegaly, metastatic involvement may be present. One characteristic feature is the tendency for the patient to seek relief of pain (if present) by assuming a sitting position with the spine flexed. Recumbency, on the other hand, worsens the discomfort. As previously mentioned, this sign may also be seen in patients with chronic pancreatitis. Onset of diabetes mellitus in the previous 2 years is an early manifestation in 20% of patients.

Approximately **45% of patients with pancreatic cancer who present with jaundice also experience itching (pruritus)**. This figure is based on a large retrospective series that specifically examined the prevalence of pruritus in patients with neoplastic (malignant) obstructive jaundice, which includes pancreatic cancer. The underlying reason for pruritus in this context is *cholestasis due to biliary obstruction by the tumor, leading to the accumulation of pruritogenic substances in the plasma.* While the precise mediators are not fully elucidated, recent evidence implicates lysophosphatidic acid (LPA) and its generating enzyme autotoxin as key contributors, with serum autotoxin activity correlating with itch intensity in cholestatic patients. Other proposed mediators include bile acids, bilirubin, and endogenous opioids, but their direct causative roles remain less certain. The pathophysiology involves activation of specific sensory neurons in the skin by these circulating pruritogens, resulting in the sensation of itch. Biliary drainage remains the most effective therapy for pruritus associated with malignant biliary obstruction, as it addresses the underlying cholestasis.

Elevated liver function tests reflect common duct obstruction and/or hepatic metastases. Neoplastic obstruction results in the bilirubin level averaging 20 mg/dL, much higher than seen with benign biliary obstruction. Serum levels of the tumor marker **CA19-9** are elevated in 85% of patients with pancreatic cancer but the *sensitivity in resectable lesions is too low (50%) to serve as a screening tool.* CA 19-9 levels also rise from biliary obstruction so a "normalized" value (total bilirubin <2.0) should be assayed. Elevated levels also occur with other gastrointestinal cancers. One usefulness of CA 19-9 measurements may be in following the treatment results and surveillance. After complete resection of a tumor, elevated levels should normalize but may rise again if recurrence.

CT scans show a pancreatic mass in 95% of cases, generally with a central area of diminished attenuation. Fine cut (≤3-mm slices) "pancreatic protocol" CT with both arterial and venous phases is required to evaluate the mass' relationship to vascular structures to assess resectability. The pancreatic duct is dilated in 70% of patients; the bile duct is dilated in 60%. The presence of both bile duct and pancreatic duct dilation ("double duct" sign) is compelling evidence for pancreatic cancer even in the absence of a mass. Findings suggesting unresectability include local tumor extension (e.g., behind the pancreas; into the liver hilum), contiguous organ invasion (e.g., duodenum, stomach), distant metastases, involvement of the superior mesenteric or portal vessels, or ascites. CT scans using dynamic scanning techniques are as accurate as angiography in assessing vascular involvement. Magnetic resonance cholangiopancreatography (MRCP) provides similar information to conventional CT and may help delineate relationship to vascular or surrounding structures.

ERCP isn't always necessary in patients with a typical clinical history and a pancreatic mass on CT, but does have an important role in diagnosis and treatment. In the absence of a mass, an ERCP is indicated. **It is the most sensitive test (95%) for detecting pancreatic cancer, though specificity in differentiating between cancer and chronic pancreatitis is low.** It may assist in diagnosis of a mass poorly seen on CT or when tissue diagnosis is necessary (e.g., diagnostic uncertainty, prior to initiation of neoadjuvant therapy). ERCP can also assist in biliary drainage for patients with biliary obstruction at the time of diagnosis (Fig. 10.4). Preoperative biliary stenting is indicated for patients with obstruction as preoperative cholangitis is associated with increased mortality,

A pancreatogram should be obtained early in cases where the existence of a pancreatic lesion is suspected but unproved. Worrisome findings consist of stenosis or obstruction of the pancreatic duct. Adjacent lesions of the bile duct and pancreatic duct are highly suggestive of neoplastic disease, especially if the biliary involvement is focal.

Percutaneous aspiration biopsy of pancreatic mass lesions is positive in 85% of malignant tumors. Although the procedure is relatively safe, there is a risk of spreading a resectable tumor, so it is contraindicated in patients who are candidates for surgery. Percutaneous aspiration biopsy is principally of value to verify a presumptive diagnosis of adenocarcinoma of the pancreas in patients with radiographic evidence of unresectability such a liver metastasis. Cytologic proof is important as treatment decisions should not be made solely based on radiologic findings.

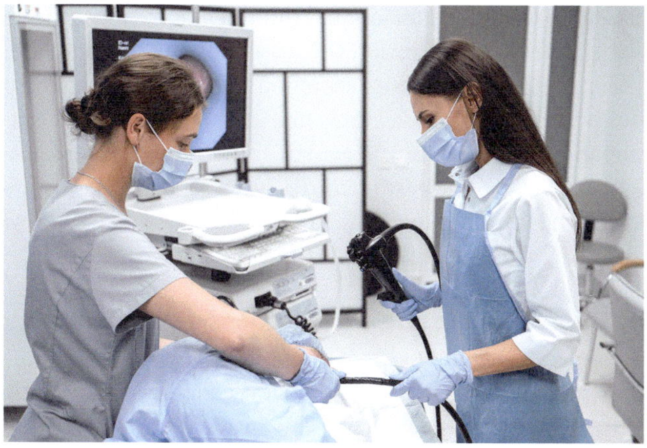

Fig. 10.4 Endoscopic retrograde cholangiopancreatography (ERCP) is an *endoscopic procedure* that enables both therapeutic biliary decompression and tissue sampling in patients with pancreatic cancer presenting with obstructive jaundice and pruritus. ERCP uses an endoscope, just like the ones used for more routine upper endoscopy—as shown here. ERCP can *relieve biliary obstruction by placing a stent across the malignant stricture, which rapidly reduces serum bilirubin and alleviates pruritus, improves hepatic function, and allows for the initiation of systemic therapy or palliation.* The American Society of Clinical Oncology recommends self-expanding metal stents as the preferred option for durable biliary drainage in patients with locally advanced or unresectable pancreatic cancer, while plastic stents may be considered for those with a limited life expectancy or planned short-term interventions. For tissue diagnosis, ERCP allows for **brush cytology and forceps biopsy** of biliary strictures. However, ERCP-based tissue sampling is limited, especially for pancreatic masses, and is generally inferior to endoscopic ultrasound-guided fine-needle aspiration/biopsy (EUS-FNA/B). ERCP is a procedure and should not be confused with **magnetic resonance cholangiopancreatography (MRCP)** which is imaging that is especially well suited for the biliary tree. Note that while ERCP has an important role as therapeutic intervention for cholestasis and issues of the biliary tree (e.g., CBD obstruction, chole**docho**lithiasis), it is not used to treat problems of the gallbladder proper (e.g., acute cholecystitis, symptomatic cholelithiasis)

Routine staging laparoscopy remains an area of debate. It is used routinely at certain centers and may decrease the rate of nontherapeutic laparotomy and assist in selection for neoadjuvant therapy in patients with borderline resectable or locally advanced cancer. Based upon imaging findings, national guidelines categorize pancreatic cancer as resectable, borderline resectable, or locally advanced. Borderline resectable patients will undergo neoadjuvant chemotherapy to convert the tumor to resectable. Approximately 30–50% of patients with borderline resectable pancreatic cancer will achieve surgical resection after undergoing neoadjuvant chemotherapy. This percentage can vary based on factors like the specific treatment regimen, tumor characteristics, and patient response. There is also evidence that neoadjuvant therapy also improves overall survival.

Resection for pancreatic cancer is appropriate only if all gross tumor can be removed with a standard resection. The pancreas is adjacent to the portal vein and the superior mesenteric vessels so these structures may be involved early. Only about 20% of cancers of the head of the pancreas can be resected, but because of local and distant spread, this is rarely possible for lesions of the body and tail. For curable lesions of the pancreatic head, pancreaticoduodenectomy (Whipple procedure) is required. The ***Whipple procedure*** *requires en bloc resection of the* ***head of the pancreas, distal common bile duct (CBD), duodenum, proximal jejunum, and gastric antrum*** (Fig. 10.5) with reconstruction via gastrojejunostomy, hepaticojejunostomy, and pancreaticojejunostomy. Pylorus-sparing Whipple procedures are usually performed.

When the procedure is performed by experienced surgeons, the operative mortality rate is less than 3%. Postoperative deaths are due to complications such as pancreatic and biliary fistulas, hemorrhage, and infection. For unresectable lesions, palliative bypasses of the bile duct and stomach are performed endoscopically or surgically. Surgical choledochojejunostomy provides relief of jaundice and pruritus. Percutaneous or endoscopically placed biliary stents also provide effective palliation and are preferable to surgical biliary decompression if the lesion is proven unresectable. Gastrojejunostomy is considered if the tumor obstructs the duodenum. Distal pancreatectomy with splenectomy is used for malignant lesions of the body and tail.

Laparoscopy can be a useful first step in patients scheduled for a Whipple procedure. About 15% of patients thought to have localized disease from preoperative studies are found to be unresectable at laparoscopy. The Whipple procedure is now becoming a minimally invasive procedure with extensive training. Ideal candidates for minimally invasive pancreatic surgery typically include those with early-stage disease, good overall health, and tumors that are accessible through small incisions. Open surgery is recommended for patients with advanced disease, complex tumor locations, or those requiring extensive resection. It is also preferred when minimally invasive surgery is technically challenging or when the surgeon assesses that the outcomes may be compromised with a minimally invasive approach. Minimally invasive pancreatic surgery offers benefits such as reduced postoperative pain, shorter recovery times, and fewer complications related to wound healing. The choice between minimally invasive and open surgery depends on the individual patient's condition, the specifics of the disease, and the surgeon's expertise.

The mean survival following palliative therapy is 7 months. Following a Whipple procedure, survival averages 18–24 months. Poor prognostic factors associated with tumor recurrence and shorter survival include lymph node involvement, tumor size over 2.5 cm, vascular invasion, and amount of blood transfused. If the margins are clear, about 20% of patients live more than 5 years. Overall, 5-year survival is about 13%, but only 60% of these patients are free of

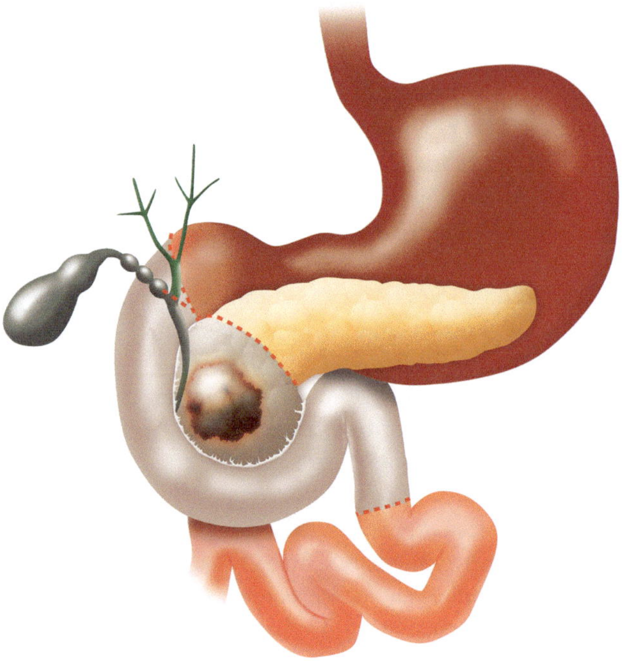

Fig. 10.5 During a **Whipple operation** (**pancreaticoduodenectomy**) for pancreatic cancer, the following anatomical structures are typically removed: the head of the pancreas, the uncinate process, the duodenum (usually the first and second portions, sometimes extending to the proximal jejunum), the distal common bile duct, the gallbladder, and often the gastric antrum (in the classic Whipple, but not in pylorus-preserving variants). The main pancreatic duct and the common bile duct are transected, and the gallbladder is removed to allow for complete excision of the biliary drainage pathway from the liver to the duodenum (red dashed lines) This resection is dictated by the close anatomical relationship of these structures, as *the pancreatic head is intimately associated with the duodenum,* and the distal common bile duct traverses the pancreatic head before entering the duodenum at the **ampulla of Vater**. The operation also includes regional lymphadenectomy (not illustrated)

tumor. Most patients undergo adjuvant chemotherapy or radiotherapy, but nearly 30% of patients fail to undergo adjuvant therapy secondary to surgical complications or slowed recovery.

Pancreatic adenocarcinoma is the most common malignancy causing biliary obstruction, but other peri-ampullary tumors must be kept in the differential diagnosis. These include distal bile duct tumors, or cholangiocarcinoma, cancer of the ampulla of Vater, and duodenal adenocarcinoma. Adenoma and adenocarcinoma of the ampulla of Vater account for about 10% of neoplasms that obstruct the distal bile duct. One-third are adenomas and two-thirds adenocarcinomas. Extra-pancreatic periampullary tumors tend to have a higher resectability rate as well as an overall higher 5-year survival rate.

Complications (morbidity) from a Whipple procedure are seen in 50–60% of patients. The most discussed is **pancreatic fistula**, seen in 20–25%. The diagnosis of a postoperative pancreatic fistula is clinical, predicated on the detection of pancreatic secretions draining from an abnormal site, usually an abdominal drain. Patients may present with abdominal drainage of fluid that is high in amylase, indicative of pancreatic secretions. CT scans can help delineate the fistula's anatomy and identify associated complications such as abscesses or fluid collections. Management of a postoperative pancreatic fistula entails conservative and interventional methods. The conservative approach includes:

1. Bowel Rest: The patient is kept NPO (nil per os) to reduce pancreatic secretions.
2. Octreotide: Somatostatin analogue decreases pancreatic exocrine secretion and supports fistula closure.
3. Nutritional Support: We prefer enteral feeding, if possible, over total parenteral nutrition (TPN) to ensure adequate nutrition and mitigate pancreatic stimulation.
4. Drainage: Interventional radiology (IR), or rarely surgical, placement of drains near the fistula to control pancreatic fluid drainage.

If conservative measures fail, or if the fistula is complex, other interventions may be tried, such as endoscopy to place stents or perform papillotomy to enable fistula closure. In cases of persistent or complex fistulas, surgical intervention to repair or resect the affected area may be required.

Delayed gastric emptying is seen in 20% of patients and managed conservatively with appropriate decompression and watchful waiting. Surgical site infections are seen in 10–15%. Hemorrhage (<10%) is relatively rare but contributes significantly to postoperative death and is most commonly due to gastroduodenal artery stump bleeding or pseudoaneurysm formation. This complication is managed with angiography and embolization.

Intraductal Papillary Mucinous Neoplasms (IPMN)

Intraductal papillary mucinous neoplasm (IPMN) of the pancreas is a type of pancreatic tumor characterized by the proliferation of mucin-producing epithelial cells within the pancreatic ducts. IPMNs are significant due to their potential to evolve into invasive pancreatic cancer, making early detection and management crucial. IPMNs are classified based on their location within the pancreatic ductal system and their histological features. They comprise nearly one-half of resected cystic neoplasms. They can be categorized into three categories:

- Main Duct IPMN: Involves the main pancreatic duct and is associated with a higher risk of progression to invasive cancer.
- Branch Duct IPMN: Occurs in the smaller branches of the pancreatic duct system. Less aggressive than main duct

IPMNs, they still have a potential for malignant transformation. Specific indicators include cyst diameter > 3 cm, duct dilation, mural nodules, or symptomatic.
- Mixed-Type IPMN: Exhibits characteristics of both main and branch duct types.

Histologically, IPMNs are characterized by the presence of papillary projections and mucin-secreting cells lining the ducts. They often exhibit various degrees of dysplasia, from low-grade to high-grade, with higher grades indicating a greater risk of progression to invasive cancer. Molecular genetic studies have identified mutations in genes such as KRAS, GNAS, and TP53 in IPMNs, providing insight into their pathogenesis and aiding in diagnosis. Cyst fluid analysis reveals viscous fluid with elevated CEA and amylase. Elevated CA19-9 in the cyst may indicate malignancy. IPMNs can be asymptomatic, especially in the early stages, which complicates diagnosis. Symptoms include abdominal pain, weight loss, jaundice, or pancreatitis. The presentation often varies depending on the tumor's location and the degree of duct obstruction.

Management of IPMN depends on several factors, including the type, size, and presence of high-grade dysplasia or invasive components. Treatment options include:

- Surveillance: For asymptomatic, low-risk IPMNs (most side-branch IPMNs) regular monitoring with imaging and clinical evaluations is often recommended.
- Surgical Resection: Considered for IPMNs with high-risk features, such as main duct involvement or high-grade dysplasia. The extent of surgery depends on the tumor's location and involvement of surrounding structures.
- Endoscopic Procedures: In some cases, endoscopic approaches may be used to manage symptoms or perform biopsies.

The prognosis of IPMN largely depends on the tumor's type, degree of dysplasia, and whether invasive cancer has developed. Generally, branch duct IPMNs have a better prognosis compared to main duct IPMNs.

Pancreatic Cystic Neoplasms

Cystic neoplasms of the pancreas are pancreatic tumors distinguished by their cystic nature. They are classically divided into mucinous cystic neoplasms (MCNs) and serous cystic neoplasms (SCNs). Cystic neoplasms of the pancreas usually present with abdominal pain, a mass, or jaundice and are diagnosed from the findings on CT scans.

Serous cystadenomas are usually microcystic adenomas and are well-circumscribed lesions consisting of multiple small cysts ranging in size from microscopic to about 2 cm. They occur commonly in females typically in fifth to seventh decade of life. The cut surface has the appearance of a honeycomb. The multicystic nature of the lesion is usually evident on CT scans and may demonstrate calcifications. The epithelium, flat to cuboidal, has no malignant potential. Treatment is usually observation, but resection is considered if symptomatic or uncertain diagnosis. An occasional serous cystadenoma will consist of one or more large cysts, or macrocystic SCN. SCNs are thought to be low or no malignancy risk and therefore no surveillance and no intervention is required except for lesions that can be symptomatic (obstruction, pain) or the inability to rule out malignancy.

Mucinous cystadenomas (macrocystic adenomas) are much more common in middle-aged women than in men and are usually multilocular lesions that have a smooth lining with papillary projections. The septate appearance on CT scans is characteristic. The lesions are usually in the body or tail. The cystic spaces measure 2–20 cm in diameter and contain mucus. The lining consists of tall columnar and goblet cells, often arranged in a papillary pattern. Cyst fluid analysis demonstrates viscous fluid. Mucinous cysts do not connect with the pancreatic duct system so fluid amylase levels are low, and the tall columnar epithelial cells can produce CEA so the lesions may have high CEA levels.

In time, most mucinous cystadenomas will evolve into cystadenocarcinomas, so total excision is the required treatment. Resection is recommended at the time of identification due to the risk of invasive cancer (10–40%). A greater malignancy risk is associated with size >4 cm and age < 55. Cystadenocarcinomas invariably present as a focus of malignancy within an existing mucinous cystadenoma. The tumors may be very large (10–20 cm) at the time of diagnosis. Metastases are seen in about 25% of cases. Complete excision results in a 5-year survival rate of 70%. An uncommon lesion, referred to as solid and papillary or papillary-cystic neoplasm of the pancreas, occurs almost exclusively in young women (under age 25 years). The tumor is usually large. It may be locally invasive, but metastases are uncommon, and cure is to be expected after resection.

Pancreatic Neuroendocrine Tumors

Pancreatic neuroendocrine tumors (pNET) are rare neoplasms of the pancreas, at less than 5% of all pancreatic malignancies. Pancreatic neuroendocrine tumors (pNETs), formerly known as *islet cell tumors*, are a heterogeneous group of tumors that arise from the endocrine tissue of the pancreas. They are rare, with increasing detection over time due to improved imaging techniques. Ten percent are associated with familial endocrine tumor syndromes. PNETs are defined by the hormones they secrete as functional and nonfunctional. PNETs may be functioning (i.e., hormone-producing) or nonfunctioning, malignant or nonmalignant. The hormones secreted by (functional) pNETs include *insulin, gastrin, glucagon, and somatostatin.*

***Insulinoma**, the **most common functioning islet cell neoplasm**, arises from beta cells and produces insulin and symptoms of hypoglycemia.* Tumors of the D cells produce **gastrin** and the **Zollinger–Ellison syndrome**. Alpha cell neoplasms may produce excess glucagon and hyperglycemia. Non-beta islet cell tumors may also secrete serotonin, ACTH, MSH, and kinins (and evoke the carcinoid syndrome).

Laboratory evaluation may reveal elevated hormone levels. PNETs also secrete the peptide, **Chromogranin A**, whose levels are generally used to monitor recurrence after resection. Most pNETs are malignant tumors of the head of the gland. If non-functional, they present with abdominal and back pain, weight loss, and a palpable abdominal mass in advanced cases. Jaundice may be present. CT scans reveal a hypervascular pancreatic mass and has lower sensitivity than EUS or DOTATATE positron emission tomography (PET). DOTATATE PET uses radioisotopes that bind to the somatostatin receptor and are highly sensitive for the detection of pNETs. They are well circumscribed, homogeneously enhancing, and hypervascular. EUS/fine needle aspiration (FNA) is indicated to establish tissue diagnosis or if tumor was not well visualized by CT.

The histologic pattern on biopsy specimens is diagnostic of islet cell tumor, but a lesion's malignancy is based on evidence of invasiveness or metastases, not the cellular appearance. Immunohistochemical staining of the tissue is positive for chromogranin and neuron-specific enolase. Metastases are present at the time of diagnosis in 80% of patients. Resection of all gross tumor is the preferred treatment but is feasible in less than half of patients because of local extension or distant metastases.

Insulinomas are solitary and benign; less than 10% are malignant.

The symptoms (related to cerebral glucose deprivation) are bizarre behavior, memory lapse, or unconsciousness. Patients may be mistakenly treated for psychiatric illness. There may be profuse sympathetic discharge, with palpitations, sweating, and tremulousness. Hypoglycemic episodes are usually precipitated by fasting and are relieved by food, so weight gain is common. The classic diagnostic criteria (**Whipple triad**) are present in most cases: (1) *hypoglycemic symptoms produced by fasting,* (2) *blood glucose below 50 mg/dL during symptomatic episodes, and* (3) *relief of symptoms by intravenous administration of glucose.*

Localization of the tumor may be difficult. CT and MR scans are successful in demonstrating about 40% of tumors. EUS may be able to show a much higher percentage. EUS is more sensitive than any preoperative test. Surgical resection is recommended. If benign, enucleation is acceptable. Patients with insulinoma associated with MEN-1 usually have multiple lesions. Patients with sporadic insulinomas lead a normal life after the tumor has been removed. The outcome is less predictable in patients with MEN-1, who may have several insulin-producing tumors.

Gastrinomas are neuroendocrine tumors that primarily secrete gastrin, a hormone that stimulates the production of stomach acid. These tumors typically arise in the pancreatic islets or the duodenum and can lead to a condition known as **Zollinger-Ellison syndrome**, characterized by *excessive gastric acid secretion*. The majority of gastrinomas are found in the "gastrinoma triangle," an area bounded by the duodenum, pancreas, and bile ducts. However, these tumors can also occur in other parts of the gastrointestinal tract. Gastrinomas are usually malignant and have a propensity for metastasizing to the liver and lymph nodes. The clinical presentation of gastrinomas is defined by excessive acid production. This often results in severe peptic ulcers, which are resistant to treatment. Patients may experience symptoms such as abdominal pain, diarrhea, and gastroesophageal reflux disease (GERD). The high levels of gastric acid can lead to complications such as chronic gastritis, diarrhea, and erosive esophagitis.

Elevated fasting serum gastrin levels are indicative of gastrinomas, but they must be interpreted in the context of other conditions that can also cause high gastrin levels. Additional diagnostic modalities include endoscopic evaluation, imaging studies such as computed tomography (CT) or magnetic resonance imaging (MRI), and somatostatin receptor scintigraphy.

Surgical resection is the primary treatment for localized gastrinomas and can be curative if the tumor is confined and localized. Surgery may not be feasible if the tumor is metastatic. In such cases, treatment focuses on controlling symptoms and slowing tumor progression. Pharmacologic management includes *proton pump inhibitors (PPIs)* and/or *histamine receptor antagonists* to reduce gastric acid secretion and alleviate symptoms. *Somatostatin analogues* are also used as they can inhibit gastrin release and have been shown to reduce tumor size in some patients. Chemotherapy and targeted therapies may be employed for advanced cases, depending on the tumor's genetic profile and behavior.

Factors influencing gastrinoma prognosis include the tumor's size, location, metastatic potential, and the patient's overall health. The 5-year survival rate for patients with localized gastrinomas is relatively high, but it drops significantly for those with advanced disease.

Glucagonomas arise from alpha islet cells. Most are large at the time of diagnosis and about 25% are confined to the pancreas. The remainder has metastasized by the time of diagnosis. Glucagonoma syndrome is characterized by migratory necrolytic dermatitis (usually involving the legs and perineum), weight loss, stomatitis, hypoaminoacidemia, anemia, and mild to moderate diabetes mellitus. The condition is more common in women. The diagnosis may be suspected from the distinctive skin lesion; in fact, the presence of a prominent rash in a patient with diabetes mellitus should be enough to raise suspicions.

Surgical removal of the primary lesion and resectable secondaries is indicated if technically feasible. If the tumor is confined to the pancreas, cure is possible.

Most cases of pancreatic "cholera" are caused by a nonbeta islet cell tumor of the pancreas that secretes vasoactive intestinal peptide (VIP), a "vipoma." The syndrome is characterized by profuse watery diarrhea, massive fecal loss of potassium, low serum potassium, and extreme weakness (WDHA Syndrome: Watery Diarrhea, Hypokalemia, & Achlorhydria). Stool volume averages about 5 L/d during acute episodes and contains over 300 mEq of potassium (20 times normal). Severe metabolic acidosis frequently results from loss of bicarbonate in the stool. Many patients are hypercalcemic, possibly from secretion by the tumor of a parathyroid hormone-like substance.

Approximately 80% of the VIP tumors are solitary, located in the body or tail, and can be removed easily. About half of the lesions are malignant, and three-fourths of those have metastasized by the time of exploration. Even if all the tumors cannot be removed, resection of most of it ("debulking") alleviates symptoms in about 40% of patients even though the average survival is only 1 year.

Somatostatinomas are characterized by diabetes mellitus, diarrhea and malabsorption, and dilation of the gallbladder (usually with cholelithiasis). The syndrome results from a somatostatinoma, half of which are malignant and accompanied by hepatic metastases. The lesion is usually large and readily demonstrated by CT scan. The diagnosis may be made by recognizing the clinical syndrome and measuring increased concentrations of somatostatin in the serum. Often, however, the somatostatin syndrome is unsuspected until histologic evidence of metastatic islet cell carcinoma has been obtained. When the disease is localized, resection can cure about 50% of cases. Enucleation is inappropriate for these tumors.

Selected Readings

1. McDermott J, Kao L, Keeley J, Nahmias J, de Virgilio C. Management of gallstone pancreatitis. JAMA Surg. 2024;159:818–25.
2. Kolbeinsson HM, Chandana S, Wright GP, Chung M. Pancreatic cancer: a review of current treatment and novel therapies. J Investig Surg. 2023;36(1):2129884. https://doi.org/10.1080/08941939.2022.2129884.
3. van Beek DJ, Verschuur AVD, Brosens LAA, Valk GD, Pieterman CRC, Vriens MR. Status of surveillance and nonsurgical therapy for small nonfunctioning pancreatic neuroendocrine tumors. Surg Oncol Clin N Am. 2023;32(2):343–71. https://doi.org/10.1016/j.soc.2022.10.010. PMID: 36925190 Review.
4. Szatmary P, Grammatikopoulos T, Cai W, Huang W, Mukherjee R, Halloran C, Beyer G, Sutton R. Acute pancreatitis: diagnosis and treatment. Drugs. 2022;82(12):1251–1276. https://doi.org/10.1007/s40265-022-01766-4. Epub 2022 Sep 8. PMID: 36074322.
5. Banks PA, Bollen TL, Dervenis C, Gooszen HG, Johnson CD, Sarr MG, Tsiotos GG, Vege SS; Acute Pancreatitis Classification Working Group. Classification of acute pancreatitis—2012: Revision of the Atlanta classification and definitions by International Consensus. Gut. 2013;62(1):102–11. https://doi.org/10.1136/gutjnl-2012-302779. Epub 2012 Oct 25. PMID: 23100216.
6. Ma ZY, Gong YF, Zhuang HK, Zhou ZX, Huang SZ, Zou YP, Huang BW, Sun ZH, Zhang CZ, Tang YQ, Hou BH. Pancreatic neuroendocrine tumors: a review of serum biomarkers, staging, and management. World J Gastroenterol. 2020;26(19):2305–22. https://doi.org/10.3748/wjg.v26.i19.2305. PMID: 32476795.
7. Colvin SD, Smith EN, Morgan DE, Porter KK. Acute pancreatitis: an update on the revised Atlanta classification Abdom Radiol (NY). 2020;45(5):1222–31. https://doi.org/10.1007/s00261-019-02214-w. PMID: 31494708 Review.
8. Forsmark CE, Vege SS, Wilcox CM. Causes of acute pancreatitis. N Engl J Med. 2016;375(20):1972–81. https://doi.org/10.1056/NEJMc1616177. PMID: 28177868 No abstract available.
9. Gardner TB, Adler DG, Forsmark CE, Sauer BG, Taylor JR, Whitcomb DC. ACG clinical guideline: chronic pancreatitis. Am J Gastroenterol. 2020;115(3):322–39. https://doi.org/10.14309/ajg.0000000000000535. PMID: 32022720.
10. Tanaka M, Fernández-Del Castillo C, Kamisawa T, Jang JY, Levy P, Ohtsuka T, Salvia R, Shimizu Y, Tada M, Wolfgang CL. Revisions of international consensus Fukuoka guidelines for the management of IPMN of the pancreas. Pancreatology. 2017;17(5):738–53. https://doi.org/10.1016/j.pan.2017.07.007. Epub 2017 Jul 13. PMID: 28735806.
11. Garajová I, Peroni M, Gelsomino F, Leonardi F. A simple overview of pancreatic cancer treatment for clinical oncologists. Curr Oncol. 2023;30(11):9587–601. https://doi.org/10.3390/curroncol30110694. PMID: 37999114.
12. Gardner TB, Park WG, Allen PJ. Diagnosis and management of pancreatic cysts. Gastroenterology. 2024;167(3):454–68. https://doi.org/10.1053/j.gastro.2024.02.041. Epub 2024 Mar 3. PMID: 38442782 Review.
13. Lai ECH, Ung AKY. Update on management of pancreatic cancer: a literature review. Chin Clin Oncol. 2024;13(3):41. https://doi.org/10.21037/cco-23-94. Epub 2024 May 17. PMID: 38769794.
14. Karunakaran M, Barreto SG. Surgery for pancreatic cancer: current controversies and challenges. Future Oncol. 2021;17(36):5135–62. https://doi.org/10.2217/fon-2021-0533. Epub 2021 Nov 8. PMID: 34747183 Review.
15. Szako L, Gede N, A. Aradi A., et al. Early occurrence of pseudocysts in acute pancreatitis- a multicenter international cohort analysis of 2275 cases. Pancreatology. 2021;21(6):1161–72. https://doi.org/10.1016/j.pan.2021.05.007.

Functional Pancreatic Endocrine Neoplasia Syndromes

11

Colette Brottman and Jeffrey Matthews

Pancreatic endocrine neoplasms are rare tumors that are considered functional or non-functional. Functional pancreatic endocrine neoplasms secrete peptide products leading to excess hormone levels that produce symptomatic clinical syndromes. Unfortunately, some endocrine neoplasms exhibit malignant behavior, although in general they carry a more favorable prognosis than cancers of the exocrine pancreas (Source: Brunicardi [1]).

The basis of diagnosing neoplasms of the endocrine pancreas consists of confirmation of elevated serum levels of hormone, localization of the tumor, and surgical or pharmacological intervention for symptom control. Preferred imaging modality is computed tomography (CT) with contrast and consideration of endoscopic ultrasound (EUS) (Source: Gheorghe [2]) (Fig. 11.1).

If a patient presents with an islet cell tumor, it is important to rule out multiple endocrine neoplasia (MEN) syndromes.

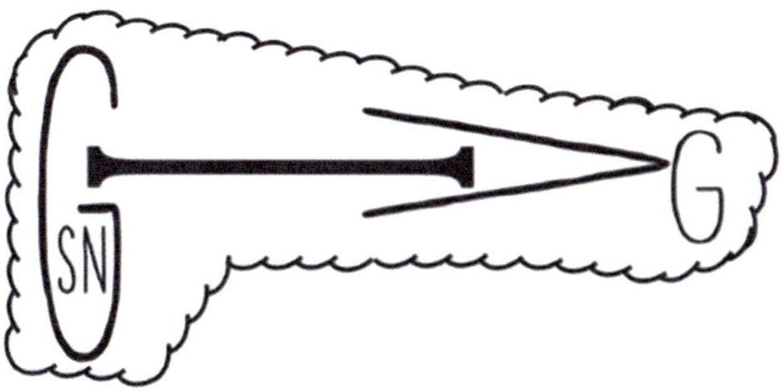

Fig. 11.1 Letters representing the most common pancreatic distribution. Gastrinoma, Somatostatinoma, Non-functional, Insulinoma, VIPoma, Glucagonoma. (Source: Hubbs and Fahey [3])

MEN1 Syndrome

Multiple Endocrine Neoplasia, type 1 (MEN 1) is a syndrome defined by the development of pancreatic endocrine neoplasms, pituitary tumors, and/or parathyroid hyperplasia. Most patients with MEN1 will present with ***hyperparathyroidism****, manifesting as asymptomatic hypercalcemia*. Some patients will present with renal colic or renal stones. Pancreatic endocrine tumors may develop, *most commonly **gastrinoma***, followed by insulinoma. ***Pituitary tumors***, such as prolactinomas, are often more aggressive for those with MEN 1 (Source: Hodgson [4]).

If patient notes a family history of renal colic or renal stones, hypercalcemia, or other MEN1-associated tumors, genetic testing is recommended. Patients with MEN 1 should undergo frequent screening imaging and labs for tumors related to the syndrome.

Insulinoma

Insulinomas are the *most common* functional neoplasm of the endocrine pancreas derived from *islet cells.* Most insulinomas are benign and solitary. Patients present with ***Whipple's triad*** which includes *symptomatic fasting hypoglycemia, serum glucose less than 50 mg/dL and resolution of symptoms with glucose intake*. (Source: Oleinikov [5]) Patients may also present with other symptoms including syncope, frequent eating, confusion, visual changes, palpitations, diaphoresis, and tremors (Fig. 11.2).

C. Brottman · J. Matthews (✉)
Department of Surgery, University of Chicago—Medicine, Chicago, IL, USA
e-mail: cbrottman@uchicagomedicine.org; jmatthews@uchicago.edu

S. Atallah, J. Dragoljevic (eds.), *Fundamentals of Surgery for Physician Assistants*, https://doi.org/10.1007/978-3-032-21069-2_11

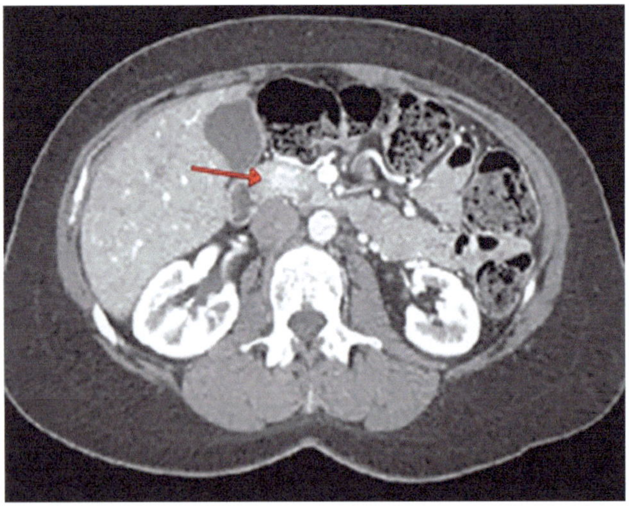

Fig. 11.2 CT scan demonstrating a 1.4 cm hypervascular mass in the pancreatic head, diagnosed as insulinoma. (Source: Sakr [8])

Laboratory findings typically demonstrate *low blood glucose, elevated serum insulin, and an elevated C-peptide.* To confirm diagnosis, it is advised that patients undergo a closely monitored fast in which the blood glucose and serum insulin are drawn every 4–6 h until the patient becomes symptomatic (Source: Oleinikov [5]). If insulinoma is suspected from the laboratory findings, then *CT with contrast* is used to localize the tumor.

Surgical resection of insulinoma is usually curative. Based upon the tumor's location and size, enucleation or distal pancreatectomy/pancreaticoduodenectomy are the preferred procedures.

Following resection, it is recommended to undergo a detailed history and physical exam with surveillance imaging within 1 year to exclude recurrence.

Gastrinoma

Gastrinomas are well-differentiated neuroendocrine tumors that secrete excess gastrin leading to a pattern of clinical symptoms known as **Zollinger–Ellison Syndrome**. They are most commonly diagnosed between ages 20 and 50 with a higher incidence in males. Most gastrinomas are located within Passo's triangle which contains the pancreatic head, duodenum, and posterior and superior lymphatic bed of the duodenum. Nearly 50% of gastrinomas are malignant with metastasis most commonly seen in the liver and bone (Source: Jenson [6]). Pancreatic gastrinomas are more likely to metastasize than other primary locations.

Zollinger–Ellison Syndrome presents as *abdominal pain, diarrhea, heartburn from hypersecretion of acid, peptic ulcers, and severe esophagitis.* Generally, patient's symptoms do not resolve with the simple use of antacids or the usual dose strength of over-the-counter antisecretory medicines (Source: Brunicardi [1]).

The diagnosis of gastrinoma is strongly suggested by a highly *elevated fasting serum gastrin level (>1000 pg/mL) (Source: Jenson [6]).* It is recommended that proton pump inhibitors are held before this test because these medications independently elevate serum gastrin. Additionally, a gastric pH level < 2 supports the diagnosis. If the findings are non-diagnostic but concern remains, a *secretin stimulation test* may be performed. To localize the tumor, *somatostatin receptor (SSTR) scintigraphy with CT* is recommended, often followed by EUS, for further localization.

The basis of treatment for gastrinoma is symptom control with high dose proton pump inhibitors (PPI). Once symptoms begin to improve, dosing can be cautiously reduced. For those on long term PPI, B12 monitoring is recommended. If gastrinoma is diagnosed before there is evidence of metastasis, surgical exploration may be considered, with the option of enucleation for tumors in the pancreatic head or duodenum. For those with limited hepatic metastases, additional liver resection may be warranted. Bilobar liver metastases or widespread metastasis can be symptomatically managed by octreotide or other somatostatin analogs. Of note, even those with curative surgery may continue to experience symptoms associated with excess gastrin production (Fig. 11.3).

Surveillance CT chest abdomen pelvis is recommended every 6–12 months for 10 years following curative treatment. Additionally, serum gastrin levels may be drawn to monitor for recurrence.

Treatment options in advanced metastatic disease include symptom control with somatostatin analogs, cytoreductive surgery, and local (liver-directed) ablative therapies including embolization, chemoembolizaton, cryotherapy, and radiofrequency ablation. ***Traditional forms of chemotherapy are generally ineffective.*** Peptide radioreceptor therapy

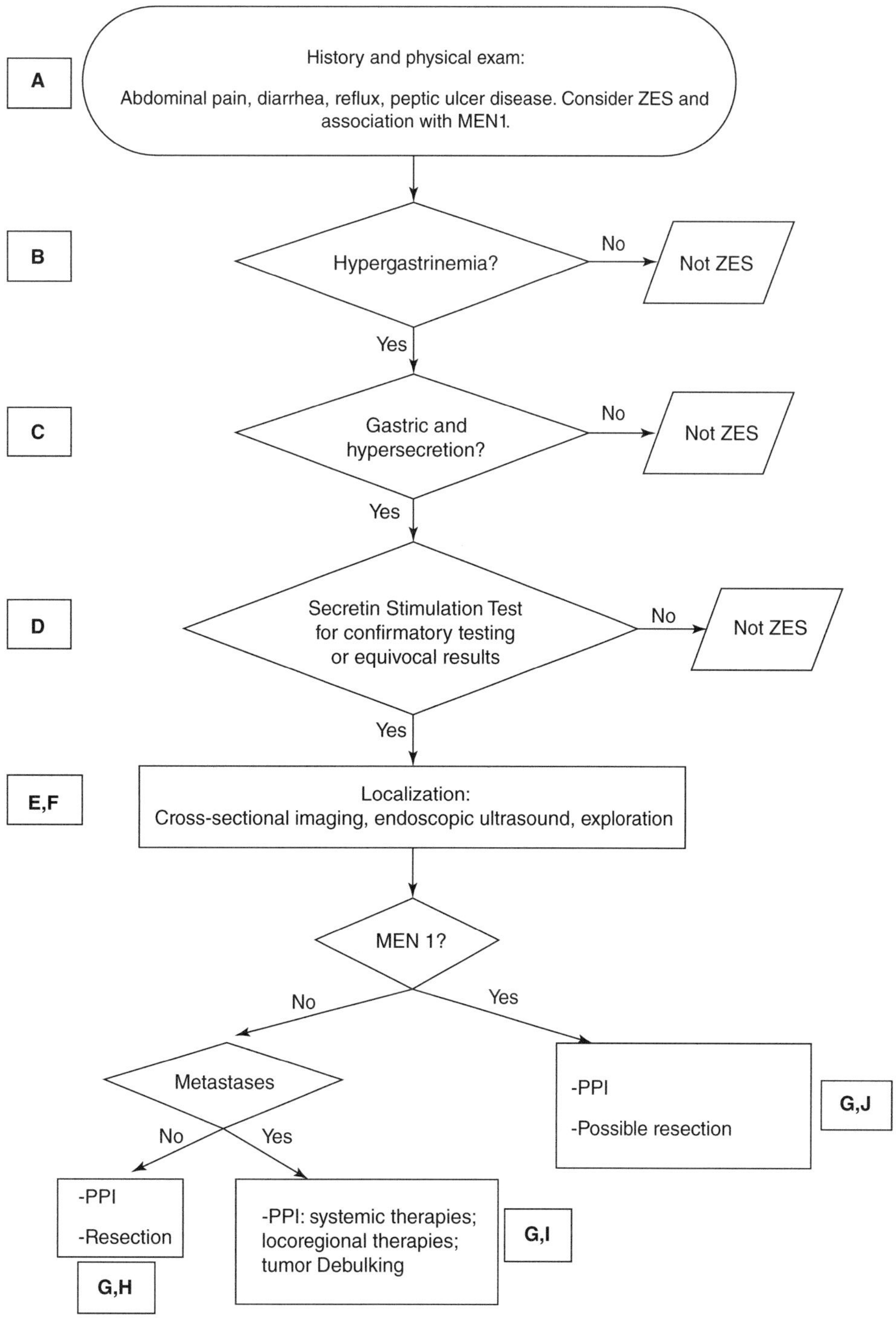

Fig. 11.3 Workup and Management of Gastrinoma. (Source: Simpson and James [7])

(PRRT) using radiolabeled somatostatin analogues has had mixed results. The occasional patient may be a candidate for liver transplantation.

Vasoactive Intestinal Peptide-Producing Tumor

Most VIPomas are found in the pancreatic body and tail. Common presentation includes ***severe watery diarrhea (>5 L per day) and weakness from fluid and electrolyte losses.*** (Source: Sakr [8]) Laboratory findings will demonstrate ***hypokalemia*** due to excess potassium in diarrhea and ***hypochlorhydia*** due to inhibited gastric acid secretion.

An *elevated fasting plasma VIP level* will confirm suspicion of VIPomas in addition to hypokalemia and hypochlorhydia. Hyperglycemia and hypercalcemia are often commonly noted. CT is used to localize the tumor (Fig. 11.4).

It is important to prioritize correction of *electrolyte disturbances* in the management of VIPomas. The addition of

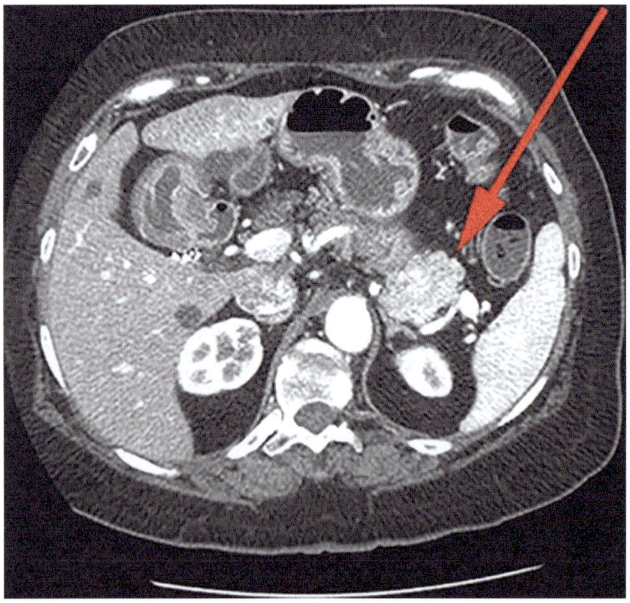

Fig. 11.4 CT scan of hypervascular tumor in distal pancreas, demonstrating VIPoma. (Source: Sakr [8])

somatostatin analogues can be helpful in decreasing diarrhea and therefore correcting other metabolic imbalances. Surgical resection can be curative, although palliative debulking with post-operative octreotide can help to manage symptoms.

Glucagonoma

Glucagonoma are predominately malignant, often unresectable, tumors that secrete excess glucagon leading to ***skin rashes, diabetes mellitus (type 2), and weight loss***. For resectable tumors, surgery is considered curative.

A characteristic rash termed **necrolytic migratory erythema (NME)** presents as a *multifocal, migrating lesions with spreading margins and healing centers.* (Source: Li [9]). They most commonly are found on the low abdomen, perineum, perioral area, and feet. Patients will also note an enlarged tongue. In addition to hyperglycemia, weight loss is another common symptom (Fig. 11.5).

Diagnosis is made by identifying an *elevated plasma glucagon level (>1000 pg/mL).* CT is used for tumor localization.

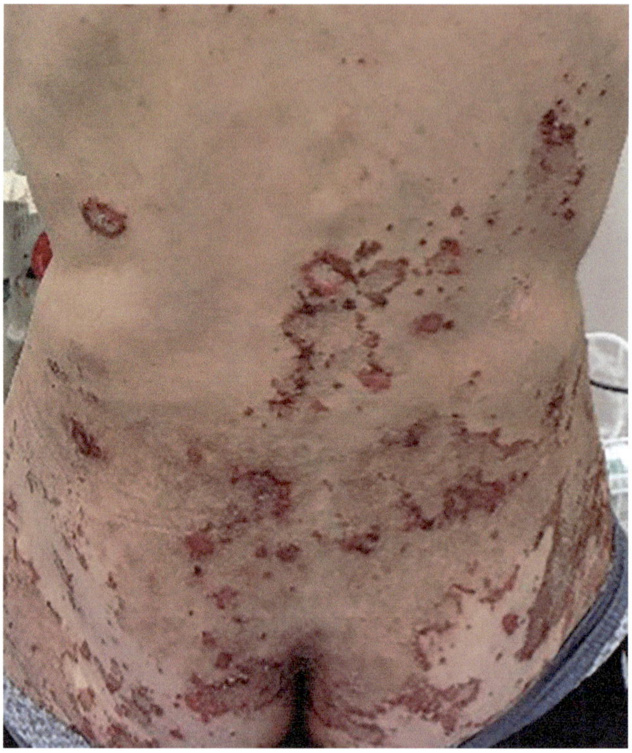

Fig. 11.5 NME of glucagonoma. Unclear boundary of rash. (Source: Li et al. [9])

If surgical resection is feasible, pre-operative management of diabetes in addition to nutritional support is crucial. Given that most tumors are found in the body and tail of the pancreas, distal pancreatectomy with splenectomy is recommended. For those with metastatic disease, chemotherapy can be considered in addition to octreotide for symptom control.

Somatostatinoma

Somatostatinomas *inhibit pancreatic and biliary secretions* leading to a syndrome of ***steatorrhea, diabetes, and gallstones***. They are rare tumors with equal distribution in male and females and are most commonly found in the pancreaticoduodenal groove (Source: Brunicardi [1]). Excessive somatostatin causes *biliary stasis, slowed gut motility and decreased acid secretion, pancreatic enzyme secretion, and intestinal absorption*. Diagnosis is made by *elevated soma-*

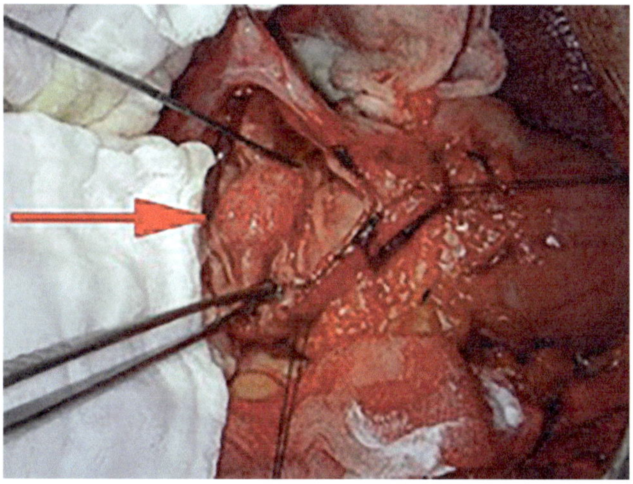

Fig. 11.6 Typical location of somatostatinoma at the second portion of the duodenum adjacent to the ampulla of Vater. (Source: Sakr [8])

tostatin levels (>10 ng/mL). CT or MRI aid in localization and EUS can provide tissue diagnosis. Unfortunately, somatostatinomas have often metastasized by the time of diagnosis but for solitary lesions, surgical resection plus cholecystectomy are recommended (Fig. 11.6).

References

1. Brunicardi F, Anderson DK, Billiar TR, Dunn DL, Hunter JG, Matthews JB, Pollock RE, editors. Schwartz's principles of surgery, 10e. McGraw-Hill Education.
2. Gheorghe EC, Săftoiu A. Pancreatic neuroendocrine tumors. In: Săftoiu A, editor. Pocket guide to advanced endoscopy in gastroenterology. Cham: Springer; 2023. https://doi.org/10.1007/978-3-031-42076-4_42.
3. Hubbs D, Fahey T. Evaluation and diagnosis of pancreatic and gastrointestinal neuroendocrine tumors. In: Gartland RM, Lee JA, editors. Endocrine surgery clerkship. Contemporary surgical clerkships. Cham: Springer; 2024. https://doi.org/10.1007/978-3-031-62091-1_2.
4. Hodgson A, Pakbaz S, Mete O. Multiple endocrine neoplasia type 1 (MEN1). In: La Rosa S, Uccella S, editors. Endocrine pathology. Encyclopedia of pathology. Cham: Springer; 2022. https://doi.org/10.1007/978-3-030-62345-6_5223.
5. Oleinikov K, Gross DJ, Jacob H, Mazeh H, Grozinsky-Glasberg S. Insulinoma. In: Yalcin S, Öberg K, editors. Neuroendocrine Tumours. Cham: Springer; 2024. https://doi.org/10.1007/978-3-031-56968-5_12.
6. Jensen RT, Ito T. Gastrinoma. [Updated 2023 Sep 27]. In: Feingold KR, Anawalt B, Blackman MR, et al., editors. Endotext [Internet]. South Dartmouth (MA): MDText.com, Inc.; 2000. Available from: https://www.ncbi.nlm.nih.gov/sites/books/NBK279075/
7. Simpson RE, James BC. Management of Gastrinoma. In: Docimo Jr S, Pauli E, editors. Clinical algorithms in general surgery. Cham: Springer; 2019. https://doi.org/10.1007/978-3-319-98497-1_115.
8. Sakr M. Pancreatic neuroendocrine tumors. In: Sakr M, editor. Head and neck and endocrine surgery. Cham: Springer; 2024. https://doi.org/10.1007/978-3-031-64102-2_20.
9. Li, W., Yang, X., Deng, Y. *et al.* Necrolytic migratory erythema is an important visual cutaneous clue of glucagonoma. Sci Rep 12, 9053 (2022). https://doi.org/10.1038/s41598-022-12882-2 https://creativecommons.org/licenses/by/4.0/

Management of GI Stromal Tumors

12

Haley Harris, Brian Untch, and Heather Yeo

Introduction

GISTs are a rare type of sarcoma, arising from *Interstitial cells of Cajal*. In the United States, an estimated 5000 to 6000 new cases are diagnosed annually, with a global annual incidence of 10 cases per million population [1]. These tumors represent approximately 1–2% of all gastrointestinal (GI) tumors and typically originate in the stomach and small intestine, though they can arise anywhere along the gastrointestinal tract [2]. Although relatively rare, the incidence of GISTs has increased over the last two decades across almost all major organ sites [3]. Therefore, the ability to accurately diagnose and effectively manage these tumors is becoming increasingly important.

Patient Presentation

GISTs affect males and females at similar rates and most commonly occur in adults aged 65 years and older. While occurrence in children is very rare, with less than 1% of tumors occurring in individuals younger than 20 years, pediatric GISTs can occur [4]. These tumors have distinct molecular and clinical profiles from adult tumors and more often occur in female patients.

GISTs can occur throughout the GI tract, with the majority occurring in the ***stomach*** (50–60%) and ***small intestine*** (25–35%) [1, 5, 6]. Other locations include the colon, rectum, mesentery, and omentum, and in rare cases, extra-GI GISTs have been described outside of the GI tract within the abdominal cavity. Tumor size varies significantly, ranging from smaller than 1 cm to more than 40 cm, with an average size of 5–6 cm in diameter [7].

Tumors may present with or without clinical symptoms, and approximately 18% of diagnosed cases are asymptomatic and are discovered incidentally, often during endoscopy or imaging studies such as computed tomography (CT) scans [2]. When symptoms are present, they typically include GI bleeding and anemia. Larger tumors may present with abdominal pain and a palpable mass, and it is not uncommon for small GISTs to remain asymptomatic for an extended period until an acute event such as a hemorrhage or rupture occurs. Presentation of symptoms may be associated with the location of the tumor. For example, rectal GISTs are more likely to present with pain, difficulty having a bowel movement, and bleeding. Esophageal and gastro-esophageal tumors rarely have symptoms but can potentially cause dysphagia or reflux-like symptoms.

Histopathologic Findings

GISTs originate from interstitial cells of Cajal (ICC), which function as the pacemakers for peristaltic contractions along the GI tract. Tumors are typically well circumscribed with fleshy pink or tan surfaces; however, areas of hemorrhagic necrosis and cystic degeneration are sometimes visible.

CD34 is expressed in 70% of GISTs and was the first immunohistochemical marker to help distinguish GISTs from other GI tumors. Identification of **KIT (CD117)** and **DOG1 (ANO1)** mutations has significantly improved the accurate identification with positive staining in more than 95% of GISTs. These markers are unique to GIST and are not commonly found in other mesenchymal tumors such as leiomyomas and leiomyosarcomas.

H. Harris · H. Yeo (✉)
Department of Surgery, NewYork-Presbyterian Hospital, Weill Cornell Medicine, New York, NY, USA
e-mail: hey9002@med.cornell.edu

B. Untch
Department of Surgery, Memorial Sloan Kettering Cancer Center, New York, NY, USA

S. Atallah, J. Dragoljevic (eds.), *Fundamentals of Surgery for Physician Assistants*,
https://doi.org/10.1007/978-3-032-21069-2_12

In tumors lacking KIT, mutations in the **platelet-derived growth factor receptor alpha (PDGFRA)** may be seen. PDGFRA mutant tumors are more likely to occur in the stomach and are generally associated with lower malignancy potential and favorable responses to treatment [8].

Tumors that lack variants in KIT and PDGFRA are known as "wild-type" tumors. These tumors are rare and may include NF1 mutant tumors or succinate dehydrogenase (SDH)-deficient tumors. Pediatric GISTs are more likely to be wild-type tumors than adult GISTs [9]. These tumors can be challenging to treat given the lack of non-surgical treatment options for tumors without mutations. However, wild-type GISTs are generally slow-growing and have good outcomes with surgery, even after recurrence [10].

Diagnostic Workup

Asymptomatic, submucosal lesions under 2 cm can be managed with regular surveillance using EUS or CT scans, depending on the location [9]. If the lesion grows or the patient presents with symptoms, a biopsy or excision should be done.

In cases where a lesion is greater than 2 cm in size, a histological diagnosis should be made. For gastric tumors, this can be done by fine needle aspiration or core needle biopsy under EUS. In some cases, characteristic findings on imaging and concern for seeding may preclude biopsy. When a biopsy is not possible—such as with lesions in the small intestine—excisional resection is often the standard. It is crucial to minimize the risk of peritoneal contamination and seeding during any procedure.

CT- or ultrasound-guidance biopsy can also be used for tumors greater than 10 cm where there is not a clear diagnosis. Diagnostic laparotomy or laparoscopy is generally unnecessary for patients with obvious metastatic disease, as a biopsy of a metastatic site is usually sufficient. The diagnosis is then made through morphological assessment and the presence of KIT or DOG1 immunopositivity. If a GIST is confirmed, mutational analysis **should** be done to assess the likelihood of response to **imatinib** and guide targeted therapy [9].

Risk Assessment

Mitotic rate, **tumor size**, and **organ site** are the key prognostic indicators.

The National Institutes of Health (NIH) released the first GIST classification in 2002 and determined the risk of recurrence by assessing the size and mitotic rate of the tumor [11]. High risk of recurrence was classified for tumors greater than 5 cm with a mitotic count higher than 5/50 high power fields (HPF) and tumors greater than 10 cm with any mitotic rate [11].

Since then, there have been multiple validated stratification tools developed to estimate risk of recurrence. These different predictive models are largely considered equivalent, but there are differences in factors and cutoff values such that it may be useful to consult multiple classification systems if the mitotic count or tumor's diameter is close to a method's cutoff value.

Modified NIH criteria[a]			
Risk category	*Tumor size (cm)*	*Mitotic count (per 50 HPF)*	
Very low risk	<2	<5	
Low risk	2–5	<5	
Intermediate risk	<5	6–10	
	5–10	<5	
High risk	>5	>5	
	>10	Any mitotic rate	
	Any size	>10	
Modified AFIP criteria[b]			
Risk category	*Tumor size*	*Mitotic rate*	*Tumor site*
None	<2 cm	<5	Any
Very low	>2 & ≤5	≤5	Gastric
Low	>2 & ≤5	≤5	Jejunal and Ileal
	>2 & ≤5	≤5	Duodenal
	>2 & ≤5	≤5	Rectal
	>5 & ≤10	≤5	Gastric
Moderate	>5 & ≤10	≤5	Jejunal and Ileal
	>10	≤5	Gastric
	>2 & ≤5	>5	Gastric
High	>2	>5	Jejunal and Ileal
	>2	>5	Duodenal
	>2	>5	Rectal
	>5	>5	Gastric
Modified Joensuu criteria[c]			
Risk category	*Tumor size*	*Mitotic index*	*Tumor site*
Very low	<2	≤5	Any
Low	2.1–5	≤5	Any
Intermediate	2.1–5	>5	Gastric
	<5	6–10	Any
	5.1–10	≤5	Gastric
High	Any	Any	Tumor rupture
	>10	Any	Any
	Any	>10	Any
	>5	>5	Any
	2.1–5	>5	Non-gastric
	2.1–5	>5	Non-gastric
	5.1–10	≤5	Non-gastric

[a]Adapted from Fletcher et al. [11]
[b]Adapted from Miettinen and Lasota [12]
[c]Adapted from Joensuu [13]

There are several validated online nomograms that have been developed to calculate the risk of survival without recurrence and risk of recurrence following surgery. Memorial Sloan Kettering (MSK) Cancer Center has developed two validated and publicly available GIST risk assessment tools based on patient data from MSK and at 80 sites comprising the Spanish Group for Research in Sarcomas [14].

Management

GISTs are inherently resistant to both standard chemotherapies and radiation, which has driven a focus on developing targeted therapy options. Treatment paradigms depend on multiple factors including the size and location of the tumor, age and comorbidities of the patient, and the presence or absence of clinical symptoms.

Localized GISTs

Standard treatment of *localized* GISTs is ***surgical resection***, with approximately 60% of patients with localized GISTs cured with surgery [7]. For histologically confirmed gastric tumors that are 2 cm and larger, surgery should be considered for patients who are fit with **the goal of achieving an R0 resection (e.g., no visible or microscopic tumor left behind)**. However, a conservative strategy of surveillance can be considered if the tumor is in an anatomically complex location (i.e., GE junction), or if the patient has significant comorbidities. Laparoscopy or robotic surgery is recommended for patients with tumors that are smaller than 5 cm and located in the stomach or small bowel. In cases where adjacent organs are involved, en bloc resection is recommended [9]. For large and difficult to access tumors, minimally invasive approaches may not be appropriate due to the potential for tumor rupture, which is associated with a very high risk of relapse.

When an R0 resection is difficult to achieve or likely to result in major functional impairments for the patient, preoperative therapy should be considered in order to shrink the tumor as much as possible prior to surgery. While there is not an established gold-standard period of administration, *imatinib is generally administered preoperatively for at least 6 to 12 months with interval imaging to assess response to allow maximal tumor shrinkage, before being stopped prior to surgery* [9]. It should be noted that preoperative therapy will make a final pathologic risk assessment difficult and the decision for postoperative therapy may be more difficult as a result. Sometimes larger tumors may be primarily resected to avoid long term treatment which may have no benefit, this is particularly true in gastric tumors. In cases where there is a high risk of recurrence, such as in the case of intestinal and rectal tumors and specific mutational driver variants or poor prognostic factors, imatinib should be given after surgery for up to 3 years and may be administered for life for patients with tumors with very high risk of recurrence. [9]

Advanced and Metastatic GISTs

From 2000 to 2019, approximately 7%–19% of GIST patients presented with distant metastatic disease at diagnosis [3]. Historically, advanced GISTs were associated with poor survival outcomes due to their lack of response to chemotherapy and radiation. Prior to the implementation and development of targeted therapies such as **tyrosine kinase inhibitors** (TKIs), patients with advanced GISTs had an overall survival of 1.5 years, compared to recent data that show overall survival estimated to be 6–8 years [15]. **TKIs revolutionized the management of GISTs due to the finding that 80%–90% of GISTs have primary KIT mutations** [16]. KIT is a tyrosine kinase that promotes the survival and replication of the interstitial cells of Cajal, which are the cells GISTs arise from. GISTs rely on a KIT gain-in-function mutation to survive. As a result, TKIs can treat GISTs by blocking the expression of KIT.

As of 2025, there are currently five FDA-approved drugs for advanced GIST treatment, all of which are TKIs:

1. Imatinib
2. Sunitinib
3. Regorafenib
4. Ripretinib
5. Avapritinib

Imatinib is considered the ***standard first-line treatment*** and is generally the best tolerated among patients. In patients with advanced GISTs, imatinib in the adjuvant setting is associated with improved survival outcomes [2]. Some research has suggested that cytoreductive surgery to achieve either R0 or R1 disease after an initial response to imatinib may be associated with improved long-term survival. Data do not support major surgery in patients where it is likely to have an incomplete resection or suboptimal debulking.

Imatinib-Resistant Disease

Approximately 10–15% of GISTs show a primary resistance imatinib [17]. For these patients, the standard next line of treatment is **sunitinib**. It is important to confirm treatment adherence and rule out any drug interactions before claiming imatinib resistance. Before treating with sunitinib, increasing the imatinib dosage to 400 mg twice daily can be considered [7]. Even in cases of resistance, maintenance of TKIs has been shown to improve outcomes and is advised in cases where alternative therapeutic options are unavailable.

However, while TKIs benefit most patients with advanced disease, they have little efficacy in patients with certain PDGFRA mutations or patients lacking both KIT and PDGFRA mutations. In patients with the PDGFRA D942V mutations, **avapritinib** is the only approved treatment in the United States and has an overall response rate of 88% [18]. As a result, avapritinib should be introduced as the first line of treatment in GISTs with PDGFRA D942V mutations.

Recurrence

Following resection, GISTs often recur locally, spreading throughout the serosal surfaces of the abdomen, or metastasizing to the liver. For localized disease, there are limited data comparing the efficacy of different follow-up strategies. However, most recommendations advocate for adjustment to the risk of recurrence with time based on known risk factors including tumor size, location, rupture during surgery, mitotic rate, and incomplete resection. In cases of unresectable or metastatic disease, follow-up should be done every 3 months. Once the response remains beyond a 5-year period, follow-up can be prolonged to every 6 months.

Special Considerations

Although most GISTs occur in the stomach and small intestine, rare sites include the colon, rectum, esophagus, and extraintestinal areas. The College of American Pathologists provides guidelines for risk assessment of primary GISTs that originate in the gastric, duodenum, jejunum/ileum, and rectum anatomical sites. For any GISTs that occur outside of these locations, it is recommended to us the risk criteria for the jejunum/ileum.

In addition, special considerations regarding the site's anatomical characteristics may be required in treatment decisions. For example, although the standard treatment for localized GISTs is curative resection, it is difficult to achieve curative resection for rectal GISTs given the proximity to the sphincter muscle and narrow pelvis [19]. In these cases, trans-anal, trans-sacral, or trans-vaginal excision are recommended for non-high-risk GISTs, but no standard treatment has been developed for the management of rectal GISTs [19–21].

Conclusion

Management of GISTs depends on a variety of factors including, but not limited to, presence of cell mutations, anatomical location, mitotic rate, and tumor size. For localized disease, curative resection remains the standard for treatment. Prognosis has significantly improved for advanced disease over the last two decades with the advent of targeted therapies and TKIs. As of today, there are seven FDA-approved TKIs for the treatment of GISTs, and it is crucial that all confirmed tumors undergo mutational analysis in order to effectively guide disease management. As data continue to emerge and our understanding of GIST biology develops, targeted management of GISTs, especially for tumors occurring in rare anatomic sites or with TKI resistance, will only improve.

References

1. Joensuu H, Hohenberger P, Corless CL. Gastrointestinal stromal tumour. Lancet. 2013;382(9896):973–83. https://doi.org/10.1016/S0140-6736(13)60106-3.
2. Parab TM, DeRogatis MJ, Boaz AM, et al. Gastrointestinal stromal tumors: a comprehensive review. J Gastrointest Oncol. 2019;10(1):144–54. https://doi.org/10.21037/jgo.2018.08.20.
3. Alvarez CS, Piazuelo MB, Fleitas-Kanonnikoff T, Ruhl J, Pérez-Fidalgo JA, Camargo MC. Incidence and survival outcomes of gastrointestinal stromal tumors. JAMA Netw Open. 2024;7(8):e2428828. https://doi.org/10.1001/jamanetworkopen.2024.28828.
4. Raitio A, Salim A, Mullassery D, Losty PD. Current treatment and outcomes of pediatric gastrointestinal stromal tumors (GIST): a systematic review of published studies. Pediatr Surg Int. 2021;37(9):1161–5. https://doi.org/10.1007/s00383-021-04931-0.
5. Corless CL. Gastrointestinal stromal tumors: what do we know now? Mod Pathol. 2014;27:S1–S16. https://doi.org/10.1038/modpathol.2013.173.

6. Gastrointestinal Stromal Tumors Treatment (PDQ®) - NCI. March 9, 2011. https://www.cancer.gov/types/soft-tissue-sarcoma/hp/gist-treatment-pdq. Accessed 2 June 2025.
7. von Mehren M, Joensuu H. Gastrointestinal stromal tumors. J Clin Oncol. 2018;36(2):136–43. https://doi.org/10.1200/JCO.2017.74.9705.
8. Joensuu H. KIT and PDGFRA variants and the survival of patients with gastrointestinal stromal tumor treated with adjuvant imatinib. Cancer. 2023;15(15):3879. https://doi.org/10.3390/cancers15153879.
9. Judson I, Jones RL, Wong NACS, et al. Gastrointestinal stromal tumour (GIST): British Sarcoma Group clinical practice guidelines. Br J Cancer. 2025;132(1):1–10. https://doi.org/10.1038/s41416-024-02672-0.
10. Nishida T. Therapeutic strategies for wild-type gastrointestinal stromal tumor: is it different from KIT or PDGFRA-mutated GISTs? Transl Gastroenterol Hepatol. 2017;2:92. https://doi.org/10.21037/tgh.2017.11.05.
11. Fletcher CDM, Berman JJ, Corless C, et al. Diagnosis of gastrointestinal stromal tumors: a consensus approach. Hum Pathol. 2002;33(5):459–65. https://doi.org/10.1053/hupa.2002.123545. PMID: 12094370.
12. Miettinen M, Lasota J. Gastrointestinal stromal tumors: pathology and prognosis at different sites. Semin Diagn Pathol. 2006;23(2):70–83. https://doi.org/10.1053/j.semdp.2006.09.001. PMID: 17193820.
13. Joensuu H. Risk stratification of patients diagnosed with gastrointestinal stromal tumor. Hum Pathol. 2008;39(10):1411–9. doi:https://doi.org/10.1016/j.humpath.2008.06.025. PMID: 18774375.
14. Bertsimas D, Margonis GA, Tang S, et al. An interpretable AI model for recurrence prediction after surgery in gastrointestinal stromal tumour: an observational cohort study. EClinicalMedicine. 2023;64:102200. https://doi.org/10.1016/j.eclinm.2023.102200.
15. Khosroyani HM, Klug LR, Heinrich MC. TKI treatment sequencing in advanced gastrointestinal stromal tumors. Drugs. 2023;83(1):55–73. https://doi.org/10.1007/s40265-022-01820-1.
16. Zhou S, Abdihamid O, Tan F, et al. KIT mutations and expression: current knowledge and new insights for overcoming IM resistance in GIST. Cell Commun Signal. 2024;22(1):153. https://doi.org/10.1186/s12964-023-01411-x.
17. Kee D, Zalcberg JR. Current and emerging strategies for the management of imatinib-refractory advanced gastrointestinal stromal tumors. Ther Adv Med Oncol. 2012;4(5):255–70. https://doi.org/10.1177/1758834012450935.
18. George S, Jones RL, Bauer S, et al. Avapritinib in patients with advanced gastrointestinal stromal tumors following at least three prior lines of therapy. Oncologist. 2021;26(4):e639–49. https://doi.org/10.1002/onco.13674.
19. Kameyama H, Kanda T, Tajima Y, et al. Management of rectal gastrointestinal stromal tumor. Transl Gastroenterol Hepatol. 2018;3(2) https://doi.org/10.21037/tgh.2018.01.08.
20. Theodoropoulos DG. Gastrointestinal tumors of the colon and rectum. Clin Colon Rectal Surg. 2011;24(3):161–70. https://doi.org/10.1055/s-0031-1286000.
21. Guo W, Yang Z, Wei Y, et al. Radical excision versus local resection for primary rectal gastrointestinal stromal tumors. Cohort study. Int J Surg. 2020;77:190–7. https://doi.org/10.1016/j.ijsu.2020.03.068.

Appendiceal Disease

13

William Cobb, Shelby Harris, Joseph Portoghese, and Marco Swanson

Introduction

The appendix remains a subject of debate in anatomical and clinical contexts. Previously considered an evolutionary remnant without function, current research suggests it may have a role in immune regulation, particularly in maintaining gut microbiota and serving as a bacterial reservoir [1].

The appendix can also be the site of various pathological processes, including appendicitis and neoplasms. Appendiceal tumors, though rare, range from benign mucinous neoplasms to aggressive adenocarcinomas with peritoneal dissemination [2]. The classification and management of these tumors have evolved with advances in pathological and molecular characterization, influencing therapeutic strategies [3].

Embryology of the Appendix

The appendix develops as a diverticulum from the midgut during early fetal development. Around the fifth week of gestation, the midgut undergoes rapid elongation and forms a U-shaped loop, which herniates into the umbilical cord due to limited space in the abdominal cavity [4]. During the 10th week of gestation, the midgut returns to the abdomen and rotates counterclockwise around the superior mesenteric artery, a process that ensures proper anatomical positioning of the intestinal structures [5]. This rotation continues through subsequent weeks of development, resulting in the final placement of the cecum and appendix in the lower right quadrant of the abdomen [6].

The mesentery, which initially suspends the midgut loop, undergoes remodeling, leading to the fixation of the ascending colon and cecum to the posterior abdominal wall [7]. This complex series of movements is crucial in establishing the final anatomical relationships of the appendix with surrounding structures, influencing variations in its positioning observed in different individuals [8].

Anatomy of the Appendix

The appendix is a narrow, blind-ended tube that arises from the posteromedial aspect of the cecum, approximately 2–3 cm below the ileocecal valve [9] (Fig. 13.1). It varies in length, typically ranging from 5 to 10 cm, though it can be as long as 20 cm. The appendix has a variable position within the abdominal cavity, with the most common orientations being **retrocecal** (Fig. 13.2) and pelvic, followed by subcecal, pre-ileal, and post-ileal positions [10].

Histologically, the appendix shares structural features with the colon, possessing a mucosa, submucosa, muscularis propria, and serosa. However, it is distinct in its abundant lymphoid tissue within the lamina propria, contributing to its proposed immunological function [11].

W. Cobb (✉) · S. Harris · J. Portoghese
Department of General Surgery, AdventHealth Orlando, Orlando, FL, USA
e-mail: william.cobb.md@adventhealth.com; joseph.portoghese.md@adventhealth.com

M. Swanson
Dermatology and Plastic Surgery of Arizona, Tucson, AZ, USA

S. Atallah, J. Dragoljevic (eds.), *Fundamentals of Surgery for Physician Assistants*, https://doi.org/10.1007/978-3-032-21069-2_13

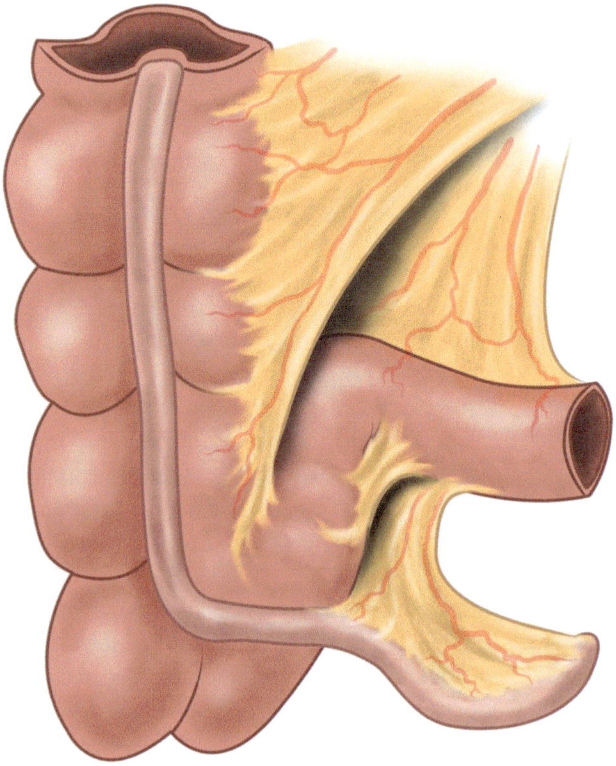

Fig. 13.1 The appendix is a narrow, blind-ended, tubular structure arising from the posteromedial wall of the cecum, typically located 2–3 cm below the ileocecal valve. Its average length is approximately 8–9 cm, but it can range from 5 to 35 cm, with a mean outer diameter of about 5.8 mm in healthy individuals; the diameter increases significantly in appendicitis. **The most common anatomical position is retrocecal** (32%), followed by pelvic (as shown here, 28%) and ileal (14%), but it can also be positioned elsewhere, contributing to variability in clinical presentation. The wall of the appendix consists of the same layers as the colon: mucosa, submucosa, muscularis propria, and serosa. The mucosa is lined by columnar epithelium with abundant goblet cells and contains numerous lymphoid follicles, **which are most prominent in childhood**, supporting its role as a **gut-associated lymphoid organ**. Functionally, the appendix is now recognized as an immunological organ, involved in the maturation of B lymphocytes, production of immunoglobulin A, and maintenance of gut microbiota by serving as a reservoir for commensal bacteria

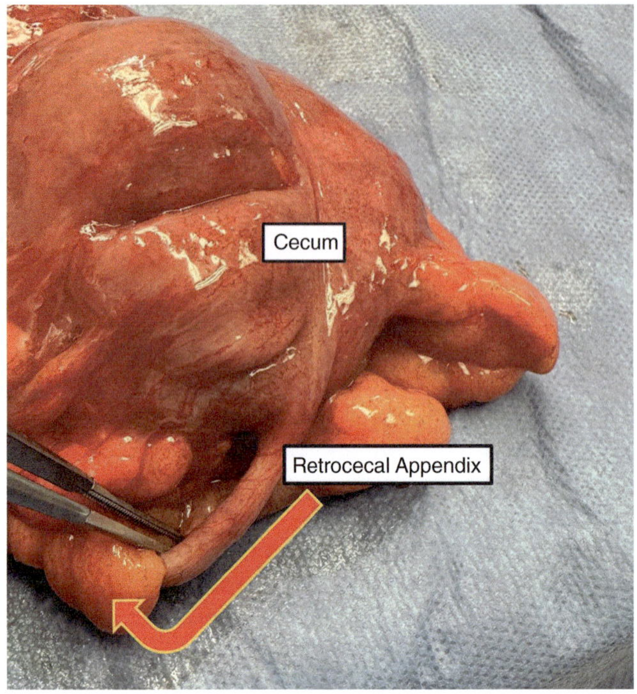

Fig. 13.2 A resected portion of bowel in its native position shows the appendix as lies "*behind" the cecum* (arrow). The **retrocecal position** of the appendix refers to the anatomical variant in which the appendix lies posterior to the cecum, often extending superiorly along the posterior abdominal wall. **This is the most common position**, with a pooled incidence of approximately 32% according to large meta-analyses of anatomical studies. The appendix in this location is typically more mobile and may be partially or completely retroperitoneal, which *influences both its clinical presentation and the spread of inflammation*. **A retrocecal appendix can lead to atypical presentations of appendicitis**. *Instead of classic right lower quadrant pain, patients may present with right flank, right upper quadrant, or even back pain, as the inflamed appendix irritates the posterior parietal peritoneum or retroperitoneal structures*. Physical findings such as localized tenderness at McBurney's point *may be absent or less pronounced*, and psoas sign may be more prominent due to proximity to the iliopsoas muscle

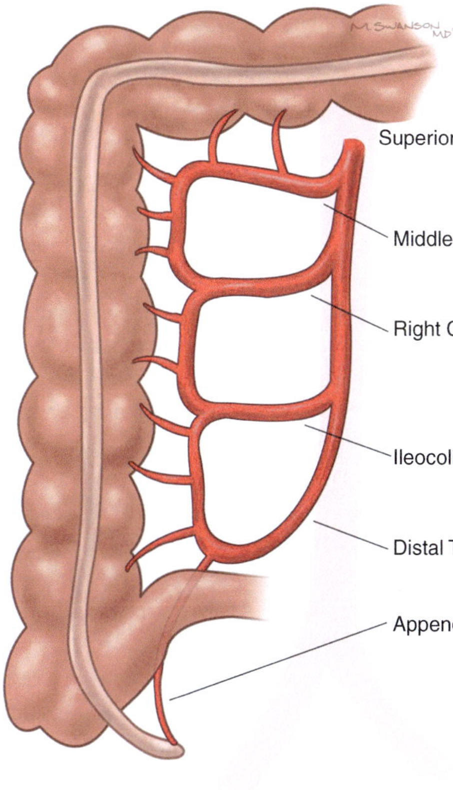

Fig. 13.3 Arterial blood supply to the appendix

Blood Supply

The primary arterial supply to the appendix is the **appendicular artery**, a branch of the **ileocolic artery**, which originates from the **superior mesenteric artery** [12]. The appendicular artery runs within the mesoappendix and is an end artery, making the appendix particularly susceptible to ischemia if the vessel is occluded [13] (Fig. 13.3).

Venous drainage occurs through the appendicular vein, which empties into the **ileocolic vein** and subsequently drains into the **superior mesenteric vein** [14].

Lymphatics

The lymphatic drainage of the appendix follows the course of the arterial supply, with lymph nodes located along the appendicular, ileocolic, and superior mesenteric pathways [15]. These nodes play a role in immune surveillance and contribute to the inflammatory response in appendicitis [16]. The appendix contains numerous lymphoid follicles within its walls, further supporting its immunological role in gut-associated lymphoid tissue (GALT) [17].

Diagnostics

The diagnosis of appendiceal pathology is primarily clinical, supplemented by laboratory findings and imaging studies [18]. Clinical assessment includes history-taking and physical examination, with key findings such as right lower quadrant tenderness, rebound tenderness, and pain migration from the peri-umbilical region being suggestive of appendicitis [19]. Physical exam findings for acute appendicitis include tenderness of **McBurney's point**, the *Rovsing sign, Psoas Sign, and Obturator sign.* McBurney's point is the most common location of the appendix located one-third of the distance from the anterior superior iliac spine to the umbilicus. Rovsing sign is right lower quadrant (RLQ) pain with palpation of the left lower quadrant (LLQ). Psoas sign is right hip extension or raising straight leg against resistance producing pain in the RLQ. Obturator sign is passive internal rotation of the right thigh producing RLQ pain [20]. Laboratory evaluation typically reveals leukocytosis with a predominance of neutrophils, and elevated C-reactive protein (CRP) levels can support the diagnosis [21]. Keep in mind that retrocecal appendicitis implies that the inflamed appendix is behind the cecum and is not able to "irritate" the sensitive *peritoneal lining*, thus ***retrocecal appendicitis may not result present with typical clinical findings***.

For appendicitis, scoring systems such as the Alvarado Score and Pediatric Appendicitis Score (PAS) have been developed to aid in the early identification and risk stratification of appendicitis.

The **Alvarado Score** consists of eight clinical and laboratory criteria, with a total possible score of 10:

- Migration of pain to the right lower quadrant (1 point)
- Anorexia (1 point)
- Nausea or vomiting (1 point)
- Tenderness in the right lower quadrant (2 points)
- Rebound tenderness (1 point)
- Elevated temperature > 37.3 °C (1 point)
- Leukocytosis >10,000/mm^3 (2 points)
- Shift to the left (neutrophilia) (1 point)

A score of 7 or higher suggests a high probability of appendicitis and may indicate the need for surgical intervention, while a score of 4–6 is considered equivocal, requiring further imaging or observation. A score below 4 is associated with a low probability of appendicitis and may warrant alternative diagnoses [2].

The **Pediatric Appendicitis Score (PAS)** is a modified scoring system designed for children between ages 3 and 18, incorporating clinical findings and laboratory markers to assess the likelihood of appendicitis:

- Right lower quadrant tenderness (2 points)
- Anorexia (1 point)
- Fever >38 °C (1 point)
- Nausea or vomiting (1 point)
- Migration of pain (1 point)
- Leukocytosis >10,000/mm^3 (1 point)
- Neutrophilia >75% (1 point)
- Cough/percussion/hopping tenderness (2 points)

PAS scores of 8–10 suggest a high likelihood of appendicitis and typically warrants surgical consultation. A score of 5–7 indicates moderate risk, requiring additional imaging such as ultrasound or CT for confirmation, while a score below 5 suggests a low probability of appendicitis and may support outpatient observation [3].

Imaging plays a crucial role in appendiceal pathology. **Computed tomography (CT)** is the preferred imaging modality in adult patients due to its high sensitivity and specificity [19]. CT findings indicative of appendicitis include an enlarged appendix (>6 mm in diameter), wall thickening, periappendiceal fat stranding, and the presence of an appendicolith [2]. However, CT is generally avoided in pregnant patients and children due to concerns regarding radiation exposure [3]. **Ultrasound** and **magnetic resonance imaging (MRI)** may also be used in diagnosis.

Pathology

Acute appendicitis is the most common pathological condition affecting the appendix, characterized by inflammation due to luminal obstruction, bacterial overgrowth, and ischemia [18]. The obstruction is often caused by **lymphoid hyperplasia**, fecaliths, foreign bodies, or, in rare cases, neoplasms. This leads to increased intraluminal pressure, venous congestion, and subsequent ischemia, which fosters bacterial proliferation and an inflammatory response. The inflammatory cascade progresses from mucosal involvement to transmural inflammation, *potentially resulting in perforation if left untreated* [19].

Histologically, acute appendicitis is marked by neutrophilic infiltration of the appendiceal wall, beginning at the mucosa and progressing outward. Early changes include mucosal ulceration, edema, and congestion, while severe cases exhibit full-thickness necrosis and fibrinopurulent exudates within the peritoneal cavity [21]. Complications include gangrenous appendicitis, perforation, and abscess formation, each carrying an increased risk of peritonitis and sepsis [2].

Chronic appendicitis, though less common, presents with recurrent or prolonged symptoms due to partial obstruction, recurrent episodes of inflammation, or underlying pathology such as endometriosis or appendiceal diverticulosis. Histological features include fibrosis, mononuclear infiltration, and residual neutrophilic presence within the appendiceal wall [3].

Appendiceal neoplasms represent a diverse group of pathological entities ranging from benign to highly malignant tumors. The most common are neuroendocrine tumors (NETs), mucinous neoplasms, and adenocarcinomas [4].

Neuroendocrine tumors (NETs), previously referred to as carcinoid tumors, arise from enterochromaffin cells and constitute the most frequently encountered appendiceal neoplasm. They are often found incidentally during appendectomy. These tumors typically exhibit a well-differentiated architecture with uniform round nuclei and a salt-and-pepper chromatin pattern. While most NETs are indolent, those larger than 2 cm, those invading the mesoappendix, or those displaying high mitotic activity carry a greater risk of metastasis and may require additional surgical management [5].

Mucinous neoplasms of the appendix (Fig. 13.4) encompass a spectrum from low-grade **appendiceal mucinous neoplasms** (LAMNs) to mucinous adenocarcinomas. LAMNs are characterized by well-differentiated mucin-producing epithelium with minimal cytologic atypia but have the potential for peritoneal dissemination, leading to pseudomyxoma peritonei (PMP) [6]. Mucinous adenocarcinomas, on the other hand, display more aggressive features such as infiltrative growth, cellular atypia, and increased mitotic activity. Tumor rupture and peritoneal dissemination can result in mucinous ascites, significantly impacting morbidity and prognosis [7].

Non-mucinous adenocarcinomas, including signet-ring cell carcinoma, are rare but highly aggressive. These tumors often present at an advanced stage with peritoneal spread and carry a poor prognosis due to limited treatment options and resistance to conventional therapies [8].

Other rare appendiceal malignancies include goblet cell adenocarcinomas, which exhibit features of both adenocarcinomas and neuroendocrine tumors, and appendiceal lymphoma, which remains exceedingly uncommon but can present with acute appendicitis-like symptoms [9].

Surgical excision remains the cornerstone of treatment for appendiceal pathology. The extent of resection depends on the underlying diagnosis, with simple appendectomy often sufficient for NETs and early-stage LAMNs, while right hemicolectomy may be required for invasive adenocarcinomas or large neuroendocrine tumors. Histopathologic evaluation is critical in determining the appropriate therapeutic approach and long-term management [10].

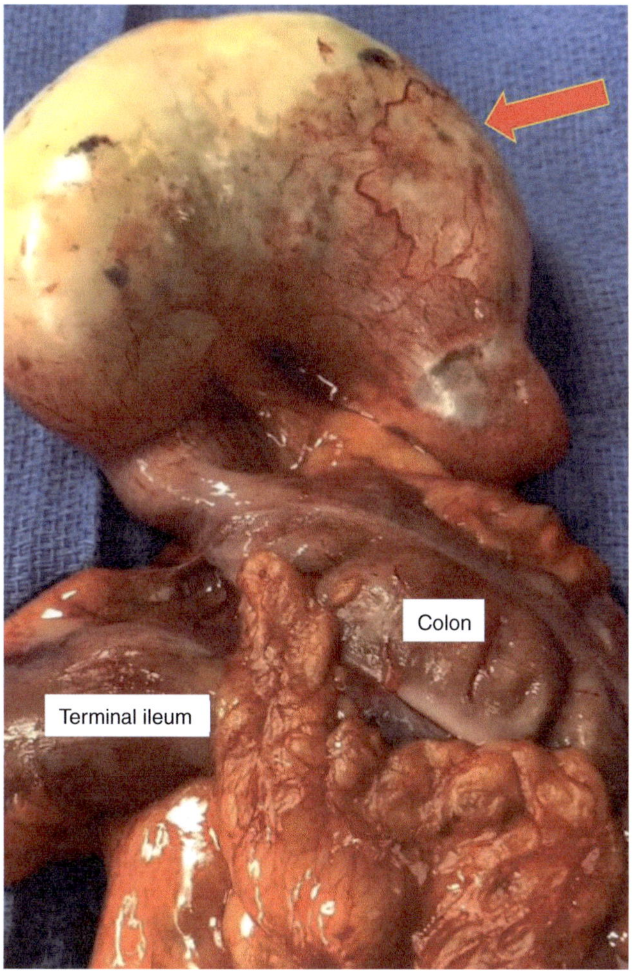

Fig. 13.4 An **appendiceal mucocele** in a resected portion of ileocolic bowel is shown, here measuring 7 cm (arrow). A mucocele is defined as a pathological dilatation of the appendix due to **intraluminal accumulation of mucinous material**. Anatomically, this results in a grossly distended, cystic, tubular structure arising from the cecum, often exceeding the normal appendiceal diameter. Clinically, appendiceal mucoceles are rare, accounting for 0.2–0.7% of appendiceal pathologies, and may present with right lower quadrant pain, a palpable mass, or be discovered incidentally on imaging or colonoscopy. The most **significant clinical concern is the risk of rupture, which can result in dissemination of mucin-producing cells into the peritoneal cavity**, leading to **pseudomyxoma peritonei,** a potentially fatal condition characterized by progressive intraperitoneal accumulation of mucin. Management is primarily surgical, with appendectomy indicated for benign lesions and more extensive resection (e.g., right hemicolectomy) for malignant or high-risk neoplastic mucoceles, as was the case here

Non-operative management of Acute Appendicitis: Antibiotics and Image-Guided Drainage

Acute appendicitis is a common surgical emergency characterized by peri-umbilical pain migrating to the right lower quadrant, nausea, vomiting, and anorexia [18]. Advances in imaging modalities such as ultrasound and computed tomography (CT) have improved diagnostic accuracy, reducing unnecessary appendectomies [19].

Uncomplicated appendicitis can be successfully managed with antibiotics alone in selected patients. Recent studies have shown that up to 90% of select patients can be treated with antibiotics and avoid surgery [21, 22]. Careful patient selection and strict evaluation of patients' response to treatment are critical to obtain success. The first-line antibiotic regimen is amoxicillin/clavulanic acid. The second-line treatment is piperacillin/tazobactam [23]. CRP levels below 60 g/L, white blood cell count below 12,000, and age under 60 years are predictors of success of antibiotic management [21]. Low modified Alvarado score (less than 4) and imaging-confirmed uncomplicated appendicitis were also more likely to achieve success with antibiotic management. The presence of an appendicolith has been recognized as a prognostic risk factor for failure of antibiotic management and its presence is associated with higher risk of perforation [21]. Patients with complicated appendicitis such as gangrenous appendicitis, perforated appendicitis, intra-abdominal abscess, and/or diffuse peritonitis should be excluded from consideration of antibiotics alone management [21]. Salminen et al. showed that within 5 years of non-operative management of appendicitis, recurrence was 39.1% [24]. Follow-up data for trials conducted in Sweden in the 1990s show the cumulative risk of appendectomy at 25 years is 40% for those initially treated with non-operative management [25, 26].

If imaging studies demonstrate an intra-abdominal or pelvic abscess, **CT- or ultrasound-guided drainage** can often be performed percutaneously or transrectally. Studies suggest that percutaneous drainage of appendiceal abscesses results in fewer complications and shorter overall length of stay than surgical drainage. It also allows inflammation to subside before appendectomy, thereby negating the need for larger operations or possible bowel resection in some cases [27]. Typically, if patients undergo image guided drainage, they will undergo interval appendectomy 6–8 weeks later.

Surgical Management of Acute Appendicitis

The first appendectomies were performed in an open technique (OA). An open incision, known as the Rockey–Davis incision, in a transverse manner across the RLQ is made and after delivery of the tip of the cecum, the mesoappendix is divided, then the base is clamped and ligated with a simple throw of the knot, and the appendix is amputated [22, 28]. OA is only performed in select patients now, typically patients who are unable to tolerate the physiology effects of pneumoperitoneum.

Laparoscopic appendectomy (LA) is the recommended treatment for acute uncomplicated appendicitis. LA is a minimally invasive technique involving three small incisions, typically at the umbilicus, the left lower quadrant, and suprapubic region. The abdomen is insufflated with carbon dioxide creating a pneumoperitoneum and the appendix is isolated and removed from its base. Historically, acute appendicitis was deemed an emergency but more recently, LA is safe within 24–36 hours of hospital presentation within selected patients and is not associated with an increased rate of infectious complications [22]. Prophylactic antibiotics prior to surgery are important for preventing wound infection and intra-abdominal abscess following appendectomy. The flora of the appendix reflects that of the colon and includes gram-negative aerobes and anaerobes [29]. LA has become the standard treatment and current evidence confirms that LA is superior to OA in adult patients, as it is associated with better postoperative outcomes and faster recovery [21]. Postoperative complications are lower in LA than in conventional OA and laparoscopic surgery is associated with fewer readmissions and fewer additional interventions than non-operative treatment with a comparable hospital length of stay [30].

Single-incision laparoscopic surgery (SILS) is an alternative minimally invasive technique for appendectomy. SILS is performed through only the umbilical incision and would presumably reduce surgical trauma, improve cosmetic results, and leave the patient with only a single incision [31]. Due to advances in technology, **robotic appendectomy (RA)** has emerged as a new option for minimally invasive surgery. Results demonstrated that LA and RA had a similar frequency and profile of complications [32].

Complications from Acute Appendicitis and Surgical Intervention

The mortality rate in simple acute appendicitis is approximately 0.1% and has not changed significantly since 1930. Progress in preoperative and postoperative care has reduced mortality from perforation to about 5%. Nonetheless, postoperative infections still occur in 30% of cases of complicated appendicitis. Although the cases may be more technically challenging, obese patients have similar rates of complication, length of stay, and readmission. The substantial increase in tubal infertility that follows perforation in young women is avoidable using early appendectomy. If the entirety of the appendix is not removed, stump appendicitis can occur in the residual appendix [33].

Pediatric Appendicitis

Appendicitis is a common cause of abdominal pain in pediatric populations and is commonly caused by **lymphoid hyperplasia**. *Note well:* The most common cause of appendicitis in **adults** is luminal obstruction by a **fecalith**, whereas in the **pediatric population**, the most common cause is obstruction by **hypertrophied lymphoid tissue**.

Typical presentation includes generalized abdominal pain that migrates to the right lower quadrant and can be associated with fever, chills, nausea, anorexia, emesis, and diarrhea [34, 35]. In pediatric patients, ultrasound is the first-line imaging modality to minimize radiation exposure [4]. A positive ultrasound finding includes a noncompressible, tubular structure in the right lower quadrant with a diameter greater than 6 mm, hyperemia on Doppler imaging, and periappendiceal fluid [5]. If ultrasound results are inconclusive, CT imaging or clinical observation may be warranted.

Studies have demonstrated that reducing the number of CT scans in pediatric patients significantly decreases cumulative radiation exposure without compromising diagnostic accuracy. Implementing ultrasound-first strategies and clinical scoring systems can lead to a substantial reduction in unnecessary CT scans, thereby lowering radiation risks in children [15, 16]. First-line treatment for appendicitis in the pediatric population is LA. Mortality from appendicitis in the pediatric population is less than 0.2% and overall complications rates vary from 5% to 10%. Nonoperative management in select pediatric populations is possible [34, 35].

Appendicitis During Pregnancy

The rate of appendicitis in pregnancy is like that in the nonpregnant female population and occurs in approximately 1 in 500 pregnancies per year. Appendicitis occurs more frequently in the second trimester than in the first or third. Preoperative diagnosis of AA can be difficult in pregnancy, and a low threshold for surgical intervention has traditionally been recommended, as complicated appendicitis is associated with a higher rate of fetal loss and increased maternal morbidity [22]. The American College of Obstetricians and Gynecologists recommend ultrasound or magnetic resonance imaging for pregnant patients with concern for appendicitis. Where emergency access to such imaging is not possible and there remains a high suspicion of appendicitis, surgery should not be delayed.

Many reports have demonstrated **LA to be a safe and effective procedure during pregnancy**. Surgical intervention for appendicitis during pregnancy was historically recommended to occur during the second trimester, but new data are suggesting laparoscopy can be performed in other trimesters as well [36]. With modification of port positions, the laparoscopic approach has even been reported during the third trimester [22]. Gravid patients should be positioned in the left lateral recumbent position to minimize compression of the vena cava and aorta. Supine positioning decreases venous return resulting in maternal hypotension, reduced cardiac output, and decreased placental perfusion during surgery [36].

Elderly

One in every 2000 adults over age 65 will develop appendicitis annually, making appendicitis an important cause of abdominal pain in this age group. Older adults tend to have a diminished inflammatory response, resulting in fewer cases of leukocytosis and less remarkable findings on history and physical examination. For these reasons, older patients often delay seeking medical care, and, as a result, they have a considerably higher rate of perforation at the time of presentation. Laparoscopic appendectomy is safe in this population [37–39].

Immunocompromised

Immunocompromised patients including organ transplant recipients, immunosuppressive therapy for autoimmune diseases, cancer, and acquired immunodeficiency syndrome (AIDS) are susceptible to infection. The immune response in these patient populations is blunted due to immunosuppressive medication or disease. As a result, they may not exhibit the typical signs and symptoms of appendicitis and may have only mild tenderness on examination. In addition, laboratory and radiological tests may not show the expected level of inflammation. An expanded differential diagnosis includes but is not limited to opportunistic and viral infections, fungal infections, secondary malignancies such as lymphoma or Kaposi's sarcoma, and typhlitis. Because of the broad differential diagnoses, there is often a delay in reaching the diagnosis and presentation to surgical evaluation, which can increase the risk of perforation [40–42]. Laparoscopic appendectomy is safe in this population.

Role for Colonoscopy

Patients who recover from non-operative treatment of acute appendicitis or who have a diagnosis of appendiceal mass should undergo colonoscopy or barium enema to detect any underlying diseases and to rule out coexistent colorectal cancer [30]. Multiple studies have emphasized the importance of screening colonoscopy following appendectomy *particularly in patients over the age of 40* due to the increased risk of colon cancer as a potential underlying cause of appendicitis with the reported incidence ranging from 0.7% to 2.9% [43–45].

References

1. Smith HF, et al. A review of the function and evolution of the cecal appendix. Anat Rec (Hoboken). 2023.
2. Hoehn RS, et al. Current management of appendiceal neoplasms. ASCO Educ Book. 2021;41:1.
3. Hissong E, Yantiss RK. The Frontiers of appendiceal controversies: mucinous neoplasms and pseudomyxoma peritonei. Am J Surg Pathol. 2022;46:e27.
4. Barlow M, et al. Developmental anatomy of the appendix and its variations. J Pediatr Surg. 2021.
5. Constantin M, et al. The vermiform appendix and its pathologies. Cancers. 2023;15.
6. Panarelli NC. Inflammatory disorders of the appendix. In: Odze and Goldblum surgical pathology. 2023.
7. Schlottmann F, et al. Surgical approaches to acute appendicitis. Curr Probl Surg. 2024.
8. Goldblum JR, et al. The appendix and its diseases. Surg Pathol. 2023.
9. Pai SA, Mannan R. Nonneoplastic pathology of the appendix. Am J Clin Pathol. 2024.
10. Lamps LW. Pathology of the appendix: a review. Surg Pathol Clin. 2021.
11. Drake FT, et al. Outcomes of nonoperative management of appendicitis. JAMA Surg. 2020.
12. Varadhan KK, et al. Antibiotic therapy versus appendectomy for acute appendicitis: a meta-analysis. BMJ. 2012.
13. Humes DJ, Simpson J. Acute appendicitis. BMJ. 2006;333:530.
14. Gorter RR, et al. Diagnosis and management of acute appendicitis. Best Pract Res Clin Gastroenterol. 2014.
15. Bhangu A, et al. Acute appendicitis: modern understanding of pathogenesis, diagnosis, and management. Lancet. 2015;386:1278.
16. Puylaert JB, et al. Imaging and intervention in patients with acute appendicitis: a review. Am J Roentgenol. 2020.
17. Andersson RE. Meta-analysis of the clinical and laboratory diagnosis of appendicitis. Br J Surg. 2004.
18. Sanchez SE, Burke PA. Current diagnosis & treatment: surgery. McGraw Hill; 2020.
19. Cho JH, et al. Features on computed tomography that correlate with acute appendicitis. Am Surg. 2023;89:2876.
20. Rentea RM, St. Peter SD. Pediatric appendicits. Surg Clin Noth Am. 2017;97(1):93–112.

21. Casas MA, et al. Medical and surgical treatment of acute appendicitis: past, present and future. Curr Probl Surg. 2024;61:101458.
22. Paterson HM, Deans C. Chapter 15—Acute conditions of the small bowel and appendix. In: Core topics in general and emergency surgery. 2024. pp. 153–70.
23. Yu CH, Chang CN, Wang CC. Causative microbes and antibiotic susceptibility of acute appendicitis in adults and children. Pediatr Neonatol. 2024;65(2):159–64.
24. Salminen P, Paajanen H, Rautio T, Nordström P, Aarnio M, Rantanen T, et al. Antibiotic therapy vs appendectomy for treatment of uncomplicated acute appendicitis: the APPAC randomized clinical trial. JAMA. 2015;313(23):2340–8.
25. Eriksson S, Granström L. Randomized controlled trial of appendicectomy versus antibiotic therapy for acute appendicitis. Br J Surg. 1995;82:166.
26. Styrud J, Eriksson S, Nilsson I, et al. Appendectomy versus antibiotic treatment in acute appendicitis. A prospective multicenter randomized controlled trial. World J Surg. 2006;30:1033.
27. Fujikawa T, Ando K. Safety of laparoscopic surgery in digestive diseases with special reference to antithrombotic therapy: a systematic review of the literature. World J Clin Cases. 2018;6:767.
28. Ajao OG. Abdominal incisions in general surgery: a review. Ann Ib Postgrad Med. 2007;5(2):59–63.
29. Andersen BR, Kallehave FL, Andersen HK. Antibiotics versus placebo for prevention of postoperative infection after appendicectomy. Cochrane Database Syst Rev. 2005;2005:CD001439.
30. Hori T, Machimoto T, Kadokawa Y, Hata T, Ito T, Kato S, Yasukawa D, Aisu Y, Kimura Y, Sasaki M, Takamatsu Y, Kitano T, Hisamori S, Yoshimura T. Laparoscopic appendectomy for acute appendicitis: how to discourage surgeons using inadequate therapy. World J Gastroenterol. 2017;23(32):5849–59.
31. Pisanu A, Porceddu G, Reccia I, Saba A, Uccheddu A. Meta-analysis of studies comparing single-incision laparoscopic appendectomy and conventional multiport laparoscopic appendectomy. J Surg Res. 2013;183(2):e49–59.
32. Becker T, DeLeon G, Rao V, Pei KY. A comparison of outcomes between laparoscopic and robotic appendectomy among ACS-NSQIP hospitals. Laparosc Endosc Robot Surg. 2023;6(2):39–42.
33. Doherty GM. Chapter 30: Appendix. In: Current diagnosis and treatment surgery. 15th ed. 2020. pp 1–7.
34. Grosfeld JL, O'Neil JAJ, Fonkalsrud EW, et al. Pediatric surgery. 6th ed. Philadelphia: Mosby; 2006.
35. Arensman RM, Bambini DA, Molloy M, et al. Pediatric surgery. 2nd ed. Austin: Landes Bioscience; 2009.
36. Jackson H, Granger S, Price R, Rollins M, Earle D, Richardson W, Fanelli R. Diagnosis and laparoscopic treatment of surgical diseases during pregnancy: an evidence-based review. Surg Endosc. 2008;22(9):1917–27.
37. Antoniou SA, Mavridis D, Kontouli KM, et al. EAES rapid guideline: appendicitis in the elderly. Surg Endosc. 2021;35:3233.
38. Fan SM, Grigorian A, Smith BR, et al. Geriatric patients undergoing appendectomy have increased risk of intraoperative perforation and/or abscess. Surgery. 2020;168:322.
39. Watters JM, Blakslee JM, March RJ, Redmond ML. The influence of age on the severity of peritonitis. Can J Surg. 1996;39:142.
40. Flum DR, Steinberg SD, Sarkis AY, Wallack MK. Appendicitis in patients with acquired immunodeficiency syndrome. J Am Coll Surg. 1997;184:481.
41. Bova R, Meagher A. Appendicitis in HIV-positive patients. Aust N Z J Surg. 1998;68:337.
42. Whitney TM, Macho JR, Russell TR, et al. Appendicitis in acquired immunodeficiency syndrome. Am J Surg. 1992;164:467.
43. Chang HS, Yang SK, Myung SJ, Jung HY, Hong WS, Kim JH, Min YI, Ha HK, Kim JC, Yu CS, Kim HC, Kim JS. The role of colonoscopy in the diagnosis of appendicitis in patients with atypical presentations. Gastrointest Endosc. 2002;56(3):343–8.
44. Dhadlie S, Mehanna D. Rates of colorectal cancer detection in screening colonoscopy post appendicectomy in patients 50 years and over. Ann Med Surg (Lond). 2018;(36):239–41.
45. Jolly S, McCullough T, Gunning T, Maddern G, Wichmann M. The role of screening colonoscopy after appendicitis in patients over 40 years of age. ANZ J Surg. 2023;93(3):602–5.

Idiopathic Thrombocytopenic Purpura (ITP) and Thrombotic Thrombocytopenic Purpura (TTP)

14

Mariem Galuia, Mohamed El Khourassani, and Ahmed Zakari

Introduction

Platelets are the smallest and the most frequent cells in blood circulation, with an average count of ***150–450 × 10^9/L*** in healthy individuals [1]. Their central role in hemostasis and coagulation is long-established and has been extensively studied since the nineteenth century. Upon vascular injury, platelets instantly adhere to the exposed collagen and tissue factor from the subendothelial matrix, resulting in platelet activation and aggregation to form a hemostatic plug that temporarily stops the bleeding while the coagulation cascade prepares to take action [1]. Recent research efforts have led to a better understanding of a wider range of platelet functions besides hemostasis and coagulation. In fact, there is growing evidence that platelets are pivotal players in tissue repair and regeneration of damaged tissues [2, 3]. During tissue injury, for example, caused by trauma or in context of surgery, the process of wound healing is initiated by platelets who aggregate at sites of the vessel disruption, get activated, and release various biological mediators, such as cytokines and growth factor (namely platelet-derived growth factor PDGF) into the microenvironment, therefore promoting a healthy inflammatory response leading to tissue remodeling and wound healing [4]. Therefore, the role of platelets in the peri-operative setting is dual:

The platelet plug formed by platelet activation and aggregation stops the bleeding during and after surgery, and additionally, they support adequate wound healing by promoting tissue regeneration, stimulating collagen deposition and angiogenesis. In summary, a normal platelet count and function is crucial for optimal surgical outcomes.

Platelets are typically biconvex discoid, lens or plate-shaped, anuclear, measuring 2 μm in greatest diameter when inactivated [5]. Platelets derive from megakaryocytes in the bone marrow. Once they reach the blood circulation, they have a lifespan of about 7–10 days, after which they are removed from the bloodstream mainly in the spleen. Their cytoskeleton is made of highly contractile actin and tubulin polymers, which mediate their rapid change in shape during their activation. On a cellular level, platelet membrane plays a pivotal role in their function in hemostasis [6]. The interaction of platelet membrane glycoproteins with the extracellular matrix initiates clot formation after blood vessel injury. The binding of von Willebrand Factor (vWF) results in conformational changes within the GPIb-V–IX complex, therefore activating GPIIb/IIIa membrane glycoprotein to bind to fibrinogen, which serve as a "glue" that will interconnect the platelets. This phenomenon is called platelet aggregation [7]. In addition to their role in primary hemostasis, platelets act directly and indirectly during coagulation as well as the repair and regeneration of damaged tissues. In fact, platelets secrete factors that mediate inflammation, promote wound healing (platelet-derived growth factor, PDGF), and stimulate angiogenesis (vascular endothelial growth factor, VEGF) [7, 8].

Thrombocytopenia is defined by platelet count below the lower limit of the reference range ***< 150,000/microliter*** (<150 × 109/L) and is a common hematologic finding with variable clinical presentation ranging from asymptomatic to life-threatening bleeding [9]. It presents significant challenges in terms of both bleeding risk and surgical outcomes for patients undergoing surgery. Perioperative management of thrombocytopenia often involves a multidisciplinary team and a close collaboration between surgeons, hematologists, and nursing staff to assess the risk of bleeding and the urgency of treatment, determined by the underlying etiology. Ultimately, we need to balance the risks of the clinical presentation based on the severity of thrombocytopenia with the risks of delaying or avoiding surgery.

This chapter reviews the clinical manifestations and the recommended approach to the diagnosis and management of *two of the most important etiologies of thrombocytopenia,*

M. Galuia · M. El Khourassani · A. Zakari (✉)
AdventHealth – Orlando, Department of Medical Oncology, Orlando, FL, USA
e-mail: ahmed.zakari.md@adventhealth.com

S. Atallah, J. Dragoljevic (eds.), *Fundamentals of Surgery for Physician Assistants*,
https://doi.org/10.1007/978-3-032-21069-2_14

idiopathic thrombocytopenic purpura (ITP) and ***thrombotic thrombocytopenic purpura (TTP)***, with specific considerations related to the perioperative setting.

Idiopathic Thrombocytopenic Purpura

Definitions and Terminology

Immune thrombocytopenic purpura (ITP) is an *autoimmune condition* defined by an *isolated decrease in platelet count (<100 × 10 ⁹/L) in the absence of other causes of thrombocytopenia* [10]. ITP, also known as idiopathic thrombocytopenic purpura, is an acquired condition, with heteregenous clinical presentation ranging from asymptomatic to life-threatening bleeding, depending on the severity of the disease [10, 11].

Although it is one of the most common causes of thrombocytopenia in adults, *the diagnosis of ITP remains one of exclusion*. A thorough clinical evaluation, laboratory tests, and sometimes a bone marrow biopsy may be necessary to rule out the large number of other potential conditions causing thrombocytopenia before considering ITP as a diagnosis.

ITP can present as idiopathic or can be associated with other autoimmune conditions such as systemic lupus erythematosus (SLE), as well as infections including hepatitis-C, HIV, or *Helicobacter pylori* [12–14]. The term secondary ITP refers to all forms of immune-mediated thrombocytopenia excluding primary ITP. This concept should not be confused with nonimmune causes of thrombocytopenia. All these considerations make the diagnosis of ITP extremely challenging.

ITP can also be classified based on its severity or chronicity of symptoms. The American Society of Hematology (ASH) provides detailed management guidelines that are based on a grading system for severity of ITP [15, 16].

Newly diagnosed ITP occurs suddenly and *may affect children following a viral infection*. It is usually a *self-limiting* condition, with *spontaneous resolution* within weeks. However, adults often times require immediate intervention to obtain remission.

Persistent ITP refers to ITP that lasts *more than 3 months* and has not met the threshold of 12 months.

Chronic ITP is more common in adults and persists for *12 months or longer*. Up to 60% of adult patients with ITP may develop chronicity. In children, only 20% will present with chronic ITP. Management of chronic ITP is more challenging and may require ongoing treatment to maintain platelet levels (Table 14.1).

Table 14.1 Phases of ITP

Newly diagnosed ITP:	Within 3 months from diagnosis
Persistent ITP:	Between 3 and 12 months from diagnosis
Chronic ITP:	Lasting for more than 12 months

The Pathogenesis of ITP

The pathogenesis of ITP has been extensively studied over the past two decades. A better understanding of the underlying pathology has led to the development of several new targeted therapies which seem to result in a significant improvement in patients' quality of life. The principal mechanism of ITP involves ***autoimmunity***, with the ***development of specific autoantibodies targeting platelet membrane components***, such as the ***glycoproteins GPIb/IX*** and ***GPIIb/IIIa*** [17]. The loss of tolerance reduces the platelets lifespan. The autoantibody-coated platelets are mainly cleared by the spleen for most individuals. This explains the fact that splenectomy is one of the most efficient treatments of ITP after failure of steroids [17–19]. Furthermore, ITP may relapse and become refractory to splenectomy because platelets are cleared at a lesser extent in other organs of the endothelial reticular system such as the bone marrow and the lymph nodes.

Although antibodies directed again platelet membrane are the main pathophysiologic driver of the disease, these antibodies have *low sensitivity and specificity*. In more than 50% of patients, these antibodies are not demonstrable and therefore are *not* useful for diagnosis confirmation or disease monitoring.

In **primary ITP**, autoimmunity is an *isolated,* de novo *finding* and is not driven by any concurrent pathologic process. Conversely, autoantibody production in **secondary ITP** is caused by the disruption of immune homeostasis, *usually driven by infections, vaccines, autoimmune diseases, or hematologic malignancies*. Viral infections are more commonly associated with ITP than bacterial infections, where antibodies against viral proteins cross-react with normal platelet antigens, therefore causing a peripheral loss of tolerance. Infection with *hepatitis-C, HIV, cytomegalovirus, and Helicobacter pylori* are the most common infections associated with secondary ITP [12–14, 20]. Additionally, chronic autoimmune conditions such as SLE can cause ITP in up to 30% of patients [21]. There are also certain malignancies associated with autoimmune cytopenia including ITP, such as chronic lymphocytic leukemia (CLL) and Waldenstrom macroglobulinemia. In fact, up to 5% of CLL patients will be diagnosed with ITP, and the association may be correlated with poor prognosis [22].

Initial Evaluation of ITP

Clinical Manifestations of ITP

Some patients with ITP are diagnosed incidentally on complete blood counts (CBCs) performed for other causes and are found to have chronic, isolated asymptomatic thrombocytopenia.

When symptomatic, ***the main symptom of ITP is bleeding***, which can be life-threatening, depending on its severity and location.

Mucocutaneous bleeding is the *most common manifestation* and usually presents as follows [23]:

- **Petechiae**: This is defined as pinpoint nonblanching spots that measure less than 2 mm, usually occurring in dependent areas of the body.
- **Purpura**: Purpura is defined by coalition of multiple petechiae. It is important to clinically differentiate between thrombocytopenic purpura, seen in ITP and other conditions associated with thrombocytopenia, and vasculitic pupura secondary to vasculitis (inflammation of the blood vessels). ***Thrombocytopenic purpura*** is ***nonpalpable*** and ***occurs in dependent areas of the body***. In contrast, vasculitic purpura is palpable and does not accumulate in dependent areas.
- **Epistaxis**: This can be minimal or more important requiring intervention with nasal packing or cauterization.
- **Severe or life-threatening bleeding**: As defined by the American Society of Hematology [15], severe bleeding in ITP is one that occurs in a critical anatomical site such as intracranial, intraspinal, intraocular, retroperitoneal, pericardial, or intramuscular with compartment syndrome; or an ongoing bleed that results in hemodynamic instability or respiratory compromise. This type of bleeding warrants urgent treatment to prevent early mortality.

  Some factors that increase the risk of severe bleeding include advanced age, prior bleeding, female sex, and exposure to NSAIDs [24]. It is important to note that we did not cite the degree of thrombocytopenia, as ***there is no correlation between the platelet count and the risk of bleeding unless the platelet count is less than 10 × 10⁹/L*** [15].

Laboratory Testing

A thorough clinical evaluation including an exhaustive history taking, a complete review of the patient's medications, and a full medical examination are necessary to guide the clinician to the possible cause of the thrombocytopenia.

Once other conditions associated with thrombocytopenia have been excluded, there exists a minimum diagnostic investigation that should be done in all patients suspected of having ITP. The first essential step is to ***repeat and review the CBC*** and ***perform a peripheral blood smear*** to confirm that thrombocytopenia is real and not false thrombocytopenia (pseudothrombocytopenia) due to platelet clumping and that there are no morphologic platelet abnormalities suggesting a hereditary platelet disorder. After confirming the reality of the thrombocytopenia, ***the diagnosis of ITP is made after excluding all other potential causes of thrombocytopenia***. Antiplatelet antibodies are not useful for diagnosis as they have very low sensitivity and specificity for ITP [25]. *It is recommended that all patients with suspected ITP are tested for* ***HIV*** *and* ***hepatitis C virus (HCV) infection***, as low platelet count is common in those infections and resolves when the infection is controlled on antiviral treatment [15, 26]. Other laboratory tests can be ordered depending on the clinical presentation, for instance, SLE antibodies and *Helicobacter pylori* testing.

Bone marrow biopsy is usually ***not*** indicated during the initial workup of new ITP. However, there are exceptions such as atypical presentation in children, refractory ITP, or when we suspect hematologic malignancy or failure to respond in patients 60 years or older.

Management of ITP

The goal of treatment of ITP varies depending on the presence and severity of bleeding, platelet count, bleeding risk, and any previous treatments. Many patients who are asymptomatic at diagnosis and who remain with stable, non-life-threatening platelet levels can be observed without intervention.

If bleeding occurs, based on our experience, we recommend ***platelet transfusion with IVIG and steroids***. If the bleeding is minor, treatment should be maintained until the platelet count is >50,000. In the event of major bleeding or high risk for fatal bleeding, the recommendation is to treat with goal of platelet count 100,000, and we usually suggest maintaining it for at least 1 week. With minor bleeding and platelet count over 30,000, we initiate corticosteroids without blood products support.

Transfusing platelets serves as a temporary treatment to acutely raise platelets, and multiple platelet transfusions may be necessary while waiting for intravenous immunoglobulins (IVIG) and steroids to take effect and counteract the autoimmune phenomenon. However, ***if there is no bleeding and platelet count is ≥ 30,000***, we recommend ***close observation and monitoring with serial hemograms*** [24].

First-Line Therapy

Corticosteroids

We anticipate a response with rise in platelet count within 2–5 days. However, at times, we may see delayed response up to 14 days post treatment.

Pulse dexamethasone: Our recommendations follow the American Society of Hematology guidelines. We use dexamethasone 40 mg daily for 4 days. The regimen may be repeated if there is no response.

Prednisone: We recommend 0.5–2 gm/kg with close monitoring of response. The duration of prednisone treatment should be *no longer than 6 weeks with a tapering off process*. Patients with ITP lasting ≥3 months who are corticosteroid-dependent or have no response to corticosteroids are treated with second-line therapies: thrombopoietin receptor agonist (eltrombopag or romiplostim), rituximab, or splenectomy.

IVIG

Our recommendation is to initiate IVIG in patients with severe thrombocytopenia, high risk of bleeding, patients who do not respond immediately to corticosteroids, or patients that may not be candidates for long-duration corticosteroids. We do anticipate a response within 24 h. The standard dose is 1gm/kg for 1–2 days or alternative dose 0.4 gm/kg for 5 days.

Anti-D immunoglobulin is an alternate treatment to IVIG in RhD-positive patients. The standard dose is 75 mcg/kg. However, potential downsides to anti-D immunoglobulin include lack of response in patients with splenectomy and high risk of hemolytic transfusions reactions.

Second-Line Therapy

Rituximab

Rituximab is a monoclonal antibody that binds to B cell lymphocyte CD20 surface antigen, depleting antiplatelet antibodies and thus countering the main pathophysiological mechanism of thrombocytopenia in ITP. Studies showed that the overall initial response to rituximab used as second- or further-line of therapy ranges between 52% and 73%. The standard dose is 375 mg/m^2 weekly for 4 weeks.

Thrombopoietin receptor agonists TPO-RA

- Romiplostim [25]: Romiplostim has been studied and shown to increase and sustain platelet counts in patients with ITP with minimal adverse reactions and lower rates of both treatment failure and splenectomy for up to 5 years. The standard dose is weekly subcutaneous 1–10 mcg/kg.
- Eltrombopag [26]: An oral agent approved for patients with relapsed or refractory ITP. In fact, based on published data, by day 15 of treatment, more than 80% of patients receiving 50 or 75 mg/day of eltrombopag had a good response and increased platelet count.
- Fostamatinib: A spleen tyrosine kinase (Syk) inhibitor approved in 2018 as treatment of chronic immune thrombocytopenia (ITP) in patients without response to at least 1 prior line of therapy. The recommended dose is 100 mg po twice a day for 30 days, which may be increased to 150 mg twice a day if platelet count remains below 50,000.

Splenectomy

Splenectomy is an effective treatment option for steroid-refractory or dependent immune thrombocytopenia (ITP). However, with the advent of new agents as second-line therapy such as rituximab, thrombopoietin receptor antagonists, and spleen tyrosine kinase inhibitors, the use of splenectomy has declined significantly and is generally reserved for patients that fail multiple medical therapies. The spleen is the primary site of platelet clearance and autoantibody production; thus, splenectomy offers the highest rate of durable response (50–70%) compared with other ITP treatment options.

We reserve ***splenectomy as last resort*** to go to in case of persistent refractoriness or inability to receive other lines of therapy.

Therapeutic Abstinence

In many situations, in children, therapeutic abstinence is also an option, especially when the various treatments fail (side effects of corticosteroids, recurrence after IVIG, etc.) and more so, when the patient does not have severe hemorrhagic signs. Platelet counts even below 10,000/mm^3 may not cause bleeding. Children may not develop bleeding despite platelet counts being too low. We can educate patients and parents and know how to reassure them in these situations.

Considerations to the Peri-Operative Management of ITP

Urgent surgeries or surgeries with increased bleeding risk Patients undergoing urgent surgeries (appendectomy for example) or procedures with increased bleeding risk (cardiothoracic, vascular, obstetric surgeries) need to have platelets transfused prior to their surgeries to transiently increase the platelet count and decrease the risk of bleeding during the procedure. Thus, ***glucocorticoids*** and/or ***IVIG*** should be administered for a durable and specific effect.

Recommended platelet count thresholds used for some common procedures are listed below. Platelet transfusion may be considered when the patient's platelet count is below the threshold for the corresponding procedure.

- Neurosurgery or ocular surgery: <100,000/microL
- Most other major surgeries: <50,000/microL
- Endoscopic procedures: <50,000/microL
- Central line placement: <20,000/microL [27]
- Bone marrow aspiration/biopsy: <20,000/microL

Table 14.2 Summary of goal-directed therapies

Goal of therapy	Clinical indication	Treatment options
Immediate rise (24–48 h) in platelet count	Treatment of serious bleeding, in preparation for emergency surgery	IVIg, high-dose corticosteroids, high-dose platelet transfusions
Rapid rise (1–2 weeks) in platelet count	In advance of planned surgical operations or invasive procedures	TPO receptor agonists, high-dose corticosteroids
Obtain remission	Patients at a relatively early stage of disease	Rituximab, TPO-RA, spleen tyrosine kinase inhibitor
Maintain a stable, hemostatic platelet count	Refractory patients, frequent bleeding complications, or reduced quality of life	TPO receptor agonists, combination immunosuppressant drugs, splenectomy

Abbreviations: *IVIG* intravenous immunoglobulin, *TPO* thrombopoietin

Patients undergoing elective surgeries
Patients who do not achieve satisfactory platelet counts with glucocorticoids or IVIG are treated with TPO receptor agonist, high-dose corticosteroids, or second-line agents as described above. Therapies usually achieve a rise in platelet counts within 2 weeks of the first administration (Table 14.2).

Prognosis

Most adults with ITP will eventually reach a stable, safe platelet count, either due to spontaneous remission or therapy. Spontaneous remissions occur in up to 20–45% of adults with ITP, most often within the first 6 months [27, 28]. Some patients may require additional second-line or other therapies. The mortality rate in people with ITP is similar to or only marginally higher than an age-matched population, despite the possibility of fatal hemorrhage from thrombocytopenia or infection in the setting of therapies that cause immunosuppression. In children, persistent severe thrombocytopenia without bleeding signs is also possible and compatible with normal life. There are some cases in which patients have thrombocytopenia despite continuous platelet production, due to accelerated kinetics and a shorter platelet lifespan. The platelet count obtained in a lab test (in vitro) does not always reflect the actual number of platelets circulating in the body (in vivo). These patients must be monitored but also be reassured. ***Regardless of what triggers ITP, treatment focuses on preventing or controlling major bleeding rather than achieving a normal platelet count.***

Thrombotic Thrombocytopenic Purpura

Definition

Thrombotic thrombocytopenic purpura (TTP) is a thrombotic microangiopathy (TMA) caused by the adhesion of platelet-rich thrombi in the small vasculature system causing thrombocytopenia and ***microangiopathic hemolytic anemia (MAHA)***, which may be associated with organ damage (primarily ***kidney*** and ***CNS***) [29]. **TTP is a medical emergency that warrants prompt initiation of treatment to prevent early mortality due to end-organ damage**. Mortality rate may be as high as 90%, but with appropriate treatment with plasma exchange, mortality is reduced to 10–20% [30].

TTP is mainly seen in the adult population (about 90% of all cases), with a median age of 40 years and is twofold more frequent in women. Childhood-onset TTP only represents less than 10% of all cases [31]. TTP is believed to be mainly caused by an acquired autoimmune mechanism; however, rare inherited forms are described during early childhood [29].

Pathophysiology of TTP

von Willebrand factor (vWF) is a very large glycoprotein produced by endothelial cells in the blood stream that plays an essential role in the blood clotting pathway, specifically ***platelet adhesion during primary hemostasis***. It acts as a "bridge" between the platelets and the damaged subendothelial collagen, therefore promoting platelet adhesion to damaged blood vessel walls and facilitating the formation of a thrombus. In physiologic conditions, vWF is produced as ultralarge multimers that are subsequently cleaved by an enzyme, **ADAMTS13 (A Disintegrin and Metalloprotease with Thrombospondin Type 1 Motif, member 13),** synthesized in the liver, into smaller VWF multimers, less adhesive to platelets. Hence, ***ADAMTS13*** *regulates the activity of vWF to maintain proper hemostasis and prevent abnormal clot formation* [32].

The hallmark of TTP is ADAMTS13 deficiency. This deficiency is most frequently acquired via *ADAMTS13 autoantibodies*, and in rare circumstances (infections, inflammation or pregnancy), it may also be inherited via mutations of the ADAMTS13 gene [33]. In the absence of functional ADAMTS13, ultralarge VWF multimers are not cleaved, and not released into circulation, thus binding to circulating

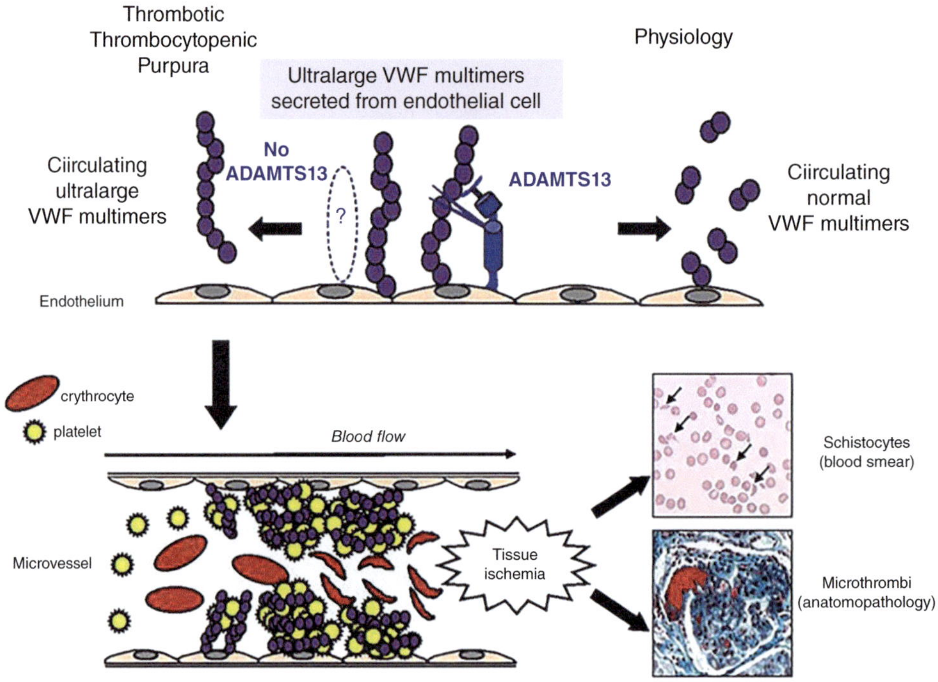

Fig. 14.1 Pathophysiology of TTP. Role of ADAMTS13 in cleavage of ultralarge VWF multimers into circulation. Absence of ADAMTS13 leading to platelet aggregation, MAHA, microthrombi, and tissue ischemia. *(Published in Frontiers In Immunology, 11 Apr 2022, Vol. 13, Molecular Diagnosis Is Vital to the Accurate Classification and Management of Thrombotic Thrombocytopenic Purpura in Children. Copyright © 2022 Karsenty, Kirk, Helber, Esquilin, Despotovic and Grimes)*

platelets and forming multiple platelet-rich microthrombi within the micro vessels. *The VWF–platelet aggregates lead to platelet consumption, causing thrombocytopenia* (Fig. 14.1). Another consequence is formation of microthrombi in the small vessels inducing tissue ischemia [32]. When a small blood vessel is partially thrombosed, the increased shear force on red blood cells can cause them to fragment, leading to microangiopathic hemolytic anemia (MAHA). The physically damaged RBCs are better appreciated in the peripheral smear of patient with a TTP as ***schistocytes*** (fragmented RBCs) among others.

Table 14.3 Clinical presentation at diagnosis according to the Oklahoma Registry

Symptoms at the time of diagnosis	Proportion of patients
Gastrointestinal symptoms	69%
Weakness	63%
Bleeding or purpura	54%
Major neurologic symptoms: coma, stroke, seizure, transient ischemic attack	41%
Minor neurologic symptoms: headache, confusion	26%
Fevers, chills	10%
Classic pentad: hemolytic anemia, thrombocytopenia, fever, acute kidney injury, and neurologic findings	<5%

Clinical Manifestations of TTP

Historically, TTP was defined by a clinical "pentad" consisting of ***microangiopathic hemolytic anemia, thrombocytopenia, neurological deficits, fever, and renal insufficiency***. **<u>This pentad is no longer up to date</u> since the establishment of plasma exchange therapy as an effective treatment of TTP**. It is estimated that <5% of patients exhibit all five symptoms. The presence of thrombocytopenia and MAHA alone should prompt consideration of the diagnosis of TTP [29, 33–35].

The Oklahoma Registry is one of the largest and is the most cited epidemiologic study that reviews presenting signs and symptoms of TTP [36]. Initial symptoms include ***fatigue, dyspnea, petechiae, or other bleeding***. Symptoms of TTP vary in location and severity and are related to organ ischemia due to microthrombi formation. ***Neurologic symptoms*** are the most common and can present as headaches, focal neurologic deficits, seizures, confusion, and vertigo. The second most common symptom was reported to be ***abdominal pain***. ***Bleeding*** was present in only 10% of the patients and kidney involvement is uncommon although classically cited in the pentad. Patients with TTP can also have cardiac involvement—in the Oklahoma series, 22% of patients had chest pain. Elevated serum troponin is independently associated with mortality and is associated with a negative prognosis [36] (Table 14.3).

Laboratory Studies

The hallmark laboratory findings in TTP are ***MAHA, thrombocytopenia, and decrease in ADAMTS13 activity***. Review of the ***peripheral blood smear*** is an essential step in diagnosing TTP. Blood smear review will confirm thrombocytopenia, exclude pseudothrombocytopenia, and confirm findings consistent with MAHA.

MAHA is characterized by prominent ***schistocytes, helmet cells and triangular cells***. These ***fragmented*** or ***irregularly shaped red blood cells*** are key findings of ***hemolysis*** that occurs in TTP due to mechanical damage when they pass through the narrowed or occluded blood vessels [37]. Other laboratory findings in patients with TTP are those found in most hemolytic anemias including a low hemoglobin concentration, elevation of the serum indirect bilirubin, and decrease in the serum haptoglobin concentration. The reticulocyte count is generally increased as the bone marrow tries to compensate for RBC destruction. The serum lactate dehydrogenase (LDH) is elevated.

The diagnostic confirmation of TTP is made with an ADAMTS13 activity level of less than 10% in patients with evidence of hemolysis and thrombocytopenia. The PLASMIC score is a clinical scoring system used to help diagnose TTP patients at higher risk for TTP, especially in the absence of all the classic symptoms of the disease [38, 39]. Schistocytes are a prerequisite to prompt using the score; however, they are not included in the score.

The PLASMIC score is based on clinical and laboratory findings intended to be used in patients with thrombocytopenia and evidence of MAHA (schistocytes) on peripheral smear, as a predictor of severity of ADAMTS13 deficiency and thus the diagnosis of TTP. A high score suggests a greater likelihood of TTP; hence the score aids in determining the urgency of intervention, as TTP requires prompt treatment (Tables 14.4 and 14.5).

Table 14.4 The PLASMIC score parameters

Parameter	Points
Platelet count <30 × 10^9/L	1
Hemolysis (reticulocyte count >2.5%, haptoglobin undetectable, or indirect bilirubin >2.0 mg/dL)	1
No active cancer	1
Treated for cancer within the past year	1
No history of solid-organ or stem-cell transplant	1
MCV <90 fL	1
INR <1.5	1
Creatinine <2.0 mg/dL	1

Table 14.5 The PLASMIC score interpretation

PLASMIC score	Interpretation
0–4	Low risk for ADAMTS13 deficiency
5	Intermediate risk for ADAMTS13 deficiency
6–7	High risk for ADAMTS13 deficiency

Management of TTP

TTP is a medical emergency that requires urgent management, usually in intensive care units, in order to prevent irreversible end-organ damage, which includes *neurologic debilitation, irreversible kidney failure, myocardial ischemia, and ultimately death* [40].

In patients with high suspicion of TTP, *treatment is often started based on clinical presentation and basic laboratory testing alone* prior to the confirmatory ADAMTS13 testing. All patients with unexplained hemolytic anemia and thrombocytopenia with a normal coagulation profile should have a treatment plan promptly started without delay by ADAMTS13 level result, although it is still required to confirm the diagnosis [41].

The goal of the management of TTP is to achieve clinical remission, which is defined by a ***sustained platelet count > 150,000, LDH < 1.5 ULN***, and the ***absence of new end-organ symptoms for over 30 days*** [42]. A complete ADAMTS13 remission is defined by ADAMTS13 activity above the lower normal limit values. An exacerbation of TTP is defined by a platelet count <150 × 10^9/L (with other causes of thrombocytopenia excluded) within 30 days after the last plasma exchange or anti-VWF therapy. After clinical remission, a clinical relapse of TTP is defined by a platelet count <150 × 10^9/L without another explanation [42]. The latter should be confirmed by severe ADAMTS13 deficiency. Disease monitoring therefore consists of serial clinical examinations, hemogram, LDH level, and ADAMTS13 activity.

1. *Total plasma exchange*
   The mainstay of treatment in TTP is total plasma exchange (TPE) with *fresh frozen plasma (FFP)* replacement in association with high-dose corticosteroid therapy [41, 43]. *Plasma exchange removes both ultralarge VWF multimers and the ADAMTS13 autoantibodies and repletes ADAMTS13*. The recommended volume of exchange is one estimated plasma volume (usually 40 mL/kg of body weight) with each treatment [41, 43, 44]. Plasma exchange is repeated daily and can be stopped abruptly when remission is achieved, or an alternative diagnosis has been established.
2. *Steroid therapy*
   Corticosteroids are an essential adjunctive treatment to plasma exchange and act by *decreasing autoantibody production*. High-dose methylprednisolone (10 mg/kg/day for 3 days and then 2.5 mg/kg/day) is usually preferred to the standard dose [42].

3. *Targeted therapies: rituximab, calpacizumab*
   A better understanding of the underlying pathophysiology of TTP has led to the emergence of newer, targeted treatments that are promising in terms of improving overall morbidity and mortality in patients with TTP. Rituximab is a humanized monoclonal antibody that targets CD20 antigen present on B lymphocytes, leading to depletion of B lymphocytes. Initially reserved for cases of relapsed, refractory TTP, rituximab is now being widely used as a frontline therapy in addition to TPE for acute de novo cases, as it has been shown to result in high clinical response rates and an increase in time to relapse, for example, in the Oklahoma TTP Registry [45–48].

Calpacizumab is a humanized monoclonal antibody fragment that binds von Willebrand factor (VWF) and blocks its interactions with platelet glycoproteins, thus preventing platelet adhesion to the endothelium even in the absence of ADAMTS13. This new medication was approved by the US Food and Drug Administration in 2019 for initial treatment of newly diagnosed TTP together with therapeutic plasma exchange (TPE) and immunosuppression [49].

Conclusion

TTP remains a fatal disease in the absence of establishing diagnosis and immediate intervention. The mortality rate can decreased from 90% to 10–20% with ***total plasma exchange (TPE), corticosteroids, and immunomodulator***s. There is great need of novel therapeutic agents to improve the prognosis of TTP and decrease the mortality. Management requires a multidisciplinary approach, starting in the emergency department and continuing in the intensive care unit, with involvement from a hematology consultation team.

References

1. Thon JN, Italiano JE. Platelets: production, morphology and ultrastructure. Handb Exp Pharmacol. 2012;210:3–22. https://doi.org/10.1007/978-3-642-29423-5_1.
2. Franco AT, Corken A, Ware J. Platelets at the interface of thrombosis, inflammation, and cancer. Blood. 2015;126(5):582–8. https://doi.org/10.1182/blood-2014-08-531582.
3. Gremmel T, Frelinger AL 3rd, Michelson AD. Platelet physiology. Semin Thromb Hemost. 2024;50(8):1173–86. https://doi.org/10.1055/s-0044-1786387.
4. van den Berg HM, Srivastava A. Hemostasis - a balancing act [published correction appears in N Engl J Med. 2024 Feb 8;390(6):580. https://doi.org/10.1056/NEJMx230013.]. N Engl J Med. 2023;389(9):853–6. https://doi.org/10.1056/NEJMe2304535.
5. Gremmel T, Frelinger AL 3rd, Michelson AD. Platelet physiology. Semin Thromb Hemost. 2024;50(8):1173–86. https://doi.org/10.1055/s-0044-1786387. Epub 2024 Apr 23. PMID: 38653463.
6. van den Berg HM, Srivastava A. Hemostasis - a balancing act. N Engl J Med. 2023;389(9):853–6. https://doi.org/10.1056/NEJMe2304535. Erratum in: N Engl J Med 2024;390(6):580. https://doi.org/10.1056/NEJMx230013. PMID: 37646683.
7. Sierra C, Moreno M, García-Ruiz JC. The physiology of hemostasis. Blood Coagul Fibrinolysis. 2022;33(Suppl 1):S1–2. https://doi.org/10.1097/MBC.0000000000001099. PMID: 35088768.
8. Jurk K, Kehrel BE. Platelets: physiology and biochemistry. Semin Thromb Hemost. 2005;31(4):381–92. https://doi.org/10.1055/s--2005-916671. PMID: 16149014.
9. Buckley MF, James JW, Brown DE, et al. A novel approach to the assessment of variations in the human platelet count. Thromb Haemost. 2000;83(3):480–4.
10. Rodeghiero F, Stasi R, Gernsheimer T, et al. Standardization of terminology, definitions and outcome criteria in immune thrombocytopenic purpura of adults and children: report from an international working group. Blood. 2009;113(11):2386–93. https://doi.org/10.1182/blood-2008-07-162503.
11. Lambert MP, Gernsheimer TB. Clinical updates in adult immune thrombocytopenia. Blood. 2017;129(21):2829–35. https://doi.org/10.1182/blood-2017-03-754119.
12. Kewan T, Gunaratne TN, Mushtaq K, Alayan D, Daw H, Haddad A. Outcomes and management of immune thrombocytopenia secondary to COVID-19: Cleveland clinic experience. Transfusion. 2021;61(7):2014–8. https://doi.org/10.1111/trf.16368.
13. Zhang W, Nardi MA, Borkowsky W, Li Z, Karpatkin S. Role of molecular mimicry of hepatitis C virus protein with platelet GPIIIa in hepatitis C-related immunologic thrombocytopenia. Blood. 2009;113(17):4086–93. https://doi.org/10.1182/blood-2008-09-181073.
14. Stasi R, Provan D. Helicobacter pylori and chronic ITP. Hematology Am Soc Hematol Educ Program. 2008:206–11. https://doi.org/10.1182/asheducation-2008.1.206.
15. Neunert C, Terrell DR, Arnold DM, et al. American Society of Hematology 2019 guidelines for immune thrombocytopenia [published correction appears in Blood Adv. 2020 Jan 28;4(2):252. https://doi.org/10.1182/bloodadvances.2019001380.]. Blood Adv. 2019;3(23):3829–66. https://doi.org/10.1182/bloodadvances.2019000966.
16. Strom TS. The thrombocytopenia of WAS: a familial form of ITP? Immunol Res. 2009;44(1–3):42–53. https://doi.org/10.1007/s12026-008.
17. Cooper N, Bussel J. The pathogenesis of immune thrombocytopaenic purpura. Br J Haematol. 2006;133(4):364–74. https://doi.org/10.1111/j.1365-2141.2006.06024.x.
18. Zufferey A, Kapur R, Semple JW. Pathogenesis and therapeutic mechanisms in immune thrombocytopenia (ITP). J Clin Med. 2017;6(2):16. Published 2017 Feb 9. https://doi.org/10.3390/jcm6020016.
19. Kuter DJ, Rummel M, Boccia R, et al. Romiplostim or standard of care in patients with immune thrombocytopenia. N Engl J Med. 2010;363(20):1889–99. https://doi.org/10.1056/NEJMoa1002625.
20. Bussel JB, Cheng G, Saleh MN, et al. Eltrombopag for the treatment of chronic idiopathic thrombocytopenic purpura. N Engl J Med. 2007;357(22):2237–47. https://doi.org/10.1056/NEJMoa073275.
21. D'Arena G, Guariglia R, La Rocca F, et al. Autoimmune cytopenias in chronic lymphocytic leukemia. Clin Dev Immunol. 2013;2013:730131. https://doi.org/10.1155/2013/730131.
22. https://www.uptodate.com/contents/immune-thrombocytopenia-itp-in-adults-clinical-manifestations-and-diagnosis?search=itp&source=search_result&selectedTitle=1%7E150&usage_type=default&display_rank=1#references.

23. Neunert C, Noroozi N, Norman G, et al. Severe bleeding events in adults and children with primary immune thrombocytopenia: a systematic review. J Thromb Haemost. 2015;13(3):457–64. https://doi.org/10.1111/jth.12813.
24. McMillan R. Antiplatelet antibodies in chronic immune thrombocytopenia and their role in platelet destruction and defective platelet production. Hematol Oncol Clin North Am. 2009;23(6):1163–75. https://doi.org/10.1016/j.hoc.2009.08.008.
25. Provan D, Stasi R, Newland AC, et al. International consensus report on the investigation and management of primary immune thrombocytopenia. Blood. 2010;115(2):168–86. https://doi.org/10.1182/blood-2009-06-225565.
26. Stasi R, Stipa E, Masi M, et al. Long-term observation of 208 adults with chronic idiopathic thrombocytopenic purpura. Am J Med. 1995;98(5):436–42. https://doi.org/10.1016/s0002-9343(99)80342-8.
27. Schifferli A, Holbro A, Chitlur M, et al. A comparative prospective observational study of children and adults with immune thrombocytopenia: 2-year follow-up. Am J Hematol. 2018;93(6):751–9. https://doi.org/10.1002/ajh.25086.
28. Aster RH. TTP: new clues to the etiology of an enigmatic disease. N Engl J Med. 1977;297(25):1400–1. https://doi.org/10.1056/NEJM197712222972511.
29. Lotta LA, Mariani M, Consonni D, et al. Different clinical severity of first episodes and recurrences of thrombotic thrombocytopenic purpura [published correction appears in Br J Haematol. 2011 Feb;152(3):364]. Br J Haematol. 2010;151(5):488–94. https://doi.org/10.1111/j.1365-2141.2010.08385.x.
30. George JN, Al-Nouri ZL. Diagnostic and therapeutic challenges in the thrombotic thrombocytopenic purpura and hemolytic uremic syndromes. Hematology Am Soc Hematol Educ Program. 2012;2012:604–9. https://doi.org/10.1182/asheducation-2012.1.604.
31. Sadler JE. Pathophysiology of thrombotic thrombocytopenic purpura. Blood. 2017;130(10):1181–8. https://doi.org/10.1182/blood-2017-04-636431.
32. George JN. Clinical practice. Thrombotic thrombocytopenic purpura. N Engl J Med. 2006;354(18):1927–35. https://doi.org/10.1056/NEJMcp053024.
33. Zafrani L, Mariotte E, Darmon M, et al. Acute renal failure is prevalent in patients with thrombotic thrombocytopenic purpura associated with low plasma ADAMTS13 activity. J Thromb Haemost. 2015;13(3):380–9. https://doi.org/10.1111/jth.12826.
34. Imanirad I, Rajasekhar A, Zumberg M. A case series of atypical presentations of thrombotic thrombocytopenic purpura. J Clin Apher. 2012;27(4):221–6. https://doi.org/10.1002/jca.21216.
35. George JN, Vesely SK, Terrell DR. The Oklahoma Thrombotic Thrombocytopenic Purpura-Hemolytic Uremic Syndrome (TTP-HUS) Registry: a community perspective of patients with clinically diagnosed TTP-HUS. Semin Hematol. 2004;41(1):60–7. https://doi.org/10.1053/j.seminhematol.2003.10.001.
36. Mariotte E, Azoulay E, Galicier L, et al. Epidemiology and pathophysiology of adulthood-onset thrombotic microangiopathy with severe ADAMTS13 deficiency (thrombotic thrombocytopenic purpura): a cross-sectional analysis of the French national registry for thrombotic microangiopathy. Lancet Haematol. 2016;3(5):e237–45. https://doi.org/10.1016/S2352-3026(16)30018-7.
37. Paydary K, Banwell E, Tong J, Chen Y, Cuker A. Diagnostic accuracy of the PLASMIC score in patients with suspected thrombotic thrombocytopenic purpura: a systematic review and meta-analysis. Transfusion. 2020;60(9):2047–57. https://doi.org/10.1111/trf.15954.
38. Jamme M, Rondeau E. The PLASMIC score for thrombotic thrombocytopenic purpura. Lancet Haematol. 2017;4(4):e148–9. https://doi.org/10.1016/S2352-3026(17)30024-8.
39. Hanby HA, Zheng XL. Current status in diagnosis and treatment of hereditary thrombotic thrombocytopenic purpura. Hereditary Genet. 2014;3(1):e108. https://doi.org/10.4172/2161-1041.1000e108.
40. Scully M, Hunt BJ, Benjamin S, et al. Guidelines on the diagnosis and management of thrombotic thrombocytopenic purpura and other thrombotic microangiopathies. Br J Haematol. 2012;158(3):323–35. https://doi.org/10.1111/j.1365-2141.2012.09167.x.
41. Cuker A, Cataland SR, Coppo P, et al. Redefining outcomes in immune TTP: an international working group consensus report. Blood. 2021;137(14):1855–61. https://doi.org/10.1182/blood.2020009150.
42. Froissart A, Buffet M, Veyradier A, et al. Efficacy and safety of first-line rituximab in severe, acquired thrombotic thrombocytopenic purpura with a suboptimal response to plasma exchange. Experience of the French Thrombotic Microangiopathies Reference Center. Crit Care Med. 2012;40(1):104–11. https://doi.org/10.1097/CCM.0b013e31822e9d66.
43. Zeigler ZR, Shadduck RK, Gryn JF, et al. Cryoprecipitate poor plasma does not improve early response in primary adult thrombotic thrombocytopenic purpura (TTP). J Clin Apher. 2001;16(1):19–22. https://doi.org/10.1002/jca.1003.
44. Bell WR, Braine HG, Ness PM, Kickler TS. Improved survival in thrombotic thrombocytopenic purpura-hemolytic uremic syndrome. Clinical experience in 108 patients. N Engl J Med. 1991;325(6):398–403. https://doi.org/10.1056/NEJM199108083250605.
45. Zwicker JI, Muia J, Dolatshahi L, et al. Adjuvant low-dose rituximab and plasma exchange for acquired TTP. Blood. 2019;134(13):1106–9. https://doi.org/10.1182/blood.2019000795.
46. Owattanapanich W, Wongprasert C, Rotchanapanya W, Owattanapanich N, Ruchutrakool T. Comparison of the long-term remission of rituximab and conventional treatment for acquired thrombotic thrombocytopenic purpura: a systematic review and meta-analysis. Clin Appl Thromb Hemost. 2019;25:1076029618825309. https://doi.org/10.1177/1076029618825309.
47. Lim W, Vesely SK, George JN. The role of rituximab in the management of patients with acquired thrombotic thrombocytopenic purpura. Blood. 2015;125(10):1526–31. https://doi.org/10.1182/blood-2014-10-559211.
48. Kühne L, Knöbl P, Eller K, et al. Management of immune thrombotic thrombocytopenic purpura without therapeutic plasma exchange. Blood. 2024;144(14):1486–95. https://doi.org/10.1182/blood.2023023780.
49. Völker LA, Brinkkoetter PT, Knöbl PN, et al. Treatment of acquired thrombotic thrombocytopenic purpura without plasma exchange in selected patients under caplacizumab. J Thromb Haemost. 2020;18(11):3061–6. https://doi.org/10.1111/jth.15045.

Metabolic Surgery

15

Neil Floch

Introduction

The concept that **metabolic disease** can be treated and prevented with surgery has been met with doubt, stigma, and criticism, but has become increasingly acceptable in the medical community, supported by significant medical evidence. The advent of glucagon-like peptide-1(GLP-1ra) receptor agonist medications has improved numerous disease processes and further highlighted **metabolic bariatric surgery (MBS)** as the most effective treatment for obesity-related diseases. In their book published in 1978, **Dr. Henry Buchwald and Dr. Richard Varco** defined "metabolic surgery" as "the operative manipulation of a normal organ or organ system to achieve a biological result for potential health gain." Previous descriptions of these operations as bariatric or weight loss surgery are a misnomer because these procedures do not primarily cause weight loss but instead make significant physiologic changes to the human body that cause a positive effect on metabolism and related diseases. The role of this chapter is to provide a detailed, useful description of these procedures, focusing on the role of the physician assistant (PA) in delivering care.

The Role of the Physician Assistant

The PA may participate in many roles in the practice of MBS. **As an advanced practice provider (APP),** the PA may function as **an assistant in the operating room, a hospitalist caring for the patient in the post-operative period or caring for the patient in the acute care setting, focusing on the long-term care of the patient**. The roles of a PA mimic and complement those of other healthcare workers and physicians. The PA may work in one, two, or all roles. A clear understanding of all responsibilities is vital to achieving a level of expertise. It is important to understand the causes of obesity, have an appreciation of the stigma of the disease, as well as the medical, and surgical treatment of obesity.

In the office setting, the APP and PA function as an extension of both the physician and the healthcare team. They are vital in educating patients about obesity as a disease and the treatment options available to potential patients. Much of the preparation to proceed to surgery is performed by the office PA. The process for the patient begins after an introductory, educational seminar, and proceeds with initial interviews where a history and physical is performed and patients are evaluated to determine whether they are surgical candidates. They are assigned a list of tasks to perform according to the program and insurance requirements. Once complete, the patients are instructed on the preoperative diet on which they are placed on for 2 weeks before surgery. Although the surgeon takes the primary role, the office-based PA helps to follow up with the bariatric surgery patient after surgery. (See section on long-term care of the bariatric surgery patient.)

The hospitalist-based physician assistant treating the bariatric patient must be skilled at ordering the appropriate medications, tests, and being able to clinically assess patients. They must be able to detect and initially treat complications on a 24-h basis for admitted patients. **They must communicate seamlessly with the treating surgeon**, especially during critical events. It may be their role, if they are the primary in-hospital clinician, to rescue a complicated patient. In hospitals that do not have a surgery residency program, the PA may have a role at the level of a senior resident.

The third role of the MBS PA is to be a **skilled technician and assistant in the operating room**. The surgeon and the PA must establish a schedule and assign a limited number of physician assistants to ensure adequate coverage while also

N. Floch (✉)
Department of Surgery, Yale School of Medicine, New Haven, CT, USA

Greenwich Hospital, Greenwich, CT, USA
e-mail: neil.floch@yale.edu

S. Atallah, J. Dragoljevic (eds.), *Fundamentals of Surgery for Physician Assistants*, https://doi.org/10.1007/978-3-032-21069-2_15

allowing for each PA to be able to obtain enough skill to function as a helpful assistant in the OR. The PA must be skilled in all facets of bariatric surgery: open technique, laparoscopy, and robotic surgery. There is no substitute for hands-on training in the operating room to obtain these skills of camera control, knowledge of procedure steps, retraction, stapling, and sewing. Physician assistants gaining skills may attend hands-on courses to learn these skills but will also need to migrate from camera-holding/second assistant, to eventually first assistant.

Demographics

In the United States, **the American Medical Association (AMA) declared obesity a disease in 2013**, but the European medical community has yet to do the same. **As of 2022, 890 billion people globally were living with obesity [2]. In the United States, currently 73% of the population is overweight, and 42% have obesity, possibly qualifying it as the most common disease**. Despite its prevalence, governments have not established coordinated strategies to prevent and treat obesity. People with obesity remain a target for social and work discrimination. Medical insurance companies do not uniformly cover benefits for obesity treatment, leaving many patients at risk for progression and development of other diseases. Medical students, physicians, and healthcare workers receive little education on nutrition and obesity in their training. Ironically, with the advent of GLP-1 agonist medications, all clinicians are increasingly called upon to prescribe medications and treat obesity in their practices. A limit in the understanding of obesity may lead to substandard advice and an increase in stigma and discrimination. To educate physicians, the American Board of Obesity Medicine (ABOM) has developed a system of education and an accessible exam to certify physicians in obesity medicine and all facets of obesity care, including MBS. The American Board of Surgery certifies bariatric surgeons for the American Society of Metabolic and Bariatric Surgery with a focused practice designation after successfully passing an exam.

Obesity is associated with 224 medical conditions, and most improve when the obesity is successfully treated. In a sense, obesity is "the mother of all chronic diseases." The most devastating diseases include cancer, type 2 diabetes (T2DM), obstructive sleep apnea (OSA), coronary artery disease (CAD), chronic heart failure (CHF), cerebrovascular accident (CVA), stroke, and kidney disease. As the understanding of metabolic disease is changing, nomenclature is changing to better reflect the metabolic underpinnings of these diseases: non-alcoholic fatty liver disease (NAFLD), has been changed to metabolic dysfunction–associated steatotic liver disease (MASLD) and nonalcoholic steatohepatitis (NASH), has been changed to metabolic dysfunction–associated steatohepatitis (MASH). Obesity contributes to metabolic dysregulation, insulin resistance, and chronic inflammation, which if untreated, progress to MAFLD and MASH. The process involves complex interactions between metabolic, inflammatory, and genetic factors. These diseases and chronic illnesses are debilitating, and decrease the quality and length of life. They result in the need for costly medications and treatments and drive up the strain on the healthcare system as well as the cost of healthcare. The presence and severity of obesity correlate with an increasing risk of earlier mortality. In 2021, obesity contributed to 335,000 deaths in the United States. (National-level and state-level prevalence of overweight and obesity among children, adolescents, and adults in the USA, 1990-2021, and Forcasts up to 2050, Lancet. 2024. GBD 2021 US Obesity Forcasting Collaborators.) Adolescence and adult weight gain are both related to increased risk of mortality when measured by both BMI and waist–hip ratio.

Obesity is associated with 16 different types of cancer, including breast, colorectal, endometrial, esophageal, kidney, pancreatic, liver, gallbladder, stomach, ovarian, thyroid, meningiomas, and multiple myeloma. **According to the Centers for Disease Control (CDC), 40% of all cancers are associated with obesity, and 55% of obesity-related cancers occur in women.** The highest risk for cancer occurs in endometrial cancer, which is seven times the normal risk. Esophageal cancer is the second most strongly associated cancer. Evidence supports that cancer cells are promoted by higher levels of insulin, insulin-like growth factors, and sex hormones.

Etiology

The obesity epidemic has evolved over more than three decades. **Adult obesity has doubled since 1990, and adolescent obesity has quadrupled in that time**. The prevalence of obesity rose rapidly in the 1970s. Many theories exist that explain the culprits and causes of the epidemic, which have been the subject of debate. Until recently, high-fat and high-carbohydrate diets were thought to be the main causes of obesity. Today, however, ultra-processed foods are considered the most significant contributor. Others suggest that the massive shift in weight gain of an entire population could be explained by the subsidies in the US Farm bills that stimulated the massive production of high-calorie carbohydrates and nutrient-poor, calorie-dense foods. This resulted in ample food at an affordable price and a larger baseline portion. These foods were also marketed aggressively to children and adults. A lack of physical activity and a sedentary lifestyle may be a contributing factor but cannot explain the onset of the epidemic. Genetics and epigenetics may explain a significantly increased risk, but not a direct cause of obesity. Environmental factors are more likely to influence obesity, such as exposure to endocrine disruptors and obesogenic substances.

An extensive list of likely factors have been implicated with the rise in obesity such as increased energy intake, food deserts, food prices, economic inequality, sleep deprivation, stress and mental health, cultural and social influences, medications that cause weight gain, medical conditions such as PCOS and hypothyroidism, maternal breast feeding, poor maternal nutrition, early childhood diet, low and high gestational weight, intrauterine factors such as weight gain during pregnancy, poor eating behaviors, and poor education surrounding food and nutrition. Classic thought is that weight gain and eventually obesity result directly from the consumption of food more than what can be burned in calories by the body. The simplicity of these ideals has been challenged by the knowledge that the human body can adapt metabolically to calorie intake.

Indications

Although waist circumference (WC) is more closely linked to cardiac risk and there are more accurate methods for assessing body composition, body mass index (BMI) remains the most practical and widely used tool for estimating a person's body size. BMI can be calculated by dividing weight in kilograms by the height in meters squared (kg/m^2) (see Fig. 15.1).

The categories of a person's size are as follows:

- Underweight less than 18.5 kg/m^2.
- Normal weight 18.5–24.9 kg/m^2.
- Overweight 25–29.9 kg/m^2.
- Class I obesity 30–34.9 kg/m^2.

Category	BMI (kg/m^2)
Underweight	<18.5
Normal weight	18.5–24.9
Overweight	25.0–29.9
Obesity Class I	30.0–34.9
Obesity Class II	35.0–39.9
Obesity Class III	≥40.0

Fig. 15.1 Weight classes according to BMI. (Credit: Neil Floch MD)

- Class II obesity 35–39.9 kg/m^2.
- Class III obesity 40–49.9 kg/m^2.
- Class IV obesity 50 kg/m^2 or greater.

The first indications for bariatric surgery were written by a National Institute of Health Committee, NIH, and published as a statement in 1991, and are followed by most insurance carriers in the United States that provide benefits for bariatric surgery. Patients are considered a candidate for bariatric surgery when they have failed medical management, such as dieting, exercise, and drug therapy. Candidates should have a BMI greater than 40 or a BMI greater than 35 and major comorbidity, such as type 2 diabetes (T2DM), obstructive sleep apnea (OSA), hypertension, severe cardiac disease, or degenerative joint disease (DJD). MBS is considered for patients who need joint arthroplasty, abdominal wall hernias, or transplantation of an organ before their goal procedure. Before proceeding to surgery, patients must have tried to lose weight by medical methods, be motivated, and be informed about the procedure and potential consequences. They must be an acceptable surgical risk. Patients who may not be considered for surgery include those with unstable coronary artery disease, severe CAD, pulmonary disease, portal hypertension, mental incapacity, active substance abuse, as well as those unable to carry out the necessary follow-up needed to maintain health.

These guidelines were not updated until 2022, but since 1991, a large pool of long-term data now exists to support the safety, efficacy, and durability of MBS. The guidelines were updated by the American Society of Metabolic and Bariatric Surgery (ASMBS and the International Federation for Surgery for Obesity IFSO) to include a **BMI of 35 kg/m^2 regardless of the presence or absence of comorbidities. MBS is recommended in patients with type T2DM and a BMI over 30 kg/m2 and is considered for individuals with a BMI between 30 and 34.9 kg/m^2 who have other comorbidities as listed above.** There is no upper age limit for MBS if patients are in an acceptable medical condition to tolerate the procedure. As people of Asian genetic origin are more susceptible to T2DM, the indication for surgery is greater than or equal to 27.5 kg/m2. Children and adolescents may be considered for MBS if they have a BMI greater than 120% of the 95th percentile along with a major comorbidity, or a BMI greater than 140% of the 95th percentile even without a comorbidity—provided the procedure is performed at a center with a multidisciplinary team (see Fig. 15.2).

Indication Category	2022 ASMBS/IFSO Indication	References
BMI ≥ 35 kg/m²	Surgery recommended, regardless of presence, absence, or severity of comorbidities	[1-3]
BMI 30–34.9 kg/m²	Surgery should be considered for individuals with metabolic disease (e.g., type 2 diabetes, hypertension)	[1-3]
Asian populations	BMI thresholds lowered: Clinical obesity at BMI >25 kg/m²; surgery offered at BMI >27.5 kg/m²	[1-2]
Adolescents	Appropriately selected children and adolescents should be considered for surgery	[1-2]
BMI criteria for comorbidities	No longer required for BMI ≥35 kg/m²; comorbidities not necessary for eligibility	[1-3]

1. Eisenberg D, Shikora SA, Aarts E, et al. 2022 American Society of Metabolic and Bariatric Surgery (ASMBS) and International Federation for the Surgery of Obesity and Metabolic Disorders (IFSO) Indications for Metabolic and Bariatric Surgery. Obesity Surgery. 2023;33(1):3-14. doi:10.1007/s11695-022-06332-1.
2. Eisenberg D, Shikora SA, Aarts E, et al. 2022 American Society for Metabolic and Bariatric Surgery (ASMBS) and International Federation for the Surgery of Obesity and Metabolic Disorders (IFSO): Indications for Metabolic and Bariatric Surgery. Surgery for Obesity and Related Diseases : Official Journal of the American Society for Bariatric Surgery. 2022;18(12):1345-1356. doi: 10.1016/j.soard. 2022.08.013.
3. Hsu JL, Farrell TM. Updates in Bariatric Surgery. The American Surgeon. 2024;90(5):925-933. doi:10.1177/00031348231220576.

Fig. 15.2 2022 ASMBS/IFSO Indications for bariatric surgery. (Credit: Neil Floch MD)

Medical Treatment of Obesity and Weight Loss Strategies

To qualify for bariatric surgery, patients must have attempted medical weight loss. The medical treatment of obesity involves a comprehensive, multimodal approach that includes lifestyle interventions, dietary changes, increased physical activity, behavioral therapy, and pharmacotherapy. According to the National Weight Control Registry, patients who are most successful at controlling their weight start with eating breakfast, exercising 1 h daily, eating a low-calorie, low-fat diet, monitoring their weight, and maintaining a consistent eating pattern both during the week and on the weekends.

Weight loss strategies involve a step-like approach beginning with maintaining a healthy lifestyle with diet and exercise, seeking assistance with a registered dietitian nutritionist, and when necessary, advancing to the use of anti-obesity medications or MBS. Comprehensive obesity treatment is imperative for successful results after bariatric surgery. **Although high-intensity lifestyle interventions, consisting of at least 14 sessions over 6 months, can achieve 5–10% weight loss, intense treatment is not feasible for a large scale of people.**

Dietary strategies focus on promoting health and reducing caloric intake. Diets, such as Atkins, ketogenic, Mediterranean, DASH, low-carbohydrate, and low-fat, show little advantage over one another except for slightly more weight loss with protein-dominated diets. A systematic review (SR) and meta-analysis (MA) in the *British Medical Journal* by Ge L, et al., and another in JAMA by Johnston, BC, found that low-carbohydrate and low-fat diets had similar effects on weight loss at 6 and 12 months, with both resulting in a weight loss of approximately 4.6 kg. **Among named diets, the Atkins diet showed the largest effect on weight reduction at 6 months, 5.5 kg; followed by the DASH diet, 3.6 kg; and the Zone diet, 4.1 kg.** An SR in the *Annals of Internal Medicine* showed significant weight loss at 12 months compared to control groups for commercial weight loss programs such as Weight Watchers and Jenny Craig.

When treating obesity aggressively with surgery, there is a rapid loss of both fat and fat-free mass, which requires a focused treatment on protein replacement to prevent sarcopenia. The average patient requires 60–80 g of protein a day. Vitamin supplementation is warranted, as most bariatric procedures include reduced total nutrient intake or malabsorption of micronutrients. Evidence demonstrates that exercise alone is a poor tool for weight loss. Physical activity has shown a modest 2-4 kg or 2-3% of body weight over a year when performed with intensity and consistency, although exercise is essential for weight maintenance.

Pharmacotherapy has been available for decades both over the counter and prescribed by physicians. Many medications remain on the market despite a long history of many former medications being banned by the Federal Drug Administration (FDA) for severe side effects. The advent of GLP-1 agonist medications has revolutionized the treatment of obesity. Only recently have anti-obesity medications demonstrated impactful effectiveness, which has presented a more popular, yet less effective initial option than MBS. Despite high cost, low supply, significant side effects, and the allowance of compounded medications, patients are using GLP-1 agonists and GIP at an increasing rate. A major drawback is adherence to drug usage. Medical obesity patients taking GLP-1 agonists must comply with weekly or daily injections. Although surgery patients have better results if they change their behaviors, such as diet, exercise, and follow-up with their surgeon, their compliance with the treatment is once on the day of surgery. **Medications are recommended for patients with a**

BMI ≥ 30 kg/m^2 or ≥ 27 kg/m^2 with weight-related comorbidities, in conjunction with lifestyle modifications. The indications for medication use instead of bariatric surgery and the future of comprehensive treatment are currently being defined as an ongoing process. Growing evidence about gut hormones—such as GLP-1, GIP, and potential future targets like glucagon, PYY, and amylin—has deepened our understanding of the underlying causes of obesity and how various treatments work.

Anti-obesity medications are used alongside bariatric surgery for several reasons, including achieving preoperative weight loss, serving as a neo-adjuvant to reduce surgical complications, and postoperatively to enhance overall weight loss, prevent weight regain, or treat weight regain after surgery. FDA-approved medications for long-term use for obesity treatment include GLP-1 receptor agonists: semaglutide, liraglutide, and tirzepatide. Other medications include phentermine-topiramate, naltrexone-bupropion, and orlistat.

GLP-1RA and GIP

GLP-1RA medications include **liraglutide**, which is administered as a daily subcutaneous (SQ) injection with a gradually increased dose up to a maximum of 3.0 mg. It demonstrated a mean weight loss of 8.0% over 56 weeks in patients without T2 DM. The GLP-1RA **semaglutide** was the first to be administered weekly, at a dose of 2.4 mg. **It shows a mean weight loss of up to 16.7% after 2 years**. **Tirzepatide** is a dual GLP-1 and glucose-dependent insulinotropic polypeptide (GIP) receptor agonist, administered weekly at doses up to 15 mg. **It has resulted in the highest weight loss of up to 22.9% after 3.5 years**. All medications have significant improvements in glycemic control and metabolic measures.

GLP-1RAs have demonstrated significant reductions in major adverse cardiovascular events (MACE), including myocardial infarction (MI), stroke, and cardiovascular death. The LEADER trial showed a 13% reduction in MACE with liraglutide, while the SUSTAIN-6 trial demonstrated a 24% reduction with semaglutide. GLP-1RAs, including liraglutide and semaglutide, can resolve steatohepatitis and delay the progression of liver fibrosis. They can improve OSA due to significant reductions in visceral fat, reduce blood pressure, postprandial lipemia, and contribute to overall cardiovascular health. Potential benefits also include chronic kidney disease and heart failure with preserved ejection fraction.

The most common side effects for GLP-1RAs are nausea, vomiting, diarrhea, constipation, and abdominal pain, which are usually transient. *Hypoglycemia* can occur when these agents are used in combination with insulin or sulfonylureas. *Pancreatitis* has been reported, but large trials have not supported a risk. Reported complications include *diabetic retinopathy, gallbladder disease, injection site reactions, anaphylaxis, and renal adverse events* associated with severe gastrointestinal fluid loss. The medications should not be used with a *personal* or *family history* of **medullary thyroid carcinoma** or **multiple endocrine neoplasia syndrome type 2 (MEN2)**.

Phentermine Topiramate

The combination of phentermine and topiramate (PHEN/TPM) is effective for weight loss in adults with overweight or obesity. **In the CONQUER trial, patients on the 7.5 mg/46 mg dose had 7.8%and those on the 15 mg/92 mg dose had a 9.8% total body weight loss, compared to a 1.2% in the placebo group.** Side effects include dry mouth, paresthesia, constipation, insomnia, dizziness, and dysgeusia. Patients may have mood and sleep disorders, such as anxiety and depression, which are dose-dependent. Difficulties with concentration and memory have been noted with topiramate. Less common adverse events include increased heart rate, elevated blood pressure, and kidney stones. Use is contraindicated with glaucoma, hyperthyroidism, and during pregnancy due to the risk of birth defects.

Bupropion/Naltrexone

Bupropion and naltrexone (NB) are commonly used for weight loss. **In the COR-II trial, patients treated with naltrexone 32 mg plus bupropion 360 mg lost 6.4% total body weight, compared to a 1.2% reduction in the placebo group at 56 weeks** [1, 2]. Common side effects include nausea, headache, constipation, dizziness, vomiting, and dry mouth. Nausea was the most frequent adverse event occurring in 29.8% of patients. Other side effects include transient increases in blood pressure and heart rate.

Orlistat

Orlistat results in a modest weight loss of anywhere from approximately 2.8% total body weight loss (TBWL) to 10.2% in 1 year. The side effects are caused by blocking the absorption of dietary fats and include oily spotting, flatulence with discharge, fecal urgency, and oily stools, and malabsorption of fat-soluble vitamins and medications. These side effects are bothersome and usually lead to treatment discontinuation. Rarely can patients develop a liver injury necessitating careful monitoring.

Patient Preparation

Patients interested in bariatric surgery should attend a live or virtual preliminary information session. The lecture should provide all potential procedures and the necessary steps to undergo MBS. The information discussed should include obesity and its related diseases, surgical options, risks and benefits, expected outcomes, alternatives, long-term implications on health, as well as patient and program expectations and responsibilities. Long-term follow-up should be discussed as a commitment.

An initial evaluation by the surgeon or an office-based PA is performed to determine whether the patient is an appropriate candidate for bariatric surgery and what requirements will be needed. Patients are introduced to multiple medical specialists, including a registered dietitian (RD), behavioral health specialists, and a bariatric surgeon. The office-based PA may facilitate or oversee this process. Patients are most critically assessed for nutritional and psychological issues. Patients with a previous psychological history are seen by a psychiatrist, whereas others may be evaluated by other mental health professionals. Patients will undergo evaluation by a multidisciplinary team to assess psychological readiness for the procedure. Some candidates may need further treatment with nutritional education or psychological support before undergoing surgery.

Candidates for surgery are evaluated for potential comorbidities such as CAD, pulmonary diseases, OSA, T2 DM, liver disease, and kidney disease. Patients may need to be evaluated by specialists in the medical fields specific to their disease processes. **At initial visitation by the bariatric surgeon, APP, or PA, a full history and physical should be performed**, including the patient's weight, weight gain over time, multiple weight loss attempts, and disordered eating behavior. The evaluation should also assess the patient's social support system, including involvement from family and friends, as this plays a critical role in long-term success. Patients are evaluated for their education in the disease process and the procedures used to treat it, their goals, and their motivation to proceed with MBS.

The goal of an evaluation is to medically optimize the patient for surgery and prepare them for lifestyle changes. The patient must understand the lifelong need for nutritional supplementation and follow-up. For patients who are dependent on certain medications for psychiatric illnesses, the potential for pharmacokinetic changes with each procedure should be considered. A pharmacist may be consulted for patients with polypharmacy, immunosuppression, or those who need to be changed from extended release to multiple doses to crush medications after surgery.

A history and physical should identify patients with an increased cardiac risk who need a cardiology evaluation. Bariatric surgery is an intermediate or high-risk cardiac procedure. Prior to surgery, patients will need **preoperative cardiac and pulmonary clearance** to ensure they are medically optimized. Screening for obstructive sleep apnea (OSA) is essential and is typically performed using the STOP-Bang questionnaire. A score of 4 has high sensitivity, 88%, whereas a STOP-Bang score of 6 is specific, 85.2%, for identifying severe OSA. If OSA is diagnosed, patients should be treated with continuous positive airway pressure (CPAP) or bilevel positive airway pressure (BiPAP) and demonstrate compliance with therapy before proceeding with surgery. Patients will also undergo optimization of glycosylated hemoglobin and smoking cessation if necessary. Patients with type 1 and T2 DM with poorly controlled hyperglycemia may require an endocrinology consult. An HbA1c level below 8% is recommended prior to MBS; however, it should not be considered a strict barrier to surgery, as bariatric procedures often lead to immediate improvements in blood glucose control.

Cigarette smoking cessation is required for at least 6 weeks preoperatively but may be longer depending on the program. Patients are also advised to stop vaping, as growing evidence shows it can have harmful health effects. Nicotine replacement therapy is safe and can be used before surgery to help patients stop smoking. Preoperative evaluation includes screening for alcohol and substance abuse, and if present, formal counseling, monitoring by testing, and abstinence are required. Although controversial, patients should be screened for marijuana usage and should be encouraged to stop before surgery if it is not used for medical reasons.

Esophagogastroduodenoscopy (EGD) is suggested when it is believed to alter treatment. It may be used in patients with severe gastroesophageal reflux disease (GERD), *Helicobacter pylori*, or a suspected hiatal hernia. Upper gastrointestinal series (UGI) can be performed to complement or as a substitute for EGD in patients with GERD or prior bariatric surgery. Manometry or 24-h pH testing may be used if motility issues are a concern or if further testing is needed to diagnose the presence of GERD. Ultrasound is performed for symptoms of biliary disease, elevated liver function tests, or when there is clinical suspicion of MASH or MAFLD. A fibro scan can also be performed to assess the liver. Colonoscopy assesses lower gastrointestinal symptoms before surgery. Dual-energy X-ray absorptiometry (DEXA) scan is selectively used in patients with concerns about low bone density. A patient should have a venous-thromboembolic (VTE) risk assessment before surgery, and patients at increased risk should undergo additional postoperative chemoprophylaxis. Risk is assessed according to BMI and the presence of prior VTE, age, gender, immobility, and the expected operative time.

Selective testing may include an electrocardiogram (EKG) based on risk and chest X-ray (CXR) for active cardiopulmonary disease. Blood tests include CBC, chem-21, vitamin levels including B-vitamins, calcium, magnesium, phosphorus, copper, zinc, selenium, vitamins ADEK, TSH, T4, PTH, and glycosylated hemoglobin levels. Routine cancer screenings should be coordinated through a primary care provider. Recommendations include prostate cancer screening starting at age 50 for men, cervical and breast cancer screenings beginning at age 25, and colon cancer screening starting at age 45. Screening should not prevent bariatric surgery from being performed but should be scheduled afterward.

Bariatric medicine can play a key role in preoperative management by using medication to help reduce BMI prior to surgery. Operating on patients at a lower BMI may reduce the risk of complications and decrease the recovery time. Although a tedious process, preoperative preparation is necessary to achieve the best short- and long-term results while attempting to prevent perioperative complications. Long-term results are most successful with continuous clinical follow-up, participation in organized support groups, and the support of family members.

Determining Which Bariatric Procedure Is Optimal

Achieving normal glycemic control after bariatric surgery depends on the preoperative duration of T2DM, BMI, preoperative fasting blood glucose levels, and preoperative HbA1c. **Patients with more severe diabetes may be candidates for RNY, DS, or the SADI-S, single anastomosis duodenal-ileal bypass with sleeve gastrectomy**. Dr. Ali Aminian at the Cleveland Clinic developed a calculator based on medical evidence to determine which procedures to use for individual patients. For example, HTN and dyslipidemia are more likely to resolve after RNY than SG. GERD will more frequently resolve after RNY and may become worse after SG. Patients with severe GERD and especially Barrett's esophagus should be strongly considered for RNY instead of SG. Patients with inflammatory bowel disease can undergo RNY when ulcerative colitis (UC) is stable. SG is recommended in Crohn's disease patients to avoid small bowel complications that can occur with an RNY. Further research is needed to determine which procedures are preferred for transplant candidates. There is no increased risk of ulcer formation in patients on chronic low-dose aspirin treatment, but there is little data for patients on high-dose treatment. Chronic steroid use1 increases the post-operative risk of complications after MBS, but it is unclear which operation to recommend, as more research is needed. A patient's BMI should not be a deciding factor in determining which procedure to use for a patient. A patient with a very high BMI may undergo staged procedures. An SG is performed initially, reserving a RNY or SADI as a future, separate procedure if the patient does not achieve their medical or weight loss goals. The strategy is to reduce operative and postoperative risk for the patient. Indirect calorimetric studies are not useful in determining which procedure should be performed. Patients who require chronic NSAID treatment are at risk of delayed ulcer healing. Patients who stop smoking within 1 year before surgery have a greater than 50% chance of smoking again in the next 7 years and may be high-risk candidates to develop marginal ulcers if they have an RNY, and therefore, an SG may be a better choice. Ultimately, determining which procedure to perform is a shared decision between the surgeon, providers, and the patient.

Restriction, Malabsorption, and Metabolic Surgery

Weight Loss Procedures that Function by Restriction

In the past, bariatric surgical procedures were classified according to the concepts of restriction and malabsorption, as these were believed to be the only mechanisms involved in causing weight loss and the secondary benefits that led to improvement and resolution of medical issues. The restrictive procedures limited caloric intake by creating a smaller stomach pouch. Although the restrictive portion of procedures accounts for a significant portion of initial weight loss, they do not directly cause changes that improve metabolic disease. The metabolic effects of restriction are secondary to weight loss only.

The vertical banded gastroplasty, VBG, was conceived by Edward E. Mason in 1982 as the first restrictive procedure for weight loss that preserved normal digestion and absorption. It was popular in the 1980s and 1990s due to its simplicity and initial promising results. The procedure is performed in the upper cardia of the stomach, by stapling a donut hole and then partitioning the stomach with a vertical staple line. The outlet at the donut hole is then encircled with a piece of mesh or a band to maintain the durability of the non-adjustable aperture. Patients are satiated when the pouch is full, but further eating may result in vomiting if the pouch is not allowed to empty. The procedure was initially introduced with the open technique and then adjusted to a laparoscopic technique. Weight loss occurs directly from decreased caloric intake of solid food. Excess weight loss (EWL) is as much as 66% at 2 years and 55% at 9 years. The ability to consume high-calorie liquid meals and sweets, the gradual increase in pouch capacity caused by overeating, and severe

GERD are major disadvantages. The VBG was largely replaced after the introduction of the adjustable gastric band. The VBG combined the disadvantages of a higher complication rate and the inability to adjust the band. The revision rate ranged from 20% to 56%, resulting mainly from staple line disruption, weight regain, stomal stenosis, band erosion, band disruption, pouch dilatation, vomiting, and GERD. Due to these complications and the advent of newer, more effective bariatric procedures, VBG has been replaced in contemporary bariatric practice. Many VBG patients will undergo conversion to SG or gastric bypass.

The Polish-born surgeon **Lubomyr Kuzmak** emigrated to America and developed the **open adjustable band in 1983**. He obtained the original patent for the device. **He published the research paper on the procedure in 1986 and the 7-year results in 1991**. The laparoscopic adjustable band, or Lap-Band®, was originally developed by BioEnterics Inc. The rights were sold to Allergan Inc., then Apollo Endosurgery Inc., Reshape Lifesciences, Inc., and now reside with Advanced Surgical Solutions. Favretti and Cadiere **developed the LAGB, laparoscopic adjustable band, AGB, Lap-Band technique in 1992, and later**, with Belgian surgeons M. Belachew and M. Legrand, they were placed in 1993 in Belgium, then extensively in Europe and Australia starting in 1994. The FDA approved its use in the United States in 2001. A second band, Realize Band® by Ethicon, was later approved by the FDA in 2007. Both bands were composed of (1) a silicone band with a balloon inner tube that wraps around the stomach, (2) a Port-A-Cath that lies under the skin on the rectus muscle for access, and (3) tubing to connect the two.

The virtual pouch in the adjustable gastric band was created by wrapping the band around the gastric cardia, partitioning the stomach into a small 2–3 cm portion above the band, leaving the remainder of the stomach below the band. The band is adjusted by inserting saline into the port 4 weeks after surgery, which increases the compression and reduces the passage of nutrients between the upper and lower stomach. The band can be adjusted in subsequent office visits until maximal weight loss is achieved while being careful not to overfill the band and cause obstructive symptoms of esophageal reflux and vomiting.

The AGB was widely used because of its easy placement, quick recovery, outpatient or 1-day hospital stay, and lower complication rate. After its introduction, the adjustable band replaced the VBG as the dominant, restrictive procedure. The advantages of the AGB included no stapling of bowel and a 0–0.5% mortality rate. It was adjustable, causing minimal vitamin and nutrient deficiencies. The band is reversible because it can be removed, but patients may develop adhesions and chronic esophageal dilatation with dysmotility and GERD. American results revealed an EWL of 45–75% at 24 months. Weight loss after AGB occurs gradually compared with malabsorptive procedures. Successful weight loss is more likely when patients are committed to close follow-up with a surgeon or PA, capable of adjusting the band by filling to achieve adequate restriction or urgent removal of fluid to relieve an obstruction. AGB is associated with the improvement of comorbidities, such as T2 DM, asthma, OSA, and HTN, while improving quality of life. These results depend on weight loss to improve metabolic conditions, whereas metabolic procedures directly improve metabolic mechanisms.

The AGB was popular, but inconsistent results over 10 years led investigators to look for a procedure with better results. The band required a less favorable diet consisting of mostly softer foods and higher carbohydrates. **Side effects such as chronic GERD and complications such as band slippage, erosion, and aspiration pneumonia led to the eventual disfavor of the procedure**. The development of the SG introduced a low-risk, metabolic operation that had more favorable results, causing the AGB to lose its dominance as the entry-level restrictive bariatric procedure.

Although considered a metabolic procedure, the SG involves reduction in stomach volume by removing the fundus of the stomach, which has been argued to be a form of restriction. These patients achieve fullness sooner, which may be attributed to the restrictive component. **As a DS and SADI-S also involve the creation of a GS, some weight loss can be attributed to the restrictive component**. The primary concept of restriction depends solely on limiting caloric intake of the quantity of food alone and is therefore a slower process. The RNY also involves a component of restriction as the small stomach pouch limits the intake and emptying of food content. Repeat studies have revealed that a small gastric pouch alone cannot contribute to significant, sustained weight loss.

Malabsorption for Weight Loss

The second traditional categorization of bariatric surgery procedures is malabsorption. In these procedures, various quantities of the stomach, duodenum, jejunum, and ileum are diverted to limit exposure to food and digestive substances. The concept depended upon the food and digestive juices meeting relatively distally within the small bowel lumen, and therefore, the food consumed has a smaller length of combined exposure to an absorptive surface area. **The first malabsorption procedure was the jejunoileal bypass (JIB), reported in 1962 after being developed by Howard Payne and Leonard T. Dewind**. The procedure bypassed the proximal jejunum to the distal ileum to create malabsorption and weight loss. Although it gained popularity in the 1960s and 1970s, it was associated with severe complications, including malnutrition, liver dysfunction, renal failure, and electrolyte disturbances. In most patients, it led to the need to reverse the procedure to avoid significant morbidity and eventual mortality.

After the JIB, other more effective procedures with less complications were developed such as the BPD, DS, and SADI-S.

The RNY combines features of both restriction and malabsorption with the creation of a small stomach pouch and a 25–30% functional small-bowel bypass. The mechanisms that cause weight loss also led to metabolic changes that alter the body in a manner that can improve diseases such as diabetes, hypertension, hyperlipidemia, and high cholesterol. In the past, the focus of bariatric surgery was to lose weight. MBS focuses on resolving over 224 diseases associated with obesity. In 2007, the ABS, American Bariatric Society, changed its name to emphasize its goal and became the ASMBS, American Society of Metabolic and Bariatric Surgery.

Metabolic Bariatric Surgery

The treatment of metabolic disease with surgery was first described by Henry Buchwald and Richard Varco in 1970. **In 1995, Walter Pories recognized the ability of RNY to treat T2 DM, "Who would have thought it? An operation proves to be the most effective therapy for adult-onset diabetes mellitus."** Despite understanding the metabolic changes after MBS, little was known about the causative mechanisms responsible for these substantial benefits to patients' health until recently. Multiple mechanisms have been elucidated, first in mice and then in humans, but their relative contribution to weight loss and metabolic changes remains to be clarified.

Gut Hormones

Although each type of MBS has different levels of effect on gut hormone alterations, several patterns are consistent with most procedures. In untreated patients, ghrelin, or growth hormone release–inhibiting peptide, peaks before meals to stimulate or initiate eating and may be responsible for "food noise" that patients describe. **After bariatric surgery, ghrelin levels decrease significantly—especially following SG, where most ghrelin-producing cells in the stomach's fundus are removed**. However, a small number of ghrelin-producing cells remain in other tissues, including the duodenum, small intestine, lungs, pancreatic islets, gonads, adrenal cortex, placenta, kidney, and hypothalamus. Ghrelin is also reduced following other types of MBS. **RNY causes a postprandial blood elevation of GLP-1, and peptide YY (PYY), from the L-cells in the ileum.** Both gut hormones decrease the desire to eat. Both GIP and GLP-1 increase insulin and decrease glucagon secretion by the pancreas after injection of glucose, an effect muted in T2 DM patients that improves after MBS. The AGB is not considered a metabolic, operation and shares a similar gut hormone stimulatory profile as dieting, which is a short-term increase in ghrelin, but no sustained changes in blood levels of ghrelin, GLP-1, and PYY.

Bile Acids

Studies in rodents have revealed that bile acids increase energy production via GLP-1 secretion. The mechanism has only been isolated in rodents. Bile acids attenuate thyroid hormone production after binding to the G-protein-coupled bile acid receptor 1, TGR5 receptors in muscle cells. **Bile acids have also been found to increase mucosal absorption of nutrients and increase energy expenditure by affecting the farnesoid X nuclear receptor (FXR) receptor pathway.** In humans, both the RNY and BPD/DS have caused an increase in circulating levels of bile acids, which have also resulted in an increased diversity of microbiota. It is unclear whether the increase in humans is directly due to an increase in endogenous bile acids by the liver.

Microbiome

Bariatric surgery induces significant changes in the gut microbiome, which are associated with metabolic improvements and weight loss. The most notable changes include a decrease in Firmicutes and an increase in Bacteroidetes in the bowel. **There is an increase in beneficial bacteria such as *Akkermansia muciniphila*.** Post-surgery, microbial diversity decreases initially but returns to baseline over time. Shifts in microbiota composition are associated with reduced inflammation, improved insulin resistance, and weight loss. Bariatric surgery increases the production of short-chain fatty acids (SCFAs) and bile acids, which assist in modulating metabolism and energy expenditure. The changes in gut microbiota and diversity alter gut hormone levels such as ghrelin, leptin, GLP-1, PYY, and CCK, contributing to enhanced satiety and reduced hedonic eating.

Neurologic

Eating is regulated by the central nervous system (CNS). Peripheral control occurs via the vagal nervous system. **In rodents and humans, ligation of vagal parasympathetic afferents and efferent nerves results in alterations of food**

preference away from high-density foods such as fats and high carbohydrates toward low-density foods such as proteins. The sympathetic efferent nervous system arises from the celiac and mesenteric ganglia and maintains control of some gut enzyme release, as well as decreasing peristalsis. The smooth muscle cells of the GI tract are also innervated in the submucosa. **There is a large neural component in the muscles of the gastric fundus, which is removed during an SG and BPD/DS and may account for a decrease in the desire to eat and an increase in fullness sensation. In RNY and BPD/DS, there is usually ligation of the vagal afferent and efferent nerves, leading to a dominant, maintained sympathetic output.** Neural stimulation of the stomach has not resulted in weight loss. Animal studies have demonstrated that vagal stimulation can influence both insulin and glucagon output and resultant blood sugar levels.

The Roux-en-Y Gastric Bypass

The RNY is the second most common surgical procedure for weight loss in the United States, accounting for 30% of cases. The original RNY procedure was first developed in animals and then in humans in 1966 by Edward E. Mason and Chikashi Ito, which included a partial gastrectomy and loop gastrojejunostomy. It was originally performed after the observation that patients lost weight after gastric ulcer surgery. The procedure was modified by John Griffen in 1977 to include a smaller gastric pouch and an RNY. **The first laparoscopic RNY was performed by Alan Wittgrove in 1994 with a 150-cm Roux limb and a 70-cm biliopancreatic limb.** Laparoscopy lowered the incidence of incisional hernias and wound infections, led to faster recovery, and led to a more rapid return to work than open surgery. The application of laparoscopy to bariatric surgery was revolutionary because it allowed significantly better access to large patients in whom open surgery was difficult and resulted in higher morbidity and mortality. The recovery from a large incision was difficult, resulting in poor wound healing and secondary complications from immobility, pain, and a complicated recovery. Laparoscopy reduced complications, recovery was faster, and morbidity decreased significantly.

In the past, weight loss after RNY was believed to be attributed to anatomical restriction and nutrient malabsorption. As described previously, other metabolic mechanisms have now been attributed to cause weight loss. RNY results in more significant weight loss averages than restrictive procedures such as AGB, VBG, and SG. In the RNY, a 30-mL gastric pouch is created as it is separated from the gastric remnant, resulting in a smaller reservoir for food and more rapid emptying. The pouch is connected by a stoma to the small bowel, creating an RNY segment. The remnant stomach and duodenum empty gastric acid, pancreatic enzymes, and bile through a 30-cm to 50-cm biliopancreatic limb, connected to the "food" or RNY limb at 75–150 cm distally. At this location, significant digestion begins. A short Roux limb will not add to the benefit of malabsorption. Roux limbs longer than 200 cm in long-limb bypass may lead to decreased absorption of vitamins and nutrients and complications of malnutrition.

The gastrojejunostomy may cause "dumping," which results in rapid emptying of concentrated contents into the small bowel and symptoms of lightheadedness, nausea, diaphoresis, abdominal pain, and diarrhea. Some patients develop a negative conditioned response to eating concentrated foods and therefore avoid them to prevent these symptoms. Ghrelin is a peptide hormone secreted in the stomach and duodenum that stimulates people to eat. Its response to eating is inhibited by the RNY and the SG. An exaggerated response of PYY may also contribute to loss of appetite. Early weight loss is rapid but reaches a plateau after 18 months, after which patients tend to gain weight if behavior modification is not instituted.

Sleeve Gastrectomy

The SG evolved as a stand-alone procedure in 2000 (Fig. 15.3). **Although many surgeons contributed to its development, possibly its most vocal advocate was Michel**

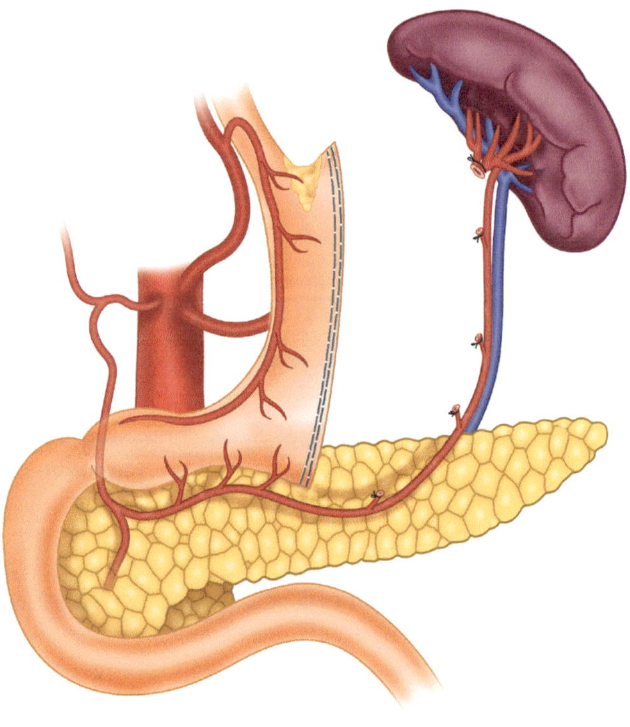

Fig. 15.3 Sleeve gastrectomy with divided stomach that is removed and portion that remains. (Credit: Neil Floch MD)

Gagner. The SG was developed by Doug Hess and others in 1988 as the gastric portion of the DS, duodenal switch operation. After increased complications following DS, Gagner proposed separating the procedure into two stages to lower the mortality rates seen in higher BMI patients undergoing BPD-DS. SG has since become stand-alone and the most common bariatric surgery in the United States and the world, comprising 70% of all procedures for weight loss. It entails the creation of a stomach tube from the cardia to the antrum that involves the removal of the fundus and body of the stomach along the greater curvature. The procedure is performed laparoscopically or robotically with multiple stapler cartridges and a single stapled technique. The staple lines may be left with or without reinforcement material or oversewn. The antrum is left intact. Analysis of the cause of weight loss in sleeve gastrectomy is well-documented by Seeley et al., and others: Restriction of food intake by a smaller pouch, hormonal changes with decreased ghrelin by removal of almost all producing cells in the fundus, increased GLP-1 and PYY levels, increased fullness, improved glucose metabolism, accelerated gastric emptying, changes in food preference, reduced inflammation in white adipose tissue, increased brown adipose tissue, and alterations in the microbiome diversity leading to decreased inflammation and improved metabolism. Patients who reach a plateau or who regain weight may choose to have their SG converted to an RNY, BPD, or SADI-S.

Biliopancreatic Diversion and Duodenal Switch

The original BPD was developed by Scopinaro et al. in 1979 in response to the poor results with jejunoileal bypass. The BPD involves a partial gastrectomy that is anastomosed distally to the ileum. There is a long segment of Roux limb and a short common channel where the food and biliopancreatic juices meet to allow absorption. **The process results in significant malabsorption and 72% EWL up to 18 years postoperatively.** The procedure is now performed laparoscopically with similar results. Unique disadvantages of BPD include mortality of 1% and high incidence of protein malnutrition, anemia, diarrhea, and stomal ulceration.

The BPD with duodenal switch (BPD/DS) is a BPD that differs by creating a partial SG with preservation of the pylorus. The BPD/DS was developed by Picard Marceau and his colleagues in the early 1990s. The intention was to reduce the incidence of postoperative complications such as dumping syndrome, diarrhea, and anastomotic ulcerations while maintaining effective weight loss and metabolic benefits. As part of the procedure, a Roux limb with a short common channel is also created. The BPD/DS has been recommended for patients with super morbid obesity, a BMI greater than 50. Unfortunately, the higher mortality rate has led to the practice of staging the procedures by performing the gastric sleeve first and the BPD later if more weight loss is necessary. BPD/DS results in less stomal ulceration and diarrhea than BPD and can be performed laparoscopically. It is not performed routinely because of high morbidity and mortality.

SADI-S

In attempts to create a procedure that resulted in more weight loss and fewer complications, **the SADI-S was developed by Antonio Sanchez-Pernaute in 2007.** It is a simplified modification of the DS. **It involves creating a traditional SG after which a modified duodenal-ileal bypass is performed by transecting the duodenum just distal to the pylorus, and an end-to-side anastomosis is created between the duodenum and the ileum, typically 200–300 cm from the ileocecal valve.** This bypasses a significant portion of the small intestine, reducing nutrient absorption. The mechanisms of weight loss and metabolic disease improvement occur as the SG component restricts food intake, while the DIB, duodenal-ileal bypass, reduces nutrient absorption. The SG and DIB components induce changes in gut hormones, including reductions in ghrelin and increases in GLP-1 and PYY, enhancing satiety and improving glucose metabolism.

The SADI-S results in similar but more significant improvements in metabolic disease than other MBS procedures. The recovery and complications from SADI-S may be less than traditional DS but greater than almost all other MBS procedures. Unique complications of SADI-S include **nutritional deficiencies of fat-soluble vitamins (A, D, E, K), zinc, and folic acid.** Lifelong supplementation with vitamins is needed, and monitoring of blood levels of vitamins is recommended every 6–12 months. A minority of patients may experience significant malabsorption, leading to protein-calorie malnutrition. **Vitamin deficiencies and hypoproteinemia may lead to the need to lengthen the common channel of the bowel greater than 200–300 cm.**

One Anastomosis Gastric Bypass

The **one anastomosis gastric bypass (OAGB)**, or mini-gastric bypass, was introduced by **Dr Robert Rutledge** in 1997 as a simpler alternative to the traditional RNY with a single anastomosis between a long, narrow gastric pouch and a jejunum limb 200 cm from the ligament of Treitz. The procedure avoids a second anastomosis between the biliopancreatic limb and common channel and is considered safer than an RNY. OAGB is effective in achieving significant weight loss and improving obesity-related comorbidities, such as T2 DM, HTN, and dyslipidemia, but with a higher incidence of bile reflux and micronutrient deficiencies compared to RNY. The ASMBS has approved OAGB as an accepted bariatric procedure because of its safety and efficacy.

Endoscopic Procedures

Multiple intragastric balloons (IGBs) have been produced by companies with various designs. All remain temporary, having only modest weight loss results. Most types are placed endoscopically, while others can be swallowed. There are variations in the shape and sizes, which may be round or bilobed, and can be a single balloon or an option to place multiple balloons. The soft balloon is inserted into the stomach and inflated with saline. The distended device fills the stomach and induces satiety while causing restriction. This mechanical restriction is the main driver of weight loss. Additionally, IGBs can slow gastric emptying, which prolongs the feeling of fullness. Hormonal changes are less pronounced than with SG and other bariatric surgeries, and the primary effect is mechanical; therefore, IGBs are not considered a metabolic surgery.

IGBs result in a %TBWL of 10–15% at 6 months; however, weight regain is common after balloon removal. Adverse events include nausea, vomiting, and abdominal pain, with a small risk of serious complications such as gastric perforation. While this procedure appeals to individuals seeking moderate weight loss, its greatest benefit may be as an initial step for superobese, high-risk patients, helping them lose enough weight to be considered lower-risk candidates for definitive bariatric procedures. With the advent of significant weight loss with GLP-1RA medications, the role of gastric balloons has become more limited.

Laparoscopic or Robotic Bariatric Surgery

Robotic-assisted surgery was developed and initially became an accepted technology for clinical use, with evidence demonstrating an advantage for patients undergoing prostate surgery. Several companies produced robot technology that amplifies human participation in laparoscopy but does not replace it, but only one company currently dominates the market. Robotic surgery allows surgeons to reach difficult locations in the abdomen, using a grasper that can move 360°, with two-endoscope and camera visualization in three dimensions. The most advanced model, the DaVinci 5™, provides surgeons with tactile feedback sensing.

The location of the prostate gland, low in the pelvis, along with limited experience with minimally invasive techniques, created a situation where this organ could be approached easily, and surgeons had outstanding visualization and dexterity. The robotic technique was then used and accepted by gynecologists and colorectal surgeons. General surgeons have traditionally been most deft with minimally invasive techniques and have been the last to utilize the robot as a tool. In the past several years, bariatric surgeons have increasingly utilized robot technology to perform bariatric surgery. In the past, medical evidence has not revealed an advantage of using robot technology over traditional laparoscopy. A recent study supports the benefit of using the robot for RNY, but no advantage for SG.

The robotic technique for SG usually involves five incisions: one for the liver retractor, but this may be eliminated by suture retracting devices used by placing a suture in the crura of the diaphragm and the abdominal wall and slinging the liver upward. The other four incisions are placed horizontally across the abdomen, 23 cm from the xiphoid and approximately 8 cm apart. Robotic and laparoscopic procedures result in similar weight loss, but the robotic technique requires more time for setup, resulting in a higher cost. A recent study demonstrated fewer complications with the laparoscopic SG. The robot staplers can sense pressure and provide more compression to improve the stapling created. It can also stop stapling if there is too much pressure, so that a larger stapler cartridge may be used. The assistant needs to know how to use the robot and place staplers, sutures, and change instruments, eliminating the need for a more skilled bariatric assistant. The robot is less physically demanding on the surgeon, who can sit during the procedure. The robotic technique can be applied to all laparoscopic bariatric procedures.

Treatment of Weight Regain

Neo-adjuvant, Adjuvant, Weight Regain Medications

The treatment for weight regain after MBS includes dietary and behavioral counseling, pharmacotherapy, and possibly endoscopic or surgical revision procedures (see section on anti-obesity medications).

Revisions

An AGB can be replaced, but most are now being removed as patients are increasingly choosing to attempt GLP-1 agonist medications or another bariatric surgery. Reasons for removal include patients who fail to lose weight, regain weight, or have band slippage, erosion, dilatation of the esophagus, GERD, or Barrett's esophagus. **An AGB can be converted to an SG, RNY, BPD/DS, or SADI-S.** The timing of the revision is controversial; although some advocate for a combined removal of the band and conversion to another procedure, others recommend staging the procedure or performing each separately. Waiting 3 months can allow inflamed and fibrotic tissue to soften and provide an easier dissection.

After SG, up to 20% of patients may require revisional surgery due to inadequate weight loss or weight regain. Other patients may have severe GERD or develop Barrett's esophagus. **Revisional procedures after failed SG include re-sleeve gastrectomy, RNY, BPD/DS, and SAD-S.** BPD/DS and SAD-S provide superior weight loss compared to RNY and re-sleeve gastrectomy but result in higher rates of late morbidity and complications. BPD/DS has the highest long-term weight loss at 1 and 3 years %TWL: 12 and 28, the SADI-S: 9 and 19, and RNY: 4.7 and 7 compared to re-sleeve gastrectomy. Re-sleeve has a higher leak and complication rate with inferior results; it is rarely recommended.

Anatomical failures of **RNY** may occur from stretching of the gastric pouch or gastrojejunal anastomosis or poor eating behavior. Development of a fistula between the gastric pouch and the remnant stomach can be closed surgically or endoscopically. Options to induce further weight loss have been studied in meta-analyses and include **APC is an incisionless, minimally invasive technique that aims to reduce the GJA by endoscopic circumferential ablation**. BMI at revision of 37 kg/m^2 and %TWL was 6, 11, and 5 after 12, 24, and 36 months, respectively. **TORe is an endoscopic technique in which the pouch and/or the GJA is reduced by sutured plications.** Pooled BMI at revision was 37.9 kg/m^2, and %TWL during follow-up was minimal at best: 5.0, 1.8, after 12 and 48 months, respectively. **TORe + APC combined** with a pooled analyses starting at a BMI at revision of 40.0 kg/m^2 and %TWL reduction showed modest results at 8, 7, and 7 after 12, 24, 36, and 60 months, respectively. Laparoscopic surgical approach to reducing the **Pouch or GJ revision** after RNY involves reducing the size of the pouch and or the GJA diameter. In multiple studies, the pouch was revised in all cases after calibration with a 32 or 34 Fr boogie. Pooled BMI at revision was 37.8 kg/m^2, and %TWL was significantly better than endoscopic approaches with a %TWL of 17, 14 18, and 16 after 12, 24, 36, and 60 months, respectively. **LGB placed over an RNY pouch** has been largely abandoned but with a pooled BMI at revision of 39.0 kg/m^2, and %TWL was 21, 15, and 17 after 12, 24, and 36 months; this procedure has had successful weight loss but the disadvantages of having an adjustable band. **Distalization of an RYGB or a "long-limb bypass"** is performed by lengthening the biliopancreatic limb and shortening the common channel where nutrients are absorbed. Two techniques are described: by taking down either the Roux limb (type 1) or the Y limb (Type 2). Pooled BMI at revision was 41.4 kg/m^2, and %TWL was 20, 24, 23, 24, and 22 after 12, 24, 36, 48, and 60 months, respectively. To avoid nutritional deficiencies, the total alimentary limb (TALL) should not be less than 300 cm. **Conversion of RNY to DS** with a BMI at revision of 45.6 kg/m^2 and %TWL was 20 and 34 after 12 and 24 months, respectively.

ERAS—Enhanced Recovery After Surgery

Enhanced recovery after surgery (ERAS) protocols have been developed for bariatric surgery. **They are designed to optimize perioperative care and improve outcomes.** The protocols are broken down into preoperative, intraoperative, and postoperative phases.

In the preoperative phase, the goal is to optimize comorbidities and as described previously and ensure that conditions such as T2 DM, HTN, OSA, and others are well-managed. Patients are educated and counseled on the preoperative nutrition requirements, procedures before surgery and patients and their families are informed about the surgical process and recovery expectations. Before surgery, patients are prescribed a high-protein liquid diet for 2 weeks preoperatively to reduce the size of their liver, with a secondary benefit of weight loss. Shortened fasting times have been helpful to prevent dehydration before surgery. Patients are allowed clear fluids up to 2 h before anesthesia induction. Certain medications should be stopped prior to surgery. Direct oral anticoagulants (DOAC) should be stopped 3 days prior to surgery. Bridging is dependent upon the disease process. Angiotensin-converting enzyme (ACE) inhibitors and angiotensin receptor blockers (ARBs) should not be taken on the morning of surgery as they may irreversibly lower blood pressure during general anesthesia. Beta-blockers and calcium channel blockers are continued. NSAIDs such as aspirin and ibuprofen are stopped 8 days before surgery. GLP-1RA protocols have been changing rapidly, but at the time of publication of this book, they should not be taken the day before surgery and patients must remain on a clear liquid diet for 48 h prior to any surgical procedure involving anesthesia (Fig. 15.4).

In the intraoperative phase, anesthesiologists aim for standardization by utilizing multimodal anesthesia to minimize opioid use and enhance pain control. Anesthesiologists or surgeons may provide local anesthesia by transversus abdominis plane (TAP) block. There is an effort to avoid invasive devices such as nasogastric tubes, urinary catheters, and drains. Minimally Invasive laparoscopic and robotic techniques are strongly recommended to reduce surgical stress and promote faster recovery.

In the postoperative phase, early mobilization is encouraged by the surgery team, as ambulation soon after surgery

Yale New Haven Health ERAS Bariatric Pathway

Procedures: Lap Roux-en-Y gastric bypass, Gastric Sleeve, and Duodenal switch

ERAS Bariatric Pre-Op Order set

Pre-Op Visit

Surgeon:
- Explain ERAS, LOS expectations
- Caprini Score - discuss Enoxaparin on discharge
- Patient optimization: Smoking / ETOH/ drug cessation. No alcohol at least 1 week pre-op
- Stop smoking at least 2 months pre-op
- Referrals as needed

Anesthesia:
- Phone screen or in-person visit
- Electrolyte drink / drink instructions
- Oral hygiene
- Chlorhexidine gluconate wash

Nursing:
- Social work / nutrition / psychiatric referrals per protocol
- Teach visit or class
- Referrals as needed
- Provide exercise physiology referrals as needed
- Carbohydrate drink instruction
- Bariatric liquid diet 2 weeks pre-op. Instruction by nutrition

Office:
- Book as ERAS

Holding Area

Surgeon:
(No specific tasks listed)

Anesthesia:
- Clear liquids up to 2 hours before hospital arrival
- Acetaminophen 1000 mg PO
- Celecoxib 200mg PO
- VTE PPX in accordance with VTE protocol (weight-based dosing)
- Consider post-operative nausea and vomiting prophylaxis per Apfel
- Scopolamine patch for all bariatric surgeries
- IV antibiotics 1 hour prior to skin incision – single dose

Nursing:
- Apply warming blanket
- Document carbohydrate loading
- Chlorhexidine mouthwash
- Chlorhexidine skin wipes
- Check CBG finger stick (140–180 g/dL range)

Intra-Op

Surgeon:
- TAP blocks intra-op by bupivacaine liposome or bupivacaine
- Avoid urinary catheter or remove in OR
- Avoid prophylactic drains

Anesthesia:
- H/o PONV – IV Dexamethasone
- SQ Heparin at induction
- Induction: Consider propofol / short-acting narcotics
- Near zero fluid balance (<3 ml/kg/hour)
- Avoid long-acting narcotics, hydromorphone
- Ketamine/lidocaine/dexmedetomidine infusion
- Avoid prophylactic NG tubes

Nursing:
- SCD intra-op
- Warming devices to keep >36°C

Post-Op

Surgeon:
- POD#0, Step 1 or 2 bariatric diet
- POD#1, advance step 3 as tolerated
- Acetaminophen 975 mg Q6 ATC
- Celecoxib 200mg PO BID
- Ondansetron, Metoclopramide, Prochlorperazine, prn
- Chew gum 30 minutes, BID
- POD#1 enoxaparin sodium PPX
- Order Ensure Max shakes, TID
- Nutrition consults prior to discharge
- Colace / senna to stimulate gut function
- Weight-based VTE prophylaxis

Anesthesia:
- Minimize narcotics in PACU

Nursing:
- POD#0: (No OSA) HOB elevated, O2 via nasal cannula
- POD#0 (with OSA): Pulse ox + telemetry x 24hrs / O2 / low threshold for CPAP
- Encourage OOB POD#0, all meals in chair
- Incentive Spirometry 10x/hour
- d/c IVF < 1 night / 24hrs
- Discharge planning: 20-gram protein drink & MD f/u scheduled prior to d/c

Fig. 15.4 ERAS Protocol Yale Bariatric Surgery Program

can reduce the risk of deep vein thrombosis, atelectasis, and pneumonia. **Oral intake of clear fluids shortly after surgery**, by drinking and recording 30 cc cups, educates the patient on the rate needed to avoid dehydration. After patients tolerate the first stage, they may advance to full liquids. **A multimodal pain management strategy** is used, combining analgesics such as IV or oral Tylenol, NSAIDs, muscle relaxants, neuropathic pain agents. In addition, thromboprophylaxis is initiated before surgery with 5000 units of heparin and the use of sequential compression devices to prevent venous thromboembolism. Anticoagulation is continued while the patient remains in the hospital with heparin or enoxaparin sodium. The goal is early discharge while ensuring appropriate follow-up care.

Long-Term Treatment of the Bariatric Patient

The surgeon and PA provide long-term treatment and follow-up with the bariatric patient to maintain the best patient care. Follow-up is necessary to monitor for surgical complications, support continued weight loss or weight maintenance, and reinforce the healthy lifestyle changes patients have adopted. After-care is integral to bariatric surgery, and the bariatric surgery office PA is best suited for this role. **Lifelong follow-up is required by ASMBS/ACS-certified centers for bariatric surgery**, and this task becomes arduous for surgeons without assistance. The office PA collaborates

Postoperative Follow-up
- 2 weeks
- 2 months
- 6 months, with labs
- 1 Year, with labs
- Yearly, with labs
- Follow-up for weight gain
- Monthly Support group

Fig. 15.5 Postoperative follow-up. (Credit: Neil Floch MD)

with the surgeon, alternating appointments with the patient. The PA sees patients in the office, as the surgeon may be allocating time to performing surgery in the operating room or rounding on patients in the hospital.

At a minimum, follow-up should occur within the first 1–2 weeks after surgery, again at 8 weeks, at 6 months with nutritional lab work, and then annually for life. More frequent follow-up visits are encouraged to closely monitor the patient's progress and ensure long-term success. Patients taking anti-obesity medications will need to be seen more frequently to monitor their dosage. The office-based PA is well-positioned to promote a healthy lifestyle by encouraging proper nutrition, regular exercise, daily use of bariatric vitamins, adequate hydration, and avoidance of addictive behaviors such as smoking and excessive alcohol consumption, while also remaining vigilant for the emergence of new maladaptive behaviors (Fig. 15.5).

The long-term care of the bariatric patient requires that the PA detect the signs and symptoms of complications, weight regain, and the onset of new comorbidities. The PA may be most accessible of the healthcare team to fulfill this role. The PA must report these findings to the surgeon and team and commence appropriate therapy. The PA works by **Providing Education and Support for lifestyle changes**, such as a diet including a total of 60–80 g of protein to prevent sarcopenia, supplemented with 20–30 g per 12-ounce shake. Patients must participate in daily physical activity of 30–60 min of exercise that is specific to their ability and needs to maintain weight loss and prevent weight regain. The PA may offer continuous emotional support and counseling to help patients adhere to these changes, as mental health therapists are not always available (Fig. 15.6).

Postoperative Expectations

Closely follow dietary guidelines
- Staged diet, clear fluid, puree, soft, regular
- Minimize carbohydrates, fat
- 60-70 g of protein daily

Regular exercise (30-45 min)
- Minimum of 3-4 times week

Lifelong vitamin supplementation
- MVI, Fe, Ca, D, B-12

PPI or H-2 Blocker
- 48-64 ounces of fluid

Fig. 15.6 Daily instructions for post-operative bariatric surgery patients. (Credit: Neil Floch MD)

Monitoring levels and ensuring the use of appropriate bariatric vitamins, which are specially created for patients after bariatric surgery, is imperative to avoid nutritional complications. Each type of procedure may require different types and amounts of vitamins. **Patients who undergo RNY need a daily bariatric multivitamin, which includes orally available B-12, 1500 mg of calcium citrate given in chewable form, $FeSO_4$ 325 mg a day, and vitamin D**. Patients after an **SG** may maintain stable levels with only a multivitamin, any type of calcium, and possibly vitamin B-12. Many Americans have multiple vitamin deficiencies; PAs need to monitor patients with at least yearly blood levels. They need to be able to detect and treat vitamin deficiencies (Figs. 15.7 and 15.8). Patients undergoing BPD/DS or SADI-S should take a daily ADEK vitamin supplement as they absorb less fat-soluble vitamins.

Prevalence of Micronutrient Deficiencies Following Bariatric Surgery. (Data Given as Percentages) From: Nutritional and Micronutrient Care of Bariatric Surgery Patients: Current Evidence Update

	LAGB	LSG	RYGB	BPDDS
Thiamin (B_1)	0	0	12	10–15
Folate (B_9)	10	10–20	15	15
Piridoxine (B_6)	0	0–15	0	10
Cobalamin (B_{12})	10	10–20	30–50	22
Vitamin A	10	10–20	10–50	60–70
Vitamin D (<30 ng/dL)	30	30–70	30–50	40–100
Vitamin E	0	0–5	10	10
Vitamin K	0	0	0	60–70
Iron	0–32	15–45	25–50	25
Copper	–	10	10	70
Zinc	–	7–15	20–37	25

1.(–) indicates that data not available
2.Abbreviations: LAGB laparoscopic-assisted gastric banding, LSG laparoscopic sleeve gastrectomy, RYGB Roux-en-Y gastric bypass, BPDDS biliopancreatic diversion with duodenal switch
3.All numbers are percentages
Via, M.A., Mechanick, J.I. Nutritional and Micronutrient Care of Bariatric Surgery Patients: Current Evidence Update. *Curr Obes Re*

Fig. 15.7 Prevalence of micronutrient deficiencies following bariatric surgery. (Credit in footnotes)

Yale Medicine Bariatric Surgery
Vitamin Requirements After Sleeve Gastrectomy and Gastric Bypass

		Vitamin/Nutrient	Dose	Comments
OPTION A	1	Complete Bariatric Multivitamin with Minerals	Depends on product: SEE VITAMIN LABEL usually 1-4 pills or chewables per day	Vitamins should be chewable for the first 3 months after surgery then tablets or capsules can be used if preferred
	2	Calcium citrate (preferable) or Calcium carbonate	500-1000 mg calcium from supplements for most patients (1200-1500 mg per day from food and supplements)	The amount needed from a supplement depends on how much calcium you eat every day. *Ask your RD how much additional calcium you should take

		Vitamin/Nutrient	Dose	Comments
OPTION B	1	Non-Bariatric Multivitamin with Minerals (no gummy multivitamins)	Usually 2 per day (supplying 200% of DV for most nutrients) With most over the counter multivitamins, you will need additional supplements	
	2	Additional B vitamins (B complex)	12-50 mg of Thiamin (B1) and 350-500 mcg of B12 needed per day	
	3	Additional Iron	45-60 mg of iron (or 18 mg for most men) needed per day	
	4	Additional Vitamin D	3000 IU of vitamin D needed per day	
	5	Calcium citrate (preferable) or Calcium carbonate	500-1000 mg calcium from supplements for most patients (1200-1500 mg per day from food and supplements)	*Ask your RD how much additional calcium you should take The amount needed from a supplement depends on how much calcium you eat every day.

Fig. 15.8 Yale medicine vitamin requirements after bariatric surgery

Acute Postoperative Complications and Treatment

The Diagnosis of Acute Complication

Complications after bariatric surgery are divided into early and late. **Early complications** occur immediately after surgery and are likely present while the patient is in the hospital or early after discharge. While on call, a PA in the hospital must be aware of the presenting signs and symptoms to treat patients expeditiously. The goal is to rescue patients by recognizing problems early to prevent long-term consequences and mortality.

The PA must perform postoperative checks hours after surgery and consistent daily rounds. Signs may be present immediately after surgery or develop after days. More latent problems may occur from weeks to months after surgery. Although this section covers complications specific to bariatric surgery, a seasoned PA will also be alerted to any other complication that can occur in the postoperative period such as myocardial infarction (MI), cerebrovascular accident (CVA), Stroke, pneumonia, urinary tract infections, wound infections, rhabdomyolysis, kidney failure, transfusion reactions, medication allergic reactions, drug-induced hepatitis, among many others.

Developing a **differential diagnosis** is the first step after a history and physical when assessing a patient for a complication. The presence of **tachycardia and fever** should alert a clinician to the presence of an **anastomotic leak** or **infection,** but could also represent **atelectasis, pneumonia,** or a **pulmonary embolism. Nausea and vomiting** are encountered with an early or late **small bowel obstruction but** may be a result of a stricture at an anastomotic site. **Abdominal pain** can be a **sign of leaks, internal hernias, or bowel obstruction.** It is also possible to have peritonitis in a patient with a very elevated BMI without significant abdominal pain. Dehydration usually is a result of persistent vomiting or inadequate oral intake.

There are specific findings associated with each of the major early complications.

An early **anastomotic leak** will usually present with **fever, tachycardia, abdominal pain**, and frequently sepsis, which occurs 24–48 h after surgery and is rare compared to later leaks. Most commonly, sleeve leaks occur 8-12 days after surgery and RNY leaks occur 9.5 days after surgery. **Imaging with an upper GI contrast study (UGI) or CT**

scan is typically used for diagnosis. **Small bowel obstruction** symptoms include **nausea, vomiting, abdominal distention, and pain**. Early obstruction may be technical due to internal hernias, adhesions, or strictures, and often requires immediate surgical intervention to prevent bowel ischemia. Early postoperative reoperation can usually be performed with laparoscopy.

Acute gastrointestinal or intraperitoneal bleeding can present with hypotension, tachycardia, and signs of anemia secondary to bleeding from the bowel, blood vessels, or abdominal wall port sites. **Initially, blood levels may be normal as they are a measure of concentration and may not have time to dilute in acute bleeding**. Assessment of bleeding with repeat blood levels is acceptable depending on the rate, amount, type, and location of bleeding. **Upper endoscopy or** immediate reoperation can be performed for an endoluminal gastric source. **Surgical site infections** can present with localized pain, erythema, and discharge. Wounds should be treated by opening them, draining, and starting antibiotics.

Chronic Complications

Chronic complications present after the patient is discharged from the hospital and begin to develop months to years after surgery. They are usually first discovered when patients are seen in the office. Each procedure has both common chronic complications and those unique to the procedure. Many acute complications can also be chronic such as bowel obstructions, while others are uniquely chronic such as severe GERD and gastric ulcers. **Late complications** include anastomotic strictures or marginal ulcers. **Persistent vomiting and food intolerance** may indicate a more chronic obstruction, anastomotic ulcer, stricture, biliary disease, or severe reflux. The procedures are listed and their complications which may be acute, chronic, or could present at any time. There remain some complications common to all MBS procedures.

Complications Common to All Procedures

Deep Venous Thrombosis and Pulmonary Embolism

Common to all bariatric surgeries is the risk of deep venous thrombosis (DVT) and pulmonary embolism (PE), which may be confused with other respiratory complications, including atelectasis, pneumonia, and respiratory failure. PE can present with dyspnea, tachycardia, chest pain, hypoxia, hemoptysis, or syncope. There can be clinical findings of tachypnea, hypotension, jugular venous distention (JVD), and signs of DVT, such as swelling, pain, and redness in the lower extremities. Spiral CT scan is the diagnostic procedure of choice, which often reveals a pulmonary embolus, the most worrisome being a saddle embolism. Alternatively, a positive Doppler of the extremities reveals a high suspicion, and a V/Q scan can determine the likelihood of a PE without using IV contrast. Transthoracic echocardiography may show right ventricular (RV) dysfunction or paradoxical septal motion, indicating strain on the right side of the heart. An elevated D-dimer supports the diagnosis, but is not specific, and an arterial blood gas (ABG) may show hypoxemia and respiratory alkalosis.

Treatment for DVT and PE after bariatric surgery involves a combination of anticoagulation, mechanical interventions, and, rarely, surgical procedures in the presence of hypoxia and right heart strain. The risk of treatment must be weighed against the possibility of postoperative bleeding. Initial treatment for DVT, PE, or PVT typically begins with anticoagulation using low-molecular-weight heparin (LMWH) or unfractionated heparin, followed by a transition to a direct oral anticoagulant (DOAC), such as apixaban or rivaroxaban, for a minimum duration of 3 months post-event. After a massive PE with hemodynamic instability, systemic thrombolysis is usually administered. Inferior vena cava (IVC) Filters are used for patients with contraindications to anticoagulation or recurrent VTE despite adequate anticoagulation.

Portomesenteric Vein Thrombosis

Portal vein thrombosis (PVT) after bariatric surgery is rare but can be fatal. It has an incidence of 0.4% in SG. PVT typically presents within the first month postoperatively, with symptoms of **tachycardia, abdominal pain, fever, nausea, and vomiting**. It occurs most commonly after laparoscopic SG but can also occur after any bariatric procedure. Risk factors include severe obesity, hypercoagulability, history of DVT, liver disease, smoking, use of oral contraceptives, T2 DM, and intraoperative technical manipulation of the splanchnic vasculature. Proposed causes include ligation of the short gastric vessels and local inflammation during surgery. Patients may present with an elevated white blood cell (WBC) count. Diagnosis can be made incidentally during evaluation for other symptoms or intentionally through imaging, typically with a CT scan using IV contrast. A CT scan of the abdomen and pelvis with IV contrast most commonly demonstrates a clot in the portal vein, followed by the superior mesenteric and the splenic veins. Alternatively, a duplex ultrasound can be diagnostic.

Treatment starts with **IV anticoagulation and hydration**. In severe cases, **thrombolysis and thrombectomy** for occlusive PVT or high-grade nonocclusive PVT, thrombolytic therapy (e.g., tissue plasminogen activator (TPA)), and surgical thrombectomy may be necessary to restore portal vein patency. In select severe cases, transjugular intrahepatic portosystemic shunt (TIPS), can also be performed. Surgery is only indicated for high suspicion of bowel ischemia or necrosis. Most patients respond well to nonoperative management. Most clinicians treat with anticoagulation for 3–6 months despite limited conclusive evidence to support the treatment. Management of acute thromboembolic disease often requires collaboration between surgery, interventional radiology, critical care, pulmonary, and hematology to optimize outcomes.

Gallbladder Disease After Bariatric Surgery

The incidence of symptomatic gallstone disease post-bariatric surgery is approximately 14.5% after RNY, 4.4% after SG, and 4.1% after AGB. Rapid weight loss leads to increased cholesterol saturation in bile and gallbladder stasis. Ursodeoxycholic acid (UDCA) reduces gallstone formation prophylactically, as shown at 6 months from 22% in the placebo group to 6.5% in the treated group, but many patients fail to adhere to taking the drug [2]. **The ASMBS recommends considering prophylactic cholecystectomy in patients with known gallstones undergoing RNY to prevent the need for an ERCP postoperatively, which entails an operation to access the remnant stomach and place the endoscope** [3].

Complications Unique to Each Procedure

Each procedure has a unique set of acute and chronic complications, and the PA must be aware of and ask appropriate questions, examine patients, and perform the timely tests to detect them. Understanding the specific incidence of procedure-related complications enables the PA to better recognize relevant signs and symptoms, facilitating the development of an accurate differential diagnosis that appropriately considers likely issues. This allows for prompt ordering of t he most appropriate diagnostic test, minimizing delays in treatment.

Sleeve Gastrectomy

SG has fewer complications than other procedures, but gastric leak is the most concerning with an incidence of 0.5%. It is categorized as acute, up to 7 days, early up to 6 weeks, late from 6 to 12 weeks, and chronic extends beyond 12 weeks. Most proximal leaks occur in the acute or early period. Technical staple line leaks present immediately after surgery, while ischemic leaks, stricture, or torsion leaks occur 5–7 days postoperatively. Staple line misfiring can occur anywhere along the staple line and is uncommon, and usually noticed at the time of the event; therefore, the staple line can be oversewn and repaired. Staple line leaks can also occur from using a bougie that is too small or a staple line that is too close to a bougie. Distal leaks usually occur from technical failure, including twisting, torsion, and obstruction, or rarely, a misfire that is not detected.

Of all leaks, **80% are found on the proximal third of the staple line**, most commonly near the esophagogastric junction. Suggested reasons include potential devascularization in the area from dissection, variable perfusion in the fundus, and variable tissue thickness. Leakage can occur in the presence of ischemia, staple line hematomas, staple malfunction, and increased pressure. The combination of a long staple line of an SG, narrow tube, closed pylorus, and lower esophageal sphincter creates an increased pressure system prone to a higher leak rate than RNY, where the anastomosis is open and has limited outlet pressure. **Narrowing is most common at the "elbow" of the sleeve or incisura, where the tube turns, and there is the highest likelihood of intermittent obstruction.** The leak rates are higher for RNY, 2.4% versus SG, 0.7%.

Detection of a leak depends on clinical evaluation. Vital signs are usually the first indication of an abnormality, with tachycardia over 120 bpm being most sensitive. Patients may have epigastric pain, left shoulder pain, and fever. Laboratory tests may reveal an elevated white count (WBC) or C-reactive protein (CRP). A CT scan with oral and IV contrast is preferred to diagnose. It can identify the area of leak, fluid collections, fat stranding, and pleural effusions. A UGI study may also detect a leak, but a CT scan has higher sensitivity. The accuracy increases to 84% when both tests are used together. If there is strong clinical suspicion, exploratory laparoscopy should be performed, as 33% of patients with leaks have a false CT scan and UGI.

Management of Leaks

Management is determined by the timing of the leak, acute, or chronic. The goal is fluid resuscitation and stopping ongoing contamination. Patients should be nothing per os (NPO), but TPN should be started to establish optimal nutrition to stave off sepsis and optimize healing. Infection is treated with broad-spectrum antibiotics targeting anaerobic bacteria, along with antifungal agents to address the stomach's commensal fungi. Non-operative management is appropriate if patients do not have peritonitis and are hemodynamically stable with a small, contained leak. The least invasive technique is percutaneous drainage, which is performed by interventional radiology. Patients should be monitored with vital signs, WBC, and CRP. If their condition deteriorates or abdominal pain intensifies, surgical intervention may be necessary.

Early GI Leaks

Endoluminal stents can close a leak and protect the staple line, allowing patients to eat and obtain adequate nutrition to heal. If a leak presents in combination with a distal stenosis, the stent will also keep the stenosis open. Stents may remain in place for 3 months. Successful treatment of acute leaks with stents is greater than 90%. The most frequent complication is stent migration, warranting suture fixation, repositioning, or replacement of the stent. When leaks are large, uncontrolled, or patients are unstable, surgery is indicated for drainage. Definitive repair can be performed within the first 3 days. Inflamed, infected, friable tissues are less likely to heal, so they should be debrided back to viable tissue and covered with omentum. A classic omental patch alone is unlikely to succeed in a high-pressure system. A feeding jejunostomy should be considered for nutrition at the time of surgery.

Chronic Fistula

A chronically draining leak is less likely to close spontaneously and may warrant a multidisciplinary team of surgeon, radiologist, and gastroenterologist. Options include radiologic placement of drains, endoscopic placement of internal, and double pigtail catheters placed by EGD through the staple line defect. Although technically difficult, endoscopic placement of a vacuum sponge attached to an NG tube at the site of the fistulous tract has been successful in 80–100% of studies. Other endoscopic options include the placement of wide clips or fibrin glue.

Surgical intervention can be technically difficult and should be performed as a last resort. Surgical options include conversion of the SG to an RNY, preferably above the leak, with laparoscopic proximal gastrectomy and RNY esophagojejunostomy. Another unique technique invoves suturing a Roux limb directly to the fistulous tract, which has been proposed by van de Vrande et al., with a 100% success rate and 54% with immediate resolution.

Bleeding from SG in the Acute or Early Post-operative Phase

Bleeding occurs in 0.6–1.9% of patients after SG and is either intraluminal (IL) or extraluminal (EL). IL bleeding occurs most commonly from the staple line, whereas EL bleeding occurs not only from short gastric vessels but also from the spleen, surrounding tissues or a trocar site. The distinction is usually obvious from clinical characteristics. Contributing factors include age, HTN, history of a cardiac procedure, anticoagulation use, T2 DM, and renal disease.

Vital signs may detect bleeding, which may present with tachycardia, hypotension, oliguria, and an eventual decrease in hemoglobin and hematocrit. A hemoglobin taken immediately after clinical bleeding should NOT be reassuring because it may be normal. It takes time for the patient to equilibrate after a bleeding episode. Other clinical findings include hematemesis or melanotic stool with intraluminal bleeding. A patient may be tender on abdominal exam as blood is an irritant. A CT scan with IV contrast can be performed in a hemodynamically stable patient to detect active bleeding or a hematoma.

Management of Bleeding

The patient should be monitored closely for **hemodynamic instability**. **They should be aggressively fluid resuscitated, and anticoagulation should be stopped. Conservative management of gastric sleeve patients is successful in 47–77% but this may require a transfusion. Over 80% of acute postoperative bleeding resolves without the need for transfusion, procedural intervention, or operation**. EL bleeding rarely requires reoperation unless a patient becomes unstable. IL bleeding can result in hemodynamic instability more rapidly, as clotting from compression is less likely. If IL bleeding fails conservative treatment, *EGD should be performed acutely using thermal energy, injections, or hemostatic clips to achieve hemostasis*. With hemodynamic instability, *if EGD fails, or there is a need for multiple transfusions, laparoscopy should be performed with oversewing of the staple lines, oversewing of short gastric vessels, control of a splenic bleed, and possible splenectomy, or control of* ***trocar port site*** *bleeding*.

Stenosis or Technical Obstruction

Functional stenosis is common and transient, and usually spontaneously resolves as it occurs from edema or hematomas at the staple line. Technical problems, such as a stenosis or twist, are more involved and the cause of proximal stenosis in 0.6–4% of patients. Although the lumen may or may not be significantly narrow, angulation at the incisura can result in clinical symptoms in the patient. Stenosis may lead to a leak from increased pressure. Although usually hospitalized, patients develop symptoms of poor oral intake and tolerance of fluids, vomiting, reflux, and regurgitation. Mucus production can be white and frothy. A UGI is usually diagnostic, but EGD may further characterize a stenosis or twisting at the incisura.

Conservative Treatment

Functional obstructions are treated with IV fluids to resolve dehydration and correct electrolyte abnormalities. Patients should remain NPO on anti-emetics as they wait for edema to resolve. Patients may also benefit from limited IV steroids such as dexamethasone, starting at 4 or 10 mg as a one-time dosage, as they may limit wound healing. More prolonged technical obstruction can be treated with a fluoroscopy-guided nasogastric (NG) tube to avoid perforation of a new staple line. More prolonged obstruction may require nasogastric feeding or total parental nutrition (TPN).

Endoscopic treatment involving a multicenter study revealed that balloon dilatation succeeds 76% of the time with an average of 1.8 attempts. Patients who fail may undergo metal stent placement, which succeeds 70–88% of the time. Surgical treatment can be performed early with the removal of imbricating sutures by laparoscopy. Gastric sero-myotomy for a stenotic segment was recommended in the past with 35% success, but there was a high leak rate. A full-thickness Heineke–Mikulicz type strictureplasty can be performed. The results of other options do not compare to conversion to an RNY, which has a 91% success rate.

Roux-en-Y Gastric Bypass

Gastrointestinal Leak After RNY

Leaks after RNY have declined from 1% in 2007 to less than 0.5% of cases in 2023. (Howard R, FinksJB, Petersen S, et al. Contemporary Trends in the Incidence, Risk Factors, and Managment of Postoperative Leak After Sleeve Gastrectomy and Gastric Bypass From 2007-2023. SOARD. 2026.) The most common locations are at the gastrojejunostomy, 67%, the gastric pouch staple line, the gastric remnant staple line, and then the jejuno-jejunostomy anastomosis. Technical factors include tension on the anastomosis, active bleeding in the stable line, and tissue ischemia. Increased patient risk factors include a history of smoking, poor nutrition, or increased comorbidities. Staple line reinforcement and tissue sealants have not been effective in reducing leaks in many studies. **Routine intraoperative leak tests are performed in 82% of cases in the United States and have not demonstrated a decrease in leaks but finding a positive leak during surgery presents the opportunity to close the leak and prevent a postoperative complication.**

Management of an RNY Leak

Management of leaks after RNY varies according to the patient's presentation, location of the leak, pouch, remnant, or anastomosis, and extent of the contamination. **Initial management includes NPO, IV resuscitation, and broad-spectrum antibiotics. UGI contrast studies and CT scans are usually diagnostic.** Non-operative management is reserved for patients with small, contained leaks. Radiologic drainage of fluid collections may control a leak and provide time for healing if adequate nutrition can be established, but usually a higher level of treatment is necessary.

Endoscopic Management

A fully covered stent can be placed across the gastroduodenal defect, performed with or without surgical intervention. They are usually poorly tolerated by patients. Stent placement may need to be performed under general anesthesia with fluoroscopy. Stents can be kept for up to 3 months, enabling oral feeding. The success rate is 95% in RNY patients. The most frequent complications include stent migration; therefore, fixation, repositioning, or replacement may be necessary.

Operative Management

Emergent surgery is recommended for clinical evidence of peritonitis, large uncontained fluid collections, hemodynamic instability, or failure of nonoperative management. During open surgery, or laparoscopy, aggressive irrigation and wide drainage should be performed to control contamination from a leak. Surgical access to provide nutrition by placing a feeding tube in the gastric remnant, after RNY for proximal leaks or a distal feeding jejunostomy for a distal leak should be performed.

Primary suture closure can be performed in the first 72 h if debridement to viable, non-friable tissue can be achieved. An omental patch may be used if there is no tension and succeeds more commonly in an RNY patient compared to an SG, where there is tension.

For complex cases that fail to heal, a T-tube may be placed in the defect exterior or into a bag. The tube can be placed for 4–6 weeks, and then slowly withdrawn to create a controlled fistula, eventually collapsing the tunnel as the tube is withdrawn. Revision of the anastomosis is rarely done in the acute setting. Downstream obstructions should be corrected as they may cause the leak to persist. Causes may include obstruction at the transverse mesocolon, the jejunum, adhesions, hernias, and closure of the mesentery. A G-tube can be placed in the excluded stomach to provide nutrition.

Bleeding After RNY

Postoperative bleeding after RNY occurs in up to 4% of patients. It can be IL or EL. IL can occur from the proximal anastomosis, jejuno-jejunostomy, or the remnant stomach. EL bleeding can occur anywhere in the abdomen, including the mesenteric hernia defect closures, staple lines, or from port sites. Late bleeding is usually secondary to an anastomotic ulcer or, rarely, a gastric remnant or duodenal ulcer. Bleeding is assessed and managed in the same manner as after an SG. Upper endoscopy is the diagnostic and treatment modality of choice. **Hemostatic clips are preferred to be used instead of cautery when involving the small bowel. There is a 70–80% success rate in controlling bleeding in the gastrojejunostomy or pouch using EGD.** An excluded stomach after RNY can be examined and bleeding managed by double balloon enteroscopy or laparoscopy-assisted transgastric endoscopy.

Bowel Obstruction

Bowel obstruction can occur in as many as 15% of patients after RNY. Presentation, diagnosis, and management are dependent on the type of obstruction. **Causes may be internal herniation, gastrojejunostomy stricture, adhesions, incisional hernias, and intussusception. Dry heaving and retching are early clinical signs that warrant a CT scan.** Non-operative management may be considered in select cases involving the proximal roux-limb, that do not involve a closed-loop, obstructions secondary to blood in the postoperative period, or food that could eventually pass. In most cases, bowel obstruction is a surgical emergency as internal herniation can rapidly result in bowel ischemia.

Internal Hernia

Internal hernias account for up to 59% of all bowel obstructions after RNY. An internal hernia can occur at any time but is at an increased incidence 1–2 years after surgery when the mesenteric fat has decreased, and a defect can develop. Patients may present differently depending on the technique of RNY performed. Patients with an anti-colic anastomosis can develop a jejunojejunostomy hernia and a Peterson's hernia, the space between the Roux limb and the transverse mesocolon.

Patients who undergo a retro-colic RNY have an additional space in the mesocolon, a defect in the transverse mesocolon where the Roux limb passes into the lesser sac.

Patients with a history of RNY who present with nausea and vomiting with or without abdominal pain must be ruled out for an internal hernia. A volvulus, incarceration, or compression can result in bowel ischemia with more significant abdominal pain that is out of proportion to physical exam. A CT scan with IV contrast is the best imaging modality and may reveal the classic finding of **"swirling of the mesentery."** There may be more subtle changes, such as haziness of the mesentery or mesenteric vessels that pass behind the superior mesenteric artery, the jejuno-jejunostomy may be on the right side of the abdomen instead of the left. **Localization of the majority of the small bowel to a single abdominal quadrant may also indicate an internal hernia.** CT scan findings may be helpful but are not sensitive or specific and should not be relied upon as they may be difficult to interpret.

Treatment of Internal Hernias

If there is a high clinical suspicion, exploratory laparoscopy should be performed to rule it out. To clearly define and reduce the hernia, exploration starts at the cecum as the bowel runs from distal to proximal. Surgeons will feel a release of pressure when the hernia reduces, and the bowel may not be seen protruding through the defect. The presence of bruising in the mesentery, around the hernia defect created by pressure will confirm the diagnosis.

Mesenteric defects should be closed with non-absorbable material. The defect should be closed from the base of the mesentery to the bowel (Fig. 15.9). The distal anastomosis mesentery is best exposed by sweeping the proximal Roux limb to the right side. To visualize Peterson's defect, the Roux limb may be swept to the left, and the transverse mesocolon is retracted toward the head as the root of the mesentery is identified. Peterson's defect is open if one could see the proximal jejunum at the ligament of Treitz (Fig. 15.10). In patients with a retro-colic RNY, the mesenteric defect is also an area of possible herniation and obstruction. This defect should be closed with a non-absorbable suture, leaving only enough room to allow passage of this portion of the small bowel. During all these procedures, injection of ICG green is an option to identify ischemic bowel, which may warrant resection. Alternatively, a planned second-look operation within 48 h is required to determine bowel viability.

Although the consensus is to close all internal herniation spaces at the time of initial surgery, this recommendation is controversial because of the argument that defects can open despite closure with permanent material. A multi-center, randomized study of over 1200 patients showed that at 3 years, there was a higher risk of internal herniation in the group where the defect was left open, 9% versus the closure group 2%, but the closure group had a higher incidence of severe postoperative complications 4% versus 3%.

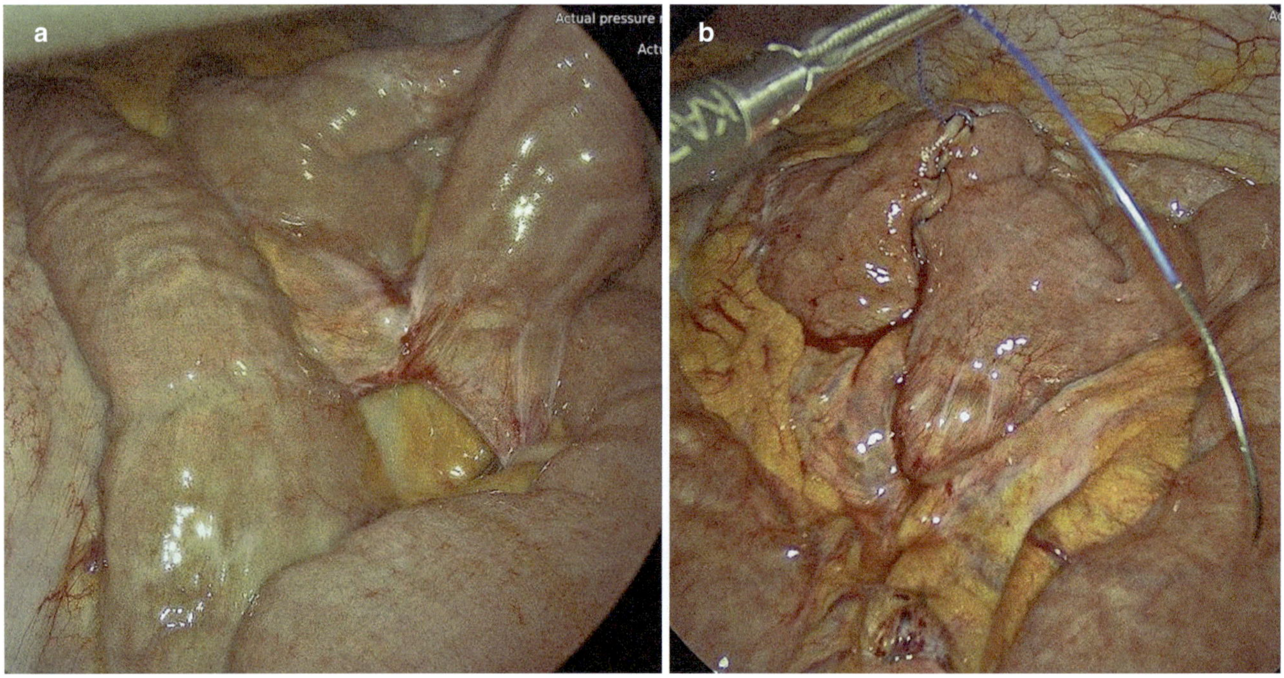

Fig. 15.9 (**a**) Jejuno-jejunostomy defect with potential hernia space. (**b**) Jejuno-jejunostomy defect closure. (Credit: Unidentified patient with permission)

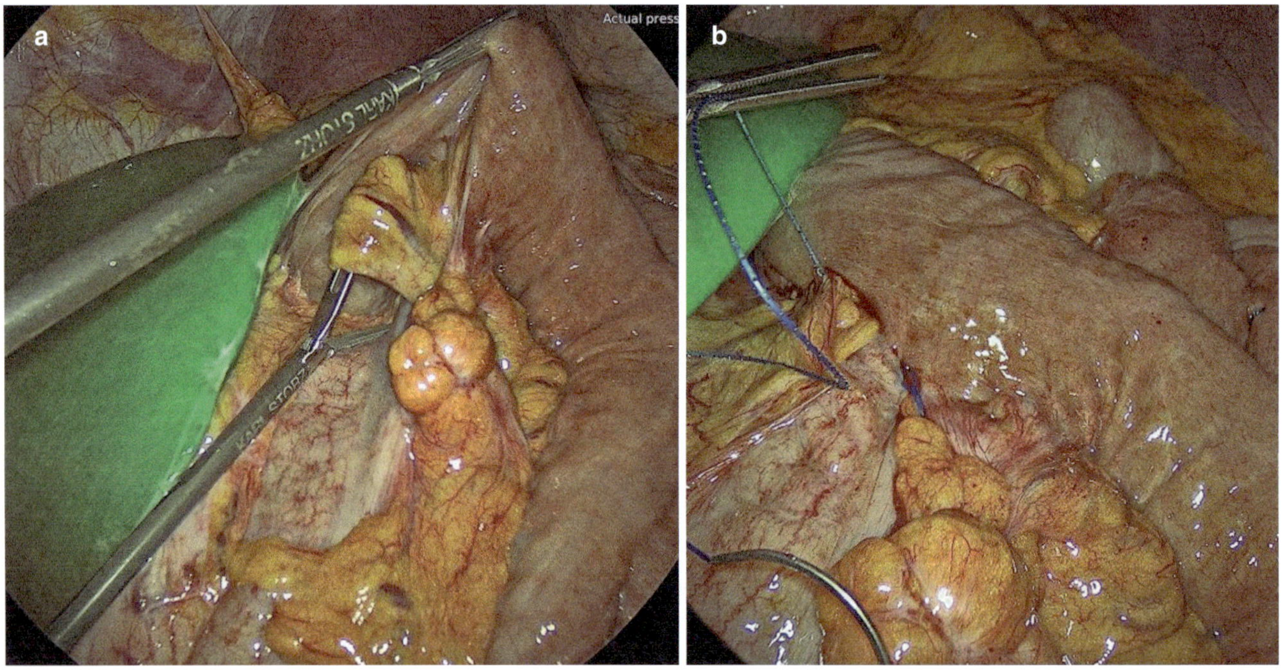

Fig. 15.10 (**a**) Peterson's defect. (**b**). Peterson's defect closure. (Credit: Unidentified patient with permission)

Gastrojejunal Anastomotic Stricture

Approximately 3–6% of patients after RNY require treatment for an anastomotic stricture. Patients present with difficulty eating solids that progress to liquid intolerance. Anastomoses with circular staplers have a higher risk compared to linear stapling or hand sewing. Larger circular staplers of 25 vs. 21 mm and smaller stapler heights are associated with lower structure rates. Strictures may also occur secondary to ischemia or marginal ulcers. At least 6 weeks after surgery, if a 10-mm endoscope cannot pass through an anastomosis, dilation is performed with the 12- to

15-mm-diameter balloon or a bougie dilator. Perforation occurs in less than 2% of patients. A single dilatation may be effective, but more may be needed.

Adhesive Small Bowel Obstruction

RNY is no different than any other abdominal surgery, where adhesions can lead to a bowel obstruction at any time. A CT scan with IV contrast is the standard for diagnosis. Patients may be treated like any other small bowel obstruction with bowel rest and IV fluids. The only exceptions are the obstruction of the biliopancreatic limb, which is a surgical emergency, and a surgeon with bariatric experience should evaluate and likely operate as an emergency. Nasogastric tube (NGT) placement should not be performed unless by radiology or by a bariatric surgeon, as the tube can perforate the small bowel at the gastrojejunal anastomosis site.

Intussusception, hemobezoar, and incisional hernias are rare causes of bowel obstruction after **RNY**. A double lumen diameter anastomosis is created at the jejuno-jejunostomy site, which is amenable to intussusception. **A CT scan may demonstrate a "target sign" where the bowel invaginates within its lumen, which is pathognomonic** (Fig. 15.11). Many intussusceptions are transient and can be found incidentally in an asymptomatic patient by CT scan. If the intussusception is long, persistent, and clinical symptoms are evident, then operative reduction to anchor, resect, or revise the anastomosis may be performed (Fig. 15.12). There is no evidence to suggest one revision operation has a benefit over another, but resection is necessary in the presence of necrotic bowel.

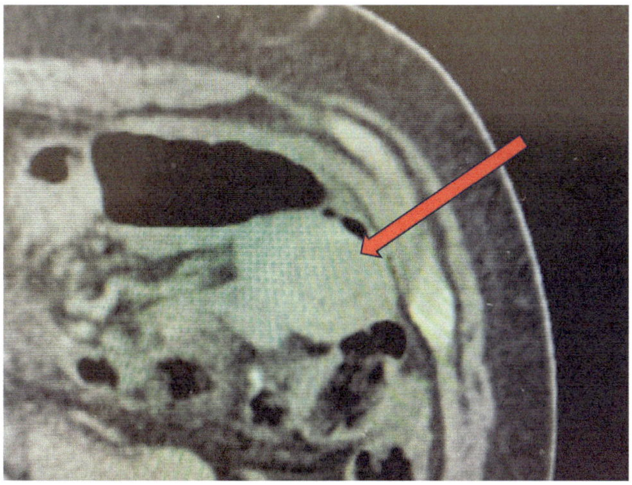

Fig. 15.11 "Target sign" found in intussusception. A black ring is seen within the dilated bowel. (Credit: Unidentified patient)

Patients may bleed at the proximal or distal anastomosis, which leads to a bowel obstruction from complete luminal obstruction by a blood clot, **hemobezoar**. A blood clot usually develops immediately postoperatively and accumulates at the distal anastomosis but can occur at the proximal gastrojejunostomy. Most resolve with hydration and waiting 48–72 h. Endoscopic intervention clearance of a proximal clot is possible, but the distal anastomosis is less amenable. Rarely is surgery indicated to clear the clot.

Incisional hernias after laparoscopic MBS require reoperation, reduction, and closure of the hernia. Closure of large port sites can decrease the incidence of internal herniation but will not eliminate the risk. At the time of initial surgery, patients may also have umbilical, ventral, inguinal, and incisional hernias, which can cause a post-operative obstruction if not closed at the time of **RNY**.

Marginal ulcers occur in 5%, most commonly presenting within the first 2 years after RNY. They are located near the gastrojejunostomy, more commonly on the jejunal side. The cause is unclear, but ischemia is suspected along with increased acid exposure and mucosal disruption. Risk factors include smoking, NSAID use, steroid use, increased pouch size, and the presence of a gastrogastric fistula. It is unclear how *H. pylori* colonization influences ulcer occurrence, but most programs attempt to detect and treat this bacterium. Circular staplers are more commonly associated with marginal ulcers than linear staplers. Prophylactic PPI use can prevent marginal ulcers, but the duration of treatment is unclear. Most programs continue PPI treatment for 1–3 months postoperatively. The risks and benefits of long-term PPI use should be weighed. Alternatively, H2 blockers may be used. Patients with marginal ulcers present with epigastric burning, nausea, and vomiting, but may also be asymptomatic. Patients may have bleeding or perforation as the initial presentation. EGD is diagnostic. Ulcers rarely occur immediately post-surgery. **A CT scan with oral contrast can detect a marginal ulcer with perforation or the presence of a gastrogastric fistula.**

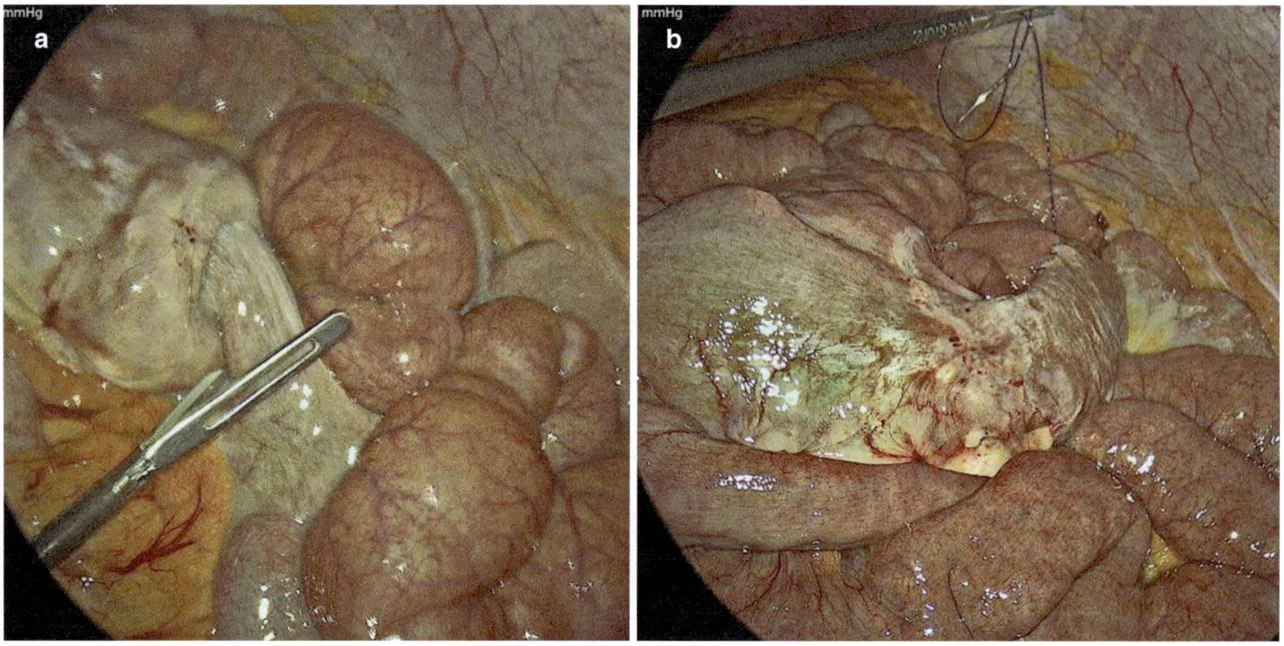

Fig. 15.12 (**a**). Intussusception of the common channel of a gastric bypass into the common channel-biliopancreatic anastomosis. (**b**). Repair of intussusception by suturing the proximal biliopancreatic limb to the distal common channel limb. (Credit: Unidentified patient with permission)

Management of Ulcers

Treatment begins with eliminating the risk factors such as smoking, NSAIDs, and steroids, and implementing IV PPI to oral, and oral sucralfate. Patients are reevaluated 2–3 months after EGD. Most patients heal with lifestyle modification alone after a year, but some fail or develop a recurrence. Surgery is limited to medical failure and involves a gastrointestinal revision by removing the previous anastomosis, making a smaller stomach, and creating a new anastomosis. Permanent sutures are avoided. A vagotomy may also be performed. The new pouch should be 20–25 cc, limiting acid-producing cells. Patients with multiple recurrences may need an RNY reversal.

Perforation is a surgical emergency and occurs in 1% of patients after gastric bypass surgery and marginal ulcers rarely perforate. Patients present without a warning sign, and 33% have no known risk factors. The goal of treatment is to control contamination with irrigation, wide drainage, and primary closure, or a Graham patch. Surgery is most effective within the first 48 h, as a delay results in suturing inflamed tissue and may have poor results. A gastrostomy tube may be placed in the remnant for oral feeding. Patients should be treated with lifestyle modification and PPI therapy afterward and possibly indefinitely.

The presence of a gastrogastric fistula can cause increased acid and marginal ulceration. This condition occurred more commonly with older staplers that stapled but did not divide the stomach. Endoscopic closure of fistulas can be performed, but recurrence rates are high. Definitive treatment is re-stapling and dividing the stomach and removing a portion of the remnant stomach. Morbidity after these procedures is high. Patients who develop bleeding from marginal ulcers should be treated by medical, endoscopic, and surgical management based on presentation as described in the section on bleeding.

Dumping syndrome occurs in 10–20% of patients after RNY, characterized by rapid emptying of hyperosmolar foods, such as sugar and carbohydrates, from the stomach into the small intestine, causing fluid shifts, cramping, and increased transit. Early dumping syndrome occurs 10–30 min after eating. The gut hormones released contribute to symptoms of tachycardia, palpitations, diaphoresis, flushing, diarrhea, nausea, and vomiting. Late dumping syndrome occurs 1–3 h after a meal, causing an exaggerated insulin response as glucose is absorbed rapidly, and patients become **hypoglycemic**. Symptoms include sweating, tremor, tachycardia, increased hunger, impaired cognition, and in severe cases, loss of consciousness and seizures. Patients are instructed to eat more frequent, smaller meals and avoid simple carbohydrates, but eat more fiber and protein. Non-responders may be prescribed **acarbose and somatostatin analogues**.

Hypoglycemia is most common after RNY, typically occurs 1–3 h after a meal high in carbohydrates. The rapid glucose absorption results in excessive postprandial secretion of **GLP-1** and other gastrointestinal peptides, resulting in overstimulation of insulin release and subsequent hypoglycemia. Symptoms range from mild: sweating, tremor, tachycardia, and increased hunger to severe: impaired cognition, loss of consciousness, and seizures. It typically presents more than 1 year after surgery. Diagnosis involves a history, records of food intake, physical activity, symptom patterns, and exclusion of other causes of hypoglycemia. Patients are guided to reduce intake of simple carbohydrates and increase protein and healthy fats. Continuous glucose monitoring may be necessary. **Acarbose, diazoxide, and GLP-1 agonists can be used for treatment.**

Endoscopic balloon dilation is the first-line treatment for RNY stenosis or strictures. Through-the-scope balloon dilators with gradual dilation over multiple sessions are performed to minimize the risk of perforation. For strictures refractory to balloon dilation, lumen-apposing metal stents (LAMS) can be used and are usually successful, although there is a risk of stent migration. LAMS can be considered early in patients requiring multiple balloon dilations. In cases where endoscopic dilation fails, laparoscopic revision of the gastrojejunostomy may be performed.

Duodenal Switch

The same complications that can occur after **RNY** and **SG** can occur after BDS, BDS/DS, and SADI-S, and are handled similarly. The **DS** is less likely to have marginal ulcers or strictures, and there is a mesenteric defect at the location of the duodenal ileostomy that must also be closed. Leakage, bleeding, bowel obstruction, and blood clots are treated like an SG and an RNY. Patients who have undergone a BDS/DS may have additional gastrointestinal symptoms when compared to other MBS surgeries. These potential issues are communicated to patients during preoperative education. Depending on the length of the common channel to the total alimentary limb, patients may have two to five bowel movements daily, which may be associated with a distinct odor. Most GI problems can be managed with dietary modification. The procedure should not be offered to patients with pre-existing bowel problems such as irritable bowel syndrome (IBS) or a prior bowel resection.

Small intestinal bacterial overgrowth, SIBO, can occur after MBS and is characterized by an excessive growth of bacteria in the small intestine due to changes in gut anatomy and motility. The prevalence of **SIBO after DS is up to 40%, with RNY ranging from 29% to 53%**, and OAGB, 37% at 6 months post-surgery. Symptoms include abdominal pain, diarrhea, bloating, nausea, and vomiting. Definitive diagnosis is made using glucose or lactulose breath tests, which measure hydrogen and methane production by bacteria in the small intestine. **Practically, many patients may be treated empirically based on a high suspicion.** Management of SIBO after BPD/DS involves antibiotic therapy, including ciprofloxacin, piperacillin-clavulanate, and metronidazole, but **the preferred antibiotic is rifaximin**. For antibiotic-resistant cases, probiotics can be given.

Nutritional deficiencies are a long-term concern with BPD/DS, as patients may develop calcium and iron deficiency. Iron deficiency can occur in up to 50% of patients and may require iron infusion. Vitamin B deficiency is more common than in RNY or a BPD because an SG is performed as part of a BPD/DS. Absorption of fat-soluble ADE and K vitamins in the terminal ileum is decreased after a BPD, BPD/DS, and SADI-S. Patients must be properly monitored for these deficiencies. If patients are lost to follow-up or do not take vitamins, they may develop osteoporosis or secondary hyperparathyroidism.

The most problematic long-term nutritional complication is protein malnutrition. Hypoalbuminemia after BDS varies from 7% to 20% because of the length of the common channel. Patients may require revisional surgery to lengthen the common channel, 4% of patients in the studies by Hess. **Limb lengthening** can be performed laparoscopically by dividing the alimentary limb proximal to the distal anastomosis and moving it more proximally to the biliopancreatic limb. There are no good studies to guide how much additional length of small bowel is appropriate.

Adjustable Gastric Banding

AGB are placed infrequently but many bands remain in place, needing maintenance in the office. Approximately 39% of patients may require multiple or excessive band adjustments. Others need removal when symptoms develop. Adjustable bands have been fraught with the need for reoperations for complications in 20–40% of patients. Interoperative **perforation of the esophagus or stomach** can occur during placement of the band. The pars flaccida technique involves a blind passage of a grasper behind the esophago-gastric junction that could travel through the stomach. Upper abdominal pain, shoulder pain, fever, tachycardia, and low oxygen saturation are all warning signs, and a CT scan or an upper GI contrast study (UGI) can detect this complication. **The most common problem is GERD,** which occurs in approximately 15% with 22.9% developing esophagitis secondary to an overinflated device, causing chronic obstruction. In the most severe cases patients can develop chronic obstruction, esophageal dysmotility, pulmonary aspiration, and pneumonia. Symptoms may resolve after deflating the band. A UGI is an initial study to detect multiple complications. First the port should be emptied of all fluid. Only after confirming a properly located band and a normal appearing esophagus, can the fluid be replaced slowly over weeks.

Adjustable Gastric Band Prolapse or Slippage

Gastric prolapse or slippage of the AGB occurs when the stomach below the band migrates through it, leaving excess stomach above the band. It may be a surgical emergency. The initial incidence was 24%, which led to fixation of the band to the stomach by creating a tunnel with three gastrogastric sutures, which reduced the incidence to 5%. Patients present with nausea, vomiting, dysphagia, and upper abdominal pain. Patients with systemic signs of tachycardia, fever, severe pain, or elevated white blood cells may have ischemia of the stomach, warranting emergent laparoscopy. Diagnosis is made by history and UGI demonstrating rotation of the band horizontally and the presence of a herniated stomach anteriorly. An upright abdominal X-ray can show a change in angulation of the band.

In a posterior prolapse, the stomach appears inferior and posterior to the band on imaging, with a vertical orientation. Posterior slippage occurs more commonly than anterior 82.4% vs 17.6% of the time. Management begins with deflating or removing fluid from the band, IV hydration, and correction of electrolytes. The band may be repositioned if it is not inflamed but with significant swelling or some ischemia. In the past, the band was either opened and left in place or removed. If necrotic stomach is present, there should be a resection.

Gastric dilatation is a more chronic problem occurring in 4–8% of patients, where the stomach slowly migrates or stretches above the band. In this situation, the band may be revised to a higher location on the stomach. With the advent of SG, many patients are encouraged to have their band removed and undergo either an SG or RNY later, as these procedures have metabolic benefits for disease treatment.

Adjustable Gastric Band Erosion

Band erosion occurs in 1–4% of patients. Potential but unproven causes may be suturing of the gastric tissue over the band buckle, micro-perforations, or a tight band. Any foreign body can erode into the bowel over time. The pars flaccida technique, where the band is wrapped around the fat on the lesser curvature, has reduced the incidence of band erosions compared to the peri-gastric technique, where the band was placed in a space created adjacent to the lesser curve of the stomach.

Erosions can present as a surgical emergency but usually are chronic and asymptomatic until signs of early satiety and nausea develop. Patients may notice erythema and pain around their port. A delayed port infection is a sign that the band eroded into the stomach and the infection has traveled along the tubing to the port. There may or may not be erosion through the tubing, which leads to detection of yellow ascitic fluid in the port or a loss of most fluid from the port. Rarely, epigastric pain and bloody vomit may indicate erosion of the band into the left gastric artery. EGD is diagnostic of an erosion. Once diagnosed, the band should be removed, which can be performed laparoscopically with suture repair of the gastric wall and drainage. In greater than 50% of patients, the buckle is eroded. Techniques have been suggested to remove a portion of the band endoscopically, after which the port and tubing are removed surgically; therefore, laparoscopic removal is recommended.

Port Complications

Port complications occur in 5–11% of patients when the tubing cracks or breaks, the port becomes detached, or flips. Tube integrity is tested by injecting contrast into the port under fluoroscopy to determine the location of a system leak. If present, replacement of the band, tubing, or port is necessary in up to 30% of patients at 10 years.

Risk of Mortality from Bariatric Surgery

A 2011 analysis by Hutter et al. compared multiple bariatric surgeries according to the Metabolic and Bariatric Surgery Accreditation and Quality Improvement Program (MBSAQIP) database. The mortality risk within 1 month for bariatric surgeries was 0.14% for **RNY**, 0.11% for **SG**, and 0.05% for **AGB**. Recently, a meta-analysis of over 3.6 million patients, including those after DS, had a 1-month mortality risk of 0.41% for **DS**, 0.09% for **RNY**, 0.05% for **SG**, and 0.03% for **AGB**. The stigma associated with bariatric surgery has led to the notion that these procedures are relatively dangerous; evidence suggests otherwise, especially compared to other procedures such as gallbladder surgery 0.52%, hip replacement 0.93%, and cardiac bypass surgery 3.30% which all have significantly higher 1-month mortality rates.

The 1-year mortality was 0.34% for **RNY**, 0.21% for **SG**, and 0.08% for **AGB**. Howard et al. found the incidence of mortality at 5 years was higher for **RNY**, 5.67%, compared to **SG**, 4.27%. Courcoulas et al. demonstrated that **postoperative RNY and SG** patients had significantly lower long-term risk of all-cause mortality compared to nonsurgical patients with severe obesity, hazard ratio (HR) = 0.43 and HR = 00.28, respectively. **A study in JAMA found that bariatric surgery, including AGB, RNY, and SG, was associated with lower all-cause mortality compared to nonsurgical obesity management.** The HR for mortality was 2.01 for **AGB**, 2.65 for RNY, and 1.60 for **SG**, OR 2.01 times, 2.65 times, and 1.6 times more likely to occur than someone with obesity who did not have surgery (Fig. 15.13).

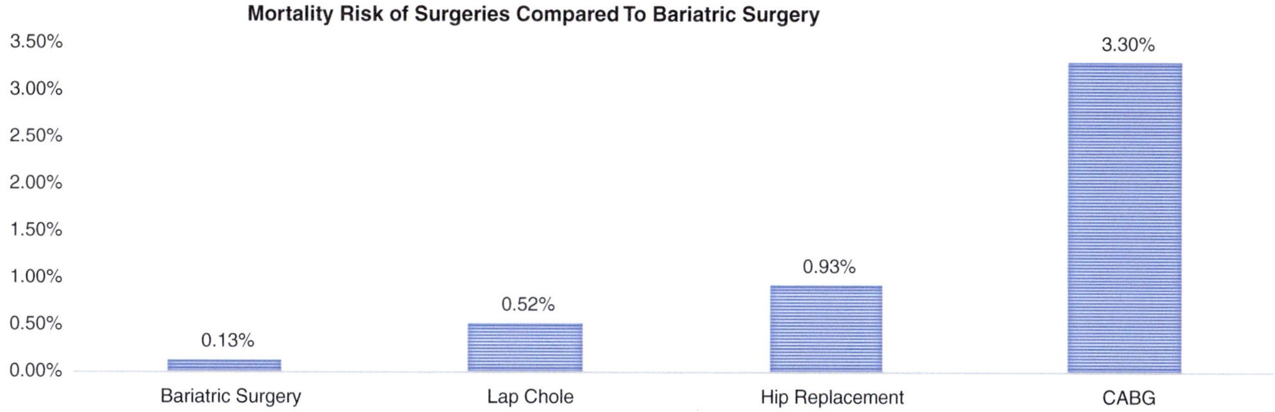

[1]Mortality rate when performed at a Bariatric Surgery Center of Excellence; Bariatric Surgery: DeMaria EJ, Pate V, Warthen M et al. Baseline data from American Society for Metabolic and Bariatric Surgery-designated Bariatric Surgery Centers of Excellence using the Bariatric Outcomes Longitudinal Database, Surgery for Obesity and Related Diseases. Article in Press.
[2]Dolan JP, Diggs BS, Sheppard BC et al. The National Mortality Burden and Significant Factors Associated with Open and Laparoscopic Cholecystectomy: 1997–2006. J Gastrointest Surg. 2009; 13:2292-2301
[3]Lie SA, Engesaeter LB, Havelin LI et al. Early postoperative mortality after 67,548 total hip replacements. Acta Orthopaedica 2002; 73(4):392-399
[4]Ricciardi R; Virnig BA, Ogilvie Jr. JW. Volume-Outcome Relationship for Coronary Artery Bypass Grafting in an Era of Decreasing Volume. Arch Surg. 2008;143[4]:338-344

Fig. 15.13 Mortality risk of bariatric surgery compared to common surgeries. (Credit: Neil Floch MD)

Outcomes

Quality of life improves significantly after bariatric surgery, both physically and mentally. Patients were satisfied to have undergone surgery 97% of the time, and more so after RNY than SG. An SR and MA with 72 studies and 9433 patients treated for obesity with bariatric surgery had an effect size of 0.88, translating to significant improvements in physical quality of life compared to mental. Long-term follow-up studies over 5 years reveal significant gains in a quality-adjusted life year (QALY) and reductions in depression scores. While quality of life improves significantly after bariatric surgery, most outcomes remain below community norms.

Weight Loss

Weight loss after bariatric surgery varies significantly depending on the type of procedure performed and the time that has passed since the procedure. Weight loss had been measured with percent excess body weight, %EBW lost by subtracting the actual weight before and after surgery divided by the total excess weight before surgery × 100. Medical weight loss has traditionally been measured in %TBW lost. With the advent of effective medical weight loss after the introduction of GLP-1RAs such as semaglutide and tirzepatide, it has now become more favorable to measure surgical weight loss with %TBW lost so that the two treatments can be compared directly. The %TBW lost is defined as the total body weight before surgery minus the weight after surgery divided by the total weight before surgery × 100.

Short-term weight loss is measured at 1 year. At this point, both duodenal switch (DS) and single anastomosis duodeno-ileostomy (SADI) procedures demonstrate the highest weight loss among bariatric surgeries. A randomized clinical trial showed comparable results between SADI and DS, with SADI achieving 81.8% %EBWL and 40.1% %TBWL, and DS achieving 84.2% %EBWL and 41.6% %TBWL. In comparison, Roux-en-Y gastric bypass (RNY) patients had an average of 77.9% %EBWL and 28.4% %TBWL, while sleeve gastrectomy (SG) patients showed approximately 50.8% %EBWL and 23.0% %TBWL at 1 year. **AGB** patients at 1 year achieve approximately 13.7% TWL and 40.8% EWL. **Intermediate weight loss is considered at around 3 years.**

Long-term weight loss is determined at 5 years. DS demonstrated superior weight loss compared to **SADI**. A multicenter prospective cohort study found that **DS** resulted in a significantly higher %EWL (80.5% vs. 68.6%), and higher %TWL (42.1% vs. 36.0%) compared to **SADI**. A 6-year study confirmed that DS patients had higher %EWL compared to SADI patients. **Weight loss is** around 21.7% TWL and 62.58% EWL for **RNY**, with durable weight loss observed up to 10 years. **SG** at 5 years, patients maintain around 16.0% TWL and 53.25% EWL. At 5 years, **AGB** patients maintain around 11.7% TWL and 47.94% EWL, with some studies reporting up to 45.9% EWL at 10 years. **When comparing the procedures RNY** consistently demonstrates higher weight loss results compared to **SG** and **AGB** in both in the short and long term. **SG** is more effective than **AGB.**

Type 2 Diabetes

The remission rates of T2 DM vary depending on the surgical procedure performed. BPD-DS demonstrates the highest long-term remission rates, reaching up to 93% in patients who were only on oral antidiabetic medications before surgery, and around 40% in those with severe T2DM. Complete remission rates can be as high as 68.1% at 10 years postoperatively. **RNY** demonstrates a 68.7% at 3 years and 86.1% remission rate of T2 DM at 5 years post-surgery. **SG has as high as a** remission rate of 38.1% at 2 years. **AGB is not an MBS and does not cause physiologic and metabolic alterations of the gut, and is only restrictive, providing a control for weight loss alone as a comparison.** The remission rates of T2DM with AGB are relatively low, at 30.2% at 3 years and 19% at 5 years post-surgery.

Two of the most recognized MBS studies were the **STAMPEDE trial** and the **SLEEVE-PASS** study which both compared **RNY** and **SG** to intensive medical therapy for T2 DM. The **STAMPEDE** trial found that, at 5 years, 29% of patients with severe insulin-dependent T2 DM who underwent Roux-en-Y gastric bypass (RNY) and 23% who had sleeve gastrectomy (SG) achieved an HbA1c of ≤6.0% and were able to discontinue all diabetes medications. In the **SLEEVE-PASS study, 47% of RNY patients and 33% of SG patients achieved DM remission with an HbA1c <6% off all diabetes medications at 5 years**. The longest RNY study: The Swedish Obese Subjects (SOS) study, prospective controlled study, found that **72% of patients with T2 DM achieved remission** as defined as a blood glucose ≤110 mg/dL without medications at 2 years post-surgery. Remission rates decreased to **30% at 15 years**.

Hypertension

A SR and MA revealed that 53.3% of patients discontinued antihypertensive medication after RNY compared to 49.4% after SG. A study by Schiavon et al. [109] found that 51% achieved HTN remission at 12 months. **Approximately 31–51% of patients achieve normal blood pressure without medications** after **RNY**. HTN resolved in 62.17% of patients and improved in 35.7% at a mean of 5.35 years of follow-up after **SG**, however, the relapse rate of HTN was 31.4% after 3 years. The **DS** remission rate is approximately **63.9%**. An SR revealed a remission rate for HTN after **SADI-S** to be **59%** at 12 months. A comparative study of **DS and SADI-S** reported remission rates of **95.2%** and **85.1%**, respectively, at 5 years, revealing the best results for the treatment of HTN among MBS procedures.

Dyslipidemia

In patients undergoing RNY, 68.5% experienced improvement or resolution of dyslipidemia compared to 48.4% of patients undergoing SG. RNY led to decreases in total cholesterol, LDL-C, and triglycerides, with 76% achieving normal total cholesterol levels. While 64.6% of patients discontinued lipid-lowering medications after RNY, unfortunately at 5 years, 46.2% restarted medications. **SG** improved dyslipidemia in 48.4% of patients, and 61.2% discontinued lipid-lowering medications, but 52.5% of these patients restarted medications within 5 years. SG increased HDL levels in 74%. The **DS and SADI-S results** in treating dyslipidemia revealed a 77.2% resolution rate by Spinos et al. at 12 months post-SADI-S, while Gebellí et al. reported a 76.4% remission rate at 5 years post-DS. At 10 years, the remission rate fell to 69.7%. Bariatric surgeries had different effects on dyslipidemia, independent of weight loss. The RNY achieved the biggest reduction in plasma lipids (TC and LDL), DS and SADI-S was next, and SG was least as demonstrated by Spivak et al.

Cardiac Disease

The impact of MBS on major adverse cardiac events (MACEs) and cardiac disease has been extensively studied. An MA by van Veldhuisen et al. found that MBS is associated with a significant reduction in **cardiovascular mortality,** HR 0.59, or 41% less risk, and incidence of **heart failure,** HR 0.50, or 50% less risk, **MI,** HR 0.58 or 42% less risk, and **stroke:** 46% less risk. Regarding medication discontinuation, Tang et al. noted that bariatric surgery leads to significant reductions in the use of medications for T2 DM and cardiovascular diseases. Aminian et al. found that 5 years after surgery, patients required fewer medications for diabetes and cardiovascular diseases, with RNY compared to SG.

Sleep Apnea

MBS improvement and resolution of OSA is well-documented. Overall, systematic review (SR) and meta-analysis (MA) reported that the remission rate of OSA after MBS, including RNY, was approximately **65%**. SG led to OSA resolution in **67.6%** of patients with an AHI ≥15. RNY led to OSA remission in **59.2%** of patients. A cohort showed that SG resulted in a **72.2%** remission rate of moderate-to-severe OSA. Long-term results after DS demonstrate the most successful rates as **90%** of patients may discontinue CPAP after surgery [5]. MBS not only reduces the severity of

OSA across all procedures but also leads to significant ability to discontinue CPAP.

Kidney Disease

Kidney disease improvement after MBS is remarkable. Meta-analyses and reviews of MBS demonstrate that **43.2%** of patients with stage 3 chronic kidney disease (CKD) improved to stage 2, and **5.1%** improved to stage 1 after MBS [1]. One meta-analysis reported a mean difference (MD) of **−0.24 mg/dL** in serum creatinine levels after bariatric surgery [2, 3]. The **Swedish Obese Subjects (SOS) study** revealed that MBS lowered the progression to end-stage renal disease (ESRD) compared medical obesity care, with an adjusted hazard ratio (HR) of **0.27** or **a 73% reduction in risk of developing ESRD.** MBS can substantially reduce the need for kidney transplants.

Liver Disease

MBS has shown significant benefits in the treatment of **nonalcoholic steatohepatitis (NASH), nonalcoholic fatty liver disease (NAFLD)**, now MASH and MAFLD. MBS can resolve NASH in 80–84% of patients at 1 year and maintain resolution up to 5 years [1]. Specifically, 25–30% had resolution of fibrosis and another 70.2% improved fibrosis, 66–88% of patients have complete resolution of steatosis, 50% had resolution of inflammation, and 49–76% had resolution of ballooning degeneration after bariatric surgery [2–4]. A recent study by Aminian found the incidence of major adverse liver outcomes, including progression to clinical or histological cirrhosis, development of hepatocellular carcinoma, liver transplantation, or liver-related mortality at 10 years, was **2.3%** in the MBS group versus **9.6%** in the nonsurgical group. **MBS** was able to reduce these major liver outcomes by 76%.

Cancers

An SR and MA by Wilson et al. [127] indicated that bariatric surgery was associated with a reduced overall incidence of cancer by 38% compared to people with obesity who did not have MBS, RR 0.62, and cancer-associated mortality decreased risk by 49%, RR 0.51. Clapp et al. [126] reported a nearly 50% reduction in the risk of non-hormonal cancers following MBS. **A study by** Aminian et al. [125] **found that MBS reduced the risk of cancer-related mortality by 48% at 10 years.**

Length of Life

The longest running MBS study, the **Swedish Obese Subjects (SOS) study** was associated with a 29% reduction in overall mortality and an increase in life expectancy compared to usual obesity care over a mean follow-up of 10.9 years, and the adjusted median life expectancy was 3.0 years longer in the surgery group compared to the control group. More recently, a meta-analysis in *The Lancet* indicated that MBS is associated with a **49.2% reduction in the risk of dying and a median life expectancy increase of 6.1** years compared to usual care.

A study of over 100,000 patients in *Annals of Surgery*, both RNY and SG were associated with significantly lower all-cause mortality compared to nonsurgical management of severe obesity [4]. **RNY** was associated with **a reduced risk of 57% and SG, 72% in reduced risk of all-cause mortality compared to nonsurgical patients at 5 years of follow-up,** RNY: HR = 0.43; SG: HR = 0.28. **RNY** was associated with a 73% lower 5-year risk of cardiovascular HR = 0.27, 46% of cancer, HR = 0.54, and 77% of diabetes-related mortality HR = 0.23. In **SG patients**, at 3 years follow-up, there was significantly 67% lower risk of cardiovascular, HR = 0.33, 74% of cancer, HR = 0.26, and 85% of diabetes-related HR = 0.15 mortality for SG patients. Despite ample evidence that MBS extends life in patients with obesity, mortality rates remain higher than those in the general population, suggesting that while bariatric surgery offers significant benefits, it does not completely normalize mortality risk.

Bariatric surgery has superior and longer-lasting results for the improvement of medical problems compared to GLP-1 RAs. Controlled trials reveal excellent results for gut hormone–based medications, at maximum dosage, in non-diabetic patients, 16% TWL on 2.4 mg of semaglutide, and 21% TWL with patients on 15 mg of tirzepatide. Real-world (RW) data of medications is significantly lower as most patients cannot obtain, stop because of side effects, or fail to adhere to medications long term. Weight regain is common upon discontinuation. **RW data on medications is more comparable to MBS weight loss results as surgery trials cannot be controlled. RW results reveal an 8.3% TBW loss for semaglutide and a 15.3% TBW loss for tirzepatide at 12 months (Semaglutide vs Tirzepatide for Weight Loss in Adults With overweight or Obesity. *JAMA Intern Medicine*, 2024 by Rodriguez PI, Goodwin Cartwright BM, Gratzi S, et al.**

Bariatric surgery achieves more sustained weight loss than GLP-1ra medications as RNY and SG have at least TWL of 23–27%. MBS is associated with higher rates of T2 DM remission, improved glycemic control, and reduced medication use. Long-term studies, such as the ARMMS-T2D pooled analysis, demonstrate superior glycemic control and T2 DM remission rates over 7–12 years compared to medical therapy, including GLP-1 RAs. Both treatments improve cardiovascular outcomes, but MBS demonstrates better improvement in MACEs. Observational data suggest that MBS reduces mortality and cardiovascular risk more effectively than GLP-1 RAs, secondary to greater sustained weight loss.

Conclusion

Metabolic and bariatric surgery is the most effective treatment for obesity. Treating the disease warrants a complete knowledge of obesity as a disease, the medications to treat it, and surgery. The PA must understand the potential short- and long-term complications of the different surgery options. Long-term patient goals include sustained weight maintenance and ongoing support—areas in which the PA plays a critical, lifelong role.

suggested Reading

The Role of the PA

1. Mechanick JI, Apovian CM, Brethauer SA, et al. Clinical practice guidelines for the perioperative nutrition, metabolic, and nonsurgical support of patients undergoing bariatric procedures—2019 update: cosponsored by American Association of Clinical Endocrinologists/American College of Endocrinology, the Obesity Society, American Society for Metabolic and Bariatric Surgery, Obesity Medicine Association, and American Society of Anesthesiologists. Obesity (Silver Spring). 2020;28(4):O1–O58. https://doi.org/10.1002/oby.22719.
2. Yuce TK, Holmstrom A, Soper NJ, et al. Complications and readmissions associated with first assistant training level following elective bariatric surgery. J Gastrointest Surg. 2021;25(8):1948–54. https://doi.org/10.1007/s11605-020-04787-0.

Demographics

3. World Health Organization. Obesity and overweight. https://www.who.int/news-room/fact-sheets/detail/obesity-and-overweight#:~:text=Worldwide%20adult%20obesity%20has%20more,16%25%20were%20living%20with%20obesity.
4. The Lancet. The global syndemic of obesity, undernutrition, and climate change: the Lancet commission report. Lancet Public Health. 2019;4(1):e1–2. https://www.thelancet.com/pdfs/journals/lanpub/PIIS2468-2667%2818%2930021-5.pdf
5. Maki KA, Sack MN, Hall KD. Ultra-processed foods: increasing the risk of inflammation and immune dysregulation? Nat Rev Immunol. 2024;24:453–4. https://doi.org/10.1038/s41577-024-01049-x.
6. Hall KD. Energy compensation and metabolic adaptation: "The Biggest Loser" study reinterpreted. Obesity (Silver Spring). 2022;30(1):11–3. https://doi.org/10.1002/oby.23308.

Etiology

7. Steele CB, Thomas CC, Henley SJ, Massetti GM, Galuska DA, Agurs-Collins T, Puckett M, Richardson LC. Vital signs: trends in incidence of cancers associated with overweight and obesity - United States, 2005-2014. MMWR Morb Mortal Wkly Rep. 2017;66(39):1052–8. Epub 2017 Oct 3
8. GBD 2015 Obesity Collaborators, Afshin A, Forouzanfar MH, Reitsma MB, Sur P, Estep K, Lee A, Marczak L, Mokdad AH, Moradi-Lakeh M, Naghavi M, Salama JS, Vos T, Abate KH, Abbafati C, Ahmed MB, Al-Aly Z, Alkerwi A, Al-Raddadi R, Amare AT, Amberbir A, Amegah AK, Amini E, Amrock SM, Anjana RM, Ärnlöv J, Asayesh H, Banerjee A, Barac A, Baye E, Bennett DA, Beyene AS, Biadgilign S, Biryukov S, Bjertness E, Boneya DJ, Campos-Nonato I, Carrero JJ, Cecilio P, Cercy K, Ciobanu LG, Cornaby L, Damtew SA, Dandona L, Dandona R, Dharmaratne SD, Duncan BB, Eshrati B, Esteghamati A, Feigin VL, Fernandes JC, Fürst T, Gebrehiwot TT, Gold A, Gona PN, Goto A, Habtewold TD, Hadush KT, Hafezi-Nejad N, Hay SI, Horino M, Islami F, Kamal R, Kasaeian A, Katikireddi SV, Kengne AP, Kesavachandran CN, Khader YS, Khang YH, Khubchandani J, Kim D, Kim YJ, Kinfu Y, Kosen S, Ku T, Defo BK, Kumar GA, Larson HJ, Leinsalu M, Liang X, Lim SS, Liu P, Lopez AD, Lozano R, Majeed A, Malekzadeh R, Malta DC, Mazidi M, McAlinden C, et al. Health effects of overweight and obesity in 195 countries over 25 years. N Engl J Med. 2017;377(1):13–27. Epub 2017 Jun 12
9. Chen C, Ye Y, Zhang Y, Pan XF, Pan A. Weight change across adulthood in relation to all-cause and cause-specific mortality: prospective cohort study. BMJ. 2019;367:l5584. Epub 2019 Oct 16

Indications

10. Eisenberg D, Shikora SA, Aarts E, et al. 2022 American Society for Metabolic and Bariatric Surgery (ASMBS) and International Federation for the Surgery of Obesity and Metabolic Disorders (IFSO): indications for metabolic and bariatric surgery. Surg Obes Relat Dis. 2022;18(12):1345–56. https://doi.org/10.1016/j.soard.2022.08.013.

Medical Treatment of the Patient

11. Elmaleh-Sachs A, Schwartz JL, Bramante CT, Nicklas JM, Gudzune KA, Jay M. Obesity Management in Adults: a review. JAMA J Am Med Assoc. 2023;330(20):2000–15. https://doi.org/10.1001/jama.2023.19897.
12. Apovian CM, Aronne L, Rubino D, et al. A randomized, phase 3 trial of naltrexone sustained release/bupropion sustained release on weight and obesity-related risk factors (COR-II). Obesity. 2013;21(5):935–43. https://doi.org/10.1002/oby.20309.
13. Lei XG, Ruan JQ, Lai C, Sun Z, Yang X. Efficacy and safety of phentermine/Topiramate in adults with overweight or obesity: a systematic review and meta-analysis. Obesity. 2021;29(6):985–94. https://doi.org/10.1002/oby.23152.

Patient Preparation

14. Kindel TL, Ganga RR, Baker JW, Noria SF, Jones DB, Omotosho P, Volckmann ET, Williams NN, Telem DA, Petrick AT, Gould JC. American Society for Metabolic and Bariatric Surgery: preoperative care pathway for laparoscopic Roux-en-Y gastric bypass. Surg Obes Relat Dis. 2021;17(9):1529–40.
15. Carter J, Chang J, Birriel TJ, Moustarah F, Sogg S, Goodpaster K, Benson-Davies S, Chapmon K, Eisenberg D. American Society for Metabolic and Bariatric Surgery position statement on preoperative patient optimization before metabolic and bariatric surgery. Surg Obes Relat Dis. 2021;17(12):1956–76. https://doi.org/10.1016/j.soard.2021.08.024.

Determining Treatment for Patients

16. Hsu JL, Farrell TM. Updates in bariatric surgery. Am Surg. 2024;90(5):925–33. https://doi.org/10.1177/00031348231220576.

Metabolic MBS

17. Evers SS, Sandoval DA, Seeley RJ. The physiology and molecular underpinnings of the effects of bariatric surgery on obesity and diabetes. Annu Rev Physiol. 2017;79:313–34. https://doi.org/10.1146/annurev-physiol-022516-034423.
18. Cummings DE, Rubino F. Metabolic surgery for the treatment of type 2 diabetes in obese individuals. Diabetologia. 2018;61:257–64. https://doi.org/10.1007/s00125-017-4513-y.
19. Xu G, Song M. Recent advances in the mechanisms underlying the beneficial effects of bariatric and metabolic surgery. Surg Obes Relat Dis. 2021;17(1):231–8. https://doi.org/10.1016/j.soard.2020.08.028.

Gut Hormones

20. Holst JJ, Madsbad S, Bojsen-Møller KN, Dirksen C, Svane M. New lessons from the gut: studies of the role of gut peptides in weight loss and diabetes resolution after gastric bypass and sleeve gastrectomy. Peptides. 2024;176:171199. https://doi.org/10.1016/j.peptides.2024.171199.
21. Perakakis N, Kokkinos A, Peradze N, et al. Circulating levels of gastrointestinal hormones in response to the most common types of bariatric surgery and predictive value for weight loss over one year: evidence from two independent trials. Metabolism. 2019;101:153997. https://doi.org/10.1016/j.metabol.2019.153997.
22. Aukan MI, Rehfeld JF, Holst JJ, Martins C. Plasma concentration of gastrointestinal hormones and subjective appetite ratings after diet or bariatric surgery: 1-year results from the DISGAP study. Int J Obes. 2025;49(2):306–14. https://doi.org/10.1038/s41366-024-01658-5.
23. Huang J, Chen Y, Wang X, et al. Change in adipokines and gastrointestinal hormones after bariatric surgery: a meta-analysis. Obes Surg. 2023;33(3):789–806. https://doi.org/10.1007/s11695-022-06444-8.
24. Gala K, Ghusn W, Abu Dayyeh BK. Gut motility and hormone changes after bariatric procedures. Curr Opin Endocrinol Diabetes Obes. 2024;31(3):131–7. https://doi.org/10.1097/MED.0000000000000860.

Bile

25. Wahlström A, Aydin Ö, Olsson LM, et al. Alterations in bile acid kinetics after bariatric surgery in patients with obesity with or without type 2 diabetes. EBioMedicine. 2024;106:105265. https://doi.org/10.1016/j.ebiom.2024.105265.
26. Wang W, Cheng Z, Wang Y, et al. Role of bile acids in bariatric surgery. Front Physiol. 2019;10:374. https://doi.org/10.3389/fphys.2019.00374.
27. Akalestou E, Miras AD, Rutter GA, le Roux CW. Mechanisms of weight loss after obesity surgery. Endocr Rev. 2022;43(1):19–34. https://doi.org/10.1210/endrev/bnab022.

Microbiome

28. Ali Ahmad M, Venema K, Ayoub Moubareck C, et al. Changes in energy homeostasis, gut peptides, and gut microbiota in Emiratis with obesity after bariatric surgery. PLoS One. 2025;20(2):e0318699. https://doi.org/10.1371/journal.pone.0318699.
29. Hamamah S, Hajnal A, Covasa M. Influence of bariatric surgery on gut microbiota composition and its implication on brain and peripheral targets. Nutrients. 2024;16(7):1071. https://doi.org/10.3390/nu16071071.
30. Juárez-Fernández M, Román-Sagüillo S, Porras D, et al. Long-term effects of bariatric surgery on gut microbiota composition and Faecal metabolome related to obesity remission. Nutrients. 2021;13(8):2519. https://doi.org/10.3390/nu13082519.
31. Luijten JCHBM, Vugts G, Nieuwenhuijzen GAP, Luyer MDP. The importance of the microbiome in bariatric surgery: a systematic review. Obes Surg. 2019;29(7):2338–49. https://doi.org/10.1007/s11695-019-03863-y.
32. Morales-Marroquin E, Hanson B, Greathouse L, de la Cruz-Munoz N, Messiah SE. Comparison of methodological approaches to human gut microbiota changes in response to metabolic and bariatric surgery: a systematic review. Obesit Rev. 2020;21(8):e13025. https://doi.org/10.1111/obr.13025.

Neurogenic

33. An Z, Wang H, Mokadem M. Role of the autonomic nervous system in mechanism of energy and glucose regulation post bariatric surgery. Front Neurosci. 2021;15:770690. https://doi.org/10.3389/fnins.2021.770690.
34. Stefanidis A, Oldfield BJ. Neuroendocrine mechanisms underlying bariatric surgery: insights from human studies and animal models. J Neuroendocrinol. 2017;29(10) https://doi.org/10.1111/jne.12534.
35. Zakeri R, Batterham RL. Potential mechanisms underlying the effect of bariatric surgery on eating behaviour. Curr Opin Endocrinol Diabetes Obes. 2018;25(1):3–11. https://doi.org/10.1097/MED.0000000000000379.
36. Gautron L. The phantom satiation hypothesis of bariatric surgery. Front Neurosci. 2021;15:626085. https://doi.org/10.3389/fnins.2021.626085.

BDS/DS

37. Marceau P, Hould FS, Simard S, et al. Biliopancreatic diversion with duodenal switch. World J Surg. 1998;22(9):947–54. https://doi.org/10.1007/s002689900498.
38. Marceau P, Hould FS, Potvin M, Lebel S, Biron S. Biliopancreatic diversion (duodenal switch procedure). Eur J Gastroenterol Hepatol. 1999;11(2):99–103. https://doi.org/10.1097/00042737-199902000-00008.

Endoscopic

39. Rapaka B, Maselli DB, Lopez-Nava G, et al. Effects on physiologic measures of appetite from intragastric balloon and endoscopic sleeve gastroplasty: results of a prospective study. Chin Med J. 2022;135(10):1234–41. https://doi.org/10.1097/CM9.0000000000002097.
40. Abu Dayyeh BK, Edmundowicz S, Thompson CC. Clinical practice update: expert review on endoscopic bariatric therapies. Gastroenterology. 2017;152(4):716–29. https://doi.org/10.1053/j.gastro.2017.01.035.

Robotic

41. Cashman CL, Shah SV, Hall AG, Walters RW, Nandipati KC. Robotic-assisted and laparoscopic bariatric surgeries still have clinically comparable outcomes. Obes Surg. 2024;34(8):2954–64. https://doi.org/10.1007/s11695-024-07368-1.
42. Tatarian T, Yang J, Wang J, et al. Trends in the utilization and perioperative outcomes of primary robotic bariatric surgery from 2015 to 2018: a study of 46,764 patients from the MBSAQIP data registry. Surg Endosc. 2021;35(7):3915–22. https://doi.org/10.1007/s00464-020-07839-3.
43. Wesley Vosburg R, Haque O, Roth E. Robotic vs. laparoscopic metabolic and bariatric surgery, outcomes over 5 years in nearly 800,000 patients. Obes Surg. 2022;32(7):2341–8. https://doi.org/10.1007/s11695-022-06082-0.

Treat Weight Regain and Revision

44. Andalib A, Alamri H, Almuhanna Y, et al. Short-term outcomes of revisional surgery after sleeve gastrectomy: a comparative analysis of re-sleeve, Roux-en-Y gastric bypass, duodenal switch (Roux-en-Y and single-anastomosis). Surg Endosc. 2021;35(8):4644–52. https://doi.org/10.1007/s00464-020-07891-z.
45. Małczak P, Shim SR, Wysocki M, et al. Comparison of different revisional surgeries after sleeve gastrectomy: a network meta-analysis. Obes Rev. 2025:e13930. https://doi.org/10.1111/obr.13930.
46. Salman MA, Salman A, Elewa A, et al. Outcomes of revisional surgery options after inadequate sleeve gastrectomy: a comprehensive network meta-analysis. World J Surg. 2024;48(9):2040–57. https://doi.org/10.1002/wjs.12293.
47. Franken RJ, Franken J, Sluiter NR, de Vries R, Euser S, Gerdes VEA, de Brauw M. Efficacy and safety of revisional treatments for weight regain or insufficient weight loss after Roux-en-Y gastric bypass: a systematic review and meta-analysis. Obes Rev. 2023;24(10):e13607. https://doi.org/10.1111/obr.13607.
48. Ghiassi S, Higa K, Chang S, et al. Conversion of standard Roux-en-Y gastric bypass to distal bypass for weight loss failure and metabolic syndrome: 3-year follow-up and evolution of technique to reduce nutritional complications. Surg Obes Relat Dis. 2018;14:554.

ERAS

49. Trotta M, Ferrari C, D'Alessandro G, et al. Enhanced recovery after bariatric surgery (ERABS) in a high-volume bariatric center. Surg Obes Relat Dis. 2019;15(10):1785–92. https://doi.org/10.1016/j.soard.2019.06.038.
50. Stenberg E, dos Reis Falcão LF, O'Kane M, et al. Guidelines for perioperative care in bariatric surgery: enhanced recovery after surgery (ERAS) society recommendations: a 2021 update. World J Surg. 2022;46:729–51. https://doi.org/10.1007/s00268-021-06394-9.

Long Term Treatment of the Bariatric Patient

51. Aarts MA, Sivapalan N, Nikzad SE, et al. Optimizing bariatric surgery multidisciplinary follow-up: a focus on patient-centered care. Obes Surg. 2017;27(3):730–6. https://doi.org/10.1007/s11695-016-2354-2.
52. Lujan J, Tuero C, Landecho MF, et al. Impact of routine and long-term follow-up on weight loss after bariatric surgery. Obes Surg. 2020;30(11):4293–9. https://doi.org/10.1007/s11695-020-04788-7.
53. O'Kane M, Barth JH. Nutritional follow-up of patients after obesity surgery: best practice. Clin Endocrinol. 2016;84(5):658–61. https://doi.org/10.1111/cen.13041.
54. Sista F, Carandina S, Andreica A, et al. Long-term results of laparoscopic gastric sleeve: the importance of follow-up adherence. Eur Rev Med Pharmacol Sci. 2022;26(18):6691–9. https://doi.org/10.26355/eurrev20220929770.

Acute Complications

55. Luo L, Li H, Wu Y, et al. Portal venous system thrombosis after bariatric surgery: a systematic review and meta-analysis. Surgery. 2021;170(2):363–72. https://doi.org/10.1016/j.surg.2021.03.005.
56. Carlin AM, Varban OA, Ehlers AP, et al. Independent predictors and timing of portomesenteric vein thrombosis after bariatric surgery. Surg Obes Relat Dis. 2022;18(12):1385–91. https://doi.org/10.1016/j.soard.2022.07.016.
57. Guzman-Pruneda FA, Garcia A, Crum RW, et al. Extended post discharge prophylaxis for venous thromboembolism prevention after bariatric surgery. Obes Surg. 2024;34(4):1217–23. https://doi.org/10.1007/s11695-024-07100-z.

Late Complications

58. Kumbhari V, le Roux CW, Cohen RV. Endoscopic evaluation and management of late complications after bariatric surgery: a narrative review. Obes Surg. 2021;31(10):4624–33. https://doi.org/10.1007/s11695-021-05603-7.
59. Larsen M, Kozarek R. Therapeutic endoscopy for the treatment of post-bariatric surgery complications. World J Gastroenterol. 2022;28(2):199–215. https://doi.org/10.3748/wjg.v28.i2.199.
60. McCarty TR, Kumar N. Revision bariatric procedures and management of complications from bariatric surgery. Dig Dis Sci. 2022;67(5):1688–701. https://doi.org/10.1007/s10620-022-07397-9.
61. Obesity and weight management for the prevention and treatment of type 2 diabetes: standards of Care in Diabetes-2025. Diabetes Care. 2025;48(Suppl 1):S167–80. https://doi.org/10.2337/dc25-S008.
62. Spota A, Cereatti F, Granieri S, et al. Endoscopic management of bariatric surgery complications according to a standardized algorithm. Obes Surg. 2021;31(10):4327–37. https://doi.org/10.1007/s11695-021-05577-6.
63. Tack J, Deloose E. Complications of bariatric surgery: dumping syndrome, reflux and vitamin deficiencies. Best Pract Res Clin Gastroenterol. 2014;28(4):741–9. https://doi.org/10.1016/j.bpg.2014.07.010.

SG

64. Goldenshluger M, Goldenshluger A, Keinan-Boker L, Cohen MJ, Ben-Porat T, Gerasi H, Amun M, Abu-Gazala M, Khalaileh A, Mintz Y, Elazary R. Postoperative outcomes, weight loss predictors, and late gastrointestinal symptoms following laparoscopic sleeve gastrectomy. J Gastrointest Surg. 2017;21(12):2009–15. https://doi.org/10.1007/s11605-017-3585-9.

RNY

65. Chahal-Kummen M, Salte OBK, Hewitt S, et al. Health benefits and risks during 10 years after Roux-en-Y gastric bypass. Surg Endosc. 2020;34(12):5368–76. https://doi.org/10.1007/s00464-019-07328-2.
66. Nielsen JB, Pedersen AM, Gribsholt SB, Svensson E, Richelsen B. Prevalence, severity, and predictors of symptoms of dumping and hypoglycemia after Roux-en-Y gastric bypass. Surg Obes Relat Dis. 2016;12(8):1562–8. https://doi.org/10.1016/j.soard.2016.04.017.
67. Griffith PS, Birch DW, Sharma AM, Karmali S. Managing complications associated with laparoscopic Roux-en-Y gastric bypass for morbid obesity. Can J Surg. 2012;55(5):329–36. https://doi.org/10.1503/cjs.002011.
68. Poitou Bernert C, Ciangura C, Coupaye M, et al. Nutritional deficiency after gastric bypass: diagnosis, prevention and treatment. Diabetes Metab. 2007;33(1):13–24. https://doi.org/10.1016/j.diabet.2006.11.004.

BPD/DS

69. Elias K, Hedberg J, Sundbom M. Prevalence and impact of acid-related symptoms and diarrhea in patients undergoing Roux-en-Y gastric bypass, sleeve gastrectomy, and biliopancreatic diversion with duodenal switch. Surg Obes Relat Dis. 2020;16(4):520–7. https://doi.org/10.1016/j.soard.2019.12.020.
70. Kitaghenda FK, Hong J, Shao Y, Yao L, Zhu X. The prevalence of small intestinal bacterial overgrowth after Roux-en-Y gastric bypass (RYGB): a systematic review and meta-analysis. Obes Surg. 2024;34(1):250–7. https://doi.org/10.1007/s11695-023-06974-9.
71. Kaniel O, Sherf-Dagan S, Szold A, et al. The effects of one anastomosis gastric bypass surgery on the gastrointestinal tract. Nutrients. 2022;14(2):304. https://doi.org/10.3390/nu14020304.
72. Dolan RD, Baker J, Harer K, et al. Small intestinal bacterial overgrowth: clinical presentation in patients with Roux-en-Y gastric bypass. Obes Surg. 2021;31(2):564–9. https://doi.org/10.1007/s11695-020-05032-y.

SADI-S

73. Sánchez-Pernaute A, Herrera MÁR, Ferré NP, et al. Long-term results of single-anastomosis Duodeno-Ileal bypass with sleeve gastrectomy (SADI-S). Obes Surg. 2022;32(3):682–9. https://doi.org/10.1007/s11695-021-05879-9.
74. Sánchez-Pernaute A, Herrera MA, Pérez-Aguirre ME, et al. Single anastomosis Duodeno-Ileal bypass with sleeve gastrectomy (SADI-S). One to Three-Year Follow-Up. Obes Surg. 2010;20(12):1720–6. https://doi.org/10.1007/s11695-010-0247-3.
75. Spinos D, Skarentzos K, Esagian SM, Seymour KA, Economopoulos KP. The effectiveness of single-anastomosis Duodenoileal bypass with sleeve gastrectomy/one anastomosis duodenal switch (SADI-S/OADS): an updated systematic review. Obes Surg. 2021;31(4):1790–800. https://doi.org/10.1007/s11695-020-05188-7.

AGB

76. Kerpel A, Klang E, Konen E, Marom EM, Amitai MM. Gastric banding: complications identified by computed tomography. Obes Surg. 2019;29(2):499–505. https://doi.org/10.1007/s11695-018-3534-z.
77. Carelli AM, Youn HA, Kurian MS, Ren CJ, Fielding GA. Safety of the laparoscopic adjustable gastric band: 7-year data from a U.S. Center of Excellence. Surg Endosc. 2010;24(8):1819–23. https://doi.org/10.1007/s00464-009-0858-8.
78. Cho EJ, Kim SM. Explantation of adjustable gastric bands: an observation study of 10 years of experience at a tertiary center. Yonsei Med J. 2019;60(8):782–90. https://doi.org/10.3349/ymj.2019.60.8.782.
79. Toolabi K, Golzarand M, Farid R. Laparoscopic adjustable gastric banding: efficacy and consequences over 13 years. Am J Surg. 2016;212(1):62–8. https://doi.org/10.1016/j.amjsurg.2015.05.021.

80. Kirshtein B, Lantsberg L, Mizrahi S, Avinoach E. Bariatric emergencies for non-bariatric surgeons: complications of laparoscopic gastric banding. Obes Surg. 2010;20(11):1468–78. https://doi.org/10.1007/s11695-009-0059-5.

Mortality

81. Robertson AGN, Wiggins T, Robertson FP, et al. Perioperative mortality in bariatric surgery: meta-analysis. Br J Surg. 2021;108(8):892–7. https://doi.org/10.1093/bjs/znab245.
82. Grieco A, Huffman KM, Cohen ME, et al. The metabolic and bariatric surgery accreditation and quality improvement program bariatric surgical risk/benefit calculator: 30-day risk. Surg Obes Relat Dis. 2021;17(6):1117–24. https://doi.org/10.1016/j.soard.2021.02.005.
83. Chaar ME, Lundberg P, Stoltzfus J. Thirty-day outcomes of sleeve gastrectomy versus Roux-en-Y gastric bypass: first report based on metabolic and bariatric surgery accreditation and quality improvement program database. Surg Obes Relat Dis. 2018;14(5):545–51. https://doi.org/10.1016/j.soard.2018.01.011.
84. Hutter MM, Schirmer BD, Jones DB, Ko CY, Cohen ME, Merkow RP, Nguyen NT. First report from the American College of Surgeons Bariatric Surgery Center Network: laparoscopic sleeve gastrectomy has morbidity and effectiveness positioned between the band and the bypass. Ann Surg. 2011;254(3):410–20.; discussion 420–422. https://doi.org/10.1097/SLA.0b013e31822c9dac.
85. Howard R, Chao GF, Yang J, et al. Comparative safety of sleeve gastrectomy and gastric bypass up to 5 years after surgery in patients with severe obesity. JAMA Surg. 2021;156(12):1160–9. https://doi.org/10.1001/jamasurg.2021.4981.
86. Courcoulas AP, Johnson E, Arterburn DE, et al. Reduction in long-term mortality after sleeve gastrectomy and gastric bypass compared to nonsurgical patients with severe obesity. Ann Surg. 2023;277(3):442–8. https://doi.org/10.1097/SLA.0000000000005155.
87. Reges O, Greenland P, Dicker D, et al. Association of bariatric surgery using laparoscopic banding, Roux-en-Y gastric bypass, or laparoscopic sleeve gastrectomy versus usual care obesity management with all-cause mortality. JAMA. 2018;319(3):279–90. https://doi.org/10.1001/jama.2017.20513.
88. DeMaria EJ, Pate V, Warthen M, Winegar DA. Baseline data from American society for metabolic and bariatric surgery-designated bariatric surgery centers of excellence using the bariatric outcomes longitudinal database. Surg Obes Relat Dis. 2010;6(4):347–55. https://doi.org/10.1016/j.soard.2009.11.015.
89. Dolan JP, Diggs BS, Sheppard BC, et al. The national mortality burden and significant factors associated with open and laparoscopic cholecystectomy: 1997–2006. J Gastrointest Surg. 2009;13:2292–301.
90. Lie SA, Engesaeter LB, Havelin LI, et al. Early postoperative mortality after 67,548 total hip replacements. Acta Orthop. 2002;73(4):392–9.
91. Ricciardi R, Virnig BA, Ogilvie JW Jr. Volume-outcome relationship for coronary artery bypass grafting in an era of decreasing volume. Arch Surg. 2008;143(4):338–44.

Outcomes

92. Fouse T, Brethauer S. Resolution of comorbidities and impact on longevity following bariatric and metabolic surgery. Surg Clin North Am. 2016;96(4):717–32. https://doi.org/10.1016/j.suc.2016.03.007.
93. Lee MMY, Sattar N, Pop-Busui R, et al. Cardiovascular and kidney outcomes and mortality with long-acting injectable and oral glucagon-like peptide 1 receptor agonists in individuals with type 2 diabetes: a systematic review and meta-analysis of randomized trials. Diabetes Care. 2025;48(5):846–59. https://doi.org/10.2337/dc25-0241.

Weight Loss

94. Arterburn DE, Johnson E, Coleman KJ, et al. Weight outcomes of sleeve gastrectomy and gastric bypass compared to nonsurgical treatment. Ann Surg. 2021;274(6):e1269–76. https://doi.org/10.1097/SLA.0000000000003826.
95. Axer S, Al-Tai S, Ihle C, Alwan M, Hoffmann L. Perioperative safety and 1-year outcomes of single-anastomosis Duodeno-Ileal bypass (SADI) versus biliopancreatic diversion with duodenal switch (BPD/DS): a randomized clinical trial. Obes Surg. 2024;34(9):3382–9. https://doi.org/10.1007/s11695-024-07421-z.
96. Finno P, Osorio J, García-Ruiz-de-Gordejuela A, et al. Single versus double-anastomosis duodenal switch: single-site comparative cohort study in 440 consecutive patients. Obes Surg. 2020;30(9):3309–16. https://doi.org/10.1007/s11695-020-04566-5.
97. Gebellí JP, Lazzara C, de Gordejuela AGR, et al. Duodenal switch versus single-anastomosis duodenal switch (SADI-S) for the treatment of grade IV obesity: 5-year outcomes of a multicenter prospective cohort comparative study. Obes Surg. 2022;32(12):3839–46. https://doi.org/10.1007/s11695-022-06317-0.
98. Maciejewski ML, Arterburn DE, Van Scoyoc L, et al. Bariatric surgery and long-term durability of weight loss. JAMA Surg. 2016;151(11):1046–55. https://doi.org/10.1001/jamasurg.2016.2317.
99. O'Brien PE, Hindle A, Brennan L, et al. Long-term outcomes after bariatric surgery: a systematic review and meta-analysis of weight loss at 10 or more years for all bariatric procedures and a single-centre review of 20-year outcomes after adjustable gastric banding. Obes Surg. 2019;29(1):3–14. https://doi.org/10.1007/s11695-018-3525-0.
100. Surve A, Cottam D, Belnap L, Richards C, Medlin W. Long-term (>6 years) outcomes of duodenal switch (DS) versus single-anastomosis Duodeno-ileostomy with sleeve gastrectomy (SADI-S): a matched cohort study. Obes Surg. 2021;31(12):5117–26. https://doi.org/10.1007/s11695-021-05709-y.

Diabetes Type 2

101. Purnell JQ, Selzer F, Wahed AS, et al. Type 2 diabetes remission rates after laparoscopic gastric bypass and gastric banding: results of the longitudinal assessment of bariatric surgery study. Diabetes Care. 2016;39(7):1101–7. https://doi.org/10.2337/dc15-2138.
102. Salman AA, Salman MA, Marie MA, et al. Factors associated with resolution of type 2 diabetes mellitus after sleeve gastrectomy in obese adults. Sci Rep. 2021;11(1):6002. https://doi.org/10.1038/s41598-021-85450-9.
103. Frenken M, Kemmet O, Frenken M, et al. Long-term remission of type 2 diabetes and patient survival after biliopancreatic diversion with duodenal switch. Obes Surg. 2022;32(10):3340–50. https://doi.org/10.1007/s11695-022-06223-5.
104. Schauer PR, Bhatt DL, Kirwan JP, et al. Bariatric surgery versus intensive medical therapy for diabetes—5-year outcomes.

N Engl J Med. 2017;376(7):641–51. https://doi.org/10.1056/NEJMoa1600869.
105. Murphy R, Plank LD, Clarke MG, et al. Effect of banded Roux-en-Y gastric bypass versus sleeve gastrectomy on diabetes remission at 5 years among patients with obesity and type 2 diabetes: a blinded randomized clinical trial. Diabetes Care. 2022;45(7):1503–11. https://doi.org/10.2337/dc21-2498.
106. Sjöström L, Peltonen M, Jacobson P, et al. Association of bariatric surgery with long-term remission of type 2 diabetes and with microvascular and macrovascular complications. JAMA. 2014;311(22):2297–304. https://doi.org/10.1001/jama.2014.5988.

Hypertension

107. Ebadinejad A, Shahshahani M, Hosseinpanah F, et al. Comparison of hypertension remission and relapse after sleeve gastrectomy and one-anastomosis gastric bypass: a prospective cohort study. Hypertens Res. 2023;46(5):1287–96. https://doi.org/10.1038/s41440-023-01180-7.
108. Schiavon CA, Bhatt DL, Ikeoka D, et al. Three-year outcomes of bariatric surgery in patients with obesity and hypertension: a randomized clinical trial. Ann Intern Med. 2020;173(9):685–93. https://doi.org/10.7326/M19-3781.
109. Schiavon CA, Bersch-Ferreira AC, Santucci EV, et al. Effects of bariatric surgery in obese patients with hypertension: the GATEWAY randomized trial (gastric bypass to treat obese patients with steady hypertension). Circulation. 2018;137(11):1132–42. https://doi.org/10.1161/CIRCULATIONAHA.117.032130.

Dyslipidemia

110. Adil MT, Perera M, Whitelaw D, et al. Systematic review and meta-analysis of the effects of laparoscopic Roux-en-Y gastric bypass and laparoscopic sleeve gastrectomy on dyslipidemia. Obes Surg. 2024;34(3):967–75. https://doi.org/10.1007/s11695-023-07022-2.
111. Esparham A, Roohi S, Ahmadyar S, et al. The efficacy and safety of laparoscopic single-anastomosis duodeno-ileostomy with sleeve gastrectomy (SADI-S) in mid- and long-term follow-up: a systematic review. Obes Surg. 2023;33(12):4070–9. https://doi.org/10.1007/s11695-023-06846-2.
112. Spivak H, Sakran N, Dicker D, et al. Different effects of bariatric surgical procedures on dyslipidemia: a registry-based analysis. Surg Obes Relat Dis. 2017;13(7):1189–94. https://doi.org/10.1016/j.soard.2017.03.013.

Cardiac

113. van Veldhuisen SL, Gorter TM, van Woerden G, et al. Bariatric surgery and cardiovascular disease: a systematic review and meta-analysis. Eur Heart J. 2022;43(20):1955–69. https://doi.org/10.1093/eurheartj/ehac071.
114. Tang B, Zhang Y, Wang Y, et al. Effect of bariatric surgery on long-term cardiovascular outcomes: a systematic review and meta-analysis of population-based cohort studies. Surg Obes Relat Dis. 2022;18(8):1074–86. https://doi.org/10.1016/j.soard.2022.05.007.
115. Aminian A, Wilson R, Zajichek A, et al. Cardiovascular outcomes in patients with type 2 diabetes and obesity: comparison of gastric bypass, sleeve gastrectomy, and usual care. Diabetes Care. 2021;44(11):2552–63. https://doi.org/10.2337/dc20-3023.

Sleep Apnea

116. Al Oweidat K, Toubasi AA, Tawileh RBA, Tawileh HBA, Hasuneh MM. Bariatric surgery and obstructive sleep apnea: a systematic review and meta-analysis. Sleep Breath Schlaf Atmung. 2023;27(6):2283–94. https://doi.org/10.1007/s11325-023-02840-1.
117. Currie AC, Kaur V, Carey I, et al. Obstructive sleep apnea remission following bariatric surgery: a national registry cohort study. Surg Obes Relat Dis. 2021;17(9):1576–82. https://doi.org/10.1016/j.soard.2021.05.021.
118. Marceau P, Biron S, Hould FS, et al. Duodenal switch: long-term results. Obes Surg. 2007;17(11):1421–30. https://doi.org/10.1007/s11695-008-9435-9.

Liver

119. Aminian A, Al-Kurd A, Wilson R, et al. Association of bariatric surgery with major adverse liver and cardiovascular outcomes in patients with biopsy-proven nonalcoholic steatohepatitis. JAMA. 2021;326(20):2031–42. https://doi.org/10.1001/jama.2021.19569.
120. Cusi K, Isaacs S, Barb D, et al. American Association of Clinical Endocrinology clinical practice guideline for the diagnosis and management of nonalcoholic fatty liver disease in primary care and endocrinology clinical settings: co-sponsored by the American Association for the Study of Liver Diseases. Endocr Pract. 2022;28(5):528–62. https://doi.org/10.1016/j.eprac.2022.03.010.
121. Rinella ME, Neuschwander-Tetri BA, Siddiqui MS, et al. American Association for the Study of Liver Diseases practice guidance on the clinical assessment and management of nonalcoholic fatty liver disease. Hepatology. 2023;77(5):1797–835. https://doi.org/10.1097/HEP.0000000000000323.

Kidney

122. Abi Mosleh K, Sample JW, Belluzzi A, et al. Bariatric surgery and the diseased kidney: a 5-year assessment of safety and postoperative renal outcomes. Surg Endosc. 2024;38(7):4014–23. https://doi.org/10.1007/s00464-024-10983-9.
123. Lee Y, Anvari S, Chu MM, et al. Improvement of kidney function in patients with chronic kidney disease and severe obesity after bariatric surgery: a systematic review and meta-analysis. Nephrology. 2022;27(1):44–56. https://doi.org/10.1111/nep.13958.
124. Shulman A, Peltonen M, Sjöström CD, et al. Incidence of end-stage renal disease following bariatric surgery in the Swedish obese subjects study. Int J Obes. 2018;42(5):964–73. https://doi.org/10.1038/s41366-018-0045-x.

Cancer

125. Aminian A, Wilson R, Al-Kurd A, et al. Association of bariatric surgery with cancer risk and mortality in adults with obe-

sity. JAMA. 2022;327(24):2423–33. https://doi.org/10.1001/jama.2022.9009.
126. Clapp B, Portela R, Sharma I, et al. Risk of non-hormonal cancer after bariatric surgery: meta-analysis of retrospective observational studies. Br J Surg. 2022;110(1):24–33. https://doi.org/10.1093/bjs/znac343.
127. Wilson RB, Lathigara D, Kaushal D. Systematic review and meta-analysis of the impact of bariatric surgery on future cancer risk. Int J Mol Sci. 2023;24(7):6192. https://doi.org/10.3390/ijms24076192.

Length of Life

128. Carlsson LMS, Sjöholm K, Jacobson P, et al. Life expectancy after bariatric surgery in the Swedish obese subjects study. N Engl J Med. 2020;383(16):1535–43. https://doi.org/10.1056/NEJMoa2002449.
129. Syn NL, Cummings DE, Wang LZ, et al. Association of metabolic-bariatric surgery with long-term survival in adults with and without diabetes: a one-stage meta-analysis of matched cohort and prospective controlled studies with 174,772 participants. Lancet. 2021;397(10287):1830–41. https://doi.org/10.1016/S0140-6736(21)00591-2.

Bariatric Surgery Versus Medications

130. Sarma S, Palcu P. Weight loss between glucagon-like Peptide-1 receptor agonists and bariatric surgery in adults with obesity: a systematic review and meta-analysis. Obesity (Silver Spring). 2022;30(11):2111–21. https://doi.org/10.1002/oby.23563.
131. Brosnihan P, Luce MS, Yetasook AK, et al. Great debates: undergoing the knife versus pill-popping—the comparative efficacy and cost-effectiveness of bariatric surgery and glucagon-like Peptide-1 receptor agonists in the management of obesity. Am Surg. 2025; https://doi.org/10.1177/00031348251337145.
132. Lah S, Hocking SL. Treatment of obesity: will Incretin agonists make bariatric surgery a thing of the past? Intern Med J. 2025;55(3):369–75. https://doi.org/10.1111/imj.16625.
133. Dicker D, Sagy YW, Ramot N, et al. Bariatric metabolic surgery versus glucagon-like Peptide-1 receptor agonists and mortality. JAMA Netw Open. 2024;7(6):e2415392. https://doi.org/10.1001/jamanetworkopen.2024.15392.

Trauma Surgery

16

Christopher Kolokythas, Tammie Trinh, Michaiah Nichole Hughes, and Rosemary Kozar

Initial Approach to Patient Assessment

The primary survey (ABCDEs) is meant to rapidly evaluate threats to life or limb in the order in which loss can occur. The traditional acronym for rapid patient assessment is "ABCDE," representing Airway, Breathing, Circulation, Disability, and Exposure, and is meant to occur simultaneously with resuscitation. During the primary survey, life-threatening conditions are identified and addressed. Once life and limb threatening injuries have been adequately temporized during the primary survey, it should be followed by the secondary survey which encompasses a complete evaluation of injuries and a history. This is meant to evaluate significant injuries. Obtain imaging as indicated, consider repeating the primary survey if clinical conditions change, and consider the need for transfer to a higher level of care.

Airway

The patency of a patient's airway can easily be assessed in awake patients by asking the patient to say their name. The ability to speak, in general, indicates a patent airway. A hoarse voice, copious oral secretions or blood, significant facial trauma including penetrating face or neck wounds, and respiratory distress can all suggest a compromised airway. Additionally, comatose patients or those with high spinal cord injuries may not be able to maintain a stable airway.

To manually open the airway, a jaw thrust is preferred over the head tilt-chin lift as trauma patients should be presumed to have an unstable cervical spine injury until imaging has been obtained. The mouth should be visually inspected and any obvious obstruction removed. Basic airway adjuncts are also options to temporize physical obstruction of the airway. Nasopharyngeal airways may be used in patients with a gag reflex, using caution with facial and head trauma. Oropharyngeal airways may be used in patients who present without a gag reflex. Avoid placing an oral airway in patients with intact gag reflexes as it may trigger emesis and aspiration.

Endotracheal intubation is the standard method for definitively securing a patient's airway. Caution should be exercised when intubating a hypotensive patient as sedation and paralytics required for rapid sequence intubation can blunt the patient's compensatory sympathetic response and lead to worsening hypotension or even cardiopulmonary collapse. Temporary airway adjuncts include the laryngeal mask airway (LMA), King airway, and iGel. The goal is to occlude the esophagus and direct airflow through the trachea into the lungs. A surgical airway may be indicated if a definitive airway is otherwise unsuccessful [1]. A surgical airway should be performed by the most experienced operator available, particularly in the event of an airway emergency. Typically a cricothyroidotomy is performed emergently and then exchanged at a later time for a standard tracheostomy.

Breathing

Once the airway is patent, assess the patient's oxygenation and ventilation. Oxygenation is the process of supplying adequate oxygen to the blood, while ventilation is the process of eliminating carbon dioxide. Methods of assessing breathing include the patient's color (pallor, cyanosis, and mottling being concerning findings), pulse oximeter reading, respiratory rate, respiratory effort, and abnormal lung sounds on auscultation. A venous or arterial blood gas may be sent to measure the patient's carbon dioxide level, acid–base status, and oxygenation. Obtaining a chest x-ray can be a valu-

C. Kolokythas · T. Trinh · M. N. Hughes
Shock Trauma Center, University of Maryland Medical Center, Baltimore, MD, USA
e-mail: Ckolokythas@umm.edu; tammie.trinh@umm.edu; Michaiah.hughes@umm.edu

R. Kozar (✉)
Shock Trauma Center, University of Marylnd School of Medicine, Baltimore, MD, USA
e-mail: rkozar@som.umaryland.edu

S. Atallah, J. Dragoljevic (eds.), *Fundamentals of Surgery for Physician Assistants*, https://doi.org/10.1007/978-3-032-21069-2_16

able means of diagnosing a structural etiology of inadequate breathing such as a hemothorax, pneumothorax, rib fractures, and severe atelectasis.

Supplemental oxygen support options include nasal cannula, oxygen mask, high flow nasal cannula, CPAP (continuous positive airway pressure), and mechanical ventilation. Ventilation support includes BiPAP (bilevel positive airway pressure), which provides set inspiratory and expiratory positive pressure, and mechanical ventilation. While a thorough discussion of mechanical ventilation is beyond the scope of this chapter, basic modes to be familiar with include assist-control volume control (AC/VC), assist-control pressure control (AC/PC), and pressure support ventilation.

Circulation

The purpose of the circulatory assessment is rapid assessment and management of obvious life-threatening circulatory derangements, which can result from a wide variety of injuries. Most commonly in the trauma patient, this compromise is due to bleeding, but can also be related to changes in cardiac output or changes in circulating blood volume. Altered level of consciousness, poor skin perfusion, or a rapid thready pulse are all potential signs of hemodynamic abnormalities that can be quickly assessed while vital signs are being obtained. Physical exam may be deceiving as neither thoracic nor abdominal hemorrhage are visible externally. Long bone fractures can be an occult source of bleeding as can retroperitoneal bleeding from pelvic fractures. Assess mental status, heart rate and rhythm, respiratory rate and effort, pulse strength and location, capillary refill time, skin temperature, and skin color.

Visible bleeding should be controlled by direct manual pressure if possible. Consider a tourniquet for control of life-threatening extremity bleeding. Place a pelvic binder if instability is suspected on exam. Look for deformities of large bones and rapidly evaluate for intra-abdominal and intrathoracic injuries with adjunctive imaging. Recent data suggests that when assessing a hemodynamically unstable patient, the first three letters are rearranged from "ABC" to "CAB" (Circulation, Airway, Breathing) to emphasize the importance of circulatory stabilization [2].

Disability

Disability is a deficit in a patient's neurological status. A quick method for assessing a patient is the Glasgow Coma Scale (GCS) which is a global assessment; patients with focal neurologic deficits (such as paraplegia following a spinal cord injury) may score GCS 15 and still have significant disability.

Exposure

Exposure serves as a reminder to fully expose the patient for a thorough exam. Even tiny puncture wounds can be signs of penetrating injury causing serious internal damage. Once thoroughly examined, patients should be covered with warm blankets to avoid the possibility of hypothermia.

Adjuncts to the Primary Survey: Imaging

Chest X-ray and a pelvic film can provide valuable information as can the extended focused assessment with sonography for trauma (eFAST) exam. All can be obtained rapidly and while the patient remains in the trauma bay.

The purpose of the FAST exam is to identify intra-abdominal free fluid, which in the trauma setting is presumed to be blood. The FAST exam is sensitive enough to identify approximately 200 cc of free fluid. To complete the FAST exam, use the cardiac or abdominal ultrasound probe and view the right upper quadrant, left upper quadrant, subxiphoid area for cardiac view, and the suprapubic view as shown in Fig. 16.1. The extended FAST also includes lung images (Fig. 16.2).

In addition to physical exam and imaging, laboratory studies should be obtained. Initial laboratory testing may include complete blood count (CBC), basic metabolic panel (BMP), lactate, coagulation panel (PT, PTT, INR, fibrinogen), type and cross, and in females of child-bearing age a pregnancy test. An arterial blood gas, liver function tests, and advanced assays of coagulation such as thromboelastography can be considered.

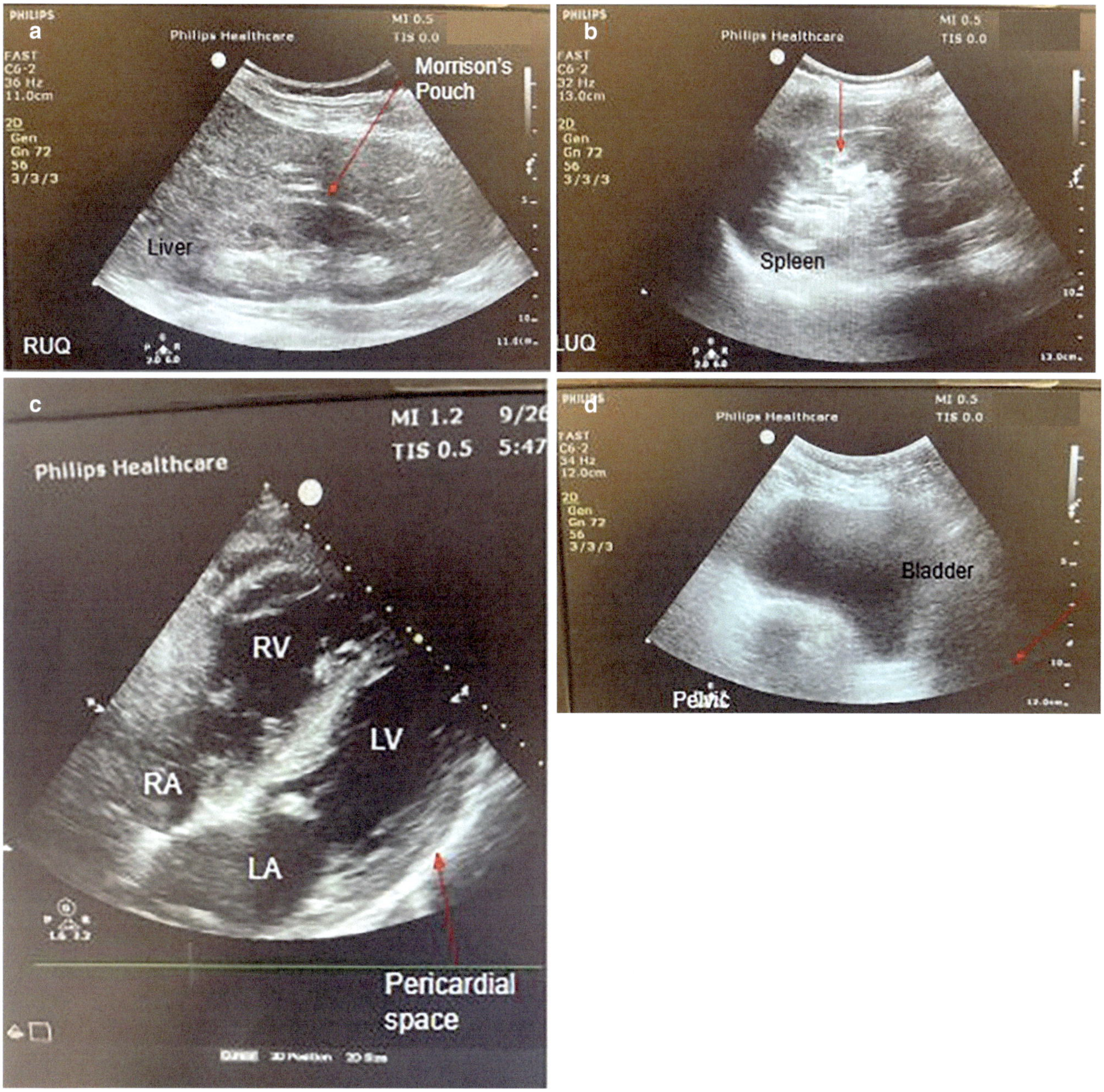

Fig. 16.1 Examples of focused assessment with sonography in trauma (FAST) images (**a**) Hepatic view—fluid stripe above liver. (**b**) Splenic view—fluid collection above the spleen. (**c**) Cardiac view—Pericardiac line. (**d**) Suprapubic view—fluid collection to the right side of the bladder wall

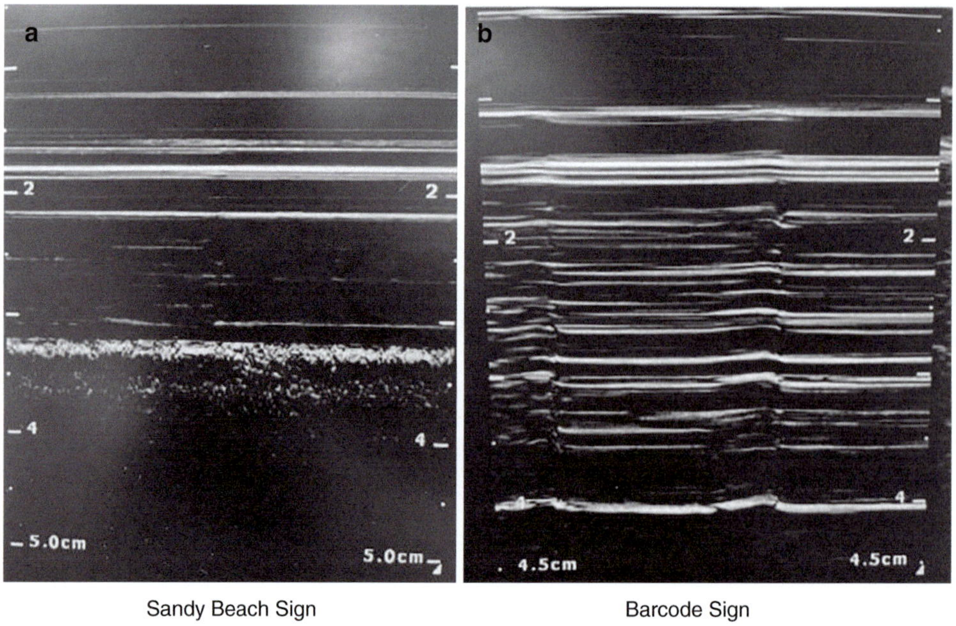

Fig. 16.2 Lung ultrasound images. (**a**) Sandy Beach Sign which represents normal motion of the lung. (**b**) Barcode Sign in which the parietal pleura is static, and suggestive of a pneumothorax

Shock

Shock is the physiologic state of inadequate perfusion. There are four broad categories of shock, including hypovolemic, obstructive, neurogenic, and cardiogenic. Although hypovolemic shock will be the most common after trauma, multiple types of shock can be present simultaneously.

Hypovolemic Shock

Hypovolemic shock is the state of inadequate circulatory volume, and in the trauma patient, it is secondary to bleeding until proven otherwise. Hemorrhagic shock is a life-threatening condition that must be identified and managed emergently. Hypotension is the classic sign of hemorrhagic shock, defined in adults as a systolic blood pressure less than 90 mm Hg and in the elderly as a pressure less than 110 mm Hg. It may be a late sign so looking for other clinical signs of hypoperfusion is important (Table 16.1). The shock index may be a more reliable indicator of shock and is defined as the heart rate divided by systolic blood pressure; 0.5–0.7 is a normal value with higher values suggesting a shock state.

The concept of damage control centers around strategies and techniques to lessen mortality and improve outcomes for injured patients in hemorrhagic shock. Damage control resuscitation (DCR) focuses on the liberal use of temporary hemorrhage-control adjuncts, early use of whole blood or balanced blood product-based transfusions, mitigation of crystalloid use, hypotensive resuscitation to promote hemostasis and decrease coagulopathy [3], and correction of ongoing metabolic derangements, followed by rapid definitive hemorrhage control [4]. Empiric administration of blood products should be followed by a more targeted strategy once lab results are available. Many centers use thromboelastography (TEG) or rotational thromboelastometry (ROTEM) for guided resuscitation. The importance of calcium administration is being increasingly recognized as an important adjunct. Calcium is a key ion in smooth muscle and cardiac muscle contractility. Hypocalcemia can be exacerbated by blood transfusion, as the preservatives in packed red blood cells chelate calcium and can lower blood calcium to dangerously low levels. As hypothermia can contribute to coagulopathy, hypothermia should be treated using external warming measures (preferably a Bair Hugger or similar device) as well as administering warmed blood products and fluids. In addition to blood product resuscitation, tranexamic acid (TXA) is an adjunctive medication for patients with hemorrhage. Anticoagulation reversal should be considered

Table 16.1 Clinical signs of hypoperfusion

Neurologic	Altered mental status (decline from baseline) *If patient is GCS < 8, consider intubation for airway protection*
Cardiac	Tachycardia (*in a patient with shock, bradycardia and hypotension is an ominous sign of decompensation and impending arrest)* Hypotension Skin color abnormalities (pallor, cyanosis, mottling) Distal pulses that are thready or not palpable Delayed capillary refill (>2–3 seconds)
Pulmonary	Tachypnea Increased work of breathing Hypoxemia
Gastrointestinal	Exam may be normal
Genitourinary	Decreased or absent urine output Metabolic acidosis (usually high anion gap metabolic acidosis due to lactic acidosis)

in patients with bleeding or at risk for bleeding that present on warfarin or direct oral anticoagulants (DOACs).

Distributive Shock

Distributive shock is inappropriately low vasomotor tone, causing hypotension and relative hypovolemia. After trauma, this is primarily due to neurogenic shock.

Cardiogenic Shock

Cardiogenic shock after trauma is rare but can stem from blunt cardiac injury and acute valve injury or an acute myocardial infarction related to the patient's preexisting cardiac disease. Combining clinical exam with a point of care ultrasound (POCUS) in the trauma bay can assist with diagnosis along with obtaining cardiac enzymes and an EKG. In the acute setting, consider a positive inotrope like epinephrine to promote cardiac contractility if the heart is hypokinetic. In the case of frank cardiac injury, emergency surgery must be considered.

Abdominal Hypertension and Compartment Syndrome

Trauma to the abdomen causes a host of hemodynamic alterations as injured visceral organs and vasculature can alter perfusion to the rest of the body. Often, the resuscitation of an acute abdominal injury requires crystalloids and blood transfusions to maintain hemodynamic goals. The increase in vascular volume can create edema within damaged organs and effusions may develop around injured organs and vasculature. Additionally, hemorrhage can contribute to any fluid collection in the abdomen, and over time, this increase in abdominal volume can build up and affect abdominal cavity pressures [5].

Normal intra-abdominal pressure (IAP) is 5–7 mmHg for critically ill adults, and < 12 mmHg is the average for most adults. Pressures greater than 12 mmHg are considered intra-abdominal hypertension (IAH), and if pressures exceed >20 mmHg with associated end-organ dysfunction, the patient is experiencing abdominal compartment syndrome (ACS). ACS, depending on the cause, can be classified as primary, secondary, or recurrent. Primary ACS is a result of a direct peritoneal or retroperitoneal injury while secondary ACS results from disease outside of the abdominal cavity. Recurrent ACS is the ongoing development of intra-abdominal hypertension despite treatment of the primary/secondary causation. Common symptoms of ACS include hypotension, persistent metabolic acidosis, respiratory failure, hypoxemia, elevated peak airway pressures, oliguria, and hyperlactemia [6].

To measure intra-abdominal pressure, a foley is placed with a closed-system pressure transducer placed at the midaxillary line at the level of the iliac crest. A normal saline bolus is infused into the bladder; 25–50 mL for adults, and pediatric patients 1 mg/kg (minimum 3 mL, maximum 25 mL). To obtain consistent measurements, it is essential that the same infusion bolus amount is applied every time and that the patient is completely relaxed and unrestricted [6, 7].

The management of ACS includes strategies that reduce abdominal pressures and decompression of the stomach and the bladder, as well as medications to relax the abdominal wall. A decompressive laparotomy is the definitive measure. With the advent of damage control resuscitation and minimization of crystalloids, the incidence of ACS has dramatically decreased [5–7].

Neurologic Injuries

Traumatic Brain Injury

Traumatic brain injury (TBI) is a major source of morbidity and mortality. Primary traumatic brain injury is caused by the initial insult, whereas secondary brain injury occurs in the hours and days following the incident. Secondary brain injury is the result of cellular damage and ischemia that can be from hypotension, hyperthermia, and hypoxia, and metabolic demand. Prevention of secondary brain injury is the ultimate goal in the management of traumatic brain injury. Grading of TBI by severity is based on the Glasgow Coma Scale which ranges from 3 to 15 with 3 being the lowest score and 15 the highest (Table 16.2) [8].

A neurological exam is part of the "disability" portion of the primary survey. It includes an assessment of level of consciousness (GCS score), pupillary reflexes, and examination of focal neurologic deficits. Noncontrast CT of the head is

Table 16.2 Glasgow Coma Scale

Glasgow Coma Scale		
Eye opening	Spontaneous	4
	To voice	3
	To pain	2
	None	1
Verbal response	Oriented	5
	Confused	4
	Incomprehensible words	3
	Incomprehensible sounds	2
	None	1
Motor response	Follows commands	6
	Localizes	5
	Withdraws	4
	Flexion	3
	Extension	2
	None	1

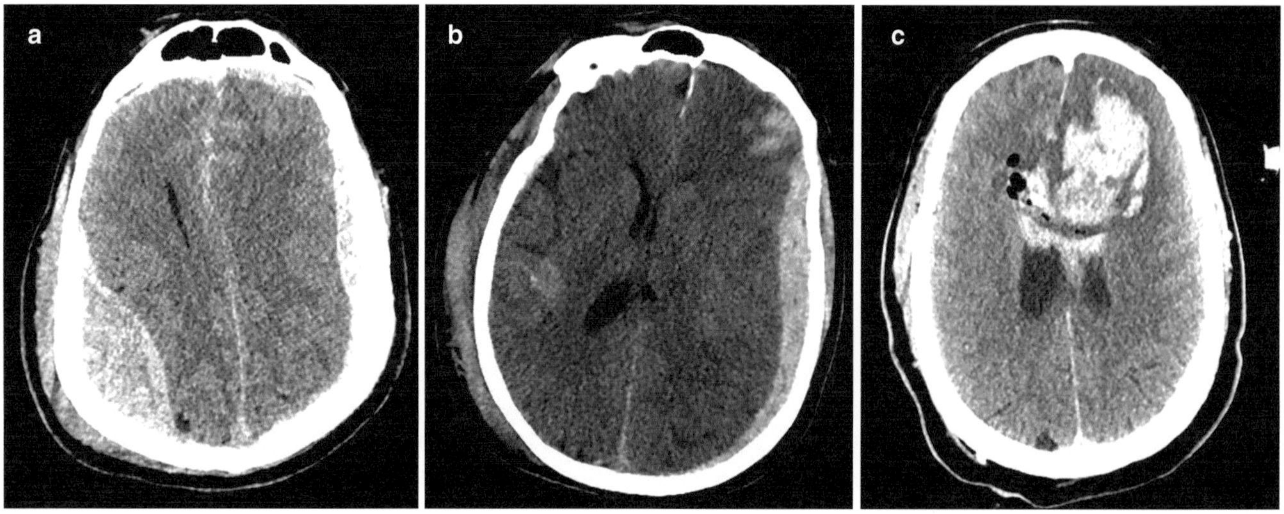

Fig. 16.3 CT images of traumatic brain injuries. (**a**) Epidural hematoma with midline shift. (**b**) Subdural hematoma. (**c**) Intracranial hemorrhage

the preferred modality of imaging for a suspected brain injury. In a normal brain, parenchyma will have distinct gray-white matter differentiation and cerebrospinal fluid of the ventricular system will appear black. Acute blood, however, will appear as bright white. Mass effect can be assessed by evaluating displacement or compression of certain anatomical structures such as the ventricles, basal cisterns, and sulci. Displacement of the lateral ventricles is referred to as midline shift (Fig. 16.3a).

Types of Brain Injuries

There are a number of different types of brain injuries. An epidural hematoma (EDH) is a hemorrhage that occurs between the skull and the dura mater. It is often secondary to a vascular disruption of the middle meningeal artery and is often associated with a skull fracture. On computed tomography (CT), epidural hematomas have a *convex* lens shape and do not cross suture lines (Fig. 16.3a). Patients presenting with an epidural hematoma may sometimes have a period of lucidity before developing neurological decompensation. Epidural hematomas frequently require surgical evacuation. Subdural hematomas (SDHs) appear as a *concave* shape hemorrhage on CT (Fig. 16.3b). They often occur as a vascular disruption to the bridging veins from the cerebral cortex to the venous sinus of the brain between the dura mater and subarachnoid space of the brain. Large SDHs that exhibit mass effect may require evacuation and decompressive craniotomy. Intracranial hemorrhages (ICHs) appear as hyperdense collections within the brain parenchyma and are often surrounded by a hypodense layer of edema (Fig. 16.3c). Traumatic subarachnoid hemorrhages (tSAHs) occur when there is disruption to blood vessels that lead to blood in the subarachnoid space. Unlike aneurysmal subarachnoid hemorrhages which are usually a hyperdense bleed near the Circle of Willis, tSAHs can be seen as a hyperdense layer of blood along the cerebral sulci, ventricular system, or adjacent to cerebral contusions. Cerebral contusions are often located in the frontal and temporal lobes of the cortex and can cause local edema and ischemia. Finally, diffuse axonal injury (DAI) is a type of injury that causes shearing to the white matter of the brain as a result of high velocity mechanisms of injury. It can appear as small petechial hemorrhages at multiple levels of the brain, commonly affecting the corpus callosum. It is best appreciated on magnetic resonance imaging (MRI). DAI should be suspected in patients with a poor neurologic exam out of proportion to the injury seen on CT scan.

Skull fractures can be categorized as linear, depressed, or basilar. Linear skull fractures are the most common and carry minimal clinical importance if not associated with an underlying brain injury. The temporal and parietal skull are the most common site of linear skull fractures. Depressed skull fractures may compress or pierce underlying brain injury and may require surgical intervention. Basilar skull fractures are the most concerning as they may indicate a dural tear and cerebral spinal fluid (CSF) leak. Two clinical signs of a basilar skull fracture include a Battle sign, ecchymosis of the mastoid process, and Raccoon sign, or periorbital ecchymosis. These patients should be monitored carefully for CSF leak [9].

Sequelae and Treatment of TBIs

Early neurosurgical consultation should be obtained for patients with a TBI. Initial management includes measures to mitigate hypotension and hypoxia as well as to optimize cerebral blood flow and reduce cerebral edema. Sequelae of traumatic brain injury may include intracranial hypertension, posttraumatic seizure, fever, paroxysmal sympathetic hyperactivity, agitation and delirium, and altered mental status. The strategies to manage these complications will be discussed below.

Intracranial hypertension is defined as an intracranial pressure (ICP) greater than 22 mm Hg for greater than 5 minutes [10]. Intracranial hypertension, if uncontrolled, can lead to brain herniation and death. When there is an increase in one intracranial component, CSF and cerebral blood flow must compensate to maintain a stable intracranial pressure. Cerebral blood flow is able to be maintained at a constant over a range of systemic blood pressure when cerebral autoregulation is intact. However, cerebral autoregulation is altered in TBI, leading to uncontrolled pressure in the cranial vault and ultimately intracranial hypertension. Cerebral perfusion pressure (CPP) can be used as a surrogate for cerebral blood flow and calculated by:

$$\text{CPP} = \text{mean arterial pressure}(\text{MAP}) - \text{intracranial pressure}(\text{ICP}).$$

Monitoring ICP can be done through various devices, such as external ventricular drains (EVDs) and intracranial bolts. EVDs are distinguished from other ICP monitoring devices for their ability to provide therapeutic drainage of CSF in addition to monitoring ICP. An EVD must be leveled at the patient's tragus, a landmark that correlates with the midbrain [10]. Drainage of CSF is done through gravity, and EVDs can be raised or lowered to hasten or slow gravity drainage. EVDs can also be clamped, continuously drained, or intermittently drained. When assessing an ICP waveform, there are three characteristic peaks that correlate to different phases of the cardiac cycle. Each peak should be lower than the last. When P2 is greater than P1, alterations in brain compliance and intracranial hypertension should be suspected (Fig. 16.4).

There are several strategies to lower elevated ICPs which include positioning (head of bed elevation), minimization of noxious stimuli (such as suctioning, turning, and frequent catheterization), sedation and analgesia, hyperosmolar therapy, optimizing ventilation, cerebral spinal fluid drainage, and decompressive craniectomy. Steroid administration is not recommended in TBI patients and has been associated with increased mortality [10, 11]. Patients should be positioned with a head of bed at 30° or higher and maintain a midline neck positioning to optimize jugular venous drainage from the brain. Sedation and analgesia can temporarily lower ICPs. Medications such as propofol, opioids, and benzodiazepines are all effective [11].

Hyperosmolar therapy is one of the most common and effective methods in lowering ICPs. There are two types of hyperosmolar therapy, hypertonic saline, and mannitol.

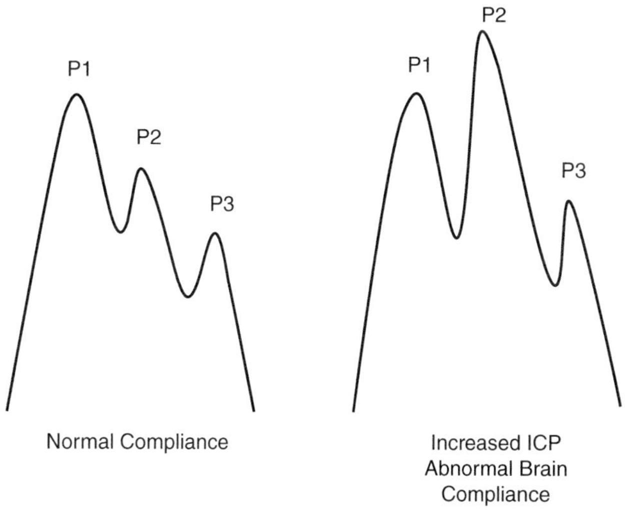

Fig. 16.4 Intracranial cerebral pressure (ICP) waveforms of normal and abnormal brain compliance

There has been no proven difference in efficacy between mannitol administration compared to hypertonic saline [10, 11]. Hypertonic saline can be readily administered and is available in several concentrations (3%, 7%, 23.4%). Mannitol can induce large volume diuresis; therefore, it is important to ensure euvolemia during administration. Targeting a CPP of 60–70 mm in patients with elevated ICPs can help maintain adequate cerebral perfusion [10]. Fluids or vasopressors can be used to reach this target.

Optimizing ventilation is another strategy that is useful in controlling ICPs. Reducing carbon dioxide causes cerebral vasoconstriction. Normocapnia is recommended for all patients with TBI. Hyperventilation to target a $PaCO_2$ of 30–35 mm Hg is recommended only as a temporizing measure in patients with refractory intracranial hypertension [10, 11].

Finally, decompressive craniectomy can be used for refractory intracranial hypertension [12, 13]. When performed early and after optimized medical management for ICPs, it has been shown to improve mortality [13].

Blood Pressure Targets

Hypotension potentiates secondary brain injury, cerebral hypoperfusion, and cerebral ischemia and therefore should be avoided. The goal is to maintain a systolic blood pressure greater than 100 mm Hg in patients aged 50–69 years and a systolic blood pressure greater than 110 mm Hg in patients aged 15–49 years or greater than 70 years old [10].

Some controversy exists regarding the management of hypertension, with targeting a systolic blood pressure below 160 mm Hg due to risk of worsening hemorrhage being a common practice.

Paroxysmal Sympathetic Hyperactivity

Paroxysmal sympathetic hyperactivity (PSH) is a phenomenon in which the injured brain releases catecholamines resulting in intermittent fever, tachycardia, hypertension, diaphoresis, and muscle rigidity. It happens as a sequela of TBI and does not immediately manifest. When diagnosing PSH, it is important to distinguish it from other conditions that may mimic its features such as sepsis [14]. Management of PSH is done through preventive and abortive medications. First-line preventive medications include bromocriptine and propranolol. Other medications that can be helpful are gabapentin, clonidine, benzodiazepine, propofol, and dexmedetomidine. Abortive medications include opioids such as intravenous morphine and benzodiazepines such as valium.

Temperature Management

Fever increases the metabolic demand of the body and is thought to deprive the injured brain of much needed cellular nutrients and oxygen. Fever should be avoided when feasible. In patients with severe TBI with intracranial monitoring in place, targeted temperature management with active cooling to normothermia especially during the first 7 days can be employed [11].

Posttraumatic Seizure

Patients with traumatic brain injury are at high risk for developing seizure especially within the first 7 days following injury during which time prophylaxis is generally recommended. Regarding the choice of antiepileptic drugs, no drug has been shown to be more effective than others but generally levetiracetam or fosphenytoin are used for prophylaxis [10].

Diabetes Insipidus

TBI can cause direct damage to the pituitary gland which results in decreased secretion of antidiuretic hormone. This leads to large volume diuresis of dilute urine, hypovolemia, and electrolyte disturbances known as central diabetes insipidus. It should be suspected in a patient with TBI and polyuria (greater than 30 mL/kg/hour or 200 mL/hour for 2 consecutive hours). The diagnosis can be confirmed by a low urine osmolality, high serum osmolality, and hypernatremia. Treatment includes fluid administration to restore euvolemia and administration of desmopressin, a synthetic analog of vasopressin [15].

Spinal Cord Injuries

Spinal cord injuries (SCIs) cause a significant amount of disability and burden upon the individual, their support system, and the healthcare system. The most common mechanisms that lead to SCI are motor vehicle collisions and unintentional falls [16, 17]. Other common mechanisms include gunshot wounds and sports injuries. Older age is considered an independent risk factor for SCI given the degenerative changes to the spine that are observed with age [16].

It is important to review the anatomy of the spinal cord in order to discuss the evaluation and management of patients with spinal cord injury, taking care to remember the functions of the different levels of the spinal cord as well as the functions of the different ascending and descending tracts of the spinal cord.

Primary spinal cord injury occurs at the time of trauma and results in direct destruction of the nervous tissue of the spinal cord. Secondary spinal cord injury is the subsequent cascade of inflammation, cellular excitotoxicity, edema, hemorrhage, and ischemia that occurs in the hours to weeks following an injury [17, 18]. Secondary spinal cord injury may lead to the manifestation of spinal cord dysfunction beyond the level of the primary spinal cord injury. Injuries to the vertebrae of the spine can lead to compression, contusion, and shearing to the nearby spinal cord. Ligamentous injury can lead to instability and lack of support to the vertebrae and also lead to misalignment and dislocation.

Diagnosis and Evaluation

SCI should be suspected in patients presenting with spinal trauma, neck tenderness, numbness, or motor deficit. Spinal precautions include placing the patient in a hard cervical collar, using a backboard for transport, and log roll technique for turns [16, 18]. Spinal precautions should be maintained until SCI can be excluded, especially for patients with altered mental status who are unable to participate in a complete exam.

The American Spinal Injury Association (ASIA) impairment scale helps communicate the degree of spinal cord dysfunction. The ASIA score is stated as a numerical number followed by an alphabetical letter. The numerical number is based on a total score of the level strength of each muscle group and sensitivity of each dermatome. The score ranges from 0 to 100, with 100 being the highest score in a neurologically intact person [16]. The alphabetic letter refers to the completeness or incompleteness of the spinal cord injury (Table 16.3) [16].

Non-contrast computed tomography (CT) is the initial diagnostic imaging of choice in suspected SCI due to its abil-

Table 16.3 ASIA Scale for spinal cord injury

ASIA Impairment Scale	
A	Complete spinal cord injury Absent motor and sensory function
B	Sensory incomplete Sensory function is preserved but not motor function
C	Motor incomplete Motor function is preserved but not sensory function Muscle strength less than grade 3
D	Motor incomplete Motor function is preserved but not sensory function Muscle strength is greater than grade 3
E	Normal sensory and motor function

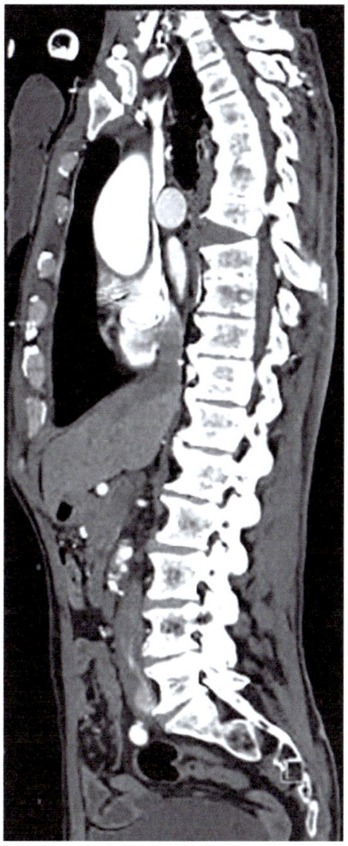

Fig. 16.5 CT image of a thoracic T7-T8 flexion extension distraction injury

ity to quickly evaluate for unstable bony fractures (Fig. 16.5). Magnetic resonance imaging (MRI) is needed to assess the spinal cord and supportive ligaments of the spine, and should be obtained urgently if there is concern for ongoing spinal cord compression [16, 18]. Prompt spine consultation should be obtained. Recent guidelines recommend patients with an acute SCI, regardless of level, undergo surgery within 24 hours after injury when medically feasible, based on data of improved functional recovery [17].

Neurogenic Shock and Spinal Shock

Neurogenic shock is a type of distributive shock associated with acute SCI and is characterized by hypotension and an absence of compensatory tachycardia. It occurs when there is a loss of regulation of the autonomic nervous system after SCI and is most frequently seen with an injury above the level of T6. Neurogenic shock should not be confused for spinal shock, which is a loss of spinal cord activity and reflexes below the level of an injury. Spinal shock can last for days to weeks and is related to the initial injury and subsequent hemorrhage, edema, and inflammation of the spinal cord. Spinal shock will recover as there is neuronal healing, collateralization, and reorganization [16]. Neurogenic shock, on the other hand, refers to a cardiovascular complication of SCI. Initial treatment is fluid to restore the relative hypovolemia with vasopressor support if further augmentation is needed. Neurogenic shock can often be accompanied by bradycardia, so when selecting a vasopressor it is important to choose a medication that has both beta- and alpha-adrenergic receptor effects such as norepinephrine.

For hemodynamically stable patients, enteral albuterol is preferred for treatment of bradycardia, but phosphodiesterase inhibitors such aminophylline or theophylline can also be considered [16]. Chronotropic intravenous medications such as atropine for the hemodynamically significant bradycardia.

Autonomic Dysreflexia

Autonomic dysreflexia is the result of a loss of regulation of the autonomic nervous system at or above the level of T6. It is characterized by an unopposed sympathetic response to stimuli below the level of spinal cord injury, such as bladder distention, gastric distention, or tight dressings and garments. Symptoms may include hypertension, tachycardia, diaphoresis, flushing, and headache. This sympathetic response can be so severe that, if uncontrolled, can lead to stroke, seizures, and myocardial infarction. Treatment of autonomic dysreflexia is to first remove the stimulus. If this does not improve, medications may be added [16].

Blood Pressure Augmentation

Practices regarding blood pressure augmentation for patients with SCI vary widely, and definitive guidelines are not established. There is some evidence to support the augmentation of blood pressure to target a mean arterial pressure (MAP) above 85 mm Hg to improve spinal cord perfusion [16, 18, 19]. This usually requires intravenous vasopressor support in the form of norepinephrine, though oral midodrine can be added to reduce intravenous requirements.

Bowel and Bladder Management

Patients with SCI may often experience neurogenic bowel and bladder dysfunction and are therefore prone to constipation and urinary retention. Regular bowel movements are important to prevent complications such as autonomic dysreflexia and ileus. It is important to institute a bowel regimen with laxatives, enemas and suppositories, and mobility early for patients with SCI to achieve a goal of regular bowel movements. Neurogenic bladder dysfunction can lead to urinary complications such as retention, urinary tract infections, and overflow incontinence. Patients who exhibit neurogenic bladder dysfunction require intermittent catheterization. Suprapubic catheters may be considered as a long-term solution when there are lower urinary tract complications (infections, abscess, skin breakdown) or anatomic abnormalities (strictures, false passages, fistulas) but are rarely required [16].

Blunt Cerebrovascular Injury

Blunt cerebrovascular injury (BCVI) is a nonpenetrating injury to either the vertebral or internal carotid arteries. The incidence of BCVI is estimated to be within 2–7% of trauma patients, although this percentage may be underappreciated due to underdiagnosis and lack of universal screening protocols. Up to 20% of patients with BCVI may develop stroke if it is not rapidly diagnosed and treated. The highest risk of stroke is within the first 72 hours. Cervical spine fractures are one of the most predictive risk factors for developing BCVI, with nearly a quarter of all patients with a cervical spine injury found to have a BCVI. Screening protocols, such as the Denver criteria or Memphis criteria, have increased the detection of BCVI. With the wide variety of identified risk factors, some institutions perform routine screening of BCVI for all major trauma patients. Computed tomography angiography of head and neck is used to both screen and diagnose BCVI. The goal of treating BCVI is to decrease the risk of stroke and its associated morbidity and mortality. It is recommended to start anticoagulation or antiplatelet therapy once diagnosis of BCVI is confirmed and deemed safe [20].

Thoracic Trauma

The thoracic cavity includes the heart, lungs, mediastinum, esophagus, trachea, pleural membranes, and diaphragm. They are protected by the rib cage, sternum, and thoracic spine. Injury can occur through either blunt or penetrating mechanisms.

Blunt Cardiac Injury (BCI)

BCI to the heart is rare, and symptoms and manifestations can widely vary. The most common mechanism for BCI is motor vehicle collision; however, BCI has also been observed in pedestrians struck by motor vehicles, falls from great height, crush injuries, assault, and sporting injuries. BCI has diverse clinical presentations, ranging from completely asymptomatic, cardiac arrhythmias, or even as life-threatening cardiac wall rupture [21].

The diagnosis of BCI can be made by electrocardiogram (ECG) and serum troponin level. ECG alone is used in many centers, but the addition of a troponin that is normal can rule out an injury. If a troponin level is elevated, it should be trended for monitoring. Echocardiogram can be added as a diagnostic evaluation for patients with hypotension or arrhythmias [22].

Management of BCI is largely supportive and varies with the etiology. Patients with any ECG changes or elevation in serum troponin level should be monitored with telemetry [22]. Surgical repair is rare and usually reserved when there is a structural defect such as valvular injury or in the rare instance of rupture, typically atrial. If a structural injury is identified on echocardiogram or clinically, emergent surgical consultation is indicated [21].

Blunt Thoracic Aortic Injury

Blunt thoracic aortic injury (BTAI) is defined as an injury to the aorta due to shearing and stretching forces. BTAI can occur anywhere along the aorta from the ascending aorta to the iliac bifurcation. The most common location is the aortic isthmus, which is thought to be an area of weakness as it is the transition point between the ascending aorta and fixed descending thoracic aorta. BTAI can lead to fatal aortic rupture with as many as 80% of patients with BTAI thought to die in the field before arriving at the hospital [23].

Mechanisms of injury leading to BTAI are usually high in energy with rapid acceleration and deceleration forces, such as motor vehicle collision, motorcycle collision, pedestrian struck, or fall from significant heights [23, 24]. Patients with BTAI may have complaints of chest pain, back pain between the scapula, trouble breathing, and dyspnea or frequently may be asymptomatic.

Early diagnosis of BTAI is crucial as the risk of aortic rupture is the highest within 24 hours of presentation [23]. Though chest X-ray may be suggestive (Fig. 16.6a), diagnosis is by computed tomography angiography (CTA) of the chest due to its high sensitivity and specificity [23, 24]. Grading of injuries and typical management is shown in Table 16.4 [23], and a CT images of a grade 3 injury is shown in Fig. 16.6b, c [24].

Medical management of BTAI consists of heart rate and blood pressure control, which decrease the shearing forces and pressure on the injured aorta. In general, targeting a heart rate of less than 100 beats per minute and a systolic blood pressure of less than 120 mm Hg is indicated [23]. Esmolol, a cardioselective beta blocker, is the drug of choice for rate control. Nonselective beta blockers can be used for blood pressure control, as well as infusions of calcium channel blockers, nitroprusside, or nitroglycerin.

There are two techniques to repair BTAI, endovascular repair or open surgery. Both carry the risk of spinal cord ischemia, resultant paraplegia, and stroke. However, thoracic endovascular aortic repair (TEVAR) is preferred over open

Table 16.4 Grading scale for blunt thoracic aortic injuries

Blunt thoracic aortic injury		
Grade 1	Intimal tear	Nonoperative management
Grade 2	Intramural hematoma	Nonoperative or operative
Grade 3	Pseudoaneurysm	Surgery indicated
Grade 4	Rupture	Emergent surgery indicated

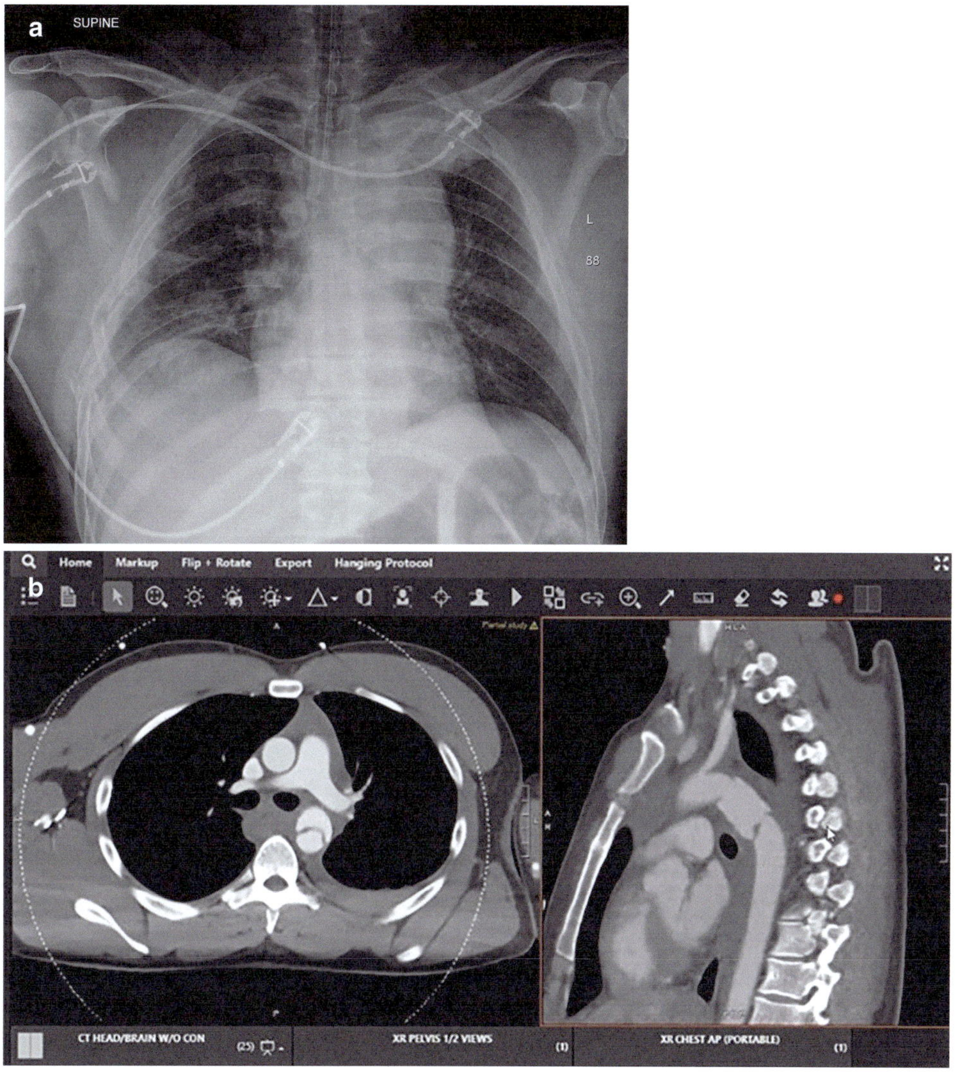

Fig. 16.6 Images of blunt aortic injuries. (**a**) Plain chest radiograph of a widened mediastinum, suggestive of a blunt aortic injury. (**b** and **c**) CT images of a grade 3 blunt aortic injury

surgical repair due to its significantly lower risks and overall lower perioperative mortality [23, 24]. TEVAR may result though in late complications such as endoleak, in-stent thrombosis, and occlusion of left carotid or left subclavian veins from graft migration [23]. Because of these complications, long-term follow-up and graft surveillance with imaging is needed.

Rib Fractures

Rib fractures are a common injury that is thought to occur in approximately 10% of all trauma patients. The mechanism of injury leading to rib fractures is usually blunt trauma [25]. Rib fractures can range from simple, nondisplaced fractures to severe flail chest, which is defined as three or more ribs broken in two or more places [26]. The result is a segment of ribs that exhibits a paradoxical movement from the rest of the chest during inspiration and expiration. Flail chest is associated with a mortality rate as high as 10–20% and can cause respiratory failure due to underlying pulmonary contusions. Rib fractures can cause pain which leads to poor inspiratory effort, atelectasis, and hypoxic respiratory failure [26]. In addition, the broken ribs can cause tears and punctures to the underlying pleura, causing pneumothorax and hemothorax. The elderly are at particular risk for respiratory failure and higher mortality following rib fractures due to the physiological changes that occur with age, such as chest wall stiffness, decreased muscle strength, decreased lung compliance, and decreased vital capacity [25, 27].

Rib fractures can be seen easily on chest radiograph (Fig. 16.7); however, CT chest is ultimately more sensitive for rib features. When identifying rib fractures, it is important to assess the number of ribs broken, the laterality of rib fractures, anterior or posterior fractures, the amount of displacement, and any associated pneumothorax, hemothorax, or pulmonary contusion.

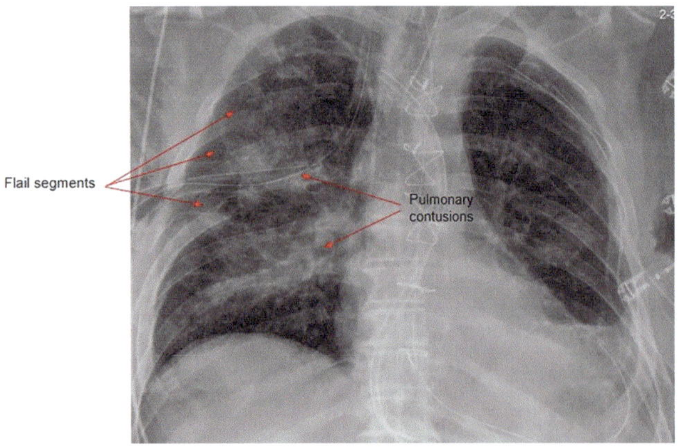

Fig. 16.7 X-ray image of bilateral rib fractures with flail segment and pulmonary contusion

Management of rib fractures is mostly supportive, with an emphasis on volume expansion and pain management. Patients who are older than 65 years old or who are considered frail with two or more rib fractures should be considered for admission to a monitored unit. Patients who are at risk for worsening respiratory failure are those who are hypoxic and require supplemental oxygen to maintain a SpO_2 greater than 92% or poor volume expansion on incentive spirometry (less than 15/kg ideal body weight). Pain control is also key to management [25, 27]. If uncontrolled, it can lead to the development of atelectasis and hypoxic respiratory failure. A multimodal pain regimen is recommended with medications such as acetaminophen, nonsteroidal anti-inflammatory medications, gabapentinoids, and antispasmodic drugs. Opioid minimization is encouraged. Regional pain management with epidurals and nerve blocks can also be employed to improve outcomes, particularly for the elderly [25, 27, 28]. Epidurals can be placed at the thoracic level of the spine to provide continuous infusion of opioids or local anesthetics. Thoracic paravertebral blockade provides unilateral segmental or sympathetic nerve blockade and can be performed as a single injection or as continuous analgesia [28]. Hypoxia can be managed with supplemental oxygen. Noninvasive positive pressure ventilation (NIPPV) with high flow nasal cannula or continuous positive airway pressure (CPAP) is reasonable in patients that have persistent hypoxia despite supplemental oxygen. There is a low threshold to proceed to intubation for patients who fail NIPPV.

Most rib fractures will be managed nonoperatively with the supportive strategies discussed above. Indications for operative stabilization are controversial but when done may be performed through a minimally invasive approach or via open thoracotomy. Some studies have reported that early operative fixation can lead to decreased complications such as days of mechanical ventilation, incidence of pneumonia, and requirement for tracheostomy [26].

Pulmonary Contusion

Pulmonary contusion, or "bruising" of the lung occurs primarily following blunt thoracic trauma and is almost always associated with rib fractures except in children who have a compliant chest wall. Pulmonary contusion is the most common blunt thoracic injury, with an incidence of approximately 30–75% of all blunt chest trauma. Contusions can trigger an inflammatory reaction in the lung that results in cytokine activation, increased neutrophil activation, and capillary leakage of fluid into the alveoli. This leads to reduced gas exchange, increased pulmonary vascular resistance, reduced lung compliance, and ultimately hypoxic respiratory failure.

It is not necessary to overly fluid restrict patients with pulmonary contusions, but it is important to avoid excessive volume administration. If there is evidence of volume overload, diuretics can be administered as appropriate. If associated hypoxia, trials of NIPPV with high flow nasal cannula or CPAP help maintain alveolar recruitment in patients with natural airways, as can positive end expiratory pressure (PEEP) if the patient is mechanically ventilated. Steroids are not helpful in the management of pulmonary contusion [29].

Pneumothorax

Pneumothorax occurs when there is accumulation of air in the pleural space. It can be seen with both blunt and penetrating trauma and is caused by any force or penetration that causes violation of the pleura. Pneumothoraxes range from being small and inconsequential to large and life-threatening, such as in the case of tension pneumothorax. Tension pneumothorax (Fig. 16.8a) is a life-threatening condition that occurs when the accumulation of air exerts a mass effect on the intrathoracic structures, resulting in compression of the vena cava and cardiac chambers that leads to hemodynamic instability. Signs of tension include hypotension, jugular vein distention, muffled heart sounds, tracheal deviation, dyspnea, and hypoxia. In an unstable patient, chest tube insertion should be immediately performed. Intervention should not be delayed while waiting for a chest radiograph if suspicion of tension pneumothorax is high. Point-of-care ultrasound can also be useful in rapidly identifying pneumothorax at the bedside by assessing lung sliding with respirations [30]. Indications for chest tube placement depend on a combination of pneumothorax size as well as the patient's respiratory status, oxygenation, and need for mechanical ventilation. Most pneumothoraxes can be managed with a small-bore tube.

Hemothorax

Hemothorax occurs when there is an accumulation of blood in the pleural space around the lungs. Hemothorax can be identified on chest radiographs; however, chest CT is more sensitive and can help estimate the volume of blood present in the chest cavity. If sizable, chest drainage is advisable (Fig. 16.8b). Indications for surgery include initial output greater than 1500 mL or greater than 200 mL per hour for 4 or more hours, though it also depends on etiology and hemodynamics. If there is inadequate drainage of blood from the pleural cavity after chest tube placement, a residual hemothorax is present. Larger volume residuals are at risk for later developing into an empyema. Early video-assisted thoracoscopic surgery (VATS) is generally indicated, and thrombolytic therapy is an alternative generally reserved for patients that are poor surgical candidates [30].

Penetrating Chest Trauma

Patients who presen with penetrating injuries that are between the nipple lines, below the sternal notch, and above the epigastric area are at risk for injury to the heart or great

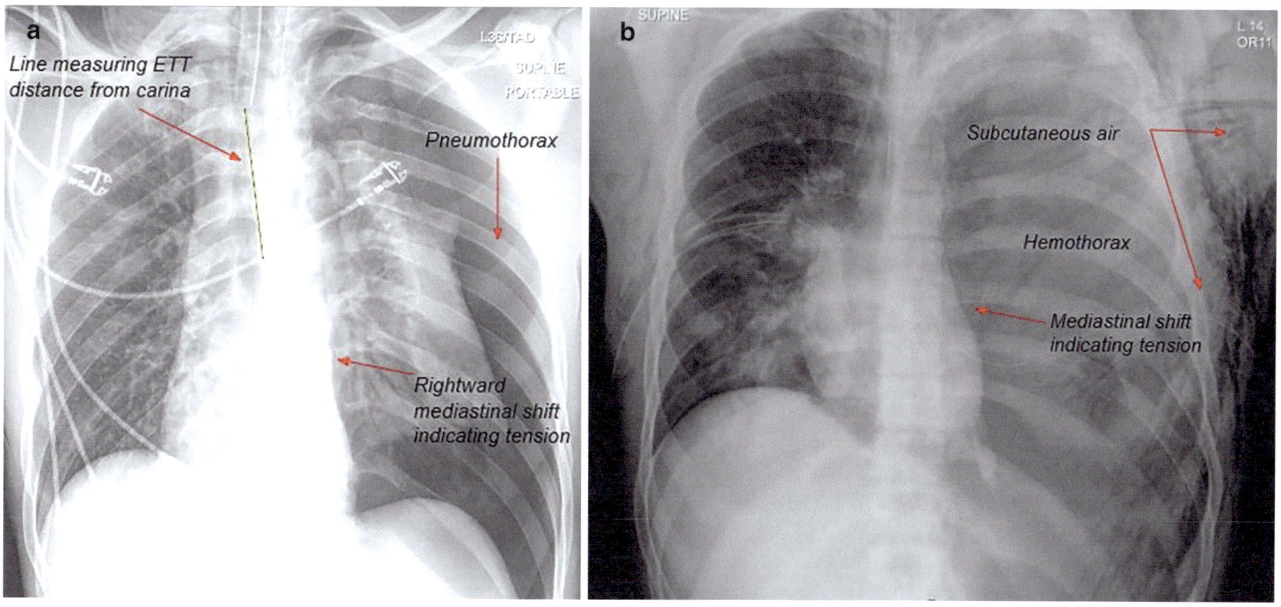

Fig. 16.8 (**a**) X-ray image of a left pneumothorax. Mediastinal shift toward the right is also demonstrated (**b**) X-ray image of a tension hemothorax. The left chest is full of blood with mediastinal shift towards the right

vessels. This area is sometimes referred to as "the danger zone" or "the cardiac box." If a patient has a penetrating injury to this central zone and is hemodynamically unstable, emergent surgery is indicated. Patients who exhibit signs of cardiac tamponade with positive findings on FAST ultrasound should be taken immediately to the operating room. Penetrating cardiac injuries will require open operative repair. It is important to understand that a penetrating cardiac injury can be present with a negative FAST of the heart if the pericardial blood has decompressed into the thoracic cavity, presenting as a hemothorax. Also, injuries to the heart can occur outside of the cardiac box. A chest X-ray and a chest CT can be used to aid diagnosis. A CT is helpful to visualize trajectory and at times diagnose injury if no pericardial blood is seen on FAST.

Diaphragmatic injuries should be suspected with injuries below the level of the nipple and maybe be difficult to see on chest CT. Laparoscopy can be performed in stable patients with a high degree of suspicion. If aerodigestive injury is suspected based on air seen on chest CT, bronchoscopy, flexible esophagoscopy, or esophagogastroduodenoscopy can be performed to evaluate for injury to the trachea or esophagus. Finally, if a patient presents with impalement from a foreign object, surgery and general anesthesia may be required for debridement and control of any hemorrhage from object removal [30].

Resuscitative Thoracotomy

A resuscitative thoracotomy is an emergency procedure done in the trauma bay in patients who present in extremis. Penetrating injuries are more likely to be intervenable with resuscitative thoracotomy than blunt injuries and therefore have a higher survival. Therefore, resuscitative thoracotomy is recommended for pulseless patients with penetrating thoracic injury and signs of life. Signs of life are defined as having pupillary response, spontaneous respirations, presence of a carotid pulse, detectable blood pressure, visible extremity movement, or electrical cardiac activity.

Extrathoracic injuries include those that involve the neck, abdomen, or extremities. Time elapsed from the last observed signs of life is very important in determining if resuscitative thoracotomy is appropriate. The longer the absence of signs of life, the poorer the prognosis and likelihood that performing resuscitative thoracotomy may be futile. Resuscitative thoracotomy is strongly recommended against pulseless patients with blunt injury without signs of life. Resuscitative endovascular balloon occlusion of the aorta (REBOA) is now being used as an alternative in patients with extrathoracic injuries [31].

Abdominal Trauma

Blunt Versus Penetrating Abdominal Trauma

Abdominal trauma can be categorized as either blunt abdominal trauma (BAT) or penetrating abdominal trauma (PAT) and should be defined by the anatomical region of the injury: peritoneal, retroperitoneal, or pelvic. Understanding the anatomical region will help the clinician evaluate specific injuries [32].

Blunt abdominal trauma can present with signs and symptoms or be asymptomatic; therefore, a high degree of suspicion is needed. External signs such as a seat belt sign can suggest intra-abdominal injury. With penetrating injuries, any wound that violates the fascia needs additional investigation. Not only should the clinician consider structural parenchymal damage, but also any contamination the site has experienced from external sources of the body, as well as internal contamination such as from the gastrointestinal tract. The degree of injury depends on the depth of penetration, the trajectory of the penetrating object, and the amount of force exerted on the body. Penetrating injuries can cause direct damage to structures in the pathway of the object as well as extended injury to surrounding organs from a blast injury in the event of firearm or explosive injuries. High velocity injuries, such as a motor vehicle collision, have a large amount of energy transference onto the body, and as a result patients will have an exponentially higher mortality rate from these types of injuries [33–35].

Typically, penetrating injuries will require a surgical consultation. Hemodynamically unstable patients should be emergently taken for an exploratory laparotomy to gain hemostatic control, stabilization, and diagnosis of the extent of injury. Hemodynamically stable patients will typically undergo a CT scan for further evaluation, though a variety of options exist [35]. For all emergent trauma procedures of the abdomen, a midline laparotomy is preferred.

Specific Abdominal Organ Injuries: Assessment and Management

Solid Organ Injuries

Solid organ injuries include injuries to the spleen, liver, kidney, and pancreas. Injuries are graded per the American Association for the Surgery of Trauma (AAST). In general, hemodynamically unstable patients with a positive FAST exam should proceed directly to the operating room. Stable patients with abdominal trauma should undergo CT angiography to diagnose and classify injuries. Dual-phase imaging to include both arterial and portal venous phases is recommended [36, 37]. New to the AAST classifications are the inclusion of vascular injuries, defined as a pseudoaneurysm or arteriovenous fistula, which appears on imaging as a focal collection of vascular contrast that decreases in attenuation with delayed imaging. Active bleeding from a vascular injury presents as vascular contrast, focal or diffuse, which increases in size or attenuation in delayed phase. Most stable patients with a solid organ injury can be managed nonoperatively. Patients with vascular injuries on CT should be considered for angioembolization.

Spleen

Injuries to the spleen can be from either blunt or penetrating injuries and are one of the most frequently injured organs in abdominal trauma. The 2018 AAST organ injury scale grading classification is shown in Table 16.5 [38], and an image of a grade V splenic injury is shown in Fig. 16.9.

Approximately 85% of blunt abdominal injury patients with splenic injuries are offered nonoperative management. Deep venous thrombosis (DVT) prophylaxis does not increase the rate of nonoperative failure. CT contrast blush alone does not mandate operative management, but angiography and embolization are frequently performed. Hemodynamically stable patients that fail nonoperative management or present with hemodynamic instability should proceed for urgent splenectomy [38]. Patients with splenectomy are at risk for overwhelming postsplenectomy infection and should receive vaccinations including against pneumococcal, hemophilus B, and meningococcal vaccines. The timing of the initial set of vaccinations is typically institution dependent but should not be given in the acute setting and typically given just prior to discharge.

Table 16.5 Splenic organ injury scaling

AAST grade	Imaging/pathologic criteria	Operative criteria
I	Subcapsular hematoma < 10% surface area	Subcapsular hematoma < 10% surface area
	Parenchymal laceration < 1 cm in depth	Parenchymal laceration < 1 cm in depth
	Capsular tear	Capsular tear
II	Subcapsular hematoma 10–50% surface area; intraparenchymal hematoma < 5 cm	Subcapsular hematoma 10–50% surface area; intraparenchymal hematoma < 5 cm
	Parenchymal laceration 1–3 cm in depth	Parenchymal laceration 1–3 cm in depth
III	Subcapsular hematoma >50% surface area; ruptured subcapsular or intraparenchymal hematoma ≥5 cm	Subcapsular hematoma >50% surface area or expanding; ruptured subcapsular or intraparenchymal hematoma ≥5 cm
	Parenchymal laceration >3 cm depth	Parenchymal laceration >3 cm depth
IV	Any injury in the presence of a splenic vascular injury or active bleeding confined within splenic capsule	Parenchymal laceration involving segmental or hilar vessels producing >25% devascularization
	Parenchymal laceration involving segmental or hilar vessels producing >25% devascularization	
V	Any injury in the presence of splenic vascular injury with active bleeding extending beyond the spleen into the peritoneum	Hilar vascular injury that devascularizes the spleen
	Shattered spleen	Shattered spleen

Reproduced with permission from publisher

Liver

The AAST classification of liver injuries is shown in Table 16.6 [38], and a CT image of a grade V liver image is shown in Fig. 16.9b. All hemodynamically stable adult patients, regardless of injury grade, should be considered for nonoperative management as long as their clinical exam, hemodynamics, and laboratory testing support injury stability. Low-grade injuries (grades I–III) have a very low incidence of complications and bleeding. Bleeding and delayed complications such as biliary leak are more common in high-grade injuries and after operative management. Bleeding associated with retrohepatic vena cava and major hepatic veins have a high associated mortality and warrant rapid mobilization of specialized teams and resources [38].

Kidney/Ureter/Bladder

Traumatic injuries to the kidneys are typically a result of blunt forces but can also be from penetrating injuries. The kidneys' anatomical location in the retroperitoneum make them susceptible to blunt forces and to acceleration–deceleration injuries. Hematuria can be present in up to 94% of cases of renal and genitourinary trauma but is not predictive of injury grade. Other symptoms to evaluate in renal trauma include costovertebral angle tenderness, abdominal pain, and rib fractures.

CT angiography with urographic delays is the gold standard in evaluating trauma to the kidneys. Injury grading is per the AAST organ injury scale (Table 16.7) [38]. The vast majority of renal injuries can be managed nonoperatively. A grade IV injury is shown in Fig. 16.9c.

Ureteral injuries are rare and typically associated with penetrating injuries. CT imaging with delayed urographic delays should be obtained in any instance where ureteral injury is suspected, and if a patient receives a laparotomy for other indications, direct evaluation of the ureters should be performed in the operating room. If a patient requires surgical repair of the ureters, a double-J stent placement is strongly advised [39].

Bladder injuries are primarily categorized as intraperitoneal or extraperitoneal injuries. Radiologic diagnosis is by

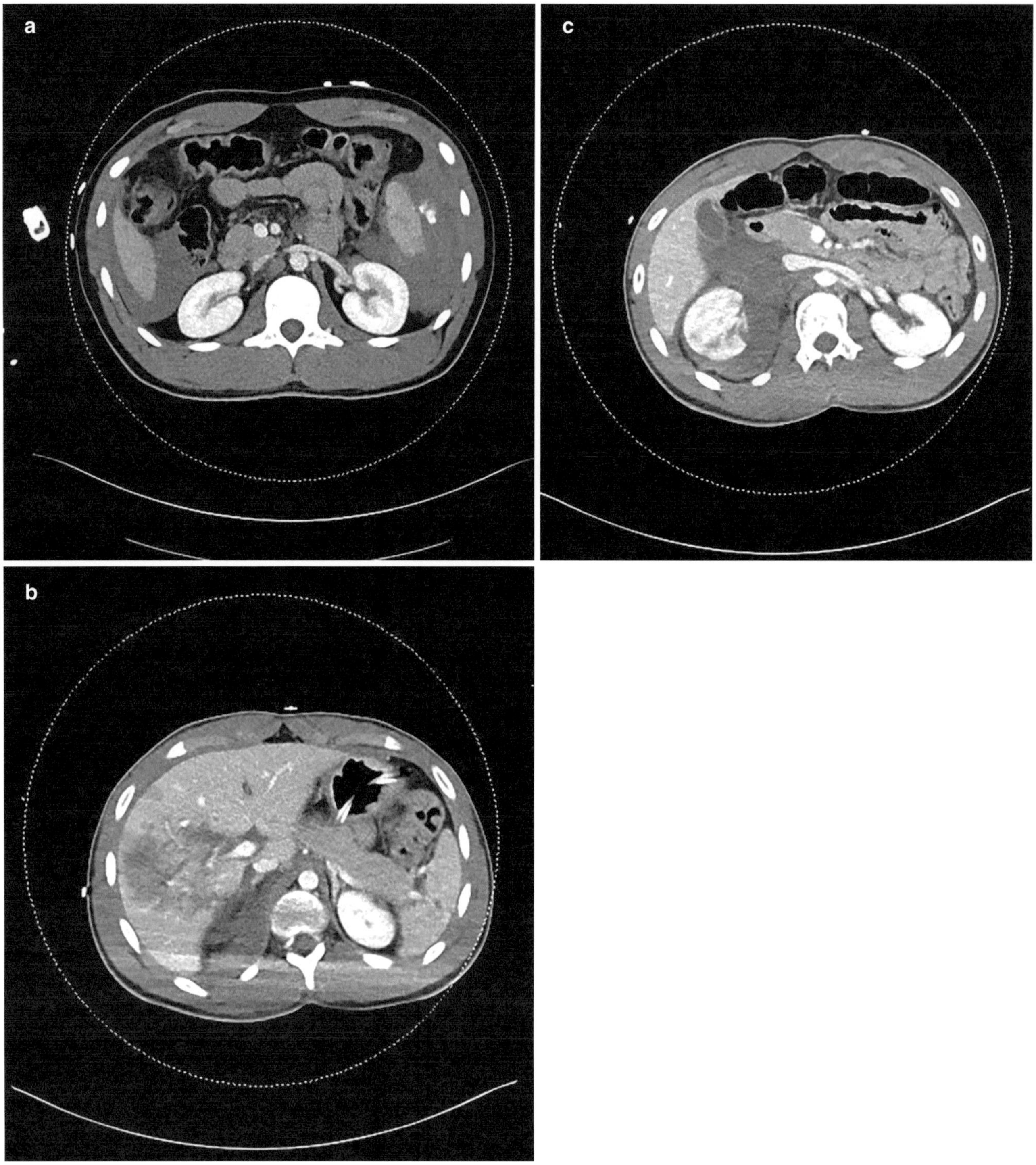

Fig. 16.9 CT images of solid organ injuries. (**a**) Grade 5 blunt splenic injury with active extravasation into the peritoneum. (**b**) Grade 5 blunt hepatic injury. (**c**) Grade 4 blunt kidney injury

Table 16.6 Liver organ injury scaling

AAST grade	AIS severity	Imaging criteria (CT findings)	Operative criteria	Pathologic criteria
I	2	Subcapsular hematoma <10% surface area	Subcapsular hematoma <10% surface area	Subcapsular hematoma <10% surface area
		Parenchymal laceration <1 cm in depth	Parenchymal laceration <1 cm in depth	Parenchymal laceration <1 cm
			Capsular tear	Capsular tear
II	2	Subcapsular hematoma 10–50% surface area; intraparenchymal hematoma <10 cm in diameter	Subcapsular hematoma 10–50% surface area; intraparenchymal hematoma <10 cm in diameter	Subcapsular hematoma 10–50% surface area; intraparenchymal hematoma <10 cm in diameter
		Laceration 1–3 cm in depth and ≤10 cm length	Laceration 1–3 cm in depth and ≤10 cm length	Laceration 1–3 cm depth and ≤10 cm length
III	3	Subcapsular hematoma >50% surface area; ruptured subcapsular or parenchymal hematoma	Subcapsular hematoma >50% surface area or expanding; ruptured subcapsular or parenchymal hematoma	Subcapsular hematoma >50%-surface area; ruptured subcapsular or intraparenchymal hematoma
		Intraparenchymal hematoma >10 cm	Intraparenchymal hematoma >10 cm	Intraparenchymal hematoma >10 cm
		Laceration >3 cm depth	Laceration >3 cm in depth	Laceration >3 cm in depth
		Any injury in the presence of a liver vascular injury or active bleeding contained within liver parenchyma		
IV	4	Parenchymal disruption involving 25–75% of a hepatic lobe	Parenchymal disruption involving 25–75% of a hepatic lobe	Parenchymal disruption involving 25–75% of a hepatic lobe
		Active bleeding extending beyond the liver parenchyma into the peritoneum		
V	5	Arenchymal disruption >75% of hepatic lobe	Parenchymal disruption >75% of hepatic lobe	Parenchymal disruption >75% of hepatic lobe
		Juxtahepatic venous injury to include retrohepatic vena cava and central major hepatic veins	Juxtahepatic venous injury to include retrohepatic vena cava and central major hepatic veins	Juxtahepatic venous injury to include retrohepatic vena cava and central major hepatic veins

Vascular injury is defined as a pseudoaneurysm or arteriovenous fistula and appears as a focal collection of vascular contrast that decreases in attenuation with delayed imaging. Active bleeding from a vascular injury presents as vascular contrast, focal or diffuse, that increases in size or attenuation in delayed phase. Vascular thrombosis can lead to organ infarction.

Grade based on highest grade assessment made on imaging, at operation or on pathologic specimen.

More than one grade of liver injury may be present and should be classified by the higher grade of injury.

Advance one grade for multiple injuries up to a grade III.

Table 16.7 Kidney organ injury scaling

AAST grade	AIS severity	Imaging criteria (CT findings)	Operative goals	Pathologic criteria
I	2	Subcapsular hematoma and/or parenchymal contusion without laceration	Nonexpanding subcapsular hematoma	Subcapsular hematoma or parenchymal contusion without parenchymal laceration
			Parenchymal contusion without laceration	
II	2	Perirenal hematoma confined to Gerota fascia	Nonexpanding perirenal hematoma confined to Gerota fascia	Perirenal hematoma confined to Gerota fascia
		Renal parenchymal laceration ≤1 cm depth without urinary extravasation	Renal parenchymal laceration ≤1 cm depth without urinary extravasation	Renal parenchymal laceration ≤1 cm depth without urinary extravasation
III	3	Renal parenchymal laceration >1 cm depth without collecting system rupture or urinary extravasation	Renal parenchymal laceration >1 cm depth without collecting system rupture or urinary extravasation	Renal parenchymal laceration >1 cm depth without collecting system rupture or urinary extravasation
		Any injury in the presence of a kidney vascular injury or active bleeding contained within Gerota fascia	–	
IV	4	Parenchymal laceration extending into urinary collecting system with urinary extravasation	Parenchymal laceration extending into urinary collecting system with urinary extravasation	Parenchymal laceration extending into urinary collecting system
		Renal pelvis laceration and/or complete ureteropelvic disruption	Renal pelvis laceration and/or complete ureteropelvic disruption	Renal pelvis laceration and/or complete ureteropelvic disruption
		Segmental renal vein or artery injury	Segmental renal vein or artery injury	Segmental renal vein or artery injury
		Active bleeding beyond Gerota fascia into the retroperitoneum or peritoneum	Segmental or complete kidney infarction(s) due to vessel thrombosis without active bleeding	Segmental or complete kidney infarction(s) due to vessel thrombosis without active bleeding
		Segmental or complete kidney infarction(s) due to vessel thrombosis without active bleeding		
V	5	Main renal artery or vein laceration or avulsion of hilum	Main renal artery or vein laceration or avulsion of hilum	Main renal artery or vein laceration or avulsion of hilum
		Devascularized kidney with active bleeding	Devascularized kidney with active bleeding	Devascularized kidney
		Shattered kidney with loss of identifiable parenchymal renal anatomy	Shattered kidney with loss of identifiable parenchymal renal anatomy	Shattered kidney with loss of identifiable parenchymal renal anatomy

Vascular injury is defined as a pseudoaneurysm or arteriovenous fistula and appears as a focal collection of vascular contrast that decreases in attenuation with delayed imaging. Active bleeding from a vascular injury presents as vascular contrast, focal or diffuse, that increases in size or attenuation in delayed phase. Vascular thrombosis can lead to organ infarction.

Grade based on highest grade assessment made on imaging, at operation or on pathologic specimen.

More than one grade of kidney injury may be present and should be classified by the higher grade of injury.

Advance one grade for bilateral injuries up to Grade III.

Reproduced with permission from publisher

cystogram or CT cystography and can be suspected on FAST or CT imaging with free fluid and no associated solid organ injury. Extraperitoneal rupture is typically associated with pelvic fractures and can be managed nonoperatively in the majority of cases with foley drainage alone. Intraperitoneal injuries can be from blunt rupture, typically associated with a full bladder at the time of impact, or from penetrating trauma. Both require surgical repair [40]. Urethral injuries are frequently associated with bladder injuries. The classic signs are blood at the urethral meatus, perineal ecchymosis, and a high riding prostate on rectal exam. Patients with penetrating injuries to the perineum and blunt trauma patients with pelvic fractures, especially associated with a widened pubic symphyses, should be suspected to have a urethral injury. Definitive diagnosis is by retrograde urethrogram.

Pancreas

Traumatic injuries to the pancreas are typically rare and usually coincide with other injuries from abdominal trauma. Pancreatic injuries can also be difficult to diagnose upon initial presentation. Symptoms are often nonspecific and generalizable to diffuse abdominal trauma, including radiating back pain, nausea, vomiting, and abdominal bruising. Complications of missing a pancreatic injury include hemorrhage, pancreatic leakage, fistula formation, abscess, acute pancreatitis, and peritonitis. Hemorrhage is the leading cause of mortality after pancreatic trauma [41].

An abdominal CT scan is the preferred imaging modality for the initial evaluation of a pancreatic injury in hemodynamically stable patients. Of note, CT imaging can appear normal in an injured pancreas for up to 12 hours after pancreatic injury. Secondary signs of injury include peripancreatic fat stranding or fluid collections, hematoma formations, and injuries to adjacent structures. If further imaging is required to make the diagnosis or to better assess the integrity of the pancreatic duct, the use of magnetic resonance cholangiopancreatography (MRCP) can provide more sensitive imaging, as can endoscopic retrograde cholangiopancreatography (ERCP). Hemodynamically stable patients with low-grade injuries can typically be managed nonoperatively. Considerations of the pancreatic ductal integrity and location of the injury in relationship to the superior mesenteric vessels are major factors in deciding if operative exploration is needed. A recently updated AAST organ injury scaling has a larger focus on duct integrity [42].

Stomach

The stomach has a flexible parenchymal structure surrounded by the rib cage, making it less common to become injured in blunt abdominal incidents. When the stomach is injured in a blunt force injury, it is often associated with other abdominal injuries. Due to the rich blood supply and highly resilient tissue of the stomach, the standard treatment for traumatic gastric perforation is primary surgical repair [43].

Bowel, Mesenteric, and Rectal Injuries

Bowel injuries are observed after both blunt and penetrating trauma. Diagnosis of these injuries can be challenging as symptoms may initially be minimal and early radiologic studies can miss injuries. On physical exam, signs include abdominal distention, tenderness on palpation, abrasions and ecchymosis across the lower abdomen (seatbelt sign), periumbilical ecchymosis, abdominal guarding, and rebound tenderness. The presence of a seatbelt sign is associated with a 12% incidence of bowel injury. Physical exam may be complicated by distracting injuries or concomitant head or spine injury, limiting the accuracy of exams. Additionally, small perforations or hypoperfused injuries of the bowel and mesentery can have delayed presentations, taking hours to days to identify the source of peritonitis [44].

A negative CT scan does not entirely rule out bowel injury. Features of bowel and mesenteric injury that can be evaluated by a contrasted CT study could include hematoma development, pneumoperitoneum, hemoperitoneum, bowel wall contusion or thickening, bowel discontinuity, mesenteric stranding, and active arterial extravasation. Blunt versus penetrating injuries have different CT findings as described in the 2020 AAST bowel organ injury scaling scores. Mesenteric injuries can range from small contusions to evidence of active bleeding and associated bowel hypoperfusion (Table 16.8) [45].

Operative management options for bowel injuries include primary repair or bowel resection with anastomosis or stoma. Most bowel injuries can be primarily repaired or resected with anastomosis. Higher-grade injuries are associated with a higher likelihood of resection with anastomosis and/or diversion, need for damage-control laparotomy, and higher incidence of complications [45].

Suspicion of a rectal injury should occur with blood on digital rectal examination, blunt mechanism with associated pelvic fracture or peritoneal wounds, or penetrating mechanism with appropriate trajectory. In stable patients with blunt injury and certain penetrating patients, CT scanning with intravenous contrast can assist in the diagnosis. Rectal contrast is generally not recommended due to the insertion of catheters and balloons into the injured rectum obscuring injury imaging, increasing the contamination of rectal wounds, and overall having poor sensitivity for injury scoring. Patients with penetrating injuries and blood per rectum should undergo sigmoidoscopy.

Table 16.8 Mesenteric injury scale

AAST grade	Imaging criteria [12]	Operative criteria	Pathologic criteria
I	Isolated mesenteric contusion and no abdominal free fluid (except for physiologic small volume pelvic free fluid)	Isolated mesenteric contusion without associated bowel wall thickening	Isolated mesenteric contusion without associated bowel wall thickening
II	Mesenteric hematoma less than 5 cm without associated bowel wall thickening or adjacent interloop fluid collection	Mesenteric hematoma less than 5 cm without associated bowel wall thickening	Mesenteric hematoma less than 5 cm without associated bowel wall thickening
III	Mesenteric hematoma greater than 5 cm without associated bowel wall thickening or adjacent interloop fluid collection	Mesenteric hematoma greater than 5 cm without associated bowel wall thickening	Mesenteric hematoma less than 5 cm without associated bowel wall thickening
IV	Mesenteric hematoma or contusion with associated bowel wall thickening OR	Mesenteric hematoma or contusion with associated bowel wall thickening OR	Mesenteric hematoma or contusion with associated bowel wall thickening OR
	Abrupt termination of mesenteric vessel	Full thickness mesenteric injury with associated viable bowel	Full thickness mesenteric injury with associated viable bowel
V	Active mesenteric intravenous contrast extravasation OR	Active mesenteric bleeding OR	Full thickness mesenteric injury with associated devascularized nonviable bowel
	Nonenhancement of associated bowel wall	Full thickness mesenteric injury with associated devascularized nonviable bowel	
Mesenteric contusion: haziness or opacity within the bowel mesentery; inhomogeneous fluid density within the mesenteric fat [13].			
Mesenteric hematoma: discrete, measurable soft tissue density within bowel mesentery [11].			
Interloop fluid collection: collection of free fluid, frequently triangular in shape, within the mesentery and/or between loops of bowel [12].			

Reproduced with permission from publisher

Management of rectal injuries depends on the location. If the injury is low and amenable to repair, this should be performed and generally will not require diversion. In destructive extraperitoneal injuries or injuries not amenable to direct repair, proximal diversion is indicated. The placement of presacral drains are no longer recommended for all rectal injuries but can be considered for posterior injuries [46].

Vascular Trauma

Large vessel thoracic and abdominal vessel injuries are generally associated with massive bleeding as are penetrating injuries to large extremity vessels such as femoral, popliteal, or brachial arteries. Emergent intervention is required. Tourniquets can be placed above the level of injury in bleeding extremity wounds.

Assessment of peripheral vascular injuries includes hard and soft signs of injury. Hard signs of vascular injury include expanding hematoma, bruit, thrill, pulsatile bleeding, pallor, lack of pulses, paresthesia, pain, or paralysis. Soft signs of injury include neurologic deficit in a nerve near an artery with suspected injury and an injury or non-pulsatile hematoma near a suspected arterial injury. Traditionally, any patient with one hard sign should immediately have a surgical evaluation. Recent data, however, has questioned this dictum and suggests hemorrhagic and ischemic signs of vascular injury are of greater clinical utility. With any suspected vascular injury, a pulse assessment should be performed with palpation. A palpable pulse can still be present and does not rule out vascular injury. Measurement of Ankle-Brachial Index (ABI), CT arteriogram, or conventional angiogram can be obtained to evaluate for arterial injury.

Operative management can include endovascular approaches or open surgery with primary vessel repair, resection and anastomosis, interposition autogenous grafting, or polytetrafluoroethylene grafting. Soft tissue coverage is recommended after definitive repair. Complications can include graft thrombosis, ischemia, compartment syndrome, and potential necrosis and limb loss. Close postoperative monitoring and management are indicated [47–49].

Trauma Orthopedic Injuries

In the assessment of traumatic orthopedic injuries, the initial step is to examine the affected area, assessing for swelling, bruising, punctures, lacerations, deformity, edema, active and passive mobility and pain, distal pulses, and neurologic function. Patients with high potential of decompensation include unstable pelvic fractures, multiple long bone fractures, or dislocation with absent distal pulses [50].

A fracture is considered open when a piece of bone penetrates the skin. The bone may be visible externally or suspected with a wound in the vicinity of a fracture. The Gustilo

Classification is a scale used to grade the complexity of open fractures [50, 51] (Table 16.9). A type I injury includes an open fracture with a clean wound less than 1 cm. A type II injury is an open fracture without extensive soft tissue injury and a wound greater than 1 cm. A type III injury is a segmental fracture with a wound more than 10 cm and has extensive soft tissue injury or an amputation. An injury is considered a type III-A if it has adequate soft tissue coverage. A type III-B injury has significant soft tissue loss with exposed bone and would require a soft tissue graft for adequate coverage. A type III-C injury has a vascular injury and would require a significant repair for limb salvage. The type of open fracture dictates antibiotic coverage. All grade injuries should be covered with intravenous antibiotics targeted at gram-positive organisms upon diagnosis. Higher-grade injuries with associated soft tissue injuries may also need gram-negative coverage. Antibiotics should be continued for at least 24 hours and potentially longer for highly contaminated wounds. Tetanus toxoid vaccination should also be considered or a tetanus booster if not received in the last 10 years. If there is uncertainty in the immunization history, then an additional dose is recommended. Fractures should be reduced and splinted pending management decisions [52, 53].

Other aspects of orthopedic surgery in trauma patients are the concepts of damage control surgery and limb salvage. Damage control surgery in orthopedics is similar to the general trauma surgery concept, where the goal is not necessary to repair and accomplish definitive fixation in the primary surgery, but rather to identify and stabilize injuries as quickly as possible while supporting hemodynamics, correcting metabolic dysfunction, and salvaging the limb for definitive repair. To temporarily stabilize orthopedic injuries, measures such as external fixators can be used to support the orthopedic injuries until the patient is clinically stable enough to tolerate definitive repair [52].

In instances where a patient is clinically deteriorating from an orthopedic injury, there is consideration of limb salvage versus amputation. A mangled extremity is defined as having injury to three of the four limb components: soft tissue, nerve tissue, vascular tissue, and skeletal tissue. If there is reasonable expectation that a limb will be intact for meaningful use then measures should be implemented to salvage the limb, but only if limb salvage will not compromise patient survival [52].

Table 16.9 Gustilo classification of open fracture

Gustilo classification of open fractures	
Type I:	Open fracture, skin wound < 1cm in length and clean
Type II:	Open fracture, laceration > 1cm in length, without extensive soft tissue damage, flaps, or avulsions
Type III:	Open segmental fracture, wound > 10 cm, extensive soft tissue injury or a traumatic amputation
III-A:	Adequate soft tissue coverage
III-B:	Significant loss of soft tissue with exposed bone, requiring soft tissue transfer to achieve coverage
III-C:	Associated vascular injury, requires repair for limb preservation

With any concern for limb malperfusion, the clinician should consider evaluating for the development of compartment syndrome. Compartment syndrome is described as increased pressurization inside of a closed fascial space that restricts the perfusion. Typically seen in the extremities, compartment syndrome can occur within any fascial space in the body. From an orthopedic perspective, it is commonly seen in arm and leg injuries after massive trauma. Edema accumulates in the soft tissues, which overtime will start to restrict the blood flow to the extremity. Hypoperfusion will cause ongoing tissue damage, causing increased amounts of edema and further impair perfusion. This can ultimately lead to limb loss and is considered a true surgical emergency. Clinical assessment should include the evaluation of early "P" symptoms of paresthesia, pain out of proportion to the injury, with passive stretching, and poikilothermia (inability to thermoregulate). Late "P" signs include paralysis, pallor, and pulselessness. Other assessment strategies can include the measurement of compartment pressures, where the difference between the diastolic blood pressure and the compartment pressure is less than 30 mmHg. When the pressure difference is less than 30, surgical management is indicated. Operative management includes prompt fasciotomies in an attempt to release compartment pressures and restore perfusion pressures [52].

Pelvic fractures vary in type complexity but can pose a serious risk acutely when associated with bleeding. Anatomic identification of pelvic injuries helps to also identify classification of injuries. Anatomic injury categories include anteroposterior compression (APC), lateral compression (LC), vertical shearing (VS), and combined mechanisms (CM). While open book pelvic fractures (Fig. 16.10) are typically the type of fracture associated with bleeding, all fracture patterns have the potential. Initial management includes evaluation and stabilization of hemodynamic status while providing mechanical stability for the pelvis and reducing hemorrhage. Stabilization devices like a pelvic binder or a tightly wrapped bed sheet can be applied to externally fixate the pelvis until definitive management is planned. In a hemodynamically stable patient, X-ray imaging can be performed for the initial evaluation of the injury type. CT angiography is helpful in identifying the extent of the fracture but also in detecting bleeding. Extraperitoneal bleeding is primary venous, but arterial bleeding can occur and appears as a contrast blush. In unstable patients or patients with evidence of ongoing bleeding, pelvic packing and/or embolization is indicated. Rectal and vaginal injuries should be considered in patients with pelvic injuries [54].

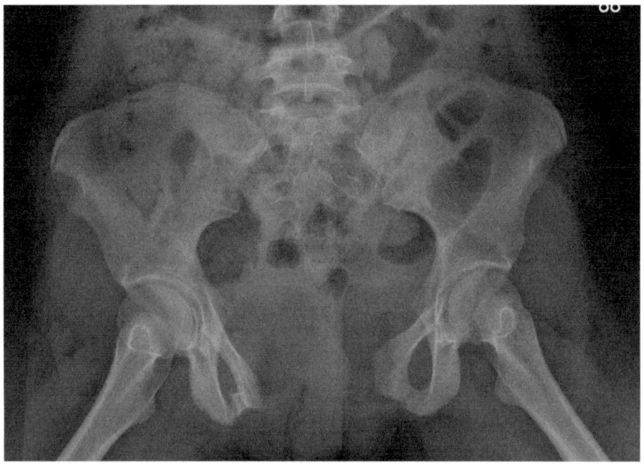

Fig. 16.10 Pelvic X-ray of an open-book pelvic fracture

References

1. Eugene V, Hutzler J, Kempema J, Bradford J, Carlos. The difficult airway in trauma: what you need to know. J Trauma Acute Care Surg. 2024; https://doi.org/10.1097/ta.0000000000004402.
2. Ferrada P, Dissanaike S. Circulation first for the rapidly bleeding trauma patient-it is time to reconsider the ABCs of trauma care. J Am Med Assoc Surg. 2023;158(8):884–5. https://doi.org/10.1001/jamasurg.2022.8436.
3. Buzzard L, Schreiber M. Trauma-induced coagulopathy: what you need to know. J Trauma Acute Care Surg. 2023;96(2):179–85. https://doi.org/10.1097/ta.0000000000004170.
4. Lammers DT, Holcomb JB. Damage control resuscitation in adult trauma patients: what you need to know. J Trauma Acute Care Surg. 2023;95(4):464. https://doi.org/10.1097/TA.0000000000004103.
5. Nasa P, Wise RD, Smit M, Acosta S, D'Amours S, Beaubien–Souligny W, et al. International cross-sectional survey on current and updated definitions of intra-abdominal hypertension and abdominal compartment syndrome. World J Emerg Surg. 2024;19(1):1–14.
6. Jang H, Lee N, Jeong E, Park Y, Jo Y, Kim J, Kim D. Abdominal compartment syndrome in critically ill patients. Acute Crit Care. 2023;38(4):399–408. American Association for the Surgery of Trauma. Injury Scoring Scale.
7. Vatankhah S, Sheikhi RA, Heidari M, Moradimajd P. The relationship between fluid resuscitation and intra-abdominal hypertension in patients with blunt abdominal trauma. Int J Crit Illn Inj Sci. 2018;8(3):149–53. https://doi.org/10.4103/IJCIIS.IJCIIS_17_18.
8. Teasdale G, Jennett B. Assessment of coma and impaired consciousness. A practical scale. Lancet. 1974;304(7872) https://doi.org/10.1016/S0140-6736(74)91639-0.
9. Herring W. Learning radiology: recognizing the basics. 5th ed. Elsevier; 2023.
10. Carney N, Totten AM, O-Reilley C, et al. Guidelines for the management of severe traumatic brain injury. 4th ed. Updated September 30, 2016. Accessed 28 Nov 2024. https://braintrauma.org/coma/guidelines/guidelines-for-the-management-of-severe-tbi-4th-ed.
11. Ratcliff J, Morrison C, Tran D, Ruzas C. Emergency neurological life support intracranial hypertension and herniation protocol. [Version 4.0]. Updated March 2020. Accessed 28 Nov 2024. https://www.neurocriticalcare.org/Portals/0/Docs/ENLS/ENLS_V_4_0_Protocol_ICP_FINAL.pdf.
12. Bullock M, Chestnut R, Ghajar J, et al. Guidelines for the surgical management of traumatic parenchymal lesions. Neurosurgery. 2006;58(3) https://doi.org/10.1227/01.NEU.0000210365.36914.E3.
13. Hawryluk GWJ, Rubiano A, Totten AM, et al. Guidelines for the Management of Severe Traumatic Brain Injury: 2020 update of the decompressive craniectomy recommendations. Neurosurgery. 2020;87(3):427–34. https://doi.org/10.1093/neuros/nyaa278.
14. Meyfroidt G, Bagueley I, Menon D. Paroxysmal sympathetic hyperactivity: the storm after acute brain injury. Lancet Neurol. 2017;16(9) https://doi.org/10.1016/S1474-4422(17)30259-4.
15. Capatina C, Paluzzi A, Mitchell R, Karavitaki N. Diabetes insipidus after traumatic brain injury. J Clin Med. 2015;4(7) https://doi.org/10.3390/jcm4071448.
16. American College of Surgeons. Best practice guidelines: spine injury. Published March 2022. Accessed 2 Dec 2024. https://www.facs.org/media/k45gikqv/spine_injury_guidelines.pdf.
17. Fehlings MG, Tetreault LA, Wilson JR, et al. A clinical practice guideline for the management of acute spinal cord injury: introduction, rationale, and scope. Glob Spine J. 2017;7(3_suppl):84S–94S. https://doi.org/10.1177/2192568217703387.
18. Ahuja C, Nori S, Tetreault L, Wilson J, Kwon B. Traumatic spinal cord injury- repair and regeneration. Neurosurgery. 2017;1(80) https://doi.org/10.1093/neuros/nyw080.
19. Evaniew N, Mazlouman SJ, Belley-Côté EP, Jacobs WB, Kwon BK. Interventions to optimize spinal cord perfusion in patients with acute traumatic spinal cord injuries: a systematic review. J Neurotrauma. 2020;37(9):1127–39. https://doi.org/10.1089/neu.2019.6844. Epub 2020 Mar 11. PMID: 32024432.
20. Kim D, Biffl W, Bokhari F, et al. Evaluation and management of blunt cerebrovascular injury: a practice management guideline from the Eastern Association for the Surgery of Trauma. J Trauma Acute Care Surg. 2020;88(6) https://doi.org/10.1097/TA.0000000000002668.
21. The American Association for the Surgery of Trauma. (2013). Blunt cardiac injury. Accessed 3 Dec 2024. https://www.aast.org/resources-detail/blunt-cardiac-injury.
22. Clancy K, Velopulos C, Bilaniuk J, et al. Screening for blunt cardiac injury: an Eastern Association for the Surgery of trauma practice management guideline. J Trauma Acute Care Surg. 2012;73(5) https://doi.org/10.1097/TA.0b013e318270193a.
23. Mouawad N, Paulisin J, Hofmeister S, Thomas M. Blunt aortic injury - concepts and management. J Cardiothorac Surg. 2020;15(62) https://doi.org/10.1186/s13019-020-01101-6.
24. Fox N, Schwartz D, Salazar J, et al. Evaluation and management of blunt traumatic aortic injury: a practice management guideline from Eastern Association for the Surgery of Trauma. J Trauma Acute Care Surg. 2015;78(1) https://doi.org/10.1097/TA.0000000000000470.
25. Mukherjee K, Schubl S, Tominaga F, et al. Non-surgical management and analgesia strategies for older adults with multiple rib fractures: a systematic review, meta analysis, and practice management guideline. J Trauma Acute Care Surg. 2020. https://www.east.org/education-resources/practice-management-guidelines/details/nonsurgical-management-and-analgesia-strategies-for-older-adults-with-multiple-rib-fractures-a-systematic-review-metaanalysis.
26. Kasotakis G, Hasenboehler E, Streib E, et al. Operative fixation of rib fractures after blunt trauma: a practice management guideline from the Eastern Association for the Surgery of Trauma. J Trauma Acute Care Surg. 2020;82(3) https://doi.org/10.1097/TA.0000000000001350.
27. Brasel K, Moore E, Albrecht R, et al. Western Trauma Association critical decisions in trauma: management of rib fractures. J

Trauma Acute Care Surg. 2016;82(1) https://doi.org/10.1097/TA.0000000000001301.
28. The Eastern Association for the Surgery of Trauma. Thoracic trauma, blunt, pain management of - practice management guideline 2016;81(5):936–51. https://www.east.org/education-resources/practice-management-guidelines/details/thoracic-trauma-blunt-pain-management-of
29. Simon B, Ebert J, Bokhari F, et al. Management of pulmonary contusion and flail chest: an Eastern Association for the Surgery of trauma practice management guideline. J Trauma Acute Care Surg. 2012;73(5) https://doi.org/10.1097/TA.0b013e31827019fd.
30. Karmy-Jones R, Namias N, Coimbra R, et al. West Trauma Association critical decisions in trauma: penetrating chest trauma. J Trauma Acute Care Surg. 2014;77(6) https://doi.org/10.1097/TA.0000000000000426.
31. Seamon M, Haut E, Van Aredonk K, et al. An evidence-based approach to patient selection for emergency department thoracotomy: a practice management guideline from the Eastern Association for the Surgery of Trauma. J Trauma Acute Care Surg. 2015;79(1) https://doi.org/10.1097/TA.0000000000000648.
32. Hoff WS, Holevar M, Nagy KK, Patterson L, Young JS, Arrillaga A, et al. Practice management guidelines for the evaluation of blunt abdominal trauma: the East practice management guidelines work group. J Trauma Acute Care Surg. 2002;53(3):602–15.
33. Akeel AS, Mahdi BA, Alshammasi ZA, et al. Emergency assessment and management of abdominal trauma. 2021. https://www.ecronicon.com/ecmi/pdf/ECMI-17-01041.pdf. Accessed 20 May 2024.
34. Diercks DB, Mehrotra A, Nazarian DJ, Promes SB, Decker WW, Fesmire FM. Clinical policy: critical issues in the evaluation of adult patients presenting to the emergency department with acute blunt abdominal trauma. Ann Emerg Med. 2011;57(4):387–404.
35. Como JJ, Bokhari F, Chiu WC, Duane TM, Holevar MR, Tandoh MA, et al. Practice management guidelines for selective nonoperative management of penetrating abdominal trauma. J Trauma Acute Care Surg. 2010;68(3):721–33.
36. American Association for the Surgery of Trauma. Injury scoring scale. 2024. https://www.aast.org/resources-detail/injury-scoring-scale. Accessed 2 July 2024.
37. Richards JR, McGahan JP. Focused assessment with sonography in trauma (FAST) in 2017: what radiologists can learn. Radiology. 2017;283(1):30–48.
38. Kozar RA, Crandall M, Shanmuganathan K, Zarzaur BL, Coburn M, Cribari C, et al. Organ injury scaling 2018 update: spleen, liver, and kidney. J Trauma Acute Care Surg. 2018;85(6):1119–22.
39. Coccolini F, Moore EE, Kluger Y, Biffl W, Leppaniemi A, Matsumura Y, et al. Kidney and uro-trauma: WSES-AAST guidelines. World J Emerg Surg. 2019;14:1–25.
40. Yeung LL, McDonald AA, Como JJ, Robinson B, Knight J, Person MA, et al. Management of blunt force bladder injuries: a practice management guideline from the Eastern Association for the Surgery of Trauma. J Trauma Acute Care Surg. 2019;86(2):326–36.
41. Ho VP, Patel NJ, Bokhari F, Madbak FG, Hambley JE, Yon JR, et al. Management of adult pancreatic injuries: a practice management guideline from the Eastern Association for the Surgery of Trauma. J Trauma Acute Care Surg. 2017;82(1):185–99.
42. Dave S, Toy FK, London S. Pancreatic trauma. In: StatPearls [Internet]. StatPearls publishing; 2023.
43. Aboobakar MR, et al. Gastric perforation following blunt abdominal trauma. Trauma Case Rep. 2017;10:12–5.
44. Weinberg JA, Peck KA, Ley EJ, Brown CV, Moore EE, Sperry JL, et al. Evaluation and management of bowel and mesenteric injuries after blunt trauma: a Western Trauma Association critical decisions algorithm. J Trauma Acute Care Surg. 2021;91(5):903–8.
45. Tominaga GT, Crandall M, Cribari C, Zarzaur BL, Bernstein M, Kozar RA, AAST Patient Assessment Committee. Organ injury scaling 2020 update: bowel and mesentery. J Trauma Acute Care Surg. 2021;91(3):e73–7.
46. Schellenberg M, Koller S, De Moya M, Moore LJ, Brown CV, Hartwell JL, et al. Diagnosis and management of traumatic rectal injury: a Western Trauma Association critical decisions algorithm. J Trauma Acute Care Surg. 2023;95(5):731–6.
47. Huber GH, Manna B. Vascular extremity trauma. In: StatPearls. Treasure Island: StatPearls Publishing; 2023. PMID: 30725610.
48. Fox CJ, Feliciano DV, Hartwell JL, Ley EJ, Coimbra R, Schellenberg M, et al. Extremity vascular injury: a Western trauma association critical decisions algorithm. J Trauma Acute Care Surg. 2023;96:10-1097.
49. Romagnoli AN, DuBose J, Dua A, Betzold R, Bee T, Fabian T, Morrison J, Skarupa D, Podbielski J, Inaba K, Feliciano D, Kauvar D, AAST PROOVIT Study Group. Hard signs gone soft: a critical evaluation of presenting signs of extremity vascular injury. J Trauma Acute Care Surg. 2021;90(1):1–10. https://doi.org/10.1097/TA.0000000000002958.
50. Gustilo RB, Anderson JT. Prevention of infection in the treatment of one thousand and twenty-five open fractures of long bones: Retrospective and prospective analyses. J Bone Joint Surg Am. 1976;58:453–58.
51. Yim GH, Hardwicke JT. The Evolution and Interpretation of the Gustilo and Anderson Classification. J Bone Joint Surg Am. 2018;100(24):e152. https://doi.org/10.2106/JBJS.18.00342. PMID: 30562299.
52. TQIP A. Best practices in the management of orthopaedic trauma. ACS Committee on Trauma; 2015. p. 3–37.
53. Hoff WS, Bonadies JA, Cachecho R, Dorlac WC. East Practice Management Guidelines Work Group: update to practice management guidelines for prophylactic antibiotic use in open fractures. J Trauma Acute Care Surg. 2011;70(3):751–4.
54. Coccolini F, Stahel PF, Montori G, Biffl W, Horer TM, Catena F, et al. Pelvic trauma: WSES classification and guidelines. World J Emerg Surg. 2017;12:1–18.

Recommended Reading

Cooper DJ, Rosenfeld J, Murray L, et al. Decompressive craniectomy in diffuse traumatic brain injury. N Engl J Med. 2011;364(16) https://doi.org/10.1056/NEJMoa1102077. The DECRA Trial.

Dankiewiez J, Cronberg T, Lilja G, Jacobsen, J, et al. Hypothermia versus normothermia after out-of-hospital cardiac arrest. N Engl J Med. 2021;384(24). https://doi.org/10.1056/NEJMoa210059. TTM2 Trial.

Hutchinson P, Kolias A, Timofeev IS, et al. Trial of decompressive craniectomy for traumatic intracranial hypertension. N Engl J Med. 2016;375(12) https://doi.org/10.1056/NEJMoa1605215. The RESCUE- ICP Trial.

Nielsen N, Wetterslev J, Cronberg T, et al. Targeted temperature management at 33°C versus 36°C after cardiac arrest. N Engl J Med. 2013;369(23) https://doi.org/10.1056/NEJMoa1310519. TTM 1 Trial.

Shock

17

Paula Ferrada and Jonathan Messing

Introduction

Shock is a critical medical condition characterized by inadequate tissue perfusion, leading to cellular hypoxia and organ dysfunction [53]. There are four primary categories of shock, each with different causes and indicated treatment modalities. Hypovolemic, cardiogenic, distributive, and obstructive shock states demand early recognition and intervention to avoid death. Despite advances in medical science, shock remains a significant cause of morbidity and mortality worldwide. This chapter aims to provide a comprehensive overview of shock, including its epidemiology, recognition, classification, diagnosis, and management strategies.

Epidemiology

Common in medicine, the recognition of shock can often be attributed to the Greeks, but it was in the 1700s when clinicians started applying the term, particularly around combat injuries [30]. While shock's prevalence may vary based on geographic location, demographic factors, and healthcare resources, it is essential to highlight its significance as a life-threatening condition requiring prompt recognition and management.

The breadth of shock states can make it challenging to fully describe its global prevalence and outcomes. One Danish study reviewed 438,191 emergency department patients over a 12-year period to identify 1553 patients exhibiting a shock state with mortality rates ranging from 12.7% to 34.6% at 7 days [19]. An Australian study examining nontraumatic shock over a 4-year period found an incidence of 76 per 100,000 persons with a 30-day mortality rate of 32.8% [6]. A systematic review of six observational studies described a range of 9.5–19 persons per 1000 with prehospital nontraumatic shock and a mortality of up to 52% [24]. With each shock class, the frequency and mortality vary, as does the outcome related to critical modifiers such as age, comorbidities, and socioeconomic status, to name a few.

P. Ferrada · J. Messing (✉)
Inova Health System, Fairfax, VA, USA
e-mail: Jonathan.Messing@inova.org

Recognizing Shock

Clinical manifestations

Shock may present with a spectrum of clinical manifestations, including tachycardia, hypotension, altered mental status, cool and clammy skin, and oliguria [53]. Timely recognition of these symptoms is essential to avoiding an irreversible state of shock and complete circulatory collapse. Often, a subtle change may be an early indication of a patient entering a shocked state, necessitating treatment before diagnosis. New oliguria, confusion, and skin mottling are all classic findings that can be easily overlooked, particularly in patients with preexisting conditions. This has led some clinicians to refer to the renal, dermatologic, and neurologic systems as the body's "windows" [53]. One can appreciate how a patient with baseline dementia, peripheral vascular disease, or chronic kidney disease may further obscure a clinician's ability to detect the presence of shock.

Other subtle clinical manifestations of shock include initial vasoconstriction and profuse diaphoresis, which can be early signs that are often overlooked [8]. While hypotension and tachycardia are commonly associated with shock, they are not always reliable indicators, particularly in the initial phase of the condition. Vasoconstriction manifests as cool and pale extremities, reflecting the body's attempt to preserve core organ perfusion by reducing blood flow to the skin and peripheral tissues [12]. Diaphoresis, when present, is driven by the sympathetic nervous system's activation. These early signs precede the more obvious indicators of hypotension and tachycardia, underscoring the importance of thorough and vigilant clinical assessment to detect shock before it progresses to more advanced stages.

S. Atallah, J. Dragoljevic (eds.), *Fundamentals of Surgery for Physician Assistants*,
https://doi.org/10.1007/978-3-032-21069-2_17

Simultaneous management initiation and source identification

The first step is recognizing that the patient is in shock by identifying impaired end-organ perfusion. In doing so, treatment must coincide with developing a differential and ultimately achieving a diagnosis. Context matters, which includes methodically obtaining a history, performing a physical examination, and employing appropriate diagnostic studies while treatment is initiated. If a patient presents hypotensive and tachycardic following a high-speed motor vehicle crash, the resuscitation team will have an elevated suspicion for hemorrhagic shock, a form of hypovolemic shock, mandating blood transfusion while preparing the patient for hemorrhage control. A Focused Assessment with Sonography in Trauma (i.e., FAST exam) may reveal free fluid in Morrison's pouch, supporting a diagnosis of hemoperitoneum. If a neutropenic oncology patient develops hypotension and confusion, the team may obtain specimen cultures and initiate broad-spectrum antibiotics before knowing the specific source or microbial to treat. Fluid resuscitation and vasopressors may commence early before an exact source is known.

Many standard laboratory values might be helpful based on clinical suspicion but should not delay intervention. Much like one does not delay the administration of antibiotics in the septic shock patient pending final culture results, one does not await the hemoglobin and hematocrit to treat acute blood loss anemia in the hemorrhagic shock patient. One lab of particular value for trending is lactic acid, although not without controversy [54]. Lactic acidosis, commonly defined as greater than 2 mmol/L, including by the Third International Consensus Definitions for Sepsis and Septic Shock, is a "sensitive…nonspecific" marker of impaired tissue perfusion when elevated [46]. Identifying and trending lactic acidosis may inform the care team about the patient's progress, although its elevation can be from other sources. Nevertheless, persistent and uptrending lactic acidosis is commonly associated with increased mortality. Weinberger et al. [54] nicely summarize the many studies, noting reductions in lactic acid align with mortality improvements while also addressing limitations and controversies.

Hemodynamic monitoring

Hemodynamic monitoring is critical in managing shock patients by providing real-time cardiac function, fluid status, and tissue perfusion data. Various modalities, including invasive and noninvasive techniques, can guide resuscitative efforts and optimize patient outcomes. Common tools include continuous telemetry, pulse oximetry, and blood pressure monitoring. Prompt electrocardiograms (ECGs) can help identify acute myocardial infarction or lethal arrhythmias leading to cardiogenic shock [49]. Many patients, particularly those with persistent hypotension and vasopressor use, require arterial blood pressure monitoring for truly continuous readings. Arterial lines also offer the advantage of readily available arterial blood sampling and blood gas interpretation. Central venous catheters provide a means for administering vasopressors and trending central venous pressures (CVP) but carry increased risks of bloodstream infection and iatrogenic injury. The presence of a central venous catheter was once a mainstay of treatment in shock and continues to be a commonly applied tool, but it is not an absolute necessity. Lower dose vasopressors can be safely administered short-term peripherally, for example, and two large bore peripheral intravenous catheters are often preferable when initiating a massive transfusion protocol for hemorrhagic shock [17, 34, 40]. Trending of CVPs can help measure preload and determine congestion, but preferably when done continuously and while accepting limitations around inaccurate readings [20]. A central venous catheter can also facilitate the measurement of central venous oxygen saturations, which, when low, may indicate decreased cardiac output [20].

Pulmonary artery catheters (PACs) have existed in critical care for over 50 years, offering insights into cardiac output, pulmonary artery pressures, wedge pressures, and mixed venous gas sampling [2]. They carry known risks of migration and pulmonary artery rupture, with other tools regularly emerging that can approximate PAC findings without the invasiveness of PACs, particularly when fewer clinicians are familiar with their insertion, waveform analysis, and interpretation [13]. They are often best reserved case-by-case for patients in mixed-shock states, major cardiothoracic surgery, or cardiogenic shock [2].

Echocardiography offers a noninvasive and repeatable heart examination with increasing point-of-care utilization. Obtaining an echocardiogram early in the evaluation and management of shock may illuminate hyper or hypodynamic states, valvular abnormalities, pulmonary hypertension, pericardial tamponade, vegetations, volume status, and ejection fraction, all at the bedside [33]. Its value in diagnosing the class of shock and response to treatment cannot be overstated.

Expanding on point-of-care ultrasound, or POCUS, is the ability to evaluate further intravascular volume, cardiac contractility, and sources of shock. The FAST exam, mentioned earlier, is a useful strategy in identifying intrabdominal free fluid and pericardial tamponade. The extended FAST exam includes a chest wall assessment for the presence of lung sliding, which, in its absence, suggests pneumothorax. The Rapid Ultrasound in SHock exam, also known as the RUSH exam, involves evaluating cardiac contractility, the pericardium for the presence of tamponade, the inferior vena cava for volume status, an extended FAST exam, and evaluation of the thoracic and abdominal aorta [38]. A recent meta-analysis supports the RUSH exam as a highly sensitive and specific tool for detecting shock [27]. Ultimately, ultrasound is famously user-dependent but carries the advantage of being radiation-free and repeatable.

Finally, minimally invasive monitoring devices can perform waveform analysis of a patient's arterial line to deliver continuous stroke volumes, stroke volume variation, cardiac output, cardiac index, systemic vascular resistance, and mean arterial pressure measurements [28]. These data points can assist in diagnosing and managing patients in shock states.

Classes of Shock

- Hypovolemic shock:
  Hemorrhagic: This is characterized by acute blood loss, often secondary to trauma, gastrointestinal bleeding, or obstetric emergencies. Uncontrolled hemorrhage can lead to rapid instability and death. Nearly two million people die from hemorrhagic shock each year [9].
  Nonhemorrhagic: This occurs due to fluid losses from other sources, such as dehydration, burns, or third-spacing.
- Distributive shock:
  Septic: This is caused by a dysregulated host response to infection, leading to systemic inflammation, vasodilation, and distributive hypoperfusion, it is the most common form of shock encountered [53].
  Neurogenic: This condition results from disruption of the sympathetic nervous system's control, often seen in spinal cord injury above the T6 level, leading to loss of vascular tone. These patients frequently present hypotensive and bradycardic [11].
  Anaphylactic: Triggered by a severe allergic reaction, leading to widespread vasodilation, bronchoconstriction, and airway compromise [32].
- Cardiogenic shock:
  Acute myocardial infarction (AMI): This occurs due to myocardial ischemia or infarction, leading to impaired cardiac function and decreased cardiac output. 5–10% of patients may develop cardiogenic shock after AMI and often experience severe left ventricular dysfunction, with a 30-day mortality rate reaching 40% [43].
  Valvular disruption: This may result from acute valvular regurgitation or stenosis, leading to hemodynamic instability [5].
- Obstructive shock:
  Cardiac tamponade: Compression of the heart by pericardial fluid, impairing cardiac filling and output [1].
  Tension pneumothorax: Accumulation of air within the pleural space, leading to mediastinal shift and impaired venous return [41].
  Pulmonary embolism: Occlusion of pulmonary arteries by thrombus, leading to increased pulmonary vascular resistance and right ventricular strain [39].
  Constrictive pericarditis: Fibrotic thickening of the pericardium, restricting cardiac filling and output due to autoimmune, infectious, noninfectious, and frequently idiopathic causes [10].
  Severe pulmonary hypertension: Elevated pulmonary arterial pressures leading to right heart failure and systemic hypoperfusion [3].
- Mixed shock:
  Some patients may exhibit features of more than one type of shock, necessitating a multifaceted approach to management (Tables 17.1 and 17.2).

Table 17.1 Classes of shock

Hypovolemic	Cardiogenic	Distributive	Obstructive
Hemorrhagic fluid third spacing Burns Pancreatitis Dehydration Hyperemesis gravidarum	Acute myocardial infarction Acute valvular disruption	Sepsis Anaphylaxis Neurogenic	Tension pneumothorax Cardiac tamponade Pulmonary embolism Constrictive pericarditis Severe pulmonary hypertension

Note. A fifth class of mixed shock can include any combination of the above

Table 17.2 Hemodynamic profiles of shock

	Hypovolemic	Cardiogenic	Distributive	Obstructive
CO	↓	↓	↑	↓
HR	↑	↑	↑ or ↓	↑
MAP	↓	↓	↓	↓
PAWP	↓	↑	↓	↑ or unchanged
SVR	↑	↑	↓	↑ or unchanged

Note. *CO* cardiac output, *HR* heart rate, *MAP* mean arterial blood pressure, *PAWP* pulmonary artery wedge pressure, *SVR* systemic vascular resistance

Diagnosis

Accurately diagnosing shock involves history building, clinical assessment, laboratory studies, and imaging modalities [26]. Key diagnostic considerations include identifying the underlying etiology, assessing the severity of hemodynamic instability, and evaluating end-organ perfusion, all while initiating treatment.

Point-of-care ultrasound (POCUS) emerged as a valuable tool for diagnosing the causes of hypotension in various clinical settings in the 1980s, with its popularity only increasing [36]. Its portability, real-time imaging capabilities, and ability to provide immediate diagnostic information make it particularly well-suited for acute care settings, such as emergency departments, intensive care units, and prehospital environments [36]. With POCUS, clinicians can quickly assess cardiac function, evaluate for signs of hypovolemia or fluid overload, and identify potential sources of obstructive or distributive shock, all of which can contribute to hypotension [21]. By visualizing the heart, great vessels, and other relevant anatomical structures directly at the bedside, POCUS enables clinicians to make rapid and accurate diagnoses, guiding subsequent resuscitative efforts and treatment decisions [7, 18, 38].

Moreover, POCUS facilitates a dynamic and tailored approach to hemodynamic assessment, allowing for serial evaluations and adjustments based on patient response. In cases of undifferentiated hypotension, where the underlying etiology may be multifactorial or unclear, POCUS can provide valuable diagnostic insights in real-time, guiding further diagnostic testing and therapeutic interventions [15, 38]. Additionally, POCUS can aid in the identification of potentially reversible causes of hypotension, such as cardiac tamponade, tension pneumothorax, or acute decompensated heart failure, where prompt recognition and intervention are paramount [38]. Early application, such as in trauma bay patients, has demonstrated advantages in fluid resuscitation, triage, and time to ICU admission [16]. Studies support that integrating POCUS into the initial evaluation of patients presenting with acute distress leads to earlier diagnosis and intervention, often influencing improved outcomes [4, 56].

Hemodynamic monitoring tools are essential in diagnosing different types of shock by providing clinicians with real-time data on cardiac function, fluid status, and tissue perfusion. For example, hemodynamic monitoring can reveal decreased preload and cardiac output in hypovolemic shock, indicating insufficient circulating volume [45]. By assessing parameters such as central venous pressure (CVP) and stroke volume variation (SVV) with techniques such as central venous catheterization and pulse contour analysis, clinicians can quantify the degree of hypovolemia and guide fluid resuscitation efforts appropriately [45]. These data, such as CVP, are not without controversy, with some suggesting they should no longer be monitored [31, 45]. Similarly, in distributive shock, hemodynamic monitoring can help identify the vasodilatory state characteristic of conditions such as septic shock. Measurements such as mean arterial pressure (MAP), systemic vascular resistance (SVR), and mixed venous oxygen saturation (SvO2) can provide insights into the extent of vasodilation and tissue hypoperfusion, guiding the titration of vasoactive medications and volume resuscitation, but should be used carefully and in the global context of the patient's state rather than in isolation [45, 46, 48].

In cardiogenic shock, hemodynamic monitoring allows for assessing cardiac function and identifying underlying myocardial dysfunction. Parameters such as cardiac output (CO), cardiac index (CI), and pulmonary artery wedge pressure (PAWP) can aid in differentiating between cardiogenic shock and other etiologies, such as hypovolemic or distributive shock, particularly when applied early [49, 51]. Additionally, hemodynamic monitoring techniques such as echocardiography provide valuable information on ventricular function, volume status, valvular abnormalities, and pericardial effusion, facilitating the timely diagnosis of conditions such as acute myocardial infarction or cardiac tamponade [51]. By integrating hemodynamic monitoring tools into the diagnostic evaluation of shock, clinicians can tailor management strategies to address the specific pathophysiology underlying each patient's presentation, ultimately optimizing resuscitative efforts and improving outcomes.

Management

Management of shock revolves around a systematic approach aimed at restoring tissue perfusion, optimizing cardiac function, and addressing the underlying cause. This may involve a combination of thoughtful fluid resuscitation, vasopressor support, inotropic agents, and targeted interventions based on the specific type of shock. These patients require critical care management and admission to the intensive care unit (ICU). In the case of hypovolemic shock, management includes volume replacement and stopping the source of volume loss. Hypovolemic shock from hemorrhage benefits from years of data supporting a balanced resuscitation using blood products and rapid control of hemorrhage [25]. Clinicians must be careful to avoid large-volume crystalloid resuscitation, which can lead to the dilution of clotting factors and propagation of the lethal triad in trauma (coagulopathy, acidosis, and hypothermia) [9, 47]. The PROMMTT and PROPPR trials famously supported resuscitation hemorrhagic shock patients with a 1:1:1 formula, entailing 1 unit of packed red blood cells for every unit of fresh frozen plasma and platelets [22, 23]. To combat hyperfibrinolysis, the CRASH-II trial strengthened support of tranexamic acid administration early [44]. Technology, such as thromboelastography, allows clinicians to tailor blood product utilization more directly to the pathophysiology, which may be platelet dysfunction, hyperfibrinolysis, or prolonged clotting time [55]. In recent years, a growing body of evidence supports treating hemorrhagic shock with whole blood over component therapy, which better matches the fluid composition lost by these patients [35].

Cardiogenic shock presents myriad challenges, with the underlying etiology dictating the necessary treatment, which may not always be easily identifiable. Regionalized systems provide the infrastructure for accessing appropriate, specialized care [49]. Within the system, immediate electrocardiogram interpretation may reveal an acute myocardial infarction warranting prompt percutaneous coronary intervention. Early use of a pulmonary artery catheter can offer insightful data points around volume status, cardiac output, mixed venous gas, and heart pressures. These data points may indicate the need for vasopressors, inotropic agents, or mechanical circulatory support. Mechanical circulatory support ranges from intra-aortic balloon pumps to axial flow devices and extracorporeal membrane oxygenation [49, 51].

Septic shock and neurogenic shock, two forms of distributive shock, warrant volume resuscitation and vasopressors. The Surviving Sepsis Campaign emphasizes using tools such as the Modified Early Warning Score to identify patients, obtain early cultures, administer antimicrobials within 1 hour of identification, and admit patients to the ICU [14]. The 2021 guidelines offer clinicians over 90 recommendations for management, including gradations of available evidence for everything from initial resuscitation, infection management, hemodynamic monitoring, mechanical ventilation, and other therapies such as corticosteroids [14]. Neurogenic shock, on the other hand, necessitates fluid resuscitation, vasopressors, and emergent neurosurgical consultation.

Obstructive shock often stems from a mechanical complication impeding cardiac output and cardiac contractility [29]. A tension pneumothorax compresses the vena cava and the right atrium so blood cannot readily return to the heart [41]. Needle decompression or finger thoracostomy, followed by chest tube placement, should release the intrathoracic pressure obstructing blood return [41, 42]. If cardiac tamponade is identified, a pericardiocentesis or pericardial window can remove the fluid lodged in the pericardium that restricts contractility [1, 52]. If from trauma, these patients often warrant emergent surgical intervention [37]. A massive pulmonary embolism often requires embolectomy and anticoagulation, but often after initial fluid resuscitation due to the diminished preload [50].

In conclusion, understanding the recognition, classification, diagnosis, management, and prevention of shock is essential for healthcare providers across various specialties. Shock is a complex and multifaceted condition that demands prompt and accurate identification to mitigate its potentially devastating effects. By recognizing early and subtle signs, such as vasoconstriction and diaphoresis, clinicians can intervene more effectively before the condition escalates to critical stages characterized by overt hypotension and tachycardia. Implementing a systematic approach ensures that all potential causes are considered and addressed, tailoring the treatment to the specific type of shock, whether hypovolemic, cardiogenic, distributive, or obstructive. This comprehensive strategy not only improves patient outcomes but also supports a more efficient use of healthcare resources.

Moreover, integrating evidence-based interventions into managing shock is crucial for optimizing patient care. Advances in medical research continually refine our understanding of shock pathophysiology and treatment modalities, providing clinicians with robust guidelines and protocols. These evidence-based practices, such as the early administration of fluids, vasopressors, and appropriate diagnostic imaging, enable healthcare providers to stabilize patients swiftly and effectively. Continuous education and training on the latest developments in shock management are imperative for maintaining high standards of care. By fostering a culture of vigilance and preparedness, healthcare systems can significantly reduce the mortality and morbidity associated with shock, ultimately improving the quality of life for affected patients.

References

1. Appleton C, Gillam L, Koulogiannis K. Cardiac tamponade. Cardiol Clin. 2017;35(4):525–37. https://doi.org/10.1016/j.ccl.2017.07.006.
2. Arias-Ortiz J, Vincent JL. The pulmonary artery catheter. Curr Opin Crit Care. 2023;29(3):231–5. https://doi.org/10.1097/mcc.0000000000001040.
3. Bartolome SD, Torres F. Severe pulmonary arterial hypertension: stratification of medical therapies, mechanical support, and lung transplantation. Heart Fail Rev. 2016;21(3):347–56. https://doi.org/10.1007/s10741-016-9562-7.
4. Ben-Baruch Golan Y, Sadeh R, Mizrakli Y, Shafat T, Sagy I, Slutsky T, Kobal SL, Novack V, Fuchs L. Early point-of-care ultrasound assessment for medical patients reduces time to appropriate treatment: a pilot randomized controlled trial. Ultrasound Med Biol. 2020;46(8):1908–15. https://doi.org/10.1016/j.ultrasmedbio.2020.03.023.
5. Bertini P, Guarracino F. Pathophysiology of cardiogenic shock. Curr Opin Crit Care. 2021;27(4):409–15. https://doi.org/10.1097/mcc.0000000000000853.
6. Bloom JE, Andrew E, Dawson LP, Nehme Z, Stephenson M, Anderson D, Fernando H, Noaman S, Cox S, Milne C, Chan W, Kaye DM, Smith K, Stub D. Incidence and outcomes of nontraumatic shock in adults using emergency medical services in Victoria, Australia. JAMA Netw Open. 2022;5(1):e2145179. https://doi.org/10.1001/jamanetworkopen.2021.45179.
7. Blum M, Ferrada P. Ultrasound and other innovations for fluid management in the ICU. Surg Clin North Am. 2017;97(6):1323–37. https://doi.org/10.1016/j.suc.2017.07.009.

8. Bonanno FG. Clinical pathology of the shock syndromes. J Emerg Trauma Shock. 2011;4(2):233–43. https://doi.org/10.4103/0974-2700.82211.
9. Cannon JW. Hemorrhagic shock. N Engl J Med. 2018;378(4):370–9. https://doi.org/10.1056/NEJMra1705649.
10. Chiabrando JG, Bonaventura A, Vecchié A, Wohlford GF, Mauro AG, Jordan JH, Grizzard JD, Montecucco F, Berrocal DH, Brucato A, Imazio M, Abbate A. Management of acute and recurrent pericarditis: JACC state-of-the-art review. J Am Coll Cardiol. 2020;75(1):76–92. https://doi.org/10.1016/j.jacc.2019.11.021.
11. Dave S, Dahlstrom JJ, Weisbrod LJ. Neurogenic shock. In: StatPearls. StatPearls Publishing Copyright © 2024, StatPearls Publishing LLC.; 2024.
12. Dumas G, Lavillegrand JR, Joffre J, Bigé N, de Moura EB, Baudel JL, Chevret S, Guidet B, Maury E, Amorim F, Ait-Oufella H. Mottling score is a strong predictor of 14-day mortality in septic patients whatever vasopressor doses and other tissue perfusion parameters. Crit Care. 2019;23(1):211. https://doi.org/10.1186/s13054-019-2496-4.
13. Evans DC, Doraiswamy VA, Prosciak MP, Silviera M, Seamon MJ, Rodriguez Funes V, Cipolla J, Wang CF, Kavuturu S, Torigian DA, Cook CH, Lindsey DE, Steinberg SM, Stawicki SP. Complications associated with pulmonary artery catheters: a comprehensive clinical review. Scand J Surg. 2009;98(4):199–208. https://doi.org/10.1177/145749690909800402.
14. Evans L, Rhodes A, Alhazzani W, Antonelli M, Coopersmith CM, French C, Machado FR, McIntyre L, Ostermann M, Prescott HC, Schorr C, Simpson S, Wiersinga WJ, Alshamsi F, Angus DC, Arabi Y, Azevedo L, Beale R, Beilman G, et al. Surviving sepsis campaign: international guidelines for management of sepsis and septic shock 2021. Intensive Care Med. 2021;47(11):1181–247. https://doi.org/10.1007/s00134-021-06506-y.
15. Ferrada P. Image-based resuscitation of the hypotensive patient with cardiac ultrasound: an evidence-based review. J Trauma Acute Care Surg. 2016;80(3):511–8. https://doi.org/10.1097/ta.0000000000000941.
16. Ferrada P, Evans D, Wolfe L, Anand RJ, Vanguri P, Mayglothling J, Whelan J, Malhotra A, Goldberg S, Duane T, Aboutanos M, Ivatury RR. Findings of a randomized controlled trial using limited transthoracic echocardiogram (LTTE) as a hemodynamic monitoring tool in the trauma bay. J Trauma Acute Care Surg. 2014;76(1):31–7; discussion 37-38. https://doi.org/10.1097/TA.0b013e3182a74ad9.
17. Galvagno SM Jr, Nahmias JT, Young DA. Advanced trauma life support(®) update 2019: management and applications for adults and special populations. Anesthesiol Clin. 2019;37(1):13–32. https://doi.org/10.1016/j.anclin.2018.09.009.
18. Ghane MR, Gharib MH, Ebrahimi A, Samimi K, Rezaee M, Rasouli HR, Kazemi HM. Accuracy of Rapid Ultrasound in Shock (RUSH) exam for diagnosis of shock in critically ill patients. Trauma Mon. 2015;20(1):e20095. https://doi.org/10.5812/traumamon.20095.
19. Gitz Holler J, Jensen HK, Henriksen DP, Rasmussen LM, Mikkelsen S, Pedersen C, Lassen AT. Etiology of shock in the emergency department: a 12-year population-based cohort study. Shock. 2019;51(1):60–7. https://doi.org/10.1097/shk.0000000000000816.
20. Hamzaoui O, Boissier F. Hemodynamic monitoring in cardiogenic shock. J Intensive Med. 2023;3(2):104–13. https://doi.org/10.1016/j.jointm.2022.10.003.
21. Hashim A, Tahir MJ, Ullah I, Asghar MS, Siddiqi H, Yousaf Z. The utility of point of care ultrasonography (POCUS). Ann Med Surg (Lond). 2021;71:102982. https://doi.org/10.1016/j.amsu.2021.102982.
22. Holcomb JB, del Junco DJ, Fox EE, Wade CE, Cohen MJ, Schreiber MA, Alarcon LH, Bai Y, Brasel KJ, Bulger EM, Cotton BA, Matijevic N, Muskat P, Myers JG, Phelan HA, White CE, Zhang J, Rahbar MH. The prospective, observational, multicenter, major trauma transfusion (PROMMTT) study: comparative effectiveness of a time-varying treatment with competing risks. JAMA Surg. 2013;148(2):127–36. https://doi.org/10.1001/2013.jamasurg.387.
23. Holcomb JB, Tilley BC, Baraniuk S, Fox EE, Wade CE, Podbielski JM, del Junco DJ, Brasel KJ, Bulger EM, Callcut RA, Cohen MJ, Cotton BA, Fabian TC, Inaba K, Kerby JD, Muskat P, O'Keeffe T, Rizoli S, Robinson BR, et al. Transfusion of plasma, platelets, and red blood cells in a 1:1:1 vs a 1:1:2 ratio and mortality in patients with severe trauma: the PROPPR randomized clinical trial. JAMA. 2015;313(5):471–82. https://doi.org/10.1001/jama.2015.12.
24. Holler JG, Bech CN, Henriksen DP, Mikkelsen S, Pedersen C, Lassen AT. Nontraumatic hypotension and shock in the emergency department and the prehospital setting, prevalence, etiology, and mortality: a systematic review. PLoS One. 2015;10(3):e0119331. https://doi.org/10.1371/journal.pone.0119331.
25. Kalkwarf KJ, Cotton BA. Resuscitation for hypovolemic shock. Surg Clin North Am. 2017;97(6):1307–21. https://doi.org/10.1016/j.suc.2017.07.011.
26. Kashani K, Omer T, Shaw AD. The intensivist's perspective of shock, volume management, and hemodynamic monitoring. Clin J Am Soc Nephrol. 2022;17(5):706–16. https://doi.org/10.2215/cjn.14191021.
27. Keikha M, Salehi-Marzijarani M, Soldoozi Nejat R, Sheikh Motahar Vahedi H, Mirrezaie SM. Diagnostic accuracy of Rapid Ultrasound in Shock (RUSH) exam; a systematic review and meta-analysis. Bull Emerg Trauma. 2018;6(4):271–8. https://doi.org/10.29252/beat-060402.
28. Lamia B, Kim HK, Severyn DA, Pinsky MR. Cross-comparisons of trending accuracies of continuous cardiac-output measurements: pulse contour analysis, bioreactance, and pulmonary-artery catheter. J Clin Monit Comput. 2018;32(1):33–43. https://doi.org/10.1007/s10877-017-9983-4.
29. Leech C, Turner J. Shock in trauma. Emerg Med Clin North Am. 2023;41(1):1–17. https://doi.org/10.1016/j.emc.2022.09.007.
30. Manji RA, Wood KE, Kumar A. The history and evolution of circulatory shock. Crit Care Clin. 2009;25(1):1–29, vii. https://doi.org/10.1016/j.ccc.2008.12.013.
31. Marik PE, Baram M, Vahid B. Does central venous pressure predict fluid responsiveness? A systematic review of the literature and the tale of seven mares. Chest. 2008;134(1):172–8. https://doi.org/10.1378/chest.07-2331.
32. McHugh K, Repanshek Z. Anaphylaxis: emergency department treatment. Emerg Med Clin North Am. 2022;40(1):19–32. https://doi.org/10.1016/j.emc.2021.08.004.
33. McLean AS. Echocardiography in shock management. Crit Care. 2016;20:275. https://doi.org/10.1186/s13054-016-1401-7.
34. Munroe ES, Heath ME, Eteer M, Gershengorn HB, Horowitz JK, Jones J, Kaatz S, Tamae Kakazu M, McLaughlin E, Flanders SA, Prescott HC. Use and outcomes of peripheral vasopressors in early sepsis-induced hypotension across Michigan hospitals: a retrospective cohort study. Chest. 2024;165(4):847–57. https://doi.org/10.1016/j.chest.2023.10.027.
35. Ngatuvai M, Zagales I, Sauder M, Andrade R, Santos RG, Bilski T, Kornblith L, Elkbuli A. Outcomes of transfusion with whole blood, component therapy, or both in adult civilian trauma patients: a systematic review and meta-analysis. J Surg Res. 2023;287:193–201. https://doi.org/10.1016/j.jss.2023.02.010.
36. Osterwalder J, Polyzogopoulou E, Hoffmann B. Point-of-care ultrasound-history, current and evolving clinical concepts in emergency medicine. Medicina (Kaunas). 2023;59(12) https://doi.org/10.3390/medicina59122179.
37. Pendleton AC, Leichtle SW. Cardiac tamponade from blunt trauma. Am Surg. 2022;88(6):1319–21. https://doi.org/10.1177/0003134820942170.

38. Perera P, Mailhot T, Riley D, Mandavia D. The RUSH exam: rapid ultrasound in SHock in the evaluation of the critically Ill. Emerg Med Clin North Am. 2010;28(1):29–56, vii. https://doi.org/10.1016/j.emc.2009.09.010.
39. Piazza G. Advanced management of intermediate- and high-risk pulmonary embolism: JACC focus seminar. J Am Coll Cardiol. 2020;76(18):2117–27. https://doi.org/10.1016/j.jacc.2020.05.028.
40. Prasanna N, Yamane D, Haridasa N, Davison D, Sparks A, Hawkins K. Safety and efficacy of vasopressor administration through midline catheters. J Crit Care. 2021;61:1–4. https://doi.org/10.1016/j.jcrc.2020.09.024.
41. Roberts DJ, Leigh-Smith S, Faris PD, Blackmore C, Ball CG, Robertson HL, Dixon E, James MT, Kirkpatrick AW, Kortbeek JB, Stelfox HT. Clinical presentation of patients with tension pneumothorax: a systematic review. Ann Surg. 2015;261(6):1068–78. https://doi.org/10.1097/sla.0000000000001073.
42. Robitaille-Fortin M, Norman S, Archer T, Mercier E. Prehospital decompression of pneumothorax: a systematic review of recent evidence. Prehosp Disaster Med. 2021;36(4):450–9. https://doi.org/10.1017/s1049023x21000509.
43. Samsky MD, Morrow DA, Proudfoot AG, Hochman JS, Thiele H, Rao SV. Cardiogenic shock after acute myocardial infarction: a review. JAMA. 2021;326(18):1840–50. https://doi.org/10.1001/jama.2021.18323.
44. Shakur H, Roberts I, Bautista R, Caballero J, Coats T, Dewan Y, El-Sayed H, Gogichaishvili T, Gupta S, Herrera J, Hunt B, Iribhogbe P, Izurieta M, Khamis H, Komolafe E, Marrero MA, Mejía-Mantilla J, Miranda J, Morales C, et al. Effects of tranexamic acid on death, vascular occlusive events, and blood transfusion in trauma patients with significant haemorrhage (CRASH-2): a randomised, placebo-controlled trial. Lancet. 2010;376(9734):23–32. https://doi.org/10.1016/s0140-6736(10)60835-5.
45. Simmons J, Ventetuolo CE. Cardiopulmonary monitoring of shock. Curr Opin Crit Care. 2017;23(3):223–31. https://doi.org/10.1097/mcc.0000000000000407.
46. Singer M, Deutschman CS, Seymour CW, Shankar-Hari M, Annane D, Bauer M, Bellomo R, Bernard GR, Chiche JD, Coopersmith CM, Hotchkiss RS, Levy MM, Marshall JC, Martin GS, Opal SM, Rubenfeld GD, van der Poll T, Vincent JL, Angus DC. The third international consensus definitions for sepsis and septic shock (Sepsis-3). JAMA. 2016;315(8):801–10. https://doi.org/10.1001/jama.2016.0287.
47. Smith A, Hendrix V, Shapiro M, Duchesne J, Taghavi S, Schroll R, Tatum D, Guidry C. Is the "death triad" a casualty of modern damage control resuscitation. J Surg Res. 2021;259:393–8. https://doi.org/10.1016/j.jss.2020.09.018.
48. Teboul JL, Hamzaoui O, Monnet X. SvO2 to monitor resuscitation of septic patients: let's just understand the basic physiology. Crit Care. 2011;15(6):1005. https://doi.org/10.1186/cc10491.
49. Tehrani BN, Truesdell AG, Psotka MA, Rosner C, Singh R, Sinha SS, Damluji AA, Batchelor WB. A standardized and comprehensive approach to the management of cardiogenic shock. JACC Heart Fail. 2020;8(11):879–91. https://doi.org/10.1016/j.jchf.2020.09.005.
50. Trott T, Bowman J. Diagnosis and management of pulmonary embolism. Emerg Med Clin North Am. 2022;40(3):565–81. https://doi.org/10.1016/j.emc.2022.05.008.
51. Vahdatpour C, Collins D, Goldberg S. Cardiogenic shock. J Am Heart Assoc. 2019;8(8):e011991. https://doi.org/10.1161/jaha.119.011991.
52. Vakamudi S, Ho N, Cremer PC. Pericardial effusions: causes, diagnosis, and management. Prog Cardiovasc Dis. 2017;59(4):380–8. https://doi.org/10.1016/j.pcad.2016.12.009.
53. Vincent JL, De Backer D. Circulatory shock. N Engl J Med. 2013;369(18):1726–34. https://doi.org/10.1056/NEJMra1208943.
54. Weinberger J, Klompas M, Rhee C. What is the utility of measuring lactate levels in patients with sepsis and septic shock? Semin Respir Crit Care Med. 2021;42(5):650–61. https://doi.org/10.1055/s-0041-1733915.
55. Whitton TP, Healy WJ. Clinical use and interpretation of thromboelastography. ATS Sch. 2023;4(1):96–7. https://doi.org/10.34197/ats-scholar.2022-0074OT.
56. Zieleskiewicz L, Lopez A, Hraiech S, Baumstarck K, Pastene B, Di Bisceglie M, Coiffard B, Duclos G, Boussuges A, Bobbia X, Einav S, Papazian L, Leone M. Bedside POCUS during ward emergencies is associated with improved diagnosis and outcome: an observational, prospective, controlled study. Crit Care. 2021;25(1):34. https://doi.org/10.1186/s13054-021-03466-z.

Surgical Critical Care

18

Caitlin A. Fitzgerald

Background

Advanced practice providers (APPs) including nurse practitioners (NPs) and physician assistants (PAs) are an important part of the care of intensive care unit (ICU) patients. While NPs and PAs have different backgrounds and training, these types of providers are used interchangeably in a variety of ways [1–3]. In nonacademic centers, APPs often staff ICUs independently whereas in academic centers, they are often integrated into the housestaff-based team [4].

When considering outcomes in the ICU, Kleinpell et al. performed a meta-analysis of 44 studies that evaluated the care provided by both APPs and residents and found similar or better patient outcomes when being cared for by an APP [5]. In a similar fashion, a meta-analysis by Kreeftenberg et al. found no differences in ICU mortality or length of stay when comparing APP and resident management but did note improved patient satisfaction and adherence to existing protocols in the APP group [6].

There are also intangible benefits when APPs are utilized to care for ICU patients. Unlike resident providers who frequently rotate through various service lines within the hospital, APPs are a consistent part of each ICU team. This consistency not only leads to improved communication between ICU staff members and patients but also increases procedural proficiency and familiarity with ICU-specific management paradigms and interventions [7–10]. APPs are an integral part of the ICU team and play an important role in the management of critically ill patients. This chapter provides an overview of common disorders that will be seen in the SICU including information on how to both diagnose and manage them successfully.

C. A. Fitzgerald (✉)
Department of Surgery, Division of Trauma, Bariatrics, and Acute Care Surgery, Baylor College of Medicine, Houston, TX, USA

Essentials of Postoperative Critical Care

The first 24 h that a surgical patient spends in the ICU are critical and focus mainly on the initial assessment and resuscitation [11]. After a detailed sign out is given from the surgical team to the critical care team, a thorough patient assessment should occur that includes any wounds, dressings, lines, drains, or monitors. The expected postoperative course should be discussed with the surgical team along with a plan if the patient were to become hemodynamically unstable. Patients who are immediately postoperative may demonstrate altered mental status due to the anesthetic agents they were given; thus, an adequate amount of time must be given in order for these medications to wear off before an appropriate neurologic exam can be performed [12]. Patients are also often hypothermic in the immediate postoperative period and forced-air rewarming devices and warmed fluids should be utilized [13].

Many patients will present from the operating room with an endotracheal tube still in place. Prior to extubation, several factors should be considered including the emergence from general anesthesia, any plans to return to the operating room in the near future, and the ease at which the patient was intubated in the operating room [11]. If a patient is unable to be successfully extubated in the immediate postoperative period, frequent reassessments should occur to determine if and when a safe extubation can occur [11].

Most postoperative patients will require some amount of resuscitation in the ICU. This need will vary based on the patients' preoperative volume status, the length of the case, and the total blood loss during the case. Measuring markers of perfusion including urine output, base deficit, and lactate should be interpreted in the setting of each patient's current clinical status [11]. If there is a concern for postoperative bleeding, resuscitation with blood products rather than crystalloid administration is preferred [11]. Once the patient has progressed out of the resuscitative phase, diuresis may be warranted in order to improve the overall volume status of the patient.

S. Atallah, J. Dragoljevic (eds.), *Fundamentals of Surgery for Physician Assistants*,
https://doi.org/10.1007/978-3-032-21069-2_18

Nutrition is another key component in the management of a postoperative patient. Early initiation of enteral nutrition (within 48 h of surgery) is associated with decreased mortality, duration of mechanical ventilation, and various infectious complications [14]. However, many patients who have just undergone abdominal surgery cannot start enteral nutrition immediately. Thus, discussion with the surgical team regarding when the initiation of enteral nutrition is appropriate is critical. If enteral nutrition is unable to be started for an extended period of time, parenteral nutrition can be considered [14].

Once the patient is out of the acute postoperative period, the focus of the critical care team shifts to the management of any ongoing organ dysfunction and the prevention of any postoperative complications [11]. Early mobilization of the patient is essential as deconditioning can occur quickly and can lead to lifelong limitations [15]. ICU delirium is also a common complication due to the combination of a disrupted sleep/wake cycle and many of the medications given for sedation and pain. Daily assessments of a patient's pain and sedation needs can help mitigate the development of ICU delirium [16]. Finally, any evidence of a developing infection including fevers, leukocytosis, change in vital signs, or change in the appearance of the surgical incision should prompt a workup with various cultures and a discussion with the surgical team [11].

Ultimately, the role of the APP on the surgical ICU (SICU) team is to anticipate, recognize, and manage surgical patients along both their anticipated postoperative course and any deviations from this pathway. Consistent communication and collaboration with the surgical team is imperative to the successful management of these patients [11].

Management of Critically Ill Patients

Pain Control and Sedation Management

Pain is common in the SICU and can be from a variety of causes such as trauma, surgical incisions, suctioning, invasive lines and drains, or preexisting conditions [17]. Untreated pain can lead to a variety of unintended complications such as the *inability to wean from the ventilator, impaired wound healing, decreased tissue perfusion, and prolonged ICU stays* [18]. While there are various pain scoring scales available, it is important to observe both behavioral and physiologic responses to analgesia as many SICU patients are unable to fully communicate [19]. Nonpharmacologic strategies for reducing pain in the ICU include patient positioning and the proper positioning of invasives lines and tubes. Pharmacologic strategies should focus on a *multimodal approach in order to synergistically target various pain receptors at lower doses and to avoid dependence on opioids alone* [20, 21].

Sedation is often necessary in the SICU as many patients are mechanically ventilated, have significant pain, or require bedside procedures. If a patient does require sedation, a sedation scoring tool such as the Richmond Agitation-Sedation Scale (RASS) should be used in order to ensure that a patient is comfortable but not overly sedated as this can lead to ICU delirium [22]. Sedated patients should also be given *daily sedation pauses* in order to assess their mental status and to allow them to undergo a spontaneous breathing trial (SBT). This strategy has been shown to lower a patient's daily dose of medication and ultimately leads to fewer ventilator days, a shorter ICU stay, and improved overall mortality [23].

Early Mobilization

Historically, patients in the ICU were thought to not be candidates for early mobilization because they were thought to be too physiologically unstable or dependent on mechanical life support. However, more recent evidence suggests that *early mobility is not only safe but also prevents long-term morbidity and physical disability* [6].

Prolonged physical inactivity has many physiologic consequences. First, it has been shown to decrease muscle mass by 1.5%–2.0% *per day* during the first 2–3 weeks of immobility. Not only are changes in muscle mass noted, but significant muscle weakness and atrophy are also known side effects of prolonged immobility [24]. Decrease in range of motion in joints can also lead to significant contractures with the elbows and ankles being the most commonly involved joints in critically ill patients [25]. Lung compliance is also reduced during prolonged immobility with significant atelectasis noted on imaging. Decreased lung compliance also leads to an increased risk of developing pneumonia [26]. Finally, skin ulceration and thromboembolic events are more common in patients who are immobile.

In order to provide early mobilization within an ICU setting, patients should be awake and engaged and on as limited sedation as possible, and they should also require as few life-support device as possible [27]. Once patients are able to mobilize, it should occur in stages at the appropriate intensity that can range from passive range of motion exercise to ambulating with and without assistance [28]. Regardless of how patients are able to mobilize, numerous studies have been published on the *benefits of early mobilization including improved brain function, return to baseline functional status, and a decrease in both hospital and ICU lengths of stay* [29].

Intravascular Devices

Central venous catheters (CVCs) are common across all ICUs and are placed for various reasons including the administration of vasoactive medications, hemodynamic monitoring, parenteral nutrition, renal replacement therapy, fluid resuscitation, and for the establishment of long-term venous access [30]. A patient's clinical presentation typically drives which type of CVC should be placed. While the number of lumens does not affect the risk of developing an infectious complication, the minimum number of necessary lumens should be considered before placing the catheter. Once the type of CVC is selected, the anatomic position of the catheter is also important. *When comparing the femoral vein and subclavian vein sites, a randomized study found that catheters placed in the femoral vein had a statistically significantly higher rate of both infectious and thrombotic complications* [31]. However, a more recent multicenter trial comparing catheters placed into the subclavian, femoral, and internal jugular veins noted a decreased risk of bacteremia with a subclavian placed catheter but did note an increased risk of **pneumothorax** when lines were placed in this location [32]. Regardless of the anatomic location that the catheter is placed in, *maintaining sterility during placement is crucial to decrease the risk of an infectious complication.*

Historically, CVCs were placed using anatomic landmarks alone. However, more recent literature has demonstrated the benefit of using ultrasound guidance when placing CVCs. Specifically when considering placement in the internal jugular vein, a meta-analysis evaluating 35 trials noted that the use of ultrasound significantly reduced line placement complications including the number of placement attempts and the time to successful placement [33]. The use of ultrasound for catheter placement has become the standard of care and should be utilized in both the elective and emergent settings whenever possible.

Complications following CVC placement are either mechanical in nature and related to the procedure itself or are caused by the presence of the catheter within the vein. Immediate complications such as bleeding, pneumothorax, arterial puncture, and catheter misplacement occur in up to 2.1% of all insertions. Complications such vessel thrombosis and infection are seen in 0.5%–1.4% of all line placements [30]. Interestingly, complications with catheter placement have not been shown to be dependent on a provider's level of training suggesting that providers-in-training can safely place CVCs with the appropriate supervision present.

Central line-associated blood stream infection (CLABSI) is the *most common cause of nosocomial bacteremia in ICU patients* and is thought to arise from various different mechanisms. These mechanisms include the migration of *skin flora* (e.g., *Staphylococcus epidermidis*) from the external surface of the catheter, infection of the catheter hub through repeated use, or seeding of the catheter from a distant source of infection [34]. The majority of organisms causing CVC-related infections are skin flora, suggesting that the most common cause is migration of these pathogens from the insertion site [35]. There are multiple interventions that should be performed at the time of catheter insertion in order to decrease the rate of CVC-related infections including *use of sterile technique, avoiding the femoral vein if possible, and the timely removal of unnecessary catheters* [36].

Ultrasonography

The use of ultrasonography has numerous applications in the SICU. One of the main benefits of this technique is that it can be performed at the bedside and gives the provider more detailed information regarding the patient's anatomy and physiology. Another benefit is that unlike diagnostic radiology which may not be interpreted and acted upon in a timely fashion, ultrasound gives the provider the ability to make changes to the patient's management in real time [37].

When considering the various uses of ultrasound in the SICU, *vascular access is one of the most common.* When placing access, the use of ultrasound allows the provider to visualize potential contraindications to access or aberrant anatomy that was not visible on physical exam. Furthermore, the use of ultrasound not only decreases complications from line placement but also increases the rate of successful line placement [38].

Not only is the use of ultrasound helpful when placing invasive lines, but it is also utilized *to evaluate the lung and pleura for underlying pathology* [39]. Ultrasound has been shown to be superior to chest radiography and can provide similar findings that are demonstrated in chest computed tomography (CT) scans without requiring the patient to travel to the CT scanner [40]. Findings that are commonly seen on ultrasound include ***pneumothorax, parenchymal consolidation, and pleural effusions.*** Here, ultrasound is also superior in that it is both diagnostic and therapeutic, specifically if managing a pneumothorax or pleural effusion [41].

Finally, the use of ultrasound in the SICU is frequently performed in the setting of shock to assess a patient's cardiac function. A limited bedside ultrasound allows providers to quickly visualize both the anatomy and the function of the heart in an unstable patient. This examination traditionally consists of five views including a parasternal long axis, parasternal short axis, apical four chamber, subcostal long axis, and inferior vena cava long axis [42]. Using these views, both *right and left ventricular function, valve and septal abnormalities, and the presence of a* ***pericardial effusion*** can be ascertained [43]. Critical care cardiac ultrasound not only provides an acute assessment of cardiac function but can also be performed frequently over time to see trends in cardiac physiology and assess for recovery of cardiac function [41].

Organ System-Specific Pathophysiology in the ICU

Cardiovascular

The cardiovascular system functions to pump oxygen-rich blood to the body while venous return carries metabolic waste products to be excreted by the lungs, liver, and kidneys. Within this system, the arterial side demonstrates high resistance, low volume, and low compliance, whereas the venous side is low resistance, high volume, and high compliance [44]. When considering a cycle of the cardiovascular system, there are two phases of ventricular activity, active *contraction* (systole), and *relaxation* (diastole). During diastole, the mitral valve opens, and the left ventricle relaxes and becomes filled with blood. In systole, the left ventricle contracts, the aortic valve opens, and the blood is released into the arterial system. As the volume of blood decreases, the ability of the ventricle to generate pressure decreases until it falls below the arterial pressure. When this occurs, the aortic valve closes and the next cycle begins [45].

When considering cardiovascular function in a critically ill patient, it is important to take into account the **Starling curve** which estimates the **left ventricular end-diastolic pressure** (LVEDP) and its relationship to the **stroke volume** (SV). As the filling pressure of the heart increases, the volume of blood that is ejected also increases in a curvilinear fashion. This is a dependent relationship, and at higher filling pressures, there is less increase in SV for a similar increase in LVEDP. *A steeper slope indicates a decreased afterload with a greater SV at each filling pressure, whereas a lower slope suggests increased afterload with a reduced SV at each filling pressure* [46].

Diastolic dysfunction is a common cause of cardiovascular dysfunction in the SICU. Things that can restrict diastolic flow include *large pleural effusions, tension pneumothoraxes, increased intra-abdominal pressure, and high levels of* ***positive-end expiratory pressure*** *(PEEP, which is a setting on ventilators).* Despite adequate LVEDP, extrinsic forces such as those just listed increase the pressure outside the heart and serve to decrease left ventricular end-diastolic volume (LVEDV) and SV [47]. In a similar fashion, a shift in the interventricular septum from right-to-left can also restrict filling during diastole. If the right ventricle became distended, the bulging septum would *reduce the volume and compliance of the left ventricle*. Conditions that may precipitate this phenomenon include *obstructive lung disease or an acute pulmonary embolism* [48]. Treatment of acute diastolic dysfunction typically consists of *both preload and afterload reduction* while *maintaining adequate coronary blood flow*. By decreasing venous return (preload), end-diastolic volume and thus LVEDP are both reduced. Decreasing the afterload reduces myocardial oxygen consumption and increases SV. Inotropes are also frequently used which act on the myocardium to both reduce end-systolic volume and increase SV. Other treatments for diastolic dysfunction include noninvasive mechanical ventilation which lowers both preload and afterload and correction of acidosis and hypoxemia [49].

In addition to diastolic function, ***hypoperfusion*** or ***shock*** is another physiologic component to consider when evaluating a patient with cardiac dysfunction. Typically, a patient in shock will demonstrate multiple clinical findings including tachycardia, hypotension, metabolic acidosis, oliguria, tachypnea, and altered mental status. If a patient is showing signs of shock, *it is important to first determine the etiology of the shock prior to treatment*. Three of the most common causes of shock include septic shock, cardiogenic shock, and hypovolemic shock [13].

Septic shock is characterized by a high SV and a <u>decreased</u> **systemic vascular resistance** (SVR) caused by the relaxation of the arteriolar smooth muscle. *Initial therapy includes broad spectrum antibiotics, volume resuscitation, and source control* [50]. Conversely, **cardiogenic shock** is characterized by low SV and a <u>high</u> SVR. Initial treatment consists of augmentation of the ability of the heart to contract with *inotropes and preload reduction* [51]. **Hypovolemic shock** is hemorrhagic or nonhemorrhagic in nature and can be due to trauma, gastrointestinal bleeding, or fluid losses from large burns. Management of hypovolemic shock includes obtaining adequate vascular access and *resuscitation with either warmed fluids or blood products* [52]. Other common causes of shock in a critically ill patient include cardiac tamponade, anaphylaxis, adrenal shock, and neurogenic shock. *With any cause of shock, prompt diagnosis, treatment, and frequent reevaluation of the patient and their response to treatment are critical* [52].

Historically, **pulmonary artery** (Swan-Ganz) **catheters** were used to assess cardiac function. While they are still used in the setting of patients with advanced heart failure, they are not as commonly used in patients in the SICU. More recently, noninvasive measures such as bedside ultrasonography, specifically focusing on the function of the heart and the appearance of the inferior vena cava (IVC) can provide crucial information regarding an assessment of cardiac output, volume status, and volume responsiveness. These measurements along with **central venous pressure** can help guide resuscitation [53].

Pulmonary

Respiratory failure occurs when a patient is either unable to oxygenate their peripheral tissues adequately or unable to ventilate. There are four main types of acute respiratory failure. Type I is known as *acute hypoxic respiratory failure* and occurs when there is some type of shunt causing inadequate gas exchange. Common causes of this include pulmonary edema and alveolar hemorrhage. Type II respiratory failure or *hypercarbic respiratory failure* occurs when there is either hypoventilation or a ventilation/perfusion mismatch. In this state, a patient's carbon dioxide (CO_2) is elevated and they typically demonstrate a reduced respiratory drive. Causes of type II respiratory failure include things such as chronic obstructive pulmonary disease and obesity hypoventilation syndrome. Type III respiratory failure is known as *postoperative respiratory failure* and occurs when atelectasis leads to a shunt and subsequent closure of small airways. Finally, type IV respiratory failure is seen in *shock* where there is inadequate oxygen delivery due to reduced CO. This type can be seen in various types of shock including sepsis and hemorrhagic shock [54, 55].

When focusing specifically on type I and type II respiratory failure, patient presentation is different. Patients with hypoxic respiratory failure typically present with tachypnea, hypoxemia on laboratory values, and can be cyanotic, whereas patients with hypercarbic respiratory failure present with a decreased respiratory drive. Whatever the cause of respiratory failure, *management goals are focused on minimizing the patient's respiratory work with ventilatory support if needed, adding additional PEEP if necessary to improve oxygenation, utilizing lung protective ventilatory strategies to avoid barotrauma, and maximizing CO to promote increased oxygen transport to peripheral tissues* [56].

Noninvasive Ventilatory Strategies

Noninvasive ventilatory (NIV) strategies are tools that can be utilized in both hypoxemic and hypercarbic respiratory failure and have been shown to reduce the need for endotracheal intubation [57]. **High-flow nasal cannula (HNFC)** is a commonly used mode of NIV and delivers warmed and humidified oxygen at rates of up to 60 L/min through a nasal cannula. HFNC is superior to conventional nasal cannula as it minimizes the amount of room air that becomes entrapped into the oxygen mixture and delivers a more precise level of oxygen. Furthermore, HFNC does deliver a low level of PEEP, thus reducing anatomical dead space [58]. Another mode of NIV is **continuous positive airway pressure (CPAP).** During CPAP, a constant level of positive pressure is delivered during spontaneous breathing. CPAP works by decreasing intrapulmonary shunts and opening up atelectatic portions of the lung [59].

The use of NIV techniques does come with risks. Some patients cannot tolerate NIV and thus require frequent interruptions or cessation of treatment all together. The masks and cannulas used can cause skin breakdown or ulceration, and make it difficult for patients to communicate. Furthermore, abdominal distention, vomiting, and aspiration can occur due to the delivery of PEEP without a secure airway in place [60]. Perhaps the most severe complication is the potential delay of intubation. While patients may demonstrate an improvement in their hypoxemia, they may be developing worsening pulmonary muscle fatigue, worsening lung injury, and worsening organ dysfunction. Thus, *patients who are being managed with NIV require close monitoring to frequently assess for any signs of impending respiratory collapse* [61].

Airway Management in the SICU

One of the most common procedures performed in the SICU is **endotracheal intubation**. When deciding whether a patient requires intubation, it is important to synthesize all clinical, laboratory, and imaging data prior to proceeding. Common causes of intubation in the SICU include acute hypoxic respiratory failure, **acute respiratory distress syndrome** (ARDS), aspiration, or acute ventilatory failure [62]. Clinical signs that indicate that a patient is progressing toward intubation include *progressive hypercapnia or hypoxia despite maximum support, respiratory mechanics that suggest muscle fatigue or impending failure, decreasing mental status, and challenging anatomy that would make an emergent intubation challenging* [62].

Immediately prior to intubation, all patients should be managed with 100% ***FiO****2 (fraction of inspired oxygen).* Vital signs should be continuously monitored before, during, and after intubation to assess any changes in patient physiology as hemodynamic instability may arise [63]. Physiologic considerations that should be taken into account include a patient's respiratory reserve and risk for bronchospasm as both may require a more expeditious intubation. Aspiration is also a risk during intubation, and gastric decompression should be performed prior to or immediately after intubation if possible [62].

The key to a successful intubation is *having all necessary equipment readily available at the patient's bedside in an airway cart or kit* [63]. Equipment to have readily available includes a laryngoscope, facemasks, and endotracheal tubes of various sizes, suction, stylet, syringe to inflate the endotracheal balloon, ambubag, oral and nasal airways, and various medications such as sedatives, muscle relaxants, paralytics, analgesics, and vasopressors [63]. Once the decision to intubate has been made, all patients should be **preoxygenated with 100% FiO_2** given the risk of rapid desaturation. Orotracheal intubation is the preferred method performed in the SICU as it is associated with less trauma, a lower incidence of **ventilator associated pneumonia (VAP),** and has a high success rate [64]. Risks of orotracheal intubation include difficulties with oral hygiene, dental trauma, cervical trauma, and difficulties properly securing the endotracheal tube to prevent dislodgement.

Physiologic changes following intubation and the initiation of positive pressure ventilation are common. The physical presence of an endotracheal tube increases airway resistance with smaller tubes demonstrating more resistance than larger tubes. Secretions that may build up along the tube further increase airway resistance [65]. Furthermore, hypotension is common postintubation as intrathoracic pressure changes from negative to positive with the institution of positive pressure ventilation. This change decreases venous return and thus cardiac output [66]. High PEEP can also increase pulmonary vascular resistance which decreases stroke volume.

Management of the Ventilated Patient in the SICU

Once a patient is mechanically ventilated, they are at risk for various complications, most notably **ventilator associated pneumonia** (VAP) and adverse effects of prolonged sedation and immobilization [67]. ***To combat the development of VAP, the head of bed should be elevated to 30°–45° in order to prevent aspiration, and oral hygiene should be performed with chlorhexidine. Daily breaks in sedation should be undertaken to assess a patient's mental status and to perform a spontaneous breathing trial (SBT).*** Daily SBTs when feasible are important as they are indicative of when a patient may be able to be weaned from the ventilator. To combat the risk of developing venous thromboembolisms, the appropriate prophylaxis should be given [68].

The mechanics of the ventilator also predispose patients to injury. Prolonged exposure to high tidal volumes and high airway pressures can lead to inflammation and lung injury [69]. Prolonged intubation with minimal patient-driven respiratory drive can also lead to diaphragm atrophy and dysfunction, making liberation from the ventilator challenging [70].

Choosing a ventilatory mode and settings are unique to each patient and depend on the cause of the patient's respiratory failure and underlying pulmonary mechanics. Typically, patients can be separated into one of the four categories to help guide ventilator mode choice. These categories include (a) patients with normal pulmonary mechanics and gas exchange, (b) patients with ARDS, (c) patients with restrictive lung disease, or (d) patients with an airway obstruction [71]. Furthermore, despite efforts to achieve complete rest of the respiratory system, most patients will make some degree of active respiratory effort which can be minimized with different ventilator strategies.

Conventional modes of ventilation are either based on a **pressure**-target or a **volume**-target. In **pressure-targeted modes**, a fixed *inspiratory pressure* is chosen *regardless of the tidal volumes* that a patient is achieving, whereas in a **volume-targeted mode**, a *set tidal volume is chosen* and is given to the patient regardless of the pressures that are required to deliver it [72]. Mixed volume and pressure modes are also available but are not used frequently. Regardless of the ventilator mode that is chosen, the initial ventilator settings should be dependent on the patient's respiratory mechanics and ventilatory needs. Arterial blood gas (ABG) is among the **most important** tests to obtain in ventilated patients as it helps guide and optimize settings. **Chest X-rays** (CXR) are also important to obtain to determine endotracheal tube placement and to assess the pulmonary fields.

Neurologic

Delirium is common among critically ill patients, occurring in 20%–80% of patients, and is due to a combination of the patient's acute illness, preexisting comorbidities, and various ICU-specific factors. **Delirium** is associated with worse patient outcomes including *longer hospital lengths of stay, long-term cognitive deficits, need for a facility at time of discharge, and death* [73]. Based on the Diagnostic and Statistical Manual of Mental Disorders (DSM) V guidelines, a diagnosis of delirium requires five criteria: a disturbance in attention, a short time period (hours to days) with fluctuation, disturbance in cognition, evidence that the disturbance is directly related to a medical condition, medication, or multiple etiologies, and finally that the disturbance cannot be explained by another neurologic disorder [73]. Delirium can be further classified into hypoactive, hyperactive, and mixed. Hyperactive delirium is uncommon and seen in <5% of critically ill patients. Due to the nature of this type of delirium, these patients are at high risk of injuring themselves, pulling out invasive lines and drains, falling out of bed, and self-extubating [74]. On the other hand, while hypoactive delirium is more common (45%–60% of critically ill patients), it is often missed by clinicians as patients are calm and not agitated [74].

Risk factors for delirium are multifactorial. Traditionally, patients with significant comorbidities may develop delirium with exposure to minimal insults, whereas previously healthy patients may require greater insults to become delirious [75]. While there are many risk factors that are not modifiable, those that are specific to the environment in the ICU or the acute illness are often able to be prevented or changed. Baseline risk factors for developing delirium include advanced age, history of substance or alcohol abuse, underlying dementia or other cognitive impairment, and a history of smoking. Risk factors related to the ICU in particular include a more severe illness, the need for mechanical ventilation, the use of sedative and analgesic medications, various electrolyte and metabolic derangements, sleep disturbances, and immobility [76].

Prevention and treatment of delirium are important in the SICU. Though antipsychotics are traditionally used to prevent the development of delirium, there is little evidence to support their use [77, 78]. Dexmedetomidine, an alpha-2 agonist, has also been used to combat delirium in the ICU. When compared with benzodiazepines, the use of dexmedetomidine was found to be associated with lower rates of delirium [79]. However, studies comparing dexmedetomidine with propofol had mixed results [80]. Ultimately, a multifactorial strategy to both minimize and treat risk factors for the development of delirium is the most effective.

Gastrointestinal

Gastrointestinal Hemorrhage

Gastrointestinal (GI) bleeding is separated into upper GI tract bleeding and lower GI tract bleeding. While not absolute, patients with an **upper GI bleed** tend to present with coffee ground emesis, hematemesis, or melena, whereas patients with a **lower GI bleed** tend to present with hematochezia [81]. Regardless of the source of bleeding, the initial management is the same and includes *obtaining **large bore intravenous access**, resuscitation with both **crystalloids** and **blood products, monitoring end organ perfusion**, placement of a **nasogastric tube** if an upper GI source is suspected, **acid suppression therapy**, involvement of gastroenterology for consideration of **endoscopy**, and the involvement of both **surgery** and **radiology** for the potential need for angioembolic or operative intervention* [81].

Endoscopic interventions are critical to the management of GI bleeding. If a patient is hemodynamically stable, endoscopy can be performed within 24 h. However, if a patient is hemodynamically unstable, emergent endoscopy is indicated with the intention of both identifying and controlling the source of hemorrhage [82]. Endoscopy is contraindicated in the setting of a perforation, severe coagulopathy, respiratory decompensation, and unstable angina. Furthermore, if the patient is exsanguinating, emergent angiography or surgical intervention is preferred [82].

If endoscopy is unable to determine the source of bleeding, diagnostic and therapeutic radiologic options are available. Angiography is able to diagnose a GI bleed by demonstrating the extravasation of contrast within the lumen of the intestine [82]. However, brisk bleeding (rate of 0.5–1 mL/min) must be actively occurring at the time of angiography or it will be nondiagnostic. Radionuclide scans can also be utilized to localize the source of bleeding. However, similar to angiography, the patient must be actively bleeding (0.5 mL/min) in order for the scan to be diagnostic [83].

Upper GI bleeding can be separated into variceal hemorrhage and nonvariceal hemorrhage. **Variceal hemorrhage** is seen in the setting of *decompensated cirrhosis* [84]. Management of variceal bleeding includes *resuscitation with IV fluids and blood, correction of any underlying coagulopathy, endotracheal intubation, antibiotic prophylaxis to combat bacterial translocation from the GI tract, medications such as somatostatin to reduce portal hypertension and increase splanchnic vasoconstriction, and endoscopic therapy for banding or sclerotherapy* [84]. It is important to note that varices have a high rate of rebleeding despite maximum medical and endoscopic therapy. **Nonvariceal hemorrhage** is typically related to ***peptic ulcer disease*** with up to 90% of patients demonstrating spontaneous cessation of bleeding [85]. Management is similar to variceal hemorrhage in that patients require *large bore IV access, resuscitation with fluid and blood products, and endoscopic management.* Following endoscopy, acid reducing medications should be utilized to reduce the rate of rebleeding [85]. Other causes of upper GI hemorrhage include Mallory Weiss tears and Dieulafoy lesions.

Lower GI bleeding is bleeding that is coming *distal to the ligament of Treitz*. The most typical causes of lower GI bleeding include ***diverticular disease*** and angiodysplasia. In most cases of potential lower GI bleeding, a brisk upper GI source should be considered, and thus *both upper and lower endoscopy should be performed* [86]. Colonoscopy should be performed within 24 h once a patient is hemodynamically stable and is able to undergo a rapid bowel prep [87]. Colonoscopy is diagnostic in 69%–80% of cases. However, if a both an upper endoscopy and colonoscopy are both negative, a small bowel source should be considered for which push enteroscopy or capsule endoscopy can be performed [86].

Cirrhosis

Liver failure in the SICU can be due to new onset acute liver failure, or acute on chronic liver failure in the setting of underlying cirrhosis. Acute on chronic liver failure can affect multiple organ systems, and thus a multiorgan system approach to management is critical [88]. Portal hypertension develops in cirrhosis due to the combination of increased portal inflow and the prolonged intrahepatic resistance to this flow. Subsequently, this leads to splanchnic vasodilation and the shunting of blood to the splanchnic system, leading to an effective decrease in cardiac output to other organs [89]. In the setting of acute, decompensated cirrhosis, patients may present with hepatic encephalopathy, refractory ascites, hepatorenal syndrome, and GI bleeding [89].

Hepatic encephalopathy can present in a variety of ways from mild alterations in mental status to coma. It occurs when the liver is unable to clear neurotoxins that are produced in the GI tract, specifically ammonia [90]. Diagnosis of hepatic encephalopathy requires a high index of suspicion, and management is focused on *clearance of ammonia buildup* using medications such as *lactulose* to stimulate GI tract excretion of these toxins [88].

Hepatorenal syndrome is another side effect of decompensated cirrhosis and is associated with high mortality. The diagnosis of hepatorenal syndrome is vague and is thought to occur when there is renal dysfunction in the setting of cirrhosis and portal hypertension [91]. Initial treatment is with *volume expansion with albumin* which has been shown to decrease patient mortality. However, *liver transplant is the only definitive treatment* of hepatorenal syndrome [92].

Finally, **ascites** is common in patients with decompensated cirrhosis and is due to the combination of sodium retention and portal hypertension [93]. Management of ascites includes *sodium restriction and diuretic therapy with a combination of both spironolactone and furosemide.* Unfortunately, some patients stop responding to the medical management of ascites and require intermittent drainage via a *transabdominal paracentesis.* Patients with *refractory ascites* can also be evaluated for consideration of a *transjugular intrahepatic portosystemic shunt (TIPS)* where blood is shunted from the portal to the hepatic system in order to decrease portal hypertension [92]. Regardless of the volume of ascites, all patients presenting with ascites should undergo a *diagnostic paracentesis* to assess for the presence of **spontaneous bacteria peritonitis (SBP)**. If positive (or if the suspicion for SBP is high), patients should be managed with a third-generation cephalosporin until culture results return and the antibiotic choice can be narrowed [94].

Acute Mesenteric Ischemia

Acute mesenteric ischemia (AMI) is a difficult diagnosis to make as the symptoms can be attributed to multiple illnesses and are nonspecific and vague [95]. Because diagnosis is often delayed, AMI is associated with patient mortality upward of 50% [96]. AMI can be caused by an acute arterial embolus, an arterial thrombosis, a mesenteric venous thrombosis, and can be nonobstructive in nature with the ***most common causes being an acute arterial embolus*** or thrombus. Patients with AMI tend to be *older (median age 74)* and often have multiple medical comorbidities including diabetes, hypertension, obesity, coronary artery disease, and a history of smoking [97]. Nonobstructive mesenteric ischemia (NOMI) is traditionally seen in low cardiac output states and is not directly related to a blood clot that prevents blood from reaching the intestine [98].

Clinical presentation is typically ***severe abdominal pain that is out of proportion to the exam*** but vomiting, diarrhea, and bloody bowel movements are also seen. If allowed to progress, patients will eventually develop frank peritonitis due to bowel ischemia and subsequent perforation [99]. In addition to performing a physical exam, imaging studies such as abdominal X-rays and **CT angiography (first-line study)** are often performed. Similar to the presenting symptom, CT findings are also often vague and can include dilated loops of bowel, bowel wall thickening, hypoenhancement of the bowel wall, mesenteric thickening or stranding, portal venous gas, and superior mesenteric artery (SMA) abnormalities [100]. Treatment of AMI consists of *urgent surgical consultation, fluid resuscitation, broad spectrum antibiotic coverage, and the initiation of therapeutic anticoagulation.* Both endovascular and open techniques have been described, and the decision is often based on whether or not there is bowel compromise [101].

Renal

Acute kidney injury (AKI) is common in critically ill patients but is associated with significant increases in patient morbidity and mortality. AKI is characterized by a decrease in the glomerular filtration rate (GFR) in combination with a decrease in urine output, a rise in serum creatinine, or both [102]. Currently, the Kidney Disease Improving Global Outcomes (KDIGO) guidelines define AKI as an ***increase in serum creatinine by at least 0.3 mg/dL within 48 h*** or a ***decrease in urine output of less than 0.5 mL/kg/h for 6 h or longer*** [102].

Within the ICU setting, AKI has been found to develop in approximately 57% of patients with up to 14% of patients requiring renal replacement therapy [103]. The annual incidence of AKI also continues to increase and complications include volume overload, uremia, and various electrolyte abnormalities. Despite the effect that AKI has on the kidneys themselves, *most of the attributable mortality from AKI is due to its effects on other organs* [104]. Interestingly, the main cause of death in patients who develop AKI is *sepsis*, accounting for over 40% of mortality [105]. *Pulmonary complications* are also frequent as patients with AKI are at a higher risk for developing pulmonary edema which may lead to the need for mechanical ventilation. AKI also affects the cardiovascular system and may lead to *cardiac injury* [106].

Historically, AKI has been categorized into prerenal, intrinsic renal, and postrenal. Initial workup to discern which type of AKI has developed includes urine studies evaluating the fractional excretion of sodium or urea, urine microscopy, and a renal ultrasound. **Prerenal AKI** is the *most commonly seen type of AKI in the ICU setting*. It is caused by decreased perfusion of the kidneys that leads to a decrease in GFR and is oftentimes seen after a patient develops shock. *Prerenal AKI is managed with* ***improving renal perfusion*** [107]. Conversely, postrenal AKI is much less common and is responsible for only 5% of AKI cases. Postrenal disease is due to an obstruction of urinary flow which subsequently increases the pressure within the renal tubules and decreases the GFR. Causes of postrenal AKI include renal stones, blood clots, masses, or urinary retention. Management of postrenal AKI includes removal of the source of the urinary obstruction or decompression of the renal system with percutaneous nephrostomy tube placement [108]. Intrinsic AKI is associated with direct damage to the kidneys due to acute tubular necrosis (ATN), acute interstitial nephritis (AIN), or contrast-associated AKI (CA-AKI). ATN can be further broken down into three subtypes including nephrotoxic, ischemic, and septic. Ischemic ATN is often seen after there is a prolonged decrease in renal perfusion, such as during sepsis, whereas nephrotoxic ATN results from an exogenous drug or toxin that directly causes renal toxicity [109]. Treatment of ATN is focused on improvement of renal perfusion and removal of any nephrotoxic medications.

As there are no specific therapies available to prevent the development of AKI, much of the treatment is supportive in nature and includes *managing the underlying cause of the AKI* and *if necessary, starting* ***renal replacement therapy (RRT).*** RRT is utilized in approximately 5% of all patients. Unlike patients who have developed end-stage renal disease, patients with AKI who require RRT oftentimes recover their kidney function and do not require long-term dialysis [103].

Overall, RRT is used to remove solutes and water. Within the SICU, the two most common types of RRT that will be utilized are *intermittent hemodialysis (IHD)* and *continuous renal replacement therapy (CRRT).* Through either method, the patient's blood is pumped across a semipermeable filter that is bathed in a dialysate solution that will remove certain solutes and water from the blood before the blood is pumped back to the patient [110]. Traditionally, IHD is reserved for patients who are hemodynamically stable as it requires larger volume shifts than CRRT. Indications for RRT are similar regardless of whether the therapy is intermittent or continuous. Common indications include *severe acidemia, electrolyte abnormalities such as hyperkalemia, ingestion of toxins, volume overload, or severe uremia* [111]. While multiple studies have tried to answer the question as to the optimal timing of RRT initiation, there has been no prospective trial to address this and thus no clear consensus.

Infectious Disease

Sepsis was first defined in 1992, and this definition has gone through several iterations. Most recently, in 2016, "**sepsis-3**" was defined as a *dysregulated host response to infection along with organ dysfunction, while septic shock was defined as the presence of sepsis with a lactate level of at least 2 mmol/L and a vasopressor requirement* [112]. Regardless of the nuances of how sepsis is defined, it is prevalent in critically ill patients and is associated with an increase in patient mortality [113]. Not only does sepsis increase patient mortality, but it also increases morbidity with more patients who develop sepsis requiring discharge to a facility versus patients who do not develop sepsis [114].

When considering the source of sepsis, the *most common source is the respiratory tract* which accounts for 64% of cases. Other common sources of sepsis include the GI tract, the bloodstream, and the genitourinary tract [115]. Once a patient has developed sepsis, it effects each organ system individually. From a vascular standpoint, septic shock is a *distributive* type of shock and results in pan-vessel dilatation and decreased vascular tone [116]. The cardiovascular system may demonstrate a global reduction in function with decreased contractility and a depressed response to fluids or vasopressors [117]. From a respiratory standpoint, due to the increase in pulmonary vascular permeability and inflammation, patients are at an increased risk for developing ARDS. Similarly, in the intestines, bacterial translocation can occur due to increased intestinal permeability and hypoperfusion of the bowel can lead to ischemia and necrosis [118]. The renal system may also demonstrate poor perfusion leading to the development of AKI. From an endocrine standpoint, sepsis causes dysregulation of blood sugar control and leads to hyperglycemia. And finally, septic encephalopathy is seen in up to 70% of patients with sepsis [119].

As patients with sepsis can present in a variety of different ways, a high index of suspicion is necessary to properly diagnose and treat sepsis. Once an infection is suspected, evaluation of a patient's mental status, systolic blood pressure, and respiratory rate can be used as a screening tool [112]. Diagnostic labs and imaging should then be used to target a potential source of infection prior to the initiation of antibiotics.

Once the diagnosis of sepsis is suspected or confirmed, timely management is crucial to minimizing morbidity and mortality. In 2018, the Surviving Sepsis Campaign introduced the 1-h bundle in an effort to both expedite and standardize sepsis care. The 1-h bundle includes *obtaining* ***blood cultures*** *before starting antibiotics, starting* ***broad spectrum antibiotics****, measuring a* ***lactate level****, fluid resuscitation with a* ***30 mL/kg crystalloid bolus****, and starting* ***vasopressors*** *to maintain a MAP of greater than 65 mmHg* [120]. When considering antibiotics, while the early initiation of them is important, the type of antibiotic to start with is less clear. Traditionally, an initial broad-spectrum approach is preferred until culture data returns with a specific pathogen at which time the antibiotic coverage can be safely narrowed [121]. The duration of antibiotic therapy also varies and is dependent on the type of infection, pathogen, and patient's clinical response [121].

Hematology

Anemia is very common among critically ill patients with up to 95% of patients in an ICU becoming anemic by day 3 of their ICU course [122]. While common, anemia is associated with *increased morbidity, mortality, and hospital length of stay*. Anemia is best defined as a reduction in red blood cell (RBC) mass that leads to a decrease in the delivery of oxygen to the peripheral tissues [123]. Within the setting of critical illness, patients demonstrate an underproduction anemia or an anemia of inflammation. This occurs when the patient's inflammatory response decreases iron availability and suppresses erythropoietin production and activity. When combined with the frequent blood loss critically ill patients experience for laboratory draws, this dysregulation accounts for the majority of cases of anemia in the ICU [124].

Given the high prevalence of anemia among ICU patients, it is not surprising that ICU patients receive more RBC transfusions than noncritically ill patients even in the era of more restrictive transfusion practices [125]. The first study to evaluate a restrictive versus liberal transfusion strategy was the TRICC trial published in 1999. This trial concluded that a restrictive transfusion strategy with a threshold hemoglobin of less than or equal to 7 g/dL is equivalent and possibly superior to a liberal transfusion strategy with a threshold hemoglobin of less than or equal to 10 g/dL [126]. Current guidelines suggest a transfusion threshold of less than or equal to 7 g/dL even in the setting of sepsis, GI bleeding, or trauma. Transfusion thresholds for patients with cardiovascular disease are not as clear, but current guidelines support a threshold of less than or equal to 8 g/dL [127].

Conclusion

APPs are a critical part of any ICU team and provide continuity to patients that often cannot be offered by other providers.

References

1. Hyzy R, Flanders S, Pronovost P, et al. Characteristics of intensive care units in Michigan: not an open and closed case. J Hosp Med. 2010;5(1):4–9.
2. Moote M, Krsek C, Kleinpell R, Todd B. Physician assistant and nurse practitioner utilization in academic medical centers. Am J Med Qual. 2011;26(6):452–60.
3. Riportella-Muller R, Libby D, Kindig D. The substitution of physician assistants and nurse practitioners for physician residents in teaching hospitals. Health Aff (Millwood). 1995;14(2):181–91.
4. D'Agostino R, Halpern N. Acute care nurse practitioners in oncologic critical care: the memorial Sloan-Kettering cancer center experience. Crit Care Clin. 2010;26(1):207–17.
5. Kleinpell R, Grabenkort WR, Kapu AN, et al. Nurse practitioners and physician assistants in acute and critical care: a concise review of the literature and data 2008–2018. Crit Care Med. 2019;47(10):1442–9.
6. Kreeftenberg HG, Pouwels S, Bindels A, et al. Impact of the advanced practice provider in adult critical care: a systematic review and meta-analysis. Crit Care Med. 2019;47(5):722–30.
7. Huang DT, Clermont G, Kong L, et al. Intensive care unit safety culture and outcomes: a US multicenter study. Int J Qual Health Care. 2010;22(3):151–61.
8. Dong Y, Suri HS, Cook DA, et al. Simulation-based objective assessment discerns clinical proficiency in central line placement: a construct validation. Chest. 2010;137(5):1050–6.
9. Loukas C, Nikiteas N, Kanakis M, et al. A virtual reality simulation curriculum for intravenous cannulation training. Acad Emerg Med. 2010;17(10):1142–5.
10. Mulcaster JT, Mills J, Hung OR, et al. Laryngoscopic intubation: learning and performance. Anesthesiology. 2003;98(1):23–7.
11. Nunnally M, Piper G. Principles of Postoperative Critical Care. In: Schmidt GA, Kress JP, Douglas IS, editors. Hall, Schmidt and Wood's principles of critical care. 5th ed. McGraw Hill; 2023.
12. Murphy GS, Brull SJ. Residual neuromuscular blockade: lessons unlearned. Part I: definitions, incidence, and adverse physiologic effects of residual neuromuscular block. Anesth Analg. 2010;111(1):120–8.
13. Apfelbaum JL, Silverstain JH, Chung FF, et al. Practice guidelines for postanesthetic care: a report by the American Society of Anesthesiologists Task Force on Postanesthetic care. Anesthesiology. 2013;118(2):291–307.
14. Padilla PF, Martinez G, Vernooij RW, et al. Early enteral nutrition (within 48 hours) versus delayed enteral nutrition (after 48 hours) with or without supplemental parenteral nutrition in critically ill adults. Cochrane Database Syst Rev. 2019(10):CD012340.
15. Corcoran JR, Herbsman JM, Bushnik T, et al. Early rehabilitation in the medical and surgical intensive care units for patients with and without mechanical ventilation: an interprofessional performance improvement project. PM R. 2017;9(2):113–9.
16. Ramsey SC, Lucas J, Barrett P, et al. Safe ambulation of critically ill cardiac patients with femoral balloon pumps: a case cohort study. J Card Fail. 2020;26(7):621–5.
17. Olsen BF, Valeberg BT, Jacobsen M, et al. Pain in intensive care unit patients- a longitudinal study. Nurs Open. 2021;8(1):224.
18. Desai PM. Pain management and pulmonary dysfunction. Crit Care Clin. 1999;15(1):151.
19. Kapoustina O, Echegaray-Benites C, Gelinas C. Fluctuations in vital signs and behavioral responses of brain surgery patients in the intensive care unit: are they valid indicators of pain? J Adv Nurs. 2014;70(11):2562.
20. Devlin JW, Skrobik Y, Gelinas C, et al. Clinical practice guidelines for the prevention and management of pain, agitation/sedation, delirium, immobility and sleep disruption in adult patients in the ICU. Crit Care Med. 2018;46(9):e825.
21. Shi S, Wang X, Song J, et al. Efficacy of intravenous acetaminophen in multimodal management for pain relief following total knee arthroplasty: a meta-analysis. J Orthop Surg Res. 2018;13(1):250.
22. Crippen D. Neurologic monitoring in the intensive care unit. New Horiz. 1994:107–20.
23. Kress JP, Pohlman AS, O'Conor MF, Hall JB. Daily interruption of sedative infusions in critically ill patients undergoing mechanical ventilation. New Eng J Med. 2000;342(20)
24. Adams GR, Caiozzo VJ, Baldwin KM. Skeletal muscle unweighting: spaceflight and ground-based models. J Appl Physiol. 2003;95:2185–201.
25. Clavet H, Hebert PC, Fergusson D, et al. Joint contracture following prolonged stay in the intensive care unit. CMAJ. 2008;178:691–7.
26. Brower RG. Consequences of bed rest. Crit Care Med. 2009;37(10):S422–8.

27. Ely EW, Truman B, Shintani A, et al. Monitoring sedation status over time in ICU patients: reliability and validity of the Richmond agitation-sedation scale (RASS). JAMA. 2003;298:2983–91.
28. Barber EA, Everard T, Holland AE, et al. Barriers and facilitators to early mobilization in intensive care: a qualitative study. Aust Crit Care. 2015;28:177–82.
29. Weiss CH, Moazed F, McEvoy CA, et al. Prompting physicians to address a daily checklist and process of care and clinical outcomes: a single-site study. Am J Respir Crit Care Med. 2011;184(6):680–6.
30. Farkas JC, Liu N, Bleriot JP, et al. Single-versus triple-lumen central catheter-related sepsis: a prospective randomized study in a critically ill population. Am J Med. 1992;93:277–82.
31. Merrer J, DeJonghe B, Golliot F, et al. Complications of femoral and subclavian venous catheterization in critically ill patients: a randomized controlled trial. JAMA. 2001;286:700–7.
32. Parienti JJ, Mongardon N, Megarbane B, et al. Intravascular complications of central venous catheterization by insertion site. N Engl J Med. 2015;373(13):1220–9.
33. Brass P, Hellmich M, Kolodziej L, et al. Ultrasound guidance versus anatomical landmarks for internal jugular vein catheterization. Cochrane Database Syst Rev. 2015;1(1):CD006962.
34. Raad IL, Hohn DC, Gilbreath BJ, et al. Prevention of central venous catheter-related infections by using maximal sterile barrier precautions during insertion. Infect Control Hosp Epidemiol. 1994;15:231–8.
35. Mermel LA, McCormick RD, Springman SR, et al. The pathogenesis and epidemiology of catheter-related infection with pulmonary artery Swan-Ganz catheters: a prospective study utilizing molecular subtyping. Am J Med. 1991;91:S197–205.
36. Pronovost P, Needham B, Berenholtz S, et al. An intervention to decrease catheter related blood stream infections in the ICU. N Engl J Med. 2006;355:2725–32.
37. Mayo PH, Beaulieu Y, Doelken P, et al. American College of Chest Physicians statement on competence in critical care ultrasonography. Chest. 2009;135:1050–60.
38. Troianos CA, Kuwik RJ, Pasqual JR, et al. Internal jugular vein and carotid artery anatomic relation as determined by ultrasonography. Anesthesiology. 1996;85:43–8.
39. Brenner DJ, Hall EJ. Computed tomography- an increasing source of radiation exposure. N Engl J Med. 2007;357:2277–84.
40. Lichtenstein D, Goldstein I, Mourgeon E, et al. Comparative diagnostic performances of auscultation, chest radiography, and lung ultrasonography in acute respiratory distress syndrome. Anesthesiology. 2004;100:9–15.
41. Mayo PH, Golst HR, Tafreshi M, Doelken P. Safety of ultrasound-guided thoracentesis in patients receiving mechanical ventilation. Chest. 2004;125:1059–62.
42. Viellard-Baron A, Mayo PH, Vignon P, et al. Expert round table on echocardiography in ICU, international consensus statement on training standards for advanced critical care echocardiography. Intensive Care Med. 2014;40:654–66.
43. Barbier C, Loubieres Y, Schmit C, et al. Respiratory changes in inferior vena cava diameter are helpful in predicting fluid responsiveness in ventilated septic patients. Intensive Care Med. 2004;30:1740–6.
44. Guyton AC. Determinants of cardiac output by equating venous return curves with cardiac output curves. Physiol Rev. 1955;35:123–9.
45. Sarnoff SJ. Myocardial contractility as described by ventricular function curves: observations on Starling's law of the heart. Physiol Rev. 1955;35:107.
46. Goldberg HS, Rabson J. Control of the cardiac output by the systemic vessels. Am J Cardiol. 1981;47:696–702.
47. Spencer KT, Lang RM. Diastolic heart failure. What primary care physicians need to know. Postgrad Med. 1997;101(1):63–5.
48. Hernandez G, Ospina-Tascon GA, Damiani LP, et al. Effect of a resuscitation strategy targeting peripheral perfusion status vs serum lactate levels on 28-day mortality among patients with septic shock. The ANDROMEDA-SHOCK Randomized Clinical Trial. JAMA. 2019;321(7):654–64.
49. Carroll JD, Lang RM, Neumann AL, et al. The differential effects of positive inotropic and vasodilator therapy on diastolic properties in patients with congestive cardiomyopathy. Circulation. 1986;74(4):815–25.
50. Pro CI, Yealy DM, Kellum JA, et al. A randomized trial of protocol-based care for early septic shock. N Engl J Med. 2014;370(18):1683–93.
51. Levin TN. Acute congestive heart failure. The need for aggressive therapy. Postgrad Med. 1997;101(1):97–100.
52. Munis JR, Bhatia S, Lozada LJ. Peripheral venous pressure as a hemodynamic variable in neurosurgical patients. Anesth Analg. 2001;92(1):172–9.
53. Bentzer P, Griesdale DE, Boyd J, et al. Will this hemodynamically unstable patient respond to a bolus of intravenous fluids? JAMA. 2016;316(12):1298–309.
54. Pelosi P, Cadringher P, Bottino N, et al. Sigh in acute respiratory distress syndrome. Am J Respir Crit Care Med. 1999;159(3):872–80.
55. Warner MA, Divertie MB, Tinker JH. Preoperative cessation of smoking and pulmonary complications in coronary artery bypass patients. Anesthesiology. 1984;60(4):380–3.
56. Brower RG, Matthay MA. Ventilation with lower tidal volumes as compared with traditional tidal volumes for acute lung injury and the acute respiratory distress syndrome. N Engl J Med. 2000;342(18):1301–8.
57. Mehta S, McCool FD, Hill NS. Leak compensation in positive pressure ventilators: a lung model study. Eur Respir J. 2001;17(2):259–67.
58. Ischaki E, Pantazopoulos I, Zakynthinos S. Nasal high flow therapy: a novel treatment rather than a more expensive oxygen device. Eur Respir Rev. 2017;26(145):170028.
59. Katz JA, Marks JD. Inspiratory work with and without continuous positive airway pressure I patients with acute respiratory failure. Anesthesiology. 1985;63(6):598–607.
60. Bellani G, Laffey JG, Pham T, et al. Noninvasive ventilation of patients with acute respiratory distress syndrome. Insights from the LUNG SAFE study. Am J Respir Crit Care Med. 2017;195(1):67–77.
61. Kang BJ, Koh Y, Lim CM, et al. Failure of high-flow nasal cannula therapy may delay intubation and increase mortality. Intensive Care Med. 2015;41(4):623–32.
62. Frat JP, Thille AW, Mercat A, et al. High-flow oxygen through nasal cannula in acute hypoxemic respiratory failure. N Engl J Med. 2015;372(23):2185–96.
63. Mort TC. Complications of emergency tracheal intubation: immediate airway-related consequences. J Intensive Care Med. 2007;22(4):208–15.
64. Holzapfel L, Cheveret S, Mandinier G, et al. Influence of long-term oro- or nasotracheal intubation on nosocomial maxillary sinusitis and pneumonia: results of a prospective, randomized, clinical trial. Crit Care Med. 1993;21(8):1132–8.
65. Levitan RM, Ochroch EA, Stuart S, Hollander JE. Use of the intubating laryngeal mask airway by medical and nonmedical personnel. Am J Emerg Med. 2000;18(1):12–6.
66. Franklin C, Samuel J, Hu TC. Life-threatening hypotension associated with emergency intubation and the initiation of mechanical ventilation. Am J Emerg Med. 1994;12(4):425–8.
67. Carlucci A, Richard JC, Wysocki M, et al. Noninvasive versus conventional mechanical ventilation: an epidemiologic survey. Am J Respir Crit Care Med. 2001;163:874–80.

68. Fink JB, Krause SA, Barrett L, et al. Extending ventilator circuit change interval beyond 2 days reduces the likelihood of ventilator-associated pneumonia. Chest. 1998;113:405–11.
69. Zhao T, Wu X, Zhang Q, et al. Oral hygiene care for critically ill patients to prevent ventilator-associated pneumonia. Cochrane Database Syst Rev. 2020;12:CD008367.
70. Demoule A, Jung B, Prodanovic H, et al. Diaphragm dysfunction on admission to the intensive care unit: prevalence, risk factors, and prognostic impact- a prospective study. Am J Respir Crit Care Med. 2013;188:213–9.
71. Jubran A, Mathru M, Dries D, et al. Continuous recordings of mixed venous oxygen saturation during weaning from mechanical ventilation and the ramifications thereof. Am J Respir Crit Care Med. 1998;158:1763–9.
72. Sajjad H, Schmidt GA, Brower RG, Eberlein M. Can the plateau be higher than the peak pressure? Ann Am Thorac Soc. 2018;15:754–9.
73. American Psychiatric Association DSM-5 Task Force. Diagnostic an statistical manual of mental disorders: DSM-5. 5th ed. Washington, DC: American Psychiatric Association; 2013.
74. Pandharipande P, Cotton BA, Shintani A, et al. Motoric subtypes of delirium in mechanically ventilated surgical and trauma intensive care unit patients. Intensive Care Med. 2007;33(10):1726–31.
75. Ely EW, autam S, Margolin R, et al. The impact of delirium in the intensive care unit on hospital length of stay. Intensive Care Med. 2001;27(12):1892–900.
76. Van Rompaey B, Elseviers MM, Schuumans, et al. Risk factors for delirium in intensive care patients: a prospective cohort study. Crit Care. 2009;13(3):R77.
77. Girard TD, Pandharipande PP, Carson SS, et al. Feasibility, efficacy, and safety of antipsychotics for intensive care unit delirium: the MIND randomized, placebo-controlled trial. Crit Care Med. 2010;38(2):428–37.
78. Page VJ, Ely EW, Gates S, et al. Effect of intravenous haloperidol on the duration of delirium and coma in critically ill patients (Hope-ICU): a randomized, double-blind, placebo-controlled trial. Lancet Respir Med. 2013;1(7):515–23.
79. Riker RR, Shehabi Y, Bokesch PM, et al. Dexmedetomidine vs midazolam for sedation of critically ill patients: a randomized trial. JAMA. 2009;301(5):489–99.
80. Pereira JV, Sanjanwala RM, Mohammed MK, et al. Dexmedetomidine versus propofol sedation in reducing delirium among older adults in the ICU: a systematic review and meta-analysis. Eur J Anaesthesiol. 2020;37(2):121–31.
81. Cuellar RE, Gavaler JS, Alexander JA, et al. Gastrointestinal tract hemorrhage: the value of a nasogastric aspirate. Arch Intern Med. 1990;150(7):1381–4.
82. Barkun AN. International consensus recommendations on the management of patients with nonvariceal upper gastrointestinal bleeding. Ann Intern Med. 2010;152:101–13.
83. Frossard JL, Spahr L, Queneau PE, et al. Erythromycin intravenous bolus infusion in acute upper gastrointestinal bleeding: a randomized, controlled, double-blind trial. Gastroenterology. 2002;123(1):17–23.
84. Vlavianos P, Mathuna PM, Williams R, Westaby D. Splanchnic and systemic haemodynamic response to volume changes in patients with cirrhosis and portal hypertension. Clin Sci (Lond). 1999;96(5):475–81.
85. Cook DJ, Guyatt GH, Salena BJ, Laine LA. Endoscopic therapy for acute nonvariceal upper gastrointestinal hemorrhage: a meta-analysis. Gastroenterology. 1992;102(1):139–48.
86. Jensen DM, Machicado GA. Diagnosis and treatment of severe hematochezia: the role of urgent colonoscopy after purge. Gastroenterology. 1988;95(6):1569–74.
87. Cohn SM, Moller BA, Zieg PM, et al. Angiography for preoperative evaluation in patients with lower gastrointestinal bleeding: are the benefits worth the risks? Arch Surg. 1998;133(1):50–5.
88. Sharma P, Rakela J. Management of pre-liver transplantation patient-part 2. Liver Transpl. 2005;11(3):249–60.
89. Garcia-Tsao G. Portal hypertension. Curr Opin Gastroenterol. 2006;22(3):254–62.
90. Ong JP, Mullen KD. Hepatic encephalopathy: an update of pathophysiologic mechanisms. Proc Soc Exp Biol Med. 1999;222(2):99–112.
91. Garcia N Jr, Mihas AA. Hepatic hydrothorax: pathophysiology, diagnosis, and management. J Clin Gastroenterol. 2004;38(1):52–8.
92. Runyon BA. Management of adult patients with ascites due to cirrhosis: an update. Hepatology. 2009;49(6):2087–107.
93. Moore KP, Aithal GP. Guidelines on the management of ascites in cirrhosis. Gut. 2006;55(suppl 6):vi1–vi12.
94. Sigal SH, Stanca CM, Fernandez J, et al. Restricted use of albumin for spontaneous bacterial peritonitis. Gut. 2007;56(4):597–9.
95. Wyers MC. Acute mesenteric ischemia: diagnostic approach and surgical treatment. Semin Vasc Surg. 2010;23(1):9–20.
96. Ryer EJ, Kalra M, Oderich GS, et al. Revascularization for acute mesenteric ischemia. J Vasc Surg. 2012;55(6):1682–9.
97. Dahlke MH, Asshoff L, Popp FC, et al. Mesenteric ischemia: outcome after surgical therapy in 83 patients. Dig Surg. 2008;25(3):213–9.
98. Bala M, Kashuk J, Moore EE, et al. Acute mesenteric ischemia: guidelines of the World Society of Emergency Surgery. World J Emerg Surg. 2017;12:38.
99. Sise MJ. Acute mesenteric ischemia. Surg Clin North Am. 2014;94(1):165–81.
100. Ghodasara N, Liddell R, Fishman EK, Johnson PT. High-value multidetector CT angiography of the superior mesenteric artery: what emergency medicine physicians and interventional radiologists need to know. Radiographics. 2019;39(2):559–77.
101. Acosta S, Bjornsson S, Ekberg O, Resch T. CT angiography followed by endovascular intervention for acute superior mesenteric artery occlusion does not increase risk of contrast-induced renal failure. Eur J Vasc Endovasc Surg. 2010;39(6):726–30.
102. Kellum JA, Sileanu FE, Murugan R, et al. Classifying AI by urine output versus serum creatinine level. J Am Soc Nephrol. 2015;26:2231–8.
103. Hoste EA, Bagshaw SM, Bellomo R, et al. Epidemiology of acute kidney injury in critically ill patients: the multinational AKI-EPI study. Intensive Care Med. 2015;41:1411–23.
104. Lee SA, Cozzi M, Bush EL, Rabb H. Distant organ dysfunction in acute kidney injury: a review. Am J Kidney Dis. 2018;72:846–56.
105. Selby NM, Kolhe NV, McIntyre CW, et al. Defining the cause of death in hospitalized patients with acute kidney injury. PLoS One. 2012;7:e48580.
106. Viera JM Jr, Castro I, Curvello-Neto A, et al. Effect of acute kidney injury on weaning from mechanical ventilation in critically ill patients. Crit Care Med. 2007;35:184–91.
107. Macedo E, Mehta RL. Prerenal failure: from old concepts to new paradigms. Curr Opin Crit Care. 2009;15:467–73.
108. Marshall S. Urea-creatinine ratio in obstructive uropathy and renal hypertension. JAMA. 1964;190:719–20.
109. Alge JL, Arthur JM. Biomarkers of AKI: a review of mechanistic relevance and potential therapeutic implications. Clin J Am Soc Nephrol. 2015;10:147–55.
110. Brunet S, Leblanc M, Geadah D, et al. Diffusive and connective solute clearances during continuous renal replacement therapy at

various dialysate and ultrafiltration flow rates. Am J Kidney Dis. 1999;34(3):486–92.
111. Sugahara S, Suzuki H. Early start on continuous hemodialysis therapy improves survival rate in patients with acute renal failure following coronary bypass surgery. Hemodial Int. 2004;8(4):320–5.
112. Singer M, Deutschman CS, Seymour CW, et al. The third international consensus definitions for sepsis and septic shock (sepsis-3). JAMA. 2016;315(8):801–10.
113. Rhee C, Jones TM, Hamad Y, et al. Prevalence, underlying causes, and preventability of sepsis-associated mortality in US acute care hospitals. JAMA Newt Open. 2019;2(2):e187571.
114. Kumar G, Kumar N, Taneja A, et al. Nationwide trends of severe sepsis in the 21st century (2000–2007). Chest. 2001;140(5):1223–31.
115. Vincent JL, Rello J, Marshall J, et al. International study of the prevalence and outcomes of infection in intensive care units. JAMA. 2009;302(21):2323–9.
116. Landry DW, Levin HR, Gallant EM, et al. Vasopressin deficiency contributes to the vasodilation of septic shock. Circulation. 1997;95(5):1122–5.
117. L'Heureux M, Sternberg M, Brath L, et al. Sepsis-induced cardiomyopathy: a comprehensive review. Curr Cardiol Rep. 2020;22(5):35.
118. De Winter BY, De Man JG. Interplay between inflammation, immune system, and neuronal pathways: effect on gastrointestinal motility. World J Gastroenterol. 2010;16(44):5523–35.
119. Papadopoulos MC, Davies DC, Moss RF, et al. Pathophysiology of septic encephalopathy: a review. Crit Care Med. 2000;28(8):3019–24.
120. Levy MM, Evans LE, Rhodes A. The surviving sepsis campaign bundle: 2018 update. Intensive Care Med. 2018;44:925–8.
121. Yealy DM, Mohr NM, Shapiro NI, et al. Early care of adults with suspected sepsis in the emergency department and out-of-hospital environment: a consensus-based task force report. Ann Emerg Med. 2021;78:1–19.
122. Corwin HL, Surgenor SD, Gettinger A. Transfusion practice in the critically ill. Crit Care Med. 2003;31:S668–71.
123. Corwin HL, Gettinger A, Pearl RG, et al. The CRIT study: anemia and blood transfusion in the critically ill- current clinical practice in the United States. Crit Care Med. 2004;32:39–52.
124. Weiss G, Ganz T, Goodnough LT. Anemia of inflammation. Blood. 2019;133:40–50.
125. Vincent JL, Jaschinski U, Wittebole X, et al. Worldwide audit of blood transfusion practice in critically ill patients. Crit Care. 2018;22:102–10.
126. Hebert PC, Wells G, Blajchman MA, et al. A multicenter, randomized, controlled clinical trial of transfusion requirements in critical care. N Engl J Med. 1999;340:409–17.
127. Carson JL, Guyatt G, Heddle NM, et al. Clinical practice guidelines from the AABB: red blood cell transfusion thresholds and storage. JAMA. 2016;316(19):2025–35.

Pediatric Surgical Emergencies

19

Mark Chaet and Michelle Le

Introduction

Pediatric surgical emergencies involve a vast array of medical conditions that can result in significant morbidity and mortality. From the neonatal period through adolescence, medical illnesses that most commonly affect children may be congenital or acquired and span across many organ systems: gastrointestinal, genitourinary, musculoskeletal, and integumentary. With etiologies ranging from congenital defects and anomalies to infectious to trauma, these childhood ailments require prompt and precise medical interventions to optimize patient outcomes. Understanding the epidemiology, etiology, pathophysiology, clinical manifestations, and diagnostic workup of these complex diseases is critical in managing the acutely unwell child. This chapter aims to provide a comprehensive overview of the most common pediatric surgical emergencies and serve as a resource for clinicians delivering evidence-based and interdisciplinary care in the setting of pediatric surgical emergencies.

Appendicitis

Introduction

Appendicitis, an inflammation of the appendix, is one of the most common and urgent pediatric medical conditions requiring prompt diagnosis and treatment—often through surgical intervention. Patients usually present with acute abdominal pain, nausea, vomiting, fever, and decreased appetite. If treatment is postponed, life-threatening complications such as perforation, peritonitis, and sepsis may arise. In children, appendicitis can be more challenging to diagnose, given the nonspecific nature of symptoms and the fact that younger children may not be able to clearly express their symptoms. Additionally, appendicitis in children may present differently than in adults, requiring pediatricians and emergency providers to have a high level of clinical suspicion.

Epidemiology

Appendicitis is the most common abdominal surgical emergency in children, with its incidence and prevalence varying by age, gender, and geographic region. This condition has an annual incidence of approximately 80–100 cases per 100,000 children in the general population. The condition predominantly affects children between the ages of 5 and 15 years, with a peak incidence around 10 to 12 years. Although appendicitis can occur at any age, it is relatively rare in infants and toddlers, as the appendix in these age groups is less likely to become inflamed.

The male-to-female ratio for appendicitis in children is approximately 1.5:1, with males being marginally more affected than females. However, the difference in gender may diminish in certain age groups, with females having a higher incidence of complicated appendicitis (e.g., perforated appendicitis) due to hormonal and anatomical factors that may influence the progression of the disease. Aside from age and gender, racial and socioeconomic disparities may also impact incidences and outcomes of pediatric appendicitis. Lack of timely access to healthcare and delayed diagnosis result in prolonged symptoms for these children, ultimately leading to higher rates of perforation in these populations. With prompt diagnosis and management, children with appendicitis generally have favorable outcomes.

M. Chaet (✉) · M. Le
Florida State University, Medical School, Orlando Regional Campus, Tallahassee, FL, USA
e-mail: mark.chaet@med.fsu.edu

S. Atallah, J. Dragoljevic (eds.), *Fundamentals of Surgery for Physician Assistants*,
https://doi.org/10.1007/978-3-032-21069-2_19

Pathophysiology

The appendix is a narrow, tube-like organ attached to the cecum, the first part of the large intestine. In children, the appendix is typically located in the right lower quadrant of the abdomen, near a point called McBurney's point. The size and position of the appendix vary between individuals, and in some children, the appendix may be located in atypical positions, which can complicate diagnosis. Although once thought to be vestigial with no significant function, research now suggests the appendix may play a role in immune system regulation. It contains lymphoid tissue that helps in the development of the immune system, especially during childhood. The pathophysiology of appendicitis in pediatric patients is complex, involving a range of factors from nonspecific luminal obstruction to pathogenic disruption and an impaired immune response. The stage at which appendicitis presents can also reveal different risks. Uncomplicated appendicitis encompasses acute and suppurative forms, while complicated appendicitis involves gangrene and perforation.

Because of its anatomical location and structure, the appendix can become easily obstructed, leading to inflammation, infection, and ultimately, appendicitis. **The most common cause of appendicitis is luminal obstruction due to fecalith material (more commonly in adults)**—which can also be caused by **lymphoid hyperplasia (which is particularly common in the pediatric population)**, tumors, or foreign bodies. Appendiceal luminal obstruction leads to a blockage of normal outflow, causing a buildup of mucus and other secretions within the appendix. As the distention worsens and bacteria proliferate, the intraluminal pressure increases, restricting blood flow and lymphatic drainage. Prolonged obstruction and impaired perfusion cause the appendiceal tissue to undergo ischemia. As a result, necrosis and gangrene may develop, eventually leading to perforation. Perforation results in the leakage of purulent material, bacteria, and toxins into the peritoneal cavity, leading to peritonitis, an infection of the peritoneum that can spread rapidly throughout the abdomen. If not promptly treated, this can result in sepsis, which is a life-threatening condition.

Clinical Presentation

The clinical presentation of appendicitis in children can be subtle and is often nonspecific, making it a challenge to diagnose. Symptoms generally develop over a few hours and tend to progress quickly. The classic presentation of appendicitis in children includes *anorexia, **periumbilical pain with migration to the right lower quadrant**, nausea, emesis, and fever.* **Tenderness at McBurney's point**—two-third from the umbilicus to the right anterior superior iliac spine—is a critical clinical finding. The pain usually worsens with movement or coughing. Changes in bowel habits may also occur, although they are not specific to appendicitis. However, an absence of these classic signs and symptoms in children should not definitively exclude a diagnosis of appendicitis due to differences in pediatric pathophysiology and the child's ability to express their symptoms. A physical examination showing involuntary guarding upon palpation, rebound tenderness, and positive signs of **iliopsoas** (pain with right hip extension), obturator (pain with right hip flexion and internal rotation), and **Rovsing** (pain in the right lower quadrant when palpating the left lower quadrant) may indicate localized or generalized peritoneal irritation. It is crucial to recognize that younger children, particularly infants, may not display the typical symptoms of appendicitis. Instead, they may show nonspecific signs such as irritability, poor feeding, lethargy, or a high-pitched cry.

Evaluation

While acute appendicitis is primarily a clinical diagnosis based on a detailed history and physical examination, its presentation can vary depending on the child's age and gender. Thus, diagnostic tools such as imaging, clinical scoring systems, and laboratory studies will aid in accurate identification of acute appendicitis in pediatric patients. A thorough history, including the onset and progression of symptoms, is essential. Physical findings such as *tenderness at McBurney's point, rebound tenderness, and rigidity are highly suggestive of appendicitis.*

Several scoring systems have been developed to aid in the diagnosis of appendicitis, as the condition often presents with nonspecific symptoms, making early diagnosis challenging. These scoring systems help clinicians assess the likelihood of appendicitis, guiding decision-making and potentially reducing unnecessary imaging or surgeries. One of the most widely used scoring systems is the Alvarado score, though others, like the Pediatric Appendicitis Score (PAS), are also used in pediatric populations.

The **Alvarado score** (also known as the MANTRELS score) is a clinical tool that incorporates eight clinical features of appendicitis in adults and has a maximum score of 10. These components include migration of pain to the right lower quadrant (1 point), tenderness in the right lower quadrant (2 points), nausea/vomiting (1 point), fever >37.3 °C (1 point), right lower quadrant rebound tenderness (1 point), elevated white blood cell count (>10,000/μL) (2 points), leukocytosis (1 point), and shift to the left in the white blood cell differential (1 point). A total score of 7 or more suggests a high probability of appendicitis, while a score below 4 usually suggests a lower likelihood of the condition.

The **Pediatric Appendicitis Score** (PAS) is a clinical scoring system designed to help in the diagnosis of appendicitis in children and has a maximum score of 10. It includes the following parameters: periumbilical or lower abdominal pain (1 point), right lower quadrant pain (2 points), anorexia, (1 point), vomiting (1 point), tenderness in the right lower quadrant (2 points), rebound tenderness: (1 point), guarding: (1 point), WBC >10,000/mm^3 (1 point), and neutrophils >75% (1 point). A total score of 0–3 indicates low risk, making appendicitis unlikely. Additional imaging or surgical intervention may not be required. A total score of 4–6 suggests intermediate risk, warranting further diagnostic evaluation, such as imaging, or a surgical consultation. A total score of 7 or higher indicates a high risk of appendicitis, and surgical evaluation or immediate surgery is advised.

Ultrasonography (US) and **computed tomography** (CT) are the imaging modalities most frequently utilized to confirm or exclude the diagnosis of appendicitis. Ultrasonography is oftentimes the imaging of choice as it is noninvasive, reliable, and expeditious. It can identify signs of appendicitis such as an enlarged, non-compressible appendix. When ultrasonography fails to provide a definitive diagnosis and a high clinical suspicion of acute appendicitis has been established, CT scans are utilized as they yield enhanced accuracy. Although it is more sensitive in comparison to ultrasound imaging, CT scans contain many disadvantages: lengthy time, exposure to significant radiation, and contrast. General surgery must be consulted and the patient is to be admitted for further observation and serial examinations if clinical suspicion of appendicitis is confirmed or remains high.

Management

Once appendicitis is diagnosed, prompt treatment is essential to prevent complications. **The standard treatment for appendicitis is an appendectomy**, the removal of the inflamed appendix, as it is curative and allows pathology testing. This can be performed through an open surgery or via a laparoscopic approach, the latter of which is less invasive and typically associated with quicker recovery times. Antibiotics are administered preoperatively and postoperatively to prevent infection. For selective children who present in stable condition without any risk factors for perforation, nonoperative management with antibiotics alone may be considered—though this approach remains controversial and is generally considered only in certain circumstances.

The antibiotics of choice for treating appendicitis in children typically aim to cover both *aerobic* and *anaerobic* bacteria, as the appendix contains a mixed bacterial flora. The choice of antibiotics may vary depending on the patient's clinical presentation (e.g., uncomplicated vs. complicated appendicitis), local antibiotic resistance patterns, and institutional protocols. In cases of uncomplicated appendicitis (where there is no perforation, abscess, or peritonitis), broad-spectrum antibiotics that cover common pathogens (i.e., *Escherichia coli*, *Bacteroides fragilis*, or *Enterococcus* species) are administered. These include ceftriaxone or cefotaxime plus metronidazole, ampicillin/sulbactam, or piperacillin-tazobactam. In cases of complicated appendicitis, where perforation, abscess formation, or peritonitis is present, more broad-spectrum and stronger antibiotics are often required to cover a wider range of pathogens, including multidrug-resistant organisms. Common regimens include piperacillin-tazobactam, ceftriaxone or cefotaxime plus metronidazole, meropenem or imipenem-cilastatin, levofloxacin or ciprofloxacin plus metronidazole.

After surgery, children are closely observed for signs of infection, such as fever, erythema, or mucopurulent drainage from the surgical site. Pain management, usually with acetaminophen or ibuprofen, plays a key role in the recovery process. Most children can resume normal activities within 2–4 weeks post-surgery.

Outcomes

Pediatric appendicitis, when diagnosed early and managed appropriately, typically has a good prognosis. However, outcomes can vary depending on several factors, including the timing of diagnosis, the presence of complications, and the overall health of the child. The majority of children who undergo an appendectomy recover completely and have no long-term effects. Appendectomy is generally considered a safe procedure with a low complication rate in pediatric patients. Children who experience delayed diagnosis and perforated appendicitis may face more complex and prolonged recovery periods. Complications of acute appendicitis in pediatric patients may include **perforation, abscess formation, bowel obstruction**, or psychological distress. In some cases, there may be an increased risk of long-term bowel complications or recurrent infections. Mortality from appendicitis in children is very rare, especially with prompt diagnosis and appropriate treatment. However, if untreated, perforated appendicitis can lead to ***life-threatening sepsis.*** With timely and appropriate intervention, the mortality rate for pediatric appendicitis is extremely low. Pediatricians, emergency providers, and surgeons must be aware of the unique challenges in diagnosing appendicitis in children and be prepared for rapid intervention when needed.

Necrotizing Enterocolitis

Introduction

Necrotizing enterocolitis is a life-threatening gastrointestinal condition predominantly found in neonates. It is characterized by severe inflammation and ischemic necrosis of the intestine. Progression of this disease can result in intestinal perforation in which peritonitis, sepsis, and death can result. Necrotizing enterocolitis predominantly affects **preterm infants with very low birth weight** and is associated with significant morbidity and mortality rates. Neonates presenting with signs and symptoms of abdominal distention, feeding intolerance, vomiting, lethargy, and bloody stools must be evaluated for necrotizing enterocolitis. This condition becomes a surgical emergency in cases of medical management failure, intestinal perforation, and necrosis.

Etiology

While the exact etiology of necrotizing enterocolitis is unclear, it is believed to be multifactorial. This condition involves a pathologic proliferation of intestinal bacteria altering the gut microbiome which results in inflammation and necrosis of the intestine. Preterm infants with immature digestive systems are at risk of developing this condition possibly due to inadequate bowel perfusion, poor biochemical defense mechanisms, weak structural barriers, and incapacitated intestinal digestion. Although more commonly found in premature infants, necrotizing enterocolitis can also affect full-term infants who are ill or very low weight. Infants with a birth weight of less than 1500 g are at an increased risk for developing necrotizing enterocolitis. Other risk factors for this condition include the early introduction of enteral feeding with formula rather than breast milk, systemic infections such as sepsis, prolonged use of broad-spectrum antibiotics, cardiovascular instability, and dysbiosis.

Epidemiology

Due to insufficient and inconsistent data, the true incidence of necrotizing enterocolitis is unknown. Despite global data variability, numerous studies have revealed that the overall incidence of necrotizing enterocolitis is inversely associated with gestational age and birth weight, particularly those with a birth weight of less than 1500 g. Rates increase fivefold in infants with extremely low birth weight and born at less than 28 weeks gestation. Greater than 90% of cases occur in neonates born at <32 weeks gestation with very low birth weights. The incidence in the United States has been approximated to be around 1 to 3 per 1000 live births, with rates appearing to decrease over a 10-year span from 2005 to 2014 and improvements in clinical outcomes—likely attributed to enhancements in early detection and aggressive management. The mortality rates range from 15% to 30% and are also inversely related to gestational age and birth weight. In the United States, preterm African American male infants have the highest risk of developing fatal necrotizing enterocolitis.

Pathophysiology

Necrotizing enterocolitis frequently develops when gas-producing bacteria invade the intestines, causing mucosal inflammation and cellular damage to the intestinal walls. Common bacteria implicated in the condition include *Escherichia coli*, *Klebsiella*, *Enterococcus*, and *Clostridia*. As necrotizing enterocolitis advances, intestinal hypoxia and ischemia exacerbate inflammation and cellular damage, ultimately resulting in bowel necrosis. Failure of timely treatment increases the risk of intestinal perforation, a potentially fatal complication. Microperforations can also occur which are small tears in the intestine that allow air to enter the wall of the intestine, leading to pneumatosis intestinalis. Intestinal perforations are complete ruptures that permit the leakage of bowel contents into the peritoneal cavity and can result in peritonitis and septic shock. Preterm infants and those with very low birth weights are especially vulnerable to developing necrotizing enterocolitis. Their immature gastrointestinal and immune systems increase their susceptibility to pathogenic bacterial invasion, as they lack the motility and protective mechanisms necessary for proper digestion.

Clinical Presentation

Signs and symptoms of necrotizing enterocolitis can be nonspecific and variable. Caregivers may observe decreased activity, fatigue, loss of appetite, vomiting, diarrhea, bloody stools, and abdominal bloating. **The most common sign is an acute change in feeding tolerance**, usually within the first 2 weeks of life in premature infants, though it can also develop later in full-term infants. **Bloody stools**, resulting from intestinal inflammation and necrosis, are one of the hallmark signs of this condition. On physical examination, findings may include **abdominal distention, visible intestinal loops, decreased bowel sounds, and erythema, tenderness, crepitus, and induration of the abdominal wall.** Advanced disease may present with nonspecific systemic signs, such as cyanosis, lethargy, apnea, temperature instability, or hypotension, all of which may indicate respiratory failure and circulatory collapse.

Evaluation

Necrotizing enterocolitis is often diagnosed clinically, based on the patient's history and physical examination findings. **Abdominal radiographs** are the most useful imaging technique and can reveal characteristic signs of necrotizing enterocolitis, including *intramural gas, pneumoperitoneum, or sentinel bowel loops*. Ultrasounds are occasionally utilized to assess complications such as bowel perforation or abscess formation. A definitive diagnosis is made from intestinal histologic findings of inflammation, ischemia, and necrosis. The examined specimens are retrieved either intraoperatively or postmortem, making it challenging to determine a pathologic diagnosis in children surviving this disease solely through extensive medical treatment.

Although non-specific, laboratory tests should be conducted to support the diagnosis and assess the severity of the condition. Resuscitation measures are dependent on these findings. A complete blood count showing neutropenia or leukopenia, with a white blood cell count below 1500 per microliter, is commonly seen in necrotizing enterocolitis and is typically associated with a poor prognosis, as it suggests infection or sepsis. C-reactive protein is often elevated in response to injury, inflammation, and infection. Blood cultures or cerebral spinal fluid cultures can help guide antibiotic therapy if sepsis is present. In children with thrombocytopenia or signs of bleeding, coagulation studies in severe cases often reveal disseminated intravascular coagulopathy (DIC), a life-threatening condition where widespread clotting in small and large blood vessels occurs due to systemic hypercoagulation. This can result in hemorrhage as clotting factors and platelets are depleted. Electrolyte imbalances observed in serum chemistries are nonspecific, but hyponatremia, hyperglycemia, and metabolic acidosis are commonly seen in cases of necrosis or sepsis.

Management

The first initiative in managing necrotizing enterocolitis involves supporting the patient's **airway, breathing, and circulation, while consulting the surgical team**. Patients experiencing respiratory failure may require stabilization through endotracheal intubation and mechanical ventilation. Hypotension or other signs of circulatory collapse should be addressed with intravenous fluid resuscitation. Oral intake should be discontinued once the diagnosis is suspected. Broad-spectrum intravenous antibiotics, such as ampicillin, gentamicin, and either clindamycin or metronidazole, should be administered to cover likely pathogens like *E. coli*, *Klebsiella*, and *Enterococcus*, until culture results are available.

Aggressive medical management is initially pursued for critically ill children with necrotizing enterocolitis who do not show signs of perforation. *If medical treatment fails, or if there is rapid deterioration, intestinal perforation, or evidence of necrotic bowel, emergent surgical intervention is required.* The standard surgical approach involves exploratory laparotomy with conservative resection of necrotic bowel, followed by primary anastomosis. In cases of extensive bowel necrosis or when there is concern about maintaining bowel continuity, a temporary colostomy or ileostomy may be performed to divert stool and promote bowel healing. If perforation has occurred, a peritoneal drain may be inserted to help manage peritonitis and sepsis without laparotomy. The selected surgical technique is dependent on the severity of the condition and the stability of the infant.

Post-operatively, it is important to monitor for signs of infection, electrolyte imbalances, and gastrointestinal recovery. Regular abdominal exams are necessary to evaluate for complications such as bowel obstruction, peritonitis, or recurrence of necrotizing enterocolitis. Total parenteral nutrition should be maintained until the patient is able to tolerate enteral feeds. Children with severe necrotizing enterocolitis may require ventilator support.

Outcomes

Necrotizing enterocolitis is a serious medical condition with a high risk of morbidity and mortality. Infants with low birth weight are particularly vulnerable to postoperative complications and extended hospital stays. The survival rate is higher in full-term infants when early intervention is provided and there is minimal bowel involvement. Severe cases involving sepsis, hypoxia, systemic inflammation, and the need for extensive bowel resection significantly increase the risk of long-term intestinal dysfunction such as short bowel syndrome, stunted growth, and neurodevelopmental challenges. Nearly 70.5% of patients experience postoperative complications, including **sepsis, intestinal strictures, and short bowel syndrome**. Exclusive breastfeeding, limited enteral feeding in premature infants, and strict infection control measures have been proven to lower the incidence of necrotizing enterocolitis. The prognosis for children with necrotizing enterocolitis is primarily influenced by the stage and severity at presentation, as well as early detection, supportive care, and prompt surgical intervention.

Hypertrophic Pyloric Stenosis

Introduction

Hypertrophic pyloric stenosis is one of the most common surgical conditions in infancy, characterized by an abnormal thickening of the gastric pyloric muscle leading to gastric outlet obstruction. Typically present in the first initial weeks of life, untreated pyloric stenosis can lead to severe dehydration, electrolyte imbalances, and malnutrition. Surgical intervention is the definitive treatment for hypertrophic pyloric stenosis, and the standard approach is a **pyloromyotomy**, which has a high success rate and low risk of complications.

Etiology

While the exact etiology of pyloric stenosis is not fully understood, studies have shown several risk factors in infants developing this condition. It is not uncommon for the infant to have a family history of pyloric stenosis in a parent or parent's sibling.

Epidemiology

Hypertrophic pyloric stenosis is a common gastrointestinal condition that affects infants, typically presenting within the first few weeks to months of life. It has a peak incidence in infants between 3 and 5 weeks of age with occurrence significantly declining after 12 weeks of age. The condition is more prevalent in male infants, with a male-to-female ratio of about 4:1. Hypertrophic pyloric stenosis also has a familial tendency, with an increased risk in infants who have a first-degree relative with a history of pyloric stenosis.

Pathophysiology

The pyloric sphincter muscle consists of circular and longitudinal muscles that open and close to allow partially digested food to pass from the stomach to the small intestine. This sphincter ensures that food is properly digested, prevents gastric acid from entering the intestine, and assists in signaling satiety. The hypertrophy and hyperplasia of this muscle disrupts its natural function and ultimately results in stomach dilation secondary to gastric outlet obstruction. Without a proper outlet for partially digested food in the stomach, nonbilious and projectile vomiting will result after feedings.

Clinical Presentation

The typical presentation for infantile hypertrophic pyloric stenosis is **abrupt postprandial projectile vomiting in an infant between 2 and 6 weeks of age**, which can intensify over time. Without adequate nutrient absorption, infants may develop electrolyte imbalances and weight loss. Signs of dehydration include sunken fontanelles, dry mucous membranes, decreased urination, poor skin turgor, lethargy, irritability, cyanosis, tachycardia, and disorientation. On physical examination, palpation of the **right upper quadrant** can reveal an ***"olive-like" mass*** which depicts the hypertrophic pyloric muscle. Laboratory findings may **reveal hypochloremic, hypokalemic metabolic alkalosis**. Clinicians are now taking measures in early detection with ultrasonography thus preventing laboratory abnormalities secondary to dehydration.

Evaluation

While hypertrophic pyloric stenosis has classical signs, symptoms, and lab findings, **ultrasonography** is the standard imaging technique in finalizing a diagnosis as it has a sensitivity of 97% and specificity of 100%. It is reliable, simple, and quick. Ultrasounds provide a direct visual of the pylorus where the wall thickness and diameter can be measured. Normal pyloric wall thickness and diameter in an infant is less than 2–3 mm and 10–15 mm, respectively. Measurements greater than 3 and 15 mm indicate pyloric stenosis. A **target sign** may appear as it represents *hypertrophied hypoechoic muscle surrounding echogenic mucosa.* When an ultrasound is nondiagnostic, other imaging modalities include barium upper gastrointestinal series, upper endoscopies, and abdominal x-rays. In contrast to ultrasounds, barium upper gastrointestinal series do not directly visualize the hypertrophied muscle. Instead, this study can reveal delayed gastric emptying, peristaltic waves (**caterpillar sign**), elongated pylorus with a narrowed lumen (**string sign**), and a beak-shaped pyloric entrance (**beak sign**). Abdominal x-rays are non-specific but when utilized in a patient with pyloric stenosis, findings include a distended stomach with absence of intestinal bowel gas secondary to gastric obstruction. Experienced practitioners can diagnose this condition with abdominal palpation and visualization of "marching fists" resulting from gastric contractions against the pyloric obstruction.

Management

Patients presenting to the emergency department with dehydration and electrolyte imbalances secondary to hypertrophic pyloric stenosis require immediate intervention. The first initiative is **fluid resuscitation** to correct *hypochloremic, hypokalemic metabolic alkalosis*. In cases of mild dehydration, 5% dextrose with 0.25% NaCl and 2 med KCl per 100 mL should be administered. Children with moderate to severe signs of dehydration should be given higher IVF NaCl concentrations. Hypoventilation is a risk of metabolic alkalosis and should be addressed by correcting and monitoring bicarbonate levels. A nasogastric tube may need to be placed in preparation for surgery. Once the child is stabilized, they are prepared for **laparoscopic pyloromyotomy**. The objective of this procedure is to cut into the pyloric muscle deep into the submucosa. This allows the stenosis to be loosened and permits food to easily pass into the intestine. Oral feeding can be reintroduced within 4–6 hours post-surgery. At first, infants may be given small quantities of formula or breast milk before gradually increasing to their regular feeding amounts. Patients should then be monitored for complications such as infection, bleeding, re-emergence of vomiting, wound dehiscence, or incomplete pyloromyotomy. Surgical intervention for pyloric stenosis is curative and has very low morbidity and mortality.

Outcomes

With early diagnosis and timely surgical intervention, the prognosis for children with pyloric stenosis is excellent. While uncommon, complications can arise. Gastric outlet obstruction may return if the pyloromyotomy was incomplete. Some children may experience reflux after surgery, but it generally improves with time. Most children recover well after surgery and thrive once the obstruction is relieved. The mortality rate is extremely low, and fatal complications are very rare in modern surgical practice. Outpatient follow-up care typically involves monitoring weight gain, normal feeding, and ensuring that the child is thriving postoperatively. Ongoing research in genetic factors, minimally invasive surgical methods, and better postoperative care is continually improving outcomes for children with pyloric stenosis.

Intussusception

Introduction

Intussusception is a medical condition in which a part of the intestine folds into the adjacent section, causing obstruction. It is the **most common cause of intestinal obstruction in infants and young children.** Intestinal invagination or telescoping most commonly involves the small intestine and rarely the large intestine. Symptoms include abdominal pain, bloating, vomiting, and bloody stools. If left untreated, complications such as bowel obstruction, bowel perforation, or peritonitis may result.

Etiology

Approximately 75–90% of intussusception in children have an unclear etiology, often occurring spontaneously between 3 months and 3 years of age. It is believed that intestinal lymphoid tissue or hyperplasia, such as Peyer's patches, may contribute to the initiation of intussusception. The enlargement or prominence of these tissues in the ileum or other parts of the bowel can serve as a lead point, triggering the telescoping of the intestine. Evidence has revealed that infections, anatomical pathologies, and dysfunctional intestinal motility may be contributing factors in intussusception. A lead point is a specific structural abnormality in the bowel that causes or increases the risk of intussusception. In these instances, the abnormality acts as the "point" where one section of the intestine folds into the next. Underlying disorders and abnormalities in the intestine such as Meckel's diverticulum, cystic fibrosis, intestinal malformation, lymphoid hyperplasia, polyps, cysts, tumors, hematomas, or vascular malformations can also serve as a lead point in intussusception.

Viral illnesses such as upper respiratory infections, otitis media, or flu-like symptoms occur in 30% of patients prior to the onset of intussusception. Research has shown a strong association between enteric adenoviruses, a group of viruses that cause gastrointestinal infections, and the development of intussusception. Peyer's patches, found along the antimesenteric border of the small intestine, can be stimulated by viral infections and hypertrophy—functioning as a lead point for ileocolic intussusception. Bacterial enteritis, most notably with *Salmonella*, *Escherichia coli*, *Shigella*, or *Campylobacter*, has also been associated with intussusception. Hematologic and immunologic disorders such as Henoch-Schönlein Purpura and sickle cell disease have also been correlated with intussusception.

Epidemiology

Intussusception primarily impacts infants and toddlers with the peak incidence being between 4 and 36 months of age. Mostly occurring in healthy and well-nourished children, intussusception that occurs beyond the typical age range is more likely to be associated with lead points pathologic in nature such as reactive lymphoid hyperplasia. Predominance is within males with the male:female ratio nearly at 3:2. The incidence also has seasonal peaks that coincide with viral gastroenteritis.

Pathophysiology

Intussusception is the invagination, also known as telescoping, of a proximal part of the intestine into the distal segment. The proximal portion of the intestine that is pulled into the other is known as the intussusceptum, and the distal portion that receives it is known as the intussuscipiens. Ninety percent of cases involve the ileocecal junction where the distal ileum invaginates the cecum, the connection between the small intestine and the colon. Intussusception can infrequently occur at other locations as well: ileo-ileal, ileo-ileo-colic, jejuno-jejunal, jejuno-ileal, or colo-colic intussusception. The mesentery of the small intestine is a double layer of peritoneum that anchors the small intestine to the posterior abdominal wall. It contains blood vessels, nerves, lymph nodes, and fat to carry out vital functions such as supplying blood and nutrients, draining lymph, and protecting the small intestine. In progressive intussusception, this layer is trapped in the bowel creating venous and lymphatic congestion which results in intestinal edema. Without surgical intervention, intussusception can progress to ischemia, perforation, and peritonitis. Sloughed mucosa occurs as a result of ischemia and mixes with blood and stool, creating the classic finding of red currant jelly stool that is seen in less than 25% of cases.

Clinical Presentation

The classic triad of intussusception in an infant or toddler includes **abdominal pain, vomiting, and currant jelly stools**. Patients typically present with a sudden onset of periodic severe and cramping abdominal pain, nausea, nonbilious and bilious vomiting, insoluble crying, lethargy, pallor, and drawing of the child's legs toward the abdomen. Occurring in 15- to 20-minute intervals, abdominal pain is intermittent due to the trapped bowel segment contracting and relaxing. As the pathology progresses, abdominal pain increases in severity and frequency. **In the initial stages, *non-bilious vomiting is often observed***, but as the obstruction worsens emesis becomes bilious. A **sausage-shaped mass** may be palpated on the right side of the abdomen. Red currant jelly stools are seen in a smaller number of cases, which reveals disease progression of ischemia. Although the classic triad of intussusception includes abdominal pain, a sausage-shaped abdominal mass, and currant jelly stools, up to 20% of infants do not present with pain and approximately one-third of patients do not pass stools containing blood or mucus. Fever is not a typical symptom of intussusception, but a necrotic bowel secondary to ischemia can progress to perforation and sepsis—causing the affected child to develop a fever.

Evaluation

Clinical suspicion of intussusception is often made based on a thorough history and physical examination, but a definitive diagnosis requires imaging. The imaging of choice is often affected by the child's presentation, level of clinical suspicion, and the preference of the consulting radiologist. With its reliability and ease of use, **ultrasonography** is often the imaging modality of choice. Ultrasound imaging may reveal a **target** or **bull's eye sign**, decreased blood flow in the intussusception, free fluid, or a lead point. Approximately 3 cm in diameter, the target shape is created by the hypoechoic outer edematous bowel surrounding the hyperechoic core of the bowel and mesentery. **Contrast enema is the gold standard** as it is *diagnostic and therapeutic* but is **contraindicated in cases of perforation**.

Management

Prior to any procedure, patients must be stabilized and given intravenous fluid resuscitation. Children presenting with typical signs of intussusception and imaging confirmation who are clinically stable are candidates for nonoperative reductions performed by interventional radiology. Nonoperative reductions performed under fluoroscopic guidance utilize either hydrostatic (saline or contrast) or pneumatic (air) enema to induce pressure and reduce the intussuscepted intestine. A resolution of symptoms and free flow of contrast or air into the small intestine indicate a successful fluoroscopic reduction. In some instances, contrast may not flow freely into the small bowel despite a complete reduction; thus, it can also be suggested when the cecum is free of a filling defect. A repeat contrast study or surgical intervention may be required when there is a suspicion for focal lead points. Sonographic-guided reductions avoid the use of ionizing radiation by utilizing a hydrostatic technique to generate retrograde pressure to reduce the intussusception. Success is determined by the disappearance of the intussusception and visualization of water and bubbles in the terminal ileum on ultrasound.

Nonoperative reductions, whether guided by fluoroscopy or ultrasound, possess high success rates ranging from 80% to 95%. The consulted surgical team should be prepared to respond when nonoperative reductions fail or complications arise. **Intussusception with sequelae** (i.e., necrosis, peritonitis, sepsis, or perforation) and **failed nonoperative reduc-**

tions require immediate surgical intervention. Most surgical reductions are successfully performed laparoscopically, which is minimally invasive, safe, effective, and associated with rapid recovery. Intraoperative manual reductions are attempted in most cases, but pediatric surgeons may need to resort to resection with primary anastomosis when manual reductions cannot be accomplished, or pathologic lead points are discovered. After surgery, the child is closely monitored for complications such as infection, anastomotic leaks, or recurrence.

Outcomes

Delayed detection and intervention increase the risk of *intestinal ischemia and necrosis, peritonitis, and sepsis*— worsening morbidity and mortality. Postoperative complications are rare and the recurrence rate in children is approximately 5–10%, especially within the first 24–48 hours post-reduction. Children who undergo bowel resection may have a slightly increased risk of developing short-bowel syndrome, particularly if a large portion of the bowel is removed. The overall prognosis of intussusception is exceptional if detected and managed with urgency. The vast majority of children recover fully after successful treatment, with a low risk of sequelae.

Intestinal Volvulus

Introduction

Intestinal volvulus is a *life-threatening* medical condition commonly found in infants in which a loop of the intestine and its supporting structure, the mesentery, twists upon itself ultimately leading to bowel obstruction. *Without swift intervention, vascular compromise can result in ischemia, necrosis, peritonitis, and perforation of the intestines*. Congenital intestinal malrotations, where intestines rotate improperly during fetal development, predispose the development of intestinal volvulus in infancy. Children often present with abdominal pain, distention, nausea, vomiting, and obstipation. With high sensitivity and specificity, a computerized tomography scan is the preferred diagnostic imaging tool. Volvulus is a **surgical emergency** and can result in significant morbidity or mortality if not promptly addressed.

Etiology

In pediatric patients, the causes of intestinal volvulus are often related to *anatomical and developmental abnormalities* such as *malrotation, intestinal atresia, or duodenal obstruction;* although other factors such as genetic disorders, trauma, and infections can also contribute. Congenital malrotation of the intestine, which affects the normal positioning or rotation of the intestines, is the leading cause of intestinal volvulus in neonates and infants. In older children, volvulus can occur due to *adhesions from prior surgeries*, mesenteric cysts, or trauma from motor vehicle accidents, falls, or blunt abdominal trauma. Pediatric volvulus is also often observed in association with certain genetic disorders or syndromes, including Hirschsprung disease, cystic fibrosis, and Trisomy 21.

Epidemiology

While intestinal volvulus is relatively rare, it is a significant surgical emergency in pediatric patients. The epidemiology of pediatric intestinal volvulus varies based on factors such as age, underlying anatomical abnormalities, and geographic location. Intestinal volvulus occurs in approximately 1 in every 6000 live births. The condition is most commonly seen in neonates and infants under 1 year of age, with a peak incidence between 1 and 3 months. Although occurrence decreases beyond 12 months of age, older children and adolescents may also present with this condition.

Pathophysiology

The most common cause of intestinal volvulus in neonates is ***malrotation***, a condition where the midgut does not rotate correctly during embryonic development. This results in a narrow mesenteric base and lack of the normal fixation of the large intestine to the posterior peritoneum. Embryological development of the gastrointestinal tract occurs in three divisions: foregut, midgut, and hindgut. Normal development results in a wide mesentery that attaches to the ligament of Treitz in the left upper quadrant to the ileocecal valve in the right lower quadrant.

The most common anomalies of midgut rotation are categorized as nonrotation and malrotation. Nonrotation is the return on the primary loop into the abdomen without the additional rotation of 180°. In malrotation, the duodenojejunal limb fails to rotate and the cecocolic limb only partially rotates. Nonrotation does not present the risk of volvulus that exists with malrotation.

Clinical Presentation

Bilious vomiting, indicating an obstruction below the level of the ampulla of Vater, is the hallmark symptom of intestinal volvulus in infants, especially within the first few days of life. Depending on the stage of intussusception, children may present with *non-bilious or bilious vomiting, abdominal pain out of proportion to examination, abdominal distention, hemodynamic instability, peritonitis, and/or hematochezia.* Although less common, other presentations may include failure to thrive, persistent diarrhea, solid food intolerance, malabsorption, pancreatitis, biliary obstruction, or intestinal motility disorders.

Evaluation

Infants presenting with ***bilious vomiting, duodenal obstruction, abdominal tenderness, and hemodynamic instability*** should raise clinical suspicion for intestinal malrotation. Children in this state require **immediate intervention** and cannot afford to await diagnostic confirmation prior to initiating management. These children are stabilized and rapidly admitted **for exploratory surgery**. In some cases, imaging may be obtained prior to surgery but is not required. In stable patients, the diagnosis should first be confirmed with imaging prior to surgical intervention. An **upper gastrointestinal series with contrast**, considered the **gold standard** for diagnosing intestinal malrotation and volvulus, can reveal the position of the duodenojejunal junction, abnormal placement of the small bowel, and a **corkscrew appearance** in cases of volvulus. Plain radiographs may showcase a **"double bubble" sign** indicating distention of the stomach and proximal end of the duodenum due to a partial obstruction of the duodenum. Ultrasonography can identify bowel distension, and in some cases, signs of bowel ischemia, but is not as specific for volvulus.

Management

Any acutely ill infant with bilious vomiting and peritoneal signs requires an immediate consultation with the pediatric surgery team. Cases in which there is a high clinical suspicion of malrotation or volvulus, whether or not confirmed with imaging, warrant an **emergency laparotomy.** *Intravenous fluid resuscitation* and *treatment of septic shock* should be initiated without delay. In preparation for emergency surgery, a *nasogastric tube* should be placed to decompress the bowel and *empiric broad-spectrum antibiotics* with bowel flora coverage must be administered. Piperacillin-tazobactam or ceftriaxone and metronidazole are often antibiotics of choice.

If a volvulus is discovered upon surgical exploration, **manual counterclockwise detorsion** is executed to resolve the intestinal malrotation and prevent or halt ischemia of the bowel. The **Ladd's procedure** is then performed to secure the bowel in a more stable position, preventing the recurrence of volvulus. This operation involves lysing the Ladd's bands—abnormally fixed fibrous peritoneal tissue that connects the cecum to the duodenum facilitating the twisting of intestines—and any adhesions between the duodenum and cecum to widen the base of the mesentery. This relieves pressure from the superior mesenteric artery and allows the duodenum to be positioned in the right lower quadrant and the cecum in the left lower quadrant. If vascular integrity of the bowel is uncertain, the surgery is concluded and the bowel will be surgically re-evaluated in 24–36 hours. In cases of bowel necrosis or perforation, bowel resection of the affected bowel is performed conservatively to prevent short bowel syndrome—a condition where significantly shortened or damaged intestines result in poor nutrient absorption.

After surgery, patients are closely monitored for complications such as *infection, anastomotic leaks, and bowel function.* Feeding is gradually reintroduced, beginning with intravenous nutrition and advancing to oral feeding as bowel function improves. Long-term follow-up is necessary to ensure normal growth and development and to monitor for any delayed complications.

Outcomes

Intestinal volvulus is a potentially life-threatening condition with outcomes contingent on the timeliness of diagnosis and intervention. Complications may include ***bowel necrosis, peritonitis, short bowel syndrome, or recurrent volvulus.*** Early surgical intervention, before significant bowel ischemia develops, results in an excellent prognosis. Approximately 89% of patients undergoing surgical intervention experience resolution of symptoms. The overall mortality is 3% to 10% and increases in patients experiencing intestinal necrosis. Early detection and surgical intervention are imperative in decreasing morbidity and mortality.

Irreducible Inguinal Hernia

Introduction

A hernia is a condition in which a portion of an organ or tissue protrudes through an abnormal weakness in the wall of muscle or connective tissue that contains it. Hernias present as visible and palpable abdominal bulges, and when they can be easily returned to the abdominal cavity with physical manipulation or decreased intra-abdominal pressure, they are termed reducible hernias. **Non-reducible hernias** are known as ***incarcerated hernias***. **Surgical emergencies arise when hernias become *strangulated***—a medical complication in which vascular compromise of the herniated contents arise as a result of progressive edema secondary to venous and lymphatic obstruction in incarcerated hernias. These defects can occur in various portions of abdominal wall, with the most common hernias affecting children being *inguinal* and *umbilical* hernias. Children with strangulated inguinal hernias may present with severe abdominal pain, abdominal distention, inconsolable crying, vomiting, tachycardia, fever, leukocytosis, or discolored swelling in the groin or scrotum.

Etiology

The etiology of strangulated inguinal hernia in children is multifactorial, involving a combination of congenital anatomical factors, increased abdominal pressure, delayed diagnosis or intervention, and mechanical factors such as incarceration. Although most inguinal hernias are not strangulated, **strangulation constitutes a surgical emergency**. The primary congenital factor in the development of an inguinal hernia is the presence of a *patent processus vaginalis*. Increased intra-abdominal pressure (such as during crying or straining) can cause a loop of intestine or omentum to protrude through the patent processus vaginalis.

Premature infants have a higher incidence of inguinal hernias, particularly on the right side. Prematurity may also be linked to underdeveloped abdominal wall structures, which increases the risk of both herniation and strangulation. Inguinal hernias are more common in males than females, with a male-to-female ratio of approximately 4:1. This is due to the normal descent of the testes and anatomical differences in the inguinal canal. Certain genetic or syndromic conditions, such as Down syndrome and Ehlers–Danlos syndrome, may predispose children to inguinal hernias and raise the risk of strangulation.

The most common trigger for the development of a strangulated hernia in children is ***increased abdominal** pressure from excessive crying, coughing, straining, or vomiting*. This raises intra-abdominal pressure, pushing abdominal contents through the hernia sac and heightening the risk of incarceration and strangulation. Children with chronic constipation may also face an increased risk of strangulation, as the straining during bowel movements can elevate intra-abdominal pressure, further increasing the likelihood of hernia incarceration. Larger hernia contents, especially in older children, are more prone to incarceration and strangulation.

Epidemiology

Risk factors of childhood inguinal hernias include ***preterm birth, very low birth weight, male gender, and family history.*** The incidence in preterm newborns is 9–11% with the frequency increasing in significantly premature infants with very low birth weights. The incidence is approximately three to four times greater in males than females. Right-sided inguinal hernias are more common in both males and females. The incidence of incarceration ranges from 14% to 31% with up to 85% occurring before reaching 1 year of age. Incarcerated inguinal hernias usually involve intestines in males and ovaries in females. Other risk factors of inguinal hernias in children also include conditions that create abdominal wall defects, increase intra-abdominal pressure, connective tissue disorders, and abnormalities in the genitourinary system.

Pathophysiology

Understanding normal inguinal anatomy is critical in recognizing the various types of inguinal hernia that children may present with. Types of inguinal hernias include indirect, direct, and femoral. The **inguinal canal** is an oblique channel containing the **spermatic cord in males** and **round ligament in females** that passes through the lower abdominal wall and into the scrotum or labia majora, respectively. The boundary of the inguinal canal is formed by several anatomical structures: the external oblique aponeurosis forms the anterior wall, the transversus abdominis muscle and internal oblique muscle form the posterior wall, the inguinal ligament forms the superior wall, and the pubic bone forms the inferior wall. The inguinal canal has two openings: the deep inguinal ring situated laterally to the inferior epigastric vessels serves as an entrance for the spermatic cord or round ligament and the superficial ring situated at the medial border of the external oblique aponeurosis above the pubic tubercle serves as an exit for the spermatic cord or round ligament. **Hesselbach's triangle**—medial to the deep inguinal ring and bordered by the ***inferior epigastric vessels, inguinal ligament, and the rectus sheath***—is a clinically significant anatomical region as *its weakness can lead to **direct** inguinal hernias.* Infants, especially premature infants, are at risk of inguinal hernias as their normal anatomy includes a short inguinal canal that is positioned more perpendicularly rather than obliquely which places the external and internal rings directly over one another.

Among the three types of inguinal hernias, *indirect inguinal hernias are more common in children.* The incomplete embryonic closure of the processus vaginalis predisposes children to indirect inguinal hernias. This occurs when herniated material protrudes through the deep inguinal ring by way of a patent processus vaginalis and into the inguinal canal. Direct and femoral inguinal hernias are rare in children.

Furthermore, hydroceles can occasionally be confused with inguinal hernias, as both conditions lead to swelling in the scrotum or groin of children, particularly in infancy or early childhood. *Hydroceles* result from serious fluid accumulation within the tunica vaginalis surrounding the testicle, leading to *painless scrotal swelling*, ***while scrotal swelling in inguinal hernias arises from the protrusion of abdominal contents***. Both hydroceles and inguinal hernias can result from the congenital incomplete closure of the processus vaginalis, a passage that should close after the testicles descend into the scrotum. In some instances, a communicating hydrocele and an inguinal hernia can occur concurrently, and the presence of a hydrocele should raise clinical suspicion of a potential inguinal hernia. Distinguishing between the two conditions is essential for appropriate treatment.

Clinical Presentation

Children with **reducible inguinal hernias** may present with a *painless, reducible bulge in the groin* that becomes more prominent with increased intra-abdominal pressure such as coughing and straining. In contrast, children with **incarcerated inguinal hernias** are typically *irritable, crying, and vomiting*. A key physical exam finding of **strangulated inguinal hernias** include a *firm, erythematous, tender, and non-reducible inguinal mass* that may extend into the scrotum or labia majora upon palpation along the groin.

Evaluation

Inguinal hernias are diagnosed clinically and do not require imaging or laboratory evaluation. The initial step involves a comprehensive examination of the groin to observe for a bulge or swelling, which may be reducible or non-reducible. A ***non-reducible mass*** accompanied by ***tenderness*** strongly indicates ***incarceration and the possibility of strangulation***. Equivocal exam findings may necessitate ultrasound confirmation which has a diagnostic accuracy of 93%. Ultrasonography has a sensitivity of 90% in detecting a patent processus vaginalis.

Management

The clinical suspicion of **strangulated inguinal hernia** should prompt **immediate surgical consultation** to prevent bowel necrosis, sepsis, and other complications. The goals of surgical intervention are to *reduce the hernia, restore blood flow to the ischemic bowel, and excise any necrotic bowel*. The initial management of strangulated inguinal hernias involves timely resuscitation with intravenous fluids and electrolytes to address dehydration and stabilize hemodynamics. Patients should be kept NPO (nothing by mouth) until the surgical plan is determined.

In cases of **incarcerated inguinal hernias**, **manual reductions** may be attempted *if the child is free of peritoneal signs, intestinal obstruction, or toxicity*. Manual reduction of incarcerated hernias is effective in the vast majority of children. Asymptomatic hernias diagnosed in the outpatient setting do not require emergent surgery but should be evaluated for possible elective repair to prevent incarceration or strangulation.

Outcomes

Strangulated inguinal hernia is a pediatric surgical emergency that requires prompt recognition, resuscitation, and surgical intervention. Complications associated with strangulated inguinal hernias include *bowel infarction, peritonitis, short bowel syndrome, and recurrence*. Most children who undergo surgical hernia repair experience positive outcomes, with postoperative infections being rare, occurring in less than 1% of cases. **Bowel infarction** is the most serious complication and *can develop within 2 hours of incarceration*. While intestinal resection may be required if severe bowel necrosis is found, this is rare in young infants. Ischemic necrosis and atrophy of the testis, as well as injury to the vas deferens, may occur in male patients, while ovarian torsion can affect female patients. With early detection and timely surgical intervention, the prognosis for children with strangulated inguinal hernia is generally favorable. However, those who require bowel resection may face long-term gastrointestinal complications. Ongoing follow-up is essential to monitor for potential issues, such as hernia recurrence, bowel function, and growth.

Testicular Torsion

Introduction

One of the most common causes of sudden scrotal pain in male neonates and adolescents is testicular torsion. This condition is characterized by the pathologic twisting of the spermatic cord—which houses the blood and lymph vessels, nerves, and vas deferens that connect to the testes in the scrotum—which *compromises blood flow to the testicle*. Patients typically present with **abrupt unilateral scrotal pain, scrotal swelling and erythema, abdominal pain, nausea, and vomiting**. Testicular torsion is a serious pediatric surgical emergency that can result in irreversible ischemia and necrosis of the testis if detection and intervention are delayed.

Etiology

Although testicular torsion can occur spontaneously, certain anatomical abnormalities such as the **Bell clapper deformity** and **cryptorchidism**, as well as environmental factors such as trauma, puberty, and physical activity, greatly heighten the risk of developing this condition. The Bell clapper deformity, present in 80–90% of testicular torsion cases, is the most significant anatomical cause of testicular torsion. Normally, the testicle is secured to the scrotal wall by a fibrous band, but in Bell clapper deformity, this band is either absent or poorly developed, predisposing the testicle to twisting. Neonates with cryptorchidism, a condition in which one or both of the testes fail to descend properly into the scrotum, are at an increased risk of testicular torsion due to the mobility of the testicles. Adolescents experiencing changes in scrotal anatomy and testicular enlargement during puberty also have an elevated risk of testicular torsion. Children may also sustain genital trauma in accidents, sports, or rough play, which increases the risk of testicular torsion. The etiology of pediatric testicular torsion is multifactorial.

Epidemiology

Testicular torsion is a relatively uncommon but serious condition, occurring in about 1 in 4000 to 1 in 5000 live births. The annual incidence of testicular torsion in children and adolescents is approximately 1.2 per 100,000 boys, with nearly 65% of cases occurring between the ages of 12 and 18 years. Testicular torsion follows a bimodal distribution, with the first peak occurring in the first year of life and the second peak during puberty. Neonatal testicular torsion is primarily linked to *maldescent of the testicle* and can occur either in utero or shortly after birth. Adolescents are believed to be at an elevated risk for testicular torsion because of the rapid testicular growth in size and weight that occurs during puberty. Testicular torsion occurs globally, without any significant geographical differences in incidence. However, regions with better access to healthcare and quicker surgical intervention tend to have lower rates of testicular loss, as prompt treatment is vital for preserving the testicle.

Pathophysiology

Normal testicular anatomy includes fixation of the posterolateral aspect of the testis to the tunica vaginalis which allows the spermatic cord to remain immobile and in proper position. Defects of the tunica vaginalis increase the risk of testicular torsion. The Bell clapper deformity, a congenital condition in which the tunica vaginalis has a high attachment to the spermatic cord instead of the testis causing the testicle to be mobile and occupy a transverse position, is the most common abnormality seen in testicular torsion. This hypermobility of the testicle predisposes the patient to testicular and spermatic cord torsion. The spermatic cord, which houses the testicular artery, veins, lymphatics, and nerves, has a vital role in providing blood supply to the testicle. *Intravaginal torsion*—where the spermatic cord is twisting within the tunica vaginalis—***leads to venous compression, testicular and spermatic cord edema, arterial occlusion, and ultimately, ischemia of the testicle.*** As the testicle and spermatic cord continue to twist, venous flow is compromised leading to venous congestion and testicular ischemia. The testicular artery will then become compromised, cutting off blood supply to the testicle, and ultimately causes necrosis of the testicle. The testicle increasingly becomes edematous, erythematous, and tender as a result. In most cases, the testicle rotates between 90° and 180° in the setting of neurovascular compromise. **Ischemia may develop within *4 hours* of torsion and is nearly inevitable after 24 hours**.

Clinical Presentation

Classically, patients present with **sudden and severe unilateral scrotal pain, nausea, and vomiting**. The severity of testicular or scrotal pain often awakens the child from their sleep, and in a minority of cases, abdominal or inguinal pain may precede testicular pain. Torsion of the testicle causes the pain to occur constantly, and in situations where the pain is intermittent, the testicle may be twisting and untwisting alternatively. Upon visual inspection, the scrotum may appear *edematous, erythematous, and indurated* with a *high-riding, transverse testicle* while palpation reveals *significant testicular tenderness and swelling*. The elevated position of the testicle is a result of a shortened spermatic cord from the twisting. The most reliable physical exam finding in testicular torsion is **the absence of the cremasteric reflex**, which is the natural elevation of the testis when the cremasteric muscle contracts in response to stroking the proximal medial thigh. Although the absence of this reflex is highly sensitive, it does not yield a definitive diagnosis. **Prehn's sign**, which involves pain relief upon elevating the affected testicle, is another clinical test that can be used during the examination of the patient. *In cases of testicular torsion, lifting the testis does* ***not*** *relieve pain,* whereas in other conditions such as epididymitis, pain relief may occur. While Prehn's sign can be a useful clinical test, it is not entirely reliable. Testicular torsion is a time-sensitive surgical emergency. The pain typically starts abruptly, is intense, and persists. ***Without treatment, the testicle will become progressively ischemic and may suffer irreversible damage within 4–6 hours.***

Evaluation

Testicular torsion is a clinical diagnosis. The **sudden onset of scrotal pain, absent cremasteric reflex, and high-riding testicle** should immediately raise clinical suspicion for testicular torsion. When evaluating children with testicular pain, the TWIST scoring system is often utilized to determine the likelihood of testicular torsion. This tool considers testicular swelling (2 points), hard testis (2 points), nausea or vomiting (1 point), retractile testis (1 point), and an absent cremasteric reflex (1 point). A score greater than or equal to 5 significantly increases the probability of testicular torsion. Any child presenting with a history and physical examination consistent with testicular torsion and pain less than 6 hours must undergo early surgical consultation and exploration immediately.

Although studies have shown that testicular torsion is a clinical diagnosis and may be excluded with a TWIST score less than 2, equivocal cases require further testing with ultrasonography to achieve diagnostic certainty. In these clinical scenarios, the surgical team should still be consulted and inspection of both the affected and unaffected testicle through **color Doppler ultrasonography** should be obtained expeditiously. Evaluating the unaffected testicle allows the clinician to gain a sense of normal structure and vascularity in the patient. In cases of testicular torsion, ultrasonography may reveal reduced or absent testicular perfusion, twisting of the spermatic cord, enlarged testis and epididymis, reactive hydrocele, reactive thickening of the scrotal layers, and/or peripheral testicular neovascularization. Homogenous echotexture is an early finding preceding necrosis.

Management

As testicular torsion is a time-sensitive condition, the primary objective is immediate detection and surgical intervention to salvage the testicle. **Surgical detorsion and orchiopexy** is the treatment of choice. It is also universally recommended to *prophylactically perform an orchiopexy in the contralateral scrotum* to reduce the risk of testicular torsion recurrence. Orchiectomy is required if a nonviable testicle is detected intra-operatively. The ability to salvage the affected testicle is directly impacted by the lapsed time between symptom onset and detorsion as testicular viability drastically decreases with time: 4–6 hours (97–100%), >12 hours (20–61%), and >24 hours (0–24%). **Surgical intervention should be performed within 6 hours of symptom onset to** optimize the likelihood of testicular preservation.

The scrotum is first incised to allow exploration of the affected testicle. The testicle is then assessed for viability, and if twisted, it is untwisted and examined for signs of ischemic damage. Following detorsion, the testicle is typically anchored to the scrotal wall with sutures to prevent future torsion. This procedure, known as orchiopexy, is usually performed on both sides, as torsion can recur on the contralateral testicle, particularly in patients with a Bell clapper deformity. The discovery of a non-viable testicle due to prolonged ischemia requires orchiectomy.

If surgical intervention is not readily available, clinicians in the emergency department may attempt **manual detorsion** under the surgeon's discretion. Although manual detorsion is not routinely performed, it can lead to better outcomes in testicular salvage if done properly. *Improper manipulation may worsen the condition; thus, it should be attempted with extreme care and diligence.* The alleviation of symptoms following outward rotation of the testis and the restoration of blood flow, as seen on a repeat Doppler ultrasound, suggest a successful manual detorsion. If there is persistent clinical suspicion of incomplete detorsion, the maneuver can be repeated with additional ultrasounds for confirmation. The success of this procedure can be challenged by the patient's discomfort and the possibility of maneuvering the testicle in the wrong direction. Thus, achieving adequate pain control and administering intravenous fluid resuscitation prior to intervention is essential. Whether manual detorsion is successful or not, **surgery remains the only definitive treatment for testicular torsion**, and surgical exploration should still be performed following manual detorsion.

Post-operatively, patients are closely monitored for infection, wound dehiscence, and torsion recurrence. Ongoing follow-up is essential to monitor recovery, evaluate fertility, and identify complications such as testicular atrophy or psychological impacts related to the loss of a testicle.

Outcomes

Testicular torsion is a medical emergency, and the outcomes are highly dependent on the timing of treatment and the extent of testicular ischemia. Timely intervention can help preserve testicular viability and improve patient outcomes, whereas delayed treatment may result in serious complications, such as *testicular loss or atrophy, cosmetic deformities, infertility, or psychological repercussions.* If surgery is performed within 6 hours of symptom onset, there is a high likelihood of preserving the affected testicle, with 80–90% of testicles being successfully salvaged when treated promptly within this time frame. Mortality in pediatric patients with testicular torsion is very rare. However, fatality can occur in cases of bilateral torsion, sepsis subsequent to untreated torsion, or peritonitis, although these scenarios are extremely uncommon. With prompt attention and care, the prognosis of testicular torsion in pediatric patients is generally favorable.

Spontaneous Pneumothorax

Introduction

Pneumothorax, the abnormal accumulation of air in the pleural space between the lungs and the chest wall causing lung collapse, can occur spontaneously or traumatically. Spontaneous pneumothorax, without a clear etiology, is classified into two types: primary spontaneous pneumothorax (occurring without evidence of underlying pulmonary disease) and secondary spontaneous pneumothorax (occurring with evidence of underlying pulmonary disease). *If left untreated, spontaneous pneumothorax can progress to* ***tension pneumothorax****, a life-threatening condition that compromises both pulmonary and cardiac function.* Common symptoms include dyspnea, tachypnea, tachycardia, sudden chest pain, cough, and dizziness. The diagnosis is confirmed through chest radiography. Management is determined by the extent of the condition. If conservative management fails or the condition recurs, emergent surgical intervention is required.

Etiology

The etiology of spontaneous pneumothorax in children can be broadly categorized into primary and secondary types. Primary spontaneous pneumothorax occurs in otherwise healthy children without any underlying lung disease. While the exact cause remains unclear, factors such as congenital weakness in the lung tissue, family history, and growth spurts during puberty are believed to contribute. In contrast, secondary spontaneous pneumothorax occurs in the presence of underlying pulmonary conditions that impact lung structure or function, including asthma, cystic fibrosis, connective tissue disorders, interstitial lung disease, pneumonia, tuberculosis, pulmonary abscesses, malignancy, and foreign body aspiration. Additional risk factors include tobacco use, increased intra-abdominal pressure, and activities that involve rapid changes in atmospheric pressure, such as diving or hiking at high altitudes.

Epidemiology

Pediatric spontaneous pneumothorax is a rare but serious condition with varying incidence depending on age, sex, and the presence of underlying pulmonary pathology. It is more prevalent in *males*, especially those between the ages of 10 and 20 years. *Primary spontaneous pneumothorax is most common in adolescence*, while secondary spontaneous pneumothorax typically occurs at an older age, often due to smoking or the development of conditions such as chronic obstructive pulmonary disease. In the United States, the incidence of primary spontaneous pneumothorax among children and adolescents is about 4 per 100,000 in males and 1.1 per 100,000 in females, with peak incidence occurring between the ages of 16 and 24 years. Symptomatic pneumothoraces occur in nearly 2 in 10,000 live births, with a higher incidence in premature or larger infants. Meconium aspiration, the inhalation of meconium during labor or delivery, also increases the risk of secondary spontaneous pneumothorax in infants. Additionally, in neonates, pneumothorax can also develop as a complication of respiratory distress syndrome or mechanical ventilation. Overall, the mortality rate for pediatric spontaneous pneumothorax is very low and the prognosis is generally good. However, complications such as tension pneumothorax or severe underlying lung conditions can increase the risk of long-term lung dysfunction, hospitalizations, and mortality.

Pathophysiology

Pneumothoraces can result as air leaks into the pleural space through either the visceral or parietal pleura. In spontaneous pneumothorax, *sudden increases in transpulmonary pressure and defects in the visceral pleura are strongly associated with alveolar rupture.* Extensive increases in transpulmonary pressure lead to alveolar distention and possible rupture, resulting in large pressure shifts. The rupture of superficial alveoli may lead to the formation of subpleural blebs, or small air pockets, which can then rupture into the pleural space, causing a pneumothorax. The accumulation of air in the pleural space exerts pressure on the affected lung, causing it to collapse. This limits the lung's ability to expand fully, thereby *impairing ventilation and gas exchange.* As pressure increases, air may travel along tissue planes in the pericardium, abdomen, and subcutaneous tissue, potentially resulting in pneumopericardium, pneumoperitoneum, or subcutaneous emphysema. As the pressure increases, **tension pneumothorax** may develop a one-way valve mechanism in which inspired air cannot escape. This condition causes a *mediastinal shift to the contralateral side, compression of blood vessels, and impaired venous return*, making it a **surgical emergency** due to the risk of cardiovascular collapse.

Clinical Presentation

The clinical presentation of spontaneous pneumothorax is influenced by factors such as the volume of air and tension in the pleural space, the extent of lung collapse, the patient's respiratory reserve, and age. It commonly presents insidiously at rest or with minimal exertion, often with an unremarkable examination. In neonates, pneumothorax may manifest as *respiratory distress, nasal flaring, grunting, or difficulty feeding*. Patients affected with large pneumothoraces often experience *sudden-onset dyspnea and sharp pleuritic chest pain on the affected side, which may radiate to the ipsilateral shoulder*. The pain is aggravated with breathing or coughing. Characteristic exam findings include decreased or absent breath sounds, hyperresonance on percussion, and decreased tactile fremitus on the affected side. Additional findings may include reduced chest wall movement, tachycardia, pulsus paradoxus, and jugular vein distention. **Tension pneumothorax** should be suspected if *tracheal deviation, diminished heart sounds, tachycardia, hypotension, and cyanosis are observed*. At this stage, urgent decompression is necessary.

Evaluation

Chest radiographs confirm the diagnosis of pneumothorax by revealing a thin, sharp white line indicating the visceral pleural outline, with absent lung markings outside this line and increased lucency in the pleural space compared to the unaffected lung. In cases of **tension pneumothorax**, *mediastinal and tracheal shifts to the contralateral side* can be observed. Radiographs in infants are typically obtained in the supine position, which can create challenges in detecting a pneumothorax as air tends to accumulate anteriorly. Positioning the patient in lateral decubitus with the affected side facing up may improve the visibility of the pneumothorax on radiographs. The size of the pneumothorax, as measured on the chest radiograph, significantly influences the treatment plan: a pneumothorax that occupies more than 30% of the hemithorax is considered large. In some instances, **point-of-care ultrasound** can quickly diagnose a pneumothorax by revealing the absence of lung sliding or the presence of the **"lung point" sign**. This highly specific diagnostic sign appears as a point on the ultrasound where the visceral pleura of the lung begins to separate from the parietal pleura of the chest wall at the edge of the pneumothorax. CT scans may be utilized in complex cases or when there is concern for underlying lung pathology, such as cystic fibrosis or lung malformations.

Continuous pulse oximetry is useful in monitoring the patient's stability. If signs of hypoxia or respiratory distress arise, arterial blood gas measurements are necessary to assess the patient's metabolic state and guide treatment. Blood gas analysis may reveal respiratory alkalosis due to hyperventilation, or respiratory acidosis in severe cases of hypoxemia.

Management

The management of pneumothorax in children depends on the size and symptoms of the pneumothorax, as well as the presence of any underlying pathology. The goals of treatment are to ***stabilize the patient, remove the air from the pleural space if necessary, and prevent recurrence.***

Clinically stable patients with *small, uncomplicated pneumothoraces* (less than 2 cm) confirmed by chest radiograph *can be managed conservatively with analgesics, antitussives, supplemental oxygen* via *non-rebreather mask, and close monitoring in the emergency department for at least 12 hours*. Administering 100% oxygen can aid in accelerating the absorption of air from the pleural space, thereby decreasing the size of the pneumothorax. In neonates, oxygen use should be avoided unless necessary, and the duration of oxygen therapy should be limited to 47–72 hours to prevent toxicity. If patients show improvement on follow-up chest radiographs, are free of respiratory distress or pain, and are able to walk comfortably, they may be deemed stable enough for discharge with anticipatory guidance and arrangements for outpatient follow-up. In many instances, small and stable primary pneumothoraces heal spontaneously with supportive care. Children under 12 years require an extended observation period before discharge. After 12 hours of monitoring, patients who show no signs of improvement or worsening pneumothorax should undergo needle aspiration or thoracostomy tube placement within 24 to 48 hours.

Patients with *moderately sized* or *small, but symptomatic pneumothoraces* causing *dyspnea, hypoxemia, or pain* require **needle aspiration**. This procedure involves inserting a needle or catheter between the ribs, typically in the **second intercostal space**, to access the pleural space and aspirate the excess air into a syringe. Performed under local anesthesia, needle aspiration is a minimally invasive procedure that typically leads to shorter hospital stays and quicker recovery times, and is often associated with successful outcomes in children.

Thoracostomy is required in cases of *moderate to large pneumothoraces, severe symptoms such as respiratory distress, or if needle aspiration is unsuccessful*. During this procedure, appropriate sedation and pain management are provided, and a chest tube connected to a drainage system is inserted through a surgical incision in the chest wall to remove excess air from the pleural space and allow for lung reexpansion. The tube is usually left in place for 24–48 hours or until the pneumothorax resolves and no further air leakage is detected. Following thoracostomy, continuous monitoring for potential complications, such as infection or re-expansion pulmonary edema, is essential.

Surgical intervention is imminent in cases of *primary spontaneous pneumothorax recurrence, secondary spontaneous pneumothorax, or if conservative treatment, needle aspiration, or thoracostomy fails* (especially after 5–7 days of thoracostomy drainage). Hospitalization for observation and management of underlying pulmonary conditions associated with secondary spontaneous pneumothorax is essential for achieving successful outcomes. Patients with conditions such as cystic fibrosis with recurrent large pneumothoraces, bullous lung disease, or bronchopleural fistulas resulting from necrotizing pneumonia should undergo lung expansion through thoracostomy followed by surgical intervention. Surgical approaches for spontaneous pneumothorax include **VATS (video-assisted thoracic surgery), mini-thoracotomy**, or **conventional thoracotomy**. VATS is a minimally invasive surgical procedure that enables surgeons to access the chest cavity through small incisions. It is typically preferred because it has a lower morbidity rate compared to traditional thoracotomy. For children with recurrent pneumothorax, ***VATS* in combination with *pleurodesis*** is recommended. This procedure helps prevent future recurrence by either *mechanically or chemically sealing the visceral and parietal pleura, effectively eliminating the pleural space*. Follow-up chest x-ray imaging is necessary after treatment to confirm resolution of the pneumothorax and verify that the lung has fully re-expanded.

Outcomes

The prognosis for children with spontaneous pneumothorax is generally favorable, especially when the condition is detected early and treated effectively. Preventing risk factors such as smoking and managing pre-existing lung conditions can help reduce the risk of pneumothorax. However, recurrence is possible, particularly in children with underlying lung diseases or those who lack adequate follow-up care. Case studies on recurrence rates have shown that adolescents with primary spontaneous pneumothorax have a 21% recurrence rate over 2 years. The risk of recurrence increases to 50–60% if primary spontaneous pneumothorax is managed non-operatively. Children with pneumothorax related to cystic fibrosis may have recurrence rates ranging from 50% to 80%, whereas VATS with pleurodesis significantly reduces the likelihood of recurrence. The mortality rate for pediatric spontaneous pneumothorax is low, especially in children without major underlying lung conditions, and most pneumothoraces resolve without leading to long-term complications.

Burns

Introduction

Burn injuries are among the leading causes of accidental death in children aged 5 to 9 and result in considerable morbidity within the pediatric population globally. The severity and nature of the burn impact the associated mortality and morbidity. Children with burn trauma require urgent, multidisciplinary medical care. Due to differences in physiology, anatomic characteristics, and responses to injury, pediatric patients require specialized, age-appropriate burn care.

Etiology

Burn injuries can result from various sources, including thermal, chemical, electrical, or radiation exposure. Thermal burns occur from heat sources such as hot liquids, flames, or direct contact with hot objects. In children, common causes of thermal burns include scalds from hot liquids, steam, cooking appliances, stovetops, or accidental fires. Inhalation or contact chemical burns can result from exposure to strong acids or alkalis, which are found in household cleaning products. Electrical burns can occur if a child comes into contact with electrical outlets or exposed wires, potentially causing both internal and external injuries as the electrical current flows through the body.

Children are especially susceptible to burn injuries due to their innate curiosity and inability to recognize or understand the hazards present in their environment. The most common types of burns in children are scalds, contact burns, and flame burns. Pediatric burn injuries can also result from neglect and abuse, often manifesting as the deliberate immersion of a child in hot liquids or the direct application of flame to the child's skin.

Epidemiology

Pediatric burn injuries represent a significant public health issue, as they are among the leading causes of morbidity and mortality in children worldwide. The incidence of pediatric burns varies by region, but it is generally estimated that approximately 1 in 200 children will experience a burn injury annually. The prevalence of burn injuries is notably higher in infants and toddlers, with males being more commonly affected than females. Socioeconomic and environmental factors play a major role in a child's risk of sustaining burn injuries. Children from lower socioeconomic backgrounds are at greater risk due to factors such as poor housing conditions, overcrowded living spaces, inadequate home safety measures, limited access to healthcare, and insufficient supervision. Scald burns from hot drinks and cooking liquids are the most common cause of burns in children under 5 years old, accounting for 69% to 88% of all pediatric burn cases.

Pathophysiology

Burn injuries in children can range in severity and lead to significant consequences due to the unique anatomy and physiological response of their bodies. In young children, the epidermal and dermal layers of skin are thinner than in adults, making them more susceptible to deeper burns. The depth of the burn is impacted by the intensity and duration of exposure. The loss of skin as a protective barrier can result in bacterial colonization and increase the risk of sepsis. Direct energy from thermal, chemical, electrical, or radiation exposure causes protein denaturation and coagulation in the skin, leading to irreversible tissue damage and prolonged reduced blood flow in the affected area. In response to the injury, the child's body releases vasoactive mediators from the damaged tissue. Key mediators such as histamine, bradykinin, cytokines, prostaglandins, and oxygen radicals increase capillary permeability, resulting in significant fluid shifts and loss of intravascular fluid. *This imbalance in fluids and electrolytes can result in hypovolemia, dehydration, and edema.* A systemic inflammatory response may ensue, potentially leading to burn shock in cases of severe burns covering large surface areas. Once resuscitation is achieved for severe burns, children may develop a prolonged hypermetabolic state. A surge in catecholamines, glucagon, and cortisol contributes to significant energy expenditure at rest and catabolism of muscle proteins—leading to a loss in lean body mass and bone mineral density. While metabolism and catabolism are heightened, anabolic hormones such as human growth hormone and insulin-like growth factor are suppressed for several weeks—hindering the recovery process. *Severe burns may result in life-threatening complications such as acute kidney injury, pulmonary dysfunction, and multi-organ failure.*

Clinical Presentation

It is essential to gather detailed historical information from the caregivers of pediatric burn patients. Identifying the cause of the burn injuries helps guide the development of a personalized assessment and management plan. Gathering vital signs—such as pulse oximetry, blood pressure, heart rate, respiratory rate, temperature, and weight—is critical in assessing the acuity of the patient. *Extensive burns can impair the body's ability to regulate temperature, increasing the risk of* ***hypothermia***, particularly in younger children. ***Hypovolemic shock***, which may result from burns affecting more than 20% of the body surface area, presents with symptoms such as *pale or cool skin, tachycardia, low blood pressure, and altered mental status*. Severe burns may also lead to secondary infections, potentially resulting in *life-threatening* ***sepsis***, *marked by fever, tachycardia, hypotension, and altered mental status.* Pain is a common feature of all burns, particularly in the early stages. In deeper burns, the child may experience numbness or reduced sensation in the affected area due to neurovascular damage. The skin may appear red, white, or black, depending on the burn's depth and severity, and swelling (edema) can develop, especially with second-degree burns and more severe injuries. Clinical signs such as upper airway obstruction, hoarseness, and singed nasal hair may indicate upper airway burns, while respiratory distress could suggest chemical or smoke inhalation injury. *In cases of repeated or patterned burns, such as those from cigarette burns or scalds with distinct borders,* ***child abuse should be suspected.*** Burns caused by abuse often exhibit unique patterns or lack consistent explanations.

Evaluation

Evaluating the size (percentage of total body surface area) and depth (superficial, superficial partial-thickness, deep partial-thickness, full-thickness, or deeper) of the burn injury is crucial for determining the appropriate treatment plan. These assessments help guide fluid resuscitation protocols and inform the decision of whether the patient should be transferred to a specialized burn care facility. The percentage of total body surface area affected by burns is typically calculated using the **Lund–Browder chart** or the "**Rule of Nines**." Superficial burns are generally not included in these calculations. ***The Lund–Browder chart is considered the most accurate method for children***, as it accounts for their relatively larger heads and smaller lower extremities, which change with growth across different age groups. For instance, the body surface area percentages for burns in an infant (head: 9.5%, neck: 1%, trunk: 13%, upper arm: 2%, forearm: 1.5%, hand: 1.25%, thigh: 2.75%, leg: 2.5%, foot: 1.75%, buttock: 2.5%, and genitalia: 1%) differ from those of a 5-year-old (head: 6.5%, neck: 1%, trunk: 13%, upper arm: 2%, forearm: 1.5%, hand: 1.25%, thigh: 4%, leg: 2.5%, foot: 1.75%, buttock: 2.5%, and genitalia: 1%).

Cutaneous burn designations are based on the depth of injury, which affects the patient's healing potential and dictates management approaches. Burns are classified as superficial, superficial partial-thickness, deep partial-thickness, and full-thickness. **Superficial burns**, commonly caused by sunburns, affect only the epidermal layer of the skin and have excellent healing potential. These burns are typically *painful, erythematous, blanchable, dry, and free of blisters.* **Superficial partial-thickness burns** involve both the epidermis and parts of the dermis. They appear *erythematous, painful, weepy, and classically develop blisters within 24 hours*. This type of burn may incur delayed healing, but are typically void of functional impairment or hypertrophic scarring. **Deep partial-thickness burns** involve the epidermis and extend deeper into the dermis, damaging hair follicles and glandular tissue, and may lead to scarring. These burns are *painful only when pressure is applied, may appear blistered or have a wet or waxy dry look, and feature erythema with white patches.* **Full-thickness burns** penetrate all layers of the epidermis and may damage the subcutaneous tissue. These burns present with *eschar, loss of sensation, non-blanchable skin, and a waxy white or leathery gray appearance*. Blisters typically do not form, and without surgical intervention, patients face a high risk of severe scarring and skin contractures. A **fourth-degree burn**, which extends beyond the epidermis into deeper tissues such as muscles, tendons, and bones, is the most severe type of burn. It requires **immediate surgical intervention** and can result in serious complications, including infection, contractures, disfigurement, and even amputation.

Laboratory studies should also be obtained in children with severe burns to assess their clinical condition and promptly address any life-threatening concerns. A complete blood count helps identify signs of inflammation, infection, and trauma. A baseline basic metabolic panel is useful for monitoring the child's metabolic changes and fluid shifts associated with severe burns. To assess for **rhabdomyolysis**, a common burn complication, tests such as creatine kinase, urinalysis, and urine myoglobin can be ordered. Additionally, if there is suspicion of carbon monoxide or cyanide poisoning, tests such as arterial or venous blood gas, carboxyhemoglobin, and serum lactate may be necessary.

Management

Mild burns can be managed at home with pain relief, topical antibiotics, and careful monitoring, while moderate to severe burns require hospitalization for specialized care. Upon the patient's arrival at the emergency department, an immediate initial assessment should be conducted to identify any life-threatening conditions, followed by prompt stabilizing treatment. The **primary survey** involves evaluating and securing the patient's *airway, breathing, and circulation*. A *neurological assessment* should then be performed to assess disability, followed by a *rapid full-body examination* to gauge the size and severity of the burns. The **secondary survey** includes gathering a *detailed trauma history* and conducting a *thorough physical examination* to determine the depth, extent, and location of the burns.

Supplemental oxygen should be provided to children with fire-related burns, and signs of airway trauma or respiratory distress may require early intubation. Children with severe burns require immediate pain management and fluid resuscitation, including the replacement of sodium, potassium, and other essential electrolytes. Reliable vascular access should be established, and bladder catheterization should be done to monitor urinary output, helping assess the patient's fluid status. Children burned in enclosed spaces should be evaluated and treated for carbon monoxide and cyanide poisoning without delay. Additionally, children with partial or full-thickness burns should receive Tetanus immunization if they have not received boosters within the past 5 years.

Adequate fluid resuscitation is determined by the total body surface area (TBSA) affected by the burns. The **modified Parkland formula (3 mL × % TBSA × weight (kg))** can be used to estimate the fluid requirements for the first 24 hours after the burn injury. *Isotonic crystalloid fluid is the preferred choice during the first 24 hours, followed by a shift to Ringer's lactate*. For children under 5 years old or weighing less than 20 kg, 5% dextrose is added to the maintenance fluid to prevent hypoglycemia. *Within the first 24 hours, 50% of the total fluid is administered during the first 8 hours, and the remaining 50% is given over the next 16 hours.* Intravenous fluid resuscitation may be adjusted based on the patient's changing volume status.

Burn wounds should be cleaned with gentle soap and water, as disinfectants are avoided to prevent hindering the healing process. Devitalized tissue, such as ruptured blisters, should be carefully debrided using sterile saline-soaked gauze to minimize the risk of secondary infections. For patients needing urgent transfer to burn centers, dry sterile dressings should be applied to cover the burn wounds.

Circumferential partial and full-thickness burns can result in severe complications, such as worsening edema, compromised blood flow, and impaired muscle function at the burn site, which may lead to compartment syndrome, gangrene, and respiratory distress if the burn affects the chest. In such cases, an emergency escharotomy and fasciotomy, a procedure that involves creating deep incisions in the thickened eschar tissue and fascia to alleviate pressure and restore circulation, may be required to prevent permanent muscle damage or loss of limb function. Patients recovering from severe burn trauma may require physiotherapy and occupational therapy to restore function and prevent contractures. Partial-thickness and full-thickness burns may also require skin grafting, along with subsequent reconstructive surgery to release scar contractures and improve cosmetic appearance. Burn trauma can lead to considerable psychological distress, with children frequently experiencing anxiety, depression, and post-traumatic stress disorder following their injury. Ongoing follow-up care and psychological support are essential for burn survivors.

Outcomes

The prognosis for pediatric burn injuries is generally positive. Children with burns affecting less than 60% of their total body surface area have survival rates exceeding 90%. Those with severe burns face a survival rate of nearly 50%. With advancements in modern medicine and burn management, the overall mortality rate has decreased significantly. However, severe burns in young children still pose life-threatening risks. Long-term challenges for burn survivors may include scarring, disfigurement, impaired function, as well as psychological effects such as post-traumatic stress disorder, anxiety, and depression. Early prevention, awareness, and prompt access to emergency medical care are crucial for minimizing incidents and optimizing outcomes.

Caustic Ingestion

Introduction

Accidental ingestion of caustic substances is a major public health concern among young children. Caustic substances such as cleaning agents and beauty products are highly acidic (i.e., hydrochloric acid) or alkaline (i.e., sodium hydroxide) chemicals that can cause significant damage to the digestive system if ingested. Immediate medical intervention upon discovery of accidental caustic ingestion is critical to minimize serious complications such as perforation, stricture formation, and systemic toxicity. Patient outcomes are markedly influenced by the type, amount, and concentration of the ingested substance, as well as the time that passes prior to medical intervention.

Epidemiology

Pediatric poisoning secondary to accidental caustic ingestion is a global concern. In developing countries, caustic substances may be more readily accessible or stored incorrectly, resulting in a higher incidence of accidental ingestions. In contrast, developed nations have implemented stringent regulations and safer product packaging, which have contributed to a decrease in caustic ingestion rates. According to the National Poison Data System, in 2022, nearly 40% of the 2.1 million toxic exposures reported in the United States involved children aged 5 and younger. Caustic ingestion is most often observed in children aged 1 to 3, with boys making up 50% to 62% of cases, primarily due to their natural curiosity and limited awareness of environmental dangers. However, older children and adolescents may also consume caustic substances, often intentionally, as in the case of suicide attempts. Environments without adequate safety precautions or adult supervision increase the likelihood of accidental caustic ingestion in pediatric patients. The most commonly ingested caustic substances include household cleaning products such as bleach and drain cleaners, industrial products such as oven cleaners, and rust removers, battery acid, medications, and cosmetic items.

Pathophysiology

Caustic agents possess strong acidic or alkaline properties that have the potential to burn and corrode organic tissue within the gastrointestinal system through various mechanisms. Both alkaline and acidic caustic substances can cause immediate or delayed life-threatening injuries upon contact, with alkaline substances typically resulting in more severe and deeper damage than acidic substances. The severity of the injury is impacted by various factors such as the type, concentration, and volume of the ingested substance, as well as the duration of exposure.

Alkaline substances such as sodium hydroxide (NaOH), potassium hydroxide (KOH), ammonium hydroxide (NH4OH), and sodium hypochlorite (NaClO) commonly found in drain/oven cleaners or hair relaxers, industrial cleaners, disinfectants or laundry detergents, and bleach, respectively, generally have a pH above 12. When these substances come into contact with mucosal tissue, they trigger fat saponification—the degradation of lipids within cell membranes causing cell lysis and deep tissue penetration—and subsequent *liquefaction necrosis*, which destroys the epithelial layers, submucosa, and muscle. The concentration of alkali and the duration of exposure significantly affect the severity of mucosal injury and can lead to perforation. Studies have revealed that as much as 1 minute of contact with solutions containing 10% sodium hydroxide can cause deep mucosal burns, while just 1 second of contact with 30% sodium hydroxide can cause transmural esophageal necrosis. Patients may face life-threatening complications such as esophageal or gastric perforation leading to peritonitis and sepsis.

Acidic, or corrosive, substances such as hydrochloric acid (HCl), sulfuric acid (H2SO4), and phosphoric acid (H3PO4) commonly found in toilet bowl cleaners or tile cleaners, dish and laundry detergents or glue, and bathroom cleaners, respectively, generally have a pH below 2. These acidic substances cause denaturation of proteins within the mucosa, leading to *coagulation necrosis*. This can lead to superficial and localized tissue damage, forming a thick, white, leathery eschar. Severe complications seen in alkali injuries, such as deep esophageal penetration and perforation, are less common with corrosive exposure due to the protective features of the coagulum that forms and the alkaline pH of the squamous epithelium. However, upper airway damage is still common and 6% to 20% of acid ingestions result in esophageal burns.

Delayed injury can lead to ongoing tissue destruction for weeks after the initial necrosis at the time of injury. During the first week, inflammation and vascular thrombosis occur as a response to the chemical injury. Within 10 days, granulation tissue forms, causing erosion of the esophageal wall and heightening the risk of perforation. By 3 weeks, scar tissue and strictures may form, decreasing the risk of perforation but increasing the likelihood of chronic pain and gastrointestinal dysfunction.

Clinical Presentation

The clinical presentation of pediatric patients with caustic ingestion varies based on the severity of the injury to the gastrointestinal tract and upper airway. Patients with oral and oropharyngeal caustic damage may present with drooling, dysphagia, hoarseness, visible burns to the lips and oropharynx, and pain in the mouth, throat, or stomach. Respiratory involvement may elicit symptoms such as chest pain, dyspnea, stridor, wheezing, nasal flaring, and retractions. The most common symptom of gastrointestinal injury is dysphagia. In cases of severe esophageal burns, esophageal dysmotility can persist for several weeks. Other gastrointestinal symptoms may include vomiting, hematemesis, abdominal pain, and signs of peritonitis. Systemic responses to caustic toxicity such as shock, metabolic acidosis, and signs of dehydration can occur in severe cases. These patients may experience weakness, confusion, tachycardia, hypotension, tachypnea, cyanosis, thirst, dry skin, reduced urinary output, nausea, vomiting, or Kussmaul respirations.

Evaluation

The type, timing, and amount of caustic exposure should be immediately extrapolated from the patient's caregiver and utilized to guide management decisions. Intentional (i.e., suicide attempts or child abuse) and accidental caustic trauma must be differentiated. If the brand of the caustic substance is known, vital information such as the pH of the chemical should be investigated from the Material Safety Data Sheet (MSDS) or poison control center.

A prompt *neurological exam* and *vital sign assessment* must be performed urgently to identify and address clinical deterioration early. Respiratory compromise and esophageal injury should be carefully evaluated and monitored. Persistent, severe back or chest pain in the presence of fever may indicate esophageal perforation and mediastinitis. Signs of gastric perforation with peritonitis may include intense focal abdominal tenderness, rebound tenderness, rigidity, and fever. Laboratory tests such as blood gases, complete blood count, and electrolytes should be conducted to assess for metabolic acidosis, sepsis, and dehydration. Chest and abdominal radiographs should be obtained in symptomatic patients to evaluate for potential complications, such as aspiration, pneumonitis, or perforations of the esophagus or stomach. Confirmation can be achieved through esophagogastroduodenoscopy, as it is the gold standard for assessing injury within the first 24 hours of caustic ingestions.

Management

Caustic ingestion in children is a medical emergency that requires immediate intervention to minimize injury to the gastrointestinal system. Asymptomatic patients with normal swallowing and ingestion of substances of low causticity can be observed in the emergency department for several hours prior to discharge. However, symptomatic patients require hospital admission for close monitoring and intensive care.

The initial step in management is assessing and securing the patient's *airway, breathing, and circulation.* Stabilization and supportive care are individualized to the patient's clinical status. For patients presenting with signs of airway compromise, emergency endotracheal intubation or a tracheostomy is required. Intravenous fluid resuscitation should be initiated in cases of dehydration or shock. Adequate analgesia should be provided to manage pain associated with severe mucosal burns. Vomiting should never be induced and activated charcoal should be avoided, as this may cause deleterious effects.

Endoscopy should be conducted *within 24 hours* of admission for patients presenting with symptoms, oral burns, or confirmed caustic ingestion. Endoscopic evaluation is an essential diagnostic tool in cases of caustic ingestion, helping to assess the severity of mucosal injury, inform treatment decisions, and predict the prognosis. Through direct visualization of the injured mucosa, burns are graded to anticipate potential complications and guide management. Endoscopy should not be attempted in patients with hemodynamic instability, respiratory distress, perforation, or significant upper airway edema. The grading system is as follows: Grade 0 (normal mucosa), Grade 1 (mucosal edema and hyperemia), Grade 2 (friability, hemorrhages, erosions, blisters, whitish membranes, and superficial ulcerations), Grade 2A (absence of deep focal or circumferential ulcers), Grade 2B (presence of deep focal or circumferential ulcers), Grade 3 (multiple ulcerations and areas of brown-black or grayish discoloration suggesting necrosis), Grade 3A (diffuse small regions of focal necrosis), Grade 3B (extensive necrosis).

Patients with Grade 1 or 2A burns generally experience mild symptoms and do not require aggressive treatment. In contrast, those with Grade 2B and 3 injuries often present with severe complications and require interventions, including a nothing-by-mouth (NPO) status, intravenous resuscitation, broad-spectrum antibiotics, H2 blockers or proton pump inhibitors to reduce gastric acid secretion and prevent further mucosal injury, and corticosteroids to reduce inflammation and prevent strictures. Antibiotics, such as third-generation cephalosporins, and acid suppressors are typically administered for 1 week. Patients with Grade 2B burns, who show no signs of esophageal perforation, may benefit from high-dose intravenous steroids such as methylprednisolone for 3 days. For NPO patients, total parenteral nutrition should be provided to ensure adequate nutritional support until oral intake can be resumed. Extensive circumferential Grade 2B or 3 burns observed on endoscopy may require careful placement of a nasogastric tube to support nutrition and maintain a patent lumen in case of stricture development.

Patients must be urgently prepared for surgical intervention in cases of perforation, abscess formation, or severe stricture formation. Depending on the extent of the injury, esophageal reconstruction or gastrostomy tube placement may be needed. In some instances, strictures can develop weeks to months after the initial injury, requiring serial dilation or surgical intervention. Long-term follow-up care is essential in improving outcomes for survivors of caustic ingestion. This includes endoscopic monitoring for the development of esophageal or gastric strictures, speech and swallowing therapy for those experiencing dysphagia, and nutritional support in cases of severe esophageal damage or following reconstructive surgery.

Outcomes

Caustic ingestion is a significant pediatric surgical emergency. The outcomes for children who experience caustic ingestion largely depend on the severity of the injury and the interventions provided, such as airway evaluation, endoscopy, and nutritional support. Mild injuries (Grade 1 and 2A) typically result in favorable outcomes with non-invasive supportive care. These children are often discharged after endoscopy and rarely experience long-term complications. Moderate to severe injuries (Grade 2B and 3) are associated with higher morbidity and mortality rates, requiring hospitalization and aggressive supportive management. They may require urgent surgical intervention due to complications such as perforation and bleeding. These patients may also need endoscopic dilation due to the significant risk of developing **esophageal strictures**, *which is the most common long-term complication of caustic ingestion.* The prognosis for Grade 3 injuries is poor. Early endoscopy is crucial in assessing the extent of the injury and guiding management, which plays a key role in improving patient outcomes.

Foreign Body Ingestion

Introduction

Foreign body ingestion is a common clinical concern among young children that can lead to serious medical complications. Due to their natural curiosity, children often explore their environment by putting arbitrary objects in their mouths without fully understanding the potential dangers. Preschool-age children and those with mental health conditions are particularly at risk for swallowing foreign objects. In the United States, coins are the most frequently swallowed foreign object that requires medical attention. While most swallowed foreign bodies are benign and pass through the gastrointestinal tract without difficulty, the ingestion of items that become lodged damage the mucosa and may require urgent medical intervention. Accidental foreign body ingestion can result in serious health complications, with approximately 1500 deaths annually in the United States attributed to such incidents.

Etiology

The etiology of foreign body ingestion in pediatric patients is multifactorial, involving a combination of developmental behaviors and environmental factors. The foreign body ingestion of food items, toys, marbles, pins, coins, magnets, batteries, pills, or chemicals in children is primarily accidental. Infants and toddlers are particularly vulnerable due to their natural curiosity to explore their surroundings, often placing various objects in their mouths as part of their developmental process. At this stage, children lack the cognitive ability to recognize the dangers of swallowing foreign objects. Insufficient supervision, particularly in settings such as daycares, playgrounds, and large gatherings, where children are playing or eating, increases the risk of accidental ingestion. Hazards in the home, schools, or daycares also contribute to these risks. The absence of safety precautions and availability of small objects such as toys, batteries, coins, buttons, or pins within children's reach heighten the chances of swallowing foreign items. Children may also accidentally ingest food that is not properly chewed. Pre-existing medical conditions, such as developmental or cognitive delays (including autism), can lead to children placing objects in their mouths without understanding the associated dangers. Pica, a condition where children have a craving to eat non-food items, is another risk factor. Children with psychological impairments are at the highest risk for unintentionally swallowing foreign objects. Additionally, pre-existing gastrointestinal conditions, such as prior surgeries, strictures, fistulas, or motility dysfunction, can increase the likelihood of medical complications from swallowed foreign bodies.

Epidemiology

Foreign body ingestion is a widespread pediatric emergency worldwide. In the United States, over 100,000 cases of foreign body ingestion are reported each year, with more than 75% occurring in children. Hospital data indicate that foreign body ingestion is responsible for approximately 20–40% of all pediatric emergency visits related to gastrointestinal issues. The majority of these incidents involve children between the ages of 6 months and 3 years, with the highest incidence occurring around one year of age. The incidence gradually decreases after the age of 4 as children's cognitive abilities and motor control improve. Boys are slightly more affected than girls, with a male-to-female ratio of nearly 2:1. The overall number of cases has significantly increased in the past two decades, with coins being the most commonly ingested objects. There has also been a notable rise in the ingestion of batteries and magnets. Coins, which can sometimes be mistaken for button batteries on radiographs, remain the most frequently swallowed foreign body by children. With the growing presence of button batteries in everyday household and recreational items, the incidence of button battery ingestion has also increased.

Pathophysiology

The pathophysiology of foreign body ingestion in pediatric patients can range from asymptomatic passage through the gastrointestinal tract to severe complications, including airway obstruction, perforation, infection, and toxicity. These outcomes are influenced by the physical properties of the ingested object, the anatomical features of the digestive and respiratory systems, and the body's response to the foreign material. While most swallowed foreign objects pass through the system without issues, 10% to 20% of cases require endoscopic removal, and fewer than 1% necessitate emergency surgical intervention. The most common complication is esophageal obstruction, although some foreign bodies may also cause caustic injury to the gastrointestinal tract. The thoracic inlet is the most frequent site of obstruction. The severity of injury or risk of complications depends on the type of object ingested and any pre-existing anatomical abnormalities the patient may have. Commonly swallowed items include coins, button batteries, magnets, plastic toy parts, needles, paper clips, marbles, jewelry, fish bones, and food.

Once an object is swallowed, it travels through the pharynx and enters the esophagus. Due to the relatively narrow diameter of the esophagus, if the object is too large, irregularly shaped, or if the child has impaired esophageal motility, it may become stuck and cause an obstruction. Esophageal regions of physiologic narrowing (i.e., upper esophageal sphincter, level of aortic arch, lower esophageal sphincter) tend to be common areas of foreign body entrapment. The midsection of the esophagus can also be an area where foreign objects become lodged. In such cases, patients may have preexisting conditions (e.g., esophageal spasms, anastomosis, or strictures) that make them more susceptible to entrapment. If a foreign body is inhaled or aspirated into the larynx, trachea, or lungs, it can result in choking, airway obstruction, or aspiration pneumonia. Children are particularly vulnerable because of their smaller airway size. Once the foreign body reaches the stomach, the acidic environment (pH 1–3) generally does not impact most solid objects. However, caustic substances can lead to localized chemical burns or erosion of the gastric mucosa. While most objects pass through the intestines and are excreted in the stool without difficulty, large, sharp, or irregularly shaped items can cause intestinal obstruction, particularly in the small intestine or at the ileocecal valve.

Direct mucosal contact with button batteries causes serious sequelae in nearly 3% of cases. The severity of the injury is influenced by the battery's electrical charge, size, and the duration of impaction. Esophageal damage can begin as early as 2 hours after ingestion, with more severe harm occurring between 8 and 12 hours later. As the surrounding mucosa becomes increasingly edematous, the battery may adhere tightly to the mucosa, leading to ulceration and perforation. The corrosive damage to the mucosa is caused by the battery's electrical discharge, pressure necrosis, and the leakage of caustic substances. Many button batteries contain heavy metals such as mercury, silver, or lithium, as well as strong hydroxides like sodium or potassium, which can cause significant corrosion and destruction of the mucosa they contact.

Magnets are increasingly found in many toys and household items. High-powered magnets made of neodymium, a rare-earth metal present in the strongest magnets, are commonly used in toys and everyday household appliances. Accidental ingestion of these powerful magnets can lead to severe damage, particularly when multiple magnets are swallowed. The strong magnetic forces can cause the magnets to attract to each other within the gastrointestinal tract, leading to life-threatening perforations, obstructions, and infections. Most children who ingest magnets require hospitalization and endoscopy, with nearly 10% experiencing life-threatening complications.

The most commonly ingested sharp objects by children include straight pins, needles, paper clips, and fish bones. While these sharp objects usually pass through the gastrointestinal tract without causing harm, they can lead to complications if lodged in the hypopharynx, potentially resulting in retropharyngeal abscesses. Toothpicks and bones are more likely to cause perforations.

Clinical Presentation

Most children who are brought to the emergency department for witnessed or suspected foreign body ingestion are asymptomatic. If symptoms do occur, they are usually related to the location of the foreign body. For instance, if the object becomes lodged in the airway, it can cause immediate symptoms such as coughing, choking, gagging, cyanosis, wheezing, or stridor, leading to respiratory distress. This is especially common with small, round objects such as coins or marbles. Foreign bodies in the esophagus may cause dysphagia, drooling, coughing, regurgitation, chest pain, or refusal to eat. Retrosternal chest pain may suggest esophageal ulceration. Swallowed sharp objects may penetrate the esophagus, leading to neck swelling, crepitus, or pneumomediastinum. Prolonged retention of esophageal foreign bodies can result in weight loss due to decreased oral intake or aspiration pneumonia from impaired swallowing of oral secretions. Cases in which objects have successfully migrated to the stomach are generally asymptomatic. Yet, large objects may have difficulty exiting the stomach and can cause gastric outlet obstruction. In such scenarios, patients may present with nausea, nonbilious vomiting, gastric distention, and refusal of feedings. Occasionally, foreign bodies pass through the esophagus and stomach into the intestines without causing injury. However, when objects such as coins settle in the distal gastrointestinal tract, delayed complications such as pain, nausea, vomiting, abscess formation, or perforation may occur. The presence of fever, bloody stools, or severe abdominal pain in patients should raise suspicion for bowel perforation or peritonitis.

Evaluation

Children brought to the emergency department with suspected foreign body ingestion should be evaluated without delay. It is essential to secure their airway and breathing while assessing the source and location of the obstruction. A thorough history and physical examination are critical for identifying the foreign object and preventing potential complications.

Immediate surgical consultation is essential if the patient shows signs of esophageal perforation. In such cases, a visual examination of the child's neck may reveal edema, erythema, or crepitus. Surgical consultation is also required when abdominal examinations indicate signs of bowel obstruction or perforation. If a child is experiencing visible respiratory distress, such as inspiratory stridor or expiratory wheezing, it may suggest that a foreign object is lodged in the esophagus, causing tracheal compression.

Initial diagnostic testing for all children with suspected foreign body ingestion includes **radiography with anteroposterior and lateral views** of the *neck, chest, and abdomen*. Radiographs showing air-fluid levels in the esophagus suggest the presence of radiolucent objects, while free air may indicate perforation. Radiolucent foreign bodies, such as plastic, wood, thin metals, or bone, are harder to detect on radiographs, but imaging is still recommended in all cases of foreign body ingestion. Radiopaque objects, like coins and button batteries, are easily visible on conventional radiographs. *It is important to differentiate between coins and button batteries, as well as between objects located in the esophagus* versus *the trachea*. Button batteries require immediate removal, whereas coins may not. If standard radiographs do not reveal a foreign object but clinical suspicion remains high, computed tomography may be performed. Endoscopy may also be considered in the evaluation, as it serves both diagnostic and therapeutic purposes, especially if the foreign body is located in the upper gastrointestinal tract (esophagus, stomach) or if there is concern about potential damage or perforation.

Management

Asymptomatic or uncomplicated cases of foreign body ingestion can be managed conservatively with careful observation, dietary adjustments, and monitoring for spontaneous passage in the stool. Urgent intervention is necessary in cases of airway compromise, esophageal obstruction, intestinal obstruction or inflammation, magnet or battery ingestion, or the ingestion of sharp, long objects. Foreign bodies that have been lodged in the esophagus for more than 24 hours also require immediate removal to prevent complications such as erosion, perforation, and fistula formation.

Patients who have swallowed a coin without signs of dysphagia or respiratory distress can be monitored for spontaneous passage within approximately 24 hours. If the patient is symptomatic, the time of ingestion is unknown, or the coin has not passed in 24 hours, urgent removal of the coin through flexible endoscopy or rigid endoscopy. Coins that have easily reached the stomach can be managed conservatively with watchful waiting for spontaneous passage within 1–2 weeks. If 4 weeks have passed without evidence of the coin in the child's stools, endoscopic removal of the coin is then recommended.

Lodged batteries in the esophagus of children are considered a **surgical emergency**. Without timely intervention, the caustic material and electrical current from the battery can lead to liquefaction necrosis, ulceration, and perforation. Immediate consultation with the pediatric surgery team is required.

Sharp objects lodged in the esophagus represent a medical emergency due to the high risk of perforation. Immediate endoscopic retrieval of sharp objects lodged in the esophagus can be accomplished with tools such as a retrieval forceps or polypectomy snare. Flexible endoscopes can also be utilized to retrieve objects in the stomach or proximal duodenum. The ileocecal and rectosigmoid regions are the most common sites for intestinal perforation caused by sharp objects. Therefore, foreign bodies situated beyond the reach of flexible endoscopes require surgical removal.

Food impaction within the gastrointestinal tract may present as dysphagia, choking, or coughing that begins acutely while eating. In cases where the child is not in acute distress, and the bolus is small or situated in the lower esophagus, conservative management and monitoring may be sufficient. Increasing oral fluid intake may soften certain foods such as bread or chips and allow the bolus to pass on its own without further intervention. However, if the food bolus fails to pass spontaneously or if the patient develops severe symptoms, an endoscopic procedure may be necessary.

Outcomes

The outcomes of foreign body ingestion in children can vary based on factors such as the type of object ingested, its location in the gastrointestinal tract, the timing of ingestion, and how quickly treatment is provided. While foreign body ingestion remains a common and potentially life-threatening concern in pediatric patients, most cases are benign and resolve with minimal intervention. Prompt diagnosis and treatment are crucial to prevent complications.

The vast majority of children who swallow non-hazardous foreign bodies, such as coins or food-related objects, recover fully without long-term complications. The ingestion of sharp objects or magnets can result in moderate complications, such as esophageal obstruction, minor injury, or the need for endoscopic removal. Button battery ingestion, multiple magnet ingestion, and large, sharp objects that cause perforation or significant injury can lead to severe complications, including surgery, long-term damage, or even death. Early detection, careful supervision, awareness of potential hazards, and timely medical intervention play a crucial role in reducing the risk, incidence, and associated morbidity and mortality of foreign body ingestion, ultimately improving patient outcomes.

Blunt Trauma

Introduction

Blunt trauma is one of the leading causes of morbidity and mortality in children worldwide. This type of injury occurs from forceful impact without penetration, often due to motor vehicle accidents, falls, sports-related incidents, or physical abuse. Children, due to their smaller size, thinner skin, and developing organ systems, are more vulnerable to severe outcomes from blunt trauma compared to adults. A thorough understanding of the different types, causes, symptoms, diagnosis, and treatment of blunt trauma in children is crucial for improving their prognosis.

Etiology

There are several mechanisms of both direct and indirect physical injuries that lead to non-penetrating trauma in children. The primary etiological categories of pediatric blunt trauma include motor vehicle accidents, falls, physical abuse, sports injuries, recreational activities, domestic or environmental hazards, and risky behaviors. Due to their physical fragility, higher activity levels, tendency toward risk-taking, and exposure to environmental dangers, children are more prone to blunt trauma. Their risk of blunt trauma varies depending on factors such as age, socioeconomic status, and the surrounding environment.

Epidemiology

Blunt trauma is a significant cause of morbidity and mortality in pediatric populations, particularly among children aged 1 to 4 years. The nature of these injuries varies based on age, environment, and activity. Infants and toddlers are particularly vulnerable to blunt trauma from falls, often occurring from furniture, playgrounds, or stairs. Infants are also at risk for injury due to physical abuse, such as shaken baby syndrome. Older children and adolescents may suffer injuries from motor vehicle accidents, bicycle crashes, playground falls, sports activities, and other falls. Physical violence among peers and risky behaviors such as speeding or not using seatbelts become more common during adolescence. Blunt trauma tends to be more prevalent in male and adolescent groups, as males are much more likely than females to be involved in motor vehicle accidents, violent events, and high-contact sports due to their propensity to participate in risky activities and behaviors. Children in urban areas are more likely to be involved in pedestrian accidents due to greater traffic density, whereas those in rural areas may face increased risks from farm machinery and larger vehicles. Children from lower socioeconomic backgrounds are more vulnerable to blunt trauma due to factors such as limited access to protective equipment, unsafe living conditions, and a higher likelihood of physical abuse or neglect.

Pathophysiology

The unique anatomical and physiological characteristics of children make them particularly vulnerable to the mechanical forces of blunt trauma. The underdeveloped nature of their spine, bones, and organs make for dangerous medical situations in the event of such trauma. The force from falls, accidents, or physical abuse is absorbed by the impacted body part, resulting in tissue distortion and the transfer of energy to internal organs. Mechanisms of blunt trauma may involve direct impact, compression, acceleration and deceleration, as well as shearing forces.

Fractures and soft tissue injuries are frequent in children, particularly due to falls and sports-related accidents. As children's bones are still developing and are more flexible than those of adults, they are more susceptible to unique injury patterns, such as greenstick fractures and growth plate injuries. During childhood, cartilage remains softer and has not yet fully ossified, making them more vulnerable to vertebral fractures or spinal cord injuries in severe trauma. Although spinal cord injuries are less frequent in children than adults, they can occur due to falls or motor vehicle accidents and are often more severe due to the immature structure of the spine.

The chest and abdomen are critical areas affected by blunt trauma, particularly in motor vehicle accidents or cases of physical abuse, due to the lack of resilient rib protection. Rib growth persists throughout childhood, with the average rib height reaching about three-quarters of the adult average by age 3, and fully reaching adult rib height by around age 15. Thoracic injuries from blunt trauma may include *rib fractures, pneumothorax, hemothorax, lung contusions, or cardiac contusions*. Children characteristically have thin abdominal walls, with less muscle and fat, providing inadequate safeguarding for their underlying organs and increasing the risk of internal injuries upon forceful impact. Common abdominal injuries include *lacerations and hemorrhage of the spleen and liver, renal injury, and bowel perforation.*

The head is the most commonly injured body part in children, particularly in motor vehicle accidents, falls, and sports-related impacts. Due to the relatively larger size of a child's head compared to their body, softer skulls, developing brain, larger subarachnoid spaces, and weaker neck muscles, the skull and brain are highly vulnerable to significant damage. Head trauma can vary from minor injuries like scalp lacerations and mild concussions to more severe injuries such as traumatic brain injuries, cerebral contusions, skull fractures, or intracranial hemorrhages. Intracranial hemorrhaging can lead to life-threatening complications, including increased intracranial pressure and permanent brain damage.

The body's hemodynamic and systemic response to blunt force trauma depends on the magnitude of the force and the location of the injury. A serious injury can lead to hypovolemic shock from substantial blood loss or fluid shifts caused by trauma. Although children may initially compensate effectively, they may face rapid clinical deterioration without timely medical intervention. Trauma can also initiate an inflammatory response, resulting in swelling and additional tissue damage, which may degrade the overall prognosis.

Clinical Presentation

Children may not always have the ability to express the full extent of their injuries, making it crucial for clinicians to recognize the signs and symptoms of blunt trauma for accurate diagnosis and treatment. The clinical presentation can vary depending on the severity and location of the injury. It is essential to identify pain that is localized to the injured area. For instance, abdominal pain may indicate damage to an internal organ, while pain in the head or neck could suggest an injury to the skull or cervical spine. Swelling and bruising are often indicative of soft tissue damage or internal bleeding. Blunt chest or abdominal trauma can potentially harm the lungs or diaphragm, leading to respiratory distress or impairment. Neurological changes, such as confusion, loss of consciousness, or unusual behavior, may point to head trauma. Patients showing signs of tachycardia, hypotension, tachypnea, cyanosis, and cold extremities could be experiencing hemorrhagic shock due to internal bleeding. Younger children, particularly infants, may show more subtle signs of injury, including irritability, difficulty feeding, lethargy, decreased activity, poor reflexes, unusual muscle tone, or a high-pitched cry. Their inability to communicate verbally makes them vulnerable to missed diagnoses, especially in cases of internal trauma or head injuries.

Evaluation

Pediatric blunt trauma is a medical emergency that requires rapid, concurrent assessment and management to improve outcomes. Details about the mechanism of injury should be gathered from the caregiver or accompanying adult while a primary survey is expeditiously conducted to evaluate and stabilize the patient's airway, breathing, circulation, disability, and exposure. Vital signs must be stabilized, and the discovery of life-threatening injuries should trigger immediate intervention. A focused secondary survey must then be performed to systematically examine all major body systems from head to toe for additional injuries, including an assessment of neurological function, typically using the Glasgow Coma Scale. This clinical assessment tool helps healthcare teams evaluate the severity of brain injury and observe changes in consciousness over time in patients with head trauma. Effective management of the patient's pain and anxiety is also crucial in ensuring successful interventions.

Imaging and laboratory tests have a critical role in the evaluation of blunt trauma in children. Plain radiographs are frequently used to evaluate the chest for rib fractures, pneumothorax, hemothorax, and cardiac tamponade; the abdomen for bowel perforation, free air, and foreign bodies; the spine for vertebral fractures and spinal cord injuries; and the extremities for fractures or dislocations. Computed tomography (CT) imaging is an extremely sensitive diagnostic tool essential for evaluating complex and severe injuries, particularly when x-ray findings are inconclusive. Head CT is used to assess intracranial hemorrhage, cerebral contusions, and skull fractures. Abdominal CT is important for detecting damage to solid organs and free intraperitoneal air. Chest CT is valuable for identifying pneumothorax, hemothorax, and other pulmonary or cardiac injuries. Spinal CT is crucial when there is suspicion of spinal injury or neurological deficits. Ultrasonography is a useful tool for detecting internal bleeding or organ damage. A FAST (Focused Assessment with Sonography for Trauma) scan is a rapid ultrasound procedure performed at the bedside to identify free fluid in the abdominal, pericardial, and pleural cavities. Children with pelvic trauma may benefit from pelvic ultrasounds, as they can quickly detect pelvic fractures and bladder injuries. In cases of suspected cardiac injury following blunt chest trauma, an echocardiogram is recommended. Magnetic resonance imaging (MRI) may be used in complex cases where there is concern for soft tissue, brain, or spinal cord injuries or when CT scans are indeterminate.

A complete blood count (CBC) should be performed to detect signs of internal bleeding and infection, which may show low hemoglobin and hematocrit levels, along with an elevated white blood cell count. A basic metabolic panel may reveal increased creatinine or BUN levels, indicating kidney injury, or electrolyte imbalances, suggesting fluid shifts due to significant blood loss or traumatic shock. A urinalysis showing hematuria can support the clinical suspicion of renal or bladder injury. Patients with significant hemorrhage require coagulation profiles and blood typing to evaluate clotting ability and prepare for appropriate blood transfusion. Toxicology screenings should also be conducted to determine whether alcohol, drugs, or other toxins contributed to the patient's traumatic injury.

Management

The findings from the primary and secondary surveys of trauma patients are crucial in guiding treatment plans, with the main focus on stabilizing the patient's airway, breathing, and circulation while addressing life-threatening complications. Even if the child initially appears stable, some traumatic injuries can lead to a sudden deterioration. For instance, a seemingly minor head injury could lead to a delayed hemorrhage. In cases of severe trauma, children may need resuscitation with intravenous fluids, oxygen, or intubation. Pain management is also a vital part of pediatric trauma care, as children are more sensitive to pain, and their reactions may differ from those of adults.

Head and neck injuries include concussions, which necessitate rest and monitoring for neurological changes, intracranial hemorrhages that may require a craniotomy to evacuate hematomas and decrease intracranial pressure in severe cases, and cervical spine injuries that need neck immobilization. Injuries to the cervical, thoracic, and lumbar spine require close monitoring, immobilization, and possible surgical stabilization if complicated fractures or neurological deficits are present. Thoracic injuries include rib fractures, which often require pain management with opioids or local anesthesia and respiratory support; pneumothorax/hemothorax, which may need thoracostomy in severe cases; and cardiac contusions, where close monitoring of the child's cardiovascular status is essential. Abdominal trauma resulting in organ damage, bowel perforation, or pelvic fractures requires emergent surgical intervention. Significant internal bleeding or organ lacerations (such as those of the kidney, liver, or lungs) and subsequent hemorrhagic shock especially necessitates emergent blood transfusions and surgical intervention to repair or remove damaged organs and control hemorrhage. Stable fractures may be immobilized, with certain displaced fractures or dislocations may require reduction prior to immobilization. Open, displaced, unstable, or comminuted fractures require surgical fixation. Soft tissue injuries such as abrasions, lacerations, contusions, sprains, and strains can typically be treated conservatively with proper wound care, pain management, and outpatient instructions. Close observation, often in an intensive care unit, may be necessary for children with serious blunt trauma.

Outcomes

Blunt trauma is a leading cause of both morbidity and mortality in children. Traumatic brain injuries are especially common, as they can result from falls, collisions, or motor vehicle accidents. Life-threatening organ injuries, particularly to the spleen, liver, and kidneys, are common in abdominal blunt trauma. The outcomes of pediatric blunt trauma vary depending on the severity of the injury and the timeliness of medical intervention. While most children recover from minor injuries (e.g., bruises, sprains), more serious injuries (e.g., head trauma, internal bleeding) can have long-term sequelae, including physical disabilities, cognitive impairments, or even death. Blunt trauma in children presents unique challenges due to their anatomical and physiological characteristics. A thorough understanding of the mechanisms of injury, patterns of trauma, clinical presentation, and management strategies is essential for improving outcomes. Prompt recognition, careful assessment, and appropriate intervention can help mitigate the long-term consequences of blunt trauma in pediatric patients and reduce mortality.

Robotic and Minimally Invasive Surgery: Rationale and Principles

20

Oladapo O. Akinmoladun, Callan Kosnik, Sunshine Pille, and Laila Rashidi

Introduction

Let's start with some basic definitions so you have a clear understanding of this topic as it relates to abdominal surgery. In **open surgery,** usually a team of surgeons stand on either side of a very narrow operating **table** (not bed) to perform a surgical task. For example, the surgeon may stand on the patient's right side and a PA (for example) may stand on the patient's left side. Together they carry out the operation. Access is obtained via a typically large incision, and the abdominal wall is held open usually by metal retractors and other self-retaining retractor sets. Operation is carried out by *direct touch* and *direct visualization* of the anatomic target. Open surgery is sometimes called traditional surgery. It's main disadvantages are a long recovery, increased pain, and increased wound-related complications (hernia, infection).

There are two main types of **minimally invasive surgery** (MIS)—**laparoscopic** and **robotic.** In laparoscopic surgery, as compared to open surgery, the access is through small "keyhole" incisions, and a safe gas (**CO_2,** *never O2 due to its flammable nature*) is used to establish body wall retraction—the gas "pushes" the abdominal wall outwardly so that it becomes dome-like. Without this gas insufflation, it would be impossible to visualize the target anatomy. Unlike open surgery, the target anatomy is not directly visualized but instead seen as a 2D rendition on LCD monitor(s). The video image is obtained from a small diameter camera lens (5–8 mm) introduced into the abdominal cavity. In laparoscopy, the assistant may (and often is) be on the same side as the surgeon. Advanced instruments and dissectors nowadays allow an entire organ (such as the colon) to be removed without ever *directly* seeing or touching it!

Robotic surgery provides *all* the advantages of laparoscopy, but with more sophisticated techniques. It's like laparoscopy, but the surgeon operating is not standing at the bedside, but rather is seated at a surgeon console that can be in the operating theater or even in another room altogether. Usually, there is still a bedside assistant (often a PA). It's important to understand that robotic surgery does not mean "the robotic is doing the surgery for you." All current robotic platforms are master-slave systems, whereby the instrument control is "translated" to an **effector arm** by the *surgeon's* hand movement. They consist of two main parts—**(a)** a bedside cart, which includes a boom and usually four robotic arms, and **(b)** a surgeon console. Table 20.1 compares and contrasts open, robotic, and laparoscopic surgery.

Much of this chapter will focus on the robotic variant of MIS, as there is *an important role for PAs here.* For all intents and purposes, *laparoscopic and robotic surgery offer similar outcomes in experienced hands.*

The Increasing Utilization of Robotics and the Role of PAs

Among all surgical subspecialties, the adoption of robotic-assisted (RAS) and minimally invasive surgery (MIS) continues to rise. From 2012 to 2018 alone, rates of robotic utilization in robotic general surgery increased from 8.7% to 35.1%, respectively [1]. When compared to open surgery, MIS is associated with improved patient outcomes such as reduced complications, shorter hospital length of stay, lower blood loss, and decreased rates of infection [2]. Robotic surgery has additional advantages over traditional laparoscopic surgery including greater operative vision, dexterity, and increased degree of freedom of surgical instruments [3].

O. O. Akinmoladun
Madigan Army Medical Center, Tacoma, WA, USA

C. Kosnik · S. Pille · L. Rashidi (✉)
Multicare Health Network, Tacoma, WA, USA

S. Atallah, J. Dragoljevic (eds.), *Fundamentals of Surgery for Physician Assistants*,
https://doi.org/10.1007/978-3-032-21069-2_20

Table 20.1 A comparison of open, laparoscopic, and robotic surgery

Category	Open surgery	Laparoscopic surgery	Robotic surgery
Incision size	Large incisions (4–12 inches)	Small incisions (0.5–1.5 cm, multiple ports)	Small incisions, similar to laparoscopic
Visibility	Direct line-of-sight to organs	2D camera view via laparoscope	3D high-definition, magnified view with very steady camera
Surgeon control	Direct hand manipulation of instruments	Hand-held instruments	Surgeon uses robotic console to control mechanical arms
Precision	Limited by hand dexterity and visual access	More precise than open, but limited by tool flexibility	Extremely precise due to articulated robotic arms, motion scaling, and wristed instrument tips
Tactile feedback	Full (surgeon can feel tissue directly)	Some tactile feedback	No direct tactile feedback (for most), relies on visual cues
Operating time	Often faster in emergencies or routine cases	Moderate duration	Can be longer due to setup and equipment adjustments
Recovery time	Longest (4–8 weeks)	Short (1–2 weeks)	Short (1–2 weeks typically)
Hospital stay	5–10 days (procedure-dependent)	1–3 days or outpatient, depending on nature of operation	1–3 days or outpatient, depending on nature of operation
Postoperative pain	More severe due to larger incision	Mild to moderate	Mild (often least pain reported)
Scarring	Significant	Minimal, small scars, usually 5 mm ports incisions	Minimal, small scars, usually 8 mm port incisions
Bleeding risk	Higher, but easier to control	Minimal, control can be challenging	Minimal, control can be challenging
Infection risk	Higher due to open wound exposure	Low	Low
Learning curve	Standard surgical training	Moderate learning curve	Steep learning curve; requires robotic training and certification; some tasks such as suturing are much easier than laparoscopy
Cost	Lowest (no advanced equipment)	Moderate (laparoscopic tools, cameras)	Highest (robot system + maintenance + training)
Technology used	Basic surgical tools	Camera, light source, long-handled instruments	Robotic arms, console, software, 3D camera
Common uses	Trauma, open-heart surgery, large tumors	Appendectomy, gallbladder removal, hernia repair	Prostatectomy, gynecologic and colorectal surgery, complex reconstructions
Accessibility	Available in all surgical centers	Widely available in most hospitals	Available at many centers and hospitals, increasing dramatically
Advantages	Direct access, no need for tech infrastructure	Minimally invasive, quicker recovery, reduced complications	Highly precise, best for complex or delicate cases, very "stable" operating platform
Disadvantages	Long recovery, high pain, more complications	Limited flexibility, less stable optics, less precision in effector arm/instrument control	Expensive, requires high expertise, long setup time

Surgical scrub technicians "scrub techs," **advanced practice providers (APP)** (i.e., advanced practice registered nurses (APRNs) and physician assistants (PA)) play a crucial role in the safe implementation and increased usage of RAS. From 2010 to 2016, the rates of APPs integrated into surgical practices *have increased by approximately 13% with the largest increases seen in general and urologic surgical practices* [2]. Although APPs have the capacity to serve in a wide range of functions in surgical practice including outpatient care (i.e., treatment, preoperative and postoperative evaluation) and inpatient medical management, the emphasis of this chapter is on their roles in the operating room, specifically as it relates to MIS and RAS.

Professional Societies, Onboarding, and Scope of Practice

Professional membership and engagement in relevant surgical societies is an effective way to gain education, mentorship, and stay current on the most recent medical advances.

Though not an exhaustive list, societies that provide tailored educational resources, didactics, workshops, and conferences in MIS and RAS include the Society of American Gastrointestinal and Endoscopic Surgeons (SAGES), Institute for Surgical Excellence (ISR), the American Association of Surgical Physician Assistants (AASPA), and the American Association of Surgical Nurse Practitioners

(AASNP). Although membership and engagement with professional organizations can come at a cost, there are many resources that are freely available. Online modules that are free to access include, but are not limited to, the Fundamentals of Laparoscopic Surgery (FLS), Fundamentals of Robotic Surgery (FRS), and the Fundamental Use of Surgical Energy (FUSE). These didactics provide guidance on the safe handling and proper usage of laparoscopic and robotic instruments, surgical energy, optimization of robotic and other system components, patient safety, and intraoperative troubleshooting. Although there are available resources for education and training in RAS and MIS, a universal curriculum has not been established for the surgical team. Historically, bedside assistants (BA) range from attending surgeons, residents, surgical scrub technicians, operating room nurses, and APPs. Currently, the role of the bedside assistant is most commonly performed by APPs and surgical technicians [4]. Due to limitations of time, differences in state-to-state and hospital system practice patterns, monetary limitations for training courses, and lack of educational uniformity, the training of bedside assistants occurs predominantly in the operating room (OR) by experienced practitioners of all backgrounds. Despite the lack of a widely accepted robotic training curriculum, many hospitals have implemented their own multimodal training plans that improve the proficiency and comfort of the entire surgical team [5]. For example, at the author's institution, there are two separate pathways for the BA distinguished by whether or not the BA requesting privileges has experience or not. BAs with experience must have an appropriate review by a proctor on the robotic surgical committee and complete designated tasks within a 6-month time period. BAs without experience must attend the robotics pathway defined by the robotics committee including hands-on training with a da Vinci Intuitive Trainer, complete required focused case reviews with a proctor within 6 months. The entirety of the pathway has been simplified for the sake of this section.

The most common robotic surgical platform used is the da Vinci Surgical System (Intuitive Surgical Inc.), which currently allows the performance of one million robotic surgeries in the United States each year [6]. Intuitive provides online training modules, in-service training including virtual, dry, and live tissue labs, and real-time intraoperative support as well [7]. To date, the only robotic surgical platforms that are both in use and FDA-approved are the da Vinci Surgical System (various iterations of which including **Si, X, Xi, Sp, V**) and the Zeus System [8]. Many newer platforms are on the horizon and are currently being used internationally.

A comprehensive review of all robotic surgical platforms is beyond the scope of this chapter, but images and other principles will be explained primarily from the perspective of the surgeon's and APP's experience on the da Vinci Xi. The majority of technical considerations will be explained from the *vantage point of the surgical team's experience in abdominal and pelvic surgery.*

Preoperative Considerations and Contraindications

Prior to undergoing MIS, a thorough history and physical examination of all candidates of surgery should be performed. This is necessary to reveal any underlying medical conditions, especially cardiac or pulmonary diseases, that limit patient toleration of pneumoperitoneum or ***Trendelenburg*** (head-down) positioning. Pertinent surgical history aimed at any prior adverse events with anesthesia, concerns for intraabdominal adhesions in a reoperative abdomen, presence of hernias, and oncologic history (tumor location or history or chemotherapy or radiation. If available, preoperative review of imaging studies can provide additional information and aid in surgical planning [9].

Indications for MIS vary, encompassing a wide range of general, gynecologic, and urologic procedures, including cholecystectomy, colectomy, and nephrectomy. Robotic systems offer enhanced dexterity and visualization, making them advantageous in complex procedures, such as those requiring fine dissection near delicate or critical structures. Contraindications primarily center around the patient's inability to tolerate pneumoperitoneum or extremes in positioning, as seen in patients with *severe cardiopulmonary conditions.* Additionally, extensive adhesions, advanced malignancies, or unmanageable obesity may limit access and visualization, rendering minimally invasive approaches inappropriate [10].

Communication

Structured communication facilitates the sharing of critical information between disciplines, such as anesthesia, nursing, and surgery. Training programs that emphasize interdisciplinary communication skills have been shown to improve the performance of surgical teams, reinforcing the importance of constant, clear communication in maintaining patient safety [4, 11]. Since robotic surgery physically separates the surgeon, on the console, from the patient, seamless communication between the surgeon and the PA (as the bedside assist) is crucial for safe surgery. Specifically, the usage of closed-loop communication between the surgeon and the PA is essential and is an identified skill of surgical teams with high nontechnical skill scoring [12]. For example, if the surgeon on console would like to exchange an instrument, the surgeon would call out, *"Would you please remove the vessel sealer in arm three, and replace it with a Cadiere for-*

ceps?" This should be returned with a response from the bedside assistant, *"Coming out with the vessel sealer in arm 3 and replacing it with a Cadiere forceps!"* This also highlights the need for the bedside assistant/PA to be *well-versed in the robotic setup, instruments, surgical anatomy of the procedure at hand, operative steps, and the timing and critical areas that require maximal assistance during the operation.* Proactive assistance is key to ensuring safe, efficient, and timely procedures. This ensures that the surgeon on console can focus on the intricate tasks at hand.

Effective communication between surgical teams also plays a significant role in trouble shooting common intraoperative events, such as instrument malfunctions, loss of working space, or other changes that cause cases to stall. For example, the BA can assess in real time the loss of pneumoperitoneum by being aware of decreased working space, lower actual pressure, and actual flow rate as displayed on the CO_2 conditioning insufflator. In robotic-assisted surgery, tasks such as instrument exchanges, suction, and maintaining pneumoperitoneum are essential to the team's success and rely heavily on precise communication. By anticipating the needs of the console surgeon and coordinating tasks like robotic docking and instrument readiness, the bedside assistant helps streamline the surgical process. This reduces delays and optimizes the surgeon's workflow, enhancing overall team performance [7, 11].

Patient Positioning and Room SetUp

Proper patient positioning is crucial to ensure optimal access and exposure of the target anatomy and minimization of complications (Figs. 20.1 and 20.2). The *initial and anticipated patient positions should be discussed with members of the surgical and anesthesia teams prior to the operation.* For instance, in MIS colorectal surgery, the Trendelenburg position, often with a lateral tilt, is utilized to facilitate access to the pelvis by shifting the bowel away from the operative field. This allows for better visualization and prevents injury to adjacent organs [7]. Special care must be taken to prevent pressure-related injuries, and padding should be used to protect vulnerable areas such as nerves and bony prominences [7, 13]. The **peroneal nerve** (which courses lateral to the knee) is *particularly prone to injury* and can result in **foot drop.** In robotic surgery, patient positioning has added *complexities due to the docking of the robotic arms.* The da Vinci Xi system, for example, requires precise positioning to allow for smooth movement of its four arms, which *must not collide with the patient or each other.* The arms are placed after ports (trocars) are inserted into the abdominal cavity, ensuring a safe working space of **8–10 cm between ports** and adequate clearance from the patient to avoid collisions [14]. What is often understated is the maximization of space around the operating table including the docked robot.

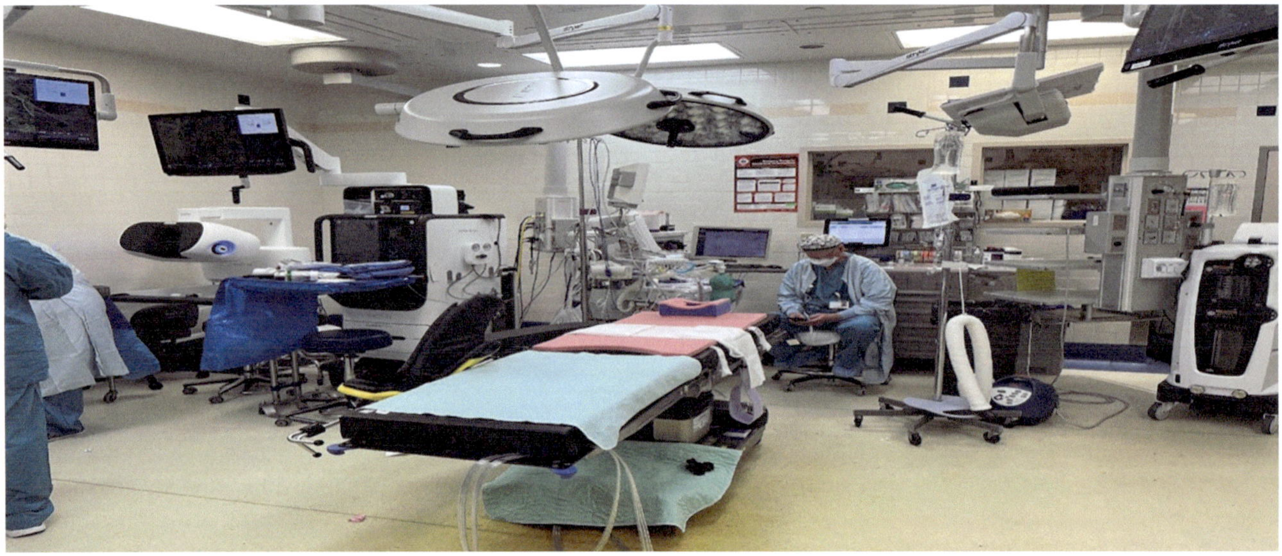

Fig. 20.1 An operating room equipped with the da Vinci V Surgical System. The console can be seen in the left corner. Remember, robotic surgery differs from laparoscopy in that the surgeon is altogether removed from the bedside. Note the LCD monitors which have been integrated into this operating theater. Although the console surgeon will be able to view image in 3D, assistants, including Pas, should be "following along" with the view seen on the monitors

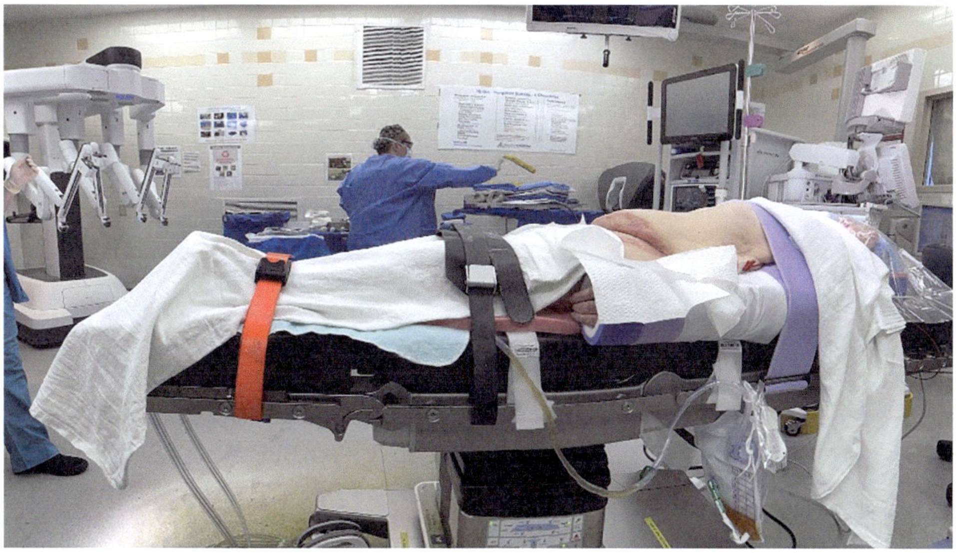

Fig. 20.2 A patient under anesthesia has been positioned supine in preparation for surgery. Note the seatbelts and straps designed to prevent the patient from slipping off of the table during various position changes, including ***"airplane"*** whereby the operating table is tilted to the left or to the right. Visible in this image is the robotic cart, with its four arms. This will be docked to the patient prior to the commencement of operation. The surgeon will be seated at a console, which is shown in the right corner, completely removed from the operating table. There are various advantages to this style of MIS surgery, one of which includes tremor cancellation—so if your hands are a bit "shaky," well, the robot corrects for that!

There should be sufficient room around the patient to allow enough space for the bedside assistant and surgical scrub technologist to interact with each other and the operative field to facilitate efficient transfer of instruments, allow the bedside assistant to insert needles and thread (for intracorporeal suturing), and provide tension and countertension for the surgeon on console. The bedside assist and surgical scrub technologist need to be able to clearly see the entirety of the patient and robotic platform in addition to the internal operative field. *Monitors should be placed to ensure that both fields can be viewed simultaneously.* The OR, if possible, should be arranged to allow a direct line of sight from the surgeon on console to the operative field to facilitate trouble-shooting of external collisions, and provide guidance to the bedside assistant should trouble arise. It's important to note that the console (operating) surgeon has her/his head in a viewfinder and is fully concentrated on the surgery itself. Thus, the surgeon will not be aware of external robotic arm collisions necessarily, and thus, it is the role of the PA/bedside assist to communicate this to the surgeon. Not infrequently, the arms have to be readjusted to prevent collision, and this is the role of the PA or other first assist.

Establishment of and Maintenance of Pneumoperitoneum

In laparoscopic and robotic surgery, initiating pneumoperitoneum is a critical step for creating the working space required for safe and efficient procedures. For both laparoscopic and robotic approaches, carbon dioxide (CO_2) is typically used to inflate the abdominal cavity, which is initiated by inserting a *Veress needle*, an *optical trocar* (Optiview®), or trocar by *direct cutdown* (**Hasson method**) to introduce CO_2 gas [14]. *Initial* insufflation pressures should be anywhere from **7 to 10 mmHg,** as higher or lower initial insufflation pressures may indicate a location that is not in the abdominal cavity (i.e., preperitoneal space or gastrointestinal lumen). Insufflation pressures around **12–15 mm Hg are typically recommended** for optimal working conditions and to reduce the risk of complications during port placement and instrument manipulation [13]. Communication with the anesthesiologist prior to and during the initiation of pneumoperitoneum is essential. ***Hypotension and especially bradycardia*** after induction of pneumoperitoneum may signify excessive **vagal stimulation** as the peritoneal cavity insufflates. If this occurs, **desufflation should commence promptly—in other words STOP the procedure** (it's the **FIRST STEP** in managing this not uncommon event). Ultimately, this may require lower initial insufflation pressures, lower peak insufflation pressure during the operation, conversion to an open procedure, or termination of the operation all together. Parasympatholytic medications such as **atropine** can also be administered.

Maintaining pneumoperitoneum throughout the surgery requires constant monitoring and adjustments to ensure safe pressure levels are sustained. Leaks around the trocar sites, issues with the insufflator, or dislodged ports are common causes of pressure loss. Troubleshooting involves first identifying the source of the issue—such as loose seals or improper trocar placement—and correcting it, often by repositioning or replacing trocars, adjusting the insufflation settings, or addressing any device malfunctions. In robotic setups, communication between the bedside assistant and the console surgeon is crucial to handle such troubleshooting effectively. The bedside assistant plays a key role in managing these situations by ensuring all ports remain sealed and actively monitoring the insufflation equipment for irregularities. In some cases, when the CO_2 is delivered via a cylinder, it may be empty leading to loss of pneumatics, and the cylinder would then need to be exchanged during the operation.

Port Placement

Proper port placement (Fig. 20.3) is critical for *optimizing access to the operative field* while *minimizing the risk of injury*. In laparoscopic surgery, ports are typically placed in a triangular fashion to allow for optimal visualization and spatial separation of manually introduced instruments, while also minimizing the risk of instrument clashing [9]. Port placement generally depends on the target anatomy and the type of procedure being performed. The distance between ports in laparoscopy may be smaller (compared to robotic trocar placement), and surgeons rely on a 2D view to navigate the instruments, which may limit the precision when compared to robotic surgery [14]. Additionally, transillumination can be used to minimize injury to abdominal wall vessels during port insertion [14].

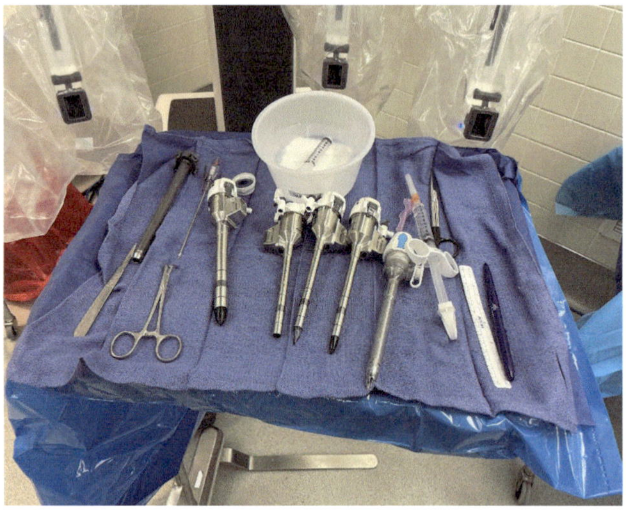

Fig. 20.3 Various robotic **trocars,** often referred to simply as **ports,** are shown. They are reusable and made of metal. Most laparoscopic ports are single-use and made of a plastic material; in many instances, an *assist port* is used, which is usually a *laparoscopic type (disposable) trocar,* which appears as the blue-capped trocar, and is in this case also used to insufflate the abdomen. The robotic arms are docked or *locked onto these metal trocars*; this essentially mates the robot to the patient. Many PAs are trained to swap out instruments through these trocars, and some are trained to place them

In robotic surgery, port placement follows similar principles, but with some additional considerations due to the use of robotic arms. In the da Vinci robotic system, the ports are positioned to *avoid arm collisions* and allow the robotic instruments to operate with *maximum range of motion* (Fig. 20.3). The camera port is typically positioned 18–20 cm from the target anatomy, with other instrument ports spaced a hand's breadth apart (around 8–10 cm). Proper spacing ensures that the robotic joints can function without external or internal clashing. For optimal efficiency, robotic ports should align in a straight line relative to the surgical workspace, ensuring that the center of the workspace is the focus of camera targeting. This configuration maximizes the working space of the robotic arms, allowing for a wider range of motion and reducing the risk of instrument collision. Robotic systems, such as the da Vinci, use a 3D stereoscopic camera that is remotely controlled by the surgeon, which (compared to laparoscopy) eliminates the need for the bedside assistant to manipulate the camera. The distance between robotic ports is generally larger, and instruments are designed to pivot around a remote center, providing greater dexterity and control, even in confined spaces. Overall, it is important to note that the surgeon is the one who will pick port placement sites, and this is not usually something a PA would be doing on their own. Still, it is good to have some knowledge regarding the rationale behind port placement!

Docking

One of the fundamental aspects of safely docking the robot is precise port placement, as stated above. Ports must align with the surgical workspace and target anatomy. The optimal configuration involves straight-line port placements (Fig. 20.4), which help maximize the workspace and mini-

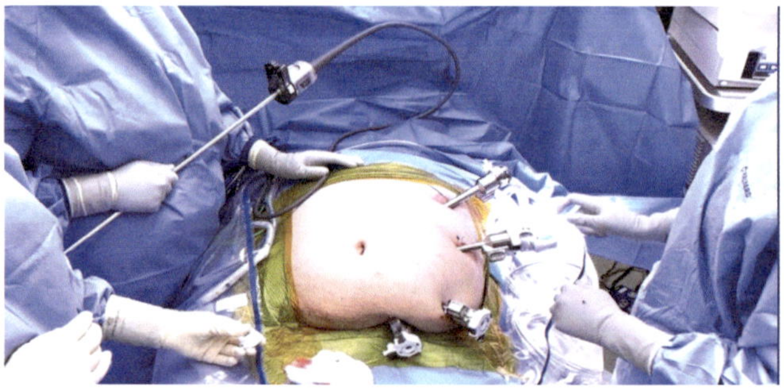

Fig. 20.4 Four trocars have been placed into the abdominal cavity in preparation for robotic surgery. Unlike laparoscopy where triangulation is important in trocar placement, the trocars here are often placed in a more linear fashion. Note that the spacing is quite wide, with ample separation between the trocars. This limited robotic arm collision, when the arms are docked to the trocars

mize the risk of collisions between robotic arms. Additionally, correct placement of the ports relative to the endoscope is essential, as the boom and robotic arms adjust during docking to provide maximum visibility and clearance while avoiding obstructions (Figs. 20.5 and 20.6). Proper docking ensures that robotic arms can move without interference, which is especially important in complex procedures where collision could result in delays or complications [13].

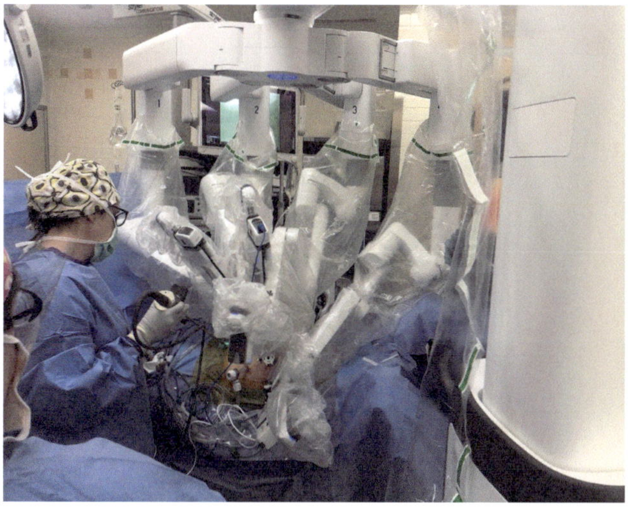

Fig. 20.5 A bedside assistant is shown holding the robotic camera and is cleaning the lens. It is common for the bedside assistant to exchange instruments and clean the camera lens if and when needed

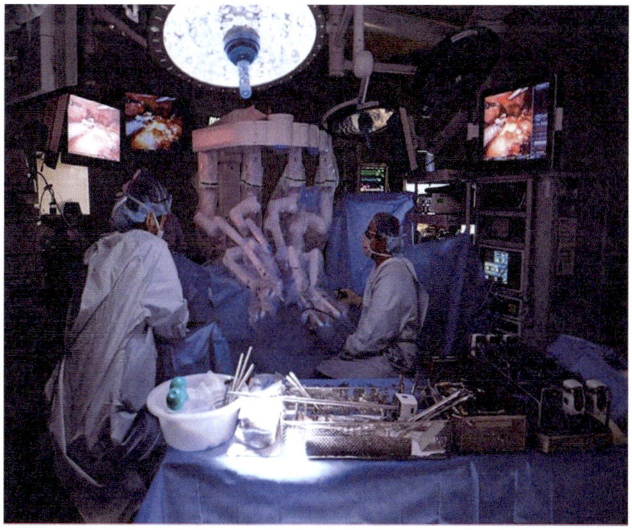

Fig. 20.6 The robotic cart has been docked to the patient and surgery is in progress. It is typical to have the "lights out" during MIS surgery, similar to how you would watch a movie. A scrub tech (left) and bedside assist (seated) are seen, but the operating surgeon is out of view. Notice that both the scrub tech and the bedside assistant are focused on the monitors which depict the operation in real-time. PAs often work as bedside assistants during robotic surgery cases

Targeting

After placing ports and identifying the abdominal quadrant of interest on the patient cart helm, a step called **targeting** is performed. Here, the cross hairs of the *targeting lines* are centered on the *camera port* (Fig. 20.7a, b). Once the camera port is docked and targeting to the center of the surgical workspace is underway, it is recommended to steady the robotic camera throughout the entirety of the targeting process. Ensure that the camera port and its associated robotic arm are in the trajectory of the target anatomy. This will serve as a guide to allow the subsequently placed robotic arms and instruments to align in the correct trajectory of the center of the operative field. Objective evidence of appropriate aligning of subsequent arms include uniformness of the top most FLEX joints of each instrument.

Making Sure the Surgical Field Is Ready for the Operation

Once alignment is ensured, and instruments are placed, ports may need to be "burped" to optimize the placement of each port as their positions may have changed during alteration of the FLEX joints and introduction of surgical instruments. Prior to placing robotic ports, it is also important to include a laparoscopic nonrobotic port for the bedside assist (when needed). The "assist port" needs to be placed in a location that maximizes the bedside assistant's comfort and maneuverability, while also ensuring that proper spacing and robotic port and instrument docking is not impaired. *If this is not correctly placed, then the bedside assistant can actually be hit by the moving robotic arms, so you have to be careful!*

The role of the surgical team, particularly those assisting in robotic docking, significantly influences the procedure's efficiency. A well-trained bedside assistant (such as a PA) can *actively manage the patient clearance joints and flex joints during docking, helping to position the robotic arms correctly to avoid collisions and improve procedural flow.* Training programs emphasize the importance of familiarizing assistants with both the system's capabilities and troubleshooting strategies. When docking issues arise, the assistant's ability to adjust the patient clearance joint or reposition the boom can prevent delays and ensure that the robotic arms can operate within the designated space *safely*.

Safe Introduction and Removal of Surgical Instruments and Foreign Bodies

The introduction of robotic and laparoscopic instruments into the abdominal cavity also involves precise setup, careful docking, and constant vigilance to minimize

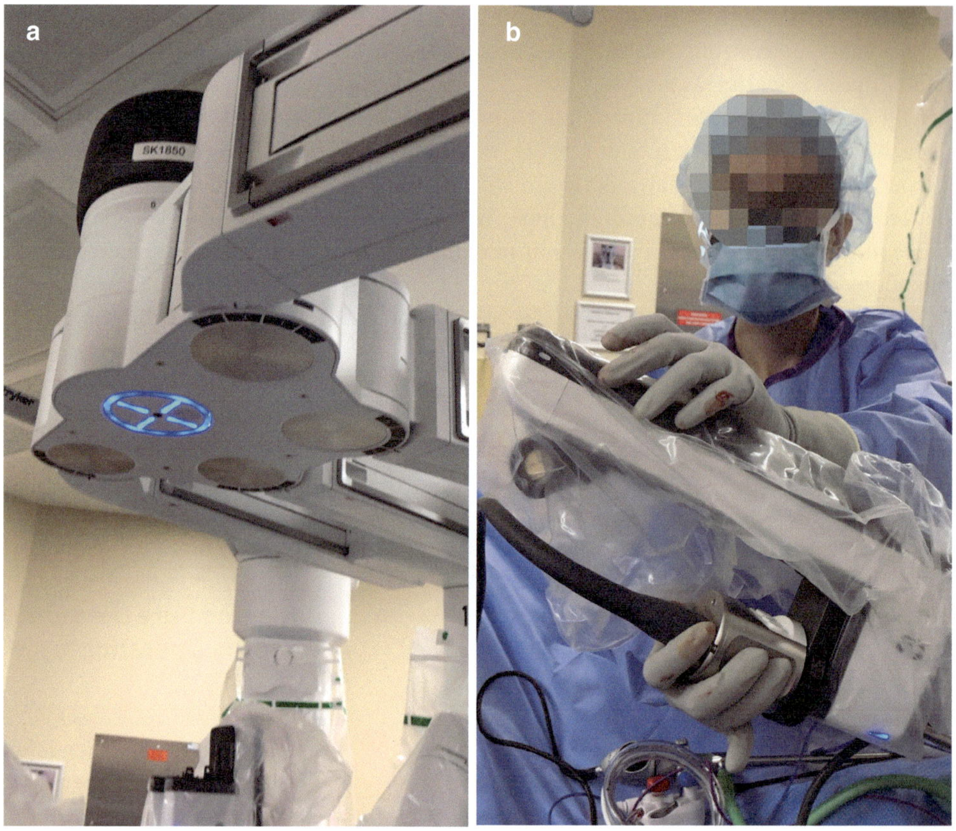

Fig. 20.7 (**a**, **b**) Using the da Vinci Surgical System, the cross hairs from a laser light integrated into the boom (**a**) are centered on the camera port. The system will then verbally direct the assistant point the scope [camera] toward the target anatomy (**b**). After this, the booms and robotic arms are essentially rotated and configured for that target anatomy automatically

patient injury (Fig. 20.8). After the establishment of pneumoperitoneum and camera placement, instruments and ports are inserted *under direct visualization*. In robotic surgery, after the robotic camera and instruments have been introduced to the center of the surgical field, the **da Vinci V** is equipped with an *internal memory of the trajectory* of that instrument if it is removed. If an instrument is reintroduced in its place, the established memory allows for a "guided-tool-change" to the location in the surgical field before the previous instrument was removed. This is indicated on the specific robotic arm in question by a flashing green light on the instrument clutch during instrument placement [2]. If the instrument clutch is *flashing blue*, this indicates an unguided instrument placement which may prompt the console surgeon to visualize the reintroduction of the instrument if needed. The bedside assistant can also use the external trajectory of the camera and other placed instruments, while also looking at the monitor to ensure safe placement. If the bedside assistant/PA is unsure of the trajectory to take when introducing a sharp instrument or needle, a simulated run can be performed with an empty blunt instrument (i.e., laparoscopic wave grasper). After a safe track is identified, the sharp instrument can be placed. The safe introduction and removal of foreign material (i.e., mesh, suture, surgical guaze, needles) during laparoscopic and robotic surgeries are crucial to minimizing complications.

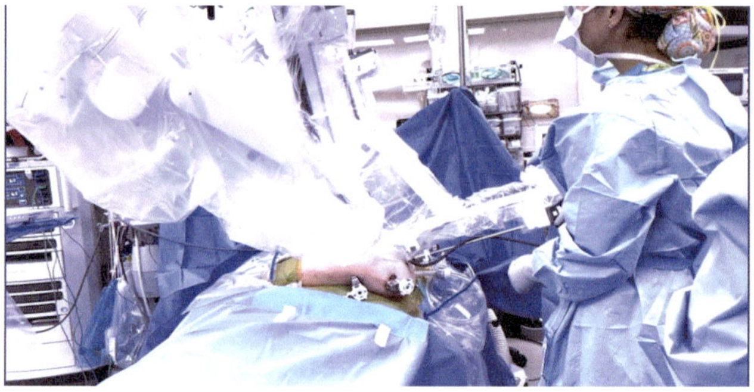

Fig. 20.8 A bedside assistant is seen introducing a robotic instrument into the abdominal cavity. Normally, the camera is the first robotic instrument to be delivered, and then subsequent instruments are directly observed (via the robotic camera) as they approach the surgical field. This *limits the risk of injury* as the instrument tip (which can be sharp) is pushed toward the target anatomy by the assistant

Instruments and foreign bodies should be introduced and removed under direct visualization. Although tissue specimens and other foreign bodies can be introduced and removed with a grasper, needles should be removed by the bedside assist with a needle driver [11]. In robotics, closed-loop communication should be utilized during instrument exchanges [11]. This is important due to the spatial relationship differences in robotic surgery where the surgeon is at the console, and not directly visually supervising instrument exchanges at the bedside. Proper coordination between the bedside assistant and the console surgeon ensures smooth instrument exchanges and reduces the risk of errors during robotic-assisted procedures.

PAs in surgery, when properly trained, perform a very critical role in robotic and MIS surgery in general. Tasks include helping with retraction which exposes the surgical field and target anatomy, suctioning to maintain a clear visual field, instrument swaps, and even clipping of vessels (Fig. 20.9). It cannot be emphasized enough: the bedside assistant/PA plays a crucial role in performing robotic surgery.

Providing Traction and Countertraction

Providing traction–countertraction by the bedside assistant while the surgeon is dissecting tissue is crucial to help the surgeon with the development and dissection of tissue planes, and to keep them open, especially when dissecting around deep structures (e.g., nerves or vessels). The bedside assistant should always be wary about how much traction and pressure they put on a particular anatomic structure. This can be assessed visually by the assistant and the console surgeon via their display, but assistants also have the ability to have haptic feedback about how "hard" they are pulling on tissue. *Constant surveillance of appropriate tissue handling during instrumentation is essential to reduce patient complications and ensure safe surgery.*

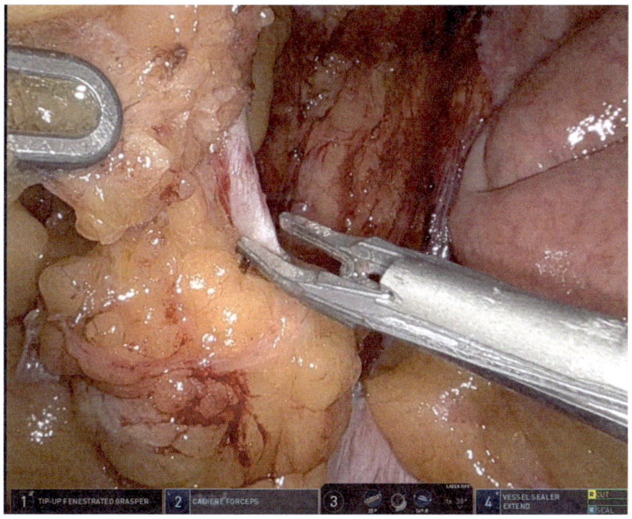

Fig. 20.9 This image is taken during live robotic surgery and is exactly what the operating (console) surgeon would see, with the exception being that the image here is in 2D, rather than 3D. This is also transmitted on an external monitor for the bedside assist and scrub tech to view. At the bottom of the screen are numbers 1 through 4, which correspond to the instrument held in each of the robotic arms; (1) tip-up fenestrated grasper, (2) Cadiere forceps, (3) camera showing that it is a 30° tip down (and includes global information about the patient position here as well, (4) vessel sealer. At this particular step, the bedside assistant, in this case a PA, has introduced a laparoscopic metal clip to be applied to the inferior mesenteric artery that has been exposed by the surgeon. In this case, it is the PA that is providing crucial assistance during one of the most important steps of this operation, a low anterior resection for rectal cancer

Evidence of tissue injury includes, but is not limited to, **bleeding,** bruising, and stretch and loss of tissue compliance leading to **tearing.** Unlike parts of our body, such as the anterior abdominal wall, that can handle substantial tugging and pulling, ***internal organs are extremely delicate and cannot handle the same level of retraction!*** To ensure concordant movements, *constant communication* with the console surgeon is required, and traction–countertraction are coordinated by the surgeon. If movements are not well coordinated, opposing forces may lead to *excessive tissue stretch, tearing, or avulsion of tissue.*

Control of Hemorrhage and Maintaining a Clear Visual Field

Although the surgeon on the console has methods to control hemorrhage including robotic instruments with bipolar or monopolar capabilities, direct pressure or application of hemostatic clips with a robotic instrument, or a robotic enabled suction and irrigation device, *the bedside assistant/PA can also play a significant role in achieving hemostasis and maintaining a clear surgical field.* Via an assist port, the assistant can *use a laparoscopic suction irrigator to remove blood or other fluid, provide manual pressure with a laparoscopic instrument or with the aid of a foreign body* (i.e., *gauze or ray-tech), stop bleeding vessels directly with a clip applier, introduce needles for suture ligation for the console surgeon, or place and instill hemostatic agents.* So it's important to know that if you are a PA in surgery assisting, you play a very important role!

Safety Checklist Prior to Removal of Ports, Undocking, and Reversal of Pneumoperitoneum

Safe removal of ports minimizes damage to internal organs and the abdominal wall. The bedside assistant plays a crucial role in retracting robotic instruments and trocars under direct visual guidance to avoid trauma to the patient. Additionally, "port hopping," where the camera is shifted between ports to enhance visibility during complex multiquadrant surgeries, helps ensure safe extraction.

The assistant must ensure that any instrument exchanges are done with precision, either using the guided-instrument-change feature that pauses the instrument's motion just before its previous position to avoid sudden jerks or damage to tissues. **A critical aspect is to verify that instruments**

and ports are completely clear of tissue before removal. Check that the surgeon has "let go" of any tissue being grasped by the robotic instruments. If needed, adjustments to positioning can be made to avoid inadvertent collisions of the robotic arms with the patient or staff during disconnection and removal of ports [14].

Before the reversal of pneumoperitoneum, a thorough safety checklist must be followed. This typically involves *deflation of the abdomen while confirming that all instruments are accounted for, and ports are safely removed under direct vision.* Ensuring that any insufflation-related devices are disconnected before deflating is crucial to avoid sudden pressure changes that could injure the patient. Additionally, the robotic system must be powered down, and the arms undocked in an orderly fashion to ensure no harm to the surrounding structures.

Constant communication between the surgeon at the console, the bedside assistant, circulating nurses, and surgical techs is vitally important to prevent retained foreign bodies and other mishaps.

Emergency Undocking Intraoperative Complications

A surgical emergency requiring conversion to an open or laparoscopic approach occurs in less than 1% of cases. As is the case in all emergent clinical situations, time to corrective interventions is key to minimizing patient decompensation or demise. When docked, robotic surgical platforms are a physical barrier to performing Advanced Cardiovascular Life Support (ACLS), a laparotomy, or other lifesaving measures. *Given the high stakes nature of surgical emergencies and the time and expertise needed to quickly and safely undock the robot, skill sessions and simulations in emergency undocking in robotic surgery protocols (EURP) should be incorporated into all robotic curricula* [12]. Hospital systems utilizing robotic surgical platforms should have a written rapid robotic undocking protocol for emergency situations.

Indications for EURP include, but are not limited to, uncontrolled hemorrhage, cardiac arrest, airway compromise, or failure or malfunction of the robotic platform [12].

The goal of surgical simulation and establishment of a rapid undocking protocol is the safe and rapid removal of the robotic platform, the establishment of thresholds for conversion to a different procedure, and the identification and role that each member in the operating theater plays. Anticipated surgical instruments needed for conversion to laparoscopy or laparotomy should be readily available for each robotic procedure. Once an indication for emergency undocking has been established and communicated between the anesthesiologist and all members of the surgical team, the console surgeon should ensure that all instruments are in the center of the operative field and ready for safe removal. The console surgeon then is available to scrub in, if indicated, for conversion to an open procedure. In the example of hemorrhage, if the console surgeon and bedside assistant can identify the source of bleeding, then the bedside assistant can **hold direct pressure** with a laparoscopic instrument, or internally placed gauze. If this is not the case, the bedside assistant removes the instruments and endoscope, followed by decannulation of the robotic arms, ports, and stowing of the robotic arms for the circulating nurse to remove the robotic patient cart away from the patient. Every effort should be made to keep the robotic patient cart and instruments sterile. If conversion to laparoscopy is anticipated, the robotic ports can be left in situ [11].

There are some surgeons who allow the ports and pneumoperitoneum to remain while converting to a laparotomy utilizing the established space between the abdominal wall and intraabdominal organs as a buffer against injury during entry. If a second bedside assistant or other personnel are in the operating room, they can obtain needed resources such as an automated external defibrillator, crash cart, or recruitment of other medical personnel from outside the OR. The location and indicated usage of one's institutional emergency resources, such as crash or malignant hyperthermia carts, fire extinguishing agents, and AEDs, are crucial for ensuring timely interventions. An example EURP protocol and simulation can be viewed Here.

Bedside Assisting in Emergent Surgical Settings

The usage of robotic surgical platforms in emergency general surgery (EGS) is an emerging area of interest. Increasing adoption has led to the creation of a position paper from the World Society of Emergency Surgery. Among other positions, the WSES recommends usage in selective clinically stable patients performed by surgeons and operating room personnel with experience in a well-equipped operating room. The most common EGS cases performed on a robotic surgical platform include cholecystectomy, colectomy, and inguinal and ventral hernia repair. When compared to laparoscopy used in the same setting, robotic surgery is associated with a significantly lower risk of conversion to an open surgical procedure. Despite this benefit, robotic surgery in EGS is associated with longer operative times, cost, and higher postoperative complications. Higher postoperative complications are seen in patients undergoing EGS due to the acuity of their presentation, nature of their and lack of ability to optimize patient comorbidities. The same principles of bedside assisting in robotic and laparoscopic surgery apply to aiding in the emergent surgical setting, but with increased urgency and vigilance in multiple domains. In acute settings, inflammation and infection pose multiple challenges. First, tissue planes may be more difficult to identify. Closer coordination between the surgeon on console and the bedside assistant/PA is essential to prevent tissue injury. If intra-abdominal perforation is present, feculent and purulent material may obscure visualization, which may require greater suctioning than normal (Fig. 20.10). Small or large bowel obstructions may make navigating the abdominal cavity more challenging due to loss of intra-abdominal domain. Introduction of needles or blunt instruments should occur under direct visualization to minimize the risk of iatrogenic injury that may cause hemorrhage or additional perforation that may prompt the conversion to an open procedure. Further studies are required to better understand the future potential of robotic surgery in EGS and the principles of surgical management for the bedside assistant.

The usage of robotic platforms in surgical subspecialties is a rapidly developing and expanding advance in surgical care. Bedside assistants play a critical role in the performance of safe and efficient robotic surgery. This requires time, varying levels of simulation, and continual quality improvement. Although challenging, bedside assisting is a rewarding and exciting occupation. This is one of the most important roles for PAs in the operating room today!

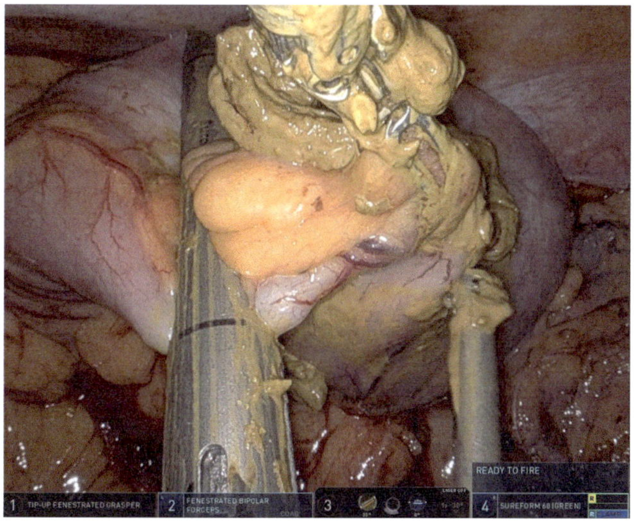

Fig. 20.10 Shown is spillage of fecal material during surgery in an unprepped colon. The console surgeon has managed to secure a robotic stapling device (left), but there is substantial spillage of stool contents. The bedside assistant is using a laparoscopic suction device (right) that has been placed through the assist port to remove the spilled fecal matter. As often is the case with robotics, the surgeon and the bedside assist mostly work in synchronicity and in cases like this in a very swift manner to deal with urgent problems such as this

References

1. Collins JM, Walsh DS, Hudson J, Henderson S, Thompson J, Zychowicz M. Implementation of a standardized robotic assistant surgical training curriculum. J Robot Surg. 2021:1–9.
2. Rivero-Moreno Y, Echevarria S, Vidal-Valderrama C, Pianetti L, Cordova-Guilarte J, Navarro-Gonzalez J, et al. Robotic surgery: A comprehensive review of the literature and current trends. Cureus. 2023;15(7):e42370.
3. Whelan RL, Fleshman JW, Fowler DL, editors. The SAGES manual of perioperative care in minimally invasive surgery: perioperative care in minimally invasive surgery. Spring, 2005; 2006.
4. Tameze Y, Low YH. Outpatient robotic surgery: considerations for the anesthesiologist. Adv Anesth. 2022;40(1):15–32.
5. Furrer MA, Omana HJ, Nair R. Assisting in robotic surgery: surgical skills for the bedside assistant. In: Costello T, editor. Principles and practice of robotic surgery. Elsevier Inc.; 2023. p. 39–46.
6. Cha JS, Athanasiadis D, Anton NE, Stefanidis D, Yu D. Measurement of nontechnical skills during robotic-assisted surgery using sensor-based communication and proximity metrics. JAMA Netw Open. 2021;4(11):e2132209.
7. McChesney S, Gahagan J, Rashida L, Steinhagen E. Robot overview. Presented at: ASCRS Residents Committee Colorectal Surgery Boot Camp Series.
8. Costello DM, Huang E, Ahlering TE, Peters JS, Tissot SJ. Robot setup. In: Md MAC, editor. Principles and practice of robotic surgery. Elsevier Inc.; 2023. p. 27–32.
9. Patel A, Oleynikov D. In: Patel A, Oleynikov D, editors. The SAGES manual of robotic surgery. 1. Springer International Publishing; 2017.
10. Jones BT, Ha JS, Lawrence C, Tsai LL, Yang SC. A dedicated robotic bedside physician assistant significantly enhances trainee console operating time in general thoracic surgery. JTCVS Open. Published online 2023. 2023; https://doi.org/10.1016/J.XJON.2023.08.024.
11. O'Sullivan OE, O'Sullivan S, Hewitt M, O'Reilly BA. Da Vinci robot emergency undocking protocol. J Robot Surg. 2016;10(3):251–3.
12. Shah SB, Chawla R, Rawal SK. Rapid undocking protocol for the da Vinci surgical robot during emergency situations. Indian J Anaesth. 2023;67(4):398–400.
13. Ballas D, Cesta M, Roulette GD, Rusnak M, Ahmed R. Emergency undocking in robotic surgery: a simulation curriculum. J Vis Exp. 2018;135 https://doi.org/10.3791/57286.
14. Lunardi N, Abou-Zamzam A, Florecki KL, Chidambaram S, Shih IF, Kent AJ, et al. Robotic technology in emergency general surgery cases in the era of minimally invasive surgery. JAMA Surg. 2024;159(5):493–9.

21 Abdominal Hernias

Sam Atallah

Introduction

Abdominal hernias in adults are a major global health issue, with over 32 million prevalent cases and 13 million new cases annually as of 2019, and the burden continues to rise due to population growth and aging despite declining age-standardized rates. The lifetime risk of developing a groin hernia is 27–42% for men and 3–5.8% for women, and the incidence of incisional hernia after abdominal surgery is approximately 11–13%. Males are disproportionately affected, with a male-to-female ratio of 6–7:1, and incidence peaks in those aged 50–69 years.

The health care burden is substantial: in the United States alone, ventral hernia repair (VHR) approaches 611,000 operations per year, with annual costs nearing $9.7 billion. Most repairs are performed electively, but emergent repairs—associated with higher morbidity and mortality—are increasing, especially among older adults. Globally, the absolute number of hernia-related deaths and disability-adjusted life years (DALYs) is rising, particularly in low- and middle-income countries, where access to timely surgery is limited, and mortality rates are higher.

Treatment options include watchful waiting for asymptomatic or minimally symptomatic hernias, but surgical repair is the definitive treatment. Tension-free mesh repair is the standard of care in adults, with both open and minimally invasive (laparoscopic or robotic) approaches available. Minimally invasive techniques are associated with reduced postoperative pain and faster recovery, but open repair remains common, especially in resource-limited settings. Mesh is used in the majority of repairs, particularly for ventral, inguinal, and incisional hernias.

Outcomes are generally favorable for elective repairs, with low rates of acute incarceration (1.8 per 1,000 patient-years for inguinal hernia), but recurrence and chronic pain remain challenges. Emergent repairs carry significantly higher risks of morbidity and mortality, especially in older adults and those with comorbidities. Ongoing research focuses on optimizing surgical techniques, reducing recurrence, and addressing mesh-related complications.

This chapter is intended as an introduction to hernias for PAs and APPs. It examines the basics of hernias, the approach to the hernia patient, and other relevant pearls. Because patients with hernias are common, it is important that all PAs who manage patients clinically, even in nonsurgical settings, be familiar with abdominal hernias, from diagnosis to treatment. Particular attention should be given to conditions that require immediate surgical consultation and intervention, as outlined herein.

Hernia Basics

Hernia surgery is among the most common operations performed by general surgeons worldwide, so it is necessary that practicing PAs and APPs have a solid grasp of the scope and nature of hernia surgery. It is important to understand that hernias can be classified by **(a) location** (Fig. 21.1) and by their **(b) clinical features**, including chronicity, symptomology (pain, intestinal obstruction).

Intestinal obstruction can be due to trapped bowel within the hernia sac, and this is known as **incarceration,** or **incarcerated bowel;** *meaning the bowel is "imprisoned" by the hernia sac* (Fig. 21.2).

Epidemiologically, the risk of incarceration in primary and incisional hernias is approximately 3.5–3.7%. Defect size (3–4 cm), peri- and infra-umbilical location, older age, higher BMI, constipation, female sex, diabetes, and higher ASA class are associated with increased risk.

Additionally, a subcategory of clinical features includes the presence or absence of intestinal **strangulation, in which the entrapped bowel "cuts off its own blood supply"**

S. Atallah (✉)
Department of Surgery, Piedmont Hospital, Mercer University School of Medicine, Macon, GA, USA
e-mail: atallah@post.harvard.edu

S. Atallah, J. Dragoljevic (eds.), *Fundamentals of Surgery for Physician Assistants*, https://doi.org/10.1007/978-3-032-21069-2_21

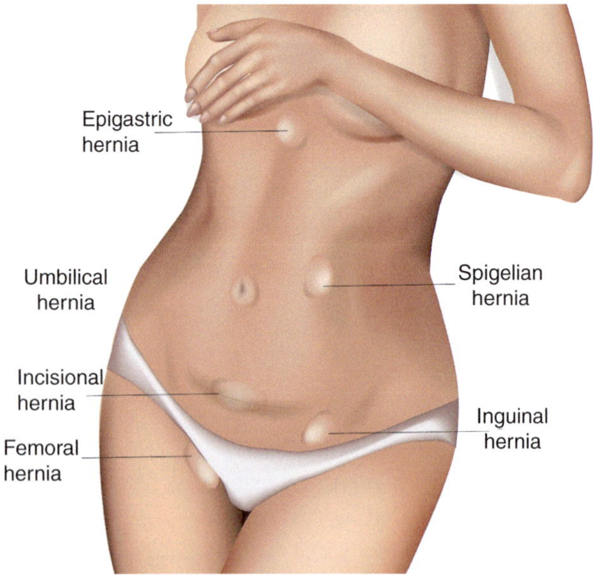

Fig. 21.1 The breakdown of abdominal wall hernias is typically based on *anatomical location* and etiology. The most common types include **umbilical hernias** (which occur at the umbilicus, often due to a congenital weakness or increased intraabdominal pressure (e.g., ascites, pregnancy, obesity); **epigastric hernias**, which occur along the linea alba between the xiphoid and umbilicus, usually containing preperitoneal fat. **Incisional hernias** develop at the site of previous surgical incisions, with risk factors including obesity, prior hernia, and increased fascial defect size (length of scar) as well as position along the abdomen. **Spigelian hernias** are relatively rare and occur through the Spigelian fascia adjacent to the linea semilunaris. Other hernias (not shown) include lumbar hernias, which are bulges through the superior or inferior lumbar triangles, representing natural weak points in the abdominal wall, and parastomal hernias, which are a subtype of incisional hernia occurring at stoma sites, particularly common in patients with ileostomies or colostomies. The American College of Radiology, in its Appropriateness Criteria, and the European Hernia Society both emphasize classification by location (midline, lateral, incisional) and size, as these factors influence management and prognosis. Noninguinal abdominal wall hernias are more prevalent in patients with higher BMI and older age, and are more likely to become incarcerated in these populations. **Groin hernias (inguinal and femoral)** are technically not classified as abdominal wall hernias but are often discussed in parallel due to their frequency and clinical overlap

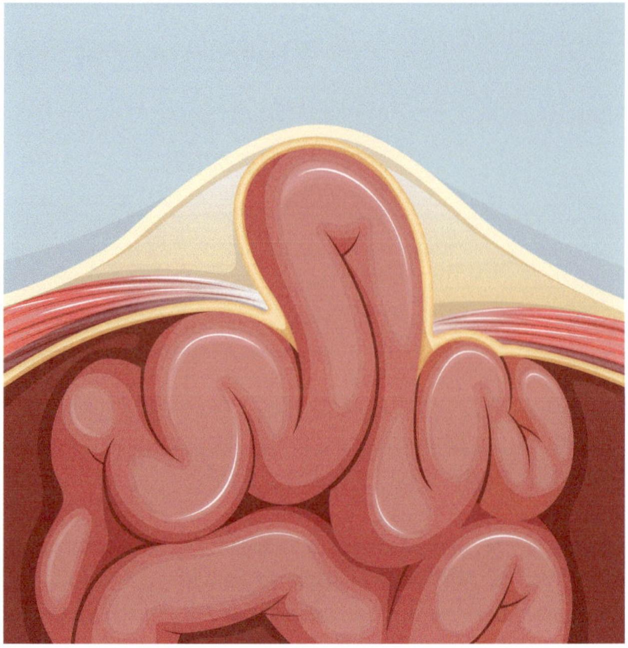

Fig. 21.2 An incarcerated hernia is illustrated. Here the small bowel is "trapped" or "jailed" within what is often a narrow neck hernia. Hernias themselves are lined by a "sac." The incarcerated bowel within the hernia sac may lead to other clinically significant conditions, most important of which are strangulation and bowel obstruction. Regardless of anatomic location, any abdominal wall hernia can be incarcerated

leading to sometimes severe ischemia and even bowel death (Fig. 21.3). Being able to identify when a hernia results in a bowel obstruction (whether partial or complete) is important, as abdominal hernias are a leading cause of small bowel obstruction (second only to adhesions).

Furthermore, it is imperative to recognize when a hernia has resulted in (bowel) strangulation. A strangulated hernia is among the most important clinical presentations for PAs and NPs to recognize because **prompt treatment is required**. Patients with strangulated bowel may present with **severe pain, erythema, and signs of bowel obstruction or peritonitis, necessitating urgent intervention. On physical exam,** *an exquisitely tender mass is appreciated, and such patients may rapidly develop signs of sepsis.* Systemic signs of illness (fever, leukocytosis) are usually present as well as an elevated lactic acid and D-dimer. CT-scans may

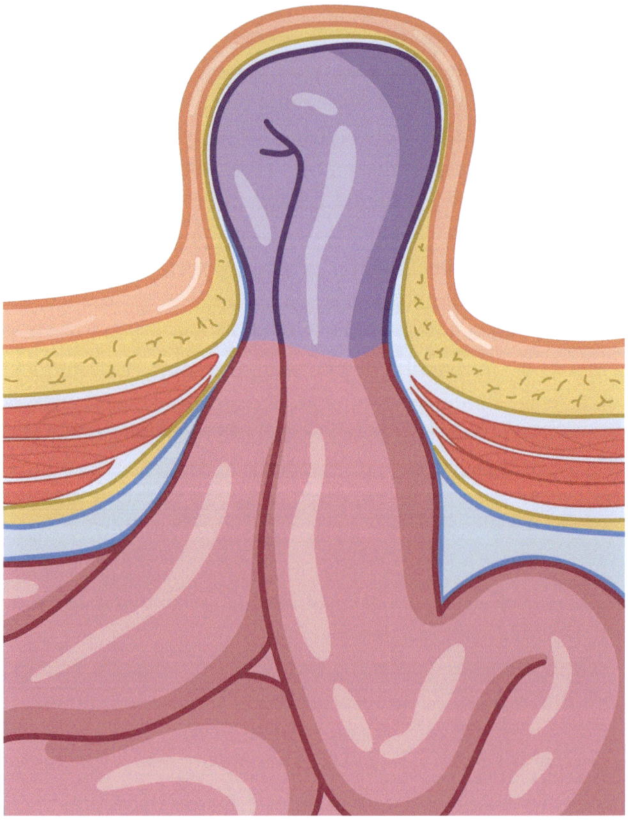

Fig. 21.3 A strangulated loop of small bowel (purple color) within a hernia is depicted. Strangulated small bowel within a hernia, sometimes referred to as a "strangulated hernia," requires emergent treatment. *Never try to manually reduce a hernia you suspect of containing strangulated bowel!*

reveal reduced wall enhancement or **pneumatosis (air in the bowel wall, classic for bowel necrosis)** which supports the diagnosis, *but early clinical suspicion is critical.* Femoral hernias, more common in women, have a particularly high risk of strangulation.

Common Hernia Locations

Inguinal hernias account for the *majority of abdominal wall hernias,* with an incidence and prevalence that far exceed those of umbilical, epigastric, incisional, Spigelian, lumbar, and parastomal hernias. According to large-scale epidemiological data, inguinal hernias represent approximately 75% of all abdominal wall hernias globally, with the remainder distributed among the other types (Fig. 21.4).

What you need to know as a PA: ***inguinal hernias*** *are the most common type of abdominal wall hernia*, accounting for **approximately 75% of cases**, with the remaining 25% distributed among umbilical, incisional, epigastric, Spigelian, lumbar, and parastomal hernias. This distribution is consistent across both global and regional data.

Femoral Hernias are most common in **elderly females.** The incidence of **femoral hernia** in adults is low, accounting for approximately 2–5% of all groin hernias in the general adult population, **but the proportion is higher in women, where femoral hernias represent up to 18.9% of groin hernias requiring repair.**

The gender breakdown is notable: ***femoral hernias are significantly more common in women than in men, with women comprising about 70–75% of femoral hernia repairs***. However, even in women, inguinal hernias remain more common overall, with a woman presenting with a groin mass being about five times more likely to have an inguinal hernia than a femoral hernia.

The demographic profile shows that femoral hernias are predominantly a disease of *older adults*, with incidence and prevalence rising steadily with age and peaking in the eighth and ninth decades of life. *Most patients presenting with femoral hernia are elderly, and the risk of incarceration or strangulation is higher in this group, leading to a greater proportion of emergency presentations and associated morbidity and mortality.*

Hernia Diagnosis

Abdominal hernias commonly **present with a visible or palpable bulge** (Fig. 21.5), localized pain or discomfort (often exacerbated by straining and/or Valsalva). In some cases, symptoms of bowel obstruction or changes in bowel habits may be present. Pain is typically dull and localized to the hernia site, with straining maneuvers accentuating symptoms.

Although hernias are diagnosed primarily clinically, radiographic **imaging** is often used adjunctively. Most commonly, **CT-body imaging of the abdomen and pelvis** is used, but other modalities, such as **ultrasound** are sometimes considered. Imaging is indicated when the diagnosis is

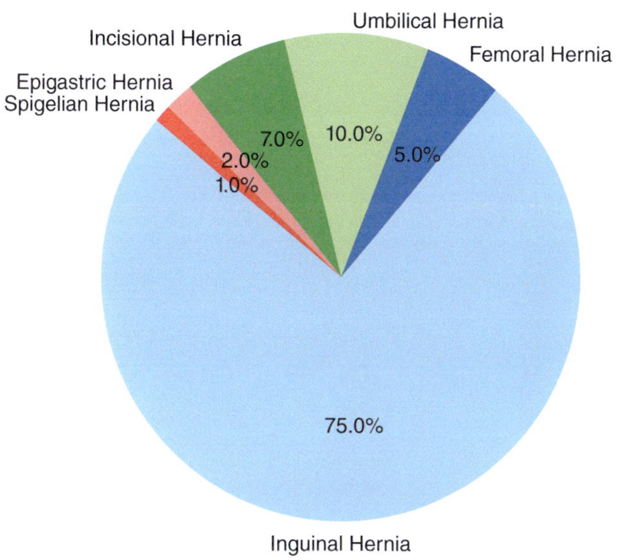

Fig. 21.4 The relative distribution of different types of abdominal hernias (including groin hernias) is shown. It is important to have an idea of which types of hernias are common, as these are the ones you are most likely to encounter clinically. You can clearly see from this graph that the vast majority of hernias (75%) are inguinal

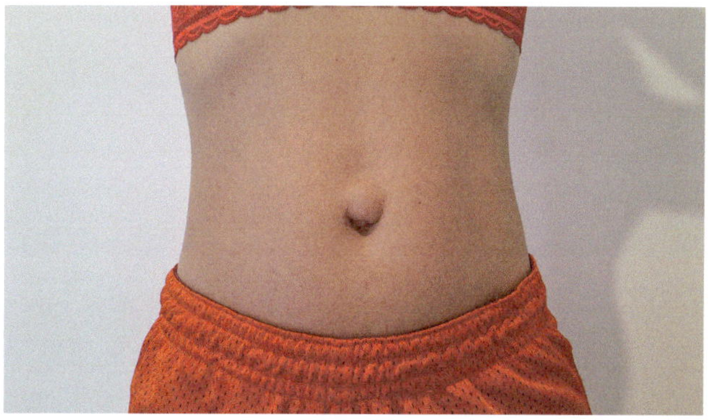

Fig. 21.5 A woman with an umbilical hernia is shown, with the classic appearance of a bulge at or near the umbilicus. The incidence of umbilical hernias in adults varies by population and risk factors. In a large Russian population-based study, the prevalence was 10.2% in adults, with higher rates in men, older individuals, those with a family history, and those with increased BMI. Risk factors include male gender, age, family history, and obesity. Umbilical hernias are also associated with conditions that increase intraabdominal pressure, such as ascites, pregnancy, and obesity. Treatment is surgical for symptomatic hernias or those at risk for complications. Elective repair is generally recommended, especially for defects ≥1 cm. Mesh repair is preferred over suture repair for defects ≥1 cm due to significantly lower recurrence rates, as supported by randomized controlled trials and registry data

uncertain, in cases of recurrent hernia, or when complications are suspected (e.g., strangulation, bowel obstruction). The American College of Radiology recommends cross-sectional imaging (CT scan) for presurgical planning and in complex cases, as discussed later.

Acute Versus Chronic Hernias

Acute abdominal hernia refers to a hernia that has become irreducible and symptomatic within hours to days, often presenting with pain, tenderness, and sometimes signs of bowel obstruction. **Chronic abdominal hernia** describes a hernia that has been irreducible for weeks to years, which may or may not be symptomatic, and often lacks acute inflammatory signs.

The clinical approach to acute hernia focuses on rapid assessment for complications. If the hernia is incarcerated but not strangulated (i.e., irreducible but without signs of ischemia or peritonitis), **manual reduction (taxis)** may be attempted within 24 hours of symptom onset, provided there are no features suggestive of strangulation such as severe pain, systemic toxicity, skin changes, or peritonitis. The World Society of Emergency Surgery (WSES) and the HerniaSurge Group both recommend that **hernia reduction should not be performed if strangulation is suspected**; in these cases, immediate surgical intervention is indicated to prevent bowel necrosis and sepsis.

For chronic hernias, the risk of acute complications is lower, and manual reduction is generally not indicated unless there is a new onset of symptoms suggestive of acute incarceration. Chronic irreducible hernias without symptoms can often be managed electively, but any new pain, tenderness, or obstructive symptoms should prompt urgent evaluation for possible acute complications.

In summary, **hernia reduction** is indicated for acute, *non-strangulated* incarcerated hernias, but is **contraindicated in cases of suspected strangulation or peritonitis**. Chronic hernias are managed electively unless they become acutely symptomatic.

Hernias: What is the Problem Exactly? How Do We Fix It?

All abdominal wall hernias represent a **defect in the fascia**. *Fascia, not muscle*, is the **strength layer of the abdominal wall** (Fig. 21.6). When a hernia repair is performed, although

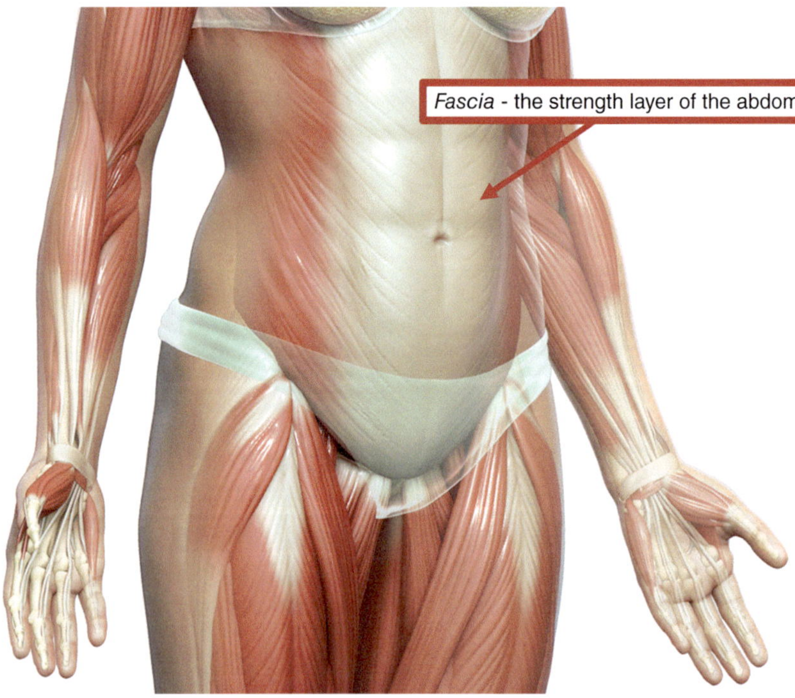

Fig. 21.6 From a surgical perspective, fascia is the single most important layer of the abdominal wall. It is composed primarily of collagen fibers, but also contains elastic fibers, fibroblasts, and varying amounts of other cell types, extracellular matrix components, and neural elements. Fascia provides mechanical support, enables force transmission, and allows for shearing and gliding between tissue layers. The fascial system is now recognized as an active participant in musculoskeletal dynamics, not merely a passive structure. Far from it, in the abdomen, the *fascia is the single most important layer providing structural support*. It is defects in the fascia (of abdominal muscle) that lead to hernia formation. Although muscle fascia is only the thickness of a few sheets of paper, it is a *very* tough material. During open surgery, you will see that fascia is often closed with a strong suture material that is long-lasting, such as #1 PDS

a multitude of techniques are used, all hernia repairs come down to one thing: **fixing the fascial defect.** This is most commonly performed using **synthetic mesh.**

Fascia is also the most important layer when considering surgery through the abdominal wall. The anterior abdominal wall consists of many layers—skin, subcutaneous fat, Camper's fascia, Scarpa's fascia, the **fascia** of the abdominal musculature, the abdominal muscles proper (e.g., rectus abdominus), preperitoneal fat, and the peritoneum. Of all these layers, after open surgery, the only layer that **requires** closure and reapproximation is the **fascia** [of the abdominal musculature]. Even the skin can be left open to heal by secondary intention, but the **fascia must be closed** [or somehow reapproximated, such as by bridging with mesh] with very few exceptions that are beyond the scope of this introductory chapter. It is the fascia—a white and strong sheath of tissue—that keeps the abdominal organs contained within the abdominal cavity. In the surgical realm, it is the **fascia** that provides strength, *not muscle*!

In some places in our abdominal, wall there are inherent "weak spots." This is especially true for areas that vessels and organ structures pass through (or at one time passed through) the abdominal wall. For example, the umbilicus is prone to herniation as it once was the point of fetal-maternal connection via the umbilical cord (the umbilical vein and arteries in utero). The inguinal canal transmits the spermatic cord and is prone to hernia formation *indirectly* (via the opening in the deep inguinal ring) or *directly* via an anatomic weak spot known as **Hesselbach's triangle** (Fig. 21.7). On physical exam, the **Valsalva maneuver** while standing and checking the scrotum and inguinal canal for a protrusion which, if identified, is highly suggestive of an inguinal hernia. There are two types of inguinal hernias — direct and indirect. The difference between **direct** and **indirect inguinal hernias** lies in their location relative to the **inferior epigastric vessels** and the pathway through which abdominal contents protrude. A useful mnemonic for remembering this is: "**MDs don't LIe**"—**M** (Medial) = Direct/L (Lateral) = Indirect. Surgical repair is standard for both, especially if symptomatic. Laparoscopic (or robotic) *vs* open techniques may be used. The differences between direct and indirect inguinal hernias are described in Table 21.1.

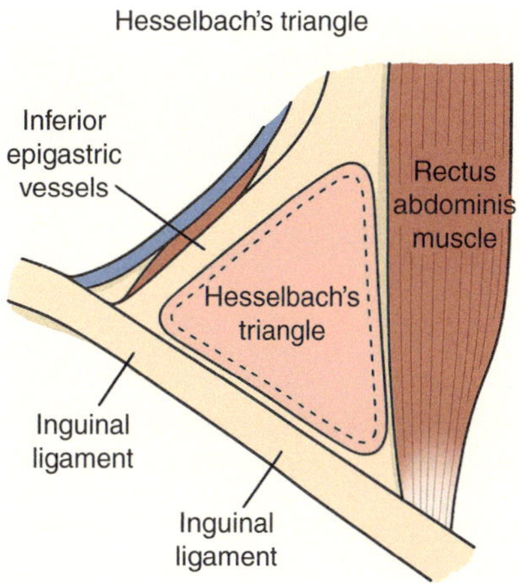

Fig. 21.7 Inguinal anatomy is somewhat complex, but PA students and PAs in practice should be knowledgeable about key anatomic landmarks. In the groin area, the site at which **direct** inguinal hernias form is within a small triangle, known as **Hesselbach's triangle**. This triangle is bordered by the lateral wall of the rectus abdominus muscle *medially,* the inferior epigastric vessels *laterally,* and the inguinal ligament *inferiorly* (the inguinal ligament is sometimes referred to by its eponym, **Poupart's ligament**). *All students on their surgery rotation should commit the boundaries of Hesselbach's triangle to memory!*

Table 21.1 Difference between direct and indirect inguinal hernias

Feature	Direct inguinal hernia	Indirect inguinal hernia
Anatomical location	Medial to the inferior epigastric vessels	Lateral to the inferior epigastric vessels
Hernia pathway	Through Hesselbach's triangle	Through deep inguinal ring, follows the inguinal canal
Cause	Weakness in abdominal wall (acquired)	Usually congenital (patent processus vaginalis)
Common in	Older men	Younger males, including infants
Sac relation to cord	Hernia sac lies beside the spermatic cord	Hernia sac lies within the spermatic cord
Risk of strangulation	Less common	More common
Exam finding	Bulge near the superficial ring, rarely into scrotum	Can extend into the scrotum in males

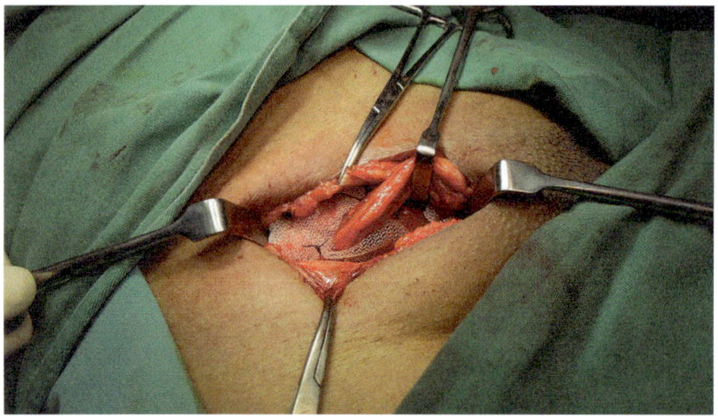

Fig. 21.8 The open repair of a right inguinal hernia in a male is shown, after placement of a synthetic mesh. Notice the spermatic cord that is allowed free passage postmesh placement. The spermatic cord contains the vas deferens and other key structures and is thus protected at operation. Synthetic mesh placement is a standard in most hernia repairs. The most significant complication of synthetic mesh is infection. As a rule of thumb, infected synthetic mesh is very difficult to treat with antibiotics alone, and infected mesh almost always requires explantation to achieve source control. Other types of mesh, referred to as biologic mesh, are sometimes used in special settings, although not routinely. Biologic mesh is very costly, but is preferred in infected fields as it tends to resist bacterial infection and may promote more autologous healing

General Guidelines for Repair

Approaches to repair include (a) open and (b) minimally invasive (laparoscopic or robotic) techniques. **Tension-free mesh repair is the standard in adults**, reducing recurrence rates (Fig. 21.8). Laparoscopic repair offers less postoperative pain and faster recovery but requires general anesthesia. Open repair may be performed under local anesthesia and is preferred in certain populations (e.g., children, resource-limited settings). In patients with cirrhosis, the American Association for the Study of Liver Diseases recommends optimizing ascites and nutrition preoperatively, with elective repair considered in *select* patients; mesh use reduces recurrence but may increase infection risk. For students and for PAs and APPs just starting their practice, *it is important to note that* ***liver cirrhosis*** *is an important risk factor, and substantially increases morbidity in patients undergoing even routine surgery.*

Complications include bowel obstruction, ischemia, necrosis, perforation, peritonitis, and sepsis. Bowel resection is required in 15–20% of strangulated cases, with a higher risk in femoral hernias (Fig. 21.9) and delayed presentations. Mortality increases significantly with delayed intervention, especially if necrosis is present.

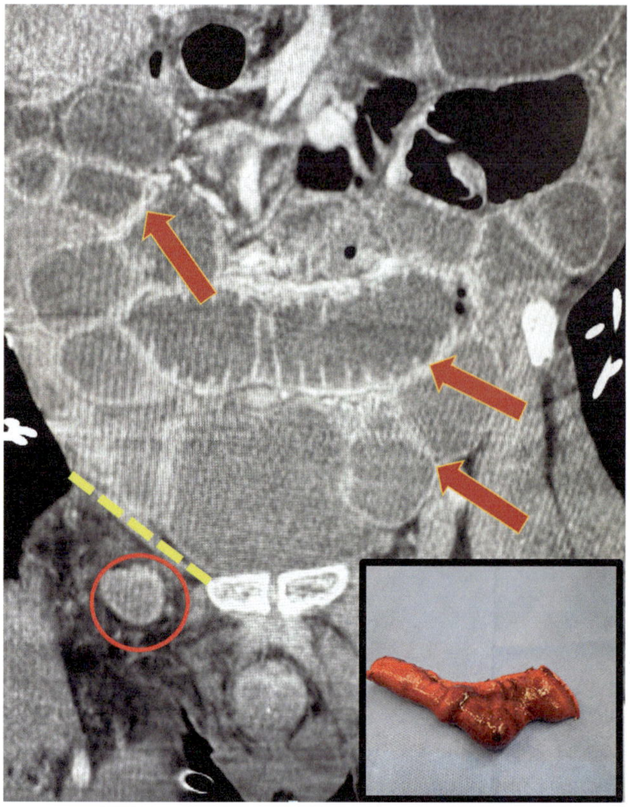

Fig. 21.9 A 74 y.o. male presented to the ED with small bowel obstruction and an incarcerated right femoral hernia. Although femoral hernias are more common in females, they still occur in males. The coronal view of a CT-scan is shown, illustrating multiple dilated loops of small intestine (red arrows). A circle highlights the cause of the small bowel obstruction: an incarcerated femoral hernia, with a loop of small bowel not only causing the obstruction, but also resulting in small bowel strangulation at the hernia site. The location of the right inguinal ligament has been depicted with a dashed yellow line. Of note, femoral hernias are located *beneath* this line. While small bowel obstruction due to adhesions is often treated first with bowel rest and nonoperative management is usually successful, here, urgent surgery is required. This patient underwent an operation, and a portion of ischemic bowel within the femoral hernia sac was resected (inset). The hernia was then repaired with a biologic mesh to minimize the risk of mesh infection

Nonoperative Management

Watchful waiting *is* appropriate for asymptomatic or minimally symptomatic inguinal hernias in men, but not for women or symptomatic patients, due to higher risks of complications, especially with **femoral hernias**.

Reducing a Symptomatic Hernia

Hernia reduction (**taxis**) is indicated for acute, nonstrangulated incarcerated hernias, particularly when surgery is not immediately available or the patient is not an optimal surgical candidate. *Manual reduction should be performed within 24 hours of symptom onset, provided there are no signs of bowel strangulation*, such as severe pain, peritonitis, systemic toxicity, or evidence of bowel ischemia (e.g., fever, tachycardia, hypotension, leukocytosis, or skin changes over the hernia). The World Society of Emergency Surgery (WSES) and the Hernia Surgery Group both state that *hernia reduction should not be performed if strangulation is suspected*, as this requires immediate surgical intervention to prevent bowel necrosis and sepsis.

The clinical approach involves **g**entle, **p**repared, and **s**afe (**GPS**) taxis, *often under conscious sedation* with individualized dosing of intravenous morphine and a short-acting benzodiazepine, titrated to effect. Ultrasound can assist in assessing bowel viability prior to reduction, especially in complex cases. After successful reduction, short-term observation is recommended, and elective hernia repair should be scheduled.

Remember: Hernia reduction is contraindicated in the presence of suspected or confirmed strangulation, peritonitis, or signs of bowel compromise. **In these cases, emergency surgery is the standard of care.** *Attempting reduction in strangulated hernias risks returning nonviable bowel to the peritoneal cavity, increasing the risk of sepsis and mortality.*

Incarcerated abdominal hernias are defined as hernias in which the contents become *irreducible*, often due to a *narrow* hernia defect or adhesions. As previously mentioned, strangulated hernias occur when the blood supply to the herniated contents is compromised, leading to ischemia and potential necrosis. Incarceration can be acute (hours to days) or chronic (weeks to years), and not all incarcerated hernias are symptomatic, especially in obese patients or those with chronic incarceration.

Clinical features of incarceration include a nonreducible, often tender mass, localized pain, and possibly symptoms of bowel obstruction (nausea, vomiting, abdominal distension, diminished flatus and/or bowel movements). **Systemic signs such as fever, tachycardia, leukocytosis, and peritonitis suggest progression to strangulation**. Strangulated hernias present with **severe, persistent pain, a tense and exquisitely tender mass, and may rapidly develop signs of sepsis** (hypotension, tachycardia). Laboratory findings such as elevated lactate or D-dimer, and imaging findings (CT showing reduced wall enhancement or **pneumatosis**) can support the diagnosis, but **early clinical suspicion is critical.**

Complications include bowel obstruction, ischemia, necrosis, perforation, peritonitis, and sepsis. Bowel resection is required in 15–20% of strangulated cases, with a **higher risk in femoral hernias and delayed presentations**. Mortality increases significantly with delayed intervention, especially if necrosis is present.

Suggested Reading

1. Biggins SW, Angeli P, Garcia-Tsao G, et al. Diagnosis, evaluation, and management of ascites, spontaneous bacterial peritonitis and hepatorenal syndrome: 2021 practice guidance by the American Association for the Study of Liver Diseases. Hepatology (Baltimore, Md.). 2021;74(2):1014–48. https://doi.org/10.1002/hep.31884.
2. East B, Pawlak M, de Beaux AC. A manual reduction of hernia under analgesia/sedation (Taxis) in the acute inguinal hernia: a useful technique in COVID-19 times to reduce the need for emergency surgery-a literature review. Hernia. 2020;24(5):937–41. https://doi.org/10.1007/s10029-020-02227-1.
3. Fitzgibbons RJ, Forse RA. Groin hernias in adults. N Engl J Med. 2015;372(8):756–63. https://doi.org/10.1056/NEJMcp1404068.
4. Garcia EM, Pietryga JA, Kim DH, et al. ACR appropriateness Criteria® hernia. J Am Coll Radiol: JACR. 2022;19(11S):S329–40. https://doi.org/10.1016/j.jacr.2022.09.016.
5. Harissis HV, Douitsis E, Fatouros M. Incarcerated hernia: to reduce or not to reduce? Hernia. 2009;13(3):263–6. https://doi.org/10.1007/s10029-008-0467-9.
6. LeBlanc KE, LeBlanc LL, LeBlanc KA. Inguinal hernias: diagnosis and management. Am Fam Phys. 2013;87(12):844–8.
7. Ma Q, Jing W, Liu X, et al. The Global, Regional, and National Burden and its trends of inguinal, femoral, and abdominal hernia from 1990 to 2019: findings from the 2019 global burden of disease study - a cross-sectional study. Int J Surg (London, England). 2023;109(3):333–42. https://doi.org/10.1097/JS9.0000000000000217.
8. Pawlak M, East B, de Beaux AC. Algorithm for management of an incarcerated inguinal hernia in the emergency settings with manual reduction. taxis, the technique and its safety. Hernia. 2021;25(5):1253–8. https://doi.org/10.1007/s10029-021-02429-1.
9. Sartelli M, Coccolini F, van Ramshorst GH, et al. WSES guidelines for emergency repair of complicated abdominal wall hernias. World J Emerg Surg. 2013;8(1):50. https://doi.org/10.1186/1749-7922-8-50.
10. Sazhin A, Zolotukhin I, Seliverstov E, et al. Prevalence and risk factors for abdominal wall hernia in the general russian population. Hernia. 2019;23(6):1237–42. https://doi.org/10.1007/s10029-019-01971-3.
11. Sneiders D, Yurtkap Y, Kroese LF, et al. Risk factors for incarceration in patients with primary abdominal wall and incisional hernias: a prospective study in 4472 patients. World J Surg. 2019;43(8):1906–13. https://doi.org/10.1007/s00268-019-04989-x.
12. SSAT Patient Care Guidelines. Surgical repair of incisional hernias. J Gastrointest Surg. 2007;11(9):1231–2. https://doi.org/10.1007/s11605-007-0200-5.
13. Zöller B, Ji J, Sundquist J, Sundquist K. Shared and nonshared familial susceptibility to surgically treated inguinal hernia, femoral hernia, incisional hernia, epigastric hernia, and umbilical hernia. J Am Coll Surg. 2013;217(2):289–99.e1. https://doi.org/10.1016/j.jamcollsurg.2013.04.020.

Complex Abdominal Wall Reconstruction

22

Danielle Kohler, Kimberly Miles, and Michael J. Rosen

Introduction

A hernia, at its most basic definition, is a weakness or defect in the abdominal wall that allows tissues or organs to protrude. Patients oftentimes complain of an associated bulge, swelling, or lump. Common locations of a hernia include groin (inguinal hernia), umbilical, hiatal or paraesophageal, ventral or incisional, or parastomal (at the site of a stoma, such as ileostomy/colostomy). Hernias may be congenital or acquired. Most hernias are acquired and may be caused by multiple factors, including obesity, causing strain to the abdominal musculature, previous surgeries causing weakness to the abdominal wall, chronic malnutrition, and the natural aging process. Ventral hernia repairs are one of the most prevalent surgeries performed by general surgeons in the United States, with approximately 325,000 surgical repairs being performed annually [1].

For the purposes of this chapter, we will focus on complex ventral abdominal wall hernias. While there is no unified definition of complex abdominal wall hernias, these are usually larger defects, in comorbid patients, and can require major surgeries for reconstruction. This provides many unique opportunities and challenges for advanced practice providers in the patients' journey of care. Ventral incisional hernias account for approximately 25% of all hernias [1]. Ventral hernias may detrimentally impact the patient, as they can cause physical pain and discomfort, negatively impact quality of life, cause psychological distress, and pose a risk for acute medical events, including incarceration or bowel strangulation or blockage. Bowel blockage or strangulation for a hernia may prompt emergent repair. Ventral hernias are electively repaired when they are symptomatic causing pain, change in bowel habits, or physical limitations. If left untreated, they can result in the bowel becoming incarcerated in the defect, which can progress to loss of the blood supply to that segment and strangulation. These result in emergency surgery with poor outcomes and significant morbidity for the patient.

The advanced practice provider (APP), which includes physician assistants (PAs) and nurse practitioners (NP), may encounter patients with complex hernias in many different aspects along the natural history of hernias. For example, they may be found incidentally on routine CT abdomen/pelvis imaging ordered for another reason, to electively when presenting to a surgeon's office, or through the emergency room after complications related to the hernia. Additionally, APPs that spend time in the operating room will often encounter repairs of patients undergoing complex abdominal wall reconstruction for their hernias. Having a working knowledge of hernias and an understanding of best practices in the management of this common surgical concern will help to provide the APP with confidence in caring for this uniquely complex patient population.

Presurgical Management

When managing complex patients undergoing a hernia repair, specifically an abdominal wall reconstruction, preoperative optimization has become an important part of practice to address modifiable risk factors and improve patient outcomes. Three frequently studied risk factors include obesity with a body mass index (BMI) > 35 kg/m^2, smoking status, and diabetes mellitus (DM).

Obesity

Obesity, affecting 40% of the United States population, is not only a risk factor for hernia formation, but also intraoperative and postoperative complications such as surgical site infections or hernia recurrence. If a patient is seen at their initial surgical consult, with a BMI >40 kg/m^2, the patient is referred to either a surgical or medical weight loss provider,

D. Kohler · K. Miles · M. J. Rosen (✉)
Department of General Surgery, Cleveland Clinic, Cleveland, OH, USA
e-mail: michael.rosen@nm.org

S. Atallah, J. Dragoljevic (eds.), *Fundamentals of Surgery for Physician Assistants*, https://doi.org/10.1007/978-3-032-21069-2_22

with an end goal of BMI <40 kg/m^2 before their hernia surgery [1]. To reduce the likelihood of patients being lost to follow-up and allow for immediate access to a medical weight loss provider, an APP can be oriented to treating patients the same day as their initial surgical consult.

During the initial evaluation, an APP should assess multiple components of the patient's history, emphasizing aspects specific to obesity. This includes gathering a baseline medical history, as well as obtaining detailed information about the patient's family, social, nutritional, behavioral, and physical activity history. Additionally, individualized laboratory testing should be conducted, and potential causes of obesity should be identified [2]. After the initial evaluation, an APP should provide nutrition and physical activity education with the plan to prioritize and encourage patient adherence. The goal for nutrition therapy is to promote a dietary intake that leads to a negative caloric balance, with a focus on adjusting the intake of carbohydrates, fats, and proteins. Depending on the APP's time and expertise, counseling can be tailored to include more specific education on nutritional patterns. However, the APP should recognize that a more detailed and individualized nutrition plan can be provided by referring the patient to a registered dietitian. In conjunction with dietary counseling, physical activity, both anerobic and aerobic, should be encouraged. It is important to emphasize that, despite having a hernia, there should be no restrictions on a patient's physical activity [3, 4]. Lastly, the patient may be started on an antiobesity medication, either FDA-approved or off-label, along with appropriate medication information. The patient should continue regular follow-up visits for weight management every 1–3 months, either in person or via telehealth, to review behavioral lifestyle changes and monitor medication progress [4]. Once the patient has reached the target BMI or goal weight, a follow-up with the surgeon may be recommended to discuss potential hernia repair options.

Smoking

Historically, active smoking was a contraindication to hernia surgery. Most large studies have indicated that smoking status significantly impacts postoperative complications following hernia surgery, such as surgical site infections (SSIs), surgical site occurrences (SSOs), and hernia recurrence. Previously, patients were provided counseling or referred for smoking cessation, with a requirement to quit for at least 4 weeks before surgery, verified through a urine test [5]. However, more recent studies have challenged this notion in elective hernia repair. Specifically, these studies have shown that while there is in fact an increase in minor wound morbidity and respiratory complications, these risks might not be prohibitive. Instead, an individualized approach is often encouraged. This can include education that smoking cessation is helpful not only for the hernia repair, but general health. However, we no longer cancel or delay surgeries for those that do not comply. While smoking cessation counseling remains important for a patient's overall health, it may no longer be a strict requirement prior to hernia surgery in all practices [6].

Diabetes Mellitus

Patients with uncontrolled diabetes mellitus (hemoglobin (Hb) A $_{1c}$ > 7.0), undergoing any surgical procedure, are found to be at an increased risk of wound infection, SSOs, and hernia recurrence. In most general surgery practices, a preoperative HbA $_{1c}$ is drawn to determine diabetic control. If the patient's HbA $_{1c}$ is found to be <9.0, the surgeon will proceed with the hernia repair but counsel the patient on healthy lifestyle changes. If the HbA $_{1c}$ is found to be >9.0, the surgery is postponed, and the patient is referred to an endocrinologist in hopes to improve wound morbidity [5].

However, most studies that have collected data on patients with uncontrolled diabetes mellitus undergoing surgery have not specifically focused on those undergoing hernia surgery. In 2024, Fafaj and colleagues collected data from the hernia-specific database, Abdominal Core Health Quality Collaborative (ACHQC), showing that there was no clinical significance in the rates of wound complications, reoperations, readmissions, length of stay, or mortality when comparing patients with HbA $_{1c}$ > 8.0 and HbA $_{1c}$ < 8.0 [6]. Given recent data, the APP and surgeon should coordinate to determine whether the patient should engage in an improved diet and exercise regimen with a referral to an endocrinologist or proceed with the hernia repair. However, it is important to note that no specific "acceptable" HbA $_{1c}$ cutoff level has been established prior to hernia surgery.

It should be emphasized that presurgical optimization will be patient-specific and involve the surgeon's careful consideration and discretion. While historically smoking, obesity, and elevated Hba1c were reasons to delay a hernia repair, recent data have questioned this paradigm. As the APP, collaboration with the surgeon and shared decision making with the patient should be adopted to carefully balance patient optimization and avoid unnecessary delays in surgical treatment.

In addition to presurgical optimization of obesity, smoking, and DM, it is recommended that a patient with comorbidities be seen by a preanesthesia clinic within 30 days of their surgical intervention. At the preanesthesia clinic, a patient may be referred to further specialists, commonly cardiologists, to diagnose an underlying condition and treat, if possible. By ensuring a preanesthesia assessment occurs within 30 days of the hernia surgery, day-of-surgery cancellations and length of hospital stay may be reduced [7].

While most hernia surgeries are considered an elective procedure and can allow for presurgical optimization, there is always a chance that a patient will undergo urgent or emergent surgery. This occurs when a patient is found to have a bowel incarceration, obstruction, and/or strangulation within the hernia. If a patient is not offered surgery at their initial consult due to a need for presurgical optimization, the patient should be educated by the surgeon or the APP on the signs and symptoms warranting an emergency department visit, such as nausea/vomiting, severe cramping abdominal pain, or obstipation [8]. Furthermore, if preoperative optimization strategies are undertaken, and a patient becomes more symptomatic, they should be offered immediate surgery to avoid an emergency operation with worse outcomes.

Intraoperative Hernia Repairs

When discussing hernia repair, a surgeon has a variety of options, which include an open or minimally invasive approach (laparoscopic or robotic), as well as decisions regarding the use, type, and placement of mesh. The decision to repair a hernia using either an open or minimally invasive approach, and whether mesh is required, depends on several factors, including the hernia location and size, the patient's history of abdominal and hernia surgeries, overall health and comorbidities, as well as the surgeon's expertise [9]. If a surgeon is using mesh, the mesh can be placed in an onlay, inlay, sublay (retromuscular or preperitoneal), or underlay (intraperitoneal) position with varying types of mesh. When to use mesh and what type of mesh to use will vary on the hernia size and complexity, resources available, case contamination, and the surgeon's expertise [10].

While new mesh options are introduced to the market, as an APP, it is important to know the three main categories of mesh being synthetic, biologic, and absorbable. Synthetic mesh is made of a permanent material and can have various pore sizes, filament diameters, and adhesive barriers. Little comparative data exists evaluating the outcomes of different materials. Absorbable mesh is made of a bioresorbable polymer that degrades at different rates. Absorbable mesh can then further be broken down into short-term absorbable mesh or long-term absorbable mesh being biologic or biosynthetic mesh [11]. Finally, biologic mesh is derived from various host materials, including human, porcine, bovine, and ovine sources. It is often processed in such a way to render them acellular and allow for purported tissue ingrowth and regeneration. These materials are typically reserved for contaminated cases when there is concern for utilizing a permanent synthetic mesh.

The surgical approach for complex incisional ventral hernias will require components of the abdominal wall to be separated, open or robotically, to relieve tension on midline fascial closure and create a large retromuscular pocket for mesh placement. While there is both an anterior and posterior component approach, the posterior component separation with a transversus abdomins release (TAR) is the most recent and widely used technique at our institution. This technique begins with a retorectus repair, also known as "Rives–Stoppa" then incises the transversus abdominis muscle proximal to the neurovascular bundles. With this release, the preperitoneal space is entered and allows for a large piece of mesh to be placed. The mesh is typically placed in a diamond fashion, extending from the xiphoid to the pubic bone, over to bilateral flanks. The benefit of a posterior component separation with a TAR allows for minimal tension with midline approximation and avoids the need for large skin flaps seen in the anterior approach, therefore minimizing the risk for wound morbidity [12].

Although the APP will not be performing the surgery, it is crucial that the APP has a comprehensive understanding of the hernia repair approaches, types of mesh, relevant abdominal wall anatomy, and vascular supply. This knowledge is essential for both assisting in the operating room and effectively managing any potential postsurgical complications.

Inpatient Postoperative Management and Care

While patients undergoing routine hernia repairs, including inguinal and small ventral hernias, are often performed as outpatient procedures, complex abdominal wall reconstructions are typically major laparotomies requiring an inpatient stay. This can involve intensive care unit level care or often on a regular nursing floor. Typically, following a standard complex ventral hernia repair, the patient will transfer from the operating room to the PACU, then a regular nursing floor (RNF) for recovery, where they are closely monitored. Continuous telemetry and pulse-oximetry monitoring are routinely ordered following surgery, and vital signs are obtained every 4 h for the first 24 postoperative hours. It is important to note that the day of surgery is considered postoperative day (POD) zero.

If close hemodynamic monitoring or ventilator weaning is required, a transfer to the surgical intensive care unit (SICU) would be warranted from the OR. This situation typically occurs when the patient has some component of loss of domain, meaning that more of the intestines are outside the abdominal cavity, in the hernia sac, than inside the peritoneal cavity. After reconstruction, the added pressure caused by returning the intestinal contents to the abdominal cavity can result in respiratory compromise. Our group has noted that, if the change in plateau pressure is more than 6 mmHg intraoperatively, as measured before and after closure of the abdominal fascia, this may be a predictor of pulmonary complications in the postoperative period, [13] so the patient may remain intubated and sedated until POD1, where ventilator weaning may occur if safe to do so. It is important to realize that this relative state of permissive intra-abdominal hypertension is temporary. Once the releases performed take effect, and the bowel edema subsides, these patients can be extubated and progress along a more typical course. However, failing to realize the potential respiratory risks associated with complex abdominal wall reconstruction can have disastrous effects on patient's outcomes and respiratory emergencies.

The average length of stay (LOS) following a transverse abdominal release (TAR) procedure is 4–6 days, [14] but the length of stay is dependent on multiple factors. Underlying chronic comorbidities, particularly diabetes mellitus (DM), COPD, and obesity, may lead to an increased length of stay and contribute to the likelihood of postoperative complications and hospital readmission. The role of the APP in the inpatient setting is to ensure the patient is successfully meeting postoperative milestones, minimizing and treating adverse events, and helping to plan for and execute a safe discharge. Oftentimes, the APP is the main point of contact amongst the surgeon, resident/fellows, case managers, nursing staff, and therapy teams. This requires strong communication skills to effectively manage the care of these complex patients.

To safely discharge a patient following an open complex abdominal wall reconstruction (AWR) surgery, it is important that they have met the following postoperative milestones: return of bowel function, adequate pain control on an oral regimen, ambulating or functioning at baseline, spontaneous voiding, and tolerating diet advancement to a gastrointestinal soft foods diet. An enhanced recovery after surgery (ERAS) protocol has been established by Colvin and colleagues to help standardize postoperative care, maximize recovery, and decrease LOS for patients undergoing elective abdominal wall reconstruction [14]. Certain factors may exclude a patient from being placed on the ERAS protocol, such as a patient with chronic pain who may require additional pain management needs, or a patient with extensive intraoperative lysis of adhesions in which a nasogastric (NG) tube is placed. When able, implementation of the ERAS protocol offers guidance and standardization for the postoperative care of AWR patients.

As a general rule, our ERAS program includes: foley catheters are placed upon induction in the operating room and removed on POD 1, the patient is placed on a clear liquid diet as tolerated on POD 0, and intravenous fluids are ordered and infused until the patient can hydrate orally. As return of bowel function is achieved, the diet is advanced to a gastrointestinal soft diet.

Early ambulation and mobilization out of bed are strongly encouraged, and patients receive preoperative education regarding the importance. Early mobilization has been shown to decrease postoperative complications, accelerate their recovery, and lead to a decrease in LOS and thereby associated costs [15]. Postoperative patients should be evaluated by physical and occupational therapy as indicated to help aid in early mobilization, determine or identify any needs for discharge, such as potential skilled nursing facility (SNF) placement, and to provide education regarding safe abdominal core exercises and precautions following surgery.

An important aspect of the ERAS protocol is the establishment of a multimodal pain regimen (MMPR) for acute postoperative pain management. A transverse abdominus plane (TAP) block is administered intraoperatively by the surgeon. The block consists of 20 cc bupivacaine diluted in 80 cc normal saline solution and is injected along the edges of the cut transverse abdominus muscle. This may offer pain control immediately following surgery and up to 12 h. So long as there are no contraindications, allergies, or underlying conditions that would discourage use, scheduled Tylenol (1000 mg every 6 h) and scheduled gabapentin is initiated (300 mg every 8 h). The patient is also started on a patient-controlled analgesia (PCA) pump with hydromorphone. The PCA is weaned with diet advancement, ideally on postoperative day 2 or 3, and discontinued when the patient is tolerating oral intake and pills. Oral oxycodone is introduced with diet advancement. The MMPR was established to decrease narcotic use and offer scheduled and consistent non-narcotic modalities for pain control. The patient is sent home with a limited supply of pain medications upon discharge, and referrals may be considered to a pain management specialist if pain persists, and it is determined there is no surgical complication contributing to these concerns.

Postoperative Complications

Given the nature of the procedure, complex ventral hernia repairs may be associated with significant postoperative complications. Patients who have undergone a recurrent ventral hernia repair are at a greater risk of complications, including prolonged operation time for repair, risk for surgical site infections (SSIs), and additional hernia recurrence [16]. Common complications in the immediate postoperative setting that may increase length of stay or alter the ERAS protocol include postoperative ileus, deep vein thrombosis (DVT) or pulmonary embolism, or surgical site infections (SSIs).

Ileus

An ileus is defined as a temporary condition in which the intestine is unable to contract normally, leading to a decrease or stopping in the movement of intestinal contents, and occurs in approximately 15–20% of patients undergoing complex abdominal wall reconstruction [17]. Indicators of postoperative ileus include nausea and vomiting, abdominal distention, absence of bowel sounds, and slow return of bowel function. It may also be identified radiographically via an abdominal x-ray or CT imaging. Treatment for an ileus may include complete bowel rest (making diet NPO), hydrating via IV fluids, and insertion of a nasogastric tube (NGT) for bowel decompression. It is worth mentioning that we have a fairly low threshold to place an NGT in patients after a complex abdominal wall reconstruction. These patients typically have a tight closure, and significant retching can disrupt the repair. In efforts to prevent this complication, the patient is encouraged to mobilize out of bed the same day as surgery, encouraged to chew gum, and is started on the ERAS protocol. If the patient does not have return of bowel function within 6–7 days following surgery, a consultation is placed with the nutrition team for consideration of peripheral parenteral nutrition. Equally important is that these patients often have a multilayered repair. Early postoperative emesis should always trigger a workup to rule out a potential interstitial hernia. This occurs when the posterior sheath repair below the mesh breaks down and bowel is incarcerated below the mesh. This is particularly problematic because there will not be signs of physical exam and can only be identified by computed tomography (CT) scans of the abdomen and pelvis. Thus, early postoperative ileus in patients after complex abdominal wall reconstruction should almost always be investigated with a CT scan.

DVT/Pulmonary Embolus

Blood clots, including deep vein thrombosis of the extremities or pulmonary embolism, are a potential adverse outcome following any operation. The risk for development of a venous thromboembolism (VTE) is dependent on the patient's personal predisposing factors (such as an age greater than 40, history of VTE, obesity, and concurrent cancer diagnosis) as well as surgical procedure performed [18]. Given the extensiveness of the operation required to reconstruct an abdominal wall, this patient population is inherently at high risk for the development of a VTE event. Literature documents that the rate of VTE in ventral hernia repairs ranges from 0.2% to 4.2% [19]. In efforts to reduce complications, VTE prophylaxis is routinely implemented following AWR procedures and includes both pharmacologic and nonpharmacological measures. VTE prophylaxis includes intermittent pneumatic stockings ordered to be worn continuously any time the patient is in bed, heparin or Lovenox injections, and frequent mobilization. Bleeding risk and intraoperative blood loss are two considerations for initiating pharmacologic VTE prophylaxis. A thorough workup is warranted if a VTE is suspected in the postoperative setting, as this reduces the risk of serious complications, including mortality.

Wound Complications

Most complex abdominal wall reconstructions are performed with a mesh prothesis. The introduction of mesh into the abdominal wall lends itself to higher rates of surgical site infections, and the patient must be diligently assessed to ensure prevention or early detection of SSIs. Underlying comorbidities, particularly current use of tobacco products, morbid obesity (defined as a BMI of 40 or greater), poor functional status at baseline, and poorly controlled type 2 diabetes mellitus are risk factors for the development of an SSI following surgery, hence supporting the importance of proper optimization for surgery in the preoperative setting. SSIs have a significant impact and detrimental consequences for both the patient and the healthcare system. They are costly to manage and put the patient at risk of undergoing additional operations, procedures, or even mesh removal or explantation.

Symptoms of an SSI may include subjective systemic complaints (fever, chills, nausea, generalized malaise) in combination with erythema, purulent drainage, or increased pain at the incision. Leukocytosis, or an increase in white blood cell counts, as well as an elevation in CRP or lactate levels may be seen on lab work. Changes in vital signs may also be indicators of infection, including hypotension or tachycardia. CT imaging of the abdomen/pelvis is ordered to investigate for any fluid collections indicating a postoperative seroma or abscess. The location, size, and presence of gas of a fluid collection on imaging will help to guide interventions for an SSI. Early detection of these signs and symptoms is important to help guide an infectious work-up and implement early interventions in efforts to prevent sepsis and decrease the need for additional surgeries, including wound debridement or infected mesh, risking mesh removal.

Treatment and management of an SSI following a complex ventral hernia repair is patient dependent. Oral antibiotics may be initiated in the outpatient setting if there is concern of a superficial SSI, presenting as minimal erythema with stable lab work and vital signs. If the patient is hemodynamically unstable, has lab work abnormalities, or if there is concern of deep surgical site infection extending into organ space or down to the mesh, then a readmission is warranted for management. CT imaging is quickly ordered to determine severity, location, and size of the infection, which will further guide the treatment plan and needs. Broad-spectrum antibiotics and IV fluids are initiated. Cultures are sent when able to appropriately guide antibiotic coverage. An infectious disease specialist may be consulted to help determine the appropriate antibiotic(s). Deep SSI management may require IR drain placement, bedside incision and drainage (I&D) with local wound care, wound vac placement, or return to the operating room for a wound washout. Often, modern meshes can be salvaged and do not require removal.

However, if the wound is not healing, at least partial mesh excision can be required.

Prior to discharge, the patient is provided with education regarding common signs and symptoms of a postoperative wound infection and coached on when to seek medical attention from his or her surgeon. For the initial 30 days following the operation, the patient is at a highest risk for the development of an SSI. At the first sign of an infection, our practice encourages the patient to follow up with a provider on our team or to present at an emergency department affiliated with our facility for workup and management. This is due to the complex nature of the procedure performed and the specialized care these patients require.

Outpatient Postoperative Care

In addition to education provided to the patient before discharge, all patients should be given a follow–up appointment for their postoperative visit in the outpatient clinic with the surgeon or APP. Typically, a patient is seen about 3–4 weeks from the date of their abdominal wall reconstruction, unless a Jackson-Pratt (JP) drain(s) were left in place. If JP drains were left in place, the patient should be seen approximately 1 week after discharge for drain removal. Most commonly, JP drains are removed when the output is <30–50 ml/day, but the specific criterion for drain removal is an area that could be further investigated [20].

At their 3–4-week postoperative visit (30-day follow-up), three important areas for evaluation are wound complications (SSI, SSO SSOPI), pain management, and physical activity.

Complications

While postoperative complications can occur while the patient is inpatient, an outpatient APP or the surgeon will oversee the management of postoperative complications that arise after discharge, including SSIs, SSOs, and SSOPIs (Surgical Site Infection, Surgical Site Occurrence, and Surgical Site Occurrence Requiring a Procedural Intervention, respectively). Depending on the severity of the complication, many can be treated by clinical examination in the clinic and outpatient therapy.

An infection that develops in the area where surgery was performed defines a surgical site infection, which can further be classified as a superficial, deep, or organ space SSI [21]. Treatment for an outpatient SSI may involve incision and drainage of infected fluid collections, typically performed with local anesthesia. This may also include obtaining a wound culture and prescribing oral antibiotics as needed [22]. Once an incision is opened in the clinic, the patient should be educated on proper wound care and dressing changes, typically wet to dry technique, to heal by secondary intention [23]. It is necessary to point out that after the APP performs an I&D, on rare occasions, the mesh used in the repair may be exposed. With exposed mesh, a close follow-up will be essential to ensure proper tissue granulation and mesh incorporation. The APP should maintain communication with the surgeon if the infection persists or if the mesh is not incorporated, as further interventions may be required. These could include imaging, such as a CT of the abdomen/pelvis with an additional incision and drainage in the clinic or readmission for IV antibiotics, debridement of infected tissue in the operating room, or in some cases, partial mesh excision [22].

The other wound complications found after a ventral incisional hernia repair include SSO and SSOPI. The definition of an SSO is any SSI as well as wound cellulitis, seroma, hematoma, wound serous drainage, development of an enterocutaneous fistula, nonhealing incisional wound, skin or soft tissue ischemia, or fascial disruption. If any of these SSOs require opening of the wound, wound debridement, suture excision, percutaneous drainage, or partial or complete mesh removal, they are defined as a SSOPI [21]. While wound cellulitis will require oral antibiotics, and serous drainage may necessitate further opening of the wound, an important surgical site occurrence to discuss in the outpatient setting is a seroma. The incidence of seromas, when clinically detected, can range from 5% to 30%, with some studies indicating that up to 10% of these cases are clinically significant. As an APP, education should be provided to the patient that most seromas are asymptomatic and will spontaneously resolve within 8 weeks. If a seroma becomes symptomatic, percutaneous drainage or surgical excision may be required [22, 24].

Pain Management

As a provider, managing pain after a ventral hernia repair continues to remain a challenge. It is shown that in patients that are opioid-naïve, 6% will continue opioids for more than 3 months after their surgery [25]. To decrease the risk of chronic opioid use, a patient is discharged home on a limited supply of narcotic medication, as mentioned earlier. An outpatient APP should continue to help decrease the amount of opioid prescription refills by focusing on multimodal analgesia regimens. Results from Desai and colleagues showed that combined nonsteroidal anti-inflammatories, acetaminophen, and methocarbamol can reduce the risk of opioid abuse while concomitantly providing adequate pain control after a ventral incisional hernia repair [26]. While not well studied but recommended in ERAS protocols for ventral hernias, an APP can recommend to a patient to use an abdominal binder for improvement of pain in the outpatient setting [20]. If the patient continues to have abdominal pain, unrelated to a surgical complication, the patient is then referred to an outpatient chronic pain provider.

Activity Restrictions

One of the most frequent questions from patients that arises after a hernia operation is related to postoperative activities, including lifting and returning to work. Following an inguinal hernia repair, current data support allowing the patient to return to their baseline level of activity as soon as possible, based on their pain level. Despite existing data for inguinal hernias, there is no conclusive data on the recommendations for activity restrictions following abdominal hernia surgery. According to a survey completed by Schaaf and colleagues, they found no justification to reduce physical activity and lifting after an incisional ventral hernia repair [27]. In our practice, patients who undergo abdominal wall reconstruction are counseled that they may return to physical activities with no restrictions and may return to work within 4–6 weeks.

A modified Delphi was completed through expert consensus showing that out of eleven clinical practice guidelines, the number one clinically relevant topic in hernia research is "activity restriction versus no activity restriction following incisional hernia repair." [28] This shows that activity restriction is a top-priority research topic requiring further high-quality evidence. As an APP in hernia surgery, contributing to activity restriction research or staying updated on the latest literature will be essential for educating postoperative patients.

If a patient is recovering well without signs of infection or delayed wound healing, they should be advised to follow up in one year with the APP or surgeon for a clinical and radiographic assessment of hernia recurrence, as well as a quality-of-life evaluation. It is important to emphasize to the patient that after an abdominal wall reconstruction, the risk of a hernia recurrence is lower than if they did not have a component separation. Fry and colleagues published results showing a hernia recurrence rate of 0.7% at 1 year, 4.2% at 3 years, and 6.8% at 5 years following a ventral hernia repair with component separation [29].

Summary

In summary, this chapter delves into the critical role of advanced practice providers (APPs) in the care of patients with hernias, in particular undergoing complex abdominal wall reconstruction. APPs work closely with general surgeons to manage preoperative optimization, intraoperative assistance, and postoperative aspects of hernia care both inpatient and outpatient. By delivering comprehensive, patient-centered care, APPs play a key role in enhancing patient outcomes, optimizing surgical procedures, and minimizing complications.

References

1. Ezeme C, Mackenzie P, Newton RC. Ventral hernias: understanding the pathogenesis, prevention and repair. Surg Oxf. 2024;42(1):22–32.
2. Ghanem OM, Orenstein S, Lloyd SJA, Andalib A, Race A, Burt HA, et al. Management of abdominal wall hernias in patients with severe obesity. Surg Endosc. 2023;37(9):6619–26.
3. Burridge K, Christensen SM, Golden A, Ingersoll AB, Tondt J, Bays HE. Obesity history, physical exam, laboratory, body composition, and energy expenditure: an obesity medicine association (OMA) clinical practice statement (CPS) 2022. Obes Pillars. 2022;1:100007.
4. Alexander L, Christensen SM, Richardson L, Ingersoll AB, Burridge K, Golden A, et al. Nutrition and physical activity: an obesity medicine association (OMA) clinical practice statement 2022. Obes Pillars. 2022;1:100005.
5. Tucker S, Bramante C, Conroy M, Fitch A, Gilden A, Wittleder S, et al. The Most undertreated chronic disease: addressing obesity in primary care settings. Curr Obes Rep. 2021;10(3):396–408.
6. Petro CC, Rosen MJ. Preoperative optimization of the hernia patient. In: Rosen MJ, editor. Atlas of abdominal wall reconstruction. 2nd ed. Philadelphia: Elsevier; 2017. p. 446–54.
7. Fafaj A, de Figueiredo SMP, Rosen MJ, Petro CC. Preoperative optimization in hernia surgery: are we really helping or are we just stalling? Hernia J Hernias Abdom Wall Surg. 2024;28(3):925–30.
8. Lamperti M, Romero CS, Guarracino F, Cammarota G, Vetrugno L, Tufegdzic B, et al. Preoperative assessment of adults undergoing elective noncardiac surgery: updated guidelines from the European Society of Anaesthesiology and Intensive Care. Eur J Anaesthesiol. 2025;42(1):1–35.
9. Alkhatib H, Fafaj A, Olson M, Stewart T, Krpata DM. Primary uncomplicated midline ventral hernias: factors that influence and guide the surgical approach. Hernia J Hernias Abdom Wall Surg. 2019;23(5):873–83.
10. Holihan JL, Nguyen DH, Nguyen MT, Mo J, Kao LS, Liang MK. Mesh location in open ventral hernia repair: a systematic review and network meta-analysis. World J Surg. 2016;40(1):89–99.
11. Ellis R, Miller BT. Mesh selection in abdominal wall reconstruction. Surg Clin North Am. 2023;103(5):1019–28.
12. Miller BT, Petro CC, Rosen MJ. Open posterior component separation: transversus abdominis release (PCS-TAR) for ventral hernia. In: Baig SJ, Bhandarkar D, Priya P, editors. Newer concepts and procedures in hernia surgery—an Atlas [Internet]. Singapore: Springer Nature Singapore; 2022. p. 45–53. [cited 2025 Feb 20]. Available from: https://link.springer.com/10.1007/978-981-19-5248-7_5.
13. Petro CC, Raigani S, Fayezizadeh M, Rowbottom JR, Klick JC, Prabhu AS, et al. Permissible Intraabdominal Hypertension following Complex Abdominal Wall Reconstruction. Plast Reconstr Surg. 2015;136(4):868–81.
14. Colvin J, Rosen M, Prabhu A, Rosenblatt S, Petro C, Zolin S, et al. Enhanced recovery after surgery pathway for patients undergoing abdominal wall reconstruction. Surgery. 2019;166(5):849–53.
15. Tazreean R, Nelson G, Twomey R. Early mobilization in enhanced recovery after surgery pathways: current evidence and recent advancements. J Comp Eff Res. 2022;11(2):121–9.
16. Holihan JL, Alawadi Z, Martindale RG, Roth SJ, Wray CJ, Ko TC, et al. Adverse events after ventral hernia repair: the vicious cycle of complications. J Am Coll Surg. 2015;221(2):478–85.

17. Venara A, Neunlist M, Slim K, Barbieux J, Colas PA, Hamy A, et al. Postoperative ileus: pathophysiology, incidence, and prevention. J Visc Surg. 2016;153(6):439–46.
18. Agnelli G. Prevention of Venous Thromboembolism in Surgical Patients. Circulation [Internet]. 2004 Dec 14 [cited 2025 Feb 20];110(24_suppl_1). Available from: https://www.ahajournals.org/doi/10.1161/01.CIR.0000150639.98514.6c
19. Andriyashkin AV, Loban KM, Kalinina AA, Ivakhov GB, Zolotukhin IA, Sazhin AV. Risk factors of venous thromboembolism after incisional ventral hernia repair. Hernia J Hernias Abdom Wall Surg. 2023;27(4):895–9.
20. Remulla D, Bradley JF, Henderson W, Lewis RC, Kreuz B, Beffa LR, et al. Consensus in ERAS protocols for ventral hernia repair: evidence-based recommendations from the ACHQC QI Committee. Hernia. 2024;29(1):4.
21. Haskins IN, Horne CM, Krpata DM, Prabhu AS, Tastaldi L, Perez AJ, et al. A call for standardization of wound events reporting following ventral hernia repair. Hernia. 2018;22(5):729–36.
22. Lu Y, Chen DC, MacQueen IT. Management of Postoperative Complications Following Ventral Hernia Repair and Inguinal Hernia Repair. Surg Clin North Am. 2021;101(5):755–66.
23. Bowman JK. Abscess incision and drainage. Prim Care Clin Off Pract. 2022;49(1):39–45.
24. Miller BT, Baier KF, Zolin SJ, Huang LC, Phillips S, Petro CC, et al. Long-term outcomes of seromas after ventral hernia repair: a propensity score-matched analysis of the abdominal Core health quality collaborative. Hernia 2022;27(2):373–378.
25. Brummett CM, Waljee JF, Goesling J, Moser S, Lin P, Englesbe MJ, et al. New persistent opioid use after minor and major surgical procedures in US adults. JAMA Surg. 2017;152(6):e170504.
26. Desai S, Carbonell C, Hoffman K, Hammond B, Crosier C, Blackhurst D, et al. Impact of methocarbamol on opioid use after ventral incisional hernia repair. Am J Surg. 2023;226(6):858–63.
27. Schaaf S, Schwab R, Güsgen C, Vilz TO, Willms A. Recommendations on postoperative activities after abdominal operations and incisional hernia repair-a national and international survey. Front Surg. 2021;8:713138.
28. Remulla D, Al-Mansour MR, Schneider C, Phillips S, Hope WW, Bradley JF, et al. Research prioritization in hernia surgery: a modified Delphi ACHQC and VHOC expert consensus. Hernia J Hernias Abdom Wall Surg. 2024;28(6):2217–22.
29. Fry BT, Schoel LJ, Howard RA, Thumma JR, Kappelman AL, Hallway AK, et al. Long-term outcomes of component separation for abdominal wall hernia repair. JAMA Surg. 2025;160(1):10.

Stoma Basics

23

Sara Myers, Jennifer S. Davids, and Samantha J. Rivard

Introduction

An **ostomy** is a surgically created connection between the bowel wall and the subcutaneous tissue or skin of the abdominal wall, and a **stoma** is the exteriorized portion of bowel. Stomas are common; in the United States, approximately 150,000 new stomas are created annually, and between 750,000 and one million individuals are currently living with stomas [1].

Stomas may be *temporary or permanent.* In the temporary setting, stomas are typically used to divert stool away from an area undergoing healing, such as an anastomosis at increased risk of anastomotic leak due to infection, immunosuppression, radiation, or distal location. Temporary stomas can also be used to divert stool away from a healing perineal wound or sacral decubitus ulcer, preventing stool from soiling the wound bed. A permanent stoma may be necessary if the anorectal sphincter mechanism is removed surgically, such as for advanced distal rectal cancer, inflammatory bowel disease, or injury from trauma. Stomas can be performed electively for fecal diversion, but may also be performed emergently due to a distal bowel obstruction, poor tissue quality, or other patient factors that increase risk of anastomotic complications.

Physiology

Within the most proximal 150 cm of the small intestine, a majority of nutrients are absorbed. The **jejunum** absorbs approximately 6 L of fluid and nutrients, while the ileum absorbs approximately 2.5 L. *The **terminal ileum** is responsible for absorbing bile acids, nutrients, and vitamins, including B12* [2]. As such, more proximal stomas such as jejunostomies often have very high output, and patients may experience vitamin deficiencies if stoma effluent is not passing through the terminal ileum.

The **colon**, *primarily responsible for water absorption,* reabsorbs 1–2 L of water from stool, such that colostomy output is *thicker and more episodic than ileostomy output* [3, 4]. However, since water gets absorbed as it passes through the colon, more proximal colostomies, including ascending and proximal transverse colostomies, produce more liquid stool, while distal transverse and descending colostomies produce more solid stool.

Types of Stomas

Ileostomy

An **ileostomy** is when the small intestine, namely the ileum, is brought out through the abdominal wall for fecal *diversion* (Fig. 23.1). An ileostomy can be temporary, as in a **loop** configuration, or permanent, generally in an **end** configuration. Liquid stool contents exit through the stoma, which is typically created to sit above the skin to prevent skin damage. Typically, ileostomies are created in the right hemi-abdomen. Small bowel stomas are smaller in caliber than colonic stomas. Given the terminal ileum's role in absorption, patients with more proximal ileostomies, particularly further than 100 cm from the ileocecal valve, are at high risk of B12 deficiency and resulting pernicious/macrocytic anemia. As the right colon is responsible for a majority of water and electrolyte reabsorption, patients with ileostomies, whose stoma contents do not pass through the colon, *are at high risk of electrolyte and fluid imbalance.* More proximal stomas such as jejunostomies may occasionally be performed for cases of extensive ileal Crohn's disease or ischemic bowel resections, but are associated with the complications of *high output.* Appropriate ileostomy output is *approximately 500–1300 ml of thick liquid per day.*

S. Myers · J. S. Davids · S. J. Rivard (✉)
Department of Surgery, Boston Medical Center, Boston University Chobanian and Avedisian School of Medicine, Boston, MA, USA
e-mail: Samantha.Rivard@bmc.org

S. Atallah, J. Dragoljevic (eds.), *Fundamentals of Surgery for Physician Assistants*,
https://doi.org/10.1007/978-3-032-21069-2_23

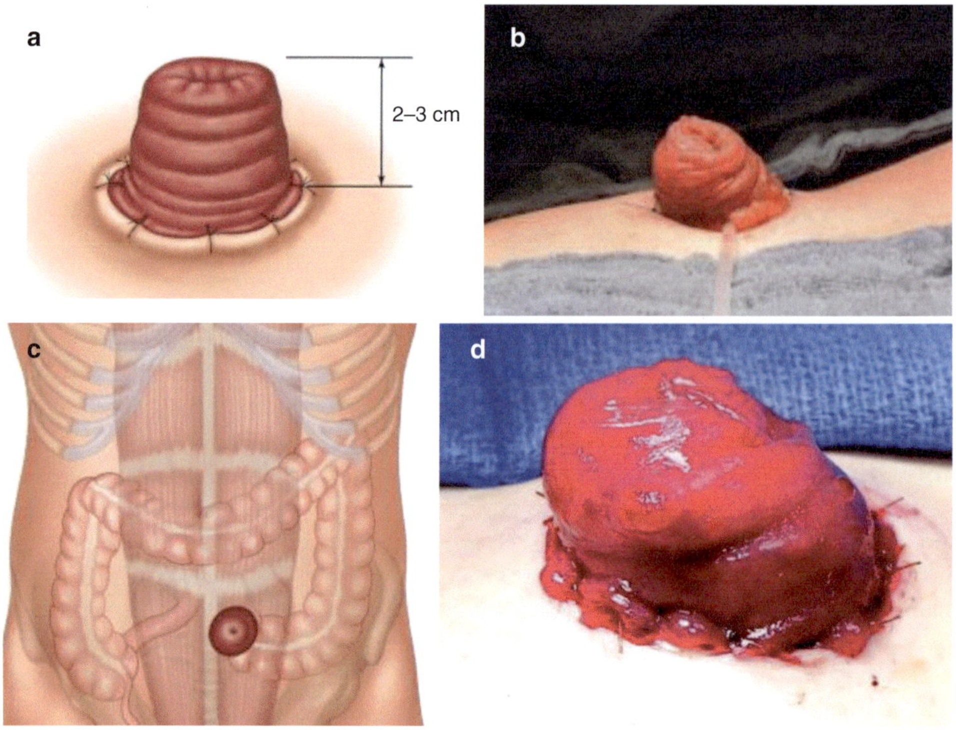

Fig. 23.1 (**a**) Illustration of an end ileostomy, which should protrude 2–3 cm from the abdominal wall at creation; (**b**) Photo of an end ileostomy; (**c**) Illustration of an end descending colostomy; (**d**) photo of an end colostomy. (Images (a and c) from "Intestinal Stoma" [30]; (b) from "Ileostomies and Colostomies," [31] (d) from "Colostomy: Types, Indications, Formation, and Reversal," [32] licenses obtained)

Colostomy

A colostomy is when the **colon,** most commonly *transverse or sigmoid/descending,* is brought through the abdominal wall for fecal diversion (Fig. 23.1c). Similar to ileostomies, colostomies can be temporary, most commonly in loop configurations, or permanent in an end configuration. *Proximal* colostomies, such as those of the *right* colon or the *proximal transverse* colon, *produce more liquid stool and gas,* while distal colostomies including those of the distal transverse, descending, and sigmoid colon produce more solid stool. This is because the stool becomes increasingly solidified (due to water resorption) as it travels through the large intestine.

Loop Configuration

In a **loop** stoma, a *loop* of bowel is brought to the abdominal wall, and the antimesenteric side of the bowel is opened such that there are two lumens sharing a back wall (Fig. 23.2). The proximal lumen is the **afferent limb,** which diverts bowel contents, while the distal lumen is the **efferent limb,** venting distal bowel and preventing a distal pressure buildup. Loop stomas are often temporary and are more commonly used to *divert succus or stool away from a healing downstream anastomosis.* By diverting stool away from a new anastomosis, the anastomosis may epithelialize without the stress of accommodating large volumes of stool. *The most common stoma in this setting is a* ***loop ileostomy.***

Loop colostomies may be particularly helpful to divert stool away from pelvic sepsis, large sacral decubitus ulcers, and perianal fistulizing disease, often in the setting of Crohn's disease. Reversal of a loop stoma is technically easier and can be performed through a local peristomal incision, avoiding a laparotomy, resulting in fewer complications. However, loop stomas may result in incomplete fecal diversion.

End Configuration

End stomas only contain one lumen that carries intestinal contents outside of the body (Figs. 23.1c and 23.2a). The single lumen of bowel is brought through the abdominal wall, opened, and the bowel wall is secured to the dermis. **End ileostomies** may be useful in clinical scenarios where the entire colon and rectum are removed, such as in the setting of a total abdominal colectomy for Ulcerative Colitis or *Clostridium difficile* toxic megacolon. **End colostomies** are used emergently in the setting of the **Hartmann procedure** (resection of sigmoid colon with construction of end colostomy) for complicated sigmoid diverticulitis. End colostomies may also be helpful among patients with anorectal sphincter absence or dysfunction, due to surgical removal in the setting of cancer or among patients with spinal cord injuries or other neurologic impairment.

While loop stomas are more often intended to be temporary, *end stomas can be temporary as well.* At the time of end colostomy creation, the proximal bowel is affixed to the abdominal wall as a stoma, while the distal bowel can be stapled off and placed back into the abdomen, available for later anastomosis. Alternatively, a **mucous fistula** can be matured, in which the *distal bowel is affixed to the subcutaneous tissue in an everted or noneverted fashion.* With a mucous fistula, *mucous produced by colonocytes can be expelled from the distal lumen rather than build up and potentially lead to perforation of the remaining intra-abdominal bowel.* Mucous fistulas may be helpful in cases of *distal obstructing tumors.*

Continent Ileostomies

Continent ileostomies, which contain an intra-abdominal reservoir for stool underneath the fascia, are emptied by patients by passing a tube into the stoma, thus avoiding an external ostomy appliance. Types of continent ileostomies include Koch pouches, Barnett continent ileal reservoirs (BCIR), and appendicostomies. However, *continent ileostomies are only performed at highly specialized centers and are associated with high complication and revision rates.*

Stoma Creation

Preoperative Considerations

The American Society of Colon and Rectal Surgeons (ASCRS) strongly recommends that patients undergoing stoma creation should receive teaching by a wound and ostomy continence nurse (WOCN), both pre- and post-operatively [1]. *Stoma teaching by a specialized provider or program has been associated with improved patient quality of life, decreased patient anxiety, reduced peristomal complications, and lower postoperative hospital length of stay* [5–9]. As some institutions do not have dedicated WOCN, physician assistants, nurse practitioners, and physicians familiar with ostomy care can provide the necessary preoperative teaching.

Preoperative **stoma marking** by a trained provider is associated with fewer ostomy-related complications and increased patient autonomy with stoma management compared to patients who do not undergo preoperative marking [1, 10–12]. While some emergency situations do not afford the time to mark patients, *preoperative marking for planned stomas is strongly recommended by ASCRS whenever possible* [1]. When selecting a site for a stoma, *the patient should be examined in multiple positions, including lying down, sitting up, and standing.* If possible, the patient should also be asked to twist to the side and bend over in order to observe the position of abdominal wall folds. Even if a patient is intubated, the head of the bed can be elevated into a seated position in order to evaluate the topography of the abdominal wall. Areas to avoid include skin folds, scars, bony prominences, the beltline, and within or underneath a pannus. While the ideal stoma site is typically within the rectus sheath between the umbilicus and the bilateral anterior superior iliac spines (ASIS), siting a stoma too low on the abdominal wall may prevent patients with panni from seeing and managing the stoma (Fig. 23.2). Instead, supraumbilical positioning, where the abdominal wall is thinner, although technically more challenging, often makes more sense for obese patients. Patients should always be advised that intra-operative findings may alter the planned site of stoma.

Operative Considerations

The **trephine**, or *aperture,* in the muscle and fascia through which the bowel is exteriorized, should be wide enough not to cause ischemia or obstruction and narrow enough to prevent parastomal hernia formation or stoma prolapse.

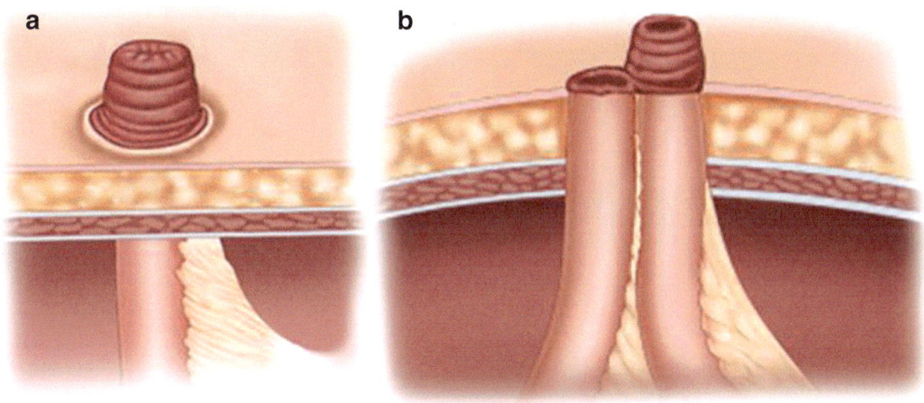

Fig. 23.2 (**a**) End ileostomy, (**b**) loop ileostomy. (Image from "Intestinal Stoma," [30] license obtained)

Typically, **this is about two-fingerbreadths** in diameter, but due to differences in surgeon hand sizes and patient anatomy, trephine size should be determined on a case-by-case basis intraoperatively (Fig. 23.3).

The stoma should be brought through the rectus muscle if possible, due to a lower risk of parastomal hernia compared to more lateral locations. If the patient also has a midline incision, the stoma should be far enough from the midline to avoid wound complications while still traveling through the rectus muscle.

Once exteriorized, the bowel wall is then everted and secured to the subcutaneous tissue circumferentially. Suturing the bowel to the epidermis can cause fistulas so dermal sutures are preferred. If there is tension on the bowel such that stoma retraction seems likely, more of the bowel should be mobilized prior to securing the stoma to the abdominal wall.

Postoperative Teaching and Support

Patients should be educated on how to change and manage their stoma appliance as soon as is feasible postoperatively. These educational sessions are ideally led by WOCN providers, but if a hospital does not have a WOCN specialist, advanced practice providers, physicians, and bedside nurses are expected provide stoma education. Family members and caregivers should be present in order to learn how to manage the stoma as well. Additionally, patients should be educated on recording the volume of stoma output, especially within the first several weeks postoperatively, when patients are at the highest risk of dehydration. Once patients leave the hospital, visiting nurses may be helpful to help keep patients on track with stoma management and troubleshoot issues that may arise. Additionally, stoma support groups may be helpful to patients in the outpatient setting.

Stoma Appliance Essentials

The stoma appliance secures onto the skin and collects gas and stool. Ideally, the system is odor-proof and leak-proof when placed onto clean, healthy, and dry skin. Two-part appliance systems have a skin barrier and a collecting bag; the skin barrier has an adhesive side, which is applied to the skin around the stoma, and the collecting bag is secured onto the barrier with a locking ring. One-piece appliances are also available. Stoma paste, skin adhesives, or a stoma barrier ring may help to create a seal between the pouch system and the skin, especially with nearby abdominal wall folds or moisture. If a seal is not achieved, effluent can leak out of the bag and irritate the peristomal skin, making a seal even more difficult to achieve. Many advances in stoma appliance technology have been made over the years to improve the quality of life of stoma patients, including opaque bags, odor filtering systems, convex shapes, and ostomy belt attachments.

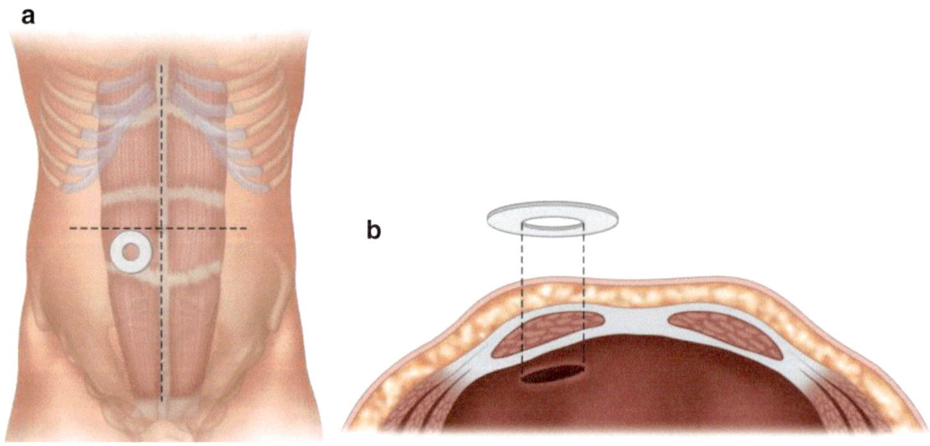

Fig. 23.3 The ideal stoma location is through the rectus muscle between the umbilicus and the bilateral anterior superior iliac spines. (**a**) External view of stoma location and size, which should be approximately the size of a quarter. (**b**) Cross-sectional view of a stoma trephine, which should be approximately two finger-breadths in diameter, and rectus muscle, through which the bowel is brought up to the abdominal wall. (Image from "Intestinal Stomas," [30] license obtained)

Stoma Complications

Early Complications

Peristomal Skin Irritation

The most common complication associated with stomas is peristomal skin irritation, aka, ***parastomal dermatitis*** (Fig. 23.4) [1, 13]. The combination of proteolytic enzymes in stoma effluent and mechanical trauma associated with removing and reapplying stoma appliances can cause a range of skin symptoms, from mild to severe dermatitis. Skin irritation can make achieving a leak-proof seal with the stoma appliance challenging, which can further worsen dermatitis, thus further worsening leakage. Covering exposed skin with skin barrier creams, stoma paste, and stoma rings can help prevent effluent from contacting the skin. Additionally, trimming long hair around a stoma may reduce irritation to hair follicles with the removal and reapplication of the adhesive side of the stoma bag.

The warm and humid environment in a stoma bag can also encourage a fungal skin infection, most commonly by *Candida albicans*. A fungal infection presents as a non-blanching erythema, a maculopapular rash, with or without satellite lesions, and patients may report itching or burning sensations [14]. Treatment involves keeping the skin clean and dry and applying nystatin powder to the lesions.

The expertise of a WOCN specialist is often invaluable in the treatment of peristomal skin irritation, as ostomy nurses may be able to creatively and safely reconfigure ostomy appliances. If peristomal skin irritation does not resolve despite best efforts, one should consider pyoderma gangrenosum as a diagnosis, particularly in patients with inflammatory bowel disease.

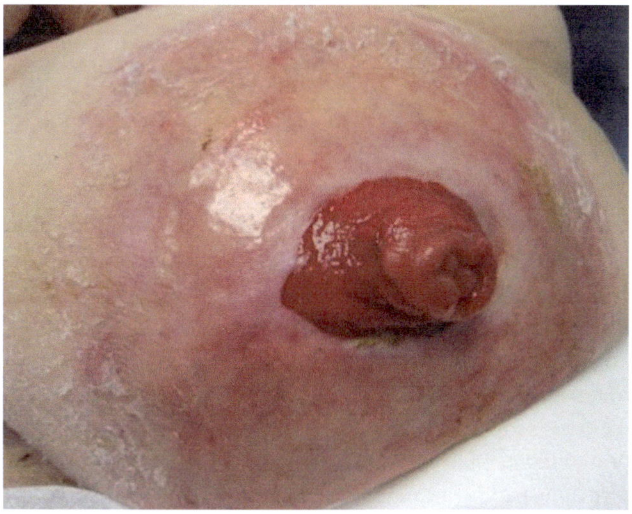

Fig. 23.4 Peristomal skin irritation, which can result from repeated application and removal of adhesive and irritation from digestive enzymes in effluent. (Image from "Local Peristomal Cutaneous Manifestations and Their Management," [33] license obtained)

Edema

In the immediate postoperative period, bowel wall edema can result in stoma swelling, which may last from days to weeks. *Stoma edema is self-limited and can be managed expectantly.* If the lumen of the bowel is significantly narrowed by the swelling, a lubricated red rubber catheter can be gently placed into the bowel lumen in order to help evacuate gas and liquid effluent. Alternatively, one can place suppositories in the stoma to encourage bowel function.

Ischemia and Necrosis

Up to 17% of stomas may exhibit signs of necrosis in the postoperative period, due to ischemia caused by a narrow trephine, minimized blood supply, or inadequate mobilization of bowel [15]. If a stoma appears ischemic or necrotic, the extent of necrosis must be determined. At the bedside, *a lubricated unlabeled test tube can be inserted into the stoma aperture,* and by shining a light into the tube, *the mucosa beyond the stoma can be examined.* If the mucosa appears healthy and necrosis appears to impact only the exterior stoma anterior to the fascia, the stoma may be observed. The mucosa may eventually turn grey and slough off. However, if the distal mucosa visible through the test tube appears necrotic as well, the patient may require emergent operative revision. Alternatively, the mucosa can be evaluated endoscopically. Of note, ischemia-related complications of small bowel stomas require more aggressive management, as small bowel effluent is more damaging to the skin. Therefore, while most colostomy ischemia complications can be observed, ileostomy ischemic complications should prompt strong consideration for operative revision.

Retraction

Stoma retraction, whereby the stoma becomes inverted to the level of the skin, can occur when there is excessive tension on the stoma due to a thick abdominal wall or inadequately mobilized bowel with a foreshortened mesentery (Fig. 23.5). If a stoma retracts but still remains above the fascia, a convex pouching system may be helpful to protect peristomal skin from effluent contents. However, if a stoma appears to retract to or *below* the level of the fascia (a rare finding), the patient will require urgent operative intervention to prevent intra-abdominal contamination and sepsis. Mobilizing additional bowel and siting the stoma in the upper abdomen in obese patients may reduce tension on the stoma.

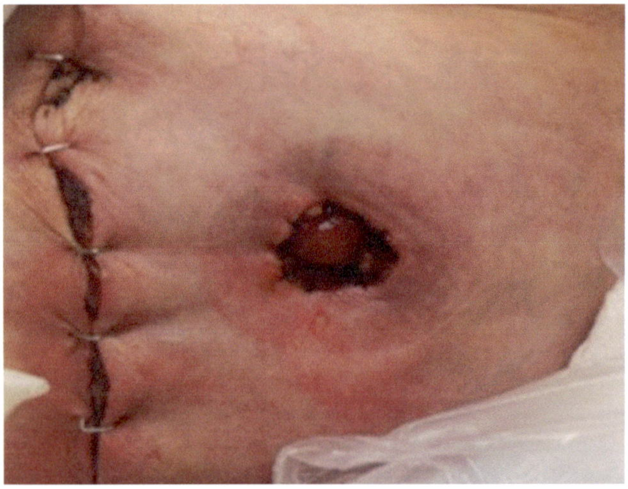

Fig. 23.5 Stoma retraction, where the stoma is pulled toward the abdomen, is most often due to tension on the stoma. (Image from "Stoma Retraction and Stenosis," [34] license obtained)

High Ileostomy Output, Dehydration, Acute Kidney Injury (AKI)

High ileostomy output can cause dehydration, electrolyte imbalances, and acute kidney injury.

Dehydration due to high ileostomy output, considered higher than 1.2–1.5 L in a 24-h period, impacts *20–30% of patients and is the primary reason patients with ileostomies get readmitted to the hospital* [16]. Initial management involves consuming smaller, more frequent meals, and consuming less insoluble fiber, such as kale, and corn and more starchy foods, such as potatoes and bananas.

If dietary changes do not reduce output, dietary ***fiber*** *(psyllium) should be introduced to bulk and thicken output.* If output does not thicken with fiber, *antimotility agents* can be added to slow stool transit time so the bowel may reabsorb more water [17]. Medications including (interestingly) **proton pump inhibitors, loperamide (Imodium), diphenoxylate and atropine (Lomotil),** and finally **tincture of opium** or **codeine** may be added in a stepwise fashion. It is important to note that each additional medication should be added to the existing regimen rather than *replacing* the prior medications. Loperamide should be initiated at 2 mg four times daily, and be cautiously titrated up to 8 mg four times daily; loperamide should be administered before meals and before bedtime. Diphenoxylate-atropine can be started at 2.5 mg Diphenoxylate/0.025 mg atropine (combined as one tablet) four times per day, and increased to 20 mg/0.2 mg daily, usually divided into two tablets four times daily, similarly given before meals and at bedtime. Tincture of opium, while used rarely, can be started at 0.3 ml and titrated up to 1 ml four times daily, again given before meals and at bedtime (Fig. 23.6).

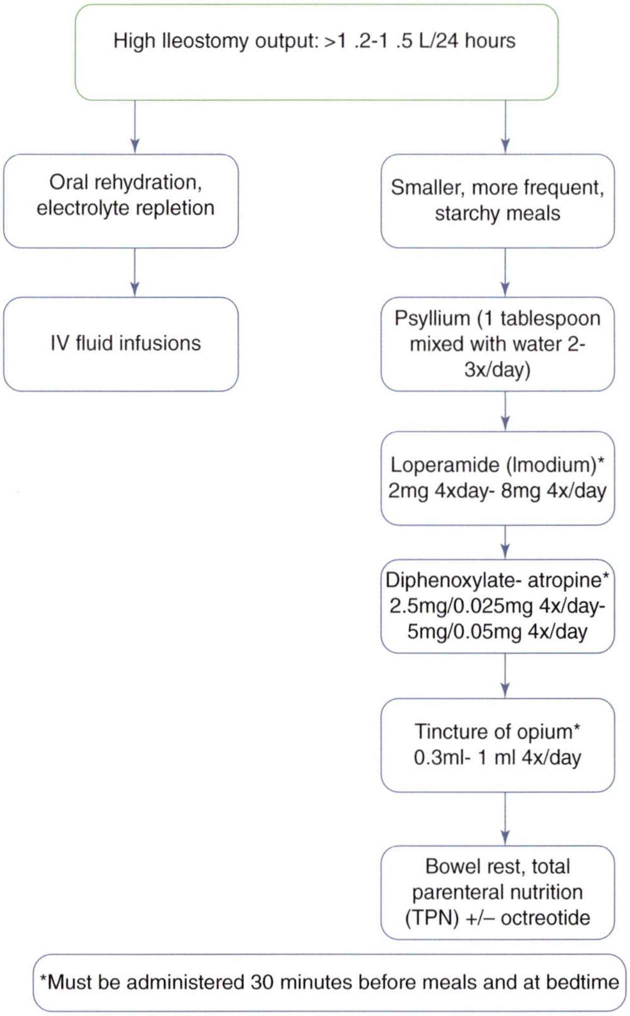

Fig. 23.6 Algorithm for treating high ileostomy output; rehydration should take place in parallel with sequentially adding medications to slow output

Rehydration should take place in parallel with the addition and titration of output-slowing medications as above (Fig. 23.6). Oftentimes, high ileostomy output in the absence of acute kidney injury (AKI) can be managed in the outpatient setting with careful recording of ostomy output and frequent communication with clinic providers. In the case of dehydration, electrolyte derangements, or AKI, readmission to the hospital may be warranted. Initial management should include intravenous and oral fluid resuscitation and correction of electrolytes. In rare instances, home intravenous fluid infusions can be arranged, or patients may be able get intravenous fluid infusions at clinics or infusion centers. Additionally, if ileostomy output does not decrease with the above interventions, patients may occasionally require bowel rest and total parenteral nutrition (TPN), with possible adjunctive **octreotide.**

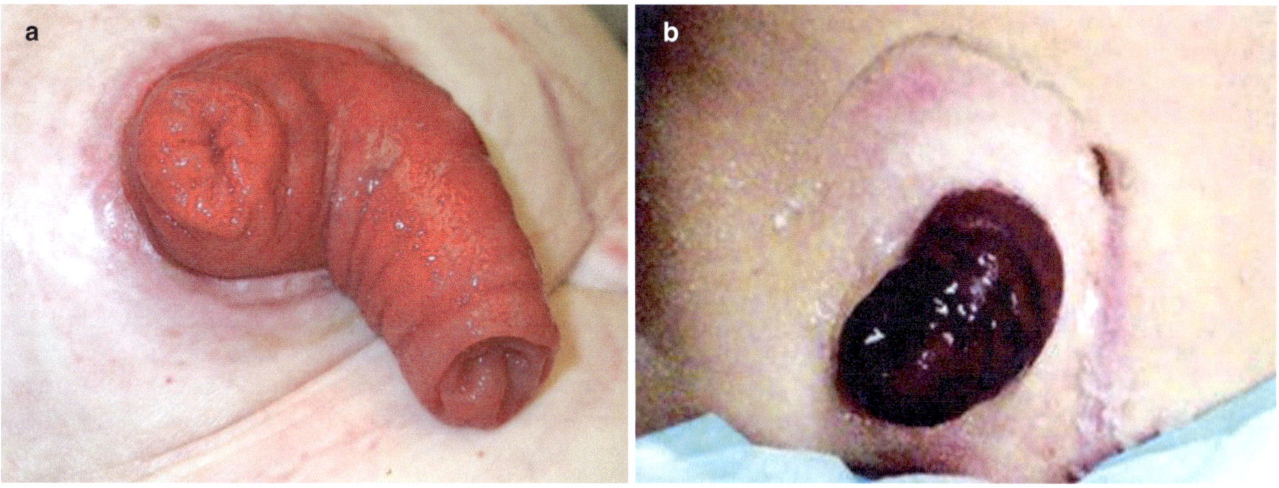

Fig. 23.7 (**a**) Prolapse of a loop stoma, without ischemia or necrosis. (**b**) Ischemic prolapsed stoma, which is a stoma emergency. (Image a from "Stoma Prolapse" [35] (2019) and b image from "Stoma Prolapse" [36] (2011), license obtained)

Late Complications

Prolapse

Stoma prolapse occurs when intra-abdominal bowel telescopes through and beyond the ***os*** (opening) of the *stoma* (Fig. 23.7). *Loop transverse colostomies have the highest risk of prolapse, and end ileostomies have the lowest risk.* Prolapse can have a range of associated complications, including pouching challenges, peristomal skin irritation, bowel wall edema, and incarceration and strangulation with mesenteric vascular compromise.

Bedside reduction of viable, prolapsed bowel can be performed with analgesia, anxiolytics, and **table sugar placed** on the bowel wall to *absorb water and reduce edema* via *an* ***osmotic gradient.*** Continuous manual pressure can be applied to the tip of the prolapsed bowel with the goal of inverting the bowel and encouraging it back into the abdomen. A stoma belt or abdominal binder may be helpful to prevent recurrent prolapse. A truly incarcerated or strangulated prolapsed stoma requires an emergent return to the operating room for either local or intra-abdominal revision, or even reversal if medically appropriate (Fig. 23.7).

Parastomal Hernia

Parastomal hernias occur when bowel not associated with the stoma protrudes through the stoma trephine, causing a bulge under the skin adjacent to the stoma (Fig. 23.8). Colostomies have a higher risk of parastomal hernia than ileostomies, but parastomal hernias are common among both; *up to 48% of patients with a stoma will develop a parastomal hernia over the course of the stoma's lifetime* [18]. Risk factors for parastomal hernias include obesity, steroid use, advanced age, and chronic cough [19]. *Parastomal hernias that are reducible and asymptomatic may be observed.* However, if patients experience symptoms or complications, including incarceration or bowel obstruction, parastomal hernia repair and resiting of the stoma elsewhere may be required.

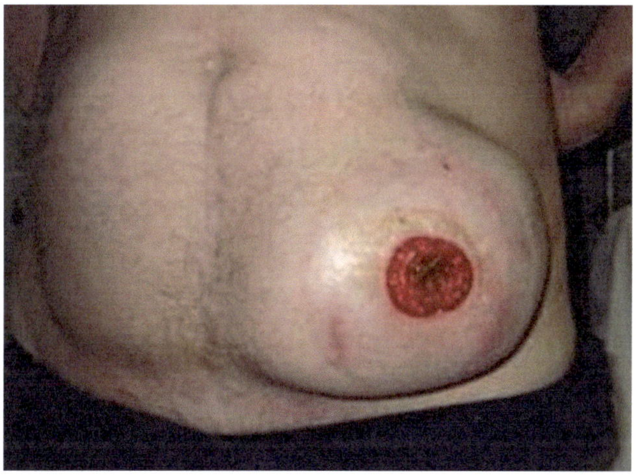

Fig. 23.8 Parastomal hernia visible as a bulge underneath the skin associated with the stoma. (Image from "Case on Parastomal Hernia Complications," [37] license obtained)

Stoma Reversal

Preoperative Planning.

Prior to loop stoma closure, the integrity of the anastomosis and distal bowel should be evaluated to assess for ongoing pathology, strictures, and leaks. Methods of examination may include digital rectal exam, rectal exam under anesthesia, proctoscopy, flexible sigmoidoscopy, and contrast enema imaging studies [20, 21]. One meta-analysis found that **contrast enema studies** had concordant results to the aforementioned examinations in 96.7% of patients, suggesting it is a reasonable and safe method to examine the distal bowel [22]. Most practitioners first evaluate the anastomosis with contrast enema studies, and if no pathology is identified, subsequently proceed to endoscopic evaluation (i.e., flexible sigmoidoscopy).

Technique

Loop stomas are closed by dissecting the bowel away from the skin, subcutaneous tissue, and fascia of the abdominal wall. The two ends of the bowel are either sewn or stapled together [23, 24]. The anastomosed bowel is then returned to the abdomen. Because both lumens of the bowel are already located at the abdominal wall, loop stomas are significantly easier to reverse than end stomas.

End stomas are reversed by freeing the stoma from the soft tissue and anastomosing to the distal bowel in the abdomen. In order to achieve this, the distal bowel must be located and dissected free from surrounding tissues laparoscopically, robotically, or with an open laparotomy incision. If the distal bowel was matured into a mucous fistula, it can be dissected free in the same manner as the end stoma. End stoma reversal can be more technically challenging and complex due to dense adhesions, intra-abdominal or pelvic inflammation, and identification and mobilization of the distal bowel. End stoma reversal is associated with more complications, including higher anastomotic leakage, than loop stoma reversal [25].

In either case, the fascia is closed, and the skin at the prior stoma site can either be closed or left open to close by secondary intention, sometimes with a purse-string suture through the dermis to approximate the skin while still leaving a central opening for potential drainage [1].

Timing

Loop stomas are typically closed at 8–12 weeks after creation, by which time the initial distal anastomosis has ideally healed, or the pelvic sepsis or wound has resolved. Additionally, adhesions from the initial operation should be less dense by this time.

The timing of end stoma reversal depends on specific patient factors and disease processes. End colostomies for complicated sigmoid diverticulitis (Hartmann procedure) can be reversed anywhere from 3 months onwards, although the literature surrounding safe timing of reversal is conflicting. Some studies demonstrate increased complications with end stoma reversal earlier than 6 months, while others demonstrate worse outcomes with reversal later than 6 months [26–29].

Postoperatively, patients are typically admitted to the hospital until they have a return of bowel function, demonstrating that gas and stool are passing through the new anastomosis without issue.

Other Stomas: Ileal Conduit

All of the foregoing stomas divert fecal matter or succus through to the abdominal wall. However, there is a special type of stoma, known as an **ileal conduit** that diverts *urine* to the abdominal wall. In this case, a portion of the ileum is surgically connected to the ureters after bladder resection (usually for bladder cancer). Bladder cancer surgery is somewhat complex and is beyond the scope of this chapter, but it involves using a "borrowed" portion of the ilium, which is removed from the gastrointestinal tract and is referred to as a **conduit** (Fig. 23.9). The ureters that drain urine from the kidneys are connected to one end of the *ileal conduit* within the abdominal cavity, and the other end is matured to the skin, usually in the right abdomen. Up close, it exactly resembles an ileostomy, *but the output is urine and not gastrointestinal contents.* You may encounter patients with ileal conduits, and it is important that you are knowledgeable about this clinical entity.

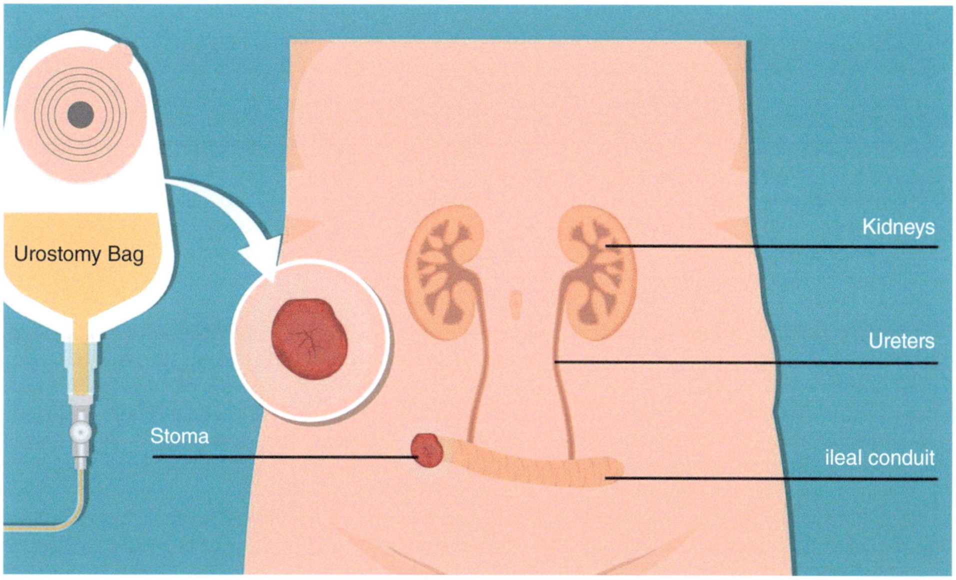

Fig. 23.9 A schematic representation of an *ileal conduit* is shown. An ileal conduit is a specialized segment of small bowel (ileum) that is used to divert urine into an appliance bag. Ileal conduits are an important way to divert urine after the bladder has been removed, often due to malignancy. The ileal conduit itself has been taken out of continuity from the gastrointestinal tract altogether, so there is no stool contents running through it

References

1. Davis BR, Valente MA, Goldberg JE, et al. The American Society of Colon and Rectal Surgeons Clinical Practice Guidelines for Ostomy Surgery. Dis Colon Rectum. 2022;65(10):1173–90. https://doi.org/10.1097/DCR.0000000000002498.
2. Kiela PR, Ghishan FK. Physiology of intestinal absorption and secretion. Best Pract Res Clin Gastroenterol. 2016;30(2):145–59. https://doi.org/10.1016/j.bpg.2016.02.007.
3. Azzouz LL, Sharma S. Physiology, large intestine. In: StatPearls. StatPearls Publishing; 2024. Accessed 5 Nov 2024. http://www.ncbi.nlm.nih.gov/books/NBK507857/
4. Kahai P, Mandiga P, Wehrle CJ, Lobo S. Anatomy, abdomen and pelvis: large intestine. In: StatPearls. StatPearls Publishing; 2024. Accessed 5 Nov 2024. http://www.ncbi.nlm.nih.gov/books/NBK470577/
5. Forsmo HM, Pfeffer F, Rasdal A, Sintonen H, Körner H, Erichsen C. Pre- and postoperative stoma education and guidance within an enhanced recovery after surgery (ERAS) programme reduces length of hospital stay in colorectal surgery. Int J Surg. 2016;36:121–6. https://doi.org/10.1016/j.ijsu.2016.10.031.
6. Harris MS, Kelly K, Parise C. Does preoperative ostomy education decrease anxiety in the new ostomy patient? A quantitative comparison cohort study. J Wound Ostomy Continence Nurs. 2020;47(2):137. https://doi.org/10.1097/WON.0000000000000623.
7. Hughes MJ, Cunningham W, Yalamarthi S. The effect of preoperative stoma training for patients undergoing colorectal surgery in an enhanced recovery programme. Ann R Coll Surg Engl. 2019;102(3):180. https://doi.org/10.1308/rcsann.2019.0145.
8. Stokes AL, Tice S, Follett S, et al. Institution of a preoperative stoma education group class decreases rate of Peristomal complications in new stoma patients. J Wound Ostomy Continence Nurs. 2017;44(4):363. https://doi.org/10.1097/WON.0000000000000338.
9. Alenezi A, McGrath I, Kimpton A, Livesay K. Quality of life among ostomy patients: a narrative literature review. J Clin Nurs. 2021;30(21–22):3111–23. https://doi.org/10.1111/jocn.15840.
10. Hsu MY, Lin JP, Hsu HH, Lai HL, Wu YL. Preoperative stoma site marking decreases stoma and Peristomal complications: a meta-analysis. J Wound Ostomy Continence Nurs. 2020;47(3):249. https://doi.org/10.1097/WON.0000000000000634.
11. Salvadalena G, Hendren S, McKenna L, et al. WOCN society and ASCRS position statement on preoperative stoma site marking for patients undergoing colostomy or ileostomy surgery. J Wound Ostomy Continence Nurs. 2015;42(3):249. https://doi.org/10.1097/WON.0000000000000119.
12. The effectiveness of preoperative stoma site marking on patient outcomes: A systematic review and meta-analysis–Kim 2021 J Adv Nurs—Wiley Online Library. Accessed 4 Nov 2024. https://onlinelibrary.wiley.com/doi/10.1111/jan.14915
13. Erwin-Toth P, Thompson SJ, Davis JS. Factors impacting the quality of life of people with an ostomy in North America: results from the dialogue study. J Wound Ostomy Continence Nurs. 2012;39(4):417. https://doi.org/10.1097/WON.0b013e318259c441.
14. Stelton S. CE: stoma and Peristomal skin care: a clinical review. AJN Am J Nurs. 2019;119(6):38. https://doi.org/10.1097/01.NAJ.0000559781.86311.64.
15. Harris D, Egbeare D, Jones S, Benjamin H, Woodward A, Foster M. Complications and mortality following stoma formation. Ann R Coll Surg Engl. 2005;87(6):427–31. https://doi.org/10.1308/003588405X60713.
16. Messaris E, Sehgal R, Deiling S, et al. Dehydration is the Most common indication for readmission after diverting ileostomy creation. Dis Colon Rectum. 2012;55(2):175. https://doi.org/10.1097/DCR.0b013e31823d0ec5.
17. Boutté HJ, Poylin V. High ileostomy output: a practical review of pathophysiology, causes, and management☆. Semin Colon Rectal Surg. 2023;34(2):100955. https://doi.org/10.1016/j.scrs.2023.100955.
18. Carne PWG, Robertson GM, Frizelle FA. Parastomal hernia. Br J Surg. 2003;90(7):784–93. https://doi.org/10.1002/bjs.4220.
19. Gillern S, Bleier JIS. Parastomal hernia repair and reinforcement: the role of biologic and synthetic materials. Clin Colon Rectal Surg. 2014;27(4):162. https://doi.org/10.1055/s-0034-1394090.
20. Lindner S, Eitelbuss S, Hetjens S, et al. Less is more-the best test for anastomotic leaks in rectal cancer patients prior to ileostomy reversal. Int J Color Dis. 2021;36(11):2387–98. https://doi.org/10.1007/s00384-021-03963-1.

21. Larsson A, Lindmark G, Syk I, Buchwald P. Water soluble contrast enema examination of the integrity of the rectal anastomosis prior to loop ileostomy reversal may be superfluous. Int J Color Dis. 2015;30(3):381–4. https://doi.org/10.1007/s00384-014-2113-6.
22. Habib K, Gupta A, White D, Mazari FAK, Wilson TR. Utility of contrast enema to assess anastomotic integrity and the natural history of radiological leaks after low rectal surgery: systematic review and meta-analysis. Int J Color Dis. 2015;30(8):1007–14. https://doi.org/10.1007/s00384-015-2225-7.
23. Hand-Sewn versus Stapled Closure of Loop Ileostomy: A Meta-Analysis | Digestive Surgery | Karger Publishers. Accessed 5 Nov 2024. https://karger.com/dsu/article/36/3/183/118294/Hand-Sewn-versus-Stapled-Closure-of-Loop-Ileostomy
24. Löffler T, Rossion I, Gooßen K, et al. Hand suture versus stapler for closure of loop ileostomy—a systematic review and meta-analysis of randomized controlled trials. Langenbeck's Arch Surg. 2015;400(2):193–205. https://doi.org/10.1007/s00423-014-1265-8.
25. Bruns BR, DuBose J, Pasley J, et al. Loop versus end colostomy reversal: has anything changed? Eur J Trauma Emerg Surg. 2015;41(5):539–43. https://doi.org/10.1007/s00068-014-0444-1.
26. Menahem B, Lubrano J, Vallois A, Alves A. Early closure of defunctioning loop ileostomy: is it beneficial for the patient? A meta-analysis. World J Surg. 2018;42(10):3171–8. https://doi.org/10.1007/s00268-018-4603-0.
27. Resio BJ, Jean R, Chiu AS, Pei KY. Association of timing of colostomy reversal with outcomes following Hartmann procedure for diverticulitis. JAMA Surg. 2019;154(3):218–24. https://doi.org/10.1001/jamasurg.2018.4359.
28. Hallam S, Mothe BS, Tirumulaju RMR. Hartmann's procedure, reversal and rate of stoma-free survival. Ann R Coll Surg Engl. 2018;100(4):301. https://doi.org/10.1308/rcsann.2018.0006.
29. Aljorfi AA, Alkhamis AH. A systematic review of early versus late closure of loop ileostomy. Surg Res Pract. 2020;2020(1):9876527. https://doi.org/10.1155/2020/9876527.
30. McGee MF, Cataldo PA. Intestinal stomas. In: Steele SR, Hull TL, Read TE, Saclarides TJ, Senagore AJ, Whitlow CB, editors. The ASCRS textbook of colon and Rectal surgery. Springer International Publishing; 2016. p. 971–1013. https://doi.org/10.1007/978-3-319-25970-3_55.
31. Weber K. Ileostomies and colostomies. In: Hohenberger W, Parker M, editors. Lower gastrointestinal tract surgery: Vol. 2, Open Procedures. Springer International Publishing; 2021. p. 183–206. https://doi.org/10.1007/978-3-030-60827-9_8.
32. Garofalo T. Colostomy: types, indications, formation, and reversal. In: Fazio VW, Church JM, Wu JS, editors. Atlas of intestinal stomas. Springer US; 2012. p. 127–45. https://doi.org/10.1007/978-0-387-78851-7_11.
33. LeBlanc K, Wiesenfeld L. Local Peristomal cutaneous manifestations and their management. In: Alavi A, Maibach HI, editors. Local wound care for dermatologists. Springer International Publishing; 2020. p. 153–62. https://doi.org/10.1007/978-3-030-28872-3_16.
34. Tankel J, Edden Y. Stoma retraction and stenosis. In: Steele SR, Maykel JA, Wexner SD, editors. Clinical decision making in colorectal surgery. Springer International Publishing; 2020. p. 623–8. https://doi.org/10.1007/978-3-319-65942-8_79.
35. Steinhagen E, Steele SR. Stoma Prolapse. In: Lee SW, Steele SR, Feingold DL, Ross HM, Rivadeneira DE, editors. Colorectal surgery consultation: tips and tricks for the management of operative challenges. Springer International Publishing; 2019. p. 217–22. https://doi.org/10.1007/978-3-030-11181-6_49.
36. Szmulowicz UM, Hull TA. Stoma Prolapse. In: Fazio VW, Church JM, Wu JS, editors. Atlas of intestinal stomas. Springer US; 2012. p. 249–72. https://doi.org/10.1007/978-0-387-78851-7_22.
37. Hansson BME. Case on Parastomal hernia complications. In: Case studies of postoperative complications after digestive surgery. Cham: Springer; 2014. p. 513–6. https://doi.org/10.1007/978-3-319-01613-9_94.

Large Bowel Versus Small Bowel Obstruction

24

Sam Atallah

Introduction

Obstruction can affect both the large and small intestine [1, 2]. Obstructions of the large intestine (colorectum) and those of the small bowel (mainly the ileum and jejunum) present quite differently and have important, clinically relevant characteristics that must be understood. In this chapter, we will discuss small bowel obstruction (SBO) and large bowel obstruction (LBO) separately. Then, we will compare and contrast the two types of obstruction to provide a clear contrast between the two. Mastery of this topic comes from being able to understand the key *differences* between them. While LBO is less common than SBO, both are important presentations that practicing physician assistants (PAs) may encounter, particularly on a surgical service and in an acute care setting.

Part I: Small Bowel Obstruction (SBO)

Anatomic Considerations

There are three segments to the small intestine: the *duodenum, jejunum,* and *ileum.* In aggregate, the length of the small intestine measures about 10 ft. (120 in/300 cm). The duodenum is the shortest segment of the small intestine and is only *rarely* the site of small bowel obstruction. The last portion of the *ileum* (just before the ileocecal valve) is referred to as the *terminal ileum*, and this segment is particularly prone to disease processes (most notably Crohn's), but it is also *often* the site of obstruction. This obstruction can be secondary to intrinsic disease of the small intestine (*e.g.,* Crohn' s-related stricture) or more classically small bowel *adhesions.* Abdominal wall *hernias* are an important cause of small bowel obstruction. **In all, hernias and small bowel adhesions are the most important causes of SBO.**

Etiology

Small bowel ***adhesions,*** often also referred to as *scar tissue*, are the most important cause of SBO in patients who have had prior surgery [3, 4]. This is particularly true for patients who have had prior *open* surgery and/or *pelvic* surgery; these tend to result in the formation of adhesions that can lead to bowel obstruction. The surgery need not be recent, and a remote history of abdominal surgery can still be the cause, so it is important to ask your patients about their complete past surgical history.

What exactly are small bowel adhesions? Adhesions are fibrous collagen bands that can take on many shapes and forms (Fig. 24.1). Interestingly, they cannot *themselves* be directly detected on plain films or even CT-body imaging. The adhesions simply do not show up. However, we can see the *effect* of the obstruction caused by these adhesions (see later).

Since you may not be familiar with adhesions, let us use a couple of analogies to improve your understanding of them. Imagine the small bowel as being slippery, and always slipping and sliding around, similar to how spaghetti slips and slides on a plate as you try to put it on your fork. That is what the small bowel is very much like normally. Now imagine that plate of spaghetti sitting out for two days, and the noodles are stuck to one another, and they no longer slip and slide freely. That is exactly how adhesions behave; they stick the loops of small bowel to one another. Note that making the intestines more "sticky" does not necessarily cause an obstruction, and most patients who have had prior surgery,

S. Atallah (✉)
Department of Surgery, Piedmont Hospital, Mercer University School of Medicine, Macon, GA, USA
e-mail: atallah@post.harvard.edu

S. Atallah, J. Dragoljevic (eds.), *Fundamentals of Surgery for Physician Assistants*,
https://doi.org/10.1007/978-3-032-21069-2_24

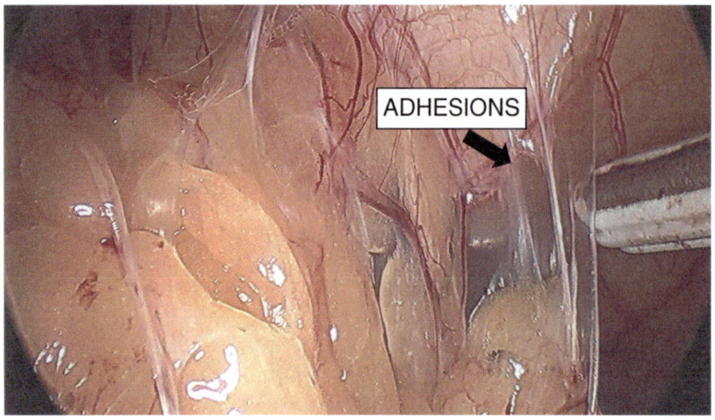

Fig. 24.1 Adhesions take on many forms and varying densities. Shown here is a laparoscopic view of "soft" adhesions from the omentum to the anterior abdominal wall. Adhesions are not *directly* visible on CT-scans or other imaging, but when they cause small bowel obstruction, the *effect* of the adhesions is clearly observed

especially minimally invasive surgery, do not go on to develop SBO.

So how exactly do adhesions cause an obstruction? For this, let us remind ourselves that the small bowel (in particular, the jejunum and *ileum*) is constantly sliding freely. Let us now imagine the small bowel is like a long garden hose moving freely along a grassy field. Imagine that a single adhesion forms a "band"—which can often resemble a tight and taut chord. This chord-like adhesion can sometimes "snag" the squirmy small bowel just like a garden hose can snag, for example, a fence post, causing the hose to kink. Anyone who has watered the lawn is familiar with this and knows the kink in the hose causes the water to suddenly stop coming out. Such kinks in the small bowel are exactly the mechanism of SBO due to adhesions.

Hernias of the abdominal wall represent defects of the abdominal wall through which small bowel can "escape" and slip into. Many times, the small bowel can be reduced back into the abdominal cavity with gentle manual pressure; in other instances, the small bowel is not reducible and is permanently "stuck" or **incarcerated** within the hernia sac. In many instances, even incarcerated small bowel, especially when it is situated within a wide-mouth hernia, will not cause an obstruction, but other times, an obstruction due to kinking of the small bowel can happen. This results in a small bowel obstruction [5].

Presenting Symptoms (General)

Regardless of etiology, all SBO patients present with the same constellation of symptoms—(**a**) bilious emesis, (**b**) decreased or absent flatus, and (**c**) decreased or absent bowel movements. Patients may also report feeling bloated with intermittent cramping abdominal pain. *These are the most important symptoms to elucidate from a patient suspected of having SBO.*

While *nausea and vomiting* are quite pedestrian complaints, encountered daily by providers, particularly in acute care settings, the type of vomiting—namely, **bilious**—*differentiates patients with obstruction from virtually all other types of patients.* Thus, for any patient with emesis who is encountered, one of the first questions about the emesis is: *what color is it?* While patients may not always be the best historians, they tend to always know the color of their emesis and are happy to report this to their healthcare provider, so do not forget to ask them!

Nonbilious emesis is usually described by patients as brown, yellow, mucus-like, containing bits of undigested food, watery, or reddish in color. In contradistinction, patients with emesis from obstruction will always describe their emesis as a **dark color green.** As a footnote, bile is actually not green but gold in color in its pure form (within the biliary tree); it turns green in color after mixing with the products of digestion within the small intestine. For all intents and purposes, bilious emesis is green, and particularly a very **dark green.** Because bilious emesis is by definition intestinal content that originates distal to the pylorus, it is often referred to as **postpyloric emesis**; emesis proximal to the pylorus is simply referred to as **gastric emesis**. These are common terms used in clinical practice.

It is important to know and document when the symptoms started, as this is an indication of when the obstruction began, which is important to surgeons. Questions include, *"when was your last bowel movement?"* and *"when was the last time you passed gas?"* In patients with emesis, it is also important to know *when* this began. The answers to these questions are **very important** to convey to the treating surgeon.

Abdominal pain is not uncommon, although severe abdominal pain is atypical for uncomplicated SBO. Patients usually describe abdominal **cramping** that comes on suddenly and occurs frequently. This is most likely related to the small bowel trying to push contents through the point of obstruction.

General Physical Exam Findings

Patients with SBO often have significant abdominal distension and sometimes tenderness upon palpation. However, peritoneal findings and severe tenderness would be *atypical* and may indicate bowel perforation and/or another, more serious condition necessitating immediate surgical consultation. As a rule of thumb, ***peritoneal findings on physical examination mandate surgical intervention.*** Stated differently, ***peritonitis implies a surgical abdomen.***

The abdomen is often *tympanic* upon percussion, and auscultation can reveal *high-pitched bowel sounds* as the fluid, known as **succus** within the intestine tries to "squeeze through" the point of obstruction.

Exam Findings Related to Hernias

Hernias are an important cause of SBO, and careful examination of the abdominal wall for hernias is an important part of the assessment, and this must include evaluation of the inguinal region bilaterally. Unlike adhesions, which cannot be seen by physical exam or even CT-body imaging, hernias are often quite visible and easily assessed by palpation. The most common hernia sites are umbilical, inguinal, and, in patients who have had prior surgery, incisional; in elderly females, ***femoral* hernias are most common**.

Imaging to Diagnosis SBO

SBO can be diagnosed with abdominal **plain films**—*i.e.*, an abdominal series. An abdominal series includes an Anterior–Posterior (AP) abdominal X-ray in the supine position, a Posterior–Anterior (PA) image with the patient erect, as well as an upright, PA chest radiograph, to check for **pneumoperitoneum**, which appears as *air under the diaphragm.* In some instances, SBO can lead to perforation of the intestine, which can be detected as pneumoperitoneum—which is a **surgical emergency.**

The pattern seen on plain films for patients with SBO is quite classic and includes *air-fluid levels* often observed in a "stair-step" or "stack of coins" pattern (Fig. 24.2). Additionally, there is an absence of gas within the rectum.

While pain films can determine *whether or not* a patient has SBO, to determine *the level* (specific point) of obstruction, a **CT-scan of the abdomen and pelvis is required**. The location of obstruction is described by radiologists as a **transition point,** whereby the proximal dilated bowel proximal to the blockage point is dilated and then it suddenly "transitions" to a normal caliber. CT-scans should be ordered with water-soluble oral contrast as well as IV contrast, assuming normal renal function and assuming the patient does not have an allergy to contrast dye or iodine.

Treatment for SBO Due to Adhesions

Nearly **80% of SBO due to adhesions will resolve with conservative therapy** (*i.e.,* nonoperative management). Conservative therapy includes discontinuing oral intake and transitioning to intravenous fluid resuscitation—typically using a maintenance crystalloid fluid, such as $D_5$1/2 Normal Saline (NS) with 20 mEq KCL, often for adults at an infusion rate of ~125 ml/hr.

In addition, a nasogastric (NG) tube should be placed to low wall suction for **decompression.** NG tubes effectively

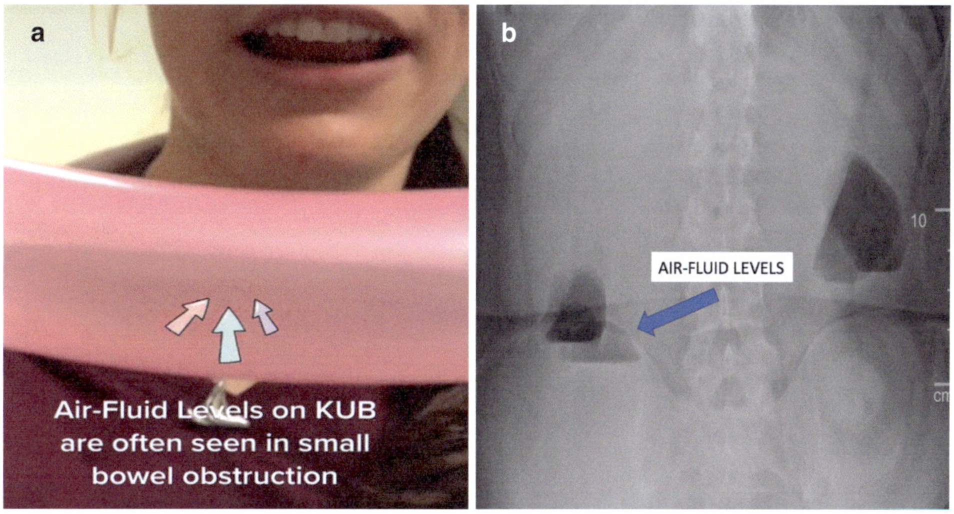

Fig. 24.2 (**a**) A party balloon is a useful analogy to understand air-fluid levels in the context of SBO. Think of the normal small bowel as a party balloon filled with water. Now imagine overfilling the balloon with air. What do you get? If you hold the balloon horizontally, due to gravity, the water layers inferiorly leaving a straight line between water and air. Thus, air-fluid levels, when observed on plain roentgenograms, are highly suggestive of a blockage. (**b**) An upright abdominal roentgenogram demonstrating air (black) fluid (white) levels with the classic *sharp horizontal line* separating the two

suction out the "backed up" bilious fluid, thus *decompressing the intestinal tract.* This backed-up fluid causes the intestines not only to "swell" or dilate, but importantly, it creates small bowel wall **edema.** When the bowel wall swells and becomes edematous, *it further narrows the lumen of the bowel at the site of obstruction, exacerbating the problem of obstruction.*

Let us use another helpful analogy. Think of a ring that is stuck on a swollen finger. You try to remove it, but every time you do, the finger just swells up even more, making it seem impossible (Fig. 24.3). The trick to getting the ring off is to decrease the swelling. The same trick is used to get rid of an obstruction, only here we are using NG tube decompression to limit bowel wall swelling. With bowel rest, hydration, NG tube decompression, and—perhaps the most important ingredient of all, *time,* SBO—can often resolve without the need for surgical intervention [6–8].

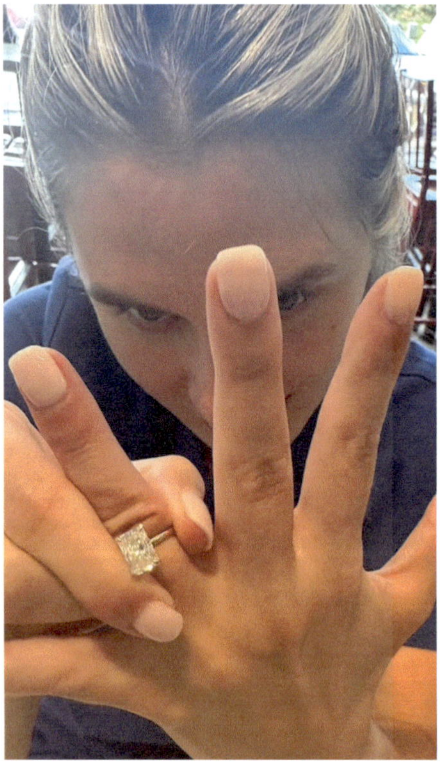

Fig. 24.3 Have you ever struggled to try to remove a ring from your finger? The more you try, the more your finger swells, and the more difficult it becomes. Just like a finger needs a "rest" to diminish the swelling, so, too, does the small intestine when it becomes swollen as a consequence of obstruction. NG tube decompression and bowel rest help reduce the bowel wall's swelling so that contents can flow through, resolving the obstruction without having to resort to surgical intervention

Treatment for SBO Due to Hernias

Remember, hernias cause SBO when a loop of small bowel slips into the hernia sac, causing it to kink. Going back to our prior analogy, this is similar to how a garden hose kinks, causing cessation of content flow and thus blockage. SBO due to hernias poses a special problem for the clinician who must determine whether or not the hernia can be manually reduced to resolve the blockage. Ideally, the hernia can just be reduced with slow, steady manual pressure and the problem solved. But there are two concerns. First, the hernia may not be able to be reduced manually, at which point surgical intervention is needed. Second, and more importantly, *the hernia may contain a strangulated loop of bowel, which should* ***not*** *be reduced.* The reason for this is that strangulated bowel may be ischemic and nonviable (Fig. 24.4). Nonviable bowel cannot be "reduced" as it will perforate and lead to other serious complications, including sepsis.

Many hernias can contain small bowel viscera, and the bowel is not threatened, even when the hernia contains loops of bowel for a long period of time—a so-called **chronically incarcerated hernia**. The hernia poses a problem when there is **obstruction,** at that time, **strangulation** has to be ruled out.

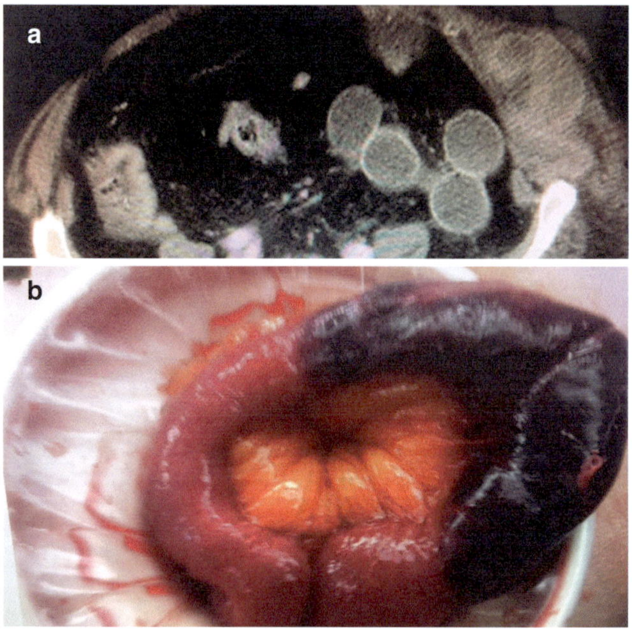

Fig. 24.4 Managing SBO due to *hernias* is different than managing SBO due to *adhesive* SBO, especially due to the risk of strangulated intestine. (**a**) An axial view from a CT-body image shows a loop of small bowel *outside* the abdominal cavity in a patient with an incarcerated and strangulated incisional hernia that has also led to SBO. (**b**) As operation, a devitalized, necrotic segment of small bowel (which had been strangulated within a narrow-neck hernia) is encountered and resected

How do hernias with strangulated loop(s) of bowel present? Strangulated small bowel often leads to *severe pain* at the hernia site along with skin changes, including *erythema* and *warmth,* and *tenderness to touch.* ***If small bowel strangulation is suspected, do not attempt to reduce the hernia. This is contra-indicated.*** Notify a surgeon immediately, as an urgent operation is required.

Conservative Therapy and Patient Management

Patients with SBO require hospital admission. The treatment, as stated, is usually conservative. Typical management on rounds for the care team includes careful evaluation of fluid Ins and Outs (I/Os) with specific attention given to the *NG tube output volume and color.* High-grade SBO is usually associated with high-output from the NG, on the order of 800 ml–1200 ml/24 hr., while low-grade pSBO and resolving SBO will usually record volumes of <400 ml/24 hr. Electrolytes should be monitored and repleted as needed, in particular **Potassium**, as patients are prone to develop a hypokalemic, hypochloremic metabolic alkalosis; the astute clinician must closely monitor and correct electrolyte derangements.

On daily rounds, patients should be asked if they have experienced flatus or have had a bowel movement, both of which are important clinical findings. In fact, they are more significant than auscultation for "bowel sounds" and even abdominal X-ray films. For example, if a patient reports having flatus and bowel movements, this means the obstruction is resolving clinically, and whether or not bowel sounds are diminished/absent and what the X-ray image appears to show is less relevant, as actual *bowel function* trumps those factors.

If the obstruction appears to be resolving clinically, the NG-output will decrease and typically become less bilious. A decision will need to be made as to when to discontinue (DC) the NG tube and resume an oral diet. There is no hard and fast rule that dictates such decisions, and generally, the surgeon will decide when and if the NG tube is ready to be discontinued and/or, in some cases, transitioned from low-wall suction to gravity, or if the tube is going to simply be DC'd altogether. Some surgeons are quite particular about how the NG tube is managed, and as a rule of thumb, **check with the surgeon and surgical team before deciding to remove the tube.**

In most instances, after the NG tube is removed, patients will be started on a diet. Here, too, there is quite a bit of variability based on surgeon and location of practice. In many instances, however, the patient will be started on a *clear* liquid diet, and if tolerating this, advanced to a *full* liquid diet. The final step is some form of a *solid* food diet, which can include a "regular" diet, a "GI soft" diet, a "cardiac" diet, a "renal" diet, as well as other formulations. **Check with the surgeon when deciding on advancing the diet,** unless you are familiar with the surgeon's routines and protocols.

During the period of diet advancement, it is important to see that the patient continues to progress clinically. Specifically, bowel function should be documented, as well as clinical findings on abdominal exam. Signs the obstruction is resolving include continued bowel movements and flatus, absence of nausea or vomiting, and tolerance for oral intake. *Ask patients about their appetite,* if they say they are hungry, this is a very good sign that the obstruction is resolving, as **patients with chronic and unresolved obstruction usually lack appetite.**

Patients do not always progress along a smooth path, and there can be ups and downs in their clinical course. Sometimes there are setbacks, for example, requiring the NG tube to be replaced after it has been removed, as the obstructive symptoms can recur. In other instances, conservative therapy can altogether fail.

Failed Conservative Therapy

While conservative therapy is effective at resolving SBO for the majority of patients, it does not always work. It is important to be alert to the signs and symptoms of your patients on rounds. **When conservative therapy fails, operative intervention is the only recourse** [9–11].

Patients who fail to progress are those who do not pass flatus or have bowel movements. On physical exam, these patients classically exhibit increasing abdominal distention with high NG output *and* they often exhibit an overall worsening clinical picture. Serial roentgenograms (*e.g.,* abdominal series) may demonstrate progression rather than improvement of the SBO. **Failure to have any flatus or any bowel movement for a 24-hr period is highly concerning, and surgical intervention should be considered.** Although in recent years there has been a paradigm shift away from prior teachings to "never letting the sun rise on a bowel obstruction" [12], **a *complete* obstruction remains of great concern,** due to potential sequelae—including but not limited to perforation.

Although rare, SBO can result in intestinal perforation. This can often be documented by an *upright chest X-ray* ***as free air under the diaphragm*** and/or *peritonitis on abdominal examination*. **Either of which is an absolute indication for emergent surgery.** *Immediately notify the surgeon and surgical team if you encounter these findings.*

Special Circumstances

Readmissions for SBO

For patients with chronic and recurrent SBO, **surgery can be considered** instead of "another round" of conservative therapy. Some patients resolve their SBO, tolerate a diet, and are discharged from the hospital, only to present with recurrent SBO requiring readmission. This scenario is actually quite common. Other patients are well enough to be discharged, but they never resolve their symptoms completely. They may, for example, be able to tolerate a diet but have cramping abdominal pain that is unresolved, and they may have CT-imaging that reveals continued, at least partial SBO (pSBO).

While there is no absolute rule about when patients with chronic and or recurrent SBO require surgical intervention, it should be considered as a method of providing more definitive therapy. As an example, patients who present with four or five admissions for obstruction over a two-month period probably warrant surgery, while patients who have three admissions for SBO over five years likely do not. The number of hospital admissions with SBO before surgery is considered arbitrary, and this is a decision best made by the surgeon, patient, and care team [7–12].

Dietary Recommendations for Patients with Adhesions and Recurrent SBO

Many patients wonder about diet and are typically concerned that "something they ate" caused the bowel obstruction, and want advice about what foods to avoid and what ones are preventative for having an obstruction. However, food does not cause SBO—hernias and adhesions do. There is no proven effect of diet on bowel obstruction. Therefore, once the blockage has resolved, patients should be able to consume all major food groups without trepidation.

Surgery for SBO Due to Adhesions

Once a decision to operate is made, either a minimally invasive (*e.g.,* laparoscopic) or open operation is performed, and adhesions are divided and released surgically using sharp dissection. Occasionally, a small bowel resection may be required, and the decision for this is individualized and often made at the time of surgery by the surgeon. Division of adhesions is called **adhesiono*lysis***, and you will often see it abbreviated as **LOA**—**L**ysis **O**f **A**dhesions.

You might be asking yourself, if LOA fixes the problem of obstruction swiftly, then why not simply operate in the first place? There are important reasons *not* to proceed with surgical LOA. First, conservative therapy is highly effective, and **the majority of SBO resolves without the need for surgery.** Second, surgery carries important risks of complications (*e.g.,* wound infections, bowel injury, and anesthetic-related complications). Third, each time a patient undergoes abdominal surgery, the risk of new adhesion formation exists—making LOA a "catch-22." That is, *the act of dividing and freeing adhesions only creates new adhesions.*

Surgery for SBO Due to Hernia

When an obstruction is secondary to small bowel entrapped within a (typically) narrow-neck hernia, surgical consultation is required urgently. If there is no clinical evidence of blood flow compromise to the entrapped loop or loops of bowel, then attempts to reduce the hernia manually with or without sedation are reasonable. *However, if the incarcerated loop of bowel is strangulated, it should <u>not</u> be reduced, and urgent surgery is indicated.* At operation, if the loop of small bowel exhibits necrosis due to prolonged compromise

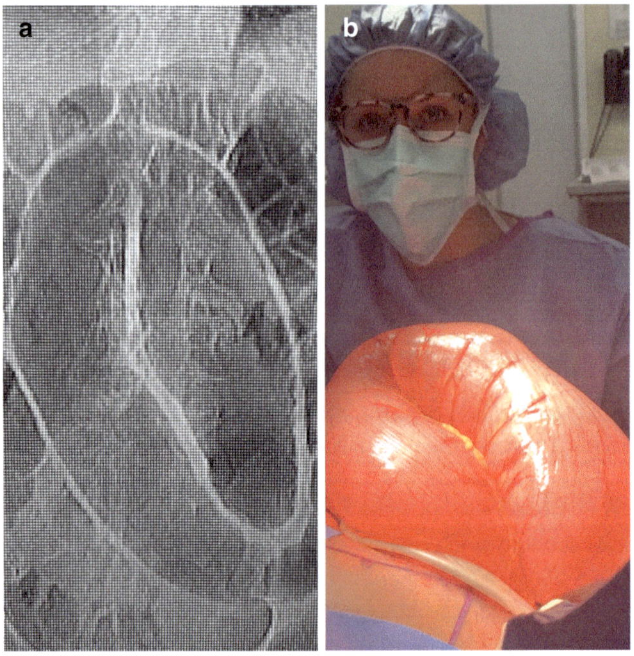

Fig. 24.5 Sigmoid volvulus, more common in the infirm and the elderly, is a twisting of the sigmoid colon upon its mesentery resulting in LBO. (**a**) An abdominal plain roentgenogram shows the silhouette of a quite dilated sigmoid colon that has volvulized. (**b**) While endoscopic decompression is the first step in management, this is not always successful, and resection is required. Shown at laparotomy in the sigmoid colon, twisted and markedly distended due to the distal obstruction

of the blood supply, then it is resected (Fig. 24.4). The hernia is also typically repaired, sometimes utilizing a biologic mesh to minimize the risk of infection if bowel resection is done at the same time. These decisions and the specifics of management are often individualized and are beyond the scope of this chapter.

Partial Versus Complete SBO

Obstructions of the intestinal tract can be partial or complete. A partial obstruction, often given the notation **p**SBO, means that some succus is making it through the point of obstruction. This is determined by the patient reporting some flatus and/or small bowel movements. Remember, *it is very important to ask about flatus as this is not something typically charted by nursing staff, and patients with flatus generally have pSBO and not complete SBO—which is more likely to resolve with conservative measures.*

"High-grade" obstructions clinically and radiographically are ominous findings and might imply the obstruction is not likely to resolve, and that surgical intervention is more probable. This is especially due to the risk of perforation of the bowel due to extreme dilation of the small intestine. *The surgeon is ultimately the one to decide whether or not to operate, and such a decision carefully examines the risk-to-benefit ratio.*

Part II: Large Bowel Obstruction (LBO)

LBO is quite different than SBO, not just by clinical findings but, importantly, by treatment and management [13, 14]. Table 24.1 highlights the important differences and similarities between the two entities. After you have read the section on LBO, spend time studying Table 24.1 by comparing and contrasting LBO and SBO to have a more complete understanding of the two.

Anatomic Considerations

Unlike the slippery and mobile "spaghetti-like" small intestine, the large intestine (colon and rectum) is *fixed* in many segments and for the most part does not move out of its place—this is particularly true for the ascending colon, hepatic flexure, splenic flexure, and descending colon which are fixed to the abdominal side wall, for example,

Table 24.1 Small bowel obstruction (SBO) versus large bowel obstruction (LBO)

Characteristic	SBO	LBO
Etiology	1. **Adhesions** (for patients with a prior surgical history) and 2. **Hernias** of the abdominal wall 3. Other causes: Small bowel tumor, Crohn's disease	Colorectal malignancy/**tumor**; less commonly, diverticular stricture and volvulus
Clinical presentation	**Bilious emesis;** diminished or no bowel activity (flatus/bowel movements); high-pitched bowel sounds on auscultation; abdominal distention; tympanic on percussion	Absent or decreased bowel activity (flatus/bowel movements); marked abdominal distention with or without tenderness; tympanic on percussion. ***Note: Emesis is not typically present***
Anatomic location of obstruction	Terminal *ileum most common*; jejunum also possible; duodenum, rare	Left side of the colon is the *most classic* (from the splenic flexure to the rectum)
Key findings on imaging	1. Plain films—dilated loops of bowel with air-fluid levels; "stack of coins"/"stair-stepping" 2. CT-imaging—Dilated loops of small bowel with a **transition point** to normal caliber	1. Plain films—colonic dilation, with **special attention to cecal diameter** 2. CT-imaging—Marked colonic dilation due to a "closed-loop"; **small bowel is normal caliber** when ileocecal valve is patent; **cecal diameter is key**
Treatment and management	1. For obstruction secondary to adhesions, **bowel rest is the rule** (nonoperative management) with IV fluid hydration, NG tube decompression, and NPO 2. For obstruction secondary to incarcerated hernia and when small bowel strangulation is suspected or present, operative intervention is mandatory; **attempts to reduce the strangulated bowel are contraindicated**	1. **Operative treatment is the rule, bowel rest does not resolve this type of obstruction;** alternatives to operative treatment include endoluminal stent placement in select settings 2. Operation may include resection of the primary tumor with diverting stoma, or just a diverting stoma initially
Utility of nasogastric (NG) tube decompression	Strongly recommended; small bowel obstruction results in HIGH bilious NG output; **decompression resolves obstruction likely by decreasing small bowel wall edema**	Low benefit, *except* in circumstances in which the IC valve is incompetent, as this can result in upstream small bowel dilation, **NG decompression will not resolve a closed-loop large bowel obstruction**
Special considerations	Excessive NG tube output can lead to **electrolyte derangements**, and monitoring with electrolyte repletion is recommended; fluid replacement should also be performed, typically 0.5 ml per 1.0 ml of NG output	***A closed-loop large bowel obstruction can lead to cecal perforation secondary to maximum wall tension (law of Laplace)***

via the *White Line of Toldt* as well as other embryonic fusion planes including attachments to the retroperitoneum. Thus, while the small bowel can twist and "kink" like a garden hose, the colon and rectum *do not generally kink and thus are not affected by adhesions (even severe ones) the way the small bowel is affected.* One important exception to this is **volvulus**, especially of the *sigmoid colon*, which can twist and kink, causing obstruction when it volvulizes (Figs. 24.5 and 24.6).

There are important and unique features of the large intestine that contribute to special problems in this portion of the alimentary tract. First, the colon is significantly wider than the small intestine, but more importantly, its diameter varies, with the *right side of the colon being wide, and the cecum being the widest.* The left side is relatively narrow, with the descending colon and sigmoid colon being the narrowest points of the large intestine before widening again as the sigmoid transitions to the rectum. Overall, **the cecum is the widest portion of the large intestine.** As we are about to see, this is a very important point that must be kept in mind in the assessment of patients with LBO.

The next important point is that the small bowel connects to the large intestine via the ileocecal (IC) valve. In the majority of patients, this valve is *competent,* allowing fluid (succus) to enter the colon in one direction, *without backflow* into the small bowel. **Thus, the IC valve behaves as a one-way valve.**

These anatomic features play an important role in our understanding of specific problems related to LBO. Specifically, these anatomic and physiologic findings will be applied to our understanding of a ***closed-loop* LBO,** *one of the most important large intestine emergencies.*

Etiology

The most likely cause of LBO is colon cancer. Tumors of the colon grow "from the inside out" as they always start on the innermost layer of the bowel, the mucosa. As tumors grow, they can narrow and obstruct the lumen of the large bowel (Fig. 24.6). In general, even large tumors of the right colon do not grow to the point of mechanical obstruction; however, when the lumen is narrower and the stool is more formed, mechanical blockage is not infrequently observed, and it can be a presenting symptom of locally advanced *left*-sided colon cancer. In particular, this includes cancers in the region of the splenic flexure, the descending colon, and the sigmoid colon.

There are other potential causes of LBO, and they include **sigmoid stricture** due to chronic and/or recurrent diverticulitis, **inflammatory bowel disease,** and rarely noncolonic primary malignancies such as lymphoma. Furthermore, in some instances, a floppy and redundant sigmoid colon can become incarcerated in an inguinal hernia, causing obstruction. As stated previously, **volvulus** of the sigmoid colon can cause the bowel to twist on itself, causing obstruction and even ischemia. Sigmoid volvulus can be recurrent, and

OBSTRUCTING COLON CANCER

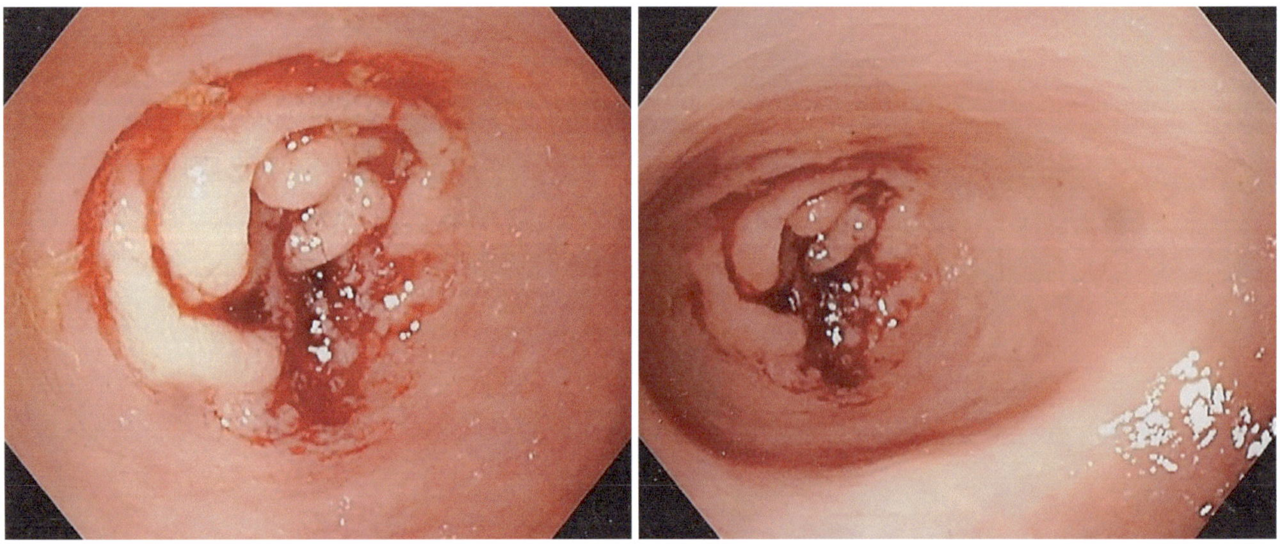

Fig. 24.6 Colonoscopic view of a large bowel obstructing cancer. The bowel is clearly distended and appears normal, up to a point that the lumen appears "sealed shut." Not only is the scope not able to advance beyond this point, but also no stool or even gas can escape, resulting in a complete LBO. This is an operative emergency (in special settings, endoluminal stenting can be considered as a bridge to surgery)

patients may present with symptoms that resolve spontaneously but tend to recur.

Presenting Symptoms

Patients with **LBO** present clinically the same as patients with **SBO**—with *one important exception.* LBO patients complain of abdominal bloating and distention, and generalized abdominal cramping pain is often reported. They, too, like their SBO counterparts, report having diminished bowel activity (*e.g.,* flatus and bowel movements). The important difference, however, is that the LBO patients do *not* typically present with nausea and bilious emesis—because, in most cases, the IC valve is competent, so there is not a backlog of small bowel contents like with SBO. Succus is able to be "forced through" the IC valve. While this is not an absolute finding, we can still say that, in general, ***patients with SBO present with bilious emesis, but patients with LBO do not.***

Physical Exam Findings

The abdomen is usually markedly distended, and overall, the abdominal exam findings are not different from those of patients with SBO, except high pitched bowel sounds are not typically auscultated. The abdomen is tympanic to percussion and mildly tender. Patients who have presented in a late state, however, may have already perforated their colon, in which case peritoneal findings are expected. Remember, *intestinal perforation represents a surgical emergency.*

Imaging

Plain films reveal moderate to severe colonic dilation, and this is also observed with CT-body imaging of the abdomen and pelvis, which will also reveal a transition point at the point of obstruction [15]. As we shall see, radiologists will always pay special attention to the amount of dilation of one part of the colon more than any other: **the cecum** [16, 17]. *The diameter of the cecum is crucial and has special implications for LBO, especially when there is a closed-loop obstruction.*

Closed-Loop LBO

One of the most important concepts in colorectal surgery to understand is the *closed-loop LBO.* This is predicated upon the anatomic findings discussed previously. Namely—(a) the

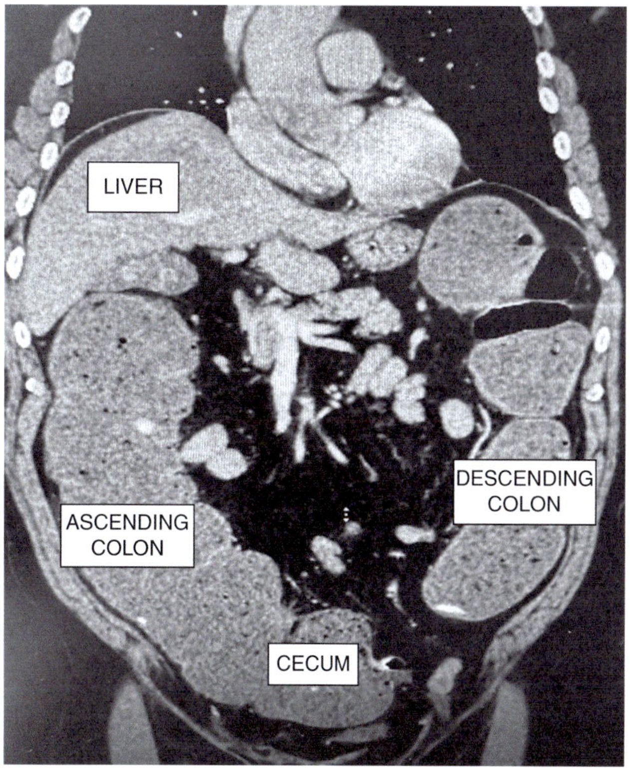

Fig. 24.7 A *closed-loop* large bowel obstruction is shown here in coronal view on CT-body imaging of the abdomen and pelvis. Note the severe dilation of the colon, but especially the cecum. Due to the competent ileocecal valve, the small bowel does not become dilated, which is why bilious emesis is not a typical symptom of LBO.

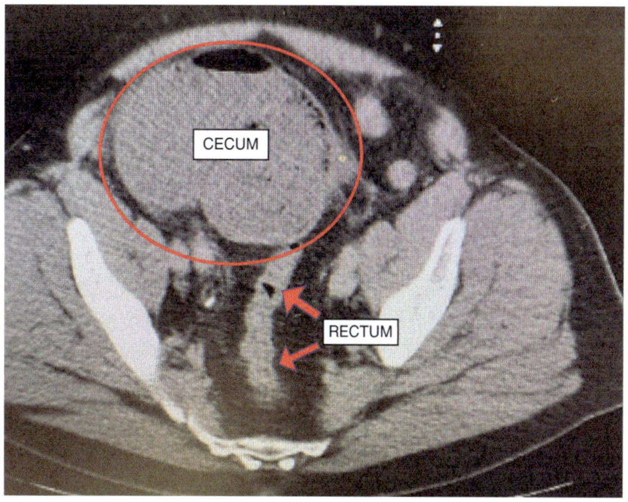

Fig. 24.8 This axial CT image from a patient with closed-loop large bowel obstruction is illustrative for two reasons. First, it shows the dramatic distension of the cecum. Second, it shows the rectum, which, in this example, is distal to the point of obstruction, so it appears not distended at all—or "decompressed." Due to Laplace's Law, the cecum is the portion of bowel most prone to perforation, even though the point of actual obstruction is at a far point, "downstream" from the cecum

cecum is the portion of the large bowel with the *widest diameter*, and (b) the IC valve functions as a *one-way* valve.

We can use an example to better understand this. Let us suppose there is a point of obstruction due to a tumor located on the left side of the large bowel. Let us suppose it is located in the descending colon and that this is completely obstructing the lumen. As the small bowel "dumps its contents" via the one-way IC valve into the colon, the wall becomes increasingly stretched and distended. Like a balloon, it expands, but not all of it expands. Only the part *up to* the tumor expands—making it a ***closed-loop*** LBO (Figs. 24.7 and 24.8). *Thus, the contents continue to build up within this "closed loop," and there is no way out.* As the colon expands, the cecum (being the largest diameter to start with) can reach a critical level of distension, potentially leading to perforation.

Why is this? We need to recall an important physics principle. Specifically, the **Law of Laplace,** which states that for a cylinder, **wall tension is proportional to the radius** [18, 19]. This can be expressed as follows:

$$\tau \propto \mathcal{R} \cdot \rho$$

Here, τ represents the *wall tension*, $\mathcal{R}$ the *radius*, ρ the *pressure gradient*. For all intents and purposes, the colon can be thought of as a cylinder. When a closed-loop LBO is present, it is the ***cecum (having the largest radius) that is at greatest risk for perforation.*** **Cecal diameter** is therefore given the <u>most attention</u> by clinicians, surgeons, and radiologists. Radiologists often *measure and record the cecal diameter* on their reports for this specific reason. Normal cecal diameter for an adult varies, but can be from **5–8 cm**; a cecal diameter of **9–12 cm** is *very* concerning and warrants careful attention and serial monitoring. Keep in mind: *the overall clinical picture is more important than the absolute numbers.*

Partial Versus Complete Obstruction

Colon cancer is the most important cause of LBO, but the obstruction is not *always* complete. The majority of patients, even those with relatively large tumors of the colon, do not present with *fully* obstructive symptoms. Even for patients with endoscopically near-complete obstruction, the treatment can be less urgent. As long as patients are able to tolerate a diet and have bowel activity, operative intervention is less urgent, and there is time to explore other modalities of cancer therapy before "rushing off" to surgery. These are complex decisions that are made by the cancer care team.

Many patients with partially obstructing tumors will present with changes in bowel habits, worsening constipation, and even diarrhea. Patients with complete LBO are patients who have no bowel activity (*i.e.,* bowel movements, flatus), and may or may not be able to tolerate oral intake. *They always require immediate surgical consultation and a swift disposition—there's no time to waste!* Complete LBO is usually determined by a combination of the CT-scan findings, clinical history, and physical exam findings. Radiologists often use the phrase *high-grade* obstruction rather than complete obstruction, because they do not have objective data about the patient *clinically.*

Treatment

As a rule, true high-grade LBO, *especially closed-loop LBO,* presents an urgent operative condition, and there is little/no benefit to conservative measures. Although adhesive SBO is managed primarily with conservative measures, this strategy will not resolve the blockage in the large bowel, especially when complete or nearly complete.

LBO requires immediate surgical consultation. The only alternative to operation is endoluminal stent placement (available only in some expert centers). Stent placement can be considered as an alternative and is mostly used as a *bridge to surgery* [20]. The decision for stenting versus surgical intervention is complex and beyond the scope of this chapter. **The key is to immediately *notify a surgeon if LBO is suspected and the patient is clinically obstructed.***

The type of operation performed for LBO is also beyond the scope of this chapter, and may include resection of the primary tumor and construction of colostomy or creation of a diverting colostomy alone. The specific etiology of LBO and its locale, as well as the patient's overall clinical condition at the time of intervention, dictate the operative approach.

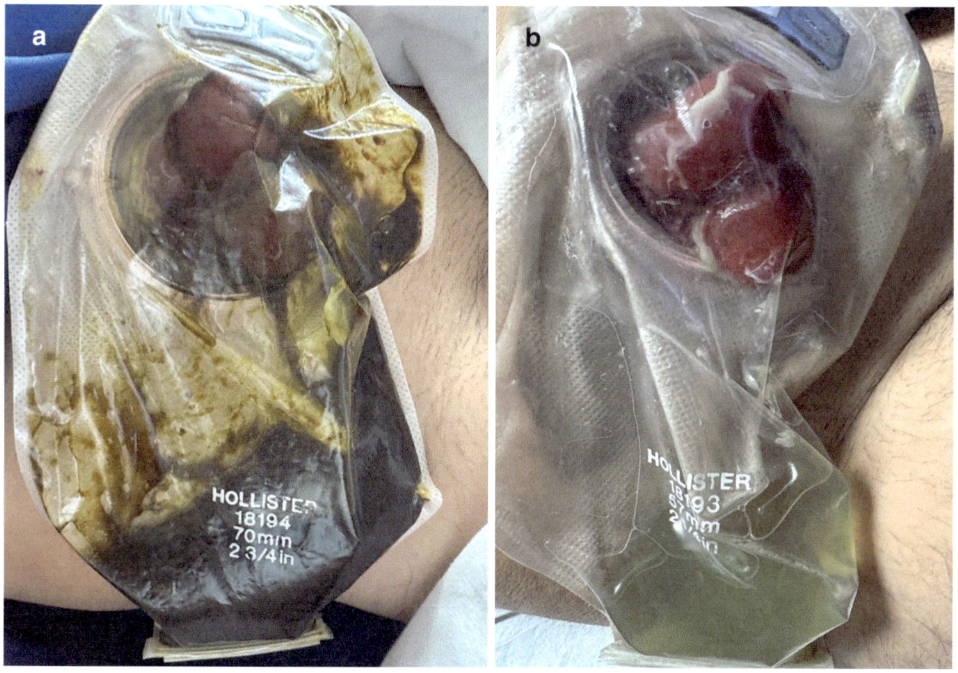

Fig. 24.9 Some patients may have an intestinal stoma or "ostomy." These can be ileostomies or colostomies. For obstructed patients who have ostomies, it is important to know how much and what type of output is being released into the stoma appliance. Gas output, bilious output (for ileostomies), and formed stool output (colostomies) should be noted. (**a**) A loop ileostomy has normal output, which appears dark green (the same color observed with bilious emesis as well). This output, together with gas in the stoma appliance, is considered normal. (**b**) A watery mucus-like output can be seen within the stoma appliance. This liquid output is *not* considered normal output and *is indicative of an ongoing bowel obstruction.* Always examine the output for character and color, do not rely on Ins/Outs charted as they can be misleading

Special Circumstances

Some patients may have a pre-existing stoma, such as an ileostomy or colostomy. For the most part, this means that rather than having stool output per rectum, the output all goes into an ostomy appliance, commonly referred to by laypeople as a "bag." For patients who have an ostomy, you want to ask them about the output and its consistency. Rather than flatus, you should ask if the stoma has had gas output. On exam, *check for visible gas within the stoma appliance.* You should also carefully check the color and consistency of the stool or succus contained within the stoma appliance.

Not all stoma output is "good output" as it depends on the quality and color. For example, if the stoma produces a watery or mucus-like clear output, this is not a sign of resolving obstruction and is usually the result of swollen and congested intestines (Fig. 24.9).

The advantage of patients with a stoma is that it is easy to monitor and even quantify both gas output and stool output. The disadvantage is that some kinds of output—watery and serosanguinous—may be charted by nursing personnel as "positive stoma output," misleading one to believe the obstruction is resolving, when in actuality it is not.

References

1. Griffiths S, Glancy DG. Intestinal obstruction. Surgery (Oxford). 2023;41(1):47–54.
2. Corral JG, Rojo CN, de la Fuente Olmos R. Bowel obstruction: signs indicating the need for urgent surgery. Radiología (English Edition). 2023;65:S92–8.
3. Köstenbauer J, Truskett PG. Current management of adhesive small bowel obstruction. ANZ J Surg. 2018;88(11):1117–22.
4. Tong JW, Lingam P, Shelat VG. Adhesive small bowel obstruction–an update. Acute Medicine & Surgery. 2020;7(1):e587.
5. Miller G, Boman J, Shrier I, Gordon PH. Etiology of small bowel obstruction. Am J Surg. 2000;180(1):33–6.
6. Hayanga AJ, Bass-Wilkins K, Bulkley GB. Current management of small-bowel obstruction. Adv Surg. 2005;39:1–33.
7. Fevang BT, Jensen D, Svanes K, Viste A. Early operation or conservative management of patients with small bowel obstruction? Eur J Surg. 2002;168(8–9):475–81.
8. Azagury D, Liu RC, Morgan A, Spain DA. Small bowel obstruction: a practical step-by-step evidence-based approach to evaluation, decision making, and management. J Trauma Acute Care Surg. 2015;79(4):661–8.
9. Diaz JJ Jr, Bokhari F, Mowery NT, Acosta JA, Block EF, Bromberg WJ, Collier BR, Cullinane DC, Dwyer KM, Griffen MM, Mayberry JC. Guidelines for management of small bowel obstruction. J Trauma Acute Care Surg. 2008;64(6):1651–64.
10. Williams SB, Greenspon J, Young HA, Orkin BA. Small bowel obstruction: conservative vs. surgical management. Dis Colon Rectum. 2005;48(6):1140–6.
11. Podda M, Khan M, Di Saverio S. Adhesive small bowel obstruction and the six w's: who, how, why, when, what, and where to diagnose and operate? Scand J Surg. 2021;110(2):159–69.

12. Zamary K, Spain DA. Small bowel obstruction: the sun also rises? J Gastrointest Surg. 2020;24:1922–8.
13. Rajan R, Clark DA. Current management of large bowel obstruction: a narrative review. Ann Laparosc Endosc Surg. 2022;30:7.
14. Johnson WR, Hawkins AT. Large bowel obstruction. Clin Colon Rectal Surg. 2021;34(04):233–41.
15. Verheyden C, Orliac C, Millet I, Taourel P. Large-bowel obstruction: CT findings, pitfalls, tips and tricks. Eur J Radiol. 2020;130:109155.
16. Saeltzer DV, Rhodes GK. Diastasic perforation of the normal cecum: resulting from obstruction of the colon. Theatr Annu. 1935;101(5):1257.
17. Lowman RM, Davis L. Roentgen criteria of impending perforation of the cecum. Radiology. 1957;68(4):542–8.
18. Basford JR. The law of Laplace and its relevance to contemporary medicine and rehabilitation. Arch Phys Med Rehabil. 2002;83(8):1165–70.
19. Srivastava A, Sood A, Joy PS, Mandal S, Panwar R, Ravichandran S, Sarangi S, Woodcock J. Principles of physics in surgery: the laws of mechanics and vectors physics for surgeons—part 2. Indian J Surg. 2010;72:355–61.
20. Kanaka S, Matsuda A, Yamada T, Ohta R, Sonoda H, Shinji S, Takahashi G, Iwai T, Takeda K, Ueda K, Kuriyama S. Colonic stent as a bridge to surgery versus emergency resection for right-sided malignant large bowel obstruction: a meta-analysis. Surg Endosc. 2022;36(5):2760–70.

25 Diverticular Disease of the Colon

Michael J. Snyder and Steven Capece

Introduction

Colonic diverticulosis is the presence of outpouchings of the colon called diverticula (Fig. 25.1). Most patients with diverticulosis are asymptomatic. Colonic diverticulitis is a condition in which a diverticulum has become inflamed and/or perforated, with symptoms that can range from mild abdominal pain to peritonitis. The management of diverticulitis has changed over the last few decades, with *surgery for uncomplicated diverticulitis becoming less common*. The variability in presentation largely dictates the treatment of the disease, with patient and physician discussion being a large part of the path toward potential elective surgical resection.

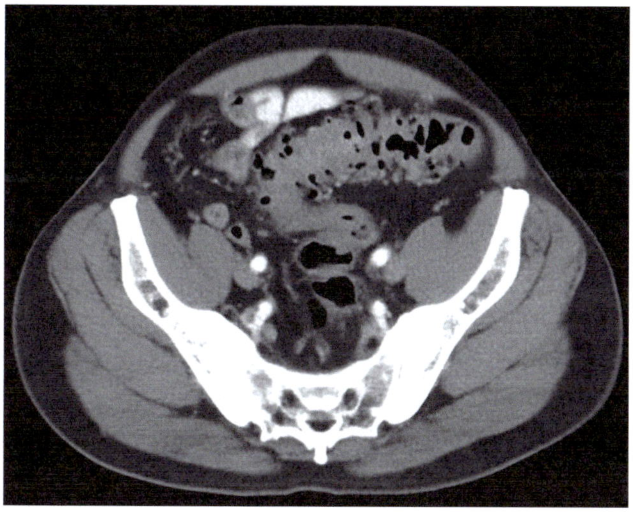

Fig. 25.1 Diverticulosis: CT depicting multiple, noninflamed diverticula, otherwise known as diverticulosis

M. J. Snyder (✉)
Section of Colon and Rectal Surgery, McGovern School of Medicine, Houston, TX, USA
e-mail: Michael.J.Snyder@uth.tmc.edu

S. Capece
Department of Colon and Rectal Surgery, Kelsey Sebold Medical Clinic, Pearland, TX, USA

Epidemiology

The presence of diverticulosis is fairly common, with an estimated incidence of at least 50% in Americans over the age of 60 years old [1]. The incidence of diverticulitis has also become more common and is responsible for over 200,000 inpatient admissions, with a significant increase in younger patients in recent years [1]. In patients under 40, there is also a significant male predominance. In addition, obesity appears to be more prevalent in younger patients with diverticulitis. The management and cost to the healthcare system are very dependent on the severity at presentation and can be quite variable. In general, diverticulitis tends to be more common in the Western population, with right-sided colonic disease more commonly seen in the Asian population [2].

History

The management of diverticulitis has evolved over the past few decades. A prior teaching included surgical resection after "x" number of episodes. *More recently, the treatment algorithm has shifted to a more patient-directed approach* [3]. Patients are currently stratified into those with *complicated* versus *uncomplicated* diverticulitis. Elective surgical resection of uncomplicated diverticulitis is more dependent on how it affects the patient's quality of life. If the patient is having multiple episodes but with minimal effect, then they may wish to forego elective resection. However, on the other end of the spectrum, the patient may have had one episode but cannot, for personal or other reasons, afford to have another, and for that reason choose to have elective resection. Furthermore, if the patient has had multiple episodes requir-

S. Atallah, J. Dragoljevic (eds.), *Fundamentals of Surgery for Physician Assistants*,
https://doi.org/10.1007/978-3-032-21069-2_25

ing hospitalization, then they may elect for resection in order to prevent further impact on their life. The general rule puts the patient at the forefront of the discussion, and how uncomplicated diverticulitis is affecting their life. Alternatively, those patients with complicated diverticulitis with obstruction, fistulae to the skin or other structures, or hemorrhage may need urgent surgery to correct the condition in an expeditious fashion. This includes those patients with uncomplicated diverticulitis who are immunosuppressed and represent a subset of patients too high-risk for a possible recurrent episode that may include overwhelming sepsis and peritonitis.

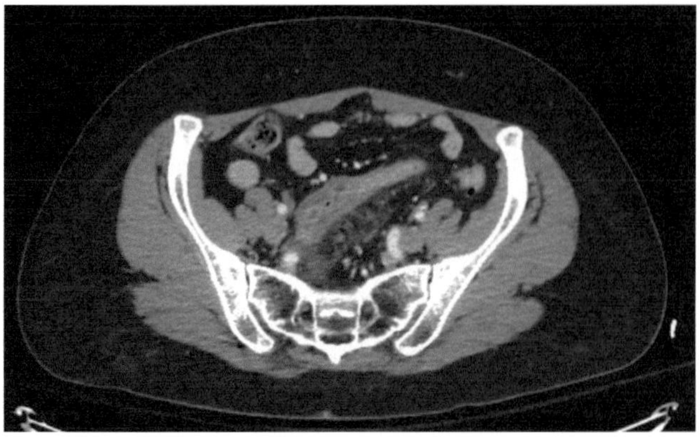

Fig. 25.2 Uncomplicated diverticulitis. CT depicting wall thickening and fat stranding seen in uncomplicated diverticulitis

Pathophysiology

There are multiple theories behind the pathophysiology of diverticulitis. The typical diverticula are herniations of the mucosa and muscularis mucosa through the colonic wall. The sites of the hernia are normal weak areas, allowing the perforation of small blood vessels that support the colonic wall. The Western-based diet with low fiber and subsequent higher colonic pressures continues to be considered as a possible culprit. Particularly, a diet high in red meat and low in fiber has been thought to be associated with the development of diverticulitis [4]. Weight loss and increased physical activity (2 h weekly), avoidance of NSAIDs and tobacco use have been shown to possibly reduce the risk of diverticulitis [3, 5]. Fiber, especially from fruits and vegetables, is felt to be protective, and there is an inverse relationship between intake of fiber and the incidence of diverticular disease. Interestingly, the old adage of not eating popcorn, nuts, and berries when you have diverticulosis has also been *refuted* with an inverse relationship with diverticular complications. The role of the microbiome has also been thought to play some role in the pathogenesis and manifestations of diverticulitis [6].

Presentation

There are three major presentations of diverticulitis, uncomplicated diverticulitis, complicated diverticulitis, and atypical diverticulitis. The typical presentation of uncomplicated diverticulitis includes a relatively sudden onset of left lower quadrant abdominal pain with possible associated fevers, chills, and changes in bowel habits. The patient may often have a history of prior episodes of diverticulitis and constipation. The history of present illness includes an evaluation of bowel function to assess for the possibility of obstruction or fistula, which may lead the patient closer to the operating room. It is also important to document a personal or family history of colon cancer and IBD due to the possibility of diverticulitis mimicking these other diseases. In that same effect, the patient's last colonoscopy and its findings are also important. A thorough surgical history is important to document, as this can help to guide surgical planning.

Physical findings of uncomplicated diverticulitis usually consist of left lower quadrant abdominal tenderness on examination without diffuse peritonitis. The patient often has a low-grade fever, but other vital signs may be normal. Laboratory evaluation may also be unremarkable except for a leukocytosis. CT scan findings often include the presence of diverticula, colonic wall thickening, and pericolic fat stranding (Fig. 25.2). There may be a small abscess also noted. Understanding the **Hinchey classification** (Table 25.1) grades I (local colonic abscess), II (distal abscess), III (purulent peritonitis), and IV (feculent peritonitis) will help guide your management, with the latter being surgical.

Complicated diverticulitis may include (a) an abscess on CT-scan (Fig. 25.3) (often requiring percutaneous drainage), (b) the formation of fistulae to the vagina, bladder, or skin, or (c) the development of focal or diffuse peritonitis due to bowel perforation. *These patients often require further interventions, either by interventional radiology to drain abscesses or urgent surgical intervention.*

Atypical diverticulitis includes a subset of patients who have chronic intermittent left lower quadrant pain. They often lack the clinical systemic manifestations of diverticulitis and have unremarkable CT scans. Many of these patients have functional bowel disorders, including irritable bowel syndrome. They may also have an atypical site of presentation, either in the ascending or transverse colon.

Table 25.1 Hinchey classifications for diverticulitis

Hinchey classification	Description
Grade 1	*Local* colonic abscess
Grade 2	*Distal* abscess
Grade 3	Purulent peritonitis
Grade 4	Feculent peritonitis

Source: Tan et al. [7]

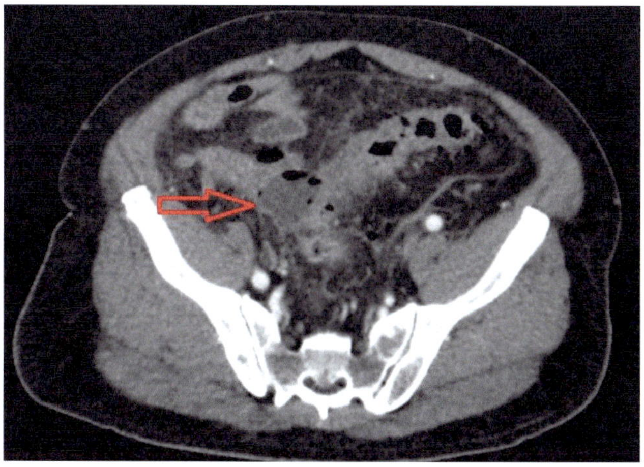

Fig. 25.3 Complicated diverticulitis. CT showing fluid collection as well as fat stranding and colon wall thickening seen in complicated diverticulitis

Work Up

A thorough history and focused abdominal exam are important. An assessment of stability and the presence of peritonitis is necessary to guide management. The typical workup should include a CBC and BMP. More particular labs, such as CRP, have been used and associated with severity [7]. If there is a concern for malignancy (i.e., presence of pericolonic lymph nodes, luminal mass [8]), a CEA can be checked. A CT scan of the abdomen and pelvis with oral and intravenous contrast is useful in identifying the location of the disease. This is especially important in patients with recurrent disease (e.g., if the episodes are in the same area each time). The use of rectal contrast for the CT scan is useful to evaluate for obstruction and possible colonic leak (ex. active extravasation), which are more likely to require surgery.

Management

The management of diverticulitis is dependent on the presentation of diverticulitis. A patient with mild left lower quadrant pain with CT showing uncomplicated diverticulitis (i.e., nonperforated) can typically be managed in the outpatient setting *with or* <u>*without*</u> *a short course of oral antibiotics* (*note well:* antibiotics are <u>**not**</u> mandatory in this setting). The use of antibiotics in mild cases has been questioned, with *evidence suggesting similar long-term outcomes in those treated without antibiotics* [9]. If antibiotics are used, typically Ciprofloxacin (Cipro) 500 mg BID in combination with Metronidazole (Flagyl) 500 mg TID is given in combination for 7–10 days. Alternatively, Augmentin 875 mg BID can be used for the same duration.

A patient with more advanced symptoms and complicated diverticulitis is usually managed as an inpatient with the use of intravenous antibiotics and the possibility of percutaneous drainage by interventional radiology if a significant intra-abdominal fluid collection (abscess) greater than 3 cm is present [10]. A patient who has peritonitis and/or hemodynamically unstable is typically managed with resuscitation and emergent operative intervention. The operative intervention in the emergent setting for sigmoid diverticulitis is typically a **Hartmann's procedure** (removal of the sigmoid colon with creation of a colostomy). An alternative option includes a primary anastomosis and diverting loop ileostomy (PADLI), but that is dependent on the patient's clinical status and the surgeon's preference.

Following an acute case of diverticulitis, *endoscopic evaluation is recommended to exclude the possibility of inflammatory bowel disease, ischemic colitis, or malignancy.* If the patient is clinically stable and able to be managed without surgery, then the current recommendation is to have a colonoscopy 6–8 weeks after resolution of the diverticulitis [11]. A repeat CT scan as follow-up is a consideration depending on the severity, presence of abscess s/p drainage, and the clinical course. The patient should be counseled on weight loss, risk factors to avoid (i.e., smoking, NSAIDs, red meat), implementation of an exercise routine, and maintaining healthy bowel habits [3]. *The discussion of elective resection is a patient-directed decision and should be individualized.*

Complications

As previously mentioned, diverticulitis can have a variety of complications that can make management more challenging. At times, when these complications are encountered, the expertise of a colorectal surgeon is often warranted.

Due to the most common location of the diverticulitis in the sigmoid colon, complications related to other pelvic organs, such as the uterus/vagina and bladder, can happen. The inflammatory and infectious conditions of diverticulitis can make fistula formation to other organs possible. A **colovaginal fistula**, or connection between the colon and vagina, can sometimes form as a consequence of diverticulitis. This typically occurs in *women who have had a hysterectomy*, and the site on the vagina is invariably the vaginal cuff. It is rare for a fistula from diverticulitis to occur in a patient who still has a uterus. In those patients, concern about inflammatory bowel disease (Crohn's disease) and malignancy is especially important. The presentation typically includes feculent vaginal discharge and possible vaginal wound infections such as labial excoriations or abscesses. The diagnosis can be made by a vaginal speculum exam. Using a rigid proctoscope in the vagina is also useful and can often visualize the opening in the vaginal cuff where stool or intestinal fluid can be seen emanating. Other adjunctive testing can include CT w/rectal contrast, barium enema, MRI, and/or colonoscopy. A colonoscopy is typically recommended to evaluate for underlying malignancy. The treatment typically will be first to stabilize and treat any signs of infection, which can include the need for debridement. After stabilization, treatment is typically dependent on the patient's clinical status and the surgeon's preference. In higher-risk patients, some surgeons will prefer a staged approach with a diverting ostomy followed by eventual resection of the diseased portion of the colon and possible vaginal repair. In lower-risk patients, some surgeons will jump straight to resection. However, the surgical pathway is typically managed with a multidisciplinary approach involving colorectal surgery and gynecology [12].

A **colovesical fistula**, or fistulous connection between the colon and bladder (Figs. 25.4 and 25.5), is managed in a similar fashion. A natural history can be multiple prior episodes of UTIs as well as *pneumaturia* ("bubbling" in the urine), and/or *fecaluria* (stool in the urine). The diagnosis is typically made with a noncontrast CT showing air in the bladder (assuming no recent prior instrumentation (ex. cystoscopy, catheterization, etc.)). Other adjunctive testing includes cystoscopy, colonoscopy, CT w/rectal contrast, and MRI. First and foremost, the patient should be resuscitated and stabilized. Urine cultures should be obtained to help guide antibiotic treatment of the underlying UTI. The surgical treatment involves resecting the diseased colon with possible bladder repair [13]. A colovesical fistula is more urgent than a colovaginal fistula because of the possibility of *urosepsis with subsequent kidney damage*. Postoperatively, a Foley is usually maintained for a short period of time for bladder decompression to prevent urine leakage.

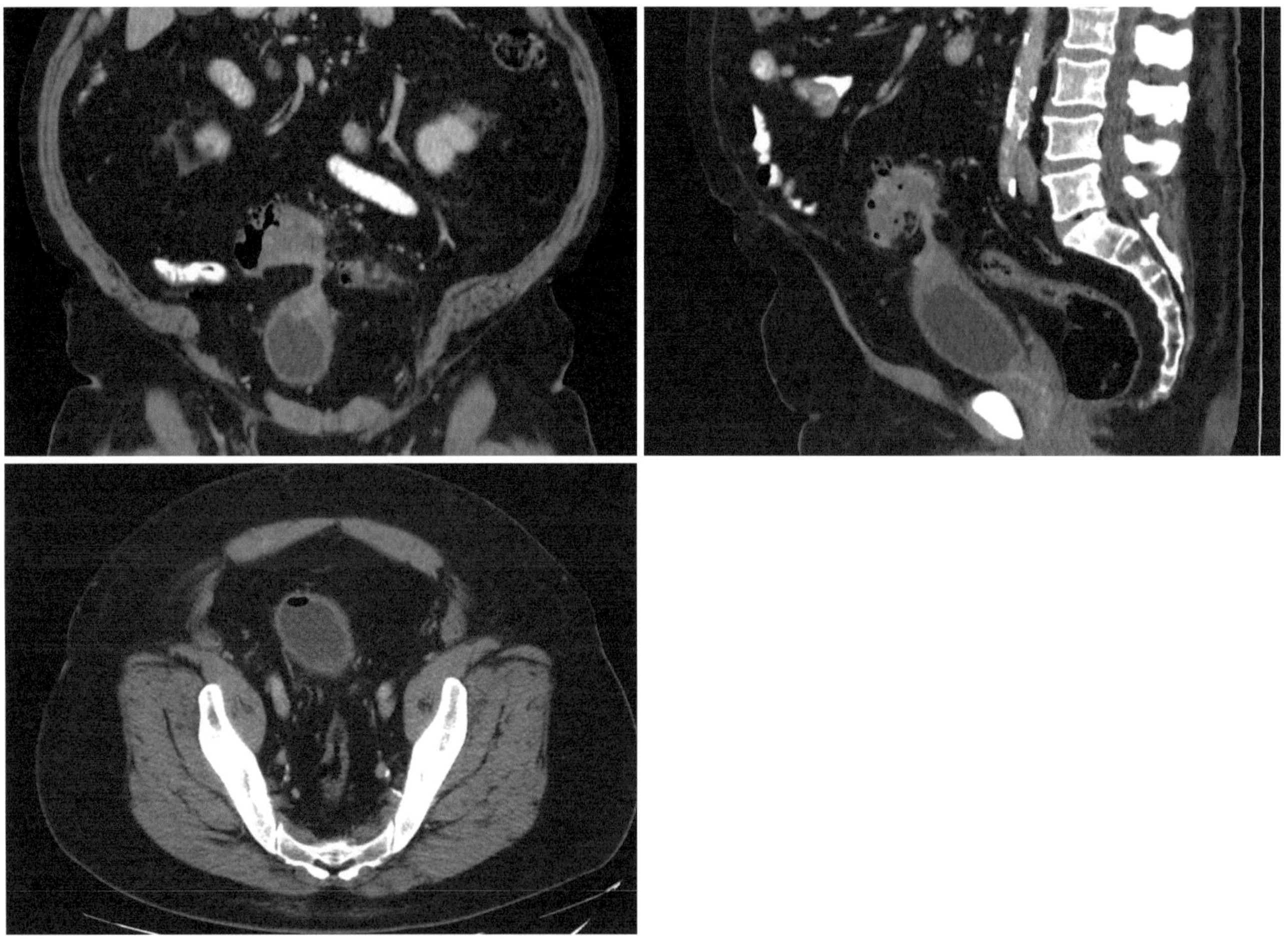

Fig. 25.4 Colovesical fistula. CT scan depicting air in the bladder as well as a fistulous tract to the bladder, concerning for a colovesical fistula

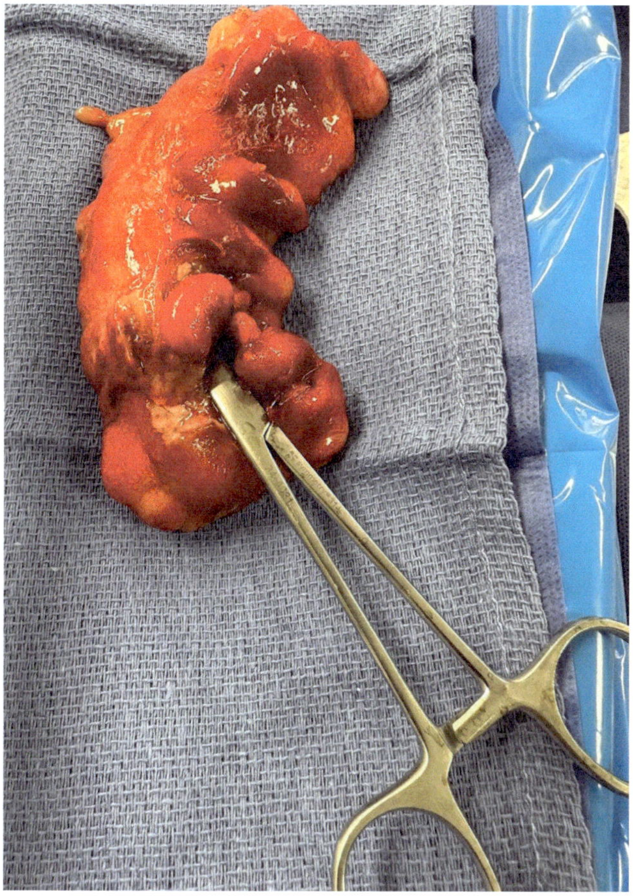

Fig. 25.5 The resected portion of the sigmoid colon is shown for a patient with colovesical fistula secondary to diverticulitis. This patient had presented with recurrent UTIs, pneumaturia, and fecaluria. In this image, a metal hemostat tip has been placed through the remainder of the fistula tract (a point of communication into the bowel lumen). Prior to resection of the sigmoid, the fistula was "taken down," meaning separated from the bladder dome. Most often, the hole on the bladder side heals itself, and does not require closure, only catheter drainage for 7–10 days postoperatively. A colovesical fistula falls into the category of *complicated* diverticulitis and mandates operative management (a fistula will not resolve with antibiotics). (Image courtesy of Sam Atallah, MD)

Red Flags

The majority of patients who suffer from uncomplicated diverticulitis will not require surgery. However, there are exceptions and red flags that you should be aware of.

Immunosuppressed Patients Those patients who are immunosuppressed, such as those on steroids, chemotherapy, or organ transplant patients, are treated differently. The possibility of a recurrent episode with a fairly precipitous development of sepsis and peritonitis is a serious possibility [14]. Some surgeons will adopt a "one strike you're out" model in which surgery is pushed sooner to prevent complications developing in these circumstances. Additionally, how they respond and heal from surgery can be more challenging, and as such, a higher index of clinical suspicion should be used when handling the postoperative care of these patients.

Smoldering Diverticulitis A recurrent, persistent episode of diverticulitis in which symptoms never truly resolve. A patient may suffer from constant pain with intermittent flare-ups, leading to repeat hospitalizations. CT scanning of the abdomen and pelvis will show the same involved segment and often a phlegmon with varying degrees of severity. These patients often require surgery and may need diversion with an ostomy.

Diverticular Stricture After an episode of diverticulitis, the inflammatory process can lead to scarring of the colonic wall. The scarring that develops from even just one episode can potentially lead to a stricture, a chronic narrowing of the colon. A diverticular stricture can cause symptoms such as bloating, abdominal pain, nausea, and constipation. The treatment for a colonic stricture typically involves surgical resection of the diseased area. However, if acute and fully obstructed, then the treatment may involve a temporary diverting colostomy to allow for decompression before resection. Other options also include endoscopic stenting, but this is typically used as a bridge to surgery or can be palliative in certain cases [15].

Diverticular Hemorrhage Diverticular bleed can be seen with or without an active episode of diverticulitis and is, in fact, most common without active diverticulitis. The importance of managing the bleeding is first *resuscitation*. The treatment to follow is largely dependent on *localizing studies* to identify the source and location of the bleed. Endoscopy, in conjunction with other studies including CT angiogram, IR angiography, and tagged red blood cell scans, can be used. *Identifying the location of the bleed is critical to guide management*. Having a bleed that is localized to the left colon can be treated with a left colectomy as opposed to a colonic bleed that is nonlocalized and may require the morbidity of a total abdominal colectomy [16]. Nowadays, most diverticular bleeding is successfully managed nonoperatively, using techniques such as embolization (via interventional radiology), and in some cases colonoscopy with clipping of the bleeding vessel (although in clinical practice this offers a low probability of success). Table 25.2 summarizes common conditions related to diverticular disease.

Table 25.2 Conditions related to sigmoid diverticulitis

Condition	CT findings	Treatment
Uncomplicated diverticulitis	Segmental colonic wall thickening, pericolic fat stranding, diverticula, no abscess or perforation	Outpatient antibiotics (***optional*** per guidelines), bowel rest, observation
Diverticular abscess	Fluid collection with rim enhancement near inflamed colon	Percutaneous drainage if >3–4 cm; antibiotics; possible surgery
Free perforation	Extraluminal air, diffuse peritonitis	Emergent surgical intervention
Colonic fistula	Air or contrast in adjacent organ (e.g., bladder)	Surgical resection and fistula repair (timing of surgery is individualized)
Diverticular stricture	Narrowed lumen with thickened segment	Elective surgery if symptomatic partial obstruction; urgent surgery if high-grade obstruction or complete obstruction
Diverticular bleeding	CT angiography shows active contrast extravasation. Tagged RBC scan (bleeding scan) can be useful to determine whether or not slow bleeding is present, but bleeding source localization is often vague	In-patient monitoring, correct coagulopathy, hold anticoagulants; endoscopic or radiologic intervention if active bleeding is persistent for source localization and control, if possible; surgery is a last resort

Source: Tan et al. [7]
Note: Management and imaging findings should always be correlated with clinical presentation and patient stability

Surgery

The surgical resection side again is largely dependent on the patient's clinical status. The goals of surgery *are not to remove all areas of diverticulosis but to remove the diseased areas and the high-pressure zone in the sigmoid colon*. During surgery, a clear delineation of a healthy vs unhealthy bowel can be seen and felt. *The diseased colon tends to have a thickened mesentery as well as bowel wall*. The resection should include the diseased areas, which typically involve the sigmoid colon down to the rectum. A distinction can be made between the sigmoid and rectum by the *splaying of the teniae and the lack of pericolic fat*. The use of ostomies (end colostomy vs diverting loop ileostomy) is typically based on the patient and their clinical status. Laparoscopic lavage has been used as a way to wash out and drain the diseased area. Primary anastomosis and diverting loop ileostomy (PADLI) has also been used, but is largely surgeon and case-dependent. A sigmoidectomy and end colostomy, otherwise known as a Hartman's procedure, is common and typically used in the acute setting [17].

Conclusion

Diverticulitis continues to provide significant challenges to both the medical system and the patient alike. The understanding of the spectrum of presentation and pathology is critical to the management. The use of surgery is typically reserved for complicated diverticulitis. Noncomplicated diverticulitis and the majority of patients can be managed as an outpatient successfully. Most importantly, prevention with increasing intake of fruits and vegetables and water is critical to educate patients who have diverticular disease but have not yet manifested diverticulitis. This will most likely be our best opportunity to intervene and diminish the incidence of diverticulitis.

References

1. Strate LL, Morris AM. Epidemiology, pathophysiology, and treatment of diverticulitis. Gastroenterology. 2019; https://doi.org/10.1053/j.gastro.2018.12.033.
2. Bhatia M, Mattoo A. Diverticulosis and diverticulitis: epidemiology, pathophysiology, and current treatment trends. Cureus. 2023; https://doi.org/10.7759/cureus.43158.
3. Hall J, Hardiman K, Lee S, et al. The American Society of Colon and rectal surgeons clinical practice guidelines for the treatment of left-sided colonic diverticulitis. Dis Colon Rectum. 2020;63:728–47. https://doi.org/10.1097/dcr.0000000000001679.
4. Carabotti M, Falangone F, Cuomo R, Annibale B. Role of dietary habits in the prevention of diverticular disease complications: a systematic review. Nutrients. 2021;13:1288. https://doi.org/10.3390/nu13041288.
5. Liu P-H, Cao Y, Keeley BR, et al. Adherence to a healthy lifestyle is associated with a lower risk of diverticulitis among men. Am J Gastroenterol. 2017;112:1868–76. https://doi.org/10.1038/ajg.2017.398.
6. Ma W, Wang Y, Nguyen LH, et al. Gut microbiome composition and metabolic activity in women with diverticulitis. Nat Commun. 2024; https://doi.org/10.1038/s41467-024-47859-4.
7. Tan JPL, Barazanchi AWH, Singh PP, et al. Predictors of acute diverticulitis severity: a systematic review. Int J Surg. 2016;26:43–52. https://doi.org/10.1016/j.ijsu.2016.01.005.
8. Chintapalli KN, Chopra S, Ghiatas AA, et al. Diveriticulitis versus colon cancer: differentiation with helical CT findings. Radiology. 1999;210:429–35. https://doi.org/10.1148/radiology.210.2.r99fe48429.
9. Daniels L, Ünlü, de Korte N, et al. Randomized clinical trial of observational versus antibiotic treatment for a first episode of CT-proven uncomplicated acute diverticulitis. J Brit Surg. 2017;104:52–61. https://doi.org/10.1002/bjs.10309.
10. Cirocchi R, Duro F, Avenia S, et al. Guidelines for the treatment of abdominal abscesses in acute diverticulitis: an umbrella review. J Clin Med. 2023;12:5522. https://doi.org/10.3390/jcm12175522.
11. Peery AF, Shaukat A, Strate LL. Aga clinical practice update on medical management of colonic diverticulitis: expert review. Gastroenterology. 2021; https://doi.org/10.1053/j.gastro.2020.09.059.
12. Berger MB, Khandwala N, Fenner DE, Burney RE. Colovaginal fistulas: presentation, evaluation, and management. Female Pelvic Med Reconstr Surg. 2016;22:355–8. https://doi.org/10.1097/spv.0000000000000289.

13. Granieri S, Sessa F, Bonomi A, et al. Indications and outcomes of enterovesical and Colovesical fistulas: systematic review of the literature and meta-analysis of prevalence. BMC Surg. 2021; https://doi.org/10.1186/s12893-021-01272-6.
14. Brandl A, Kratzer T, Kafka-Ritsch R, et al. Diverticulitis in immunosuppressed patients: a fatal outcome requiring a new approach? Can J Surg. 2016;59:254–61. https://doi.org/10.1503/cjs.012915.
15. Neale J. Surgical management of diverticular disease in the elective setting. Clin Colon Rectal Surg. 2018;31:236–42. https://doi.org/10.1055/s-0037-1607962.
16. Mohammed Ilyas MI, Szilagy E. Management of diverticular bleeding: evaluation, stabilization, intervention, and recurrence of bleeding and indications for resection after control of bleeding. Clin Colon Rectal Surg. 2018;31:243–50. https://doi.org/10.1055/s-0037-1607963.
17. Feingold D, Steele SR, Lee S, et al. Practice parameters for the treatment of sigmoid diverticulitis. Dis Colon Rectum. 2014;57:284–94. https://doi.org/10.1097/dcr.0000000000000075.

26 Colon and Rectal Cancer

Sam Atallah

Introduction

Colorectal cancer (CRC) is the third most commonly diagnosed cancer and the ***second leading cause of cancer death in the United States***, with an estimated 153,020 new cases and 52,550 deaths projected for 2023. Incidence rates are higher in men (41.5 per 100,000) than in women (31.2 per 100,000), and highest among Alaska Native, American Indian, and Black populations. While overall CRC incidence and mortality have declined over the past two decades—driven by increased screening and improved treatment—the rate of decline has slowed recently, and incidence is *rising among adults under 50 years old*. The 5-year relative survival rate for CRC has improved from 50% in the mid-1970s to 65% for cases diagnosed between 2012 and 2018, but survival is highly stage-dependent and remains poor for metastatic disease (Fig. 26.1) [1–4].

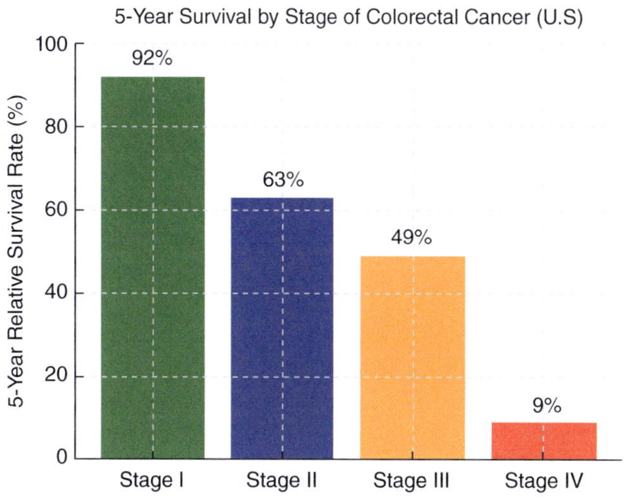

Fig. 26.1 The 5-year survival by stage is shown for the United States. Note the disparity in survival between early stage (I) and late stages (IV) of the disease. This underscores the importance of early detection and treatment, as the outcomes vary dramatically. It also emphasizes the value of colon cancer screening programs, where the objective is early detection

Comparatively, **breast cancer is <u>twice as common</u> as CRC** (an estimated 297,790 new cases) in 2023; *however,* **<u>more people die of CRC</u> annually**, based on 2023 data

S. Atallah (✉)
Department of Surgery, Piedmont Hospital, Mercer University School of Medicine, Macon, GA, USA
e-mail: atallah@post.harvard.edu

S. Atallah, J. Dragoljevic (eds.), *Fundamentals of Surgery for Physician Assistants*,
https://doi.org/10.1007/978-3-032-21069-2_26

(43,170 breast cancer-related deaths versus colon cancer 52,550). The 5-year relative survival rate for breast cancer is approximately 90%, which remains *much higher* than CRC, underscoring the need for improved early detection and treatment, as CRC tends to present at later-stages of diagnosis compared to breast cancer [1–7].

Younger Colon Cancer The median age of colon cancer diagnosis is currently 66 (which is a downward trend from 72, which represented the median age in the early 2000s). There have been increasingly more patients diagnosed with CRC who are younger than 50. This change reflects a significant epidemiological trend: *the proportion of colorectal cancer (CRC) cases diagnosed in individuals under 50 years has increased steadily over the past two decades*, now accounting for approximately 10–12% of new colon cancer cases and 25% of rectal cancer cases in the United States. This rise in early-onset CRC is particularly notable among those born after 1950, who have double the risk of colon cancer and quadruple the risk of rectal cancer compared to those born around 1950, as shown in multiple large-scale epidemiological studies and highlighted by the American Cancer Society and the American College of Gastroenterology in their guidelines.

The increase in early-onset CRC is accompanied by a higher likelihood of left-sided tumors and a more advanced stage at diagnosis in younger patients. The trend is not fully explained by hereditary syndromes, as most early-onset cases are *sporadic*. In response, the American Cancer Society and the American College of Gastroenterology have lowered the recommended age of screening for persons of average-risk for CRC from 50 to 45. It is worth noting that CRC has now emerged as the number-one cancer killer of those < 50.

Anatomic Distribution of Cancer

The anatomic distribution of colon and rectal cancer is such that a substantial portion of tumors are right-sided. Right-sided colon cancer accounts for approximately 46–52% of all colon cancers in large population-based studies from the United States and Europe, with some variation by age, sex, and ethnicity. The right colon is typically defined as the cecum, ascending colon, hepatic flexure, and sometimes the transverse colon.

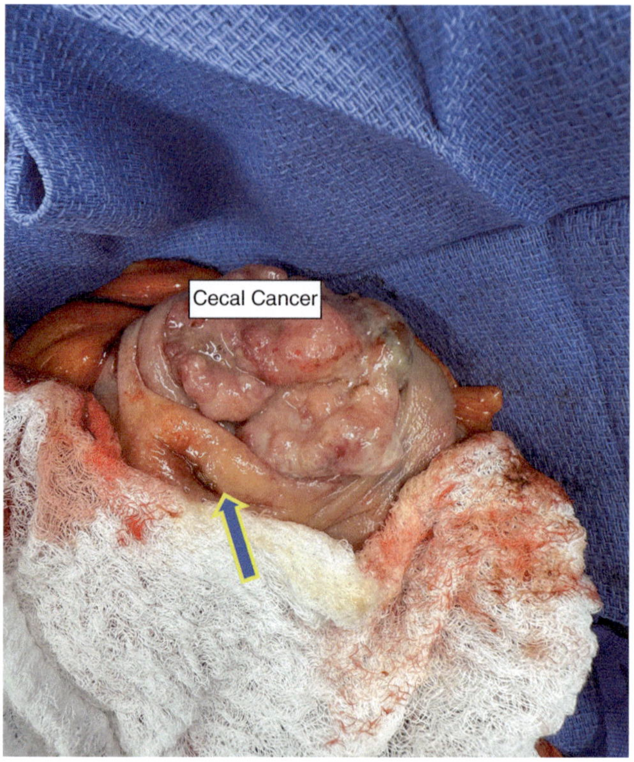

Fig. 26.2 A portion of the bowel, including the cecum, has been cut open, revealing a large cecal tumor. It is located in close juxtaposition to the ileocecal valve (arrow). Cancers of the colon are not uniform in their distribution and, statistically, a significant portion are found in the cecum (18–20%)

Cecal cancers specifically represent about 18–20% of all colon cancers. This proportion is supported by single-institution and population-based studies, which consistently report that cecal cancers comprise a substantial subset of right-sided colon cancers (Fig. 26.2). The frequency of cecal cancer increases with age, particularly in elderly women. The overall distribution of colon cancer is shown in Fig. 26.3.

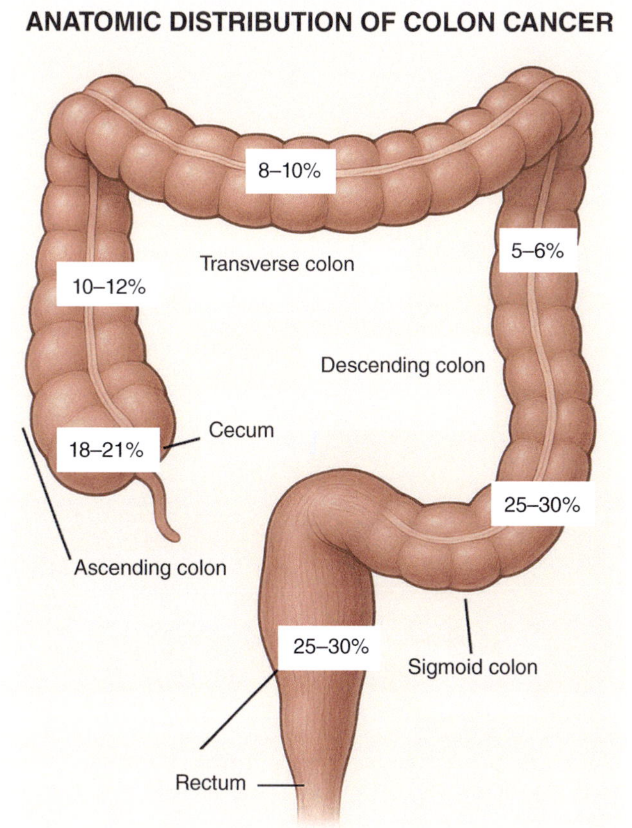

Fig. 26.3 The breakdown of colorectal cancer incidence by anatomical site, based on large population-based studies and registry data, is as follows: cecum: 18–20%; ascending colon: 10–12%; transverse colon: 8–10%; descending colon: 5–6%; sigmoid colon: 25–30%; rectum: 25–30%. These proportions are consistent across multiple large cohorts and registry analyses, including SEER and European datasets. The rectosigmoid junction is sometimes reported separately and typically accounts for an additional 5–7% of cases. Right-sided colon cancers are defined by most colorectal surgeons as *anything proximal to the splenic flexure* and include the cecum, ascending, hepatic flexure, and transverse colon. Right-sided colon cancer accounts for approximately 46–52% of all colon cancers, and cecal cancers specifically represent about 18–20% of all colon cancers. The remaining cases are distributed among the left-sided colon (descending, sigmoid) and rectum. Note: *these figures may vary slightly by population, age, and sex, but the overall distribution remains consistent in the medical literature*

Pathology 101: What's a Polyp? What's a Cancer?

Anatomy is important for all aspects of surgery, including oncologic surgery, and understanding the anatomy is crucial for staging of cancers of the colon and rectum. The bowel wall is made up of layers. From the innermost to outermost layer, they are as follows: **mucosa, submucosa** (the strongest layer), **inner circular muscle, outer longitudinal muscle**, and **serosa** (absent in some areas). Cancers of the *colorectum always begin growing from the innermost layer,* the mucosa (Fig. 26.4a, b). This is an important rule that makes screening via colonoscopy possible.

CRC starts out as a benign **polyp** (polyps are tiny, neoplastic growths on the mucosal lining). Polyps can form as a flat growth, termed a **sessile polyp**, or as a growth on a stalk, termed a **pedunculated polyp**. They simply represent two common polyp morphologies. Without going into a lot of detail, pedunculated polyps are generally easier to remove with a colonoscope, while large sessile polyps are more challenging.

The most common benign polyp is known as an **adenoma**. An adenoma is NOT a cancer. Adenomas can be subdivided into **tubular adenomas, tubulovillous adenomas,** and **villous adenomas**. There is a special category of adenomas that can behave aggressively and require careful monitoring, called a **sessile serrated adenoma** (which represents a three-fold increased risk of developing CRC). Although all of these are benign, they portend different risks of developing into a cancer over time, with *villous adenomas and sessile serrated adenomas representing the highest risk.* All adenomas should be removed during colonoscopy, as they harbor at least some risk of malignant transformation—although this is a very slow process that occurs over a period of years. It should be noted that there is a type of polyp called the **hyperplastic polyp**. Hyperplastic polyps do not turn into cancer, and we generally don't have to worry about them like we do other (adenomatous) polyps.

Colon and rectal cancer are almost always of the type known as **adenocarcinoma**. Pay careful attention to the terminology, as this is something often confused by PAs in training. Adenomas are BENIGN; adeno*carcinomas* are MALIGNANT. Any tumor with the suffix ***-carcinoma*** is synonymous with malignant, and malignant tumors are also described as **invasive** cancer (as opposed to ***pre***cancerous lesions that are described as **in situ**). Colorectal tumors are staged by the classic TNM system (Table 26.1), relating to ***t***umor characteristics, ***n***odal status, and distant organ ***m***etastasis; it correlates with cancer stage and, in turn, survival (Table 26.2).

With colon cancer, the size of the tumor is not important, but the *depth of penetration* is important; the deeper the tumor penetrates into the bowel, the higher the T stage. Size only matters if the tumor grows to a point that leads to bowel obstruction, and this is described separately in another chapter on *bowel obstruction.*

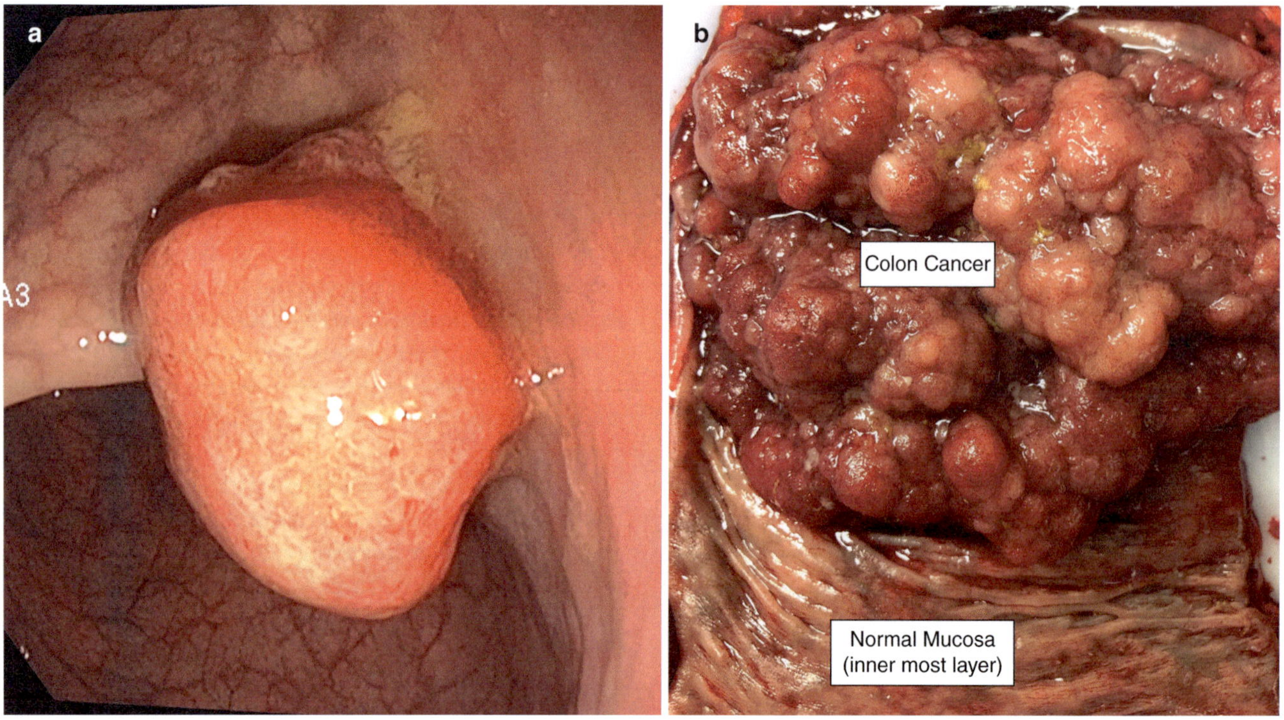

Fig. 26.4 As a rule, CRC originates from the innermost lining of the colorectum, which is the mucosa. (**a**) A colonoscopic view of an early, 2 cm rectal cancer is depicted. This represents the transformation of a benign polyp into a malignant tumor. Benign polyps can simply be removed during a colonoscopy, while cancers require more complex treatment. (**b**) A surgical specimen has been cut open to reveal a bulky colon cancer. Note that the tumor begins from the mucosal (innermost layer). For comparison, the normal colonic mucosal layer has been annotated

Table 26.1 TNM staging for colon and rectal cancer

Category	Stage	Definition
T—Primary tumor		
Tis	Carcinoma in situ	Intraepithelial or invasion of lamina propria
T1	Tumor invades submucosa	Below muscularis mucosae but not into muscularis propria
T2	Tumor invades muscularis propria	Still confined to the bowel wall
T3	Tumor invades through muscularis propria into subserosa or pericolic/perirectal tissues	Does not penetrate the visceral peritoneum or adjacent organs
T4a	Tumor penetrates to the surface of the visceral peritoneum	Serosal involvement
T4b	Tumor directly invades or is adherent to other organs or structures	Advanced local spread
N—Regional lymph nodes		
N0	No regional lymph node metastasis	
N1a	Metastasis in 1 regional lymph node	
N1b	Metastases in 2–3 regional lymph nodes	
N1c	Tumor deposit(s) without regional nodal metastases	In subserosa, mesentery, or nonperitonealized pericolic or perirectal tissues
N2a	Metastases in 4–6 regional lymph nodes	
N2b	Metastases in ≥7 regional lymph nodes	
M—Distant metastasis		
M0	No distant metastasis	
M1a	Metastasis confined to one distant organ or site	e.g., liver, lung
M1b	Metastases in more than one distant organ/site	Or peritoneum
M1c	Peritoneal metastasis	With or without other organ involvement

Table 26.2 Colorectal cancer: TNM staging, AJCC stage, and 5-year survival

AJCC stage	TNM criteria (colon/rectum)	5-year relative survival (%)
Stage 0	Tis N0 M0	~100% (carcinoma in situ)
Stage I	T1–T2 N0 M0	~91–93% (localized disease)
Stage II-A	T3 N0 M0	~66–85%
Stage II-B	T4a N0 M0	~58–72%
Stage II-C	T4b N0 M0	~37–45%
Stage III-A	T1–T2 N1 or T1 N2a M0	~71–83%
Stage III-B	T3–T4a N1 or T2–T3 N2a or T1–T2 N2b M0	~46–64%
Stage III-C	T3–T4a N2b or T4b N1–2 M0	~28–44%
Stage IV	Any T, Any N, M1 (a/b/c)	~5–13% (distant metastases)

N-stage is determined by whether or not there are lymph nodes that contain colon cancer, and the M-stage relates to whether or not there is cancer known to be in distant organs. It is not necessary that you memorize the staging criteria. We don't need to get into too many details regarding the TNM staging beyond this.

Screening for Colon Cancer

General Principles of Cancer Screening Screening programs by definition address an entire population, *not* just those at high risk (although high-risk patients are given special consideration in cancer screening programs). From a population-based, health maintenance and wellness perspective, it is important to consider *which* cancers to screen for and *when* to screen for them.

Have you ever thought about why we screen for some types of cancers, but not others? To be a "*screenable*" cancer, the cancer must satisfy these criteria: **(a)** It must occur relatively frequently (i.e., be a *common* type of cancer), **(b)** if identified early, the prognosis is significantly improved, **(c)** it must be logistically and financially suitable for healthcare implementation for the given population, and **(d)** it has to be *acceptable* to the population and not pose significant burden. CRC is exactly such a type of cancer and is very effectively screened and arguably prevented with appropriate screening. Unlike screening for breast cancer, which has the main objective of detecting early breast cancer, colon cancer screening (via colonoscopy) can be diagnostic and therapeutic, as the precursors to cancer can be removed by polypectomy.

Methods of Screening In the United States, **colonoscopy is considered the gold standard** of CRC screening; this is not how screening is carried out in many other countries, including European ones, due to differences in public perceptions and variances in healthcare infrastructure and funding. The most important advantage of colonoscopy is that it is both **diagnostic** (detects cancer) *and* potentially **therapeutic** (removes precancerous polyps before they can ever turn into cancer).

Alternatives to Colonoscopy Current methods for colorectal cancer (CRC) screening in the United States, other than colonoscopy, include **fecal immunochemical test (FIT), multitarget stool DNA-FIT (mt-sDNA), flexible sigmoidoscopy**, and computed tomography **(CT) colonography**. The American College of Gastroenterology, the American Gastroenterological Association, and the United States Preventive Services Task Force all recommend that average-risk adults **begin screening at age 45,** with the choice of modality based on patient preference, risk, and test availability. Colonoscopy is typically repeated at *variable* intervals depending on whether or not polyps are found and on the quality of the bowel preparation on the index colonoscopy (Table 26.3). The FIT test should be performed annually, the mt-sDNA every 1–3 years, flexible sigmoidoscopy every 5–10 years (with or without annual FIT), and CT colonography every 5 years [8–10].

These modern modalities contribute to early detection and improved outcomes by identifying both cancer and precancerous lesions (**adenomas**), allowing for removal before malignant transformation. Colonoscopy is unique in its ability to both detect and remove polyps in a single procedure, directly reducing CRC incidence and mortality [8, 11]. Noninvasive tests such as FIT and mt-sDNA have high sensitivity for cancer as opposed to adenomas, but carry the advantage of *ease of use, improving screening uptake*, which is critical for population-level impact [9, 11].

Compared to breast cancer screening, which primarily uses mammography to detect established cancers, CRC screening uniquely offers cancer prevention through polyp removal. This dual benefit—early detection and prevention—has contributed to the significant decline in CRC incidence and mortality in screened populations [8, 11, 12].

Table 26.3 Colonoscopy surveillance recommendations

Patient/findings at index colonoscopy	Recommended interval	Notes
Normal colonoscopy (average risk)	10 years	Start at age 45 per USPSTF/ACS unless otherwise indicated
1–2 small (<10 mm) tubular adenomas	5–7 years; shorter intervals sometimes used	Low-risk adenomas
3–4 small (<10 mm) tubular adenomas	3–5 years	Increased adenoma burden
≥5 adenomas OR any ≥10 mm adenoma	3 years	High-risk findings
Adenoma with villous features or high-grade dysplasia	3 years	Higher risk for progression to CRC
Sessile serrated lesion <10 mm without dysplasia	5–10 years	Similar to low-risk adenoma
Sessile serrated lesion ≥10 mm or with dysplasia	3 years	Treated as advanced lesion
Traditional serrated adenoma (TSA)	3 years	Higher malignant potential
Piecemeal resection of large sessile polyp (≥20 mm)	6 months–1 year	Repeat to ensure complete removal
Colorectal cancer (postresection)	1 year, then 3 years, then 5 years	Start at 1 year after surgery
IBD with colonic involvement (e.g., UC or Crohn's colitis)	Every 1–3 years	Start 8 years after onset of symptoms
First-degree relative with CRC diagnosed <60 years, or ≥2 relatives with CRC at any age	Every 5 years starting at age 40, or 10 years before earliest diagnosis in family	High-risk family history
First-degree relative with CRC ≥60 years	Every 10 years starting at age 40	Moderate risk

The Katie Couric Effect While breast cancer screening programs have traditionally been well embraced by the public, the same could not be said about colon cancer, which has suffered from a negative or "taboo" stigma. Some of these perceptions have changed over time thanks to colon cancer awareness campaigns. One landmark campaign event involved celebrity network news anchor Katie Couric, who underwent a live colonoscopy on national television (broadcast in March 2000 on the *Today* show). This led to a well-documented, immediate, and substantial increase in colorectal cancer (CRC) screening rates in the United States, a phenomenon often referred to as the "**Katie Couric effect**." Multiple analyses have shown that colonoscopy rates increased by approximately 20% in the months following the broadcast, with a sustained elevation in screening rates for at least several months to a year after the event. This effect was attributed to increased public awareness and health information-seeking behavior triggered by the high-profile media event, as supported by observational and survey data [13, 14].

The increase in CRC screening rates is clinically significant because higher screening uptake is directly associated with earlier detection, reduced incidence, and lower mortality from CRC. As demonstrated in large population studies, increased screening rates have contributed to a decline in both CRC incidence and mortality over the past two decades [15–17]. The American College of Gastroenterology specifically recommends **colonoscopy as a primary screening modality**, citing a 68–70% reduction in CRC mortality with screening colonoscopy [8]. In contrast, breast cancer screening rates have historically been higher and more stable, with less dramatic changes in response to individual media events, although media coverage can still influence mammography uptake [13, 18].

Genetic Colon Cancer

In genetics, we often consider the pattern of acquiring cancer. For some, there is a known gene mutation that contributes to the development of cancer, such as the **p53 gene mutation** that is associated with a multitude of cancers. In other instances, a cancer may develop in someone seemingly without any gene mutation. These patients do not have a family history of colon cancer. When someone develops colon cancer for no apparent reason, we term it **sporadic**. **Most colon cancer is sporadic** (without family history and without a known gene mutation). A small subset of patients develops colon cancer that is attributable to known gene mutations. The most important of which are **Familial Adenomatous Polyposis (FAP)** and **Hereditary Nonpolyposis Colorectal Carcinoma (HNPCC)**. Both inherited via **autosomal dominant** genes, they represent the most important and best studied forms of genetic colorectal cancer.

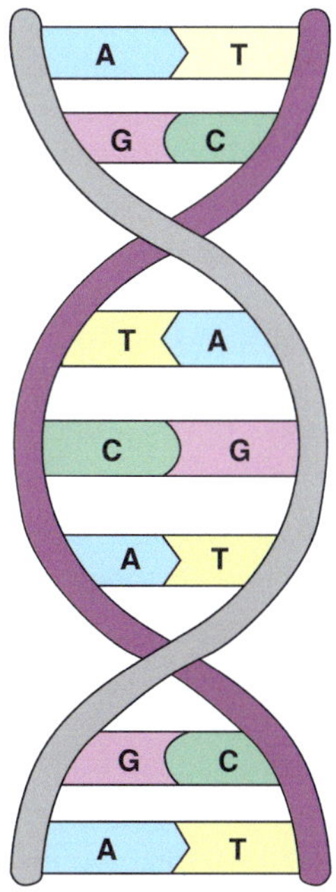

Fig. 26.5 Our genetic code (DNA) is composed of sequences of four base pairs: adenine, thymine, guanine, and cytosine. These base pairs make up the structure of DNA. They are attached in a specific way—like pieces of a puzzle. DNA obeys the rule that adenine (A) only binds to thymine (T); and cytosine (C) only binds to guanine (G), as shown in this illustration of the DNA double helix

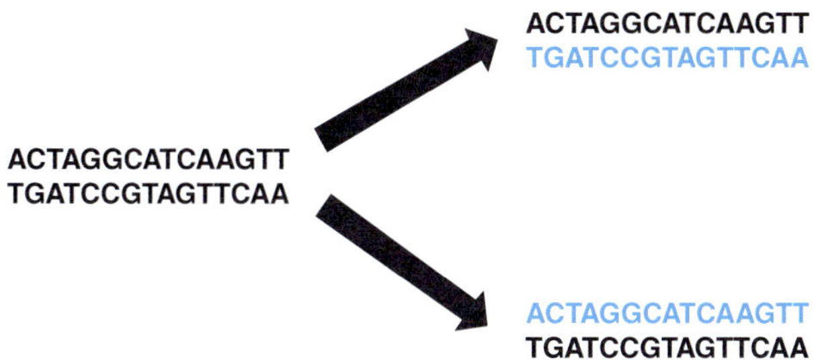

Fig. 26.6 DNA is two strands (the double helix) of code made up of A, G, C, and T. When DNA replicates, the two strands split, and each strand then serves as a template for a new strand (shown in blue). Thus, one double helix creates two new double helices that are identical. This is normal DNA replication

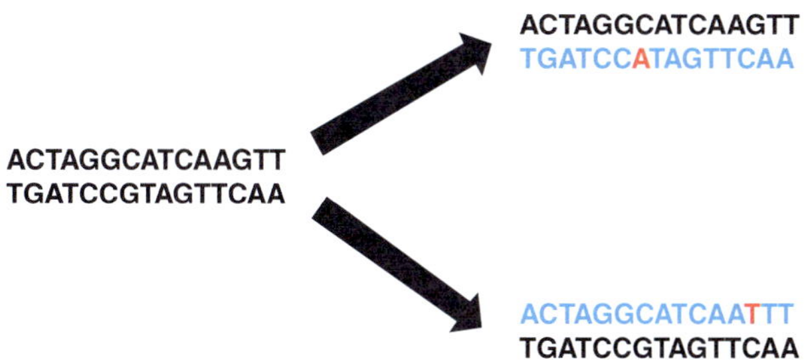

Fig. 26.7 Sometimes, during replication, a mistake is made, and the base-pairs are "mismatched." In this example, two mismatches have been made (shown in red), whereby adenine (A) has been mismatched with cytosine (C) (top replicated strand), and thymine (T) has been mismatched with cytosine (C) (bottom strand). If this error is not fixed, the integrity of the original DNA will be lost. This can eventually lead to the development of cancer. Thus, a mechanism to repair such errors in replication is necessary

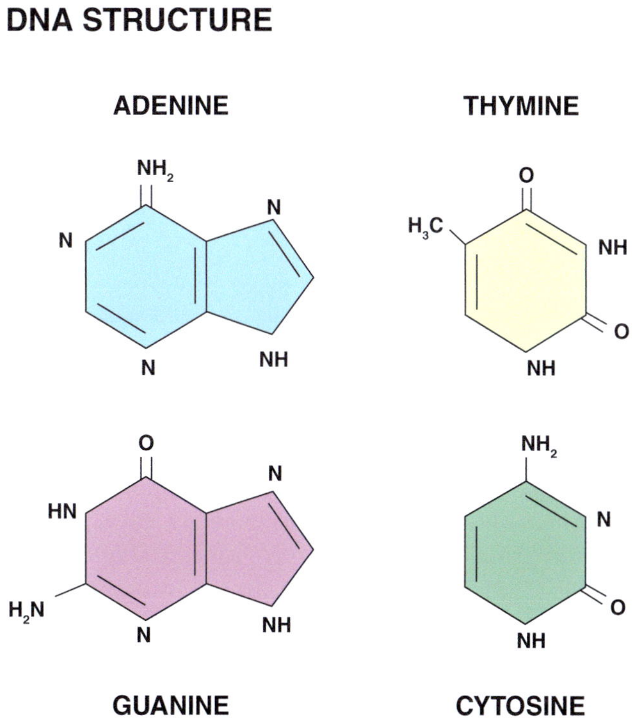

HNPCC and Lynch Syndrome Patients with HNPCC are sometimes referred to as having **Lynch syndrome**, and there are two types, *Lynch I and II*. **Lynch syndrome type I** refers specifically to families with a *predominance of colorectal cancer (CRC),* while **Lynch syndrome type II** describes families with *both CRC and a spectrum of extracolonic cancers,* most notably **endometrial,** ovarian, gastric, small bowel, urinary tract, and other malignancies. Both types are caused by germline mutations in DNA mismatch repair (MMR) genes (MLH1, MSH2, MSH6, PMS2, or EPCAM), leading to deficient mismatch repair (dMMR) and resulting in microsatellite instability-high (MSI-H) status in tumors (see next) [19–24].

Surveillance for Lynch syndrome (both types) **is more intensive than for sporadic CRC**, with *colonoscopy recommended every 1–2 years starting at age 20–25, or 2–5 years before the earliest CRC in the family*, as recommended by the American College of Gastroenterology [19]. For Lynch syndrome type II, additional surveillance for endometrial and other extracolonic cancers is indicated. The presence of dMMR/MSI-H in CRC is also predictive of better prognosis in nonmetastatic disease and, interestingly, a lack of benefit from adjuvant 5-FU (chemotherapy) in stage II CRC [21, 25].

DNA and HNPCC To best understand this genetic condition of HNPCC, we need to review the basics of DNA replication. Recall that the double helix structure of DNA is made up of four base pairs, **Adenine, Thymine, Cytosine, and**

Guanine, which are often abbreviated as **A, T, C,** and **G** (Fig. 26.5). They are matched in a *specific* way, such that **A binds to T**, and **C binds to G**, like this:

ACTAGGCATCAAGTT

TGATCCGTAGTTCAA

These DNA building blocks make up our genetic blueprint, and they are put together in a specific sequence. If the sequence isn't right, then the DNA code is not able to do what it's supposed to and becomes **mutated**. *Mutations in DNA can lead to cancer.* Every time DNA replicates, the double helix splits apart to make four daughter strands, as shown in Fig. 26.6. This is a very important process in cell division, and occurs frequently in our body, but especially in tissues with high turnover rates, such as the lining of the intestine. Therefore, it needs to happen as close to perfectly as possible. Even though replication is performed millions of times flawlessly, on occasion, there are errors in DNA replication that can lead to mutations if not corrected. These errors occur, for example, when A is **mismatched** with G or C rather than with T during replication (Fig. 26.7). Such an error in replication can lead to downstream errors in **translation** (i.e., making gene products or proteins) with untoward consequences that can lead to cancer.

Fortunately, we have a DNA proofreading system that is designed to catch these mistakes in replication during the process. It is not just one gene, but a family of genes that code for proteins whose sole purpose is to *check* the replicated DNA code for errors, *identify* the errors, and *correct* the errors so that the integrity of our DNA is preserved during this critical process (Fig. 26.8). This family of genes that codes for DNA proof-reading genes and which fix base-pair mismatches is, not surprisingly, known as DNA **Mis**match **R**epair **(MMR)** genes. If these genes are all working, and a patient develops colon cancer, we describe this as MMR *proficient,* sometimes abbreviated as **pMMR**. If any one or more of these genes (in the family of genes) is not present in the tumor of a patient with colon cancer, then it is described as MMR-*deficient,* abbreviated **dMMR**. This represents a *loss of expression* of one or more of the MMR proteins and is consistent with the diagnosis of HNPCC.

Because of the importance of therapeutic options now available to patients with dMMR, **every patient with invasive colorectal cancer (adenocarcinoma) undergoes assessment for this family of genes to determine whether or not they have an MMR mutation.**

Testing for HNPCC **Germline** (DNA) **testing** for mutations is often costly and labor-intensive. In the real world, germline testing for HNPCC is rarely performed. Instead, a pathologist assesses the cancer not for the actual DNA mutations, but rather for the *proteins* they genes code for. It would stand to reason that if the protein the DNA codes (the actual MMR protein that corrects the mismatches) is present in the tissue sample, then the gene that makes the protein is also present, and that there is no problem with the mismatch repair genes. But, if the protein is not found, it likely means there is a problem with the gene that makes the protein, and such a patient would be considered dMMR, due to loss of expression of an MMR protein(s).

But how do we know if the MMR protein is present or absent? Pathologists use special stains that are able to detect each of these proteins. They are specific histologic stains for the MMR proteins. This is done by a process known as **immunohistochemistry (IHC)**. While the exact process is beyond the scope of this chapter, it is important that clinicians who deal with colon cancer (surgery and/or oncology) be familiar with this terminology, as it is regularly included on pathology reports and has *significant implications for treatment.*

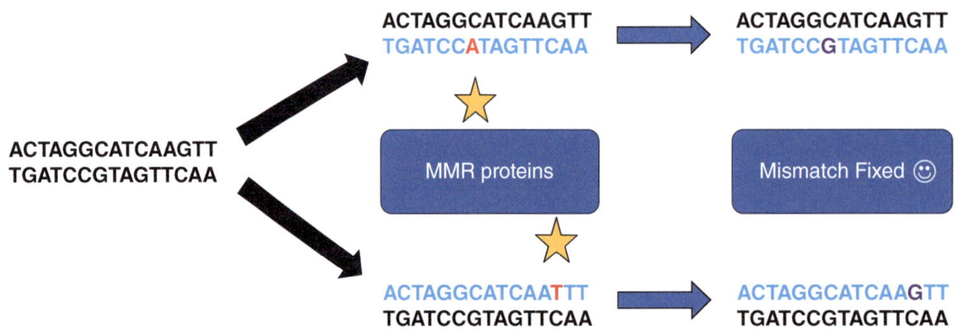

Fig. 26.8 DNA mismatches (such as the ones shown in red) can be identified and repaired. There is a family of genes that code for specific proteins that detect mismatches and restore them to the correct base-pairs, as shown here. This family of genes is known as the **MisMatch Repair (MMR) genes**. Patients with HNPCC have mutations in one or more of the MMR genes, so this repair mechanism doesn't work correctly, and the DNA ends up becoming mutated. *This is the mechanism that leads to a higher incidence of colon cancer in HNPCC*

Microsatellite Instability and dMMR DNA **microsatellite instability-high** (MSI-H) and deficient mismatch repair (dMMR) are closely related but distinct molecular features in colorectal cancer. dMMR refers to the loss of function of one or more DNA mismatch repair proteins (MLH1, MSH2, MSH6, PMS2), typically detected by IHC. MSI-H describes the phenotype of widespread length alterations in microsatellite regions of DNA, detected by PCR or next-generation sequencing, *which results from* dMMR. *In practice, these terms are often used interchangeably because* ***dMMR leads to MSI-H****, and both identify the same biologically and clinically relevant tumor subset* [26–30].

Both MSI-H and dMMR status are critical for guiding treatment decisions. The American Society of Clinical Oncology and the College of American Pathologists recommend **universal testing of all colorectal cancers for dMMR/MSI-H to identify patients eligible for immunotherapy and to screen for Lynch syndrome**. **Pembrolizumab** (Keytruda) is FDA-approved and recommended as first-line therapy for *unresectable or metastatic MSI-H/dMMR colorectal cancer,* based on superior progression-free survival and quality of life compared to chemotherapy. This benefit is <u>not</u> seen in **microsatellite stable** (MSS) or mismatch repair proficient (pMMR) tumors, which do not respond to immune checkpoint inhibitors [3, 25, 27, 29, 31–33].

In surveillance after resection, **MSI-H/dMMR tumors have a better prognosis** and lower risk of distant metastasis, *but* a higher risk of **metachronous tumors** (e.g., tumors that occur at a later point in time). This influences the intensity and duration of surveillance, and may prompt consideration of extended colectomy in hereditary cases. MSI-H/dMMR status also predicts lack of benefit from adjuvant **5-fluorouracil-based** chemotherapy in stage II disease, further impacting management [25, 29, 34–37].

Clinically, patients with HNPCC have a higher incidence of colon and rectal cancer than what is found in the general population, and they are afflicted at a younger age than what is normally observed. HNPCC tends to be more *right-sided* (defined as **proximal to the splenic flexure**); they are also associated with other cancer types, the most important of which is **endometrial cancer**. Females with proven HNPCC who have completed their family should be strongly recommended to undergo prophylactic (preventative) hysterectomy. While the extent of resection (amount of colon removed) is debated among colorectal surgeons, what is clear is that *patients with a history of HNPCC who have undergone resection require careful monitoring* or surveillance to be sure the cancer doesn't come back, or develop elsewhere in the colon. Thus, HNPCC undergo more frequent colonoscopies than other colon cancer survivors.

Familial Adenomatous Polyposis (FAP) Like HNPCC, **familial adenomatous polyposis (FAP)** is inherited in an **autosomal dominant** fashion, meaning there is a 50% likelihood that offspring will carry the gene mutation. The gene mutation is in the **APC gene**. Patients with FAP develop polyps—sometimes hundreds of them—in their teens, and 100% will go on to develop colon cancer, usually by age 40 if untreated. A **total proctocolectomy is curative** as it *removes the at-risk mucosa* and prevents cancer formation (Fig. 26.9a, b). This operation is usually performed in mid to late adolescence or early 20s, typically around the time the diagnosis is made. FAP patients are candidates for reconnection surgery, but it is somewhat more complex and requires the construction of a small bowel pouch that is connected to the anus. This **restorative procedure** allows patients to "live without a [stoma] bag" for the rest of their lives, and is known as an **ileal pouch anal anastomosis (IPAA)**. Because the small bowel pouch is fashioned to resemble the shape of the capital letter ***J***, it is often referred to as a "**J-pouch**."

FAP and HNPCC are the most important of the genetic forms of CRC, and PA students and those practicing in GI and colorectal surgery should be familiar with these important conditions (Table 26.4). Other forms of genetic CRC include **MUTYH-associated polyposis**, which is autosomal *recessive* and tends to be more attenuated (fewer polyps) than classical FAP.

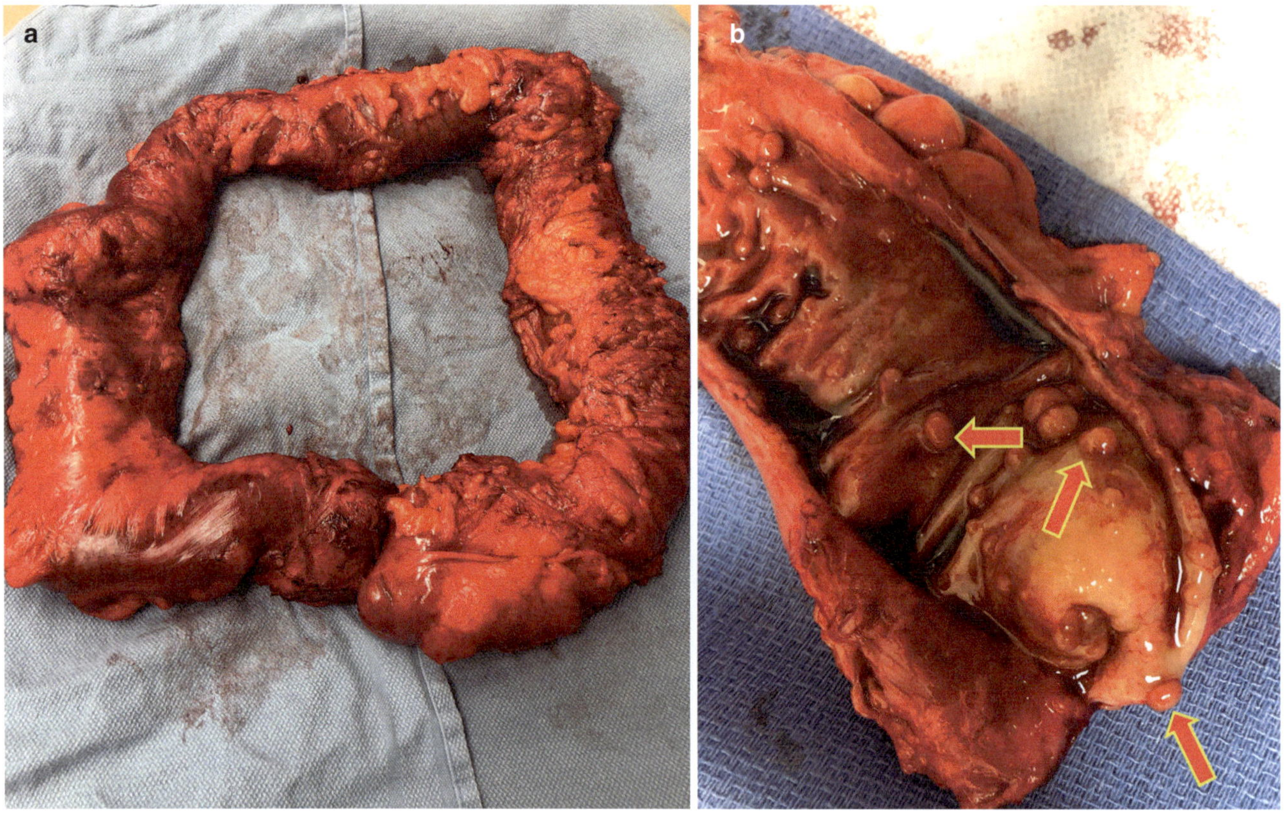

Fig. 26.9 FAP patients who undergo a prophylactic total proctocolectomy can be cured of the disease, which is marked by the formation of hundreds of polyps along the mucosal lining. (**a**) The specimen of a teenage patient who has undergone a total proctocolectomy. (**b**) The open specimen reveals numerous polyps (arrows)

Table 26.4 Comparison of FAP vs. HNPCC (Lynch syndrome)

Feature	FAP (Familial Adenomatous Polyposis)	HNPCC (Hereditary Nonpolyposis Colorectal Cancer/Lynch Syndrome)
Gene involved	APC gene (tumor suppressor) on chromosome 5q21	DNA mismatch repair (MMR) genes—most commonly MLH1, MSH2, MSH6, PMS2
Inheritance pattern	Autosomal dominant	Autosomal dominant
Colorectal cancer risk	~100% (if untreated)	~80% lifetime risk
Polyp burden	Hundreds to thousands of adenomatous polyps in colon	Few polyps (often <10), but with high malignant potential
Age of onset	Teen years to 20s for polyps; CRC in 30s–40s if untreated	CRC typically develops in 40s–50s
Extracolonic manifestations	Desmoid tumors Osteomas Congenital hypertrophy of retinal pigment epithelium (CHRPE) Duodenal/ampullary adenomas	Endometrial cancer Ovarian cancer Gastric, small bowel, biliary tract, urinary tract cancers
Screening recommendations	Colonoscopy starting at age 10–12; annual if polyps present	Colonoscopy starting at 20–25, every 1–2 years
Prophylactic surgery	Colectomy often recommended due to inevitable progression	Prophylactic colectomy is not recommended, but early screening/frequent colonoscopy indicated. Surgery needed if cancer is found; prophylactic hysterectomy/oophorectomy considered in women
Diagnosis	Genetic testing for APC mutation *or* clinical criteria	Amsterdam or Bethesda criteria, confirmed with MMR testing and microsatellite instability (MSI) testing
Syndrome subtypes	Classic FAP and attenuated FAP (fewer polyps, rectal sparing)	Lynch I (isolated CRC) and Lynch II (CRC + extracolonic cancers)

Overview of Colon and Rectal Cancer Staging Workup

Once the diagnosis of CRC has been established, clinical staging is required. The recommended staging workup for colon cancer in the United States includes **contrast-enhanced CT of the chest, abdomen, and pelvis** to assess for metastatic disease—with careful attention to the **liver** and **lung**, which are the *most common sites of distant organ metastasis*. Imaging can also be valuable in guiding the surgical plan. The American Society of Colon and Rectal Surgeons (ASCRS) recommends this approach. A **liver MRI** can be obtained *if* the findings of CT-abdomen reveal liver lesions that cannot be easily characterized, as MRI is better able to distinguish them. PET/CT is *not* routinely recommended. A baseline **carcinoembryonic antigen (CEA)** should be obtained (which is also important to follow longitudinally). **Rectal MRI** (with a special *cancer staging protocol*) is indicated for *rectal cancer*, and this can be used adjunctively with **endorectal ultrasound**.

Staging follows the **Tumor (T) node (N) metastasis (M)**, or **TNM staging** (Table 26.2). TNM can be used to define the **four cancer stages I–IV**. There is a substantial disparity in outcomes based on stage, with stage IV disease remaining associated with poor 5-year survival (Table 26.3).

Surveillance After Curative Intent Resection

After curative resection, surveillance protocols are designed to **detect recurrence** and ***meta*chronous** (*meta:* Greek meaning *later in time*) neoplasms early. The American Society of Colon and Rectal Surgeons recommends the following for stage II and III colon cancer: **(a)** history and physical examination along with **carcinoembryonic antigen (CEA)**, a protein marker used in cancer diagnosis and monitoring, every 3 months for the first 2 years (then every 6 months up to 5 years); **(b)** annual CT of the chest, abdomen, and pelvis for at least 3 years; **(c)** colonoscopy at 1 year postresection, then at 3 years, and every 5 years thereafter if normal. More intensive surveillance (e.g., more frequent imaging or CEA) does not improve overall or disease-specific survival compared to standard protocols, but may detect recurrences earlier [38–40]. Surveillance colonoscopy is associated with improved overall survival and higher rates of detection of asymptomatic recurrences, enabling more curative-intent resections, though the impact on cancer-specific mortality is less clear [41]. Most recurrences and metachronous cancers are detected *within the first 3 years postresection*, supporting the rationale for more intensive surveillance during this period [41]. These approaches, integrated with current screening practices, have contributed to declining colorectal cancer mortality in the US by facilitating early detection and intervention [12].

The Emerging Role of ctDNA **Circulating tumor DNA (ctDNA)** is a highly specific and sensitive biomarker for detecting minimal residual disease and early recurrence after curative resection of colon cancer—outperforming standard surveillance methods such as CEA measurement and providing earlier detection than imaging or colonoscopy in many cases. Postoperative ctDNA positivity is strongly associated with a markedly increased risk of recurrence, and serial ctDNA monitoring can detect recurrence a median of 3–10 months before conventional imaging or CEA elevation [42–50].

Compared to CEA, ctDNA demonstrates superior sensitivity, but not specificity for recurrence detection (sensitivity up to 66% vs. 32% for CEA; specificity ~96–98% for both) [42, 44, 48]. Imaging (CT or PET) remains more sensitive for established disease, but **ctDNA can identify molecular relapse before radiographic evidence, enabling potential earlier intervention** [42, 46, 47, 49]. However, in direct head-to-head comparisons, ctDNA does not consistently outperform the combination of imaging plus CEA in overall sensitivity for recurrence detection, and the *clinical benefit of earlier detection on survival outcomes remains under investigation* [42, 46, 51].

The American Society of Colon and Rectal Surgeons recognizes ctDNA as a promising tool for risk stratification and early recurrence detection, *but does not yet recommend it as a replacement for standard surveillance* (history, physical, CEA, colonoscopy, and CT imaging) due to the need for further validation and standardization [38]. Current evidence supports the use of ctDNA as a complementary adjunct to standard surveillance, particularly for identifying high-risk patients who may benefit from intensified follow-up or adjuvant therapy [38, 43, 45, 50, 52].

Patterns of Cancer Spread

Colon and rectal cancer spreads or **metastasizes** to certain organs preferentially. While CRC can metastasize to bone and brain, it seldom does; it favors two distant organs over all others: **1. Liver** and **2. Lung** (liver is most common). Patterns of cancer spread are closely tied to **(a)** the **lymphatic system** and **(b)** the **hematogenous route**. For left-sided tumors especially, the venous drainage is via the portal system—e.g., the **inferior mesenteric vein** (IMA) drains into the portal vein (Fig. 26.10). This is important because the first organ the por-

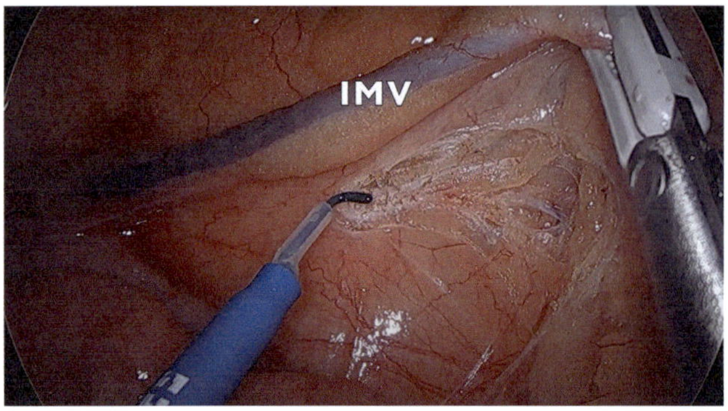

Fig. 26.10 A laparoscopic view during surgery is shown, specifically highlighting the inferior mesenteric vein (IMV). During left-sided cancer surgery, the IMV is ligated "high," which ensures that the mesentery, which includes lymph nodes, is harvested. Recall that the IMV drains into the *portal* venous circulation (not the *systemic* venous circulation) and is considered part of the portal venous system. Because the IMV drains directly into the liver, this accounts for the high incidence of liver metastatic disease in mCRC, as cancer cells spread via the hematogenous route

tal vein contents arrive at is the liver—thus tumor cells from the colon that enter the portal venous system can lodge in the liver and "set up shop" leading to metastatic growth. Tumor growth in the liver is probably also favored, as the liver provides a "fertile breeding ground" for cancer to grow.

Principles of Surgery for Colon and Rectal Cancer

One of the most important "big pictures" to grasp as a PA is that *each cancer type is treated uniquely* and is based on clinical evidence, usually from large-scale trials. As you start to learn about different cancers, you will see that the treatment and approach for each vary widely. For example, lymphoma (a type of bone marrow cancer) is treated mainly with chemotherapy, while anal cancer (a type of squamous cell cancer) is treated mainly with radiation therapy. **In the realm of colon cancer, surgery alone is used to treat about half of all CRC** (Table 26.5). **Furthermore, surgery alone is curative for the majority (80–90%) of nonmetastatic, stage I and II CRC**. Thus, surgery plays a big part in the treatment of colon cancer.

Table 26.5 Colorectal cancer treatment modalities in the United States

Treatment modality	Approx. proportion of patients	Notes
Surgery only (curative intent)	≈50% of patients with localized CRC	Surgery alone cures about half of patients with colon cancer
Surgery + Adjuvant Chemotherapy	Majority of remaining patients	Particularly, stage III colon and stage III rectal cancers
Neoadjuvant Chemotherapy + Chemoradiation *followed by* Surgery	Increasing role for locally advanced rectal cancer; various protocols termed total neoadjuvant therapy (TNT)	Standard for stage III rectal cancer; chemoradiation for recta cancer
TNT alone (no surgery)	Select cases, when a complete response occurs; only for rectal cancer	Emerging chemotherapy protocols for select rectal cancers
Inoperable/ Palliative Chemotherapy	~14–15% overall	Often due to advanced metastatic disease or comorbidities

There are essentially two kinds of operations that surgeons perform for colorectal cancer: (a) **radical resection**, also known as an **oncologic resection,** and (b) **local excision;** performed <u>*only*</u> in highly select instances. **Radical resection is the standard operative approach for the majority of colorectal malignancies**. It doesn't matter if the operation is performed via an open approach, a laparoscopic approach, or a robotic approach—**the operation is always the same**, following the same principles. The resection "template" is predicated upon the draining lymph node basin and the idea with radical resection is to **(a)** remove lymph nodes that could potentially harbor cancer that has spread, **(b)** remove a portion of bowel containing the tumor with negative margins (at least 5 cm) on either side, when possible, and **(c)** do all of this ***en bloc***—meaning "in one piece" not in fragments (Fig. 26.11). There are other guidelines for oncologic resection, but these are the most important ones. Minimally invasive approaches, namely, laparoscopic (Fig. 26.12) and robotic (Fig. 26.13a–c), provide patients and surgeons several advantages and are generally favored approaches for all elective colorectal procedures nowadays.

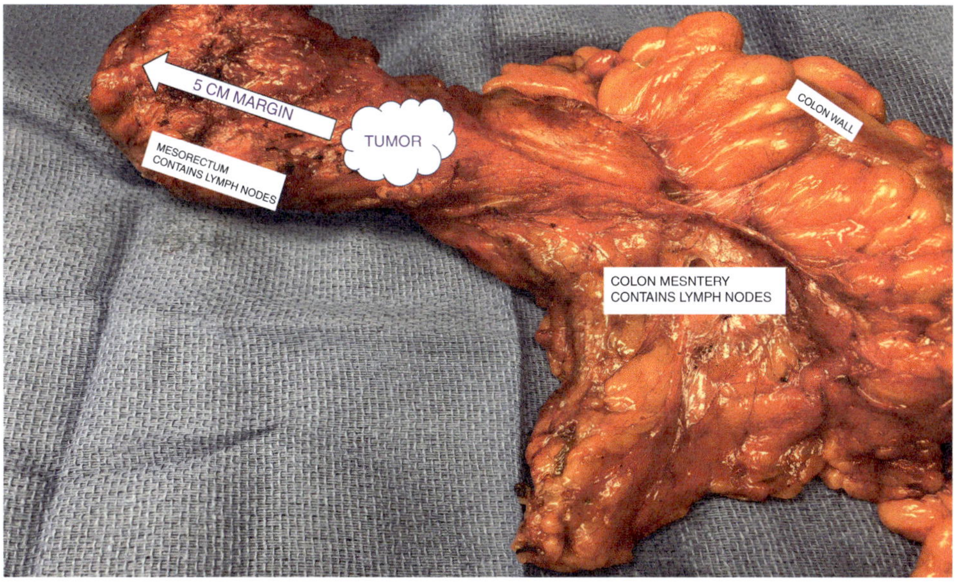

Fig. 26.11 When colon cancer surgery is performed, in many cases, the tumor itself is not seen, even after the specimen has been removed from the body. Shown here is a segment of bowel, the colorectum, that has been surgically removed and that contains the tumor within it, although it is not visible. The entire specimen includes the portion of bowel containing the tumor, as well as lymph nodes from the draining lymph node basin. The specimen is removed as one piece, which is described as *en bloc*. The principles of CRC surgery also dictate that a negative margin, from the edge of the resection to the edge of the tumor, is achieved (as shown)

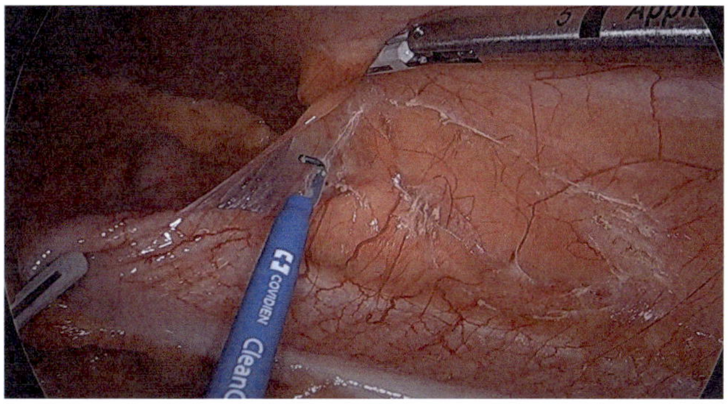

Fig. 26.12 A still view during laparoscopic colectomy is shown. Two 5 mm graspers are used to expose the plane of dissection, as electrocautery (blue, with hook tip) is used to release the lateral attachments along the descending colon, which is affixed to the abdominal sidewall, with an attachment known as the **white line of Toldt**. The white line of Toldt represents the line where the *visceral* peritoneum of the colon fuses with the *parietal* peritoneum of the abdominal wall laterally. Operation on the large bowel often requires the segment of bowel be freed from its attachments and embryonic fusion planes

One other important detail: prior to resection, and during colonoscopy, the tumor is typically **tattooed** so that it may be identified at the time of surgery (Fig. 26.14).

After resection, the specimen is collected and sent to the pathology lab for further histologic examination and final (pathologic) staging. In minimally invasive surgery, the specimen can be retrieved, for example, via a small Pfannenstiel incision—or even transrectally (and in females transvaginally) in centers with expertise in these techniques. Once this has been done, surgeons will then make a decision about *reconnection* of the two ends of bowel—termed **an anastomosis** (Fig. 26.15a, b). Sometimes anastomosis is possible, other times it is not. The most important factors that are required for constructing an anastomosis are **(a)** *good arterial blood supply*, **(b)** *no tension* on the bowel, and **(c)** an *absence of severe underlying comorbidity* or malnutrition. The most important and dreaded colorectal-specific risk of surgery is an **anastomotic leak**, which can lead to severe

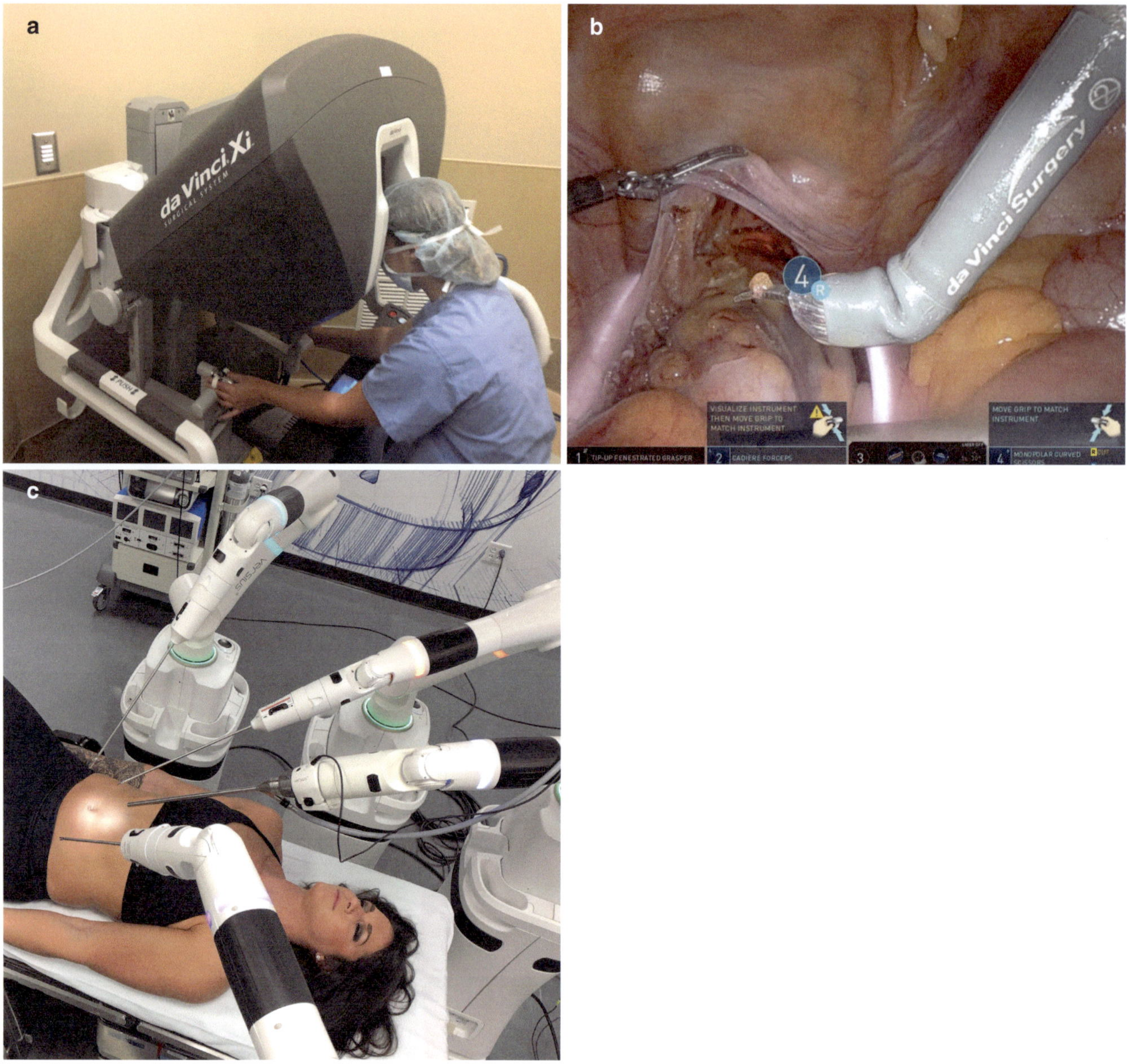

Fig. 26.13 (**a**) The surgeon console for the Xi da Vinci Surgical System (Intuitive Surgical) is shown. It is quite different from "old-fashioned" surgery in that the surgeon is not scrubbed in and instead operates remotely. (**b**) The console view is shown during colorectal surgery for cancer. Lighted stents have been placed in the ureters (visible by two white bands on either side of the colon), and the da Vinci system is being used to retract and expose the operative field. Note the information displayed at the bottom of the viewfinder that details various patient-related parameters. 3D vision, wristed instrumentation, and precision are among the advantages of robotics over laparoscopy. However, current evidence is mixed and suggests that in expert hands, laparoscopic colon surgery and robotic colon surgery have similar outcomes. (**c**) Although the robotics industry has been previously dominated by a single vendor, many new robotic systems are emerging within the global market. Shown here is a modular design by CMR Surgical (Versius®). This allows for improved flexibility and is more adaptable to laparoscopic equipment than da Vinci. A multitude of other robotic systems are emerging, and there is an increasing role for artificial intelligence applications, particularly for computer vision

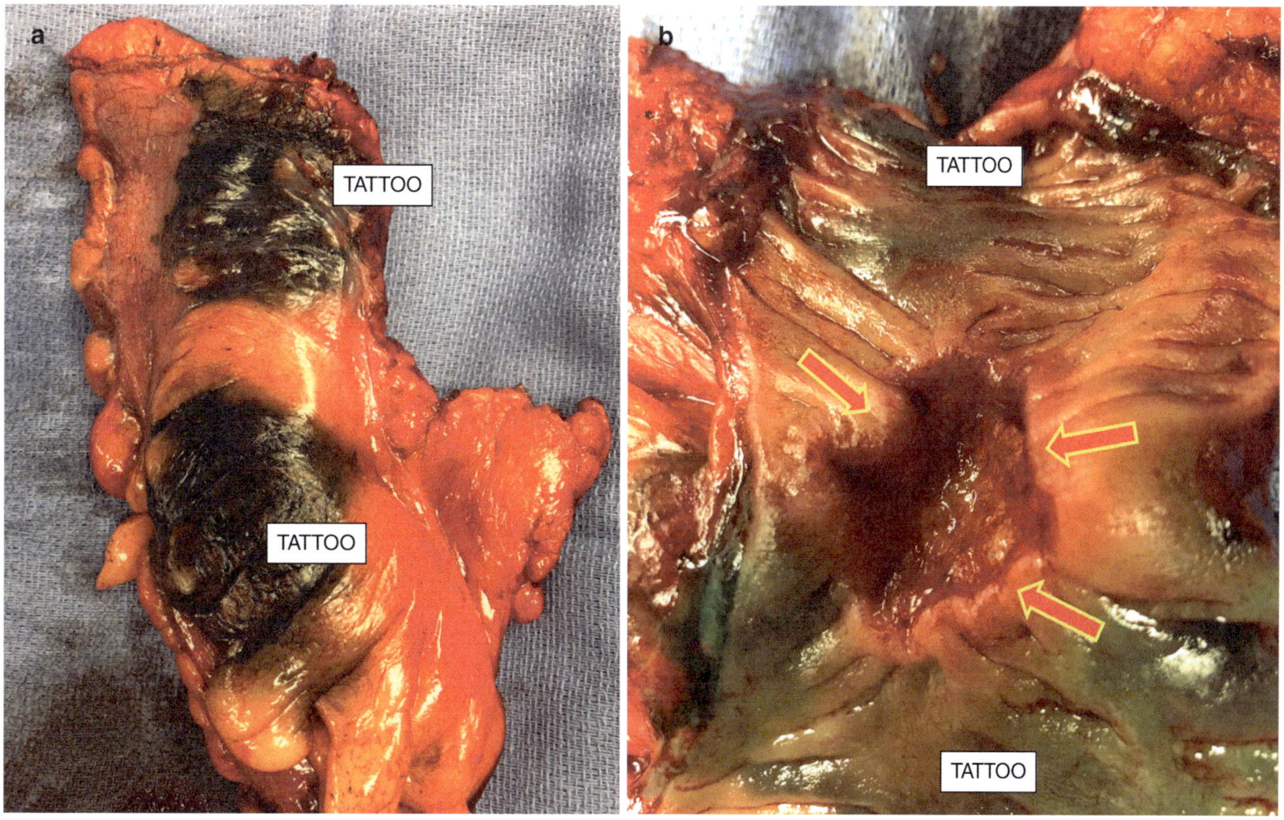

Fig. 26.14 (**a**) Two dark blue tattoos have been placed during colonoscopy, prior to surgery. They were used to locate the tumor, which is otherwise impossible to visualize. The resected specimen, shown, reveals the tattoos, but not the tumor, which is hidden deep inside. (**b**) When the specimen is opened, after it has been resected, the ulcerated cancer is clearly found, and you can see the tattoo marks that were placed endoscopically (prior to surgery). Just like you can go out and get a skin tattoo, the colon can *also* be tattooed in the same way, only the technique involves injecting ink (such as India Ink) in the submucosal plane during colonoscopy using a special injection needle. The purpose of the tattoo is so that the segment containing the tumor can be visualized, especially during minimally invasive surgery, as you cannot feel the tumor and thus may not be able to find/localize it during surgery. Remember, this is because cancers grow from the inside out, so they're not usually visible from the outside!

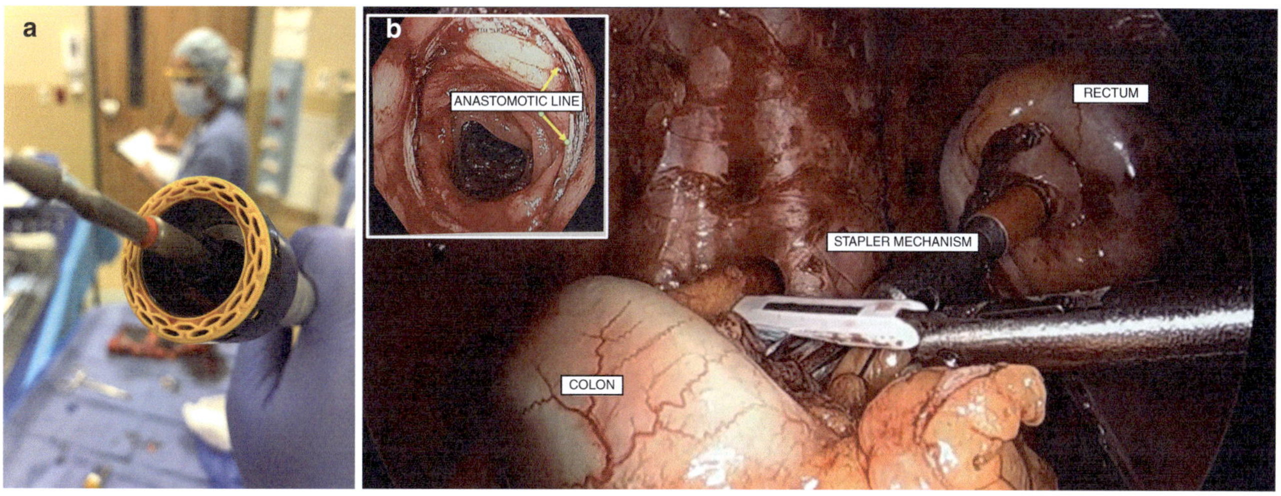

Fig. 26.15 (**a**) The arm portion of a highly specialized circular endoluminal stapler is shown with the spike deployed; the yellow circle contains two rows of staples. (**b**) This stapler arm is delivered transanally, the spike is deployed, and mated to another component called the anvil. This allows the two ends to be connected "mechanically" rather than by suturing. Stapling devices such as this one are very commonly used in gastrointestinal surgery. Inset: the anastomosis formed with the staple gun is shown via endoscopic (colonoscopic) view

sepsis and even death. When an anastomosis is deemed not suitable for the patient by the surgeon, a **stoma** is created to divert the stool. Stomas can be permanent or temporary, depending on the specifics of the case and patient. Sometimes a **diverting** or "**defunctioning**" stoma (especially an ileostomy) is made at the time of anastomosis, to allow the anastomosis a better chance at healing and/or to minimize the consequences of a leak. Whether or not to create a defunctioning stoma at the time of anastomosis is multifactorial and beyond the scope of this chapter.

Perfusion Assessment in Real-Time One important way to assess perfusion and thus ensure good healing after an anastomosis is by using a biofluorescent dye, called **indocyanine green (ICG),** which can be administered systemically (usually by the anesthesiologist during the procedure). If there is blood flow to an organ (such as the bowel), it will be rapidly detected using cameras that are capable of imaging in the near infrared spectrum (Fig. 26.16), and will appear neon green (Fig. 26.17). This tells the surgeon whether or not there is or is not adequate blood flow to attempt an anastomosis. Believe it or not, ICG biofluorescence is a complex process that utilizes principles from **quantum mechanics** (Fig. 26.18).

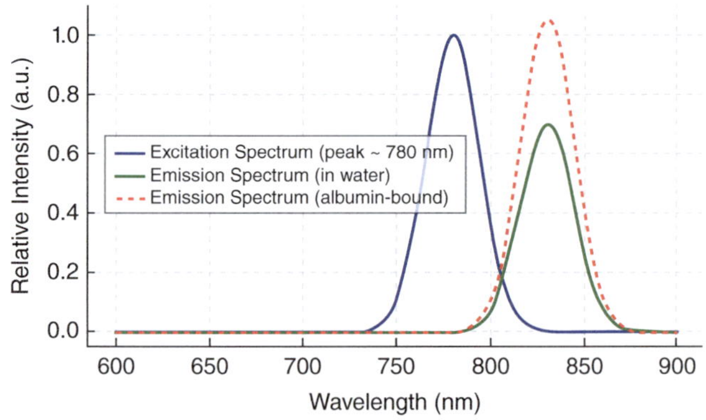

Fig. 26.16 A graph depicting the excitation and emission spectra of **Indocyanine Green (ICG)** is shown. Here, the blue curve represents excitation (peak around 780 nm), while the green curve represents emission in water (~830 nm), and the red dashed curve represents emission when bound to albumin, which *increases fluorescence intensity*. This illustrates how protein binding (e.g., to albumin in blood) enhances ICG's quantum yield and brightness—a key reason it's effective for in vivo imaging. The quantum yield of indocyanine green (ICG) depends on the environment it's in, generally speaking. When ICG binds to **plasma proteins like albumin, it** stabilizes ICG and **increases** its quantum yield. In blood, when ICG is bound to albumin, the quantum yield is approximately 2.7%. Despite its low quantum yield, ICG is widely used in surgery because it is still quite useful and results in a "bright" image that can be easily and quickly assessed intraoperatively in real-time

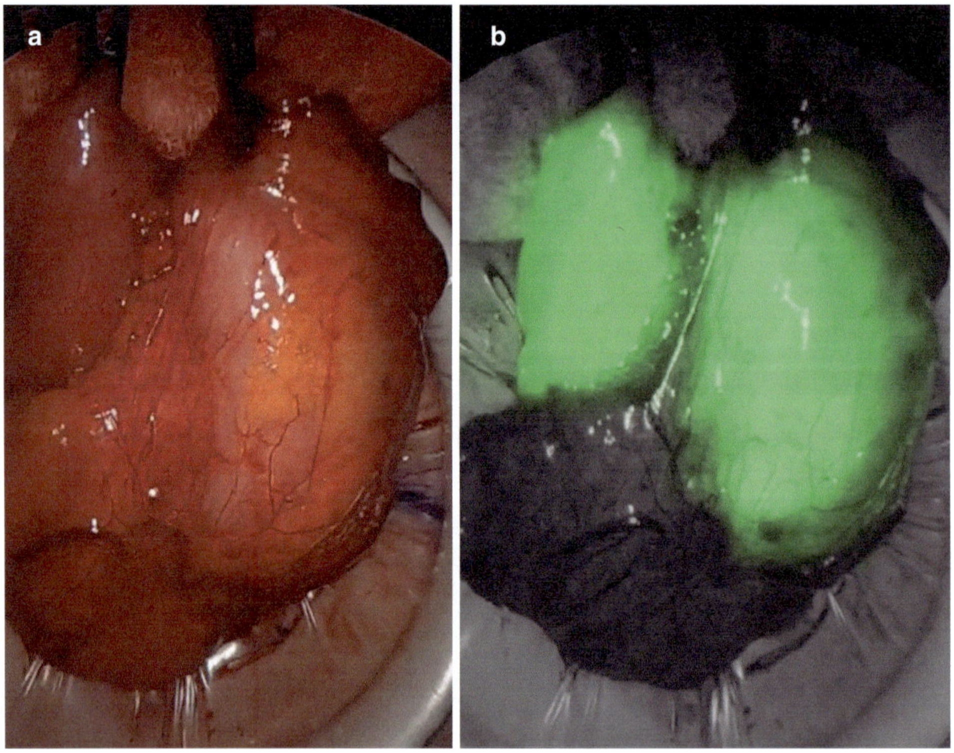

Fig. 26.17 (**a**) Two portions of bowel, small intestine on the left and large intestine on the right, are brought into juxtaposition in preparation for anastomosis. Visualized under normal white light of a standard laparoscope, it is not possible to determine whether or not the two ends are perfused (e.g., viable). (**b**) A few seconds after the systemic injection of indocyanine green (a biofluorescent dye), the bowel appears neon green under near infrared light. This confirms bowel perfusion, which is a compulsory requirement to ensure anastomotic healing

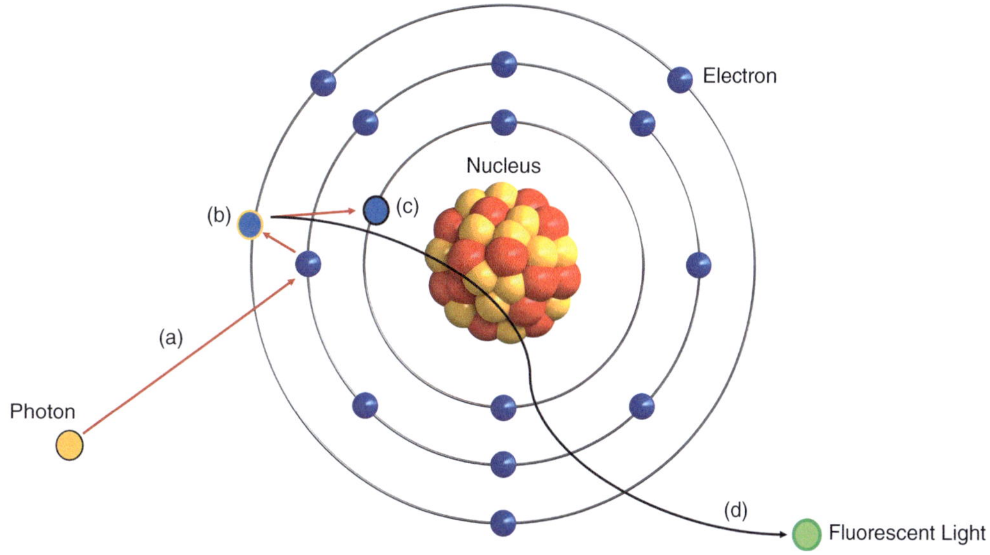

Fig. 26.18 When light behaves as a particle, we describe it as a photon (a massless packet of energy that can be quantized). That light behaves as ***both* a wave and a particle** represents a concept known as ***wave-particle duality***, which is a central idea in **quantum mechanics**. When **a photon** (white light) hits a fluorescent molecule (**a**), the **energy of that photon is absorbed** by an **electron** in the molecule. This energy **excites the electron**, causing it to jump from a **low-energy state (ground state)** to a **higher-energy state (excited state)** (**b**). Think of this like giving a child a sugar rush—*they go from calm to hyperactive (excited) quickly!* The excited electron doesn't stay excited for long (typically **nanoseconds**), and the electron **returns to its ground state** (**c**), and as it does, it **releases a photon** (**d**)—except this time the photon is **fluorescent**, and is what we end up seeing, which is what ICG is used for in the operating room to assess arterial bowel perfusion. ***Quantum yield*** (Φ) is a measure of how efficiently a photophysical process occurs—specifically, it tells you how many useful events happen per photon absorbed, and can be mathematically defined as follows:

$$\Phi = \left(\frac{\text{Number of Photons Emitted}}{\text{Number of Photons Absorbed}} \right)$$

Rectal Cancer Is Different

We often lump colon cancer and rectal cancer together, but ***they are quite different!*** While most *colon* cancer treatment follows standardized and straightforward algorithms, ***rectal* cancer treatment is *highly complex*** and may involve a combination of treatments that include surgery, chemotherapy, and radiotherapy. This strategy is commonly used for locally advanced tumors. When more than one type of cancer treatment is used in the treatment strategy for cancer, it is described as **multimodal** therapy. Since 2020, the focus has been on treating rectal cancer with *upfront* therapy, using a protocol termed **total neoadjuvant therapy, or TNT**. Here, patients with locally advanced rectal cancer receive systemic chemotherapy followed by radiation therapy (or vice versa) and *then* surgery (as the *last* step). Thus, in TNT, patients get all their [nonsurgical] treatment *upfront*. Rectal cancer cases are routinely presented at the **multidisciplinary tumor board (MDT)** for discussion and treatment disposition. MDT is a meeting in which surgeons, radiation oncologists, medical oncologists, pathologists, radiologists, geneticists, and nurse navigators meet to review patient cases and render treatment recommendations.

Radiation for Rectal Cancer

In the **field of oncology**, we often discuss cancer in terms of (a) **local control** and (b) **systemic control** (i.e., preventing/curtailing metastatic disease). While systemic chemotherapeutics address metastasis, *local control is addressed with surgery and/or radiation.*

External beam radiotherapy (XRT) can be of use as part of a multimodal approach to rectal cancer. In counter distinction, radiation is not used to treat colon cancer (with very rare exceptions). XRT is well-suited for some tissue types (the anus, prostate, rectum) but not others. For example, the small intestine is not able to tolerate XRT at all. When XRT is administered, it is usually given with a so-called radio-sensitizer. A radio-sensitizer is a low dose of chemotherapy that is often given as a pill (oral **capecitabine**, brand name **Xeloda**), but also as **infusional 5-FU**. This boosts the effect of XRT only and is nowhere near the strength of standard chemotherapy regimens. Still, because some chemotherapy is administered with XRT, it is often described as **chemoradiation** or **chemo-XRT**. This is somewhat misleading, because it is the radiation (and *not* the chemo-sensitizer) that is providing the *main effect.*

While there are many nuances to when chemo-XRT should be administered for patients with rectal cancer, one important rule is that if radiation is going to be given, it should be prior to and not after surgery. Note: giving *treatment prior to surgery* is termed ***neo*adjuvant** treatment; while administering chemotherapy or radiation *after* surgery is termed **adjuvant**. The goal of targeting a rectal tumor with radiation prior to surgery is to shrink it down so that when it comes time to operate, it will be more likely that the tumor will be removed completely. When a tumor is surgically removed without any tumor left behind, it is described as an **R0** (pronounced *R-zero*) **resection**. Patients who have an **R0 resection** have a much lower chance of having the tumor come back after resection than those who do have residual tumor. **The goal of every cancer surgery is an R0 resection**.

Total Mesorectal Excision for Rectal Cancer

The same principles of radical resection apply (as for colon cancer, discussed previously) with a strict focus on achieving an R0 resection. For rectal cancer specifically, much effort is given to assuring that the mesorectal envelope is removed intact and completely (Fig. 26.19). This concept was introduced in the 1980s as an important technique by Prof. Bill Heald, and is known as **total mesorectal excision,** or **TME**. **TME is the gold-standard in oncologic surgery for rectal cancer** and is universally practiced today. It has been well demonstrated that TME translates into improved clinical outcomes. TME for rectal cancer can be done open, laparoscopically, or robotically. A minimally invasive approach is generally preferred.

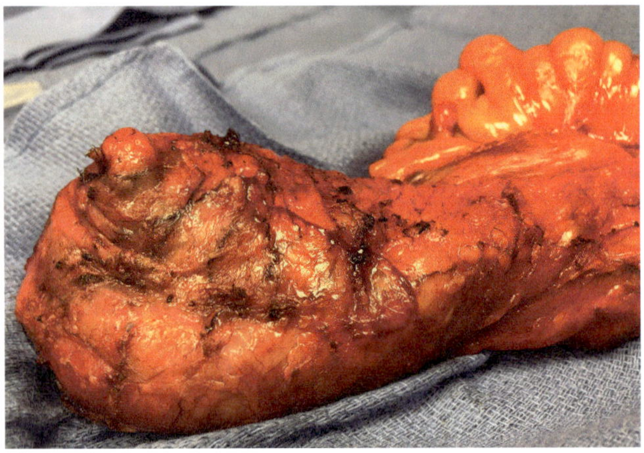

Fig. 26.19 The surgical specimen from a patient with rectal cancer is shown. The tumor is not visible from the outside, as it lies *deep inside*. Importantly, the principles of rectal cancer surgery mandate that the surrounding mesorectal envelope be removed "intact" without violation of this envelope. Removing the mesorectal envelope intact in this manner is known as **total mesorectal excision**, or **TME**. *TME is the standard approach for rectal cancer*. This image reveals an intact TME specimen, with smooth (not jagged) edges to the mesorectal envelope

Local Excision of Rectal Cancer

Although oncologic resection is the gold-standard for the surgical treatment of colorectal cancer, there are some instances when a nonradical approach—called **local excision**—is used (Fig. 26.20). Most typically, this is a strategy applied for *early-stage* **rectal** cancers T1N0M0 that are histologically "favorable" (meaning nonaggressive). It is best suited for patients with *low-lying,* early-stage rectal tumors, because doing the gold-standard operation in this case could result in a permanent colostomy, due to technical reasons, and also because rectal radical resection carries substantially more risk than **colon** radical resection for reasons that are beyond the scope of this chapter, but are mainly due to the complex location of the rectum within the pelvic cavity.

The principles of local excision are: **(a)** tumor removal *without* fragmentation, **(b)** with negative margins, and **(c)** ideally through the entire thickness of the bowel wall, which can be reapproximated via endoluminal suturing. Nowadays, most local excision is carried out using a technique called ***t****rans****a****nal* ***m****inimally* ***i****nvasive* ***s****urgery* (**TAMIS**) [54–56], which can also be performed robotically—**robotic TAMIS** (Fig. 26.21).

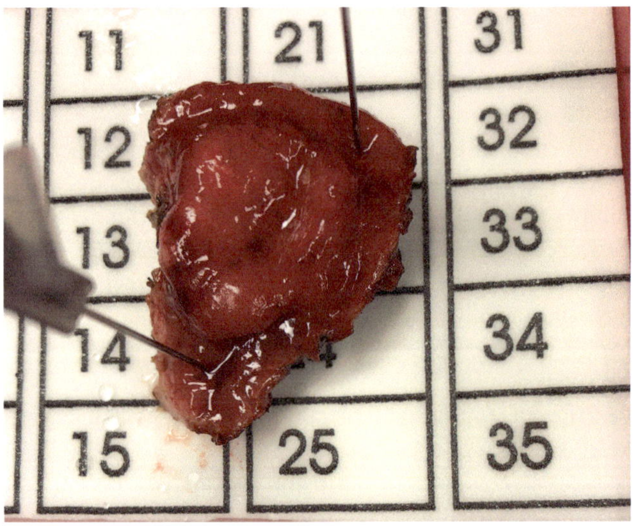

Fig. 26.20 A locally excised tumor is shown. A full-thickness local excision is a special type of operation, reserved *only* for select cases of early-stage rectal cancer. It is most typically performed using a technique called transanal minimally invasive surgery (TAMIS). The operation is performed with curative intent and spares patients the morbidity associated with radical resection

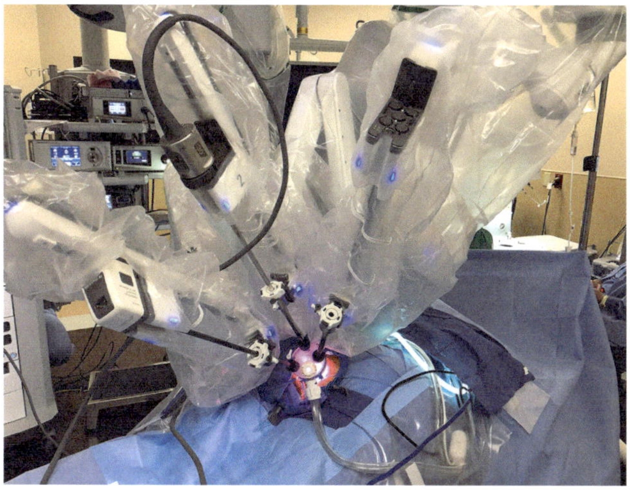

Fig. 26.21 Robotic transanal minimally invasive surgery (robotic TAMIS) is shown. This is an advanced technique that allows surgeons to remove tumors of the rectum transanally. The robotic cart has been docked transanally using a special access channel, called a "TAMIS port." Just like with laparoscopy, CO_2 insufflation allows the colorectum to be expanded, creating a working space and delineating the surgical field. TAMIS can be done with laparoscopic instruments (as it was first described) or using robotics. Precision and control are thought to improve the quality of oncologic excision; robots also simplify the task of endoluminal suturing, which is done after the excision of the tumor to reapproximate the rectal wall

Surgery for Liver and Lung Metastasis

For *some* types of cancer, once the tumor has spread to other parts of the body (stage IV), the only effective treatment is systemic chemotherapy, which is generally not curative. However, this is not always the case and is not true for all types of cancer, including metastatic CRC -- mCRC. In some cases of mCRC, it is possible to resection of the metastatic lesions with curative intent. For example, a portion of the liver (or lung) can be removed, and this has been shown to cure some patients with stage IV colon cancer. Thus, surgical removal of the metastasis, or **metastasectomy**, can be performed for curative intent for patients with stage IV CRC. *Surgical removal of all gross disease (primary tumor plus metastatic deposits) provides the best chance at cure.*

Standard Chemotherapy for Colon and Rectal Cancer

The standard chemotherapy regimens for colon cancer include **FOLFOX** (folinic acid, fluorouracil, and oxaliplatin), **CAPOX** (capecitabine and oxaliplatin), *or* **irinotecan-based regimens** such as **FOLFIRI** (folinic acid, fluorouracil, and irinotecan). FOLFOX and CAPOX are the preferred adjuvant therapies for **stage III colon cancer**, with the American Society of Colon and Rectal Surgeons recommending 3–6 months of therapy based on risk stratification and patient tolerance. In the United States, irinotecan-based regimens are less favored as first-line therapy in the **adjuvant** setting but are an option in metastatic disease, often as FOLFIRI or in triplet regimens (FOLFOXIRI) for select patients [38, 53].

In **metastatic colorectal cancer (mCRC),** these regimens are combined with targeted agents (e.g., bevacizumab, cetuximab; see next) based on molecular profiling and tumor location (see next). For patients with microsatellite instability-high (MSI-H) or deficient mismatch repair (dMMR) mCRC, the American Society of Clinical Oncology and the American Society of Colon and Rectal Surgeons recommend pembrolizumab (Keytruda) as first-line therapy, based on the KEYNOTE-177 trial, *which demonstrated superior progression-free survival and improved quality of life compared to chemotherapy* [3, 31, 38, 53]. Chemotherapy remains the standard for proficient mismatch repair (pMMR) or microsatellite stable (MSS) tumors, and for MSI-H/dMMR tumors when immunotherapy is contraindicated or not tolerated [21].

Targeted Therapies and the Changing Landscape of Colon Cancer Treatment

In the past decade, substantial clinically validated data have led to improvements in chemotherapy for CRC—most notably for mCRC and for dMMR CRC. This section highlights these findings.

It was discovered that patients with **wild-type K-*ras*** (i.e., nonmutated K-*ras* oncogene) **and** liver mCRC (especially

Table 26.6 Targeted drug therapy for colorectal cancer

Drug name	Mechanism of action	Application
Cetuximab	Blocks EGFR	Proven benefit for liver metastatic K-ras *wild type* CRC
Panitumumab	Blocks EGFR	When combined with sotorasib, improves survival for KRASG12C mutated metastatic CRC (CODEBREAK 300 TRIAL)
Revacizumab (Avastin)	Blocks VEGF	Cytostatic, used for control of liver metastatic CRC
Sotorasib	Inhibits KRASG12C	Improved survival for patients with KRASG12C mutated liver metastatic CRC (CODEBREAK 300)
Pembrolizumab (Keytruda)	Blocks PD-1 (on T-cells)	Used to treat unresectable MSI-H/dMMR CRC (KEYNOTE-177 trial)
Dostarlimab	Blocks PD-1 (on T-cells)	Cured patients with locally advanced rectal cancer with dMMR
Encorafenib	Targets BRAF V600E mutations	When combined with cetuximab showed benefit for BRAF mutant metastatic CRC (BREAKWATER TRIAL)
Nivolumab	Blocks PD-1 (on T-cells)	For dMMR nonmetastatic CRC, when combined with ipilimumab significantly down-staged CRC (NICHE I/II TRIALS)
Ipilimumab	Blocks CTLA-4 (on T-cells)	For dMMR nonmetastatic CRC, when combined with nivolumab significantly down-staged CRC (NICHE I/II TRIALS)

Legend: *EGFR* epidermal growth factor receptor, *PD-1* Programmed Cell Death, *dMMR* deficient in the mismatch repair gene, *MSI-H* microsatellite instability—*high*

unresectable tumors) benefit from adding a biologic agent—namely, **cetuximab**, a monoclonal antibody IgG to *Epidermal Growth Factor Receptor* **(EGFR)** expressing cells [57]. Cetuximab is usually given in conjunction with conventional chemotherapy. Note that many so-called *biologic drugs* are monoclonal **antibodies (ab)** to various targets, and this is why their nomenclature includes "ab,' 'such as cetuxim***ab***.

In 2025, it was shown that the doublet combination of **sotorasib** plus **panitumumab** is beneficial for refractory liver metastatic cancer who are **K-*ras* G12C** mutated [58, 59]. It was also shown that patients with unresectable liver metastasis also benefit from another type of biologic therapy called **revacizumab** (Avastin), which targets *vascular endothelial growth factor* **VEGF-A** [60]. Often, revacizumab is given in conjunction with conventional or "traditional" chemotherapeutics, although revacizumab is cyto*static* and not cyto*toxic*, so it *basically prevents disease progression,* but doesn't shrink or melt away cancer.

Recent trials (2025) have demonstrated that, for liver mCRC exhibiting **dMMR,** patients benefited from biologic therapy as *first-line treatment*—without the addition of conventional chemotherapy. The biologic agent used in these studies was **nivolumab** in combination with **ipilimumab** (**Niche I and II trials**) [61].

There have been other quite exciting developments with *programmed cell death* **(PD-1)** ***inhibitors*** for dMMR colorectal cancer. In 2022, it was shown that single-agent **PD-1 blockers** can completely cure dMMR rectal cancer *without* any other treatment at all—this was considered one of the most important studies from 2022 [62].

In 2025, the **Breakwater TRIAL** results were published [63]. Here, adding **encorafenib** and **cetuximab** to standard/conventional chemotherapy (mFOLFOX-6) in **BRAF-600** ***mutant*** **colon cancer** helped prolong survival and improve liver metastatic disease control. These trials highlight the real changes in the treatment of colorectal malignancy over recent years. Table 26.6 summarizes the use of targeted therapy in the modern treatment of CRC.

Special Circumstances: Nonoperative Management

In some cases, the tumors of the rectum are treated under a TNT protocol, receiving all treatment upfront, and the tumor melts completely away. This is known as a **complete (clinical) response, cCR**. This occurs up to 30% of the time with TNT. Prior to the 2000s, such patients routinely underwent standard resection, even though there was no cancer on pathologic examination of the specimen, a finding termed **complete pathologic response pCR** (Fig. 26.22a, b). This led to the realization that some patients can just be observed, and not undergo resection at all. Thus, when neoadjuvant therapy is given, and the tumor exhibits cCR, then patients can forgo surgery if they are willing to be enrolled in a program called **watch and wait**. In such programs, patients are carefully observed for local regrowth. If they develop regrowth, they require surgery. The majority of patients do not have regrowth, however, and remain cured without requiring surgery [64, 65].

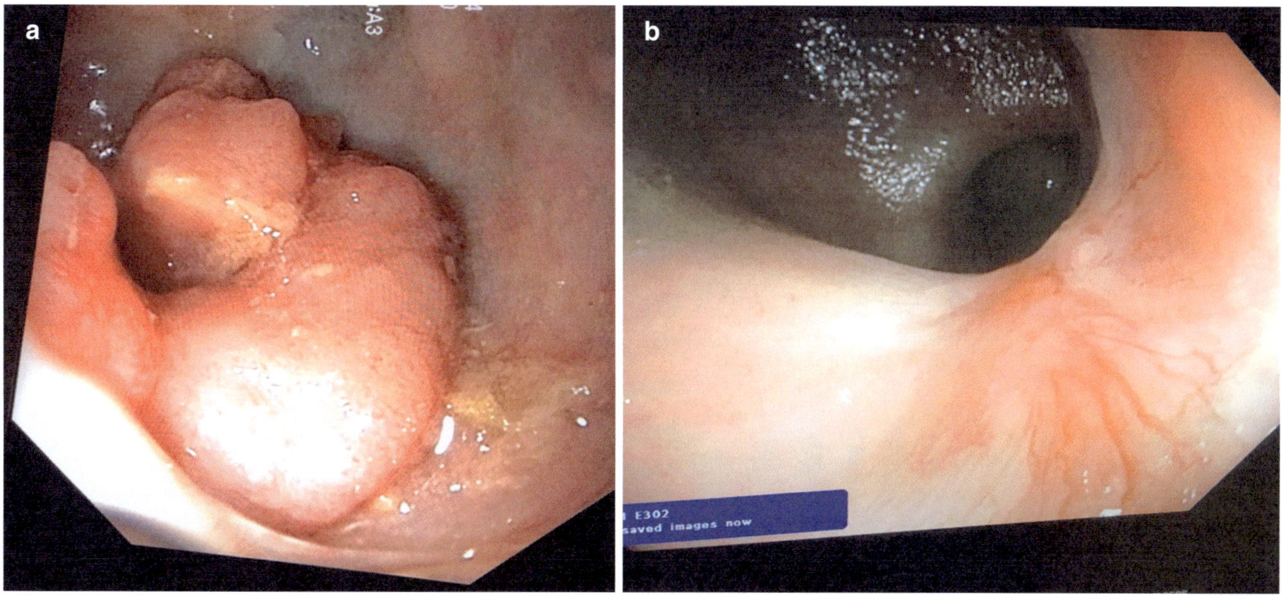

Fig. 26.22 (**a**) Endoscopic view of a rectal cancer prior to treatment, image taken at the time of diagnosis. The patient underwent neoadjuvant systemic chemotherapy followed by chemoXRT (TNT) prior to surgery. (**b**) Prior to surgery, the patient underwent flexible sigmoidoscopy to reexamine the tumor, and the endoscopic view here captures a complete clinical response, with only white scar and telangiectasias present (cCR). Rather than subject the patient to undergo radical resection of the rectum where no apparent viable tumor remains, this patient was enrolled in a program called "watch and wait," and plans for surgery are essentially put on pause

References

1. Siegel RL, Wagle NS, Cercek A, Smith RA, Jemal A. Colorectal cancer statistics, 2023. CA Cancer J Clin. 2023;73(3):233–54. https://doi.org/10.3322/caac.21772.
2. Giaquinto A, Kratzer T, Minihan A, et al. Colorectal cancer facts & figures. American Cancer Society; 2025.
3. Morris VK, Kennedy EB, Baxter NN, et al. Treatment of metastatic colorectal cancer: ASCO guideline. J Clin Oncol. 2023;41(3):678–700. https://doi.org/10.1200/JCO.22.01690.
4. Tan JY, Yeo YH, Ng WL, Fong ZV, Brady JT. How have US colorectal cancer mortality trends changed in the past 20 years? Int J Cancer. 2024;155(3):493–500. https://doi.org/10.1002/ijc.34926.
5. Giaquinto AN, Sung H, Miller KD, et al. Breast cancer statistics, 2022. CA Cancer J Clin. 2022;72(6):524–41. https://doi.org/10.3322/caac.21754.
6. Caswell-Jin JL, Sun LP, Munoz D, et al. Analysis of breast cancer mortality in the US-1975 to 2019. JAMA. 2024;331(3):233–41. https://doi.org/10.1001/jama.2023.25881.
7. DeSantis CE, Ma J, Gaudet MM, et al. Breast cancer statistics, 2019. CA Cancer J Clin. 2019;69(6):438–51. https://doi.org/10.3322/caac.21583.
8. Shaukat A, Kahi CJ, Burke CA, et al. ACG clinical guidelines: colorectal cancer screening 2021. Am J Gastroenterol. 2021;116(3):458–79. https://doi.org/10.14309/ajg.0000000000001122.
9. Issaka RB, Chan AT, Gupta S. AGA clinical practice update on risk stratification for colorectal cancer screening and post-polypectomy surveillance: expert review. Gastroenterology. 2023;165(5):1280–91. https://doi.org/10.1053/j.gastro.2023.06.033.
10. Davidson KW, Barry MJ, Mangione CM, et al. Screening for colorectal cancer: US preventive services task force recommendation statement. JAMA. 2021;325(19):1965–77. https://doi.org/10.1001/jama.2021.6238.
11. McCabe MA, Mauro AJ, Schoen RE. Novel colorectal cancer screening methods - opportunities and challenges. Nat Rev Clin Oncol. 2025;22(8):581–91. https://doi.org/10.1038/s41571-025-01037-7.
12. Smith RA, Andrews KS, Brooks D, et al. Cancer screening in the United States, 2019: a review of current american cancer society guidelines and current issues in cancer screening. CA Cancer J Clin. 2019;69(3):184–210. https://doi.org/10.3322/caac.21557.
13. Li W, Watts J, Tan N. From screen to screening: entertainment and news television media effects on cancer screening behaviors. J Health Commun. 2019;24(4):385–94. https://doi.org/10.1080/10810730.2019.1607954.
14. Liu J, Niederdeppe J, Tong C, et al. Associations between news coverage, social media discussions, and search trends about celebrity deaths, screening, and other colorectal cancer-related events. Prev Med. 2024;185:108022. https://doi.org/10.1016/j.ypmed.2024.108022.
15. Montminy EM, Karlitz JJ, Landreneau SW. Progress of colorectal cancer screening in United States: past achievements and future challenges. Prev Med. 2019;120:78–84. https://doi.org/10.1016/j.ypmed.2018.12.004.
16. Yang DX, Gross CP, Soulos PR, Yu JB. Estimating the magnitude of colorectal cancers prevented during the era of screening: 1976 to 2009. Cancer. 2014;120(18):2893–901. https://doi.org/10.1002/cncr.28794.
17. Levin TR, Corley DA, Jensen CD, et al. Effects of organized colorectal cancer screening on cancer incidence and mortality in a large community-based population. Gastroenterology. 2018;155(5):1383–1391.e5. https://doi.org/10.1053/j.gastro.2018.07.017.
18. Liu J, Niederdeppe J. Effects of communicating lifetime risks and screening rates of colorectal cancer and breast cancer. Risk Anal. 2023;43(12):2581–96. https://doi.org/10.1111/risa.14109.
19. Syngal S, Brand RE, Church JM, et al. ACG clinical guideline: genetic testing and management of hereditary gastrointestinal cancer syndromes. Am J Gastroenterol. 2015;110(2):223–62; quiz 263. https://doi.org/10.1038/ajg.2014.435.
20. Tiwari AK, Roy HK, Lynch HT. Lynch syndrome in the 21st century: clinical perspectives. QJM. 2016;109(3):151–8. https://doi.org/10.1093/qjmed/hcv137.

21. Sinicrope FA. Lynch syndrome–associated colorectal cancer. N Engl J Med. 2018;379(8):764–73. https://doi.org/10.1056/NEJMcp1714533.
22. Durno C, Boland CR, Cohen S, et al. Recommendations on surveillance and management of biallelic mismatch repair deficiency (BMMRD) Syndrome: a consensus statement by the US multi-society task force on colorectal cancer. Am J Gastroenterol. 2017;112(5):682–90. https://doi.org/10.1038/ajg.2017.105.
23. Sinicrope FA. Increasing incidence of early-onset colorectal cancer. N Engl J Med. 2022;386(16):1547–58. https://doi.org/10.1056/NEJMra2200869.
24. Carethers JM, Stoffel EM. Lynch syndrome and lynch syndrome mimics: the growing complex landscape of hereditary colon cancer. World J Gastroenterol. 2015;21(31):9253–61. https://doi.org/10.3748/wjg.v21.i31.9253.
25. Sepulveda AR, Hamilton SR, Allegra CJ, et al. Molecular biomarkers for the evaluation of colorectal cancer: guideline from the American Society for Clinical Pathology, College of American Pathologists, Association for Molecular Pathology, and the American Society of Clinical Oncology. J Clin Oncol. 2017;35(13):1453–86. https://doi.org/10.1200/JCO.2016.71.9807.
26. Awosika JA, Gulley JL, Pastor DM. Deficient mismatch repair and microsatellite instability in solid tumors. Int J Mol Sci. 2025;26(9):4394. https://doi.org/10.3390/ijms26094394.
27. Bartley AN, Mills AM, Konnick E, et al. Mismatch repair and microsatellite instability testing for immune checkpoint inhibitor therapy: guideline from the College of American Pathologists in Collaboration with the Association for Molecular Pathology and Fight Colorectal Cancer. Arch Pathol Lab Med. 2022;146(10):1194–210. https://doi.org/10.5858/arpa.2021-0632-CP.
28. Ambrosini M, Manca P, Nasca V, et al. Epidemiology, pathogenesis, biology and evolving management of MSI-H/dMMR cancers. Nat Rev Clin Oncol. 2025;22(6):385–407. https://doi.org/10.1038/s41571-025-01015-z.
29. Chakravarty D, Johnson A, Sklar J, et al. Somatic genomic testing in patients with metastatic or advanced cancer: ASCO provisional clinical opinion. J Clin Oncol. 2022;40(11):1231–58. https://doi.org/10.1200/JCO.21.02767.
30. Yoshino T, Pentheroudakis G, Mishima S, et al. JSCO-ESMO-ASCO-JSMO-TOS: International expert consensus recommendations for tumour-agnostic treatments in patients with solid tumours with microsatellite instability or NTRK fusions. Ann Oncol. 2020;31(7):861–72. https://doi.org/10.1016/j.annonc.2020.03.299.
31. André T, Shiu KK, Kim TW, et al. Pembrolizumab in microsatellite-instability–high advanced colorectal cancer. N Engl J Med. 2020;383(23):2207–18. https://doi.org/10.1056/NEJMoa2017699.
32. Lizardo DY, Kuang C, Hao S, et al. Immunotherapy efficacy on mismatch repair-deficient colorectal cancer: from bench to bedside. Biochim Biophys Acta Rev Cancer. 2020;1874(2):188447. https://doi.org/10.1016/j.bbcan.2020.188447.
33. Williams CJM, Peddle AM, Kasi PM, et al. Neoadjuvant immunotherapy for dMMR and pMMR colorectal cancers: therapeutic strategies and putative biomarkers of response. Nat Rev Clin Oncol. 2024;21(12):839–51. https://doi.org/10.1038/s41571-024-00943-6.
34. Cavestro GM, Mannucci A, Balaguer F, et al. Delphi initiative for early-onset colorectal cancer (DIRECt) international management guidelines. Clin Gastroenterol Hepatol. 2023;21(3):581–603.e33. https://doi.org/10.1016/j.cgh.2022.12.006.
35. Sun CY, Chiang JM, Chen TC, Hung HY, You JF. Different surgical outcome and follow-up status between dMMR and pMMR colorectal cancer patients who fulfilled with Amsterdam-Ii criteria. World J Surg Oncol. 2020;18(1):195. https://doi.org/10.1186/s12957-020-01976-8.
36. Zhao K, Pang W, Liu X, et al. Mismatch repair status and lymph node ratio in survival prediction of Stage II/III rectal cancer patients: a comprehensive analysis of a multi-center retrospective study. Cancer Med. 2025;14(7):e70756. https://doi.org/10.1002/cam4.70756.
37. Johannet P, Rousseau B, Aghajanian C, Foote MB, Diaz LA. Therapeutic targeting of mismatch repair-deficient cancers. Nat Rev Clin Oncol. 2025;22(10):734–59. https://doi.org/10.1038/s41571-025-01054-6.
38. Vogel JD, Felder SI, Bhama AR, et al. The American Society of Colon and Rectal Surgeons clinical practice guidelines for the management of colon cancer. Dis Colon Rectum. 2022;65(2):148–77. https://doi.org/10.1097/DCR.0000000000002323.
39. Hardiman KM, Felder SI, Friedman G, et al. The American Society of Colon and Rectal Surgeons clinical practice guidelines for the surveillance and survivorship care of patients after curative treatment of colon and rectal cancer. Dis Colon Rectum. 2021;64(5):517–33. https://doi.org/10.1097/DCR.0000000000001984.
40. Kahi CJ, Boland CR, Dominitz JA, et al. Colonoscopy surveillance after colorectal cancer resection: recommendations of the US multi-society task force on colorectal cancer. Am J Gastroenterol. 2016;111(3):337–46; quiz 347. https://doi.org/10.1038/ajg.2016.22.
41. Fuccio L, Rex D, Ponchon T, et al. New and recurrent colorectal cancers after resection: a systematic review and meta-analysis of endoscopic surveillance studies. Gastroenterology. 2019;156(5):1309–1323.e3. https://doi.org/10.1053/j.gastro.2018.12.006.
42. Dawood ZS, Alaimo L, Lima HA, et al. Circulating tumor DNA, imaging, and carcinoembryonic antigen: comparison of surveillance strategies among patients who underwent resection of colorectal cancer-a systematic review and meta-analysis. Ann Surg Oncol. 2023;30(1):259–74. https://doi.org/10.1245/s10434-022-12641-7.
43. Negro S, Pulvirenti A, Trento C, et al. Circulating tumor DNA as a real-time biomarker for minimal residual disease and recurrence prediction in Stage II colorectal cancer: a systematic review and meta-analysis. Int J Mol Sci. 2025;26(6):2486. https://doi.org/10.3390/ijms26062486.
44. Duffy MJ, Crown J. Circulating tumor DNA as a biomarker for monitoring patients with solid cancers: comparison with standard protein biomarkers. Clin Chem. 2022;68(11):1381–90. https://doi.org/10.1093/clinchem/hvac121.
45. Chidharla A, Rapoport E, Agarwal K, et al. Circulating tumor DNA as a minimal residual disease assessment and recurrence risk in patients undergoing curative-intent resection with or without adjuvant chemotherapy in colorectal cancer: a systematic review and meta-analysis. Int J Mol Sci. 2023;24(12):10230. https://doi.org/10.3390/ijms241210230.
46. Wang Y, Li L, Cohen JD, et al. Prognostic potential of circulating tumor DNA measurement in postoperative surveillance of nonmetastatic colorectal cancer. JAMA Oncol. 2019;5(8):1118–23. https://doi.org/10.1001/jamaoncol.2019.0512.
47. Henriksen TV, Tarazona N, Frydendahl A, et al. Circulating tumor DNA in stage III colorectal cancer, beyond minimal residual disease detection, toward assessment of adjuvant therapy efficacy and clinical behavior of recurrences. Clin Cancer Res. 2022;28(3):507–17. https://doi.org/10.1158/1078-0432.CCR-21-2404.
48. Symonds EL, Pedersen SK, Murray D, et al. Circulating epigenetic biomarkers for detection of recurrent colorectal cancer. Cancer. 2020;126(7):1460–9. https://doi.org/10.1002/cncr.32695.
49. Schøler LV, Reinert T, Ørntoft MW, et al. Clinical implications of monitoring circulating tumor DNA in patients with colorectal cancer. Clin Cancer Res. 2017;23(18):5437–45. https://doi.org/10.1158/1078-0432.CCR-17-0510.

50. Kotani D, Oki E, Nakamura Y, et al. Molecular residual disease and efficacy of adjuvant chemotherapy in patients with colorectal cancer. Nat Med. 2023;29(1):127–34. https://doi.org/10.1038/s41591-022-02115-4.
51. Fakih M, Sandhu J, Wang C, et al. Evaluation of comparative surveillance strategies of circulating tumor DNA, imaging, and carcinoembryonic antigen levels in patients with resected colorectal cancer. JAMA Network Open. 2022;5(3):e221093. https://doi.org/10.1001/jamanetworkopen.2022.1093.
52. Malla M, Loree JM, Kasi PM, Parikh AR. Using circulating tumor DNA in colorectal cancer: current and evolving practices. J Clin Oncol. 2022;40(24):2846–57. https://doi.org/10.1200/JCO.21.02615.
53. Grothey A, Venook AP. Optimizing adjuvant therapy for localized colon cancer and treatment selection in advanced colorectal cancer. J Natl Compr Canc Netw. 2018;16(5S):611–5. https://doi.org/10.6004/jnccn.2018.0038.
54. Atallah S, Larach SW. Transanal minimally invasive surgery. JAMA Surg. 2021;156(1):92–3.
55. Atallah S, Albert M, Larach S. Transanal minimally invasive surgery: a giant leap forward. Surg Endosc. 2010 Sep;24(9):2200–5.
56. Kızıltoprak N, Aaron J, Diez C, Atallah S. TAMIS: new horizons in modern colorectal surgery. Turk J Colorectal Dis. 2025;35(2):33–40.
57. Karapetis CS, Khambata-Ford S, Jonker DJ, O'Callaghan CJ, Tu D, Tebbutt NC, Simes RJ, Chalchal H, Shapiro JD, Robitaille S, Price TJ. K-ras mutations and benefit from cetuximab in advanced colorectal cancer. N Engl J Med. 2008;359(17):1757–65.
58. Yaeger R. Combination therapy and appropriate dosing to target KRAS in colorectal cancer. N Engl J Med. 2023;389(23):2197–9.
59. Kim TW, Price T, Grasselli J, Strickler JH, Masuishi T, Kwok GW, Yalcin S, Obiozor CC, Chan E, Gokani P, Sunakawa Y. A phase 3 study of first-line sotorasib, panitumumab, and FOLFIRI versus FOLFIRI with or without bevacizumab-awwb for patients with KRAS G12C–mutated metastatic colorectal cancer (CodeBreaK 301).
60. Gruenberger T, Bridgewater J, Chau I, Alfonso PG, Rivoire M, Mudan S, Lasserre S, Hermann F, Waterkamp D, Adam R. Bevacizumab plus mFOLFOX-6 or FOLFOXIRI in patients with initially unresectable liver metastases from colorectal cancer: the OLIVIA multinational randomised phase II trial. Ann Oncol. 2015;26(4):702–8.
61. Chalabi M, Verschoor YL, Tan PB, Balduzzi S, Van Lent AU, Grootscholten C, Dokter S, Büller NV, Grotenhuis BA, Kuhlmann K, Burger JW. Neoadjuvant immunotherapy in locally advanced mismatch repair–deficient colon cancer. N Engl J Med. 2024;390(21):1949–58.
62. Cercek A, Lumish M, Sinopoli J, Weiss J, Shia J, Lamendola-Essel M, El Dika IH, Segal N, Shcherba M, Sugarman R, Stadler Z. PD-1 blockade in mismatch repair–deficient, locally advanced rectal cancer. N Engl J Med. 2022;386(25):2363–76.
63. Elez E, Yoshino T, Shen L, Lonardi S, Van Cutsem E, Eng C, Kim TW, Wasan HS, Desai J, Ciardiello F, Yaeger R. Encorafenib, cetuximab, and mFOLFOX6 in BRAF-mutated colorectal cancer. N Engl J Med. 2025;392(24):2425–37.
64. Renehan AG, Malcomson L, Emsley R, Gollins S, Maw A, Myint AS, Rooney PS, Susnerwala S, Blower A, Saunders MP, Wilson MS. Watch-and-wait approach versus surgical resection after chemoradiotherapy for patients with rectal cancer (the OnCoRe project): a propensity-score matched cohort analysis. Lancet Oncol. 2016;17(2):174–83.
65. Fernandez LM, São Julião GP, Figueiredo NL, Beets GL, van der Valk MJ, Bahadoer RR, Hilling DE, Kranenbarg EM, Roodvoets AG, Renehan AG, van de Velde CJ. Conditional recurrence-free survival of clinical complete responders managed by watch and wait after neoadjuvant chemoradiotherapy for rectal cancer in the International Watch & Wait Database: a retrospective, international, multicentre registry study. Lancet Oncol. 2021;22(1):43–50.

Anal Cancer

27

Steven D. Wexner and Marcus Oosenbrug

Introduction

Anal cancer is a rare disease, accounting for 2.8% of all gastrointestinal (GI) tract malignancies and 0.5% of all new cancer cases in the United States [1, 2]. To put it into perspective, there are approximately 153,000 new *colorectal* cancers diagnosed annually in the United States, compared to ~9700 new cases of *anal* cancer. In certain high-risk populations, however, the incidence is significantly higher [3, 4], and continues to rise, having risen by 2.7% per year from 2001 to 2015 in patients 50 years and older [5]. While anal malignancies reflect the multiple histologic subtypes found in the anal canal and include adenocarcinomas and malignant melanomas, the large majority are ***squamous cell carcinomas (SCC)***, and these are the focus of this chapter.

Epidemiology and Risk Factors

Analogous to cervical, vulvar, and penile cancers, anal SCC is a human papillomavirus (HPV)-associated malignancy, and risk factors relate directly to either ***exposure to the HPV virus*** or ***immunodeficiency***. HPV is the most common sexually transmitted infection in the United States, with 13 million Americans becoming infected every year [6]. HPV infection typically manifests grossly as the condyloma acuminatum (anal wart) (Fig. 27.1); however, chronic infection is associated with the development of precancerous lesions and malignancy. Over 450 serotypes of HPV have been identified [7], and those with a predilection for anogenital epithelium are classified according to their risk of oncogenicity. For example, low-risk ***HPV 6 and 11 are associated with benign anogenital warts***, while high-risk ***HPV 16 and 18 are associated with the development of precancerous lesions and anal SCC*** [8]. Transmission of the virus occurs through direct skin-to-skin contact or anoreceptive intercourse; however, autoinoculation from other genital lesions has been described [9]. Additional HPV exposure-related risk factors include men who have sex with men (MSM), a history of multiple sexual partners, sexually transmitted infections, and prior HPV-associated gynecological precancerous lesions or cancer [10–13].

Most HPV infections are cleared by the cell-mediated immune response within 12 months [14]. However, the virus may also persist as a subclinical infection, enter a latent phase, or even undergo future reactivation [15]. In the setting of ***immunodeficiency***, the risk of anal SCC is significantly elevated due to persistent infection or impaired ability to clear the virus. As such, human immunodeficiency virus (HIV) infection and solid organ transplant recipients are independent risk factors for the development of HPV-associated benign and malignant lesions [8, 16]. Patients with autoimmune diseases, including Crohn's disease and ulcerative colitis, have also been shown to have an increased risk of developing anal cancer [11]. Additionally, cigarette smoking has been shown to be associated with anal cancer [17], as has female sex [5]. No such correlation exists between anal SCC and colorectal cancer.

Benign manifestations of HPV infection include ***condylomata acuminata*** (note, **condyloma acuminatum** is the *singular* form, and should not be confused with **condyloma *latum*,** which is a cutaneous manifestation of secondary syphilis), or anal warts, which are raised, fleshy, cauliflower-like lesions and are often associated with itching. Treatment options include patient-applied topical agents such as imiquimod, 5-fluorouracil (5-FU), provider-applied trichloroacetic acid (TCA), cryotherapy (e.g., topical liquid nitrogen), and surgical ablation for larger or more extensive lesions. Importantly, ***warts have no malignant potential***. The ***Buschke–Löwenstein tumor*** (Fig. 27.2), or giant condyloma, is a rare, slow-growing, exophytic cauliflower-like

S. D. Wexner (✉) · M. Oosenbrug
Department of Colorectal Surgery, Medstar Georgetown University Hospital, Washington, DC, USA
e-mail: steven.d.wexner@medstar.net; marcus.oosenbrug@medstar.net

S. Atallah, J. Dragoljevic (eds.), *Fundamentals of Surgery for Physician Assistants*,
https://doi.org/10.1007/978-3-032-21069-2_27

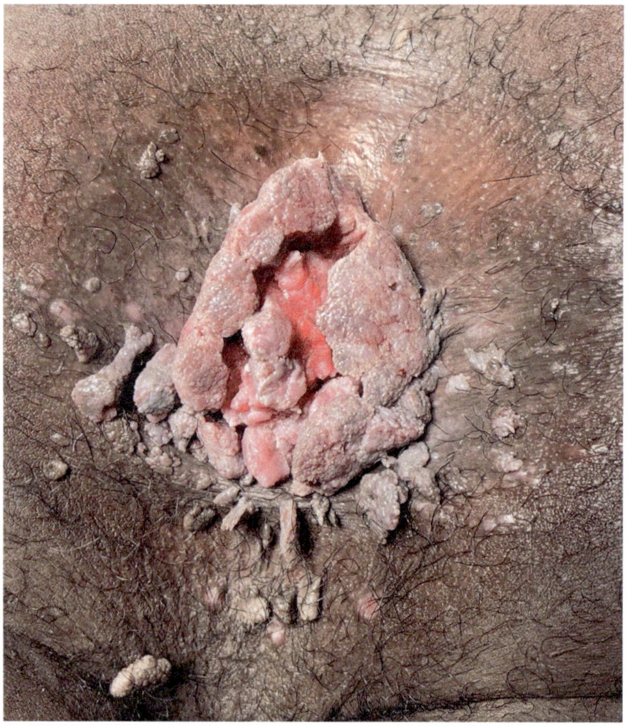

Fig. 27.1 Extensive circumferential condylomata acuminata (anal warts), with characteristic cauliflower appearance. (Courtesy: Dr. Juan J. Nogueras)

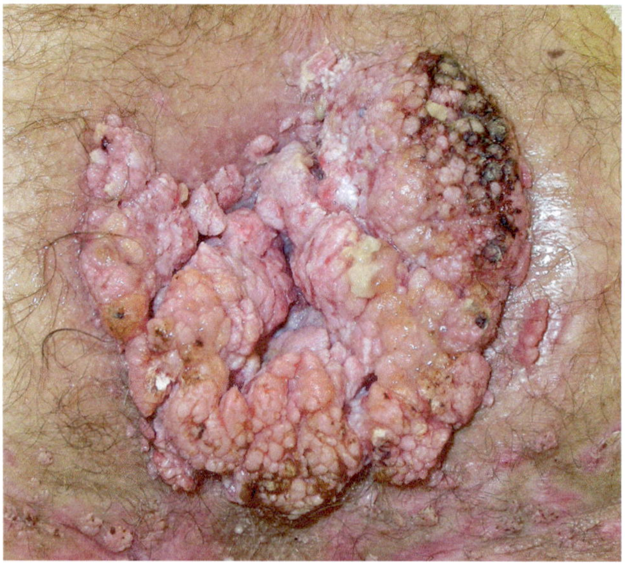

Fig. 27.2 Buschke–Löwenstein tumor harboring squamous cell carcinoma. (Courtesy: Dr. Juan J. Nogueras)

lesion. Although it has a tendency to spread laterally and can be locally destructive, it lacks basement membrane invasion and ***should also be considered a benign lesion***. Nevertheless, it does carry a risk of malignant transformation in over 50% of cases [18]. Treatment is surgical, with wide local excision being the mainstay of treatment, reserving abdominoperineal resection (APR; resection of the anus and rectum with creation of a permanent colostomy) for rare cases of sphincter involvement.

Anal Squamous Intraepithelial Lesions

Anal cancer is preceded by the development of precancerous lesions termed ***anal squamous intraepithelial lesions (SIL)***. Historically, these dysplastic lesions in the anal canal and perianal skin were termed anal intraepithelial neoplasms (AIN) and divided into three grades, reflecting the degree of morphologic change toward invasive cancer: AIN-1, -2, and -3. More recently, this terminology was simplified to distinguish the biology of transient, often spontaneously regressing HPV infection from persistent precancerous lesions, termed low- or high-grade squamous intraepithelial lesions (LSIL or HSIL, respectively) [19]. ***LSIL corresponds to either raised, exophytic warts or to flat lesions (AIN-1)***, reflecting a self-limited HPV infection. ***HSIL refers to AIN-2 and AIN-3*** (Fig. 27.3), lesions more likely to progress to invasive cancer. Immunohistochemical staining for p16, a biomarker of HPV-associated cell proliferation, classifies intermediate lesions (AIN-2) as LSIL or HSIL.

Although patients with anal SIL may present with symptoms of rectal bleeding or discharge, itching or pain, most individuals are asymptomatic, and diagnosis is most often made incidentally after anorectal surgery, or as part of screening for anal cancer. While guidelines are evolving, screening is recommended for all groups at high-risk for developing anal cancer. These include ***people living with HIV, people with a history of vulvar or cervical cancer, solid organ transplant recipients, HIV-negative MSM, and other immunocompromised persons without HIV infection***. Anal cancer screening is not recommended in the general population [20]. Screening is performed through anal **cytology** via cotton swab (with or without testing for HPV) and/or using ***high-resolution anoscopy (HRA)*** to obtain a tissue biopsy. A cytology result showing LSIL or HSIL should be referred for HRA. HRA is an office-based procedure used to assess the lining of the anal canal for dysplastic changes, and is analogous to colposcopy in screening for cervical and vulvar cancer. Under magnification of the anal canal, ***3% acetic acid solution*** is applied to the mucosa, and acetowhite staining correlates with dysplastic areas. HSIL-specific changes include a punctate appearance and mosaicism of the vasculature, as well as honeycombing and hyperpigmentation of the epithelium. ***Lugol's iodine solution*** is next applied, which causes brown staining of normal mucosa and yellow staining of HSIL. HRA allows for targeted biopsies of the anal mucosa, as well as simultaneous ablative treatment.

In general, LSIL may be observed, while HSIL is treated. While no clear surveillance guidelines exist, given the low risk of disease progression to invasive cancer, observation of LSIL with digital rectal examination (DRE) and HRA every 6–12 months is generally sufficient. In contrast, the recent landmark ANCHOR trial showed that treatment of HSIL has been shown to reduce the risk of anal cancer in high-risk patients, compared to observation alone [21]. The modality of treatment is guided by the anatomical location and extent of disease, cost and availability, and patient preference. Like the treatment of benign warts, patient-applied topical options include immunomodulators such as imiquimod, 5-FU, and podophyllotoxin. HRA-guided ablative treatments include TCA application, electrocautery, radiofrequency ablation, and infrared coagulation. Regardless of the chosen treatment method, patients should be surveilled every 6–12 months in the setting of dysplasia [22, 23].

Given the direct link between HPV infection and the development of anal cancer, significant efforts have been made at primary prevention, before the onset of sexual activity. As such, the Centers for Disease Control (CDC) currently recommends a ***two- or three-dose vaccination schedule for all individuals at age 11 or 12 years old, through to age 26***. There is no role for vaccination for secondary prevention in patients with HPV-associated lesions. Additionally, safer sex practices such as condom use should be advocated [24], and smoking cessation should be encouraged in all patients.

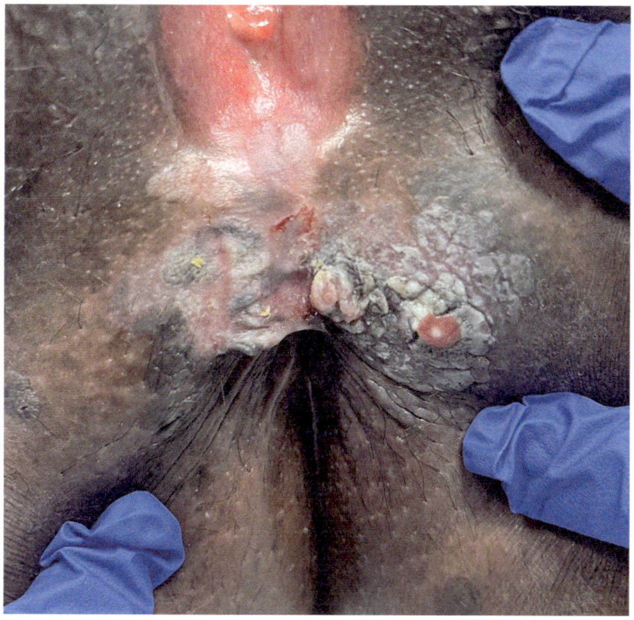

Fig. 27.3 Anal condylomata with a focus of HSIL. (Courtesy: Dr. Juan J. Nogueras)

Evaluation and Workup

The evaluation of a suspected anal cancer is highly dependent on the location of the lesion and requires an appreciation of its anatomic landmarks and histologic features. The anus comprises both the anal canal and the perianal skin. The "surgical" anal canal extends from the top of the anal sphincter complex proximally to the anal margin distally. The anal canal is lined by several types of mucosa, with proximal glandular/columnar mucosa (similar to that in the colon and rectum), a middle segment of transitional epithelium at the anal transition zone (ATZ), followed by distal squamous epithelium. An anal cancer is classified as an ***anal canal*** cancer if the lesion cannot be fully visualized with gentle traction of the buttocks. The perianal skin extends 5 cm radially from the anal margin and is lined with epidermis. ***Perianal cancers*** are those that can be fully visualized with gentle traction of the buttocks (Fig. 27.4) [25]. Lesions further than 5 cm from the anal margin are classified as ***skin cancers***, rather than anal cancers, and are staged and managed according to a separate algorithm.

Nearly half of patients with anal SCC present with bleeding, and *many report symptoms of anal pain* (one third), itch-

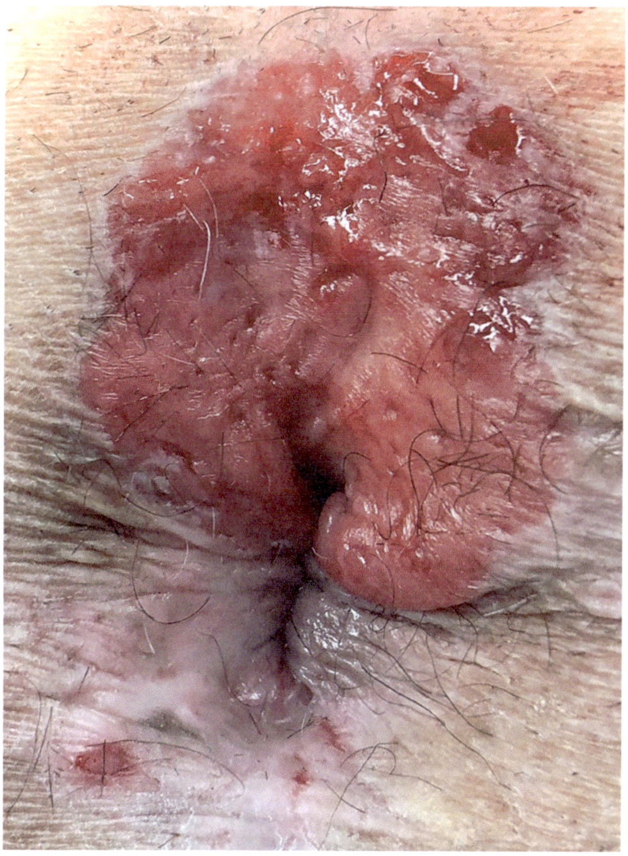

Fig. 27.4 Anal canal squamous cell carcinoma (note that the lesion is not fully visualized with gentle traction of the buttocks). (Courtesy: Dr. Juan J. Nogueras)

ing, mucus seepage, or a palpable mass. In contrast, 20% of patients are asymptomatic [13]. **Diagnosis is frequently delayed because these nonspecific symptoms may be easily attributed to common benign conditions such as hemorrhoids, fissures, and fistula-in-ano** [26, 27]. Half of patients present with local disease at diagnosis, while a further 29% present with locoregional node involvement [28].

In addition to the above symptoms, a thorough evaluation involves eliciting a sexual history, as well as a prior history of HPV-related lesions and HPV vaccination status. Physical examination includes inspection of the genitalia and perineum for the presence and distribution of warty lesions, as well as a careful digital rectal exam (DRE). Unlike hemorrhoids, anal canal tumors are usually firm to the touch. Anoscopic evaluation is paramount to assess the size, extent, and distribution of lesions present in the anal canal, as well as their relationship to the vagina and sphincter muscles. Given the lymphatic drainage pattern in the anal canal distal to the dentate line, ***examination of the bilateral inguinal lymph node basins is mandatory***. Diagnosis is confirmed on histology, and a tissue biopsy may be obtained in the office or in the operating room. Palpable groin lymphadenopathy or radiographically suspicious lymph nodes should undergo fine needle aspiration. *If you are a clinical practitioner and you are uncertain about the clinical and physical exam findings,* ***refer the patient to a colorectal surgeon for evaluation***.

Staging investigations include pelvic magnetic resonance imaging (MRI) to assess for locoregional disease, and a computed tomography (CT) scan of the chest, abdomen, and pelvis is the primary test for metastatic disease. Positron-emission tomography (PET) may also be performed to evaluate pelvic lymphadenopathy. Although there is no direct association with colorectal cancer, recent guidelines do recommend colonoscopy, as a significant number of patients have been shown to have synchronous colorectal neoplasms at diagnosis [27]. HIV testing should also be performed if the patient's status is not known. ***The TNM staging system for anal SCC is based on the size of the primary lesion and the presence of nodal metastasis*** [25], unlike in colorectal cancer, where T staging is based on the depth of invasion into the layers of the bowel wall.

Management: Chemoradiotherapy

The management of anal SCC has shifted from radical surgery toward nonoperative management. Standard of care for any new diagnosis now involves evaluation and joint decision-making by surgeons, medical and radiation oncologists, radiologists, and pathologists at a multidisciplinary cancer conference. ***Chemoradiotherapy (CRT) is the mainstay of management***, and ***surgery is typically reserved for cases of persistent or recurrent disease after nonoperative management***.

Definitive concurrent chemotherapy with mitomycin C and 5-fluorouracil (5-FU), with radiotherapy of 45–50.4 Gy, is now the first-line treatment for all anal canal SCC and most perianal SCC. Historically, anal SCC was definitively treated with abdominoperineal resection; however, this led to unacceptably high rates of local recurrence and poor overall survival (OS), in addition to significant morbidity. Preoperative chemoradiation was first described in 1974, and patients were found to have significant rates of complete response on pathologic specimens, leading to its use as the sole treatment for anal SCC without surgery. This approach is still commonly referred to as the ***Nigro protocol***, despite changes that have been made to the regimen since its original description [29]. CRT is associated with an **80–90% complete response (cure) rate** [30, 31]. *Thus, the vast majority of patients with (nonmetastatic) anal cancer are cured with chemoradiation alone.* Part of the reason for this is that SCC is highly ***radiosensitive***.

Current guidelines recommend repeat evaluation at 8–12 weeks after the completion of chemoradiation with DRE, anoscopy, and inguinal lymph node examination [27]. It is important to note, however, that tumor regression is slow and that ***treatment response can continue for several months beyond the completion of CRT***; in fact, nearly one third of patients may not achieve a complete clinical response until 26 weeks [31]. As such, patients may be monitored at 3-month intervals for up to 6 months after completion of CRT [27]. Any evidence of disease progression or persistence beyond this point should undergo targeted biopsy, repeat staging with CT/PET and pelvic MRI, and referral for salvage surgery. Once a complete clinical response is achieved, patients should undergo surveillance examinations every 3–6 months for 5 years. Importantly, ***routine biopsy of a complete response is unnecessary***, and doing so in radiated tissue may be associated with poor healing of the biopsy site. Patients with T3 and T4 tumors should also undergo CT scans of the chest, abdomen, and pelvis at least every 3 years.

Management: Surgery

The primary indication for surgery is in persistent or locally recurrent disease after CRT. The operation performed is typically an ***abdominoperineal resection, or APR,*** *which is a radical resection of the entire anus and rectum with permanent colostomy.* Despite the efficacy of CRT, between 20% and 30% of patients have persistent or recurrent disease after treatment [32]. Patients treated with salvage APR have been shown to have a 5-year OS of up to 60% [33–36]. It is important to note that radical surgery in the setting of previously radiated tissues poses unique challenges and is associated with poor wound healing and significant morbidity, particularly in comparison to APR performed for rectal adenocarcinoma. Many patients require reconstruction with muscle flaps, including gluteal, gracilis, or vertical rectus abdominus muscle (VRAM) flaps. The latter is often preferred and has been shown to have lower rates of wound complications, including dehiscence [37].

While surgery is typically reserved for cases of persistent or recurrent disease after nonoperative management, there are two scenarios where upfront surgery may be indicated. ***Patients with early-stage (T1), node-negative, moderately to well-differentiated tumors involving the perianal skin*** (rather than the anal canal) may be managed with **local excision alone,** as long as 1 cm margins may be obtained. In this selected group, an excellent 5-year OS of 85.3% has been shown, with no significant difference compared to CRT [38]. The other involves patients with ***superficially invasive squamous cell carcinoma (SISCCA)***. These often incidentally found lesions are defined as anal cancer that has been completely excised, with less than or equal to 3-mm basement membrane invasion and maximal horizontal spread of less than or equal to 7 mm. It is important to note that persistent or recurrent HSIL is more common after local excision of anal SCC, compared to CRT, and patients should continue HRA-guided surveillance [39].

Management: Metastatic Disease

Ten to twenty percent of patients present with distant metastatic disease, with the most common sites being the liver, lungs, and extrapelvic lymph nodes [40]. Chemotherapy is the primary treatment in the setting of metastatic disease, and carboplatin with paclitaxel is recommended as the first-line regimen [27]. However, locoregional treatment with palliative CRT to the primary site may also be offered, and is associated with increased overall survival compared to chemotherapy alone [41]. The role of immunotherapeutic agents such as nivolumab and pembrolizumab is also currently being investigated [42, 43].

Summary

- Risk factors for the development of anal SCC relate directly to either exposure to the HPV virus or to immunodeficiency.
- Anal squamous intraepithelial lesions are precancerous lesions and are classified as LSIL or HSIL, based on their risk of developing into anal cancer.
- Screening high-risk patients with anal cytology and/or HRA is recommended, and treatment of HSIL reduces the risk of anal cancer.
- HPV vaccination is recommended for all individuals at age 11 or 12 years of age, through to age 26.
- Definitive CRT (external beam radiation in combination with 5-FU and mitomycin) is the mainstay of management of anal cancer.
- Treatment response can continue for several months after CRT, and routine biopsy of a complete response is unnecessary.
- Salvage APR is reserved for persistent or recurrent disease, and local resection is an option for small, early-stage tumors.

Disclosures Dr. Wexner is a consultant for ActivSurgical, Arthrex, Baxter, Becton, Dickinson and Co., Glaxo Smith Kline, Intuitive Surgical, OstomyCure, Polypid, Seikagaku, and Takeda, receives stock options for consulting from Polypid and OstomyCure, and receives royalties from Intuitive Surgical, Karl Storz Endoscopy America Inc., and Unique Surgical Solutions, LLC.

References

1. SEER cancer stat facts: anal cancer. National Cancer Institute. Bethesda, MD. https://seer.cancer.gov/statfacts/html/anus.htm.
2. Siegel RL, Miller KD, Wagle NS, Jemal A. Cancer statistics, 2023. CA Cancer J Clin. 2023;73(1):17–48.
3. Colón-López V, Shiels MS, Machin M, et al. Anal cancer risk among people with HIV infection in the United States. J Clin Oncol. 2018;36(1):68–75.
4. Hernández-Ramírez RU, Shiels MS, Dubrow R, Engels EA. Cancer risk in HIV-infected people in the USA from 1996 to 2012: a population-based, registry-linkage study. Lancet HIV. 2017;4(11):e495–504.
5. Deshmukh AA, Suk R, Shiels MS, et al. Recent trends in squamous cell carcinoma of the anus incidence and mortality in the United States, 2001–2015. J Natl Cancer Inst. 2020;112(8):829–38.
6. Centers for Disease Control and Prevention. Human Papillomavirus (HPV). https://www.cdc.gov/hpv/about/index.html. Accessed 25 Jan 2025.
7. McBride AA. Human papillomaviruses: diversity, infection and host interactions. Nat Rev Microbiol. 2022;20(2):95–108.
8. Lin C, Franceschi S, Clifford GM. Human papillomavirus types from infection to cancer in the anus, according to sex and HIV status: a systematic review and meta-analysis. Lancet Infect Dis. 2018;18(2):198–206.
9. Goodman MT, Shvetsov YB, McDuffie K, et al. Sequential acquisition of human papillomavirus (HPV) infection of the anus and cervix: the Hawaii HPV cohort study. J Infect Dis. 2010;201(9):1331–9.
10. Stier EA, Lensing SY, Darragh TM, et al. Prevalence of and risk factors for anal high-grade squamous intraepithelial lesions in women living with human immunodeficiency virus. Clin Infect Dis. 2020;70(8):1701–7.
11. Clifford GM, Georges D, Shiels MS, et al. A meta-analysis of anal cancer incidence by risk group: toward a unified anal cancer risk scale. Int J Cancer. 2021;148(1):38–47.
12. Frisch M, Glimelius B, van den Brule AJ, et al. Sexually transmitted infection as a cause of anal cancer. N Engl J Med. 1997;337(19):1350–8.

13. Ryan DP, Compton CC, Mayer RJ. Carcinoma of the anal canal. N Engl J Med. 2000;342(11):792–800.
14. Giuliano AR, Lu B, Nielson CM, et al. Age-specific prevalence, incidence, and duration of human papillomavirus infections in a cohort of 290 US men. J Infect Dis. 2008;198(6):827–35.
15. Doorbar J. The human Papillomavirus twilight zone - latency, immune control and subclinical infection. Tumour Virus Res. 2023;16:200268.
16. Chin-Hong PV, Kwak EJ. AST Infectious Diseases Community of Practice. Human papillomavirus in solid organ transplantation. Am J Transplant. 2013;13(Suppl 4):189–200.
17. Daling JR, Madeleine MM, Johnson LG, et al. Human papillomavirus, smoking, and sexual practices in the etiology of anal cancer. Cancer. 2004;101(2):270–80.
18. Chu QD, Vezeridis MP, Libbey NP, Wanebo HJ. Giant condyloma acuminatum (Buschke-Lowenstein tumor) of the anorectal and perianal regions. Analysis of 42 cases. Dis Colon Rectum. 1994;37(9):950–7.
19. Darragh TM, Colgan TJ, Thomas Cox J, et al. The Lower Anogenital Squamous Terminology Standardization project for HPV-associated lesions: background and consensus recommendations from the College of American Pathologists and the American Society for Colposcopy and Cervical Pathology. Int J Gynecol Pathol. 2013;32(1):76–115.
20. Barroso LF, Stier EA, Hillman R, Palefsky J. Anal cancer screening and prevention: summary of evidence reviewed for the 2021 centers for disease control and prevention sexually transmitted infection guidelines. Clin Infect Dis. 2022;74(Suppl_2):S179–92.
21. Palefsky JM, Lee JY, Jay N, et al. Treatment of anal high-grade squamous intraepithelial lesions to prevent anal cancer. N Engl J Med. 2022;386(24):2273–82.
22. Alam NN, White DA, Narang SK, Daniels IR, Smart NJ. Systematic review of guidelines for the assessment and management of high-grade anal intraepithelial neoplasia (AIN II/III). Color Dis. 2016;18(2):135–46.
23. Spindler L, Etienney I, Abramowitz L, et al. Screening for precancerous anal lesions linked to human papillomaviruses: French recommendations for clinical practice. Tech Coloproctol. 2024;28(1):23.
24. Baldwin SB, Wallace DR, Papenfuss MR, Abrahamsen M, Vaught LC, Giuliano AR. Condom use and other factors affecting penile human papillomavirus detection in men attending a sexually transmitted disease clinic. Sex Transm Dis. 2004;31(10):601–7.
25. Goodman KA, Gollub MJ, Eng C, et al. AJCC cancer staging system, version 9: anus. American College of Surgeons; 2020.
26. Klas JV, Rothenberger DA, Wong WD, Madoff RD. Malignant tumors of the anal canal: the spectrum of disease, treatment, and outcomes. Cancer. 1999;85(8):1686–93.
27. Stewart DB, Gaertner WB, Glasgow SC, et al. The American Society of Colon and Rectal Surgeons clinical practice guidelines for anal squamous cell cancers (revised 2018). Dis Colon Rectum. 2018;61(7):755–74.
28. Altekruse SF, et al. SEER Cancer Statistics Review, 1975–2007. Bethesda: National Cancer Institute; 2010.
29. Nigro ND, Vaitkevicius VK, Considine B Jr. Combined therapy for cancer of the anal canal: a preliminary report. Dis Colon Rectum. 1974;17(3):354–6.
30. Bartelink H, Roelofsen F, Eschwege F, et al. Concomitant radiotherapy and chemotherapy is superior to radiotherapy alone in the treatment of locally advanced anal cancer: results of a phase III randomized trial of the European Organization for Research and Treatment of Cancer Radiotherapy and Gastrointestinal Cooperative Groups. J Clin Oncol. 1997;15(5):2040–9.
31. James RD, Glynne-Jones R, Meadows HM, et al. Mitomycin or cisplatin chemoradiation with or without maintenance chemotherapy for treatment of squamous-cell carcinoma of the anus (ACT II): a randomised, phase 3, open-label, 2 × 2 factorial trial. Lancet Oncol. 2013;14(6):516–24.
32. Roohipour R, Patil S, Goodman KA, et al. Squamous-cell carcinoma of the anal canal: predictors of treatment outcome [published correction appears in Dis Colon Rectum. 2008 May;51(5):620]. Dis Colon Rectum. 2008;51(2):147–53.
33. Pocard M, Tiret E, Nugent K, Dehni N, Parc R. Results of salvage abdominoperineal resection for anal cancer after radiotherapy. Dis Colon Rectum. 1998;41(12):1488–93.
34. Mullen JT, Rodriguez-Bigas MA, Chang GJ, et al. Results of surgical salvage after failed chemoradiation therapy for epidermoid carcinoma of the anal canal. Ann Surg Oncol. 2007;14(2):478–83.
35. Sunesen KG, Buntzen S, Tei T, Lindegaard JC, Nørgaard M, Laurberg S. Perineal healing and survival after anal cancer salvage surgery: 10-year experience with primary perineal reconstruction using the vertical rectus abdominis myocutaneous (VRAM) flap. Ann Surg Oncol. 2009;16(1):68–77.
36. Lefèvre JH, Corte H, Tiret E, et al. Abdominoperineal resection for squamous cell anal carcinoma: survival and risk factors for recurrence. Ann Surg Oncol. 2012;19(13):4186–92.
37. Sheckter CC, Shakir A, Vo H, Tsai J, Nazerali R, Lee GK. Reconstruction following abdominoperineal resection (APR): indications and complications from a single institution experience. J Plast Reconstr Aesthet Surg. 2016;69(11):1506–12.
38. Chai CY, Tran Cao HS, Awad S, Massarweh NN. Management of Stage I Squamous Cell Carcinoma of the Anal Canal. JAMA Surg. 2018;153(3):209–15.
39. Cappello C, Cuming T, Bowring J, Rosenthal AN, Chindawi N, Nathan M. High-resolution anoscopy surveillance after anal squamous cell carcinoma: high-grade squamous intraepithelial lesion detection and treatment may influence local recurrence. Dis Colon Rectum. 2020;63(10):1363–71.
40. Cummings BJ. Metastatic anal cancer: the search for cure. Onkologie. 2006;29(1–2):5–6.
41. Wang Y, Yu X, Zhao N, et al. Definitive pelvic radiotherapy and survival of patients with newly diagnosed metastatic anal cancer. J Natl Compr Cancer Netw. 2019;17(1):29–37.
42. Morris VK, Salem ME, Nimeiri H, et al. Nivolumab for previously treated unresectable metastatic anal cancer (NCI9673): a multicentre, single-arm, phase 2 study. Lancet Oncol. 2017;18(4):446–53.
43. Ott PA, Piha-Paul SA, Munster P, et al. Safety and antitumor activity of the anti-PD-1 antibody pembrolizumab in patients with recurrent carcinoma of the anal canal. Ann Oncol. 2017;28(5):1036–41.

Benign Conditions of the Anus: Hemorrhoids, Fissures, and Fistulae

28

Maura Walsh, Cynthia Araradian, and V. Liana Tsikitis

Anatomy

Hemorrhoids, fissures, and fistulae are common issues that can be painful, embarrassing, and have a profound negative impact on patients' quality of life. To understand their treatment, an understanding of anorectal anatomy is key.

There are two definitions of the anal canal: the **anatomic anal canal** and the **surgical anal canal** (Fig. 28.1). The former extends from the **dentate line** to the **anal verge**, which marks the boundary between the hairless anoderm and normal perianal skin. The **dentate line** is significant for many reasons. One is that it marks the embryologic fusion of *ectoderm* and *endoderm*, therefore resulting in a change in histology, innervation, and blood supply. Proximal to this line, innervation comes from parasympathetic and sympathetic nerve fibers, and distal to this line, sensation is somatic. *Procedures below the* ***dentate line*** *are therefore very painful without appropriate analgesia, and those above it should only be felt as a sensation of pressure*. The **dentate line** is visible on anoscopy as a ridged line demarcating a shift in color to a paler pink more distally. These ridges represent the anal crypts at the base of the columns of Morgagni, which contain the anal glands. Obstruction or infection of these glands is the etiology of most anal abscesses and fistulas [4, 11].

The **surgical anal canal** is the area from the **anorectal ring**, consisting of the upper border of the **internal anal sphincter**, the **external anal sphincter**, and the **puborectalis muscle**. Notably, the internal anal sphincter is innervated by the autonomic nervous system and is involuntary, whereas the external anal sphincter is innervated by somatic nerves and is under voluntary control [11].

M. Walsh · C. Araradian · V. L. Tsikitis (✉)
Department of Surgery, Oregon Health and Science University, Portland, OR, USA
e-mail: tsikitis@ohsu.edu

Hemorrhoids

Key Points

- First-line treatment for hemorrhoids is nonoperative treatment with dietary changes (increased water and fiber supplementation), changing toileting habits, and sitz baths.
- Patients presenting with hemorrhoids who are over the age of 45, with risk factors for colorectal cancer, or red flag symptoms (unintentional weight loss, changes in bowel habits) should be referred for a colonoscopy to rule out colorectal cancer.
- If medical treatment fails, there are many effective in-office approaches such as rubber band ligation, sclerotherapy, and energy ablation. Referral to a surgeon for excisional hemorrhoidectomy is also an option for refractory or extensive hemorrhoidal disease.

Hemorrhoids are a normal part of anorectal anatomy. They exist as submucosal arteriovenous plexuses that form cushions within the anal canal in the *left lateral, right anterior, and right posterior positions*. Their exact incidence is undefined, but are estimated to affect 4% of the US population. Risk factors include straining/chronic constipation, pregnancy, COPD, weightlifting, and other reasons for impaired venous return. They are classified as **internal** or **external** hemorrhoids based on whether they originate from above or below the dentate line, respectively. Internal hemorrhoids are further classified as *grades I-IV*, which help guide treatment selection. *Grade I* hemorrhoids do not prolapse below the dentate line but are visibly engorged. *Grade II* hemorrhoids prolapse below the dentate with bearing down or bowel movements but spontaneously reduce. *Grade III* hemorrhoids prolapse but can be reduced manually. *Grade IV* hemorrhoids are prolapsed and cannot be manually reduced [2, 6, 10].

S. Atallah, J. Dragoljevic (eds.), *Fundamentals of Surgery for Physician Assistants*,
https://doi.org/10.1007/978-3-032-21069-2_28

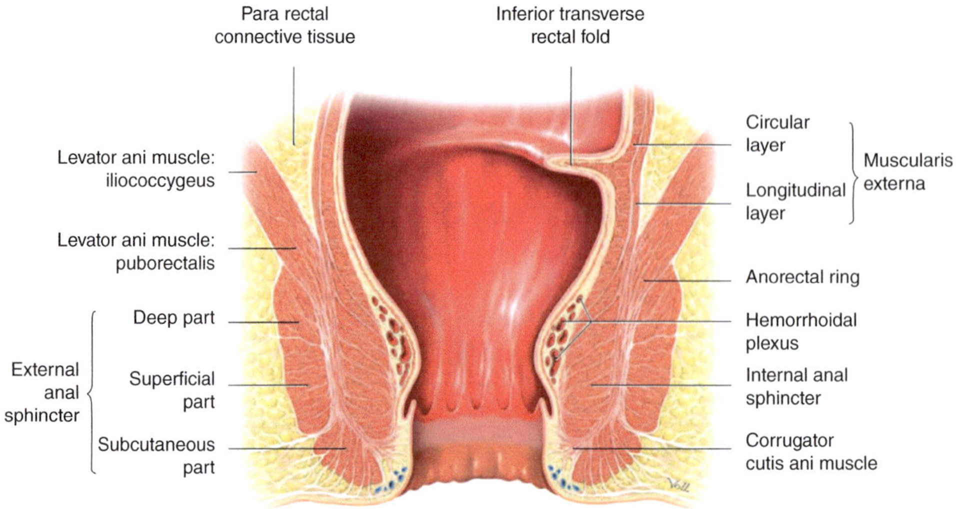

Fig. 28.1 Labeled diagram of the anal canal. (Copyright received from Thieme Publishing. Original image from Clinical Anatomy, Histology, Embryology and Neuroanatomy Textbook by Jamie Wikenheiser (2013))

Hemorrhoids may also become **strangulated**. This occurs when the blood flow to a Grade IV hemorrhoid becomes compromised, putting the tissue at risk of becoming necrosed or **gangrenous**. A **thrombosed** hemorrhoid is a very painful class of external hemorrhoids that occurs due to a clot under pressure inside it. These are typically blue- or purple-tinged and may have a tense, palpable clot within the bulge of the hemorrhoid. If these patients present within 72 h of their symptom onset, they benefit from a thrombosed hemorrhoid excision, which can be performed in the office [6].

The classic presentation of internal hemorrhoids is **painless bleeding** with bowel movements *with or without intermittent protrusion of tissue from the anus*. However, symptoms vary and may manifest as rectal pressure, mucous/stool soilage, itching, irritation, and difficulties maintaining anal hygiene. If a patient is reporting pain, the hemorrhoid is either **external** or **thrombosed**, or there may be a concurrent *anal fissure, fistula, or abscess*. Since **internal** hemorrhoids are above the dentate line, they should be painless. Patients should be questioned about the extent, duration, and severity of their symptoms, their fiber and water intake, stooling habits, issues with fecal incontinence, and any prior anorectal surgeries, obstetric history, or pelvic radiation. The physical exam includes a visual inspection of the anus and perineum, digital rectal exam (DRE) as tolerated, and anoscopy to visualize the extent and anatomic relationship of the hemorrhoids to each other and the dentate line.

*Patients often self-diagnose hemorrhoids, but they may have another etiology for their symptom*s. Alternative diagnoses include rectal varices, fissures, skin tags, melanoma, and irritable bowel disease. Importantly, **any patient with changes in bowel habits, recent unintentional weight loss, or a family history of colorectal cancer should be recommended for a colonoscopy to rule out colorectal adenocarcinoma**. **This standard is followed for patients of all ages, not just those 45 and older**. Furthermore, while bleeding is a common sign of hemorrhoidal disease, this rarely results in anemia; patients with anemia should also undergo a colonoscopy to work up an alternative etiology [10].

First-line treatment of hemorrhoids is a trial of **nonoperative management,** including increased water and fiber intake (25–50 g daily), improving bowel habits by reducing time on the toilet, and sitz baths as needed for symptomatic relief. While topical ointments such as hydrocortisone, phenylephrine, pramoxine, and witch hazel are commonly used, evidence does not support their long-term efficacy. If a patient experiences symptomatic relief, continued use carries a minimal risk and may be considered; treatment is often individualized to each patient [10].

Refractory symptoms for grade I-II and occasionally III hemorrhoids can be treated with in-office procedures such as **rubber band ligation (RBL)**, **sclerotherapy**, or **energy ablation**. **RBL** is accomplished through placing a rubber band on the redundant mucosa of the internal hemorrhoid column, *effectively cutting off the blood supply to the hemorrhoid and causing it to slough off in the following 5–7 days*. It is important to ensure that the rubber band is deployed above the dentate line; otherwise, this procedure is intolerably painful. **Sclerotherapy** is another effective technique that is preferable for patients on anticoagulation. A sclerosing agent, such as hypertonic saline or phenol in oil, is injected into the submucosa of the hemorrhoid base, causing it to fibrose. **Infrared photocoagulation** is a type of **energy ablation** technique that utilizes a heated probe to coagulate the vessels within the hemorrhoid. Patients should be counseled on the risks of postoperative complications, including pelvic sepsis, pain, bleeding, recurrence, urinary retention, and ulceration/fissure formation [2, 6, 10].

If these techniques are unsuccessful or a patient suffers from grade III-IV hemorrhoidal disease, or their hemorrhoids are incarcerated, strangulated, or gangrenous, referral to a colorectal surgeon for *operative hemorrhoidectomy is warranted.* The most common technique is an excisional hemorrhoidectomy, closing the skin (Ferguson hemorrhoidectomy) or leaving it open to heal by secondary intention (Milligan & Morgan hemorrhoidectomy). The hemorrhoidal columns are dissected and excised, utilizing suture ligation to prevent bleeding. When performing multiple columns of hemorrhoid excisions, surgeons must leave adequate skin bridges between them to reduce the risk of anal stenosis. They must also be cognizant of minimizing damage to muscle fibers to avoid issues with fecal incontinence. Postoperative management includes continuing a high-fiber diet, adequate water intake, multimodal pain control, and sitz baths for hygiene and comfort. Patients should be advised that a small amount of bleeding is normal, but they should seek immediate advice if they have excessive bleeding or insurmountable pain with fecal impaction [2, 6, 10].

Anal Fissures

Key Points

- Anal fissures are *painful* tears in the anal mucosa that can be acute (<6 weeks) or chronic (>6 weeks).
- Nonoperative management includes stool softeners, fiber supplementation, sitz baths, and topical therapies such as nitrates or calcium channel blockers.
- Botox injections are also an effective therapy, as they relax the sphincter muscle and encourage wound healing.
- Gold standard operative management is accomplished through a **lateral internal sphincterotomy**, which has high healing rates but also carries a (minimal) risk of permanent fecal incontinence.

Anal fissures are linear tears in the anal mucosa that are caused by trauma and/or irritation, often due to constipation and hard stools or frequent diarrhea. Patients with anal fissures present with painful defecation and bleeding with bowel movements and are *most often in the posterior midline of the anal canal.* If they are *lateral* in location (**atypical fissures**), *this may suggest an underlying disease state such as HIV, tuberculosis, inflammatory bowel disease, or syphilis.* The treatment of anal fissures varies depending on whether it is acute (<6 weeks) or chronic (>6 weeks). This classification is often evident upon visual inspection. A **chronic fissure** may have *indurated edges, visible* (exposed) *internal sphincter muscle fibers* (which have a classic **white** appearance), *hypertrophic papilla,* and/or a *sentinel tag/pile.* Their chronicity is theorized to be due to an abnormally high internal sphincter tone, which leads to local ischemia and impaired wound healing [7, 18].

First-line treatment is **nonoperative management** with stool softeners, fiber supplementation, sitz baths (or bathtub soaks), and lidocaine gel for symptomatic treatment. This will successfully resolve symptoms in almost half of patients with *acute* fissures. Topical therapies such as **nitrates** or **calcium channel blockers** work by relaxing the sphincter muscle tone to encourage wound healing. Both have high healing rates with chronic fissures, but *nitrates can be limited by their side effect profile of painful headaches.* For that reason, many physicians preferentially prescribe topical **calcium channel blockers** such as *nifedipine* or *diltiazem.* **Botulinum toxin injections** may also be used as a first- or second-line treatment. Patients may experience incontinence, though it is temporary and more often with flatus than stool [7, 18].

Operative management of anal fissures with **lateral internal sphincterotomy** are more effective than medical management or botox injections with healing rates reported at 88–100%, though they carry an 8–30% risk of fecal incontinence as described in the literature[7]. It is often performed after failure of nonoperative treatments, but can also be considered for patients with extreme and debilitating symptoms. It is usually offered to patients, as first-line treatment, who are unlikely to have sequelae of fecal incontinence. For example, patients without prior obstetrical injury, inflammatory bowel disease, history of anorectal surgeries, or decreased anal sphincter tone. The procedure involves incising the muscle fibers of the internal sphincter distal to the dentate line to the height of the fissure along the lateral aspect of the anus. A "tailored" approach can be used, which brings the incision to the apex of the fissure as opposed to the dentate line, as is done in the "traditional" approach. The former carries a higher risk of nonhealing than the "traditional" approach, but a lower risk of incontinence. Other operative options include local advancement flaps or fissurotomy and/or fissurectomy [7, 18]. In the postoperative period, patients should be encouraged to continue to use fiber supplementation and drink a lot of water, use stool softeners as needed, and take sitz baths as their surgical site heals.

Anal Abscesses and Fistulas

Key Points

- Identification of a perianal abscess and correct classification of the abscess can help determine management with the ultimate goal of performing an internal or external incision and drainage.
- An anal abscess is associated with an anal fistula at least 50% of the time.

- The goals for management of fistulas include *controlling sepsis and repairing (or controlling) the fistula while maintaining continence.*
- Simple, low-lying fistulas can be managed with a fistulotomy, while fistulas that encompass more than 30% of the external sphincter or more complex fistulas require a seton, endorectal advancement, or ligation of fistula tract (LIFT) in one or multistage procedures.
- Complex fistulae are often managed in a staged manner, usually after placement of a seton to control the local septic process.

Anorectal abscesses occur due to obstruction of the anal gland within the anal canal, while **anal fistulas** often occur as a result of chronic infection and epithelialization of the abscess tract [8]. The abscess occurs most commonly due to obstruction of the glands in the area of the *columns of Morgagni*. The fistula itself is an *abnormal, epithelialized connection between the rectum or anal canal and the surrounding perianal skin*. The components of the fistula include an internal opening, a tract, and the external opening. About 50% of perianal abscesses are associated with fistulas [14].

Anorectal abscesses are classified by location and management varies depending on which type of anorectal abscess one is treating. See Fig. 28.2 for locations of anorectal abscesses. The abscesses are classified into four categories:

- **Perianal**: This is the space that is continuous with the subcutaneous fat of the buttocks. An abscess here is often seen as a painful, erythematous nodule at the anal verge. These abscesses can often be drained at bedside without requiring an exam under anesthesia.
- **Intersphincteric**: These abscesses form in the area between the internal and external sphincters. This abscess cannot be seen on external exam and is often difficult to diagnose given its location. Patients will often have severe pain with a digital anorectal exam. This abscess will often require an exam under anesthesia and internal drainage.
- **Ischiorectal**: This is the space that is lateral and posterior to the anus. This abscess cannot be seen on external exam, but will be palpated with a digital anorectal exam. Rectal exams can be quite painful for these patients, and a tender swelling can be palpated. If the ischiorectal abscess extends to both sides and into the deep postanal space, this is categorized as a **horseshoe abscess**. The ischiorectal abscess will be managed with a skin incision over the area of the abscess. Horseshoe abscesses tend to be more complicated to manage and will require multiple incisions, usually with a deep postanal incision with counter incisions over bilateral ischiorectal spaces [8].
- **Supralevator**: The abscesses in this location are above the levator ani muscles. This can be due to an intra-abdominal process like Crohn's disease, diverticulitis, or an extension of an intersphincteric abscess. They are often diagnosed on imaging, like CT or MRI. The management is variable depending on the origin of the abscess.

Table 28.1 lists the prevalence of anorectal abscesses by location [15].

Depending on the type of abscess, often the patient's exam and symptoms can help determine the origin of the abscess and management. If there is confusion about the extent and location of the abscess, a CT image can be obtained.

Management of abscesses is often surgical with an **incision and drainage**, *often not necessitating antibiotics.* Antibiotics can be considered if the patient is systemically ill or is immunocompromised. A randomized, double blind, multicenter study demonstrated that antibiotics after drainage of an abscess did not change the risk of fistula formation [17]. The incision should be large enough to provide drainage but should avoid the sphincter complex if possible. If the incision is not large enough, then this will not facilitate

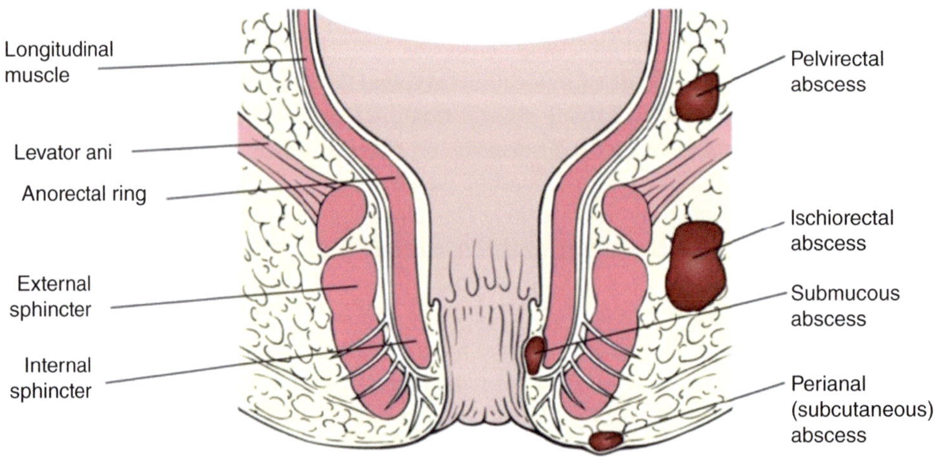

Fig. 28.2 Locations of anorectal abscesses. (Copyright obtained from Copyright Clearance Center, original image from General Surgery Lecture Notes with Wiley, 13th Edition, 2016)

Table 28.1 Prevalence of anorectal abscesses

Location	Prevalence
Perianal	42.7%
Ischiorectal	22.8%
Intersphincteric	21.4%
Supralevator	7.3%
Submucous	5.8%

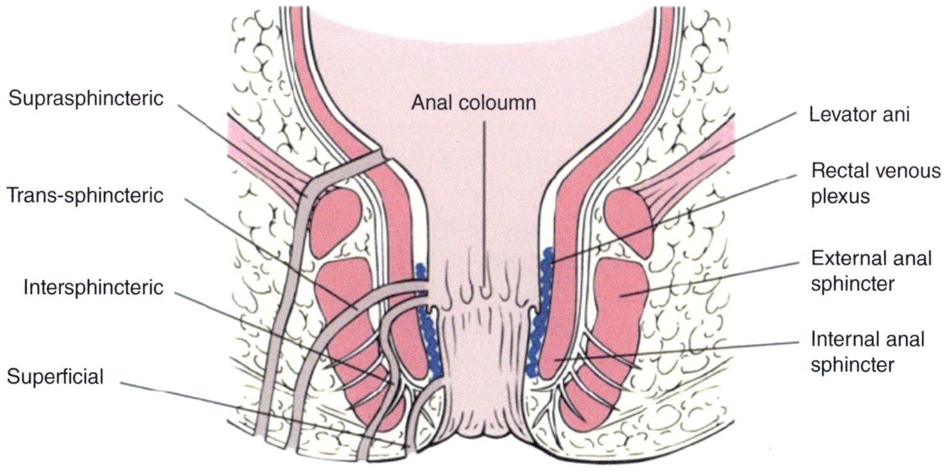

Fig. 28.3 The tracts for each of the anorectal fistulas are drawn on the left side of the image. Given that extrasphincteric tracts are more complicated, a tract is not identified in the figure. (Copyright obtained from Copyright Clearance Center, original image from General Surgery Lecture Notes with Wiley, 13th Edition, 2016)

adequate drainage and can lead to recurrence. If a fistula is encountered at the time of the incision and drainage, then the fistula should be managed per the recommendations later described in this chapter via primary fistulotomy or seton placement. Intersphincteric and supralevator abscesses tend to be the most highly associated with the incidence of fistula [15].

Fistulas are characterized based on the **Parks' classification**. See Fig. 28.3 for locations of anorectal fistulas:

- **Submucosal/Superficial**: No involvement of sphincter muscles and the fistula tract superficially courses below the anoderm.
- **Intersphincteric**: Most common type of anal fistula that is usually a result of a perianal abscess. The tract passes through the internal sphincter without involvement of the external anal sphincter. The tract is through the internal anal sphincter into the intersphincteric space to the perianal skin.
- **Transsphincteric**: The tract involves both the internal and external sphincter muscles. This is further divided into low vs high. Low fistulas involve less than 30% of the external sphincter compared to high fistulas that involve more than 30% of the external sphincter.
- **Suprasphincteric**: The tract passes through the internal anal sphincter and traverses the external sphincter and travels cephalad, coursing into the ischiorectal space.
- **Extrasphincteric**: Tract passes outside the sphincter complex through the ischiorectal fossa to the perianal skin [16]. The origin of the extrasphincteric fistula is not often cryptoglandular but may be due to the presence of inflammation or malignancy.

Patient presentations can be variable depending on the symptoms present from chronic drainage of fluid, pain, and bleeding. The differential diagnosis includes hemorrhoids, anal fissures, perianal abscesses, Crohn's disease, and malignancy. Patients should be questioned about their history of prior episodes of abscesses or fistulas, duration and severity of their symptoms, issues with fecal incontinence, obstetric history, and any prior anorectal surgeries. Anorectal exams in the office can help identify an external opening, but often the diagnosis is based on an exam under anesthesia to identify an external and internal opening. If further information is needed to characterize the type of fistula, especially when complex, an MRI can be obtained prior to the procedure.

Other differential diagnoses, besides infection for the development of anal fistulas, includes **Crohn's disease** and, rarely, malignancy. **Anal fistulas are a common manifestation in individuals with Crohn's disease, seen in 6–34% of patients**. Suspicion is raised for a Crohn's diagnosis when patients present with multiple fistulas or a fistula with an opening that is >3 cm away from the anal verge [14]. In the setting of a patient with Crohn's disease with multiple prior fistulas, an *MRI is often obtained to better characterize the course of the tract*. In Crohn's disease, fistulas are often improved with the use of a **seton and biologic agents** (e.g., infliximab). If a fistula tract does not appear to be healing and appears abnormal, malignancy should remain on the differential diagnosis, and **the tissue should be biopsied**.

An exam under anesthesia is often performed to diagnose and treat fistulas. Fistula tracts can be delineated by the external and internal openings with fistula probes. It is crucial to ensure the known fistula tract is probed and a new tract is not iatrogenically created. **Goodsall's rule** can be a helpful tip to determine the internal opening once the external opening is identified. The rule states that fistulas with an anterior external opening follow a radial tract to the internal opening, while a posterior external opening follows a curvilinear tract to the internal opening. The exception to the rule includes anterior external openings that are greater than 3 cm away from the anal margin. Another useful technique to identify an internal opening is the use of **hydrogen peroxide** injected with an angiocatheter through the external opening.

Once the fistula is diagnosed and both openings are identified, it is important to determine adequate management. Management of fistulas includes removal or unroofing of the tract and preventing recurrence, while maintaining continence. There are different procedures to perform depending on the extent of external muscle involvement. A **primary fistulotomy,** which opens up the fistula tract, can be used for simple, low-lying fistulas, like intersphincteric and transsphincteric fistulas, which encompass less than 30% of the external anal sphincter. Marsupialization of the tract, which means suturing the edges of the tract to the wound, allows for faster wound healing and less postoperative bleeding [8].

When a complex fistula is encountered with multiple openings, a transsphincteric fistula encompassing greater than 30% of the external anal sphincter, or a suprasphincteric fistula, a fistulotomy should not be performed due to the risk of complications. A **seton** is often used in this scenario to facilitate drainage of the tract and to create fibrosis, converting the fistula from a high fistula to a low one for a subsequent operation [13]. The seton is usually a vessel loop that is pulled through the fistula tract and tied together, loose enough that it will not erode through the skin but tight enough that it should not fall out. It should also be cut short enough that it won't bother the patient while sitting or get in the way of bowel movements. The setons are kept in place for a minimum of 6-weeks [3]. A second-stage procedure after seton placement can entail either a primary fistulotomy, an **endorectal advancement flap,** or a **ligation of the intersphincteric fistula tract (LIFT)**.

Endorectal advancement flap is a sphincter-preserving option for complex fistulas that are high transsphincteric or suprasphincteric. The fistula tract is initially curetted, then a full-thickness flap containing mucosa, submucosa, and a portion of the internal anal muscle from the level of the dentate line is mobilized over about 4–6 cm to cover the internal opening. It is important to preserve the blood supply to the flap, so the base of the flap should be at least twice as wide as the tip. In a retrospective analysis, the endorectal advancement flaps had a 63% success rate [5]. A **LIFT procedure** identifies the fistula in the intersphincteric space, divides it, and ligates the two ends of it, thereby avoiding the sphincter complex. The success rate of a LIFT procedure is estimated near 76% [8].

Two other methods of management include a **fibrin plug** and the use of **fibrin glue**. The **fibrin plug** is a collagen matrix that is inserted into the fistula tract. The tract is identified, and curettage is performed; then the plug is inserted and fixed at the internal opening to close it. The issues with the plug include plug dislodgement and recurrence, with recent success rates of 30–40% [5]. The benefit of the plug is the fact that it is sphincter sparing, and if it fails, other procedures can be attempted. The **fibrin glue** is a preloaded syringe of sealant that activates thrombin to form a fibrin clot within the fistula tract. Again, the benefit is that the procedure is sphincter sparing, but it has *poor* success rates over time [9].

Complications associated with these procedures include fistula recurrence, incontinence, and infections. Fistula recurrence or failure is associated with higher rates in high transsphincteric tracts, horseshoe extension, multiple tracts, and prior anal surgery [12]. Incontinence can be associated with a history of prior anorectal operations, higher fistulas with more sphincter involvement, and patients with baseline incontinence. It is crucial to obtain a thorough history from patients to assess their baseline continence prior to the exam under anesthesia. A retrospective review demonstrated a fecal incontinence rate of about 15% with higher transsphincteric fistulas, suprasphincteric fistulas, and age over 45 being independent predictors. The fistula plugs in this study were associated with the highest rates of postoperative sepsis [1].

References

1. Abbas MA, Jackson CH, Haigh PI. Predictors of outcome for anal fistula surgery. Arch Surg. 2011;146(9):1011–6. https://doi.org/10.1001/archsurg.2011.197.
2. Akinmoladun O, Oh W. Management of hemorrhoids and anal fissures. Surg Clin N Am. 2024;104(3):473–90. https://doi.org/10.1016/j.suc.2023.11.001.
3. Bolshinsky V, Church J. How to insert a draining seton correctly. Dis Colon Rectum. 2018;61(9):1121–3. https://doi.org/10.1097/DCR.0000000000001132.
4. Carmichael J, Mills S. Anatomy and embryology of the colon, rectum, and anus. 2022. Retrieved from https://www.ascrsu.com/ascrs/view/ASCRS-Textbook-of-Colon-and-Rectal-Surgery/2285001/all/Anatomy_and_Embryology_of_the_Colon__Rectum__and_Anus.
5. Christoforidis D, Pieh MC, Madoff RD, Mellgren AF. Treatment of transsphincteric anal fistulas by endorectal advancement flap or collagen fistula plug: a comparative study. Dis Colon Rectum. 2009;52(1):18–22. https://doi.org/10.1007/DCR.0b013e31819756ac.
6. Davids J, Ridolfi T. Hemorrhoids. 2022. Retrieved from https://www.ascrsu.com/ascrs/view/ASCRS-Textbook-of-Colon-and-Rectal-Surgery/2285079/all/Hemorrhoids.
7. Davids JS, Hawkins AT, Bhama AR, Feinberg AE, Grieco MJ, Lightner AL, et al. The American Society of Colon and Rectal Surgeons clinical practice guidelines for the management of

anal fissures. Dis Colon Rectum. 2023;66(2):190–9. Retrieved from https://journals.lww.com/dcrjournal/fulltext/2023/02000/the_american_society_of_colon_and_rectal_surgeons.8.aspx.
8. Gaertner WB, Burgess PL, Davids JS, Lightner AL, Shogan BD, Sun MY, Steele SR, Paquette IM, Feingold DL. The American Society of Colon and Rectal Surgeons clinical practice guidelines for the management of anorectal abscess, fistula-in-Ano, and rectovaginal fistula. Dis Colon Rectum. 2022;65:964–85. https://doi.org/10.1097/DCR.0000000000002473.
9. Haim N, Neufeld D, Ziv Y, Tulchinsky H, Koller M, Khaikin M, Zmora O. Long-term results of fibrin glue treatment for cryptogenic perianal fistulas: a multicenter study. Dis Colon Rectum. 2011;54(10):1279–83. https://doi.org/10.1097/DCR.0b013e318223c894.
10. Hawkins AT, Davis BR, Bhama AR, Fang SH, Dawes AJ, Feingold DL, et al. The American Society of Colon and Rectal Surgeons clinical practice guidelines for the management of hemorrhoids. Dis Colon Rectum. 2024;67(5):614–23. Retrieved from https://journals.lww.com/dcrjournal/fulltext/2024/05000/the_american_society_of_colon_and_rectal_surgeons.5.aspx.
11. Lee JM, Kim NK. Essential anatomy of the anorectum for colorectal surgeons focused on the gross anatomy and histologic findings. Ann Coloproctol. 2018;34(2):59–71. https://doi.org/10.3393/ac.2017.12.15.
12. Mei Z, Wang Q, Zhang Y, Liu P, Ge M, Du P, et al. Risk factors for recurrence after anal fistula surgery: a meta-analysis. Int J Surg. 2019;69:153–64. https://doi.org/10.1016/j.ijsu.2019.08.003.
13. Pearl RK, Andrews JR, Orsay CP, Weisman RI, Prasad ML, Nelson RL, et al. Role of the seton in the management of anorectal fistulas. Dis Colon Rectum. 1993;36(6):573–7; discussion 577-579. https://doi.org/10.1007/BF02049864.
14. Rakinic J, Poola VP. Hemorrhoids and fistulas: new solutions to old problems. Curr Probl Surg. 2014;51(3):98–137. https://doi.org/10.1067/j.cpsurg.2013.11.002.
15. Ramanujam PS, Prasad ML, Abcarian H, Tan AB. Perianal abscesses and fistulas. A study of 1023 patients. Dis Colon Rectum. 1984;27(9):593–7. https://doi.org/10.1007/BF02553848.
16. Shawki S, Wexner SD. Idiopathic fistula-in-ano. World J Gastroenterol. 2011;17(28):3277–85. https://doi.org/10.3748/wjg.v17.i28.3277.
17. Sozener U, Gedik E, Kessaf Aslar A, Ergun H, Halil Elhan A, Memikoglu O, et al. Does adjuvant antibiotic treatment after drainage of anorectal abscess prevent development of anal fistulas? A randomized, placebo-controlled, double-blind, multicenter study. Dis Colon Rectum. 2011;54(8):923–9. https://doi.org/10.1097/DCR.0b013e31821cc1f9.
18. Tsikitis V, Marecik S. Anal fissure and anal stenosis. 2022. Retrieved from https://www.ascrsu.com/ascrs/view/ASCRS-Textbook-of-Colon-and-Rectal-Surgery/2285004/all/Anal_Fissure_and_Anal_Stenosis.

Soft Tissue Abscess, Pilonidal Disease, & Hidradenitis Suppurativa

29

Jana Zeineddine, Liliana Bordeianou, and Holly Bonnette

Skin Abscesses

Introduction

Skin abscesses are a common skin and soft tissue infection (SSTI). In fact, the incidence of SSTIs, including skin abscesses, has been increasing over the past few years. In the United States, a study found that the annual SSTI incidence almost doubled between 2000 and 2014, reaching 4.2 million cases per year [1]. Skin abscesses are more common in certain populations than others. For example, a study found that skin abscesses constituted 7% of all SSTIs in large urban populations with high population density [2, 3]. Furthermore, within urban areas, those from disadvantaged socioeconomic groups are most affected [3]. The incidence of skin abscesses also differs between genders and age groups. Though all age groups can be affected, peak incidence occurs in adults between the ages of 30 and 50 years. Similarly, though all genders can be affected, incidence is higher in males, potentially due to increased exposure to risk factors such as trauma and intravenous drug use [4].

Presentation and Symptoms

Skin abscesses present with different severity from patient to patient. Generally, they tend to be tender, erythematous, and fluctuant swellings [5]. In some cases, skin abscesses are associated with surrounding cellulitis and are warm to the touch due to underlying inflammation [6]. In other cases, systemic symptoms occur, including fever and malaise [5]. Drainage and pus might also be present, especially when abscesses are large. Drainage helps alleviate pain and pressure but might also be a warning sign of infection progression that must be recognized and managed promptly to avoid complications and support complete resolution [7].

J. Zeineddine · L. Bordeianou · H. Bonnette (✉)
Department of General and Gastrointestinal Surgery, Massachusetts General Hospital, Boston, MA, USA
e-mail: hbonnette@mgh.harvard.edu

Diagnosis

Skin abscesses can be diagnosed clinically, though imaging modalities can be useful in some cases:

I. **Physical examination**: A healthcare provider (HCP) will first assess the shape, size, and characteristics of the abscess and evaluate for systemic symptoms.
II. **Laboratory tests**: Culture and sensitivity tests are obtained by sampling pus or drainage from the abscess. Essential for antibiotic selection [8].
III. **Ultrasonography**: In cases of complicated or unresolved abscesses, ultrasonography can be used to aid diagnosis. This enables visualization of abscess depth and guides incision and drainage if necessary [9].
IV. **CT Scans**: In more complex situations, CT scans may provide a more detailed image to assess for involvement of deeper tissues and organs [9].

Classification and Risk Factors

There are several forms of skin abscesses, each with varying underlying causes and unique characteristics. **Boils (Furuncles)** are amongst the most common [8]. They form around hair follicles and present as painful, deep nodules. Furuncles often arise from bacterial infections, most commonly Staphylococcus aureus infections [8]. **Carbuncles** form from the coalescence of multiple boils. They are larger and more severe than simple boils, capable of spreading deeper into the skin, resulting in extensive infection. **Epidermoid Cysts** are slow-growing, benign cysts originating from the epidermis. Though they are noncancerous, they have the potential of becoming infected, resulting in abscess

S. Atallah, J. Dragoljevic (eds.), *Fundamentals of Surgery for Physician Assistants*,
https://doi.org/10.1007/978-3-032-21069-2_29

formation [10]. **Hydradenitis Suppurativa (HS)** is a chronic skin disease where abscesses form in areas abundant in apocrine glands, including the armpits and groin [9]. HS patients suffer from recurrent nodules, abscesses, and sinus tracts, associated with significant discomfort. Each of the abscess types discussed presents with unique diagnostic and therapeutic challenges, requiring tailored approaches for effective management [9].

Pathogenesis

There are several underlying causes for skin abscesses. The most prevalent is bacterial infections, particularly those caused by Staphylococcus aureus or Streptococcus species [8]. These bacteria have the ability to invade the skin through minor breaches of the skin's protective barrier, resulting in local inflammation and pus formation. Abscesses can also result from blocked hair follicles, which trap sebum and bacteria, generating an environment supportive of infection and abscess formation [10]. Skin trauma is also a predisposing factor. This includes bites, cuts, or puncture wounds that directly introduce bacteria into deeper layers, bypassing the skin's natural defense system. Other risk factors include diabetes, which weakens the body's immune system, and immune disorders, which impair overall immune function, heightening abscess susceptibility. These conditions make it more challenging for the body to resolve infections, increasing the risk of severe and frequent abscess formation [9].

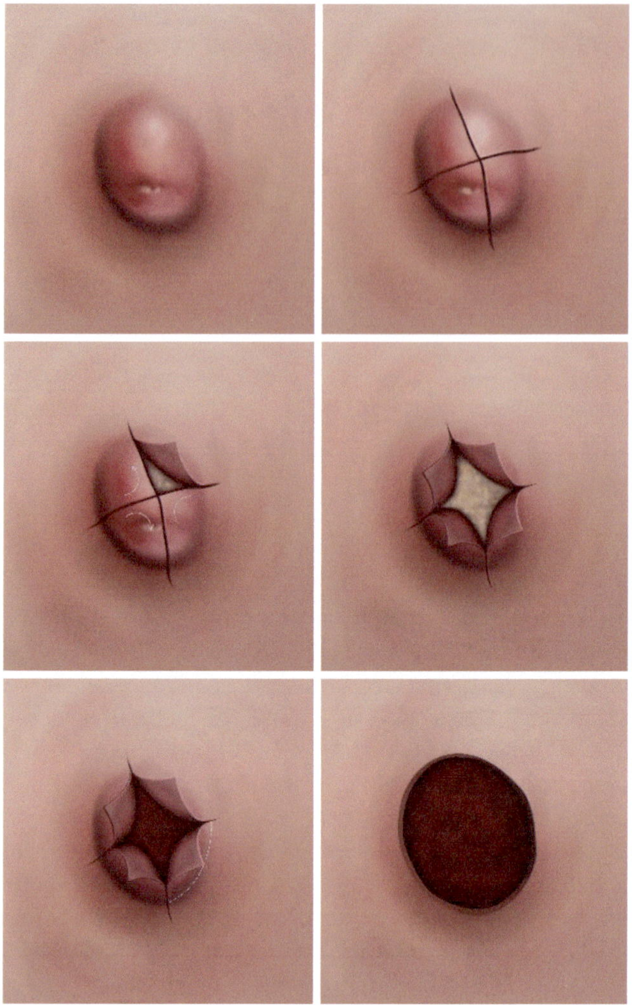

Fig. 29.1 Proper I&D of a skin abscess via cruciate incision. (*Original illustration by Jana Zeineddine, MD*)

Treatment and Management

A multifaceted approach is most effective for skin abscess treatment as it addresses both the infection and any associated symptoms. The gold standard treatment for any abscess larger than 2 cm is incision and drainage (I&D), which relieves pain and pressure while enabling accumulated pus to drain out, promoting faster healing.

Proper I&D of abscesses involves making a cruciate incision, as shown in Fig. 29.1. Two perpendicular 1 cm cuts generate skin flaps that can be folded back and excised, leaving the infected area open to heal by secondary intention. This technique provides lower rates of recurrence than the basic linear incision, which often results in "premature closure" or "reclosure," whereby the incision closes too quickly postdrainage. This allows for abscess reaccumulation and exposes the patient to unnecessary pain and avoidable repeat procedures.

Following drainage, culture results and sensitivity tests are utilized to guide antibiotic prescription [8]. This ensures that effective antibiotics are selected to minimize the risk of antibiotic resistance. Antibiotics are not required for small, uncomplicated abscesses [8]. They are indicated when there are multiple or large abscesses, rapid symptom progression or cellulitis occurs, signs of systemic infection (fever, chills) are present, underlying comorbidities or immunosuppression are present, patient lies in the extremes of age, abscess is located in an area that is hard to drain (genitalia, hands, face), inadequate response to I&D is achieved, or the patient is at high risk of MRSA or has documented MRSA infection [8].

Common antibiotics used include:

1. **Cephalexin**: Used for less severe abscesses where suspicion of Methicillin-resistant Staphylococcus aureus (MRSA) is low [6].
2. **Trimethoprim-sulfamethoxazole (TMP-SMX)**: Effective against MRSA [11].
3. **Clindamycin**: Effective against MRSA and other Gram-positives [6].

4. **Doxycycline or Minocycline**: Effective against MRSA [12].
5. **Amoxicillin-clavulanate**: Broad-spectrum antibiotic used for polymicrobial infections [6].

Warm compresses are commonly recommended as supportive therapy, which helps soften the abscess, encouraging pus to rise to the skin, facilitating drainage [9]. Pain management is another important part of treatment. Nonprescription pain medications like acetaminophen and ibuprofen are usually sufficient to alleviate pain and fever [10]. Good hygiene is also critical for preventing infection progression and aiding recovery. The affected area should be regularly cleaned to avoid further complications and support healing [13].

After I&D and/or antibiotic therapy, patients should be re-evaluated within 24–48 h to ensure clinical improvement and adequate drainage. Patients should also be educated about proper wound care and any red flags indicating worsening infection. I&D can be repeated if necessary.

Prevention

Efficient prevention strategies can help control the spread of Staphylococcus aureus infections. The foundation of prevention in this case is maintaining proper hygiene through regularly washing hands and adopting diligent skin care. This practice should be especially reinforced in environments where people are more exposed to infections, such as community spaces and healthcare facilities [13]. Another preventative measure is prompt treatment, as addressing superficial skin infections early can hinder progression into advanced infections, systemic spread, and threatening complications necessitating more intensive interventions [8]. Early treatment usually consists of wound care and topical antibiotics. It is also important to manage chronic conditions that impede healthy immune responses and wound healing. This includes immunocompromised states and diabetes. Simple medication adherence, regular check-ups, and lifestyle adjustments can significantly decrease the risk of abscess formation and progression [9].

Red Flags

Important red flags that must be promptly recognized with regard to skin abscesses include:

Red flags for abscesses that prompt immediate treatment include:

I. **Severe Pain or Tenderness**: Worsening pain should be addressed immediately [6].
II. **Rapid Swelling or Increased Size** [4].
III. **Fever or Systemic Symptoms** [5].
IV. **Redness and Warmth**: An area that is becoming increasingly red and warm to the touch signals inflammation and potentially an expanding abscess [6].
V. **Pus or Drainage**: Signals that the abscess is worsening or becoming infected [7].
VI. **Difficulty Moving or Function Loss**: Any abscess in an area that is impeding function or mobility, such as around a joint, can cause significant functional impairment and long-term complications [14].
VII. **Underlying Health Conditions**: Diabetes, immunosuppression, or chronic illness [4].
VIII. **History of Abscesses or Recurrence** [6].

Pearls and Pitfalls of Skin Abscess Management

Pearls

I. Prompt Diagnosis and Treatment can prevent complications. Ultrasound should be used to guide the diagnosis of difficult-to-assess abscesses [15].
II. Incision and Drainage (I&D) is the gold standard treatment. HCPs should ensure thorough abscess drainage utilizing local anesthesia to control patient discomfort [10]. Cruciate incisions provide lower rates of recurrence than basic linear incisions.
III. Antibiotics should be reserved for cases with particular indications (e.g., immunocompromised patients, large abscesses, systemic symptoms). Antibiotics should be selected based on local resistance patterns, culture results, and sensitivities [6, 11].
IV. Patients should not be discharged before receiving education on proper wound care and warning signs [13, 16].
V. Patients should be monitored and must return for follow-ups to ensure no complications. An I&D can be repeated if the abscess recurs or fails to resolve [5, 17].

Pitfalls

I. Failure to adequately drain an abscess increases the risk of recurrence and infection progression. Imaging should be utilized to ensure complete drainage in more complex cases [15, 18].

II. Routine use of Antibiotics for uncomplicated abscesses contributes to antibiotic resistance and should be avoided. Reserve antibiotic for cases that meet specific criteria (e.g., immunocompromised state, systemic symptoms) [6, 11].
III. Selection of ineffective antibiotics can contribute to antibiotic resistance and treatment failure. All antibiotics should be selected based on culture results, sensitivities, and local resistance patterns [13, 16].
IV. HCPs should be very vigilant for warning signs such as rapid progression of infection, systemic symptoms and severe pain. Failing to detect more complex or deeper infections (e.g., necrotizing fasciitis) can lead to severely adverse outcomes [11, 17].
V. Missing follow-up visits can lead to recurrence or missed complications. HCPs should follow up with patients to monitor healing and complications [13, 18].
VI. Poor patient education of hygiene and wound care is associated with recurrence and poor healing outcomes. Clear instructions should be provided by HCPs to ensure patient understanding [13, 16].
VII. Inadequate pain control is associated with poor patient compliance and enhanced discomfort [18, 19].

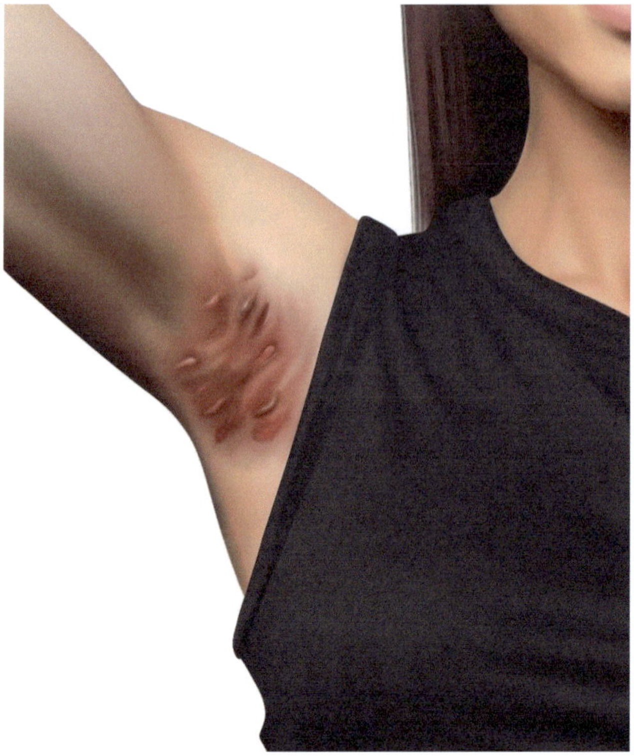

Fig. 29.2 Hidradenitis suppurativa of the axilla. (*Original illustration by Jana Zeineddine, MD*)

Hidradenitis Suppurativa

Introduction

Hidradenitis suppurativa (HS) is a chronic, inflammatory skin disorder that affects around 1–2% of the population globally [20]. It often presents in early adulthood, with peak incidence around the age of 20–40 [21]. Patients usually present with painful abscesses, nodules, and tissue destruction in areas like the groin and armpits, as shown in Fig. 29.2 [20]. The inflammatory nature of the disease generates debilitating scarring that often significantly impacts quality of life through chronic pain, mental health deterioration, mobility difficulties, and social stigmatization [20].

Pathophysiology

The pathophysiology of HS includes complex immunological pathways involving IL-17 and TNF-α. HS typically begins with keratosis and hyperplasia, which produce follicular occlusion. This activates immune responses, inflammation, and tissue destruction.

Key risk factors include:

I. **Lifestyle**: Smoking, Obesity, Stress.
II. **Genetics**: HS is sometimes familial, inherited in an autosomal dominant fashion. Mutations often affect immune function, epidermal proliferation, or ceramide synthesis.
III. **Hormones**: The disease predominantly affects females and fluctuates with hormonal changes.

Diagnosis

Different standardized techniques are available for diagnosing HS and assessing severity. Each technique provides unique insights into disease progression and patient morbidity [22]. They also help guide tailored treatment plans and monitor outcomes.

Hurley Staging

The Hurley Staging system is commonly used to classify HS severity. It divides disease progression into three stages:

I. **Stage 1**: Single or multiple abscess with no scarring or sinus tracts [22].
II. **Stage 2**: Recurrent abscesses with scarring and sinus tracts. Lesions are separated by normal skin [22].
III. **Stage 3**: Diffuse or near-diffuse involvement. Multiple interconnected abscesses and sinus tracts across a large area [22].

HiSCR (Hidradenitis Suppurativa Clinical Response)

HiSCR is used to evaluate patient response to treatment in clinical trials. It mainly assesses a reduction in the number of inflammatory nodules and abscesses [22]. A positive HiSCR refers to at least 50% reduction in overall nodule and abscess count without any increase in draining fistula or abscess count [22].

Modified Sartorius Score

The Modified Sartorius Score contributes a more in-depth assessment. It involves counting nodules, fistulas, and scars in seven well-defined anatomical regions [22]. Furthermore, it takes into account the longest distance between lesions and whether interconnections between lesions are present. Thus, this score helps determine the distribution and extent of the disease, enabling comprehensive severity evaluation [22].

HS-PGA (Hidradenitis Suppurativa Physician Global Assessment)

HS-PGA is a subjective tool that categorizes HS severity into six groups

I. Clear
II. Minimal
III. Mild
IV. Moderate
V. Severe
VI. Very severe

The patient is assigned to a group based on their number of nodules, draining fistulas, abscesses, and overall morbidity [22].

HSSI (Hidradenitis Suppurativa Severity Index)

HSSI assesses disease severity based on factors such as the number of affected sites, number of inflammatory lesions, presence of drainage, skin surface area involved, and pain level experienced by the patient [22]. HSSI provides a more holistic overview of the disease, taking into consideration both symptomatic and physical aspects.

IHS4 and IHS4–55 (International Hidradenitis Suppurativa Severity Score System)

IHS4 is a scoring system that utilizes the number of inflammatory nodules, abscesses, and fistulas to evaluate HS severity [22]. The score can be calculated by adding

- The number of nodules x1
- The number of abscesses x2
- The number of fistulas x4

With higher scores correlating with more severe disease [22].

On the other hand, the IHS4-55 is a modified version that considers additional parameters to more precisely assess patients in various contexts [22].

Nonsurgical Treatment

Topical, systemic, and surgical therapies are available, providing limited relief [20]. Currently, the anti-TNF-α antibody, Adalimumab, is the only FDA-approved biological treatment, but it was only found effective in around half of patients [20]. New research is targeting JAK/STAT and IL-17 pathways, with promising clinical trials underway [20].

Surgical Treatment

Traditionally, medical management was the first line for treating HS, with surgery left as a last resort. However, in recent years, combining medical and surgical management has been gaining popularity [23]. Surgery has been found to increase treatment effectiveness by addressing the inflammatory and structural barriers of the disease that medical treatments cannot sufficiently handle alone [23].

The surgical method selected depends on the patient's disease severity and stage. Technique options include:

I. Deroofing: Useful for mild to moderate HS. Involves removing the roof of the abscess to enable secondary healing [23].
II. Local Excision: Useful for early-stage, small-sized lesions, but associated with a high recurrence rate [23].
III. Wide Excision: Removing lesions with a clear margin, which reduces recurrence rates compared to local excision [23].
IV. Radical Excision: Extensive removal of affected tissue. Associated with the lowest recurrence rates, particularly in severe cases [23].

V. Laser Therapy: Minimally invasive neodymium-doped YAG laser, which offers effective results. Useful in cases that are refractory or do not respond to conventional therapies or for patients who are not candidates for invasive procedures [23].

In addition to basic surgical strategies, reconstructive strategies are available, including:

I. Skin Grafts and Biologics: Suitable for large defects. Utilizes techniques like skin grafting and negative pressure wound therapy [23].
II. Locoregional Flaps: Flaps match the defect tissue. Easy to perform with good results [23].
III. Perforator Flaps: Useful option for reconstructing larger defects with faster recovery and minimal functional deficits. Offers versatile, reliable options for reconstruction [23].

Surgery is often combined with biological therapies to reduce recurrence and progression, and improve outcomes. For example, Adalimumab is effective alongside surgery.

Surgical Outcomes

A systematic review of 46 studies, covering 8344 patients and 10,000 procedures, found that amongst basic surgical approaches, wide excision was the most commonly utilized [23]. Additionally, incision and drainage were linked to relatively high recurrence rates, while deroofing offered quicker recovery but higher recurrence rates as opposed to other surgical options [23]. Furthermore, with regard to wound closure, primary closure had the shortest healing time, but the highest recurrence rates in comparison to secondary intention, flaps, and grafts [23].

Prognostic factors such as patient BMI, age, smoking status, disease severity, and number of lesions were found to significantly impact surgical outcomes. The highest rates of complications and recurrences were associated with smoking and obesity [23].

Finally, adjunctive treatments like antibiotics and biologics (adalimumab, infliximab, ustekinumab) were found to be beneficial, enabling better outcomes with regard to recurrence, symptom severity, and quality of life. However, they could potentially lengthen healing time [24]. Nevertheless, a multidisciplinary approach was found to have the best long-term outcomes [24].

Management Limitations

The most significant challenges impeding HS management include delayed diagnosis, the need for well-defined disease biomarkers and phenotypes, and the lack of standardized clinical trial measures [21]. Nevertheless, ongoing research is expected to improve patient outcomes [21].

Preventing Complications

I. **Preoperative Planning**: Strong preoperative planning is required to correctly anticipate the size of the effect and potential anatomical variations, so last-minute reconstructive decisions are avoided [25].
II. **Timing**: If lesions are heavily draining and infected, it is preferable to perform the reconstruction in two or more stages [25].
III. **Monitoring**: Postoperatively, flaps should be checked every 2–4 h for the first 24 h, and patients should be monitored closely [25].
IV. **Supportive Measures**: Arm splints should be used for axillary resections, while pressure offloading should be employed for extensive gluteal/perineal reconstructions [25].
V. **Pain Management**: Non-narcotics are preferred due to the higher risk of addiction amongst HS patients [25].
VI. **Postdischarge Support**: Patients should be linked with case managers and social workers to streamline their discharge process, reduce the likelihood of readmission, and introduce patients to sources of social support postoperatively [25].

Pearls and Pitfalls

I. **Preoperative Counseling**: It is important to emphasize weight loss, tobacco cessation, wound management, and superinfection treatment preoperatively [25].
II. **Documentation**: It is useful to consistently document patient progression through tools like the Hurley stage. It is also recommended to monitor treatment response using severity scores [25].
III. **Adjuvant Therapy**: Pain management and nonsurgical therapies should be utilized alongside surgery, including preoperative adalimumab [25].
IV. **Reconstruction Planning**: For extensive or radical excisions, consider temporary diversion procedures such as cystostomy or colostomy [25].
V. **Perforator Identification**: A Doppler probe should be used to locate perforators near the defect margin [25].
VI. **Dissection Techniques**: Subfacial dissection and magnification for clear visualization should be used for distant perforators. Bipolar cautery and needle-tip bovie should be used for dissection [25].

VII. **Flap Selection**: Large perforators should be isolated but not skeletonized. Important to check vascularity when multiple perforators are available [25].

VIII. **Intraoperative Monitoring**: Perforator status should be assessed regularly using a Doppler. Peninsular flaps are preferred over island flaps due to better drainage [25].

IX. **Flap Inset**: Flaps should be Inset without tension; Flap should be delayed or supercharged if a vascularity issue occurs [25].

X. **Cultures**: Deep cultures should be obtained postresection to inform antibiotic selection. Might be necessary to resect and analyze infected lymph nodes [25].

Pilonidal Disease

Introduction

Pilonidal disease is a chronic inflammatory skin condition of the natal cleft, which is the deep groove that runs between the buttocks. It can result in painful, inflamed nodules which may progress to abscesses, sinus tracts, and scarring, as shown in Figs. 29.3, 29.4, and 29.5 [26]. The word "Pilonidal" is derived from the Latin root "pilus" meaning "hair" and "nidus" meaning "nest," translating to "nest of hairs." It was initially coined "Jeep Disease" after many U.S./soldiers who rode in Jeeps in WWII were diagnosed with this condition, which was felt to be a result of prolonged sitting and repeated rubbing of the natal cleft against the seat [26, 27]. This recurrent action results in micro-traumas to the skin, creating "pits" or pinpoint openings, which create an opening for debris such as hair follicles to become embedded under the skin. Furthermore, because of the hook morphology of hair, the sharp ends can pierce the skin while the hook ends of the hair prevent it from retracting, thus driving the hair deeper into the tissue [27]. The motion of walking also creates friction between the glutes, promoting the hairs to be driven deeper into the pit. This phenomenon results in the formation of tunnels under the skin, also known as sinus tracts. As the hairs become trapped in the sinus tracts, a foreign body reaction occurs, which can then result in the formation of a subcutaneous abscess cavity [28]. The warmth, repeated friction, and moisture in the natal cleft create an ideal environment for infection to thrive.

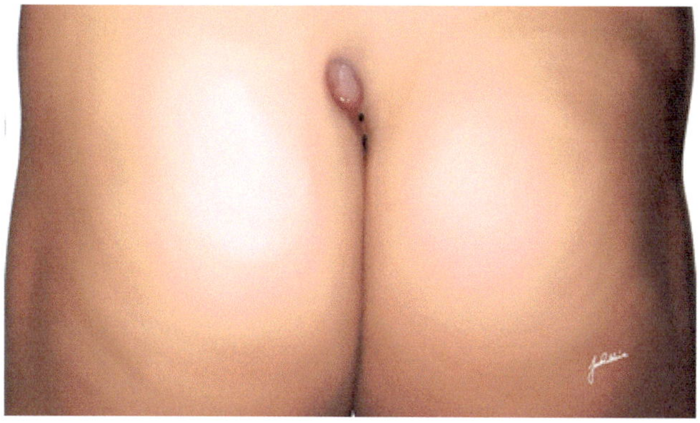

Fig. 29.3 Midline pits with abscess cavity left of midline, cephalad to natal cleft. (*Original illustration by Jana Zeineddine, MD*)

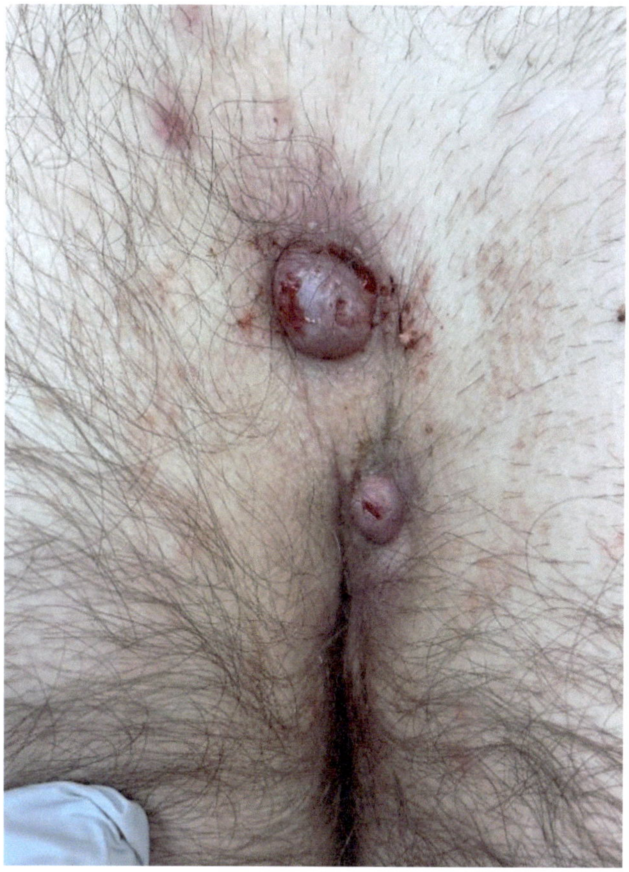

Fig. 29.4 Multiple chronic draining pilonidal abscesses. (*Photo courtesy of Holly Bonnette, NP*)

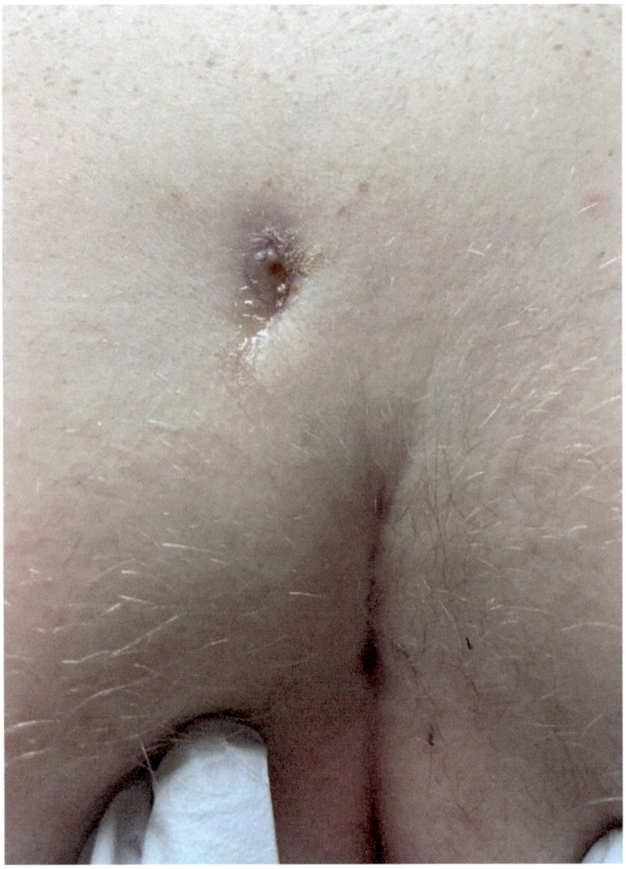

Fig. 29.5 Draining pilonidal abscess with pits in midline cleft. (*Photo courtesy of Holly Bonnette, NP*)

Pilonidal disease is a spectrum and can range from a dormant and asymptomatic disease to an active and purulent infection [26]. Words such as "cyst," "abscess," and "disease" are often used interchangeably when referring to pilonidal disease. The most appropriate terminology when referring to an active infection of the sinus or cyst is a "pilonidal abscess" [26].

Risk factors for the development of pilonidal disease include [26–28]:

I. Overweight/obesity
II. Male sex (2.2x more likely than women)
III. Family history
IV. Deep natal cleft
V. Sedentary lifestyle, occupation, or prolonged sitting
VI. Local trauma or irritation
VII. Hirsutism (thick, coarse hair)
VIII. Poor hygiene
IX. Excessive sweating

Pilonidal disease affects approximately 70,000 people in the United States annually [27].

Diagnosis

Pilonidal disease is primarily diagnosed on history and physical exam. Patients may report pain, swelling, tenderness, drainage, or bleeding. Symptoms often occur intermittently. The key with diagnosing pilonidal disease is the location at which these symptoms occur on exam—the natal cleft vs the perianal region. Differential diagnoses may include perianal abscess, anal fistula, hemorrhoids, or hidradenitis suppurativa. Examination will help rule out these other possibilities. Pilonidal abscesses are most commonly found lateral to the natal cleft, superior or cephalad to the anus. In contrast, a draining anal fistula or perianal abscess will be closer in proximity to the anal opening. An abscess related to hidradenitis will be located on the perineum or in the inguinal area as opposed to the natal cleft. A useful differentiation when the patient is experiencing bleeding is that bleeding or drainage from pilonidal disease is not linked to bowel movements, unlike hemorrhoids.

On physical exam, there will be one or more "pits" or pinpoint openings in the midline gluteal cleft from which there may be protruding hairs. With more chronic disease, these pits may connect, and the openings may result in elongated wounds. Superior to the pits, often branching off to the left or right of midline, there may be palpable lateral extensions—"tracts"—which ultimately lead to a cystic or abscess cavity. Signs suggestive of an active infection or abscess could include overlying erythema, pain or tenderness to palpation, localized warmth, fluctuance, and/or induration. Active drainage of blood or purulent material may or may not be seen. If a patient has had chronic disease or prior procedures, scarring may also be noted.

Diagnosing pilonidal disease is based on clinical evaluation, and no additional lab tests or imaging are necessary.

Nonsurgical Treatment

In patients with minimal symptoms (absence of abscess), the primary treatment of pilonidal disease consists of conservative management. This includes hair removal via laser, shaving, creams, or waxing to reduce hair burden on the back and buttocks. Treatment plans should also include adjustments to lifestyle and addressable risk factors. It is also recommended for patients to scrub their gluteal cleft with a coarse cloth like a washcloth while showering daily, to help keep pits free of debris and hair. It is helpful to counsel patients that some mild bleeding may occur with this rubbing, and that is not a cause for alarm.

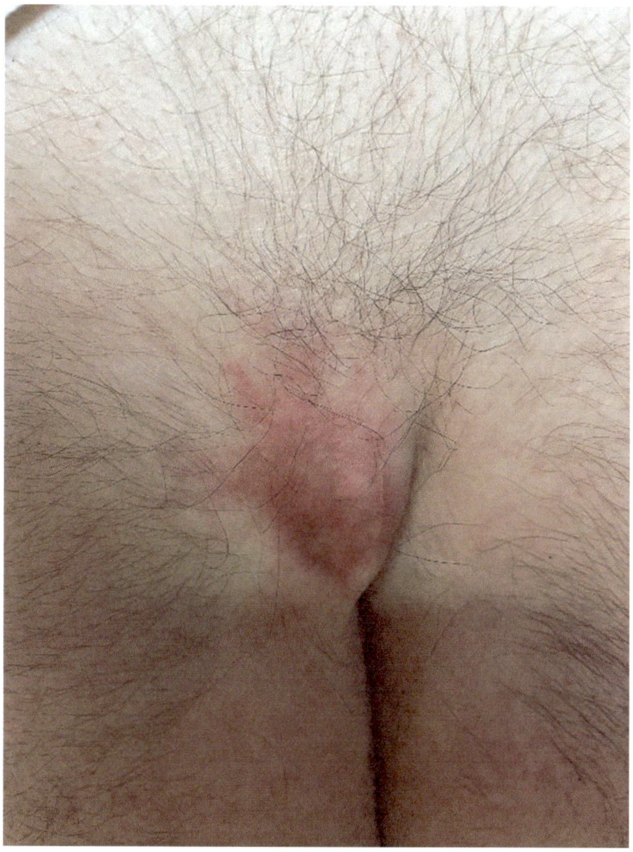

Fig. 29.6 Pilonidal abscess in need of I&D. (*Photo courtesy of Holly Bonnette, NP*)

Surgical Treatment

Acute Symptoms (Abscess)

In patients with an acute, active infection or abscess, as shown in Fig. 29.6, the primary treatment is incision and drainage (I&D), regardless of whether it is a primary or recurring episode. Grade of

Recommendation

Strong recommendation based on moderate-quality evidence [29]. I&D is typically performed at the bedside, though deeper, more indurated abscesses may require anesthesia for adequate pain control. Prior to incision, the skin overlying the abscess and the surrounding area should be prepped with chlorhexidine or iodine swabs. Local anesthetic is then injected around and under the abscess cavity. It is important to remember that the environment of an abscess is acidic, which may neutralize the effects of the anesthetic. For this reason, it is crucial to use enough anesthetic and give it time to take effect to ensure adequate pain control. Another tip is to avoid injecting directly into the abscess cavity, as this can also result in incomplete anesthesia.

Incision is achieved with a scalpel over the most fluctuant part of the abscess. It is crucial to make the opening large enough to allow for adequate drainage so that the skin does not heal over too quickly, resulting in a residual abscess cavity. The abscess cavity should be probed, and loculations should be broken up. This can be achieved with the use of Q-tips or a Kelly Clamp. Some clinicians will then choose to irrigate the cavity with normal saline.

Wound packing following I&D is a widely debated topic and is thought to aid hemostasis and prevent abscess recurrence. The patient is instructed to remove the packing 24 h later at home, which can be anxiety-provoking and painful. If the patient is noncompliant with packing removal, this can lead to further infectious complications. In a study by Leiwand et al., which followed one hundred pediatric patients with subcutaneous abscesses, they found no difference in the abscess recurrence rate between the two study groups and concluded that it was safe and effective to omit packing, which can help to minimize the painful and anxiety-provoking component of this wound care [30].

Definite treatment is usually postponed until after an acute infection or abscess has been resolved. Delaying definitive treatment by weeks has been associated with lower long term recurrence rates compared to primary surgery without I&D. A study by Doll et al. looked at 583 patients over 20 years and found a 16% recurrence rate in the I&D cohort vs a 34% recurrence rate in the primary open treatment group [31].

As noted above, the primary treatment for pilonidal abscesses is I&D, and antibiotics are generally not needed. However, in certain populations (those who are immunosuppressed, diabetics, MRSA, or high risk for endocarditis) or with findings of significant cellulitis or systemic symptoms (fevers, chills, malaise) antibiotics should be considered in addition to I&D. It is important to remember that in the presence of an active infection antibiotics should never be considered as the sole treatment—I&D is crucial. When antibiotics are warranted, the preferred choice is a first-generation cephalosporin plus metronidazole [28].

At-home wound care includes frequent warm soaks (sitz baths) to help promote drainage and covering the area with dry gauze to help catch drainage. Gauze should be changed throughout the day when wet.

Chronic Symptoms (Persistent Wound, Pain, Drainage)

In patients with persistent symptoms, there are many treatment options that exist. The decision for which to pursue should be individualized based on the patient's exam findings and goals of treatment. The most commonly offered treatments include:

I. **Phenol—**In patients with acute or chronic pilonidal disease without abscess, phenol application is an effective treatment. Grade of Recommendation: Strong recommendation based on moderate-quality evidence [29]. This procedure involves hair removal, curettage of the cyst by enlarging the cavity, and application of 1–3 mL of crystallized phenol into the cyst and associated tracts. The phenol solution causes a caustic burn and denatures the hairs though, to cause pilonidal disease. In general, 1–4 procedures are required to achieve healing. This procedure can be done under local anesthesia with overall success rates of 62–95% and low complication rates of 0–2% [26].

II. **Fibrin Glue**—In patients with acute or chronic pilonidal disease without abscess, fibrin glue may be effective as a primary or adjunctive treatment. Grade of Recommendation: Weak recommendation based on moderate-quality evidence [29]. After curette is performed to remove hair and debris from the sinus tract, fibrin glue can be instilled to fill in the remaining dead space. This, in turn, can help limit granulation tissue formation and prevent more debris from collecting. It can be utilized after excision and skin flap closure, to fill in the wound left by sinus excision (without closure), or to fill in the void left after curettage of pilonidal pits as previously noted [29]. Given the lack of high-quality evidence and long-term results, the utility of fibrin glue remains unclear [27, 31].

III. **Pit-picking**—The Bascom pit-picking procedure involves excising the pits with a knife. The healthy skin in between the pits is preserved, which helps to reduce pain and prolonged wound healing.

IV. **Surgical Excision**—In patients with chronic pilonidal disease, excision is the standard of treatment. Grade of Recommendation: Strong recommendation based on moderate-quality evidence [29]. Closure after excision can be achieved via primary closure (this includes flaps) or by secondary intention (via marsupialization). Healing via primary closure involves closing the wound in layers, whereas healing via secondary intention involves leaving the wound open to heal from the bottom up. Secondary intention is often achieved by marsupializing or sewing the wound edges to help prevent premature closure of the wound. Primary closure has been shown to result in quicker healing, less time off work, and less need for wound care (as there is no open wound) [27, 31]. However, healing by secondary intention has been shown to have a 35% less risk of recurrence compared with primary closure [32]. Curiously, surgical site infection rates are similar between primary closure and secondary intention healing, and an infection in a wound closed via primary intention does not increase the risk of long-term recurrence [33]. If a primary closure is performed, the preferred technique is to keep the closure off the midline, as this decreases the risk of surgical site infection and promotes faster healing [29, 34].

V. **Flaps**—Flap procedures can be performed in the setting of complex and recurrent chronic pilonidal disease when other techniques have failed. Grade of Recommendation: Strong recommendation based on moderate-quality evidence [29]. The goal with flaps is to provide healthy tissue coverage following wide excision of the disease. There are numerous flap techniques, including the rhomboid or Limberg flap, the Karydakis flap, the cleft-life technique or Bascom procedure, the V-Y advancement flap, and the Z-plasty technique. The details of these flaps are beyond the scope of this chapter. The decision for which technique to employ depends on the surgeon's training and is patient-dependent.

Complications

The main complications of pilonidal disease are recurrence and wound healing problems. This includes delayed wound healing and surgical site infections.

Pearls and Pitfalls

I. Pilonidal disease is an inflammatory skin condition of the natal cleft that affects approximately 70,000 people in the United States annually.

II. It is more common in hairy men, those who are overweight/obese, or with deep natal clefts. Other factors like family history, sedentary lifestyle, job, poor hygiene, or excessive sweating also increase the risk of pilonidal disease formation.

III. It is a spectrum, so some will be asymptomatic, and others may suffer from recurrent abscess and drainage.

IV. Key to diagnosing pilonidal disease is the location—look for pits in the natal cleft, and sinus tracts/abscess cavities off midline, usually superior or cephalad to the cleft.

V. In the presence of an active infection (abscess), I&D is the gold standard for treatment. Antibiotics are generally not needed, unless for certain populations (immunosuppressed, diabetics), then they may be used as an adjunct, but should never be the sole treatment.

VI. Delaying definitive treatment by weeks following an I&D is ideal, as it has been shown to be correlated with lower long-term recurrence rates.

VII. Surgical excision in patients with chronic pilonidal disease is the standard of treatment. Closure can be achieved with primary or secondary intention. If primary closure is performed, the preferred technique is to keep the closure off the midline.

VIII. Flap procedures are generally performed for complex and recurrent chronic pilonidal disease when other techniques have failed. The decision for which technique to employ depends on the surgeon's training and is patient-dependent.

References

1. Pallin DJ, Camargo CA, Schuur JD, Singer AJ. Increased US emergency department visits for skin and soft tissue infections, and changes in antibiotic choices, during the emergence of community-associated methicillin-resistant Staphylococcus aureus. Arch Intern Med. 2014;164(11):1592–7.
2. Talan DA, Mower WR, Krishnadasan A, Abrahamian FM, Moran GJ, EMERGEncy ID Net Study Group. A randomized trial of clindamycin versus trimethoprim-sulfamethoxazole for uncomplicated skin infections. N Engl J Med. 2016;374(9):823–32.
3. Hersh AL, Chambers HF, Maselli JH, Gonzales R. National trends in ambulatory visits and antibiotic prescribing for skin and soft-tissue infections. Arch Intern Med. 2008;168(14):1585–91.
4. Dryden MS. Complicated skin and soft tissue infection. J Antimicrob Chemother. 2010;65(Suppl 3):iii35–iii44.
5. Singer AJ, Talan DA. Management of skin abscesses in the era of methicillin-resistant Staphylococcus aureus. N Engl J Med. 2014;370(11):1039–47.
6. Stevens DL, Bisno AL, Chambers HF, Dellinger EP, Goldstein EJC, Gorbach SL, Hirschmann JV, Kaplan SL, Montoya JG, Wade JC. Practice guidelines for the diagnosis and management of skin and soft tissue infections: 2014 update by the Infectious Diseases Society of America. Clin Infect Dis. 2014;59(2):e10–52.
7. Sartelli M, Malangoni MA, May AK, Viale P, Kao LS, Catena F, Ansaloni L, Moore EE, Moore FA, Peitzman AB. The management of skin and soft tissue infections: expert consensus statements. World J Emerg Surg. 2018;13(1):1–24.
8. Lee MC, Rios AM, Aten MF, Mejias A, Rodriguez SA. Skin and soft tissue infections. Pediatr Rev. 2018;39(10):498–510.
9. Frew JW, Navrazhina K, Marohn M, Garzon MC. Hidradenitis suppurativa: current understanding and management. J Am Acad Dermatol. 2020;82(5):1237–50.
10. Alves P, Neves M. Management of epidermoid cysts. J Dermatol Treat. 2020;31(8):769–74.
11. Moran GJ, Krishnadasan A, Gorwitz RJ, Fosheim GE, McDougal LK, Carey RB, Talan DA. Methicillin-resistant S. aureus infections among patients in the emergency department. N Engl J Med. 2006;355(7):666–74.
12. Liu C, Bayer A, Cosgrove SE, Daum RS, Fridkin SK, Gorwitz RJ, Kaplan SL, Karchmer AW, Levine DP, Murray BE, Rybak MJ. Clinical practice guidelines by the infectious diseases society of America for the treatment of methicillin-resistant *Staphylococcus aureus* infections in adults and children. Clin Infect Dis. 2011;52(3):e18–55.
13. Cameron DR, Rybak MJ, McKinnon PS. Patient education: preventing recurrent skin infections caused by community-associated methicillin-resistant Staphylococcus aureus. Infect Control Hosp Epidemiol. 2014;35(12):1477–82.
14. Czernick M, Zane D. Skin and soft tissue infections: pathophysiology and management. Ann Emerg Med. 2013;62(4):403–14.
15. Tibbles CD, Porcaro W. Procedural applications of ultrasound. Int J Emerg Med. 2014;7(1):1–9.
16. May L, Emond JA. Delays in diagnosis and treatment of necrotizing fasciitis in the emergency department. Ann Emerg Med. 2009;54(5):684–91.
17. Miller LG, Perdreau-Remington F, Bayer AS. Clinical and molecular epidemiology of community-associated methicillin-resistant Staphylococcus aureus in an urban population. J Clin Microbiol. 2005;43(10):5246–52.
18. Stewart DB, Eachempati SR, Lysaght MJ, Hydo LJ. Surgical site infections: prevention and treatment. J Am Coll Surg. 2014;219(2):404–16.
19. Burris J, Gupta R. Loop drainage technique for abscess management in an urban community hospital: a case series. J Med Case Rep. 2016;10(1):4–9.
20. Krueger JG, Frew J, Jemec GB, Kimball AB, Kirby B, Bechara FG, et al. Hidradenitis suppurativa: new insights into disease mechanisms and an evolving treatment landscape. Br J Dermatol. 2024;190(2):149–62.
21. Pandey A. Essentials of hidradenitis suppurativa: a comprehensive review of diagnostic and treatment perspectives. Ann Med Surg. 2024;86(9):5304–13.
22. Kim Y, Lee J, Kim HS, Ko HC, Kim BS, Kim MB, Shin K. Review of scoring systems for hidradenitis suppurativa. Ann Dermatol. 2024;36(1):9.
23. Li K, Jeremian R, Bi WG, Bouadi N, Seigel K, Asgarpour J, et al. Prognostic factors in hidradenitis suppurativa surgeries: a scoping review. JAAD Rev. 2024;1:22.
24. Issa CJ, Hong AC, Lio PA. Combined biologic and surgical interventions for hidradenitis suppurativa: a systematic review. Dermatol Ther. 2024;2024(1):6637006.
25. Krajewski A, Alsayed A, Capek A, Casey K, Chandawarkar R. Surgical management of hidradenitis suppurativa. Plast Reconstr Surg Glob Open. 2024;12(6):e5860.
26. Bhama AR, Davis BR. Pilonidal disease and hidradenitis suppurativa. In: Steele SR, Hull TL, Hyman N, Maykel JA, Read TE, Whitlow CB, editors. The ASCRS textbook of colon and rectal surgery. Cham: Springer; 2022. https://doi.org/10.1007/978-3-030-66049-9_16.
27. Nixon AT, Garza RF. Pilonidal cyst and sinus. In: StatPearls [Internet]. Treasure Island (FL): StatPearls Publishing; 2020. Available from: https://www.ncbi.nlm.nih.gov/books/NBK557770/.
28. Johnson EK. In: UpToDate, Connor RF, editors. Pilonidal disease. Wolters Kluwer; 2024. Accessed on 2 Aug 2024.
29. Johnson EK, Vogel JD, Cowan ML, Feingold DL, Steele SR. The American society of colon and rectal surgeons' clinical practice guidelines for the management of pilonidal disease. Dis Colon Rectum. 2019;62(2):146–57.
30. Leinwand M, Downing M, Slater D, Beck M, Burton K, Moyer D. Incision and drainage of subcutaneous abscesses without the use of packing. J Pediatr Surg. 2013;48(9):1962–5.
31. Doll D, Matevossian E, Hoenemann C, Hoffmann S. Incision and drainage preceding definite surgery achieves lower 20-year long-term recurrence rate in 583 primary pilonidal sinus surgery patients. J Dtsch Dermatol Ges. 2013;11(1):60–4.
32. Ahmed AK, McCallum I, King PM, Bruce J. Healing by primary versus secondary intention after surgical treatment for pilonidal sinus. Cochrane Database Syst Rev. 2010;2010(1):CD006213.
33. Doll D, Matevossian E, Luedi MM, Schneider R, Van Zypen D, Novotny A. Does full wound rupture following median pilonidal closure alter long-term recurrence rate? Med Princ Pract. 2015;24(6):571–7.
34. Sewefy AM, Hassanen A, Atyia AM, Saleh SK. Karydakis flap with compressing tie-over interrupted sutures without drain versus standard Karydakis for treatment of sacrococcygeal pilonidal sinus disease. Dis Colon Rectum. 2017;60(5):514–20.

30 Inflammatory Bowel Disease

Paulo Gustavo Kotze
and Rafaela de Araújo Molteni Moretti

Introduction

Inflammatory Bowel Disease (IBD), encompassing Crohn's disease (CD) and ulcerative colitis (UC) (Figs. 30.1 and 30.2), is a chronic inflammatory condition of the gastrointestinal tract that often requires urgent medical and surgical interventions.

When IBD is suspected, treating healthcare providers want to know which *type* it is—CD or UC. These two entities are quite similar in some ways but different in others (Table 30.1). When the affected segment of bowel involves the *large intestine only,* it sometimes isn't easy to distinguish CD from UC, and making this diagnosis can be a bit tricky. This is true for a couple of reasons. First, histopathology from a biopsy, which is often a gold standard for arriving at a diagnosis, is *notoriously inaccurate or nonconclusive.* Pathologists are very good at diagnosing things like cancer with a biopsy, but for IBD, it's hard for them to tell the difference between CD and UC, as they often look the same under a microscope. Second, CD can entirely mimic UC (even though the converse is not true). Thus, if the disease happens to involve the large intestine *only* (something quite possible with CD), then we have to carefully assess ***the pattern of disease distribution.*** We can use playing cards as a useful analogy (Figs. 30.3 and 30.4).

While many patients achieve remission through pharmacological treatment (Table 30.2), acute complications such as perforation, massive hemorrhage, toxic megacolon, and

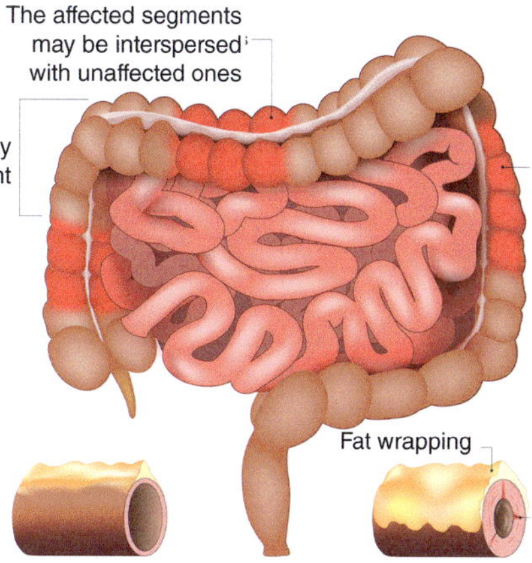

Fig. 30.1 **Crohn's disease** (CD) can involve any segment of the alimentary tract "from mouth to anus," and can affect all layers of the intestine. It often can present with interspersed segments of disease, separated by nonaffected or normal segments of bowel, as shown. Thus, Crohn's can "skip around" from one region to another, which is the reason it is sometimes also referred to as regional enteritis. Due to the **full-thickness** nature of Crohn's disease, fistulae and/or associated abscesses are often also present. The inflammation can stricture and even mechanically obstruct the intestine, especially in the terminal ileum. Although Crohn's can affect any segment of bowel, it has a strong predilection for the **terminal ileum** and **anus**. An important macroscopic feature of Crohn's disease is known as **mesenteric fat wrapping or *creeping***, whereby the mesenteric fat wraps around toward the antimesenteric side, as depicted (editor's comment)

P. G. Kotze (✉) · R. de Araújo Molteni Moretti
Pontifícia Universidade Católica do Paraná (PUCPR), Health Sciences Postgraduate Program, IBD outpatient clinics, Curitiba, PR, Brazil

S. Atallah, J. Dragoljevic (eds.), *Fundamentals of Surgery for Physician Assistants*,
https://doi.org/10.1007/978-3-032-21069-2_30

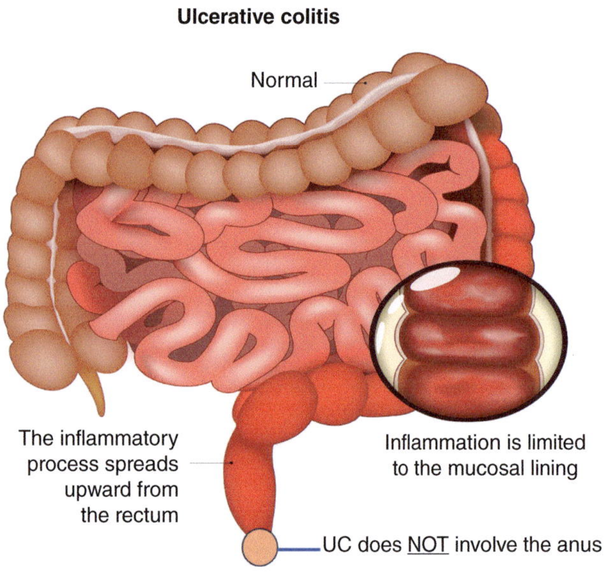

Fig. 30.2 **Ulcerative Colitis** (UC) is a mucosal disease that affects only the colon and rectum. It does not affect the anus. UC follows a specific pattern of spread that is contiguous and extends from the rectum cephalad. Unlike Crohn's disease, UC does not "skip around," and it does not affect the small bowel and/or the foregut (editor's comment)

severe obstruction may necessitate *emergent surgical management* [1, 2]. Primary care providers and emergency department (ED) ***PAs play a crucial role in recognizing these life-threatening situations to ensure timely referral and intervention.***

Acute surgical emergencies in IBD patients can arise due to disease progression, treatment failure, or postoperative complications. In CD, complications such as intra-abdominal abscesses, perforations, and strictures can lead to bowel obstruction, often requiring resection [3]. In UC, **toxic megacolon**—a *severe form of colonic distension associated with systemic toxicity*—**demands prompt recognition** and possible colectomy to prevent perforation and sepsis [4]. Delay in surgical intervention can significantly increase morbidity and mortality, highlighting the importance of early diagnosis in emergency settings. Patients with toxic megacolon are at risk for bowel perforation, sepsis, and even death. It is imperative that diagnosticians, including PAs, are knowledgeable about this condition. Common signs and symptoms are summarized in Table 30.3. **Toxic colitis** is a variant of toxic megacolon in which the colon is not dilated, but the condition still requires urgent attention. If you sus-

Table 30.1 Similarities and differences between Crohn's disease (CD) and ulcerative colitis (UC)

Characteristic	Crohn's disease	Ulcerative colitis
Age distribution	Bimodal (15–35) and (50–70)	Bimodal (15–35) and (50–70)
Etiology	Immune system related, other factors	Immune system related, other factors
Bloody diarrhea	Uncommon	Common
Cramping abdominal pain	Common	Common
Affected segment of bowel	Any	*Only* colon and rectum
Can have "skip" areas (disease is noncontiguous)	Yes	No
Most commonly affects	Terminal ileum, anus	Rectum and left side of colon
Anal disease (fistula/abscess)	Common	Never
Layers of bowel affected	All	Mucosa only
Fistula and abscess typical	Yes	No
Small bowel obstruction	Yes	No
Extra-intestinal manifestations?	Possible	Possible
Is medication the mainstay Of treatment?	Yes	Yes
When to operate	Obstruction, fistula, abscess, severe stricture, perforation, refractory symptoms	Refractory symptoms, toxic colitis, toxic Megacolon dysplasia, cancer, failed medical therapy
Is surgery curative?	No	Yes, a total proctocolectomy Is curative of the intestinal manifestations of UC

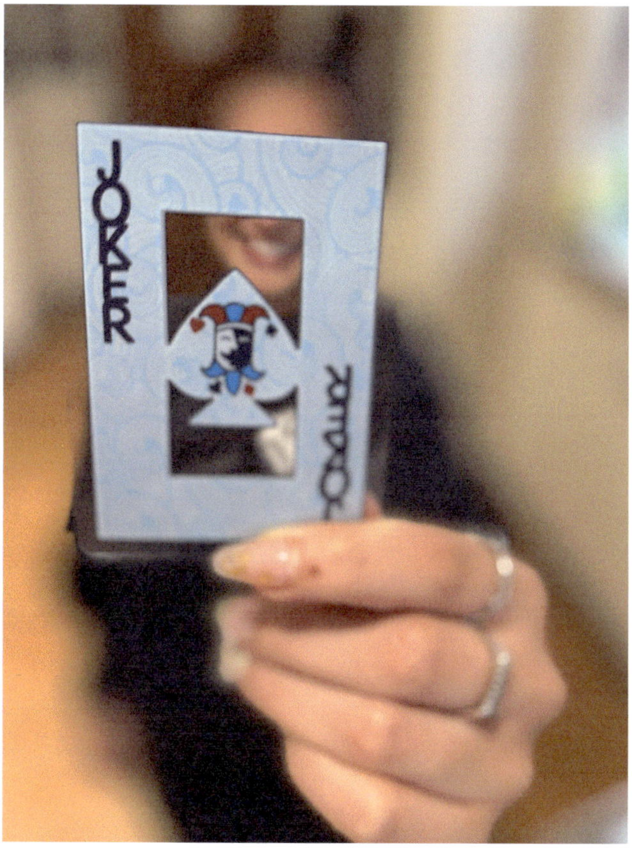

Fig. 30.3 Using playing cards as an analogy, CD is like a "wild card" or joker. Thus, CD can affect anywhere it wants to, in any pattern. It "doesn't play by the rules," and thus any pattern of disease is permissible with CD. This is entirely not the case for UC, fortunately, and this helps us distinguish the two, mainly in that it can help us exclude UC (editor's comment)

pect a patient may have toxic colitis or toxic megacolon, *notify a surgeon immediately.*

Postoperative complications also contribute to surgical emergencies in IBD patients. Anastomotic leaks, intra-abdominal abscesses, and short bowel syndrome can lead to significant morbidity and require immediate surgical or interventional radiology management. Additionally, malnutrition and immunosuppressive therapies commonly used in IBD treatment, such as corticosteroids and advanced therapies, may be related to an increased risk of postoperative infections and impaired wound healing, making close postoperative monitoring essential [1, 2].

Given the complexity of surgical emergencies in IBD, primary assistants in emergency rooms and those managing postoperative patients must be well-informed about the presentation, diagnostic approach, and initial management of these conditions. This chapter aims to provide an overview of the most common emergency situations requiring surgical intervention in IBD, with a focus on their pathophysiology, clinical manifestations, diagnostic strategies, and initial management principles. By enhancing the understanding of these emergencies, healthcare providers can contribute to improved outcomes through timely and appropriate intervention.

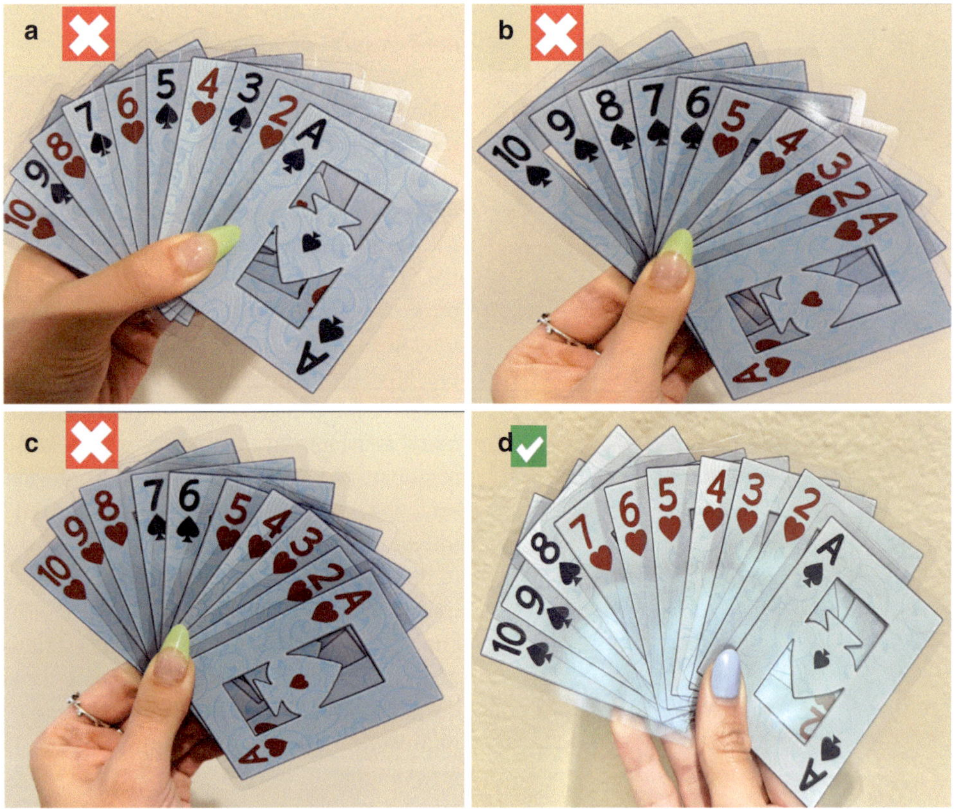

Fig. 30.4 Although CD is a "wild card" and "doesn't play by the rules," UC very much *obeys strict rules.* Most importantly, it never affects the anus and always spreads contiguously from the distal-most rectum cephalad. It may or may not affect the entire colon and does not affect the small bowel. In this playing card analogy, let's suppose red hearts denote active disease, and black spades denote normal tissue. Let's further suppose "A" denotes the anus, and that "2" represents the distal-most rectum. Now let's examine each of these patterns to understand why only one is consistent with UC. In (**a**) although the anus is spared, which would go along with UC, the pattern is noncontiguous and therefore cannot be UC; (**b**) here the pattern is contiguous, and would be consistent with UC if it was not for the anal involvement; (**c**) Here there is a normal segment between the two segments of inflammation, which is not consistent with UC, also the anus is involved; (**d**) Here the UC rules are obeyed. The pattern of spread is cephalad and contiguous. The anus is also spared. Note that the entire colon need not be affected, as long as the disease is *contiguous.* This is the only pattern that would be consistent with UC of the ones shown. Remember, because CD is a "wild card," it could theoretically be any one of those patterns (editor's comment)

Table 30.2 Common medications used to treat inflammatory bowel disease (CD and UC)

Medication class	Examples	Indication	Mechanism of action	Common side effects
Aminosalicylates (5-ASAs)	Mesalamine, sulfasalazine, Olsalazine	Mild to moderate disease, maintenance therapy	Anti-inflammatory effect in the gut via inhibition of prostaglandin synthesis	Headache, nausea, abdominal pain, rash
Corticosteroids	Prednisone, budesonide, hydrocortisone	Acute flare-ups, short-term control	Suppress inflammation by inhibiting immune cell function	Weight gain, osteoporosis, hyperglycemia
Immunomodulators	Azathioprine, Mercaptopurine, methotrexate	Steroid-sparing, long-term maintenance	Suppress immune system activity by inhibiting DNA/RNA synthesis	Leukopenia, liver toxicity, pancreatitis
Biologics (TNF inhibitors)	Infliximab, Adalimumab, Certolizumab, Golimumab	Moderate to severe disease, refractory cases	Block tumor necrosis factor (TNF), a key mediator of inflammation	Infections, infusion reactions, malignancy
Biologics (anti-integrins)	Vedolizumab, Natalizumab	Moderate to severe disease, especially with fistulas	Block integrins to prevent immune cell adhesion and migration to inflamed tissues	Headache, infections, liver dysfunction
Biologics (IL-12/IL-23 inhibitors)	Ustekinumab	Moderate to severe disease, refractory cases	Inhibit interleukin-12 and interleukin-23 pathways involved in inflammation	Headache, fatigue, upper respiratory infections
Antibiotics	Metronidazole, ciprofloxacin	Infections, abscesses, and fistulas (especially in Crohn's disease)	Antibacterial effect may help control gut flora and treat abscesses	Nausea, diarrhea, peripheral neuropathy
Probiotics	VSL#3, align, Florastor	Maintenance therapy, symptom relief in mild cases	Promote healthy gut flora, potentially modulating immune response	Mild gastrointestinal discomfort
JAK inhibitors	Tofacitinib	Moderate to severe ulcerative colitis (FDA-approved)	Inhibit Janus kinase enzymes involved in inflammatory pathways	Infection risk, liver enzyme elevation

Notes:

Corticosteroids are typically used for short-term management during flare-ups; long-term use is not recommended due to serious side effects.

Immunomodulators and **biologics** are often used for long-term control and to reduce the reliance on steroids.

Biologics (TNF inhibitors, anti-integrins, IL-12/IL-23 inhibitors) are especially useful in refractory cases of Crohn's disease and ulcerative colitis.

JAK inhibitors are a newer class and are particularly used for ulcerative colitis.

Table 30.3 Clinical findings suggestive of toxic megacolon

Clinical finding	Description
Abdominal distention	Significant enlargement of the abdomen due to colonic dilation
Severe abdominal pain	Intense cramping or diffuse pain in the abdominal region
Fever	Elevated body temperature, often >38.6 °C (101.5 °F)
Tachycardia	Increased heart rate, typically >120 bpm
Hypotension	Low blood pressure, often resulting in signs of shock
Diarrhea or bloody stools	Frequent, watery stools, sometimes accompanied by blood
Dehydration	Signs of fluid loss, such as dry mouth, decreased urine output, or dizziness
Leukocytosis	Increased white blood cell count, often >15,000/μL
Radiologic findings	Abnormal dilation of the colon (>9 cm on imaging)
Altered mental status	Confusion, agitation, or delirium, especially in severe cases
Sepsis	Systemic inflammatory response syndrome (SIRS) may progress to septic shock

Crohn's Disease

Emergent Surgical Indications in Crohn's Disease

Surgical interventions in Crohn's disease (CD) are generally reserved for patients with complications that do not respond to medical therapy. The primary indications for emergent surgery include bowel obstruction, perforation, intra-abdominal abscess, and massive gastrointestinal hemorrhage [5, 6]. Bowel obstruction, either due to inflammatory strictures or fibrotic stenosis, is a frequent surgical emergency in CD and may require diversion or bowel resection, depending on the severity and location of the lesion. In cases of perforation, surgical intervention is critical to prevent peritonitis and sepsis, and in most instances, a segmental resection with or without temporary diversion is necessary [2].

Intra-abdominal abscesses, often secondary to penetrating disease, require immediate drainage—either **percutaneously under radiological guidance** (preferable) or surgically if percutaneous drainage fails or the abscess is not accessible [2, 3]. Hemorrhage, although less common, may occur from ulcerated segments of the bowel and can lead to hemodynamic instability. Endoscopic, angiographic, or surgical interventions such as bowel resection may be necessary depending on the severity and location of bleeding. Given the relapsing nature of CD, emergency surgery should always aim to balance disease control with bowel preservation to minimize short bowel syndrome and postoperative complications [2].

Diagnosis and Management of Perianal Abscesses and Fistulizing Crohn's Disease

Perianal disease is a common manifestation of CD, with perianal abscesses being the most frequent complication of perianal fistulizing disease. These abscesses result from infection exacerbated by underlying inflammation and fistula formation. Patients typically present with severe perianal pain, swelling, fever, and purulent drainage. Diagnosis relies on clinical examination, but in cases of deep-seated abscesses, pelvic MRI or endoscopic ultrasound (EUS) may be necessary to assess the extent of the infection and associated fistulas [7].

The mainstay of treatment for perianal abscesses is urgent **surgical *incision and drainage* to prevent further tissue destruction and septic complications.** Seton placement is often performed in cases of fistulizing disease to maintain drainage and prevent premature closure, which could lead to recurrent abscesses. Broad-spectrum antibiotics covering anaerobes and enteric flora are recommended, particularly in immunosuppressed patients. Advanced therapies such as anti-TNF agents (infliximab, adalimumab) or other agents (e.g., JAK inhibitors or anti-IL-23 agents) can be beneficial in reducing fistula recurrence, but surgical intervention remains crucial for the acute management [8].

Recognition and Management of Abdominal Emergencies in Crohn's Disease

Abdominal emergencies in CD most commonly present as bowel obstruction or sepsis due to intra-abdominal abscesses or perforation. Obstruction results from either inflammatory or fibrotic strictures, with symptoms including severe cramping, abdominal distension, nausea, vomiting, and constipation. Initial management involves bowel rest, intravenous fluids, nasogastric decompression, and corticosteroids in cases of inflammatory strictures. However, fibrotic strictures rarely respond to medical therapy and often require surgical intervention, with segmental bowel resection and diversion. Endoscopic balloon dilation may be an option in short strictures without significant fibrosis or perforation risk, but are mostly done electively [2, 3].

Sepsis in CD can arise from intra-abdominal abscesses, which develop due to transmural inflammation and microperforations leading to localized infection. Symptoms include fever, localized tenderness, leukocytosis, and signs of systemic inflammatory response syndrome (SIRS). Imaging, particularly a contrast-enhanced CT scan, is crucial for identifying the abscess size and location. Management typically involves percutaneous drainage under radiological guidance, but larger or multiloculated abscesses may require open or laparoscopic surgical drainage. Antibiotic therapy should be initiated promptly, with coverage for Gram-negative and anaerobic organisms [2, 3].

If an abscess is associated with a perforation or worsening peritonitis, emergency surgical intervention is warranted. In such cases, segmental resection with primary anastomosis is preferred when feasible, although a temporary diverting ileostomy may be necessary in patients with severe sepsis or malnutrition. The use of biological therapy in these patients should be postponed until the infection is adequately controlled, as immunosuppression can worsen septic outcomes [2].

Prompt recognition and intervention are critical in these emergencies, as delayed treatment can significantly increase morbidity and mortality. ER physicians and primary care providers must be vigilant in identifying high-risk patients, ensuring early imaging and surgical consultation when needed. By optimizing acute management and coordinating multidisciplinary care, healthcare providers can improve survival rates and reduce long-term complications in CD patients.

Diagnosis and Management of Postoperative Complications in Abdominal Crohn's Disease

Surgical intervention in Crohn's disease (CD) is often necessary to **manage complications** such as strictures, fistulas (Fig. 30.5), and abscesses. However, postoperative complications remain a significant concern, with thrombotic events, intestinal obstruction, and anastomotic leaks being among the most critical. Early recognition and prompt management of these complications are essential to reduce morbidity and mortality. The risk of complications is heightened in CD patients due to chronic inflammation, malnutrition, and the frequent use of immunosuppressive therapies, which impair wound healing and immune function [2, 3].

Thrombotic complications, including deep vein thrombosis (DVT) and pulmonary embolism (PE), are particularly prevalent in IBD patients due to their hypercoagulable state. Postoperative immobilization, dehydration, and inflammatory cytokine activation further increase this risk [9]. Pharmacological thromboprophylaxis with low-molecular-weight heparin (LMWH) or direct oral anticoagulants

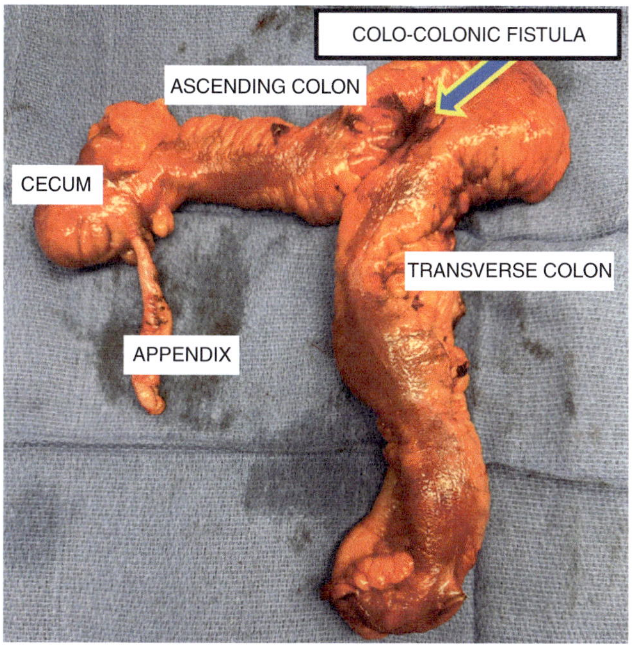

Fig. 30.5 A patient with severe Crohn's colitis underwent subtotal colectomy, with the resected specimen shown. In addition to severe pancolonic disease, a fistula (false passage) between the ascending colon and transverse colon was present (arrow). Due to the full-thickness nature of Crohn's disease, fistulas are not uncommonly observed. While the general approach is to "not operate" on Crohn's patients, there are important exceptions, which include fistulae, abscesses, severe strictures, bowel obstruction, and perforation. None of those conditions will resolve with medications, and surgery is required (editor's comment)

(DOACs) is recommended unless contraindicated by active bleeding. In patients with suspected PE—presenting with dyspnea, tachycardia, and hypoxia—immediate CT pulmonary angiography is indicated, and anticoagulation should be initiated promptly. In severe cases with hemodynamic instability, thrombolysis or surgical thrombectomy may be required [10].

Postoperative intestinal obstruction can arise due to adhesions, anastomotic edema, or residual strictures. Clinically, patients present with nausea, vomiting, abdominal distension, and failure to tolerate oral intake. Initial management involves bowel rest, nasogastric decompression, intravenous (IV) fluid resuscitation, and correction of electrolyte imbalances. In cases of complete obstruction or worsening symptoms despite conservative measures, surgical re-exploration may be necessary to relieve the obstruction and prevent ischemia [2, 3].

One of the most serious postoperative complications in CD is sepsis secondary to an anastomotic leak or intra-abdominal infection. Anastomotic leaks typically present within the first postoperative week with fever, tachycardia, hypotension, worsening abdominal pain, and signs of peritonitis. Diagnosis requires contrast-enhanced CT with oral or rectal contrast to assess for extraluminal air or fluid collections. Management includes broad-spectrum IV antibiotics (covering Gram-negative and anaerobic organisms), aggressive IV fluid resuscitation, and ICU admission for hemodynamic monitoring in severe cases. Percutaneous drainage is preferred for localized collections, but in cases of generalized peritonitis, surgical intervention with lavage, drainage, and possibly temporary stoma creation may be required [2].

By maintaining a high index of suspicion for these complications, primary assistants and emergency physicians can play a crucial role in early diagnosis and appropriate intervention, ultimately improving postoperative outcomes in Crohn's disease patients.

Ulcerative Colitis

Indications for Emergency Surgery in Ulcerative Colitis: Recognition and Initial Management

Ulcerative colitis (UC) is a chronic inflammatory disease primarily affecting the colonic mucosa, but in severe cases, it can progress to life-threatening complications requiring emergency surgical intervention [11]. The main indications for emergency surgery in UC include toxic megacolon, fulminant colitis with hemodynamic instability, massive lower gastrointestinal (GI) bleeding, and colonic perforation (Fig. 30.6a and b) [1]. These conditions often arise in patients with severe or refractory disease despite optimal medical therapy, and early recognition is crucial for preventing morbidity and mortality. The standard emergency surgical procedure for these patients is subtotal colectomy with end ileostomy, which provides rapid control of inflammation and prevents further complications [12].

Toxic megacolon, one of the most feared complications of UC, is characterized by extreme colonic dilation (>6 cm), systemic toxicity (fever, tachycardia, leukocytosis), and signs of peritonitis. Initial management includes aggressive IV fluid resuscitation, broad-spectrum antibiotics (covering Gram-negative and anaerobic bacteria), and IV corticosteroids if the patient is not already on them. Immediate surgical consultation is required, as the perforation risk is high. Similarly, fulminant colitis, defined by severe bloody diarrhea, abdominal distension, and systemic compromise, necessitates close monitoring, early total parenteral nutrition (TPN) consideration, and urgent escalation to colectomy if there is no response to medical therapy within 24–48 h [4].

Massive lower GI bleeding in UC is less common but can be life-threatening, particularly in extensive colonic involvement or superimposed **cytomegalovirus (CMV) infection.** Patients may present with hemodynamic instability, requiring fluid resuscitation, blood transfusions, and urgent colonoscopy to identify bleeding sites [1, 4]. If endoscopic and pharmacological interventions fail, total colectomy is the

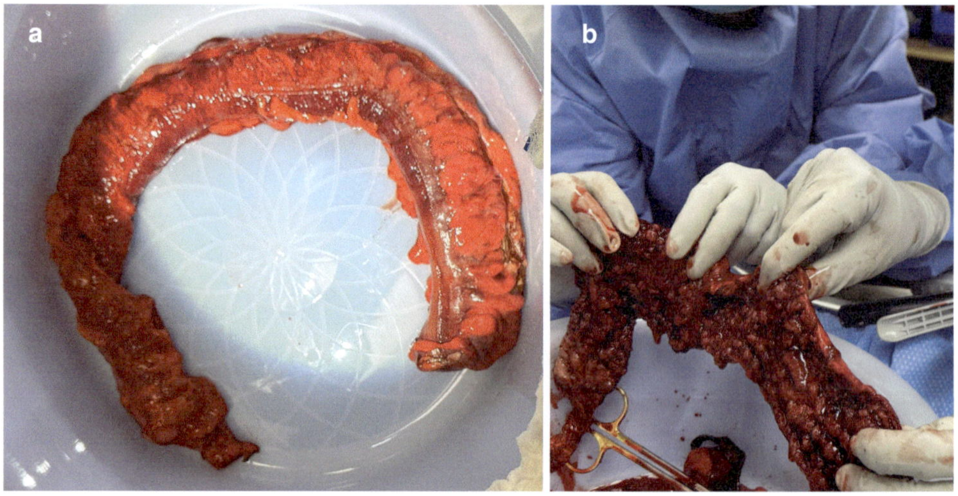

Fig. 30.6 (**a** and **b**) A patient underwent emergent subtotal colectomy for severe, refractory lower intestinal hemorrhage due to UC. (**a**) The gross resected specimen is shown. Remember, UC is a *mucosal disease,* so looking at the specimen from the *outside*, it does not look abnormal and is quite unassuming. However, when the specimen is cut open to expose the mucosa (**b**), the severe inflammatory changes consistent with UC are quite evident! (editor's comment)

definitive treatment. Colonic perforation, the most critical surgical emergency in UC, presents with severe abdominal pain, peritoneal signs, and hemodynamic collapse. A contrast-enhanced CT scan can confirm free air in the peritoneal cavity, and immediate laparotomy is required to prevent fatal sepsis [1].

For PAs in emergency departments, prompt recognition and early stabilization of these UC emergencies are critical. ***Key steps include aggressive IV hydration, electrolyte repletion, early broad-spectrum antibiotics, and avoiding antidiarrheal agents or opioids, which can worsen colonic dilation.*** Emergency surgery should be considered without delay in cases of toxic megacolon with worsening toxicity, perforation, or persistent severe bleeding. Coordination with gastroenterology and surgical teams ensures optimal management, reducing mortality and improving patient outcomes [4].

Recognition and Management of Postoperative Complications in Emergency Colectomies with Ileostomies in Ulcerative Colitis

Emergency colectomy with ileostomy is the standard surgical approach for patients with severe or refractory ulcerative colitis (UC). While this procedure is life-saving, it is associated with significant postoperative complications, including sepsis, small bowel obstruction, and dehydration due to high-output ileostomy. Early recognition and appropriate management of these complications are essential to improve patient outcomes and reduce morbidity [1].

Postoperative sepsis, often secondary to anastomotic leaks, intra-abdominal abscesses, or wound infections, presents with fever, tachycardia, hypotension, and increasing abdominal pain. Primary assistant physicians should maintain a high index of suspicion, particularly in patients with worsening inflammatory markers (leukocytosis, elevated C-reactive protein, or procalcitonin). Initial management includes broad-spectrum intravenous (IV) antibiotics covering Gram-negative and anaerobic pathogens, aggressive IV fluid resuscitation, and, in severe cases, intensive care unit (ICU) admission for hemodynamic monitoring. A contrast-enhanced CT scan with oral contrast is the preferred diagnostic modality to identify intra-abdominal collections, which may require percutaneous or surgical drainage [1, 4, 12].

Small bowel obstruction (SBO) is another common postoperative complication, typically due to adhesions, kinking of the ileostomy, or anastomotic strictures. Patients present with nausea, vomiting, abdominal distension, and reduced stoma output. Initial management includes bowel rest, nasogastric decompression, and IV fluid administration to correct dehydration and electrolyte imbalances. If there is no resolution within 48–72 h, imaging (abdominal X-ray or CT scan) should be performed to assess for a mechanical obstruction requiring surgical intervention [1, 4].

Dehydration due to high-output ileostomy (>1.5–2 L/day) is a major postoperative concern, especially in the early postoperative period. It can lead to acute kidney injury, electrolyte disturbances (hypokalemia, metabolic acidosis), and orthostatic hypotension. Management includes oral rehydration with electrolyte-rich solutions, loperamide or codeine to slow intestinal transit, and IV fluid support in severe cases. Monitoring urine output and serum electrolytes is crucial in these patients, and dietary modifications such as reducing hyperosmolar foods and increasing soluble fiber intake may also be beneficial [1].

Diagnosis and Management of Pouch Surgery Complications in Ulcerative Colitis

Not everyone with UC requires emergent or urgent surgery. Some patients may *fail medical management* or may develop *dysplasia* (abnormal colon cells) due to years of chronic disease. They may also develop *refractory symptoms.* Unlike CD, patients with UC can undergo a procedure in which the entire colon and rectum are removed. This would thus *remove all the affected colonic mucosa,* and thus removing the colon and rectum in this manner provides a **surgical cure for the intestinal manifestations of UC.** There are several associated extra-intestinal manifestations of IBD (Table 30.4) that may not resolve, however.

When the entire colon and rectum are removed, and then a portion of small bowel is made into a "pouch" and connected surgically to the anus, this is termed a **restorative proctocolectomy with ileal pouch-anal anastomosis, or IPAA.**

For patients undergoing restorative proctocolectomy with ileal pouch-anal anastomosis (IPAA), postoperative complications such as sepsis, pouch obstruction, and dehydration due to high-output ileostomy can significantly impact outcomes. These complications require early detection and timely intervention to prevent long-term morbidity.

Pouch-related sepsis can occur due to anastomotic leaks, pelvic abscesses, or pouchitis. Patients with anastomotic leaks or pelvic abscesses may present with fever, perineal or lower abdominal pain, and persistent drainage from surgical wounds. Diagnosis is confirmed with contrast-enhanced CT or pelvic MRI, and management involves IV antibiotics, percutaneous or surgical drainage of abscesses, and, in severe cases, temporary ileostomy diversion [1, 13]. **Pouchitis**, a common inflammatory complication, presents with increased stool frequency, urgency, and crampy abdominal pain. It is typically managed with a two-week course of antibiotics such as ciprofloxacin or metronidazole [14].

Table 30.4 Extra-intestinal manifestations of inflammatory bowel disease

Manifestation	Description	Prevalence
Arthritis	Joint pain or inflammation, particularly in large joints like knees and hips	10–20%
Uveitis	Inflammation of the eye, causing pain, redness, and blurred vision	2–10%
Erythema Nodosum	Painful, red nodules on the skin, often on the shins	3–10%
Pyoderma Gangrenosum	Ulcerating skin lesions, usually on the legs	1–2%
Primary Sclerosing cholangitis	Inflammation and scarring of the bile ducts, often leading to liver issues	2–5%
Gallstones	Formation of gallstones, more common in patients with primary sclerosing cholangitis	10–25%
Ankylosing spondylitis	Inflammation of the spine and sacroiliac joints, leading to stiffness and pain	2–5%
Mouth ulcers	Painful ulcers inside the mouth, often in IBD flare-ups	10–20%
Thromboembolism	Increased risk of blood clots, especially deep vein thrombosis (DVT) and pulmonary embolism	1–3%
Renal stones	Kidney stone formation, more common in patients with Crohn's disease	5–10%

Pouch obstruction can result from anastomotic strictures or adhesions, leading to abdominal pain, bloating, and difficulty evacuating stool. Digital rectal examination may help identify strictures at the pouch-anal anastomosis. Initial management includes dietary modifications, stool softeners, and, in cases of significant narrowing, endoscopic balloon dilation. If obstruction is due to adhesions, conservative management with bowel rest and IV fluids may suffice, but persistent or severe cases may require surgical intervention [14].

When the restorative proctocolectomy with IPAA operation is done, it is usually done in stages. In the first stage, there is usually a temporary ileostomy created by the surgeon to prevent contents from going downstream into the pouch (basically to give it time to heal). This is referred to by surgeons as a ***defunctioning ileostomy.*** **Dehydration** due to high-output from such an ileostomy remains a **significant risk** following IPAA, particularly in patients with short bowel syndrome or rapid intestinal transit. Patients should be monitored for signs of hypovolemia, including dizziness, tachycardia, and reduced urine output. *Management includes optimizing oral hydration with electrolyte-rich solutions, pharmacological therapy (loperamide, diphenoxylate/atropine), and IV fluid resuscitation.* Patient education on dietary modifications and hydration strategies is crucial to reducing long-term complications [1].

By recognizing these complications early, PAs can ensure timely intervention, preventing severe outcomes and improving postoperative recovery in UC patients undergoing colectomy or pouch surgery.

As a PA, if you encounter patients who have had a history of IPAA and who develop complications, consult an expert colorectal surgeon *early on,* as the management of pouch-related problems can be quite complex.

Conclusions

Primary assistant physicians in emergency departments and postoperative care settings play a critical role in the early recognition and initial management of life-threatening complications in inflammatory bowel disease (IBD). In both Crohn's disease (CD) and ulcerative colitis (UC), emergency surgical interventions may be necessary for conditions such as bowel obstruction, perforation, toxic megacolon, and massive gastrointestinal bleeding. Prompt identification of these conditions, along with appropriate resuscitation measures—including fluid resuscitation, electrolyte correction, early antibiotic administration, and timely surgical consultation—can significantly improve patient outcomes. Understanding the specific emergency indications for surgery in CD and UC enables nonspecialist physicians to provide timely and effective interventions in critical situations.

Postoperative complications following emergency colectomy with ileostomy or pouch surgery in UC, as well as abdominal surgery for CD, require careful monitoring to prevent morbidity and mortality. Sepsis, thrombotic complications, small bowel obstruction, and dehydration due to high-output ileostomy are among the most common and serious concerns. Emergency physicians and nonspecialist clinicians should be proficient in recognizing these complications early, initiating appropriate fluid and electrolyte management, and facilitating early surgical or intensive care referral when necessary. Simple interventions such as optimizing hydration, adjusting medications for bowel function, and monitoring for infectious complications can have a substantial impact on patient recovery.

Although the management of IBD and its surgical complications is complex, a structured and proactive approach by frontline healthcare providers can greatly improve outcomes. By maintaining a high index of suspicion for severe complications, coordinating closely with gastroenterology and surgical teams, and implementing evidence-based supportive care strategies, primary assistant physicians can ensure that patients with IBD receive timely and effective treatment. Continuous education on the acute management of IBD emergencies and postoperative care can further strengthen the ability of nonspecialist physicians to contribute to the multidisciplinary care of these challenging patients.

References

1. Spinelli A, Bonovas S, Burisch J, Kucharzik T, Adamina M, Annese V, et al. ECCO guidelines on therapeutics in ulcerative colitis: surgical treatment. J Crohns Colitis [Internet]. 2022 [cited 2025 Feb 24];16(2):179–89.
2. Adamina M, Minozzi S, Warusavitarne J, Buskens CJ, Chaparro M, Verstockt B, et al. ECCO guidelines on therapeutics in Crohn's disease: surgical treatment. J Crohns Colitis [Internet]. 2024 [cited 2025 Feb 24];18(10).
3. Lightner AL, Vogel JD, Carmichael JC, Keller DS, Shah SA, Mahadevan U, et al. The American society of colon and rectal surgeons clinical practice guidelines for the surgical management of Crohn's disease. Dis Colon Rectum [Internet]. 2020 [cited 2025 Feb 24];63(8):1028–52.
4. Kotze PG, Honap S, Savio MC, Araújo RMM, Quaresma AB, Peyrin-Biroulet L. Acute severe ulcerative colitis: defining the precise moment for colectomy. Expert Rev Gastroenterol Hepatol [Internet]. 2025 [cited 2025 Mar 27];19(1).
5. Maggiori L, Panis Y. Laparoscopy in Crohn's disease. Best Pract Res Clin Gastroenterol [Internet]. 2014;28(1):183–94.
6. Fowkes L, Krishna K, Menon A, Greenslade GL, Dixon AR. Laparoscopic emergency and elective surgery for ulcerative colitis. Color Dis. 2008;10(4):373–8.
7. Kotze PG, Shen B, Lightner A, Yamamoto T, Spinelli A, Ghosh S, et al. Modern management of perianal fistulas in Crohn's disease: future directions. Gut. 2018;67(6):1181–94.
8. Kotze P, Albuquerque I, Moreira A, Tonini W, Olandoski M, Coy C. Perianal complete remission with combined therapy (seton placement and anti-TNF agents) in crohn's disease: a Brazilian multicenter observational study. Arq Gastroenterol. 2014;51(4):1–7.
9. Bernstein CN, Blanchard JF, Houston DS, Wajda A. The incidence of deep venous thrombosis and pulmonary embolism among patients with inflammatory bowel disease: a population-based cohort study. Thromb Haemost. 2001;85(3):430–4.
10. Olivera PA, Zuily S, Kotze PG, Regnault V, Al Awadhi S, Bossuyt P, et al. International consensus on the prevention of venous and arterial thrombotic events in patients with inflammatory bowel disease. Nat Rev Gastroenterol Hepatol [Internet]. 2021 [cited 2025 Mar 27];18(12):857–73.
11. Kobayashi T, Siegmund B, Le Berre C, Wei SC, Ferrante M, Shen B, et al. Ulcerative colitis. Nat Rev Dis Primers [Internet]. 2020;6(1)
12. Kotze PG, Heuthorst L, Lightner AL, Damião AOMC, Bemelman WA. New insights on the surgical management of ulcerative colitis in the 21st century. Lancet Gastroenterol Hepatol [Internet]. 2022 [cited 2025 Mar 27];7(7):679–88.
13. Kotze PG, Avellaneda N, Moretti RDAM, Carvello M, Tomada EP, Campos FG, et al. Controversies in IPAA for ulcerative colitis: a systematic review of different anastomotic techniques. Dis Colon Rectum [Internet]. 2024 [cited 2025 Mar 27];67(S1):S26–35.
14. Fazio V, Kiran R, Remzi F, Coffey J, Heneghan H, Kirat H, et al. Ileal pouch anal anastomosis. Ann of Surg. 2013;257(4):679–85.

Toxic Colitis and Megacolon

31

Bhuwan Giri and Scott R. Steele

Introduction

Toxic colitis, alternatively called inflammatory colitis, fulminant colitis, or acute severe colitis, is a term used to describe severe inflammation of the colon. Clinically, patients will present with a rapid onset of symptoms such as abdominal pain, diarrhea, and systemic signs of infection or inflammation. Toxic megacolon (TM) is defined radiographically as colonic dilatation >5.5 cm without an obstructive cause in addition to clinical features of toxic colitis. A commonly described clinical criteria by Jalan and colleagues include radiologic evidence of colonic distension and three out of four features of fever >101.5 degrees (38.6° C), tachycardia greater than 120 beats per minute, leukocytosis greater than 10.5 × 10^3 cells/dL, or anemia along with at least one of the following: volume depletion, altered mental changes, electrolyte abnormalities, and hypotension [1].

The most common causes are inflammatory bowel disease (IBD)—commonly ulcerative colitis, infection (commonly *Clostridiodes difficile*), and ischemia (Table 31.1). Interestingly, despite its relative incidence, the exact mechanisms leading to toxic megacolon remain unclear. Regardless, defective smooth muscle contraction originating from mucosal inflammation leading to progressive colonic dilatation is believed to play a role in propagating colonic dilatation.

Toxic colitis with toxic megacolon is a medical and surgical emergency that requires prompt diagnosis and evaluation. Fulminant toxic megacolon can have mortality rates as high as 50% [2].

Table 31.1 Etiology and diagnostic criteria of toxic colitis and toxic megacolon

Etiology	Diagnosis
Inflammatory bowel disease *Ulcerative Colitis* *Crohn's disease*	***Toxic Colitis*** Rapid onset of symptoms such as abdominal pain, diarrhea, and systemic signs of infection or inflammation
Infections *Clostridiodes difficile* *CMV* *Campylobacter* *Shigella* *Rotavirus*	Presence of three out of four features: fever >101.5 °F, tachycardia >120 bpm, leukocytosis >10.5 × 10^3 cells/μL or anemia along with at least one of the following: volume depletion, altered mental changes, electrolyte abnormalities, and hypotension
Drug-induced colitis *Immunotherapy checkpoint inhibitors* *Chemotherapy*	***Toxic Megacolon*** Toxic Colitis with radiographic evidence of colonic dilation (>5.5 cm) without obstructive cause
Ischemic Colitis	

Which Patients Are at Risk?

Patients with inflammatory bowel disease, especially in the earlier part of their disease, are most at risk for toxic colitis. There is a higher incidence of toxic colitis in patients with ulcerative colitis compared to Crohn's disease. *Clostridiodes difficile* infection (CDI) can also lead to severe colitis in patients who are immunosuppressed, hospitalized, or have been exposed to antibiotics recently. Further, CMV colitis may occur in immunocompromised patients, neutropenic colitis in chemotherapy patients, and drug-induced colitis

B. Giri · S. R. Steele (✉)
Digestive Disease Institute, Cleveland Clinic Foundation, Cleveland, OH, USA

S. Atallah, J. Dragoljevic (eds.), *Fundamentals of Surgery for Physician Assistants*, https://doi.org/10.1007/978-3-032-21069-2_31

(most commonly immune checkpoint inhibitors) also have the potential to progress to fulminant colitis and toxic megacolon.

CMV colitis may be seen in patients with marked immunosuppression (HIV/AIDS, transplant recipients), IBD, and patients with multiorgan failure. Diagnosis relies on the endoscopic appearance of punched-out ulcers in the colon (seen in 70–80% of patients) and immunohistochemistry against CMV antigens with characteristics of owl eye inclusion bodies seen on histology.

Immune-mediated colitis is a common complication, affecting 1–25% of patients on checkpoint inhibitors, depending on the type and combination of drugs used. There is a significant overlap in endoscopic and histologic presentation between immune-mediated colitis and IBD. It typically occurs approximately 5–10 weeks after the second or third treatment dose.

Ischemic colitis can also present with bloody diarrhea and peritonitis in similar patient populations and is a significant differential to consider. This is discussed in a separate chapter.

Clinical Presentation

Patients with toxic megacolon will typically appear ill. They may present with bloody diarrhea (typically >ten times per day) with associated abdominal pain, nausea, vomiting, and altered mental status. Physical examination is essential to look for abdominal distension and tenderness. Peritonitis (i.e., diffuse tenderness, guarding, rigidity), along with fevers, altered mental status, and hypotension, may indicate the severe complication of bowel perforation. Many of these patients may be on steroids, masking some of these symptoms; thus, a high index of suspicion and close follow-up are required in immunocompromised patients. Inquiries should be made on the underlying condition's root cause, distinguishing primarily between infectious and inflammatory causes. It is important to ask about any prior diagnosis of inflammatory bowel disease. For patients without a prior diagnosis of IBD, it is essential to investigate any previous symptoms of undiagnosed IBD, like abdominal pain, diarrhea, bloody stools, or vomiting. Additionally, the potential for exposure to gastrointestinal pathogens through close contact, environmental factors, and use of recent medications such as antibiotics should be noted. Lastly, it is crucial to determine if the patient is immunocompromised due to conditions such as HIV, cancer, or chemotherapy.

Diagnosis

Patients with UC may present with acute severe ulcerative colitis (ASUC), which is a worsening of chronic inflammation seen in ulcerative colitis [3]. This diagnosis is based on the presence of more than six bloody stools per day with signs of systemic toxicity (think of tachycardia, fever, anemia, and elevated inflammatory markers like ESR and CRP). Approximately 5% of these patients may present with toxic megacolon.

ASUC patients are prone to developing *C. difficile* and should be tested on presentation. A combination of UC and *C. difficile* portends a higher risk of complications.

Patients at risk for *C. difficile* include elderly or immunocompromised patients, patients from nursing homes, those with severe baseline comorbidities, and those who have been recently exposed to antibiotics [4]. The presence of diarrhea with greater than three watery stools per day in the presence of these risk factors should be considered for *C. difficile* testing. In most hospitals, a positive initial screening test using a sensitive Glutamate dehydrogenase (GDH) test or Nucleic acid amplification testing (NAAT), followed by a specific test for *C. difficile* toxin (typically a PCR test), is confirmatory for CDI. Stratifying patients into mild/nonsevere, severe, or severe-complicated fulminant disease is helpful to triage these patients and direct therapy. The presence of leukocytosis greater than 15 × 10^3/μl or creatinine>1.5 mg/dL is defined as severe infection, and severe complicated/fulminant disease is characterized by the systemic manifestation of hypotension, sepsis, shock, ileus or megacolon, or those requiring ICU care. One of the most important caveats is that since CDI is primarily a mucosal disease, life-threatening fulminant toxic colitis may not be associated with colonic dilatation.

Radiologic Features

Toxic megacolon is the presence of toxic colitis with colonic dilation greater than 5.5 cm. This dilation is usually seen in the transverse colon and is accompanied by bowel wall edema, causing it to lose its regular haustral pattern on imaging. Patients who are suspected of having toxic megacolon should be followed with an abdominal radiograph every 12–24 h, depending on their clinical presentation.

A CT scan is helpful in revealing the extent and complications of toxic colitis. It may show colonic dilatation (Fig. 31.1) and, in cases of an acute complication, perforation, or signs of impending or occult bowel ischemia (presence of pneumatosis, portal venous gas, free air, and free fluid). The decision to operate on the patient should be driven by the patient's presentation (i.e., shock, multiorgan failure, need for vasopressors) and in patients with concerning imaging findings (free air, free fluid, persistent colonic dilation, abnormal haustral pattern, and colonic wall thinning). Toxic megacolon is less common in Crohn's disease, but the imaging findings in both UC and Crohn's disease overlap. One must remember that clinical examination alone may not be accurate enough to detect perforation in the setting of a toxic megacolon, and the first signs of this complication may be provided on a plain radiograph or a CT scan (Figs. 31.2 and 31.3).

Recommendations for complete colonoscopic examination and contrast enema studies in patients who are suspected of having toxic colitis or megacolon are controversial and

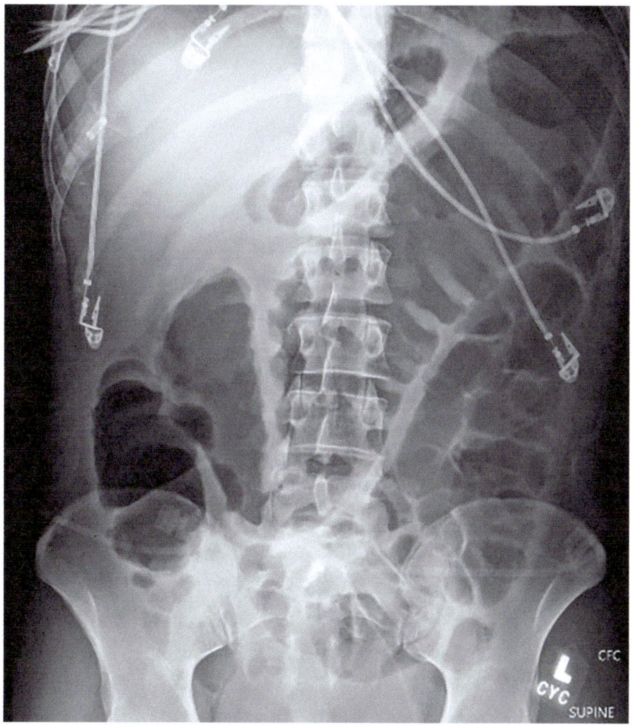

Fig. 31.1 Transverse colon dilation up to 10 cm with colonic wall thickening in a patient with toxic megacolon secondary to ulcerative colitis

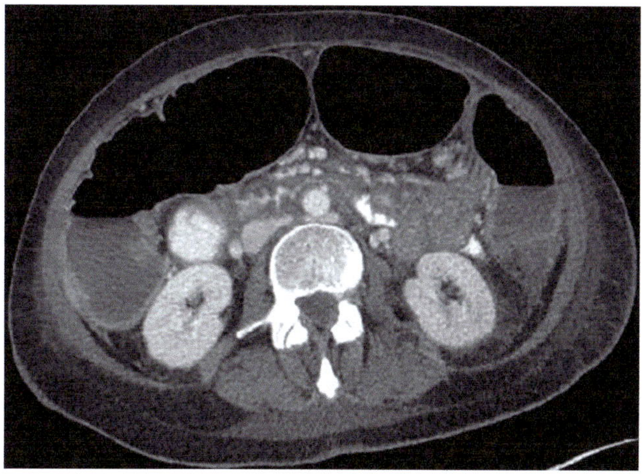

Fig. 31.2 CT scan showing pan-colonic dilatation in a patient with ulcerative colitis and toxic megacolon

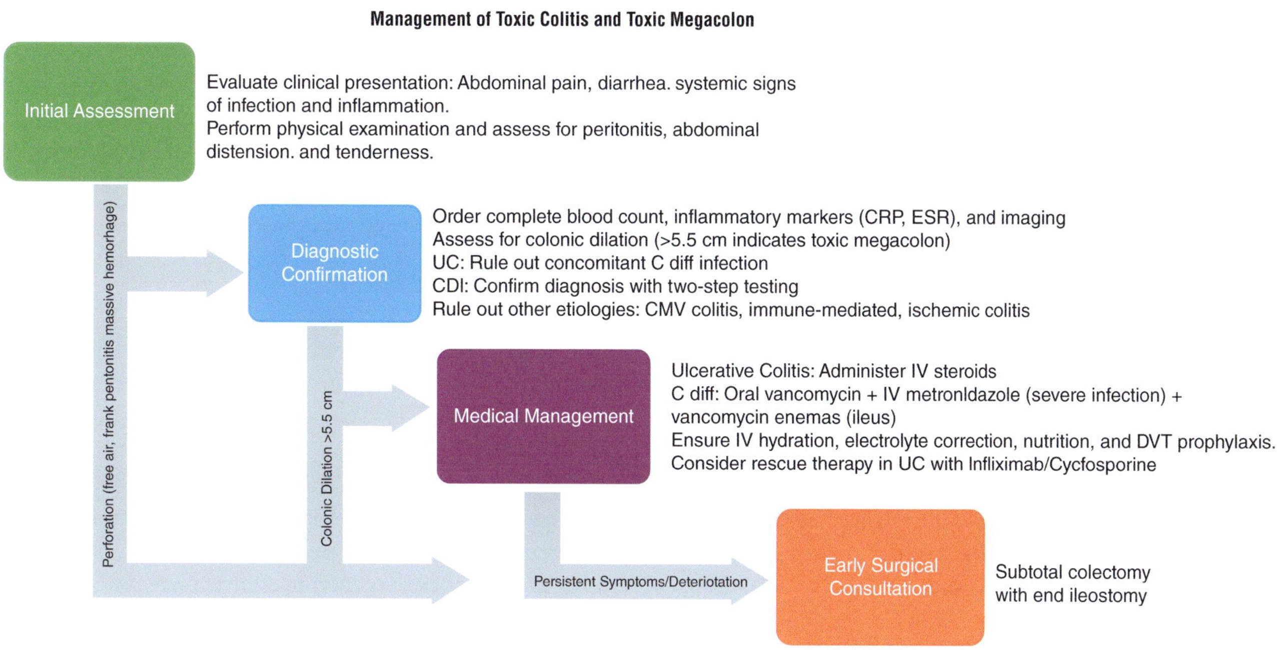

Fig. 31.3 Summary of management of toxic colitis and toxic megacolon

not typically recommended for fear of perforation. In select cases, limited flexible sigmoidoscopy without bowel preparation may be used to identify underlying pathology and direct therapy.

Management

Medical Management

In ASUC, IV steroids like methylprednisone or hydrocortisone are the first line of treatment to induce remission. Gastroenterologists and surgeons should be consulted early during their care to direct therapy and monitor response. Supportive care should include IV hydration, electrolyte correction, DVT prophylaxis, and diet as tolerated. There is no added benefit of bowel rest while patients are on IV steroids and in those who can tolerate an oral diet. Providers should monitor for signs of worsening conditions and systemic toxicity daily and consider surgical options for nonresponders. Patients should undergo *C. difficile* testing and endoscopy to assess disease severity during this time. Greater than eight bowel movements per day by the third day of steroid treatment or evidence of persistently elevated inflammatory markers in the setting of 3-to 8 bowel movements predict the need for colectomy [5]. Rescue therapy with biologics or immunomodulators (typically infliximab and cyclosporine) should be considered if there is no response to steroids within 3–5 days, and surgical options should be explored after that. If patients fail medical therapy by day 5–9 of cyclosporine or infliximab treatment, colectomy is recommended.

Relative indications for surgery include severe medically refractory ASUC, toxic megacolon, hemorrhage, or colonic perforation. As discussed above, clinical deterioration may be masked by immunosuppressive medical therapy.

Initial treatment for CDI includes discontinuing offending antibiotics if clinically feasible. The first-line treatment options for uncomplicated CDI are oral vancomycin (125 mg four times daily) or fidaxomicin 200 mg twice daily, which is somewhat limited by higher costs (Table 31.2). Previously, IV metronidazole was recommended as an alternative first-line treatment, but an increased risk of treatment failure has been seen with only IV metronidazole therapy.

In cases of severe, complicated, or fulminant *C. difficile*, patients should undergo an early evaluation by a surgeon and be upgraded to oral vancomycin 500 mg four times daily and metronidazole 500 mg IV three times daily. Vancomycin retention enemas (500 mg in 500 mL normal saline every 6 h) should be considered for patients with ileus or those with severe, complicated, or fulminant CDI.

Approximately a third of patients with fulminant or severe complicated CDI require surgery.

Table 31.2 Diagnosis and treatment of initial C. difficile infection

Severity of C. difficile infection	Diagnostic criteria	Initial treatment options	Escalation of treatment options
Mild/ nonsevere	Absence of leukocytosis and creatinine levels within normal limits	Oral vancomycin (125 mg four times daily)	Fidaxomicin (200 mg twice daily) if no response to initial therapy or Add IV metronidazole (500 mg three times daily)
Severe	Presence of leukocytosis (>15 × 10^3/ μL) or creatinine >1.5 mg/dL	Oral vancomycin (125 mg four times daily)	Add IV metronidazole (500 mg three times daily) if no response
Severe complicated/ fulminant	Presence of systemic symptoms such as hypotension, sepsis, shock, ileus, megacolon, or ICU care requirement	Oral vancomycin (500 mg four times daily) + IV metronidazole (500 mg three times daily)	Consider surgical consultation Vancomycin retention enema (500 mg in 500 mL) normal saline every 6 h)

Evidence of colonic perforation and failure to respond to medical management are indications for surgery. IBD is a significant coconspirator with CDI, and UC patients with CDI oftentimes have twice the risk of requiring a colectomy for CDI. Despite the high mortality rate for patients undergoing colectomy for fulminant *C. difficile*, many studies have shown that early surgical management improves mortality compared with patients who are on prolonged medical management [6, 7].

Management of immune-mediated colitis requires early recognition, discontinuation of offending therapy, and prompt initiation of steroids. Infliximab and vedolizumab have been described to be used in steroid-refractory instances.

Surgical Consideration

Patients with medically refractory ASUC or CDI, toxic megacolon, colonic perforation, or significant hematochezia should undergo surgery. The operation of choice for this is a subtotal colectomy with end ileostomy. This includes the removal of the majority of the colon, leaving the rectum and a portion of the distal colon in place. In patients with UC, proctectomy should be deferred to avoid the risk of postoperative complications, reduce operative time, and plan for future reconnection. A trans anal rectal tube is commonly placed for decompression to prevent complications from pelvic sepsis in case of rectal stump dehiscence. Some surgeons will elect to place the distal stump in the subcutaneous tissue or create a mucous fistula. As mentioned, since *C. difficile* is a mucosal-based disease, the severity and extent of the disease cannot be typically determined by visualizing the colon during laparotomy; thus, segmental colectomy is not usually recommended.

Another surgical option for *C. difficile* colitis includes placing a diverting loop ileostomy with antegrade colonic lavage of warmed polyethylene glycol solution via ileostomy and antegrade instillation of vancomycin. This is described as a colon-saving approach with potentially higher ostomy reversal rates and gastrointestinal continuity restoration. Still, it may lead to recurrent *C. difficile* colitis and is not widely practiced.

Conclusion

Toxic colitis and toxic megacolon are severe, life-threatening conditions that demand prompt recognition and management. Having a high index of suspicion in patients who are at risk and initiation of aggressive medical management and prompt surgical intervention when needed can significantly improve patient outcomes. For advanced practice providers, management of this condition means being vigilant for signs of systemic toxicity and rapid disease progression. Collaboration with gastroenterologists, infectious disease, and surgical teams is essential. Additionally, recognizing exacerbating factors of concomitant *C. difficile* infection can guide treatment. The goal is to stabilize the patient with medical management and prepare for potential surgery if conservative interventions fail.

References

1. Jalan KN, Sircus W, Card WI, et al. An experience of ulcerative Colitis. I. toxic dilation in 55 cases. Gastroenterology. 1969;57(1):68–82.
2. Longo WE, Mazuski JE, Virgo KS, Lee P, Bahadursingh AN, Johnson FE. Outcome after colectomy for Clostridium Difficile Colitis. Dis Colon Rectum. 2004;47(10):1620–6. https://doi.org/10.1007/S10350-004-0672-2.
3. Holubar SD, Lightner AL, Poylin V, et al. The American society of colon and rectal surgeons clinical practice guidelines for the surgical management of ulcerative Colitis. Dis Colon Rectum. 2021;64(7):783–804. https://doi.org/10.1097/DCR.0000000000002037.
4. Poylin V, Hawkins AT, Bhama AR, et al. The American society of colon and rectal surgeons clinical practice guidelines for the management of Clostridioides Difficile infection. Dis Colon Rectum. 2021;64(6):650–68. https://doi.org/10.1097/DCR.0000000000002047.
5. Travis SP, Farrant JM, Ricketts C, et al. Predicting outcome in severe ulcerative colitis. Gut. 1996;38(6):905–10. https://doi.org/10.1136/Gut.38.6.905.
6. Lamontagne F, Labbé AC, Haeck O, et al. Impact of emergency colectomy on survival of patients with fulminant Clostridium Difficile Colitis during an epidemic caused by a hypervirulent strain. Ann Surg. 2007;245(2):267–72. https://doi.org/10.1097/01.Sla.0000236628.79550.E5.
7. Ahmed N, Kuo YH. Early colectomy saves lives in toxic megacolon due to clostridium difficile infection. South Med J. 2020;113(7):345–9. https://doi.org/10.14423/SMJ.0000000000001118.

Ischemic Colitis

32

Matthew Fuglestad, Rishi Batra, and Sean J. Langenfeld

Introduction

Ischemic colitis is an important cause of morbidity in the elderly and critically ill [2, 5, 6, 15]. Successful management requires prompt recognition, early initiation of treatment, and clear communication between medical and surgical teams as a patient's clinical trajectory evolves. Ischemic colitis is frequently managed nonoperatively by correction of the inciting cause and optimization of predisposing medical comorbidities [2, 14]. However, when surgical intervention is indicated, it should be timely and definitive to avoid failure to rescue. This chapter details an approach to the evaluation and management of patients with ischemic colitis, beginning with the physiologic/anatomic basis for the disease process and extending into relevant discussions of treatment options. Furthermore, the chapter highlights important decision-making from a surgical perspective with the aim of improving outcomes in patients affected by ischemic colitis.

Ischemic Colitis: Anatomic and Pathophysiologic Considerations

Ischemic colitis results from a low-flow state creating a sustained mismatch between oxygen delivery and the metabolic demands of the colon [2, 5, 14]. This imbalance initially results in reversible mucosal ischemia, responsible for many of the presenting symptoms. Importantly, the deleterious effects of a transient low-flow state can be compounded by anatomic variations in blood supply and baseline comorbidities that predispose patients to end-organ ischemia. The early effects of ischemic colitis are often reversible and, with supportive care, will result in mucosal healing. However, prolonged or untreated ischemia can progress to full-thickness injury, resulting in a variety of acute and long-term complications.

Ischemic Colitis & Its Relationship to Acute Mesenteric Ischemia

Disambiguating **ischemic colitis** and **acute mesenteric ischemia** is important in effective communication between providers and care teams. These two disease states, though they share the end results of bowel ischemia, are *distinct clinical entities*. As opposed to ischemic colitis, acute mesenteric ischemia is a *higher acuity disease* process affecting both the small and large bowel. It is often associated with occlusion of named vessels and is *more likely to result in surgical intervention.* While ischemic colitis is a result of periods of low flow, acute mesenteric ischemia is classified according to its etiology, including nonocclusive mesenteric ischemia, arterial thrombosis, venous thrombosis, and arterial embolic disease. To avoid inadvertent confusion as to the nature of the patient's illness, these categories should *not* be applied to the term "ischemic colitis" as described above.

M. Fuglestad (✉) · R. Batra · S. J. Langenfeld
Division of Colorectal Surgery, Department of Surgery, University of Nebraska Medical Center, Omaha, NE, USA
e-mail: matthew.fuglestad@unmc.edu

S. Atallah, J. Dragoljevic (eds.), *Fundamentals of Surgery for Physician Assistants*,
https://doi.org/10.1007/978-3-032-21069-2_32

Colonic Vascular Anatomy and Watershed Areas of the Colon

Blood flow to the colon and rectum is *distributed over three interconnected vascular territories* [1, 7, 8, 11]. The **superior mesenteric artery** distribution supplies the right colon and the proximal two-thirds of the transverse colon. This is accomplished through the *ileocolic artery, right colic artery, and middle colic artery* arising off the superior mesenteric artery. The anatomy of branches off the superior mesenteric is variable and, from a technical standpoint, most patients do not possess a true right colic artery, despite this being illustrated in most anatomy books.

The **inferior mesenteric artery** distribution supplies the distal one-third of the transverse colon, left colon, and upper rectum. The internal iliac artery distribution via the **middle and inferior rectal artery** supplies the distal two-thirds of the rectum. ***At the intersection of these vascular territories, the bowel is more susceptible to ischemia.*** These **watershed areas** are eponymously known as **"Griffith's Point"** at the *splenic flexure* and **"Suddeck's Point"** at the *rectosigmoid junction*, representing the junction between the *superior mesenteric* and *inferior mesenteric* artery distribution; and *inferior mesenteric* and [branches of] the *internal iliac artery* distribution respectively.

Connecting these vascular territories are multiple arcs—aka, **vascular arcades**—that provide redundancy in the case of vascular occlusion or injury [1, 7, 11, 12]. These arcs include the **marginal artery (of Drummond),** the **Arc of Riolan,** and the **Moskowitz artery.** All serve as *a bridge between the flow of blood from the superior mesenteric artery to the inferior mesenteric artery distribution. The most well-known of these arcs is the* ***marginal artery.*** It parallels the colon wall extending along the length of the right and left colon. On average, it is located 2.5 cm from the mesenteric edge of the bowel and supplies the vasa recta to the bowel wall [12]. While considered a part of standard human anatomy, the marginal artery has been found to be incomplete in 7–12% or diminutive (< 1 mm in diameter) in over 20% of anatomic specimens [12]. Given the many variations in anatomic location and completeness, proper identification and preservation during a colectomy is essential in maintaining the viability of the colon remaining in-situ. An incomplete or diminutive marginal artery can in part explain the segmental nature of ischemic colitis and why possessing a complete marginal artery in the watershed regions is critical to maintain blood flow in a stressed state.

The Arc of Riolan and Moskowitz arteries are more variably seen, and there is some debate as to their exact definition and anatomic course. Karatay et al. found that the arc of Riolan and Moskowitz arteries are present radiographically in 27.5% and 16.5% of patients, respectively [10]. Both reside in the colonic mesentery at the splenic flexure and serve as collateral paths of blood flow outside of the marginal artery [7, 10, 12]. These vessels have become more relevant as minimally invasive approaches to colectomy increase nationally, and medial-to-lateral dissection of the colon has gained popularity. Inadvertent transection during splenic flexure mobilization or left-sided colectomy can compromise anastomotic healing or predispose patients to ischemic colitis in the future.

Presentation & Workup of Suspected Ischemic Colitis

History, Physical Exam, and Labs

Ischemic colitis commonly presents in the outpatient or emergency department setting as *bloody diarrhea and cramping abdominal pain* after a patient sustains a physiologic insult leading to hypoperfusion of the colon [2, 4, 6]. Patients may describe a preceding period of vomiting, diarrhea, poor oral intake, and/or dehydration prior to the development of abdominal symptoms. Ischemic colitis may also develop in situations of high insensible losses and/or shunting of blood away from the abdominal viscera, such as long-distance running or illicit drug use. *Patients who develop ischemic colitis in the inpatient or ICU setting are more often critically ill or with significant predisposing factors* (e.g., shock, sepsis, significant atherosclerotic vascular disease, or cardiac failure). These individuals can deteriorate rapidly, progressing to *full-thickness necrosis, perforation, and multisystem organ failure.*

A detailed history of all patients with suspected ischemic colitis can aid healthcare providers in making the diagnosis of ischemic colitis and better defining the acuity of a patient's presentation. A history of colectomy, vascular bypass, or abdominal aortic aneurysm repair alters baseline colonic blood flow and predisposes to ischemia. Less commonly, ischemic colitis can present acutely in patients who have undergone IR-based procedures (interventional radiology), open aneurysm repair, endovascular abdominal aortic aneurysm repair, and segmental colectomy.

Physical exam will vary depending on the degree of colonic ischemia, its duration, and the presence of complications related to ischemic colitis. Hemodynamic instability is uncommon in mild cases of ischemic colitis and should prompt consideration of complications of ischemic colitis, such as perforation or another diagnosis altogether.

Similarly, early in the presentation, the patient's abdominal exam commonly shows mild abdominal tenderness, distention, and the *absence* of physical findings of peritonitis. Laboratory evaluation is nonspecific but can include leukocytosis, *leftward shift* in WBC differential (namely, neutrophils), anemia, elevated lactate, and elevation in inflammatory markers. Importantly, a normal lactate does not exclude the diagnosis of ischemic colitis and needs to be interpreted within the specific clinic context. To rule out infectious colitis, rapid stool-based testing for causes of infectious diarrhea should be performed.

CT Findings

Cross-sectional imaging plays an important role in the evaluation of suspected ischemic colitis, excluding other etiologies, patients' symptoms, and evaluating for complications of ischemic colitis [3, 9]. Lacobellis et al. reviewed CT scans with IV contrast in patients with endoscopically proven ischemic colitis. In the acute phase, common findings included the presence of pericolic fluid (100%), colonic dilation (100%), signs of concurrent parenchymal ischemia in other intra-abdominal organs (85%), intra-abdominal free fluid (50%), and hyper-enhancement on noncontrasted CT (45%). While in the acute phase, patients had thin-walled dilated bowel, 100% of patients developed colonic thickening in the subacute phase, leading the authors to discuss the importance of both ischemia and reperfusion injury as a source of colonic damage in ischemic colitis [9].

Generally, there is approximately an 80:20 distribution of left-sided ischemic colitis to right-sided colitis. Common locations on the left include the splenic flexure, descending colon, and sigmoid colon. In the right colon, the cecum is commonly affected. *Pan-ischemic colitis and isolated proctitis are rare and should prompt considerations of additional diagnosis or confirmation of the diagnosis by endoscopy* [3, 4, 9]. **Stated another way, ischemic colitis is typically <u>segmental</u>, affecting the <u>watershed areas</u>, and colonoscopy would reveal unaffected segments of bowel that appear normal, because they are nonischemic.**

Pathologic Findings

Pathologic diagnosis of ischemic colitis by endoscopic biopsy or surgical resection is the standard to confirm the diagnosis of ischemic colitis if the diagnosis is in question (Fig. 32.1). Endoscopy to rule out ischemic colitis can be performed in the endoscopy suite or in the setting of ICU-level needs at the bedside. The pathognomonic histologic findings of ischemic colitis include **ghost cells** (cells without cytoplasmic contents that have maintained their cellular structure) and mucosal infarction [4]. Unfortunately, these findings are not universally found, and other nonspecific findings of mucosal/submucosal hemorrhage, edema, and capillary fibrin thrombi are more commonly seen [4]. Importantly, characteristic findings of inflammatory bowel disease, radiation colitis/proctitis, and infectious colitis are absent. Without the presence of pathognomonic features, the diagnosis is made by collating all relevant history, imaging, and endoscopic findings while at the same time confirming no other etiology of colitis is present.

Nonoperative Management of Ischemic Colitis

In many instances, ischemic colitis can be managed <u>non-operatively</u>. Nonoperative management of ischemic colitis aims to minimize the metabolic demand on the colon, restore perfusion by correcting the low-flow state, optimize medical comorbidities that contribute to poor perfusion, and monitor for clinical decline [2, 6, 15]. **<u>Initial treatment includes IV fluid resuscitation to restore any volume deficits sustained prior to presentation</u>**. During this time, patients should be made **NPO** (bowel rest) with consideration of nasogastric tube placement in the setting of ileus. *Prophylactic antibiotics* should be administered due to the compromised mucosal barrier within the colon to prevent the theoretical risk of bacterial translocation and complications associated with bacteremia.

Following initiation of treatment, *patients should be admitted to a monitored setting for serial evaluations of their clinic status and abdominal examination.* Baseline conditions such as significant anemia, heart failure, and hypoxemia should be corrected and optimized as able. With nonoperative management, improvement can be anticipated over 24–48 h and is marked by a reduction in abdominal pain, resolving hematochezia, and improvement in diarrhea. With improvement in abdominal pain and resolution of ileus, oral intake should be resumed, monitoring for recurrent symptoms. In cases of prolonged periods of inability to tolerate PO intake, parenteral nutrition should be considered. Fever, tachycardia, new hemodynamic compromise, persistent hematochezia, or development of progressive abdominal pain may indicate treatment failure and the need for surgery. In the setting of suspected treatment failure, repeat cross-sectional imaging (i.e., CT-body imaging) can be highly valuable for preoperative planning and evaluation of complications of ischemic colitis, but should not delay operative intervention in unstable patients with a clear intra-abdominal source of sepsis.

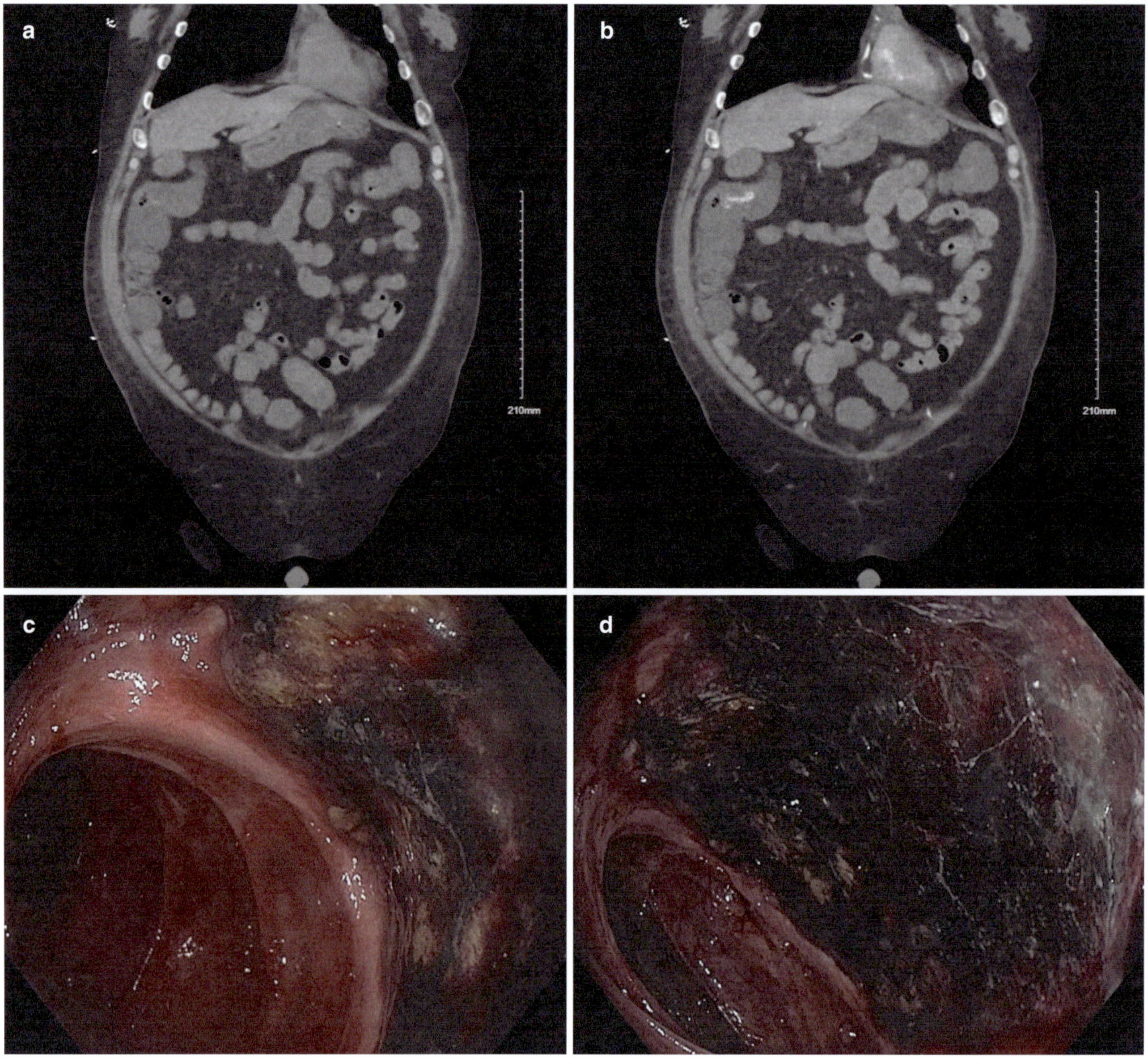

Fig. 32.1 Ischemic colitis after cardiac surgery. CT imaging and confirmatory colonoscopy demonstrated ischemic colitis in the region of the hepatic flexure. The patient underwent a right colectomy with ileostomy creation. Pathology confirmed transmural necrosis of the colon wall. (**a**, **b**) Segmental colonic thickening seen on noncontrast CT with contrast extravasation (**b**). (**c**, **d**) Endoscopic images demonstrating patchy necrosis with ulceration and active bleeding

Surgery for Ischemic Colitis

As previously discussed, **ischemic colitis is most often a segmental process** with the preponderance of cases being isolated to the left colon. As such, segmental resection of nonviable bowel is the treatment of choice in medically refractory disease. Important preoperative considerations include ostomy site marking by an entero-stomal therapist (if available), establishing secure IV access, broad-spectrum antibiotic coverage, and ensuring availability of blood products for the OR. Early communication with an ICU team about the possibility of temporary abdominal closure can prevent delays in returning to the ICU due to a lack of needed equipment. Critical to the success of the operation is rapid yet thorough evaluation of the abdominal cavity, *control of ongoing sources of sepsis,* determining the extent of resection, and deciding on the role of temporary abdominal closure.

Extent of Resection and End Ostomy Creation

In the acute setting, segmental resection of all nonviable colon, creation of an end ostomy with Hartmann's pouch, and abdominal closure is safe and definitive. The extent of resection is guided by direct visualization of the abdominal contents and adjunctive tests such as testing of the marginal artery and indocyanine green angiography. While it is essential to resect all grossly nonviable bowel, excessive resection places patients at risk for complications of a proximal stoma and may limit options for restoration of GI continuity in the future. Bowel whose viability is in question can be re-evaluated after restoration of hemodynamics intraoperatively or re-evaluated after a period of resuscitation in the ICU using a temporary abdominal closure.

Given the high mortality rate associated with surgical management of ischemic colitis, attempting a primary is generally anastomosis is not advisable. The patient-related factors that place patients at risk of ischemic colitis are the same risk factors that predispose patients to anastomotic failure. Furthermore, the addition of another source of intra-abdominal sepsis from an anastomotic leak in an already critically ill patient may very well prove fatal. Counseling patients and their families regarding the rationale for stoma creation and that significant support is available to assist in the transition to life with an ostomy can ease the discomfort patients feel as they navigate this difficult time in their lives. When feasible, preoperative stoma education and marking to optimize ostomy location should be performed, *as up to two-thirds of the stomas created will not be reversed.*

Long-Term Outcomes of Ischemic Colitis

Medically managed ischemic colitis is associated with a high rate of successful treatment. A recent meta-analysis has suggested that up to **85% of patients can be managed nonoperatively** [5, 13, 14]. Mortality in patients managed nonoperatively is estimated at 6%. Ischemic colitis that requires surgical intervention, however, is associated with a high mortality rate approaching 25–40%. Major prognostic factors include need for surgery, right-sided ischemia, end-stage renal disease, and coronary artery disease.

Recurrence after the initial episode is low overall. However, of those who develop recurrent ischemia, 20% will go on to progress to chronic ischemic colitis, characterized by persistent diarrhea, hematochezia, recurrent bouts of sepsis, and colonic strictures. Symptomatic strictures may require segmental colectomy in the future. As previously discussed, stoma reversal rates in general are low. However, in appropriately selected patients, restoration of GI continuity can be considered. Case series specifically evaluating ostomy reversal after ostomy creation for ischemic colitis have found a high utilization of intensive care and a higher incidence of mortality than elective colostomy takedown for other indications.

However, the risks associated with an attempt at colostomy takedown may be worth it to a patient in the setting of a symptomatic parastomal hernia, poor pouching, ostomy stenosis/retraction, or if the presence of a colostomy significantly affects their mental/emotional health or quality of life.

Conclusion

Ischemic colitis remains an important cause of intestinal ischemia that is benefited by a multidisciplinary approach and close communication between providers. Early recognition and treatment can prevent surgical management, which is associated with drastically higher rates of morbidity and mortality. Long-term, patients affected by ischemic colitis need to be monitored for recurrent or chronic symptoms. For those who are found to be candidates for ostomy reversal, it is feasible to consider understanding the risk profile of the patient and the procedure.

References

1. Allison AS, Bloor C, Faux W, Arumugam P, Widdison A, Lloyd-Davies E, Maskell G. The angiographic anatomy of the small arteries and their collaterals in colorectal resections: some insights into anastomotic perfusion. Ann Surg. 2010;251(6):1092–7. https://doi.org/10.1097/SLA.0b013e3181deb649.
2. Bala M, Catena F, Kashuk J, De Simone B, Gomes CA, Weber D, Sartelli M, Coccolini F, Kluger Y, Abu-Zidan FM, Picetti E, Ansaloni L, Augustin G, Biffl WL, Ceresoli M, Chiara O, Chiarugi M, Coimbra R, Cui Y, et al. Acute mesenteric ischemia: updated guidelines of the World Society of Emergency Surgery. World J Emerg Surg. 2022;17(1):54. https://doi.org/10.1186/s13017-022-00443-x.
3. Berritto D, Iacobellis F, Mazzei MA, Volterrani L, Guglielmi G, Brunese L, Grassi R. MDCT in ischaemic colitis: how to define the aetiology and acute, subacute and chronic phase of damage in the emergency setting. Br J Radiol. 2016;89(1061):20150821. https://doi.org/10.1259/bjr.20150821.
4. Brandt LJ, Feuerstadt P, Blaszka MC. Anatomic patterns, patient characteristics, and clinical outcomes in ischemic colitis: a study of 313 cases supported by histology. Am J Gastroenterol. 2010;105(10):2245–52. https://doi.org/10.1038/ajg.2010.217.
5. Demetriou G, Nassar A, Subramonia S. The pathophysiology, presentation and Management of Ischaemic Colitis: a systematic review. World J Surg. 2020;44(3):927–38. https://doi.org/10.1007/s00268-019-05248-9.
6. FitzGerald JF, Hernandez Iii LO. Ischemic colitis. Clin Colon Rectal Surg. 2015;28(2):93–8. https://doi.org/10.1055/s-0035-1549099.
7. Garcia-Granero A, Sánchez-Guillén L, Carreño O, Sancho Muriel J, Alvarez Sarrado E, Fletcher Sanfeliu D, Flor Lorente B, Frasson M, Martinez Soriano F, Garcia-Granero E. Importance of the Moskowitz artery in the laparoscopic medial approach to splenic flexure mobilization: a cadaveric study. Tech Coloproctol. 2017;21(7):567–72. https://doi.org/10.1007/s10151-017-1663-3.
8. Garćia-Ruiz A, Milsom JW, Ludwig KA, Marchesa P. Right colonic arterial anatomy. Implications for laparoscopic surgery. Dis Colon Rectum. 1996;39(8):906–11. https://doi.org/10.1007/BF02053990. PMID: 8756847.
9. Iacobellis F, Berritto D, Fleischmann D, Gagliardi G, Brillantino A, Mazzei MA, Grassi R. CT findings in acute, subacute, and chronic ischemic colitis: suggestions for diagnosis. Biomed Res Int. 2014;2014:1–7. https://doi.org/10.1155/2014/895248.
10. Karatay E, Javadov M. The importance of the Moskowitz artery as a lesser-known collateral pathway in the medial laparoscopic approach to splenic flexure mobilisation and its evaluation with preoperative computed tomography. Wideochirurgia I Inne Techniki Maloinwazyjne = Videosurg Other Miniinvasive Tech. 2021;16(2):305–11. https://doi.org/10.5114/wiitm.2020.100826.
11. Kuzu MA, İsmail E, Çelik S, Şahin MF, Güner MA, Hohenberger W, Açar Hİ. Variations in the vascular anatomy of the right colon and Implications for right-sided colon surgery. Dis Colon Rectum. 2017;60(3):290–8. https://doi.org/10.1097/DCR.0000000000000777.
12. Mann MR, Kawzowicz M, Komosa AJ, Sherer YM, Łazarz DP, Loukas M, Tubbs RS, Pasternak A. The marginal artery of Drummond revisited: a systematic review. Transl Res Anat. 2021;24:100118. https://doi.org/10.1016/j.tria.2021.100118.
13. O'Neill S, Yalamarthi S. Systematic review of the management of ischaemic colitis. Color Dis. 2012;14(11) https://doi.org/10.1111/j.1463-1318.2012.03171.x.
14. Qian W, Bruinsma J, Mac Curtain B, Ibraheem M, Temperley HC, Ng ZQ. Surgical prevalence and outcomes in ischemic colitis: a systematic review and meta-analysis. World J Surg. 2024;48(4):943–53. https://doi.org/10.1002/wjs.12123.
15. Washington C, Carmichael JC. Management of ischemic colitis. Clin Colon Rectal Surg. 2012;25(4):228–35. https://doi.org/10.1055/s-0032-1329534.

33 Benign Conditions of the Breast

Sam Atallah

Introduction

Benign disorders occur in both male and female breasts and may be categorized as infectious, cutaneous, benign, or high-risk lesions; many of these are summarized in Table 33.1. They can occur at any time during development and lifespan, with peak incidence during childbearing years in females. Although most conditions present as visible abnormalities, a variety of imaging modalities have been utilized to better characterize and facilitate management. Students and PAs should be familiar with basic breast anatomy, as shown in Fig. 33.1.

Infections and Skin Conditions

Mastitis

Mastitis with or without abscess formation is the *most common* occurring infection in breast tissue. The most frequent cause is the introduction of cutaneous flora into the breast skin or ductal tissue. Although it is more likely to be seen in *lactating females,* patients with a history of trauma (such as nipple piercing, animal scratches, etc.) or underlying chronic diseases such as diabetes, prior MRSA (methicillin-resistant *Staphylococcus aureus*) infections, broken skin from psoriasis or eczema, or immunologic disorders may develop mastitis. The most common bacteria are cutaneous flora, and thus treatment should be directed toward coverage for *Staphylococcus, Streptococcus, and diphtheroid species*. If there is an associated fluid collection, ***fine needle aspiration*** (FNA) for culture should be obtained to better guide antibiotic therapy (Fig. 33.2). For those patients who develop mastitis and are actively breastfeeding, *they should continue to pump and discard the milk while on certain antibiotics and/or pain medication so that the infant does not get exposed.*

Breast Abscess

Abscesses most often develop as a *secondary infection of trapped milk in the* ***postpartum patient who has been diagnosed with mastitis***. It may also occur postoperatively within a seroma cavity or due to secondary seeding of a hematoma following blunt or penetrating injury. Imaging with ***ultrasound*** is the best modality to determine etiology and provide a means by which ***percutaneous drainage*** may be employed for treatment. *More substantial abscesses of the breast should be treated with* ***incision and drainage****, as is the standard of care for all soft tissue abscesses* (Fig. 33.3). In certain circumstances where there appears to be a *solid component* or the abscess is not responding to appropriate antibiotic therapy, minimally invasive **core needle biopsy** (Fig. 33.4) is indicated to rule out more unusual causes of persistent infection, such as granulomatous mastitis or inflammatory breast cancer. In very rare cases, necrotizing fasciitis may be encountered, requiring extensive open debridement, but these patients also deserve an aggressive workup for other underlying systemic diseases associated with poor healing.

Hidradenitis Suppurativa

Hidradenitis suppurativa is a condition involving ***infections of the apocrine sweat glands*** (Fig. 33.5) ***located in the inframammary crease, axilla, and rarely around the areola***. Its presentation is similar to hidradenitis involving other parts of the body. Sweating and occlusion of the areas are believed to be the cause. Treatment consists of ***antibiotics***

S. Atallah (✉)
Department of Surgery, Piedmont Hospital, Mercer University School of Medicine, Macon, GA, USA
e-mail: atallah@post.harvard.edu

S. Atallah, J. Dragoljevic (eds.), *Fundamentals of Surgery for Physician Assistants*,
https://doi.org/10.1007/978-3-032-21069-2_33

Table 33.1 Benign breast conditions: summary table

Condition	Clinical presentation	Common age group	Diagnosis	Treatment
Fibroadenoma	Mobile, firm, rubbery mass; nontender	<35 years (young women)	Clinical exam, ultrasound, core needle biopsy if uncertain	Observation or surgical excision if large or symptomatic
Fibrocystic changes	Nodular, painful breasts; varies with menstrual cycle	30–50 years	Clinical exam, mammography, ultrasound	Supportive care, NSAIDs, caffeine reduction, reassurance
Breast cyst	Fluid-filled sac; can be painful	35–50 years	Ultrasound (anechoic, well-defined), aspiration for diagnosis	Aspiration if symptomatic; usually resolves spontaneously
Fat necrosis	Firm, irregular mass often after trauma	Any	Mammography (oil cysts), ultrasound, biopsy to rule out malignancy	Observation if benign confirmed; excision if symptomatic or suspicious
Intraductal papilloma	Small tumor in breast duct; may cause nipple discharge	30–50 years	Ductogram, ultrasound, core needle biopsy, nipple discharge cytology	Surgical excision due to small malignancy risk
Mastitis/abscess	Painful, red, swollen breast; often in lactating women	Postpartum women	Clinical, ultrasound (to rule out abscess)	Antibiotics (dicloxacillin), drainage if abscess
Duct ectasia	Dilated ducts; thick green or black nipple discharge	Perimenopausal women	Clinical exam, ultrasound, mammography	Warm compresses, antibiotics if infected, surgery if recurrent
Gynecomastia	Breast tissue enlargement in males	Neonates, puberty, elderly	Clinical, hormonal evaluation, ultrasound if needed	Observation, treat underlying cause, surgery if persistent or severe
Galactocele	Milk-filled cyst due to duct obstruction	Lactating women	Ultrasound (fat-fluid level), aspiration	Aspiration, supportive care; typically resolves with cessation of breastfeeding
Phyllodes tumor (benign)	Fibroepithelial tumor, may grow rapidly	30–50 years	Clinical exam, imaging, core biopsy	Wide local excision due to recurrence risk

for associated abscess, excision +/– skin grafting, and even breast reduction to reduce moisture accumulation.

More specifically, the treatment for hidradenitis suppurativa is guided by disease severity and includes a combination of medical and surgical approaches. The United States and Canadian Hidradenitis Suppurativa Foundations recommend the following stepwise management: **topical clindamycin** *is first-line therapy*, as well as adjunctive measures include weight loss, smoking cessation, *and* antiseptic washes. For patients with more extensive or refractory disease, **oral tetracyclines** (e.g., doxycycline or minocycline) are recommended for a 12-week course or as long-term maintenance when appropriate. If inadequate response, combination oral clindamycin and rifampin is effective, typically for 8–12 weeks. **Antiandrogen contraceptives**, spironolactone, metformin, and finasteride may be considered, particularly in women with features of androgen excess or polycystic ovary syndrome**. Oral retinoids** (acitretin, isotretinoin, alitretinoin) are options for refractory cases, with acitretin showing the most benefit, but teratogenicity limits use in women of childbearing potential. The *anti-TNF-α agent* ***adalimumab*** is the only biologic with robust evidence and regulatory approval for Hidradenitis Suppurativa. **Surgical intervention** is indicated for persistent nodules, abscesses, sinus tracts, or scarring, and may include local excision, *but especially* ***unroofing***, or wide excision for extensive disease.

Duct Ectasia

Drainage from the nipple, whether spontaneous or elicited with compression, is frequently cloudy, simulating pus, and many patients are placed on antibiotics unnecessarily. **Duct ectasia** is a condition that may develop in patients who *breastfeed, smoke, or have chronic inverted nipples* and is characterized by ***dilated ducts with associated cellular debris*** resulting in *thick, cheesy-like material* able to be evacuated through the larger ducts out through the nipple. Occasionally, this material will become secondarily infected, or the enlarging duct will erode/form a fistula to the surface of the periareolar skin, resulting in a chronic draining sinus tract or abscess. *Management of the ectasia is expectant, as most patients are asymptomatic with this condition.* Surgical intervention is indicated only if there is recurrent infection, fistula formation, or if an uncertain etiology exists, as in the case of a solid nodule within the duct, spontaneous nipple discharge that is clear or bloody, or ductal microcalcifications are present mammographically.

Nipple Discharge

In most cases, nipple discharge without an associated palpable mass represents a benign problem. When a patient complains of discharge, it is important to obtain a detailed history regarding color, volume, consistency, whether the

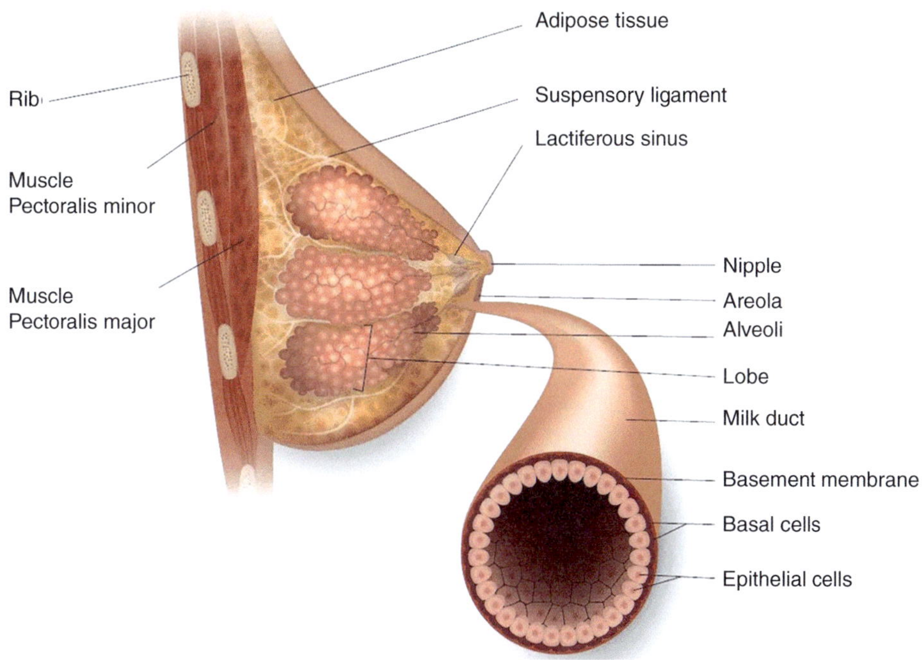

Fig. 33.1 Anatomic representation of female breast parenchyma, including relevant ductal structures. The female breast is composed of glandular, fibrous, and adipose tissue, organized into distinct anatomical structures. The glandular component consists of 15–20 lobes, each containing multiple lobules, which are the functional units responsible for milk production. These lobules drain into a branching ductal system that converges into lactiferous ducts, which open at the nipple. The ducts and lobules are embedded within a stroma of connective (fibrous) and adipose tissue, which provides structural support and determines breast size and contour. The breast is situated on the anterior thoracic wall, overlying the pectoralis major muscle, and extends from the second to the sixth rib vertically and from the sternum to the mid-axillary line horizontally. The superficial and deep layers of the superficial fascia envelop the breast, with the deep layer anchoring the breast to the pectoral fascia. Cooper's ligaments (suspensory ligaments) traverse the breast parenchyma, connecting the dermis to the deep fascia and providing internal support. The nipple-areolar complex is centrally located and contains the openings of the lactiferous ducts. The areola is pigmented and contains sebaceous (Montgomery) glands. Vascular supply is primarily from branches of the internal thoracic, lateral thoracic, and intercostal arteries. Lymphatic drainage is mainly to the axillary lymph nodes, with additional drainage to the internal mammary and supraclavicular nodes. The breast is innervated by the anterior and lateral cutaneous branches of the fourth to sixth intercostal nerves

breast or nipple had to be squeezed to bring on the discharge, current medications, and pregnancy status. **Milky discharge** may be due to pregnancy, elevated prolactin levels from medication, or a benign brain tumor (microadenoma). **Clear or bloody discharge** can be seen in patients with **papillomas**, which are growths within the ducts frequently seen with breast ultrasound if large enough, as calcifications on mammogram, or as abnormal ductal enhancement on breast MRI. ***Fibrocystic changes** (discussed later) are also a potential cause for multicolored discharge, ranging from green to yellow, blue, and even black.* Should there ever be a question as to the etiology, minimally invasive core biopsy with ultrasound, mammographic, or MRI guidance may be performed.

Sebaceous Cysts and Montgomery Tubercles

Small oil glands communicating with the periareolar and nipple skin are present to help keep the nipple and areola from drying and cracking. These glands become more prominent during puberty and occasionally become clogged, resulting in a "whitehead" appearance to the nipple or just under the areolar skin. Additionally, sebaceous or epidermal inclusion cysts can occur anywhere there is hair overlying the breast and axilla. They may be differentiated from Montgomery tubercles in that *there is usually an overlying central pore.* It is extremely rare to develop sebaceous cyst carcinoma or a cancer in these lesions, so surgery is only indicated if infected, painful, or enlarging.

Rashes

Both eczema and psoriasis may affect the breast and areolar skin. They may be mistaken for *impetigo*, which is a gram-positive (esp. *Staphylococcus*) infection, shingles (herpes zoster), ringworm, or skin cancer. The rash may be a **contact dermatitis** (e.g., wearing a new bra, jewelry piercing, change in detergent) or may represent something more ominous (such as *Paget's disease of the nipple*), but ***sparing of the nipple usually rules out this form of cancer.*** Bilateral

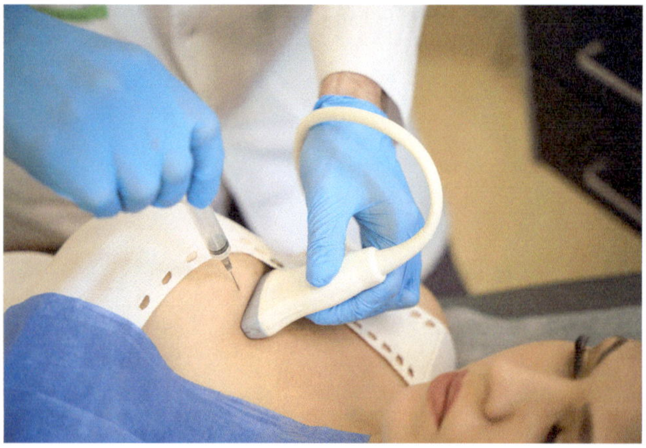

Fig. 33.2 Fine needle aspiration (FNA) is typically performed using a thin, hollow needle, most commonly in the 22- to 25-gauge range. The Society of Interventional Radiology defines FNA as using a 22-gauge or smaller needle for cytologic evaluation. The technique involves immobilizing the target lesion, inserting the needle into the lesion under palpation or image guidance (*esp.* ultrasound) as shown, and then moving the needle back and forth within the lesion to obtain cellular material. This can be done with or without the application of negative pressure (aspiration). The capillary (nonaspiration) technique involves moving the needle without suction, relying on capillary action, while the aspiration technique uses a syringe to apply negative pressure as the needle is moved. While FNA is the go-to for providing cytologic information, it does not provide histologic architecture as core needle biopsy does, and thus, FNA is not used for determining whether or not a breast lesion is malignant

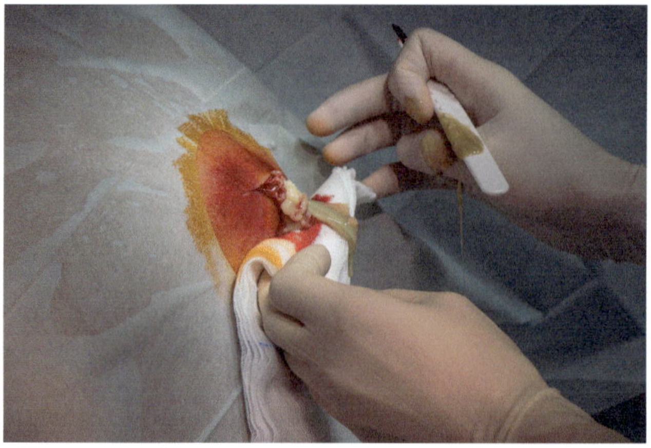

Fig. 33.3 A breast abscess may present with an area of fluctuance, as well as cellulitis changes (blanching erythema) to the surrounding dermis. Shown here is the incision and drainage of a breast soft tissue abscess, which can be incised with an 11 or 15-blade cold knife after infiltration of local anesthetic. This can be done with or without sedation or in the operating room if necessary, depending on severity and patient tolerance. Abscess cavities usually contain varying amounts of purulent fluid and debris, which is evident here. After incision and drainage, the cavity is packed with surgical gauze, or it can be left open without packing. Importantly, *the incision is not closed, but is instead left open to heal by secondary intention.* Generally, incision and drainage alone are adequate therapy, but systemic antibiotics can be administered as an adjunct, for example, if there is associated cellulitis or in patients who are immunocompromised. The fact that incision and drainage is first-line treatment for a soft tissue abscess underscores an important surgical axiom: some, *even bacterial* infections, are not treated *primarily* with antibiotics

disease is also *less likely* to represent cancer. Rashes elsewhere on the body, along with nailbed and arthritis changes, may be more suggestive of psoriasis than eczema, but a **punch biopsy** (Fig. 33.6) of the skin is the best way to determine the etiology and guide treatment. Frequent scratching while sleeping may delay healing during treatment. Once the cause is determined, then treatment with antibiotics or antifungals for infection, steroids to treat inflammation (at the lowest strength possible to prevent weakening of the subcutaneous tissue), antihistamines for itching, antivirals for shingles (herpes zoster), and biologics for eczema/psoriasis will result in more rapid healing.

Hypopigmented Skin Lesions

Skin lesions lighter than the surrounding breast skin are considered **hypopigmented** and *most represent benign conditions*. Some, however, are associated with systemic conditions requiring more aggressive treatment. As with rashes of the breast, a *punch biopsy* is the best way to determine the cause and recommend the correct therapy. *Tinea* infections can be treated with *coal tar shampoos or topical antifungals*.

Vitiligo (Fig. 33.7) is an acquired, chronic disorder characterized by well-demarcated, depigmented macules and patches resulting from the selective loss of functional melanocytes in the skin and sometimes hair or mucous membranes. The pathogenesis of vitiligo is multifactorial, with strong evidence supporting an autoimmune mechanism in which cytotoxic T cells target melanocytes. Genetic predisposition, environmental triggers, oxidative stress, and intrinsic melanocyte defects also contribute to disease development and progression. Vitiligo is frequently associated with other autoimmune diseases, such as autoimmune thyroid disease and type 1 diabetes. The condition affects approximately 0.5–2% of the global population and can have a significant psychosocial impact due to its visible nature, especially in individuals with darker skin. The course of vitiligo is unpredictable, with periods of stability and progression (spontaneous repigmentation is uncommon). Diagnosis is clinical, based on the characteristic appearance and distribution of lesions. First-line treatment for vitiligo, including when it affects the breast area in women, is topical corticosteroids for localized disease, with topical calcineurin inhibitors as an alternative, especially for sensitive areas such as the breasts, face, and intertriginous regions due to a lower risk of skin atrophy. For more extensive or refractory lesions, narrow-band ultraviolet B (NB-UVB) phototherapy is considered first-line, either as monotherapy or in combination with

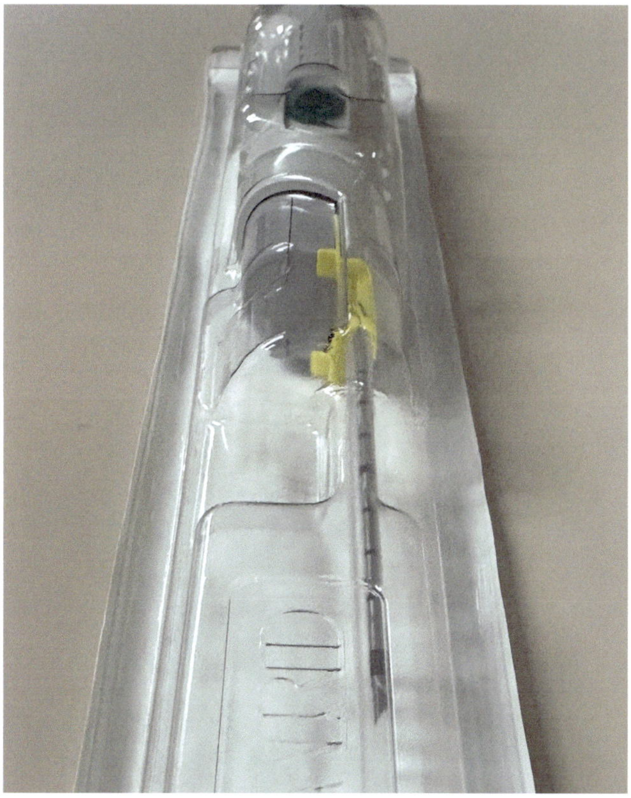

Fig. 33.4 A commercially available, single-use core needle biopsy is shown. This highly specialized needle is spring-loaded and "fired" (like a gun) into tissue using a trigger mechanism. When deployed, the needle is injected into the tissue, and a tiny cylinder of this tissue is obtained within the needle's specialized chamber. After the biopsy is obtained, the sample chamber is accessed, and the cylinder of tissue (aka, the core biopsy) is retrieved, then collected and sent to pathology for histologic interpretation. The specific core needle biopsy shown here is a 14-gauge, 10 cm needle, and the sample chamber (notch) is 1.9 cm in length. The purpose of a core needle biopsy is to provide *histologic architecture*, allowing pathologists to differentiate between invasive cancer and premalignant and/or other lesions. For this reason, *core needle biopsy is the gold-standard modality for addressing suspicious palpable breast masses*

topical corticosteroids, as combination therapy has demonstrated superior efficacy compared to monotherapy in randomized controlled trials. For localized patches, a potent topical corticosteroid (e.g., mometasone furoate 0.1%) is typically applied once daily for up to 3 months, with intermittent regimens (e.g., alternate weeks) to minimize adverse effects such as skin atrophy, particularly relevant for the breast area. Topical calcineurin inhibitors (e.g., tacrolimus 0.1% ointment) are preferred for long-term use or in areas at higher risk for steroid-induced side effects. Recent advances include the use of topical Janus kinase (JAK) inhibitors, such as ruxolitinib 1.5% cream, which has been approved for nonsegmental vitiligo in patients aged 12 years and older, offering another first-line topical option, particularly for localized disease.

Localized *scleroderma* and *morphea* usually do not require treatment, but investigation for other *non*cutaneous symptoms is necessary. **T cell lymphoma**, or *mycosis fungoides*, is a *special type of skin cancer that responds to UV light therapy* when confined to just the skin. In rare instances, a melanoma may present as a *hypo*pigmented lesion (this is termed **amelanotic melanoma**). Treatment is the same as for pigmented melanoma (wide excision, sentinel node biopsy depending on thickness, +/− radiation, biologics depending on stage).

Hyperpigmented Skin Lesions

Skin lesions that appear darker than the surrounding breast skin are hyperpigmented lesions. They may be flat (freckles or benign nevi), raised (keratoses, seborrheic dermatitis, warts/papillomas, raised moles), ulcerated (skin cancer or breast cancer eroding through the skin), or associated with a mass. As mentioned previously, ***biopsy** remains the gold standard to make the diagnosis and guide treatment.*

Fibrocystic Changes

Fibrocystic changes are extremely common, *affecting up to 50% of women over age 30*, with some studies reporting lifetime prevalence as high as 90%. The incidence rises until menopause and then declines. The term "fibrocystic changes" is used to describe a common benign (noncancerous) condition of the breast that involves two key histologic changes withing the parenchyma (Fig. 33.8): **(1)** Stromal *fibrosis*—This refers to an increase in connective tissue, which can feel *firm or rubbery* on clinical exam, and **(2)** a *cystic component* (cysts). These cysts are fluid-filled sacs that form in the breast tissue, which are often visible on breast ultrasound, and are typically characterized by *multiple cysts or varying sizes,* often with *well-circumscribed margins* that are anechoic or hypoechoic, and typically have posterior acoustic enhancement.

The etiology is multifactorial, with hormonal influences (particularly estrogen and progesterone) playing a central role. Increased percent body fat, metabolic syndrome, diabetes, and fatty liver are associated with a higher risk, while higher lean mass is protective. There is no clear association with polycystic ovary syndrome, but hypothyroidism may increase the risk. Fibrocystic changes are not considered a direct precursor to breast cancer, though certain histologic subtypes (e.g., those with atypia) may confer a modestly increased risk.

Fibrocystic changes of the breast are characterized by a combination of cyst formation, fibrosis, and epithelial hyperplasia, often presenting as breast pain, tenderness, and

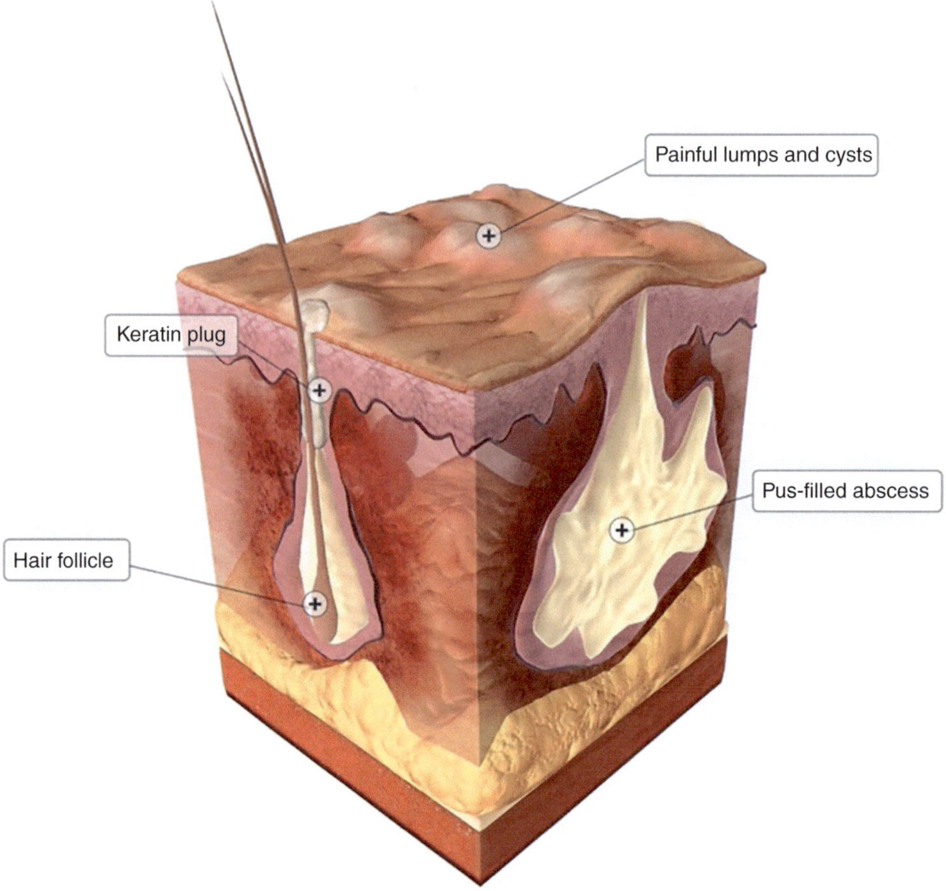

Fig. 33.5 The elements involved in hidradenitis suppurativa are shown, and include follicular occlusion and rupture. The disease initiates with hyperkeratosis and plugging of the hair follicle, leading to follicular rupture and release of keratin and bacteria into the dermis, which triggers inflammation. Chronic inflammation and tissue remodeling occur over time, and persistent inflammation leads to the formation of nodules, abscesses, draining sinus tracts (tunnels), and scarring, with involvement of fibroblasts and abnormal wound healing. Hidradenitis suppurativa, although classically described as affecting the apocrine sweat glands found in the groin and axilla, also affects other skin structures—most notably the hair follicles, which are centrally involved in its pathogenesis. The current consensus is that the disease begins with follicular occlusion and rupture within the *folliculopilosebaceous unit* (FPSU), which includes the hair follicle and its associated sebaceous and apocrine glands. This initiates a cascade of inflammation and tissue destruction. Both innate and adaptive immune responses are central, with increased activity of macrophages, neutrophils, and T cells, and elevated pro-inflammatory cytokines such as TNF-α, IL-1β, and IL-17. B cells and plasma cells also contribute, and anti-inflammatory mediators like IL-10 are present but insufficient to control inflammation. Environmental and lifestyle factors, such as obesity and smoking, are major risk factors, as are hormonal influences (e.g., puberty, menstrual cycle) modulating disease activity

nodularity, particularly in the upper outer quadrants. *These changes are most common in women of reproductive age and are typically bilateral and diffuse, though they can be focal and mimic malignancy on clinical exam or imaging.* Diagnosis is *primarily clinical*, supported by imaging (ultrasound or mammography) when indicated to exclude malignancy. *Histological confirmation* via *core needle biopsy is reserved for cases with atypical features or when malignancy cannot be excluded.* Imaging may reveal cysts, increased breast density, or areas of fibrosis. When lesions of uncertain malignant potential are found, percutaneous biopsy is recommended.

Treatment *Most cases require no specific therapy* beyond reassurance and symptomatic management. For significant pain, *first-line options include nonsteroidal anti-inflammatory drugs (NSAIDs) and supportive measures* (e.g., well-fitted bras). In refractory cases, hormonal therapies such as danazol or luteinizing hormone-releasing hormone (LHRH) analogs may be considered, with danazol shown to reduce pain and nodularity, although side effects (*esp.,* weight gain, hirsutism) limit use. Surgical intervention is reserved for dominant or suspicious masses or when malignancy cannot be excluded.

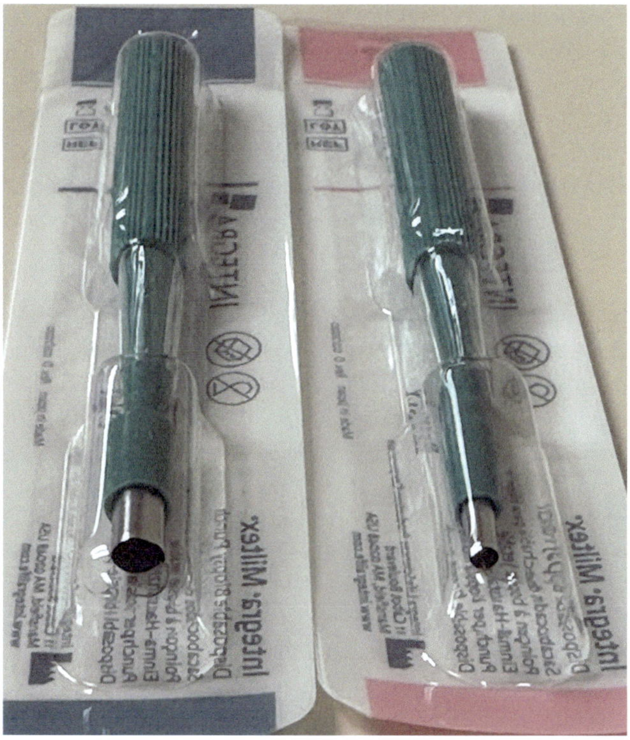

Fig. 33.6 Shown are two sizes of commercially available single-use punch biopsy tools, with different diameters—5 mm (left) and 3 mm (right). The best technique for performing a punch biopsy is to use a sterile, disposable punch tool (3–6 mm may be used depending on lesion size and location) to obtain a full-thickness cylindrical skin specimen that includes epidermis, dermis, and superficial subcutis. The biopsy should target an area that is clinically representative. After local anesthesia is administered, the skin is stretched perpendicular to the relaxed skin tension lines to facilitate an elliptical wound for easier closure, should this be required. The punch is rotated with gentle downward pressure through the dermis into the upper subcutaneous fat. The specimen is gently lifted with forceps and severed at the base with scissors to avoid a crush artifact. Hemostasis is achieved with pressure or chemical cautery, and the wound is often left open but can be closed with a suture, if necessary

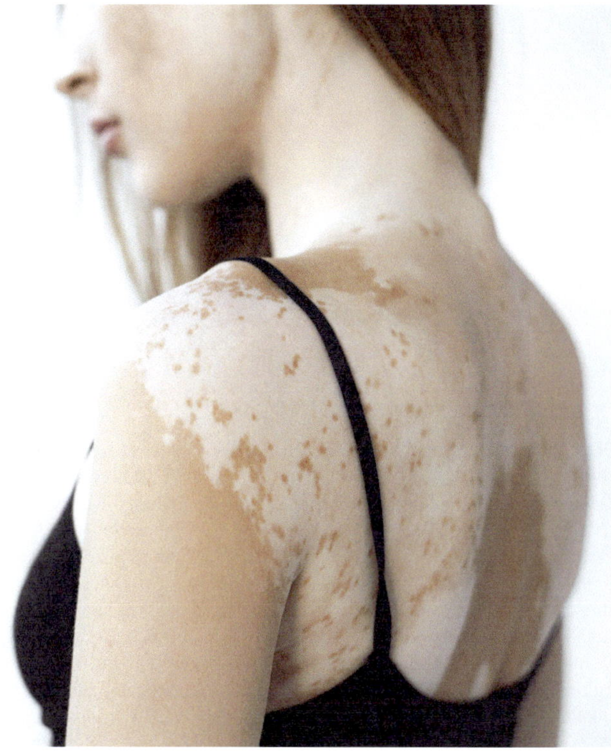

Fig. 33.7 A woman with the classic findings of vitiligo is shown, which has various topographic manifestations. The most common form is nonsegmental (generalized) vitiligo, which typically presents with symmetrical depigmented patches on the face, hands, and other body sites, while segmental vitiligo is unilateral and localized. Vitiligo can affect the breast area in women. Clinical studies of vitiligo distribution patterns have shown that the trunk, which includes the breast area, is a common site of involvement, particularly in women. Specifically, women are more likely than men to have vitiligo affecting the trunk and body folds, which encompasses the breast region

Breast Masses

Workup for the palpable breast mass involves obtaining an accurate history as well as appropriate imaging to determine whether the condition is benign or malignant. The patient should be questioned as to the onset, location, overlying skin changes (dimpling, rash, redness), and duration of the palpable finding, and whether there is a history of trauma. Pain remains a poor indicator of etiology—*both benign and malignant lesions may be painful.* Once the history is obtained and an examination is performed, imaging with ***mammography*** and ***ultrasound*** is advised. For patients who are *younger than 25* with just a cyst by ultrasound and no family history of cancer, the mammogram may be considered optional. *For all other patients, both modalities (ultrasound and mammogram) are the gold standard.* A ***breast MRI*** may be added in instances of positive family history, dense breasts by mammography, prior breast cancer history, or where the mammogram and/or ultrasound are inconclusive. If a discrete lesion is identified by any of these studies, then ***image-guided core biopsy*** is recommended. For very superficial lesions, a punch biopsy may be necessary, and for masses close to underlying/surrounding structures such as implants, ribs, or blood vessels, then image guided localization with excision in the operating room is preferable.

For patients in whom the diagnosis of a cyst is made, monitoring with follow-up studies is all that is indicated. Percutaneous drainage with ultrasound guidance may be offered for symptomatic relief. Excision is an option for recurrent fluid accumulation, secondary infection, or when a solid intracystic component is identified.

Solid masses documented by imaging frequently return ***fibroadenomas***. ***Biopsy-proven fibroadenomas do not suggest a higher risk for developing breast cancer.*** However, 1 in 40 suspected fibroadenomas will return a ***phyllodes*** *tumor* on biopsy. These tumors have a particular *frond-like*

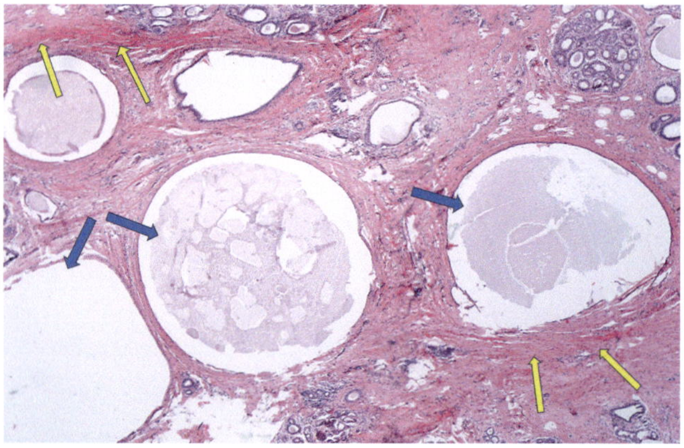

Fig. 33.8 Light microscopy depicting fibrocystic changes of the female breast. The term *fibrocystic* comes from the histologic appearance. This benign condition is characterized by both a cystic component (*blue arrows*) and a component of fibrosis (*yellow arrows*). Fibrotic stroma appears as dense pink collagen, with large fibroblasts visible on higher magnification. Fibrotic tissue is rigid and less functional, and this can be a more significant problem when fibrosis occurs in a vital organ, such as the lungs. On hematoxylin and eosin (H & E) stain, eosin stains supporting cellular structures, such as the stroma, are a pink-red color, while hematoxylin will stain cellular components, such as the nucleus, deep blue or purple. Here, large dilated ducts (appearing as cysts) are occupied by amorphous eosinophilic material in some instances, and they are juxtaposed to regions with smaller, proliferative ducts. This H & E histologic slide is classic for demonstrating fibrocystic changes of the breast

appearance under the microscope, which differentiates them from the typical fibroadenoma. Although they are usually benign, they can grow to very large sizes quite rapidly and may degenerate to become a borderline or malignant tumor, based on the number of cells seen dividing in the specimen. Management used to be wide excision with margins of at least 1 cm in any direction, but *more recent studies have demonstrated that, for the benign phyllodes lesions, just removal of the mass with close monitoring thereafter may be enough to reduce the chances of recurrence.*

Other possible benign biopsy results of solid lesions or abnormal imaging that usually do not require surgery include *proliferative breast disease* (hyperplasia, both ductal and lobular), *stromal fibrosis, sclerosing adenosis, and fibrocystic changes*. Radial scars may also be seen on biopsy, but if they are less than 1 cm, the risk of sampling error is much less, and therefore, excision of small radial scars is no longer recommended.

Some fibrocystic disease-related conditions seen on biopsy, however, do put the patient at a higher lifetime risk for developing breast cancer. The increased risk ranges from 1.7 to 5 times greater than that of the general population. These diagnoses include *atypical ductal flat atypia* (single intraductal layer of abnormal cells), *sclerosing papilloma* or *intraductal papilloma with atypia*, and *atypical lobular hyperplasia*. The likelihood of finding precancer or cancer on excision has led to recommendations of removing all these lesions in their entirety, except the atypical lobular hyperplasia. Following these diagnoses, patients are offered a higher level of surveillance with imaging and possibly genetic counseling/testing to better calculate absolute risk. Preventative medications such as **tamoxifen** may be offered to lower that risk and are usually prescribed by the medical oncologist.

Breast Pain

Many women, as well as some men, will experience breast pain at some point during their lifetime. The age at onset, characteristics of the pain, whether the pain is cyclical, current medication/supplement regimen, and other chronic diseases/conditions present may help direct imaging and provide an underlying diagnosis to explain the symptoms. ***Fibrocystic changes are the most common cause of <u>cyclical</u> breast pain***. Hormonal changes that come with the menstrual cycle, pregnancy, perimenopause, hormone treatments after menopause, hormone/endocrine therapy for breast or prostate cancer, and undiagnosed hormone deficiencies (e.g., hypothyroidism) all exacerbate breast pain. Many men on endocrine treatment for prostate cancer not only will have pain but will also have abnormal growth of their breast tissue (**gynecomastia**). *Breast pain should be worked up just like a palpable mass, with imaging and biopsy if indicated.* In addition, however, hormone levels should be measured. If a medication or supplement is identified as the cause (Table 33.2), removal will usually help with the pain. Additionally, weight loss, increased exercise, and less caffeine may also alleviate the pain. Treating hormone deficiencies will also help. First-line therapy with *evening primrose oil* or *fish oil* may benefit those with milder symptoms. In extreme circumstances, prescription treatment of the pain with bromocriptine (lowers prolactin), danazol (brings on menopause), tamoxifen (selective estrogen receptor modulator), or an aromatase inhibitor (blunts estrogen effect on breast tissue) may be indicated.

Table 33.2 Medications/supplements associated with breast pain

Hormones
Birth control pills
Replacement therapy
Infertility treatments
Cardiac medications
Diuretics
Digitalis
Methyldopa
Spironolactone
Atenolol

Gynecomastia

Men will occasionally develop enlarged breasts during their lives. During puberty, most boys will have some prominence of the subareolar breast tissue, frequently unilateral, that may become severely painful. This hypertrophy usually levels off or reverts and is asymptomatic by the early 20s. When the symptoms persist beyond this time frame, workup with hormone levels and imaging is indicated, and biopsy or excision may be offered for treatment if an underlying cause is not identified. For breast development occurring after puberty, a detailed history that includes ALL medications and supplements, as well as social history, should be obtained, as *soy intake, anabolic steroids, certain medications and hormone treatments, marijuana, and alcohol use are linked to abnormal breast growth in men* (Tables 33.3 and 33.4). Once the cause has been identified, stopping the medication/supplement/hormone/social activity should resolve the issue or at least result in regression. Surgery may be performed for persistent symptoms or cosmetic reasons.

Table 33.3 Gynecomastia-inducing drugs: known mechanism of action

Pro-estrogen drugs (bind to receptors)	**Reduced testosterone** (testicular damage)	
Topical estrogen creams	Busulfan	
Digitalis	Nitrosurea	
Clomiphene	Vincristine	
Marijuana	Ethanol	
Delousing powder		
Pro-estrogen drugs (increased synthesis)	**Testosterone or androgen blockade**	
Gonadotropins	Ketoconazole	Flutamide
Growth hormone	Spironolactone	Bicalutamide
Androgen supplements	Metronidazole	Finasteride
DHEA	Etomidate	Cyproterone
Soy	Zanoterone	Ranitidine
	Cimetidine	

Table 33.4 Gynecomastia-inducing drugs: uncertain mechanism of action

Griseofulvin	Methyldopa
Phenothiazines	Isoniazid
Reserpine	Metoclopramide
Tricyclic antidepressants	

Selected Reading

1. Mansel RE, Webster DJT, Sweetland HM, et al. Hughes, Mansel & Webster's benign disorders and disease of the breast. 3rd ed. Elsevier Limited; 2009.
2. Sars C, et al. Current clinical practice in the management of phyllodes tumors of the breast: an international cross-sectional study among surgeons and oncologists. Breast Cancer Res Treat. 2023;199(2):293–304.
3. Polat DS, Schopp JG, Arjmandi F, Porembka VS, Farr D, Xi Y, Dogan BE. Performance of a clinical and imaging-based multivariate model as decision support tool to help save unnecessary surgeries for high-risk breast lesions. Breast Cancer Res Treat. 2020;185:479–94.
4. Boughey JC, Hartmann LC, Anderson SS, Degnim AC, Vierkant RA, Reynolds CA, Frost MH, Pankratz VS. Evaluation of the Tyrer-Cuzick (international breast cancer intervention study) model for breast cancer risk prediction in women with atypical hyperplasia. J Clin Oncol. 2010;28(22):3591–6.
5. Breast pain. https://medlineplus.gov/enc/article/003152.htm.

Breast Cancer

34

Melissa Camp

Breast cancer is the most commonly diagnosed cancer in women in the United States, and second only to lung cancer as a cause of death from cancer in women. Approximately one in eight women in the United States will develop breast cancer over the course of their lifetime. In 2025, it is estimated by the American Cancer Society that there will be 316,950 new diagnoses of invasive breast cancer in US women, 59,080 new diagnoses of ductal carcinoma in situ (DCIS or stage 0 breast cancer), and 42,170 women will die from breast cancer [1]. As breast cancer is such a commonly diagnosed disease, it is an entity encountered frequently in clinical practice. Multidisciplinary treatment of breast cancer is essential and has led to improved outcomes and survival for patients.

Breast Cancer Screening

With routine screening, many breast cancers are diagnosed well before they are palpable by the patient or detected on a clinical breast exam by a provider. The age at which to begin screening mammography varies according to different guidelines as well as the risk factors of the patient. The US Preventive Services Task Force (USPSTF) (www.uspreventiveservicestaskforce.org), National Comprehensive Cancer Network (NCCN) (www.nccn.org), American College of Radiology (ACR) (www.acr.org), and the American College of Obstetricians and Gynecologists (ACOG) (www.acog.org) all recommend that average-risk women begin screening mammography at age 40. The American Cancer Society (ACS) (www.cancer.org) recommends that average-risk women begin annual mammography at age 45, with the option to begin at age 40. The NCCN, ACR, and ACOG all recommend annual mammography. The ACS recommends annual mammography from ages 45–54, with the option to continue annual mammography or switch to every 2 years starting at age 55. The USPSTF recommends mammography every 2 years. Although the guidelines do vary, a general rule is to ***consider and discuss routine screening mammography with all patients starting at age 40***.

For patients at increased risk of developing breast cancer, it may be appropriate to initiate screening for breast cancer at a younger age. A family history of breast cancer is one of the most common risk factors associated with an increased risk of developing breast cancer, and the ages at which relatives were diagnosed with breast cancer can impact screening recommendations. For example, patients with a family history of breast cancer should begin mammography screening ***10 years prior to the earliest age of breast cancer diagnosis in the family <u>or</u> at age 40, whichever comes first***. If a patient's mother was diagnosed with breast cancer at age 43 and her grandmother at age 75, then the patient should begin mammography screening at age 33. If a patient's mother and aunt were diagnosed with breast cancer in their 60s, the patient should begin mammography screening at age 40.

Some patients with a strong family history of breast cancer and/or other cancers may carry a genetic mutation associated with an increased risk of breast cancer. ***BRCA 1*** *and* ***BRCA 2*** *mutations are the most common genetic mutations associated with an increased risk of breast cancer.* Patients with BRCA 1 or BRCA 2 mutations should begin screening for breast cancer with an annual breast MRI starting at age 25, and add annual mammography beginning at age 30. Other genetic mutations that are associated with an increased risk of breast cancer include ATM, CHEK2, PALB2, PTEN, and TP53. If you suspect a possible genetic mutation due to a strong family history of breast cancer or other cancers, a referral to a genetic counselor for further evaluation and consideration of genetic testing is warranted.

In addition to a family history of breast cancer, there are a multitude of other risk factors associated with an increased risk of breast cancer. Some of these risk factors include an

M. Camp (✉)
Division of Surgical Oncology, Breast Surgery Section, Johns Hopkins University School of Medicine, Baltimore, MD, USA
e-mail: mcamp@jhmi.edu

S. Atallah, J. Dragoljevic (eds.), *Fundamentals of Surgery for Physician Assistants*,
https://doi.org/10.1007/978-3-032-21069-2_34

earlier onset of menarche, a later onset of menopause, having a first child after age 30, not having children, prolonged use of hormone replacement therapy after menopause, increased weight and BMI in women after menopause, >4–5 alcoholic drinks per week, having dense breast tissue on mammogram, and having a history of previous breast biopsies showing atypical cells. Various combinations of these risk factors can place patients in a higher risk category for potentially developing breast cancer in the future, and there are risk models that can help assess a patient's risk. The Gail model and the Tyrer-Cuzick model are two of the most common risk assessment tools. If the estimated lifetime risk of developing breast cancer exceeds 20% based on a validated risk assessment model, then additional screening may be indicated. Annual breast MRI, for example, may be recommended in addition to annual mammography.

Breast Cancer Diagnosis

If an abnormality is detected on a routine screening mammogram or if a patient presents with a concerning finding on clinical exam (a palpable breast mass, nipple discharge, breast skin changes, and/or palpable axillary lymph nodes), then further workup and diagnostic imaging are indicated. Diagnostic imaging could include additional mammographic views and a breast or axillary ultrasound to further evaluate the area of concern (Fig. 34.1a, b). Suspicious findings on diagnostic imaging should undergo a biopsy for tissue diagnosis. For breast lesions, a ***core needle biopsy*** is preferred to obtain *histologic architecture* of the tissue and provide as much information as possible from pathologic assessment. A core needle biopsy of a breast lesion is typically performed under imaging guidance. For lesions best seen on mammogram, such as calcifications, a mammogram-guided (stereotactic) core needle biopsy is performed. For lesions best seen on ultrasound, such as masses, an ultrasound-guided core needle biopsy is performed. Some breast lesions are only seen on MRI, and in those cases, an MRI-guided core needle biopsy is performed. With all core needle biopsies of the breast, a biopsy clip is placed to mark the location of the biopsy site. This biopsy clip serves as a marker to guide future surgical excision of the lesion if indicated based on pathology results, or to mark the location of a benign biopsy on future mammograms.

If cancer is identified on a core needle biopsy, the pathology results will provide information regarding in situ versus invasive cancer, the type of cancer, such as ductal or lobular, the grade of the cancer, and the receptor status (estrogen, progesterone, and HER2). **In situ** *cancer refers to cancer cells that are still* ***contained,*** *whereas* ***invasive cancer cells*** *have invaded out of the ducts or lobules of the breast and* ***into the surrounding breast tissue***. The grade of the breast cancer is based on how the cells appear under the microscope. Grade 1 refers to cancer cells that appear less aggressive and most resemble normal breast cells. Grade 2 refers to

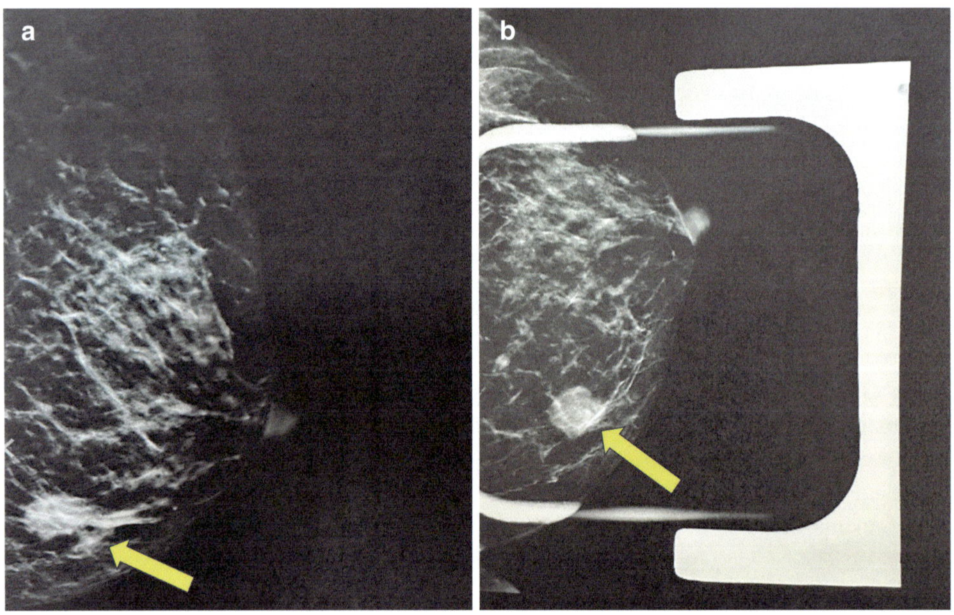

Fig. 34.1 A diagnostic mammogram from a 66 y.o. female who presented with a clinically palpable mass in the left breast at the 9 o'clock position is shown. Mammography is the standard imaging modality for breast cancer. (**a**) A 1.5 cm mass 6 cm from the nipple-areolar complex (arrow) in the left medial breast that appears radiopaque. (**b**) Spot compression view of the same breast showing the angular, radio-dense margins. These findings are suspicious for breast cancer according to the **B**reast **I**maging-**R**eporting **A**nd **D**ata **S**ystem (**BI-RADS**) assessment, and would be considered a BI-RADS category 4. While this is suggestive of malignancy, confirmation can only come from histology obtained from a biopsy. Core needle biopsy of breast lesions is the gold standard, as it preserves the histological architecture from the tissue (fine needle aspirates do not)

cancer cells that appear moderately aggressive, and Grade 3 refers to cancer cells that appear most aggressive and least resemble normal breast cells. The stage of breast cancer is based on the size of the cancer and the lymph node status. Stage 0 refers to noninvasive breast cancer, or ductal carcinoma in situ (DCIS). Stage 1 is the earliest stage of invasive breast cancer, with Stages 2 and 3 representing larger invasive cancers with increasing numbers of lymph nodes involved by cancer. Stage 4 breast cancer refers to breast cancer that has spread (metastasized) to other parts of the body, such as the liver, lungs, and/or bones. All of this information about the features of the cancer is utilized to help guide decisions about treatment.

Breast Cancer Treatment

The treatment of breast cancer is truly multidisciplinary and involves specialties such as surgery, medical oncology, radiation oncology, radiology, plastic surgery, physical therapy, and genetic counseling, among others. All of these specialties play an important role in guiding treatment decisions and ensuring the best possible outcomes for patients.

The majority of patients diagnosed with early-stage breast cancer (Stages 0, 1, and 2) will undergo surgery as the first step in treatment. There are two main options for surgical management of breast cancer: lumpectomy and mastectomy. **Lumpectomy** entails removing the portion of the breast where the cancer is located, with the goal of achieving negative margins. This approach is sometimes termed **breast-conserving surgery (BCS)**. If pathology reveals that cancer cells are present at the margin (which occurs in 10–20% of the time after lumpectomy), then additional surgery may be necessary to obtain clear margins. ***Following lumpectomy, a course of radiation is typically recommended*** to treat the remaining breast tissue and decrease the risk of local recurrence (the risk of cancer coming back in the same breast). **Mastectomy** refers to the removal of the entire breast, and this can often be performed with some type of reconstruction by plastic surgery to recreate the breast. There are different types of mastectomy including **simple mastectomy, skin sparing mastectomy, and nipple sparing mastectomy. A modified radical mastectomy includes removal of the entire breast plus an axillary lymph node dissection.** The original **radical mastectomy** proposed by Halsted, with removal of the pectoralis major and minor muscles, is no longer used, as it adds morbidity without improvement in local control.

The long-term survival is equivalent regardless of whether patients undergo (a) lumpectomy plus radiation versus (b) mastectomy. The risk of cancer recurring in the breast is a little higher after lumpectomy and radiation (approximately 5–8%) since the majority of the breast tissue remains intact, but the risk of cancer recurring in the chest wall after a complete mastectomy is not zero (the risk of local recurrence after mastectomy is approximately 2–4%) [2]. The decision-making process for choosing lumpectomy versus mastectomy can be impacted by many different factors. Sometimes a mastectomy may be necessary if the size of the cancer is large in relation to the size of the breast, if there are multiple areas of cancer in the same breast that involve a large portion of the breast, or if the patient is unable to receive radiation to the breast. If both lumpectomy and mastectomy are feasible surgical options, other factors such as a family history of breast cancer, the presence of a genetic mutation that predisposes to breast cancer (such as a **BRCA 1** or **BRCA 2** mutation, both of which are autosomal dominant), and patient preference all can affect the decision to pursue lumpectomy versus mastectomy.

In conjunction with either lumpectomy or mastectomy, axillary lymph nodes are typically removed to determine if breast cancer has spread beyond the breast. A **sentinel lymph node biopsy** *samples the first few lymph nodes under the arm that drain the breast on that side.* A tracer (technetium sulfur colloid and/or blue dye) is injected into the breast tissue on the day of surgery, and the tracer travels through the lymphatic channels in the breast to determine which lymph nodes are the first draining lymph nodes. ***If the sentinel lymph nodes are negative for cancer, it is presumed that the remaining axillary lymph nodes are negative***. If the sentinel lymph nodes are positive for cancer, then additional lymph nodes may or may not need to be removed.

For patients with multiple involved lymph nodes, an axillary lymph node dissection (removing the level 1 and 2 axillary lymph nodes) may be necessary. *The more lymph nodes removed, the greater the risk for patients to develop* ***lymphedema*** *of the arm postoperatively.* The risk of lymphedema with a sentinel lymph node biopsy (on average, removal of 1–4 lymph nodes) is approximately 5%. **Following an axillary lymph node dissection, the risk of lymphedema can approach 20–30%** [3]. If lymphedema does develop, a referral to physical therapy for manual lymphatic drainage is important for management. Patients may also need to wear a compression sleeve for the management of lymphedema. *Minimizing the risk of lymphedema by doing the lymph node dissection only if necessary is the impetus behind doing the sentinel lymph node biopsy.* In simple terms, we do not want to take out axillary lymph nodes in patients if they do not harbor cancer, because doing so can result in a higher risk of lymphedema.

Another important type of complication during breast surgery, and especially axillary lymph node dissection, is potential injury to the **long thoracic nerve**, which can lead to a **winged scapula** deformity (Fig. 34.2a, b). The incidence of long thoracic nerve injury is highest after procedures that include axillary lymph node dissection, and some data reveal the incidence to range from 8% to 28% in the early postoperative period, with most cases showing partial or complete

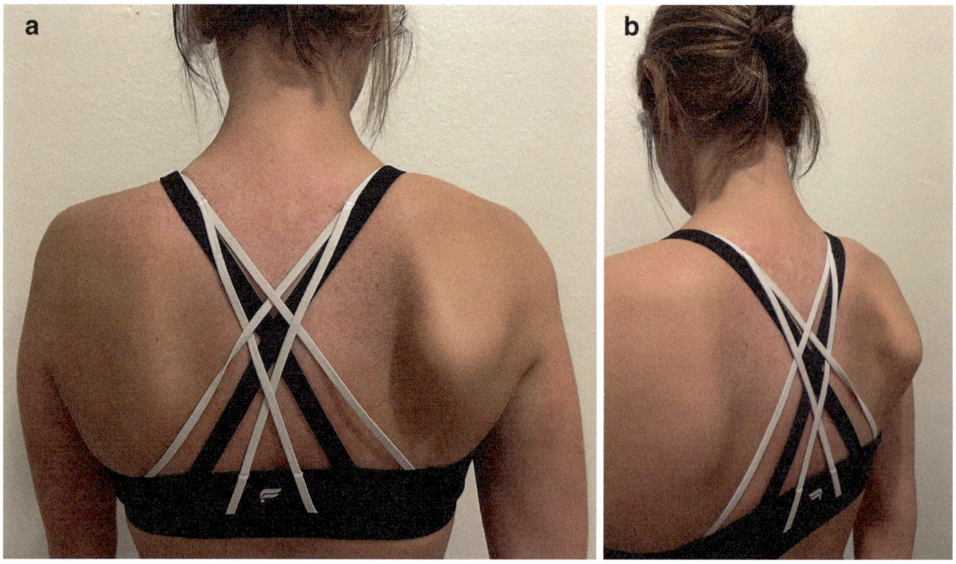

Fig. 34.2 An example of a right-sided *winged scapula* is shown here with (**a**) back and (**b**) oblique views. Note the projection of the scapula in comparison to the contralateral side. Winged scapula can result from injury to the long thoracic nerve, particularly during axillary lymph node dissection. Fortunately, most patients who have this injury recover function over time. (Photographs courtesy of Brianne Kimura, PA-C, with permission)

recovery over time. Simple mastectomy without axillary dissection is associated with a much lower risk, as the long thoracic nerve isn't exposed and thus the risk of injury is negligible.

The pathology results from surgery, including the size of the cancer and the lymph node status, will determine the staging of the cancer. The need for additional treatment after surgery (adjuvant therapy) also depends on the pathology results. In general, radiation is recommended after lumpectomy to decrease the risk of cancer recurring in the breast. Radiation is not always needed after mastectomy, but is indicated in certain situations, such as cancers larger than 5 cm and/or positive lymph nodes. Radiation typically lasts for 4–6 weeks, and occurs Monday through Friday for a few minutes per day. The decisions about systemic therapies, including chemotherapy, HER2 targeted therapy, and hormone blocking therapy, are far more nuanced. The **receptor status** of the cancer ***(Estrogen (ER), Progesterone (PR), and HER2 receptors)*** plays an important role in determining appropriate systemic therapies, as does the size of the cancer and the lymph node status. HER2-positive cancers, for example, will typically require HER2-targeted therapy plus chemotherapy. The specific regimen is dictated by the size of the cancer and the lymph node status. Chemotherapy is almost always indicated for triple-negative cancers (ER negative, PR negative, and HER2 negative), as these cancers are not responsive to HER2-targeted or hormone-blocking therapies. Hormone blocking therapy is used to treat hormone-positive cancers (ER and/or PR positive), and some hormone-positive cancers may also require chemotherapy.

For patients with more advanced cancers at the time of diagnosis (larger cancers or those with lymph node involvement, including Stage 3 and some more aggressive Stage 2 cancers), the first step in treatment is typically systemic therapy with chemotherapy. HER2 targeted therapy or immunotherapy may also be indicated for HER2-positive or triple-negative cancers, respectively. The advantages of giving systemic therapy prior to surgery (neoadjuvant therapy) are to downstage the size of the cancer in the breast as well as the axillary lymph nodes. With a good response to neoadjuvant systemic therapy, the cancer may shrink so that a smaller portion of the breast is involved, potentially allowing for a lumpectomy instead of a mastectomy. In addition, fewer lymph nodes may need to be removed from under the arm. Sometimes, all of the cancer cells that were previously in the breast and lymph nodes may be killed when chemotherapy is given prior to surgery. If pathology from surgery finds no evidence of viable cancer cells in the tissue removed (a pathologic complete response or pCR), this is indicative of improved outcomes for the patient. The pathology results from surgery, whether a pathologic complete response or a partial response, will then be utilized to inform decisions about systemic therapies given after surgery.

Patients who are diagnosed with Stage 4 breast cancer have evidence that cancer has spread to other parts of the body, such as the liver, lungs, and/or bones. For most patients with Stage 4 cancer, the most important treatment is **systemic therapy (chemotherapy, HER2 targeted therapy and/or hormone blocking therapy)** to treat the entire body. Surgery for the breast is typically not performed, except on a case-by-case basis.

Conclusions

Breast cancer is a very common disease. Appropriate initiation of screening, timely diagnosis of breast cancer, and multidisciplinary treatment all lead to improved outcomes for patients with breast cancer. Surgery, radiation, and systemic therapy are key components of breast cancer treatment.

References

1. Breast cancer statistics: how common is breast cancer? [Internet]. [cited 2025 May 17]. Available from: https://www.cancer.org/cancer/types/breast-cancer/about/how-common-is-breast-cancer.html#:~:text=The%20American%20Cancer%20Society's%20estimates%20for%20breast,42%2C170%20women%20will%20die%20from%20breast%20cancer.
2. Boughey JC, Rosenkranz KM, Ballman KV, McCall L, Haffty BG, Cuttino LW, Kubicky CD, Le-Petross HT, Giuliano AE, Van Zee KJ, Hunt KK, Hahn OM, Carey LA, Partridge AH. Local recurrence after breast-conserving therapy in patients with multiple ipsilateral breast cancer: results from ACOSOG Z11102 (Alliance). J Clin Oncol. 2023;41(17):3184–93. https://doi.org/10.1200/JCO.22.02553. Epub 2023 Mar 28. PMID: 36977292; PMCID: PMC10256355.
3. Isik A, Soran A, Grasi A, Barry N, Sezgin E. Lymphedema after sentinel lymph node biopsy: who is at risk? Lymphat Res Biol. 2022;20(2):160–3. https://doi.org/10.1089/lrb.2020.0093. Epub 2021 Jun 30. PMID: 34191608.

35 Problems in Vascular Surgery: Carotid Artery Stenosis, Diseases of the Aorta, and Peripheral Vascular Disease

Amber Amick, Trent Gabriel, Tracy Totten, and Frank R. Arko III

Carotid Artery Stenosis (CAS)

Anatomy and Physiology

The carotid arteries are the predominant vessels that supply blood to the head and neck. The right common carotid artery (RCCA) originates from the brachiocephalic artery, whereas the left common carotid artery (LCCA) originates directly from the aortic arch. Both CCAs bifurcate in the neck at the level of the carotid sinus into two branches. The external carotid arteries (ECAs) supply the neck and face with arterial blood, whereas the internal carotid arteries (ICAs) supply the brain. To further specify location, the carotid arteries are located posterior to the sternoclavicular joints and are protected as they lie within the carotid sheath, which is a fibrinous connective tissue that also contains the internal jugular veins and the vagus (tenth cranial) nerve. For most patients, the bifurcation of the CCAs into the ECAs and ICAs occurs at the level of the upper border of the thyroid cartilage and roughly the level of the fourth or fifth cervical vertebrae. At the bifurcation, there is the carotid body as well as the carotid sinus. The carotid body is a chemoreceptor that works to detect the levels of PO_2, PCO_2, and pH of the blood that passes through the bifurcation into the brain and face. This mainly works to alert the brain of the need to increase the respiratory rate. The carotid sinus is a baroreceptor that responds to changes in the stretch of the blood vessel and helps to maintain blood pressure (Fig. 35.1).

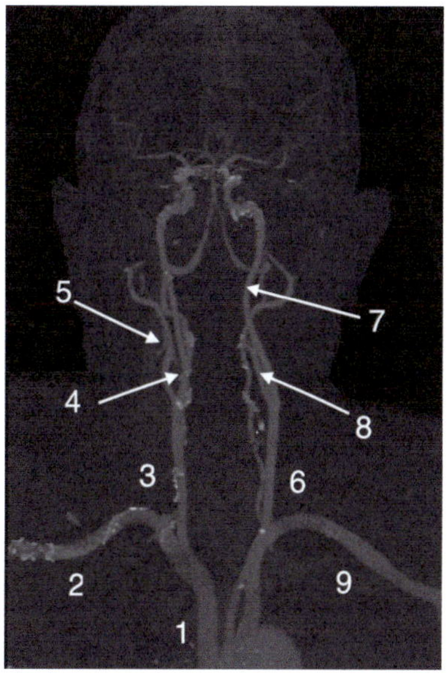

1. Brachiocephalic artery
2. Right subclavian
3. Right common carotid artery
4. Right internal carotid artery
5. Right external carotid artery
6. Left common carotid artery
7. Left internal carotid artery
8. Left external carotid artery
9. Left subclavian artery

Fig. 35.1 Carotid anatomy (with key legend)

Pathology/Pathophysiology of Carotid Artery Stenosis

There are several potential causes of CAS with the most common being the development of atherosclerosis, fibromuscular dysplasia, anatomical variances, carotid artery aneurysms, Takayasu's arteritis, radiation therapy injuries, and carotid body tumors.

Far and away the most common cause of CAS is the development of atherosclerosis. One of the prominent reasons the development of atherosclerosis can specifically

A. Amick · T. Gabriel · T. Totten
Atrium Health/Sanger Heart & Vascular Institute, Charlotte, NC, USA
e-mail: Amber.amick@atriumhealth.org; benjamin.gabriel@atriumhealth.org; tracy.totten@atriumhealth.org

F. R. Arko III (✉)
Vascular and Endovascular Surgery, Atrium Health/Sanger Heart & Vascular Institute, Charlotte, NC, USA
e-mail: Frank.Arko@atriumhealth.org

S. Atallah, J. Dragoljevic (eds.), *Fundamentals of Surgery for Physician Assistants*,
https://doi.org/10.1007/978-3-032-21069-2_35

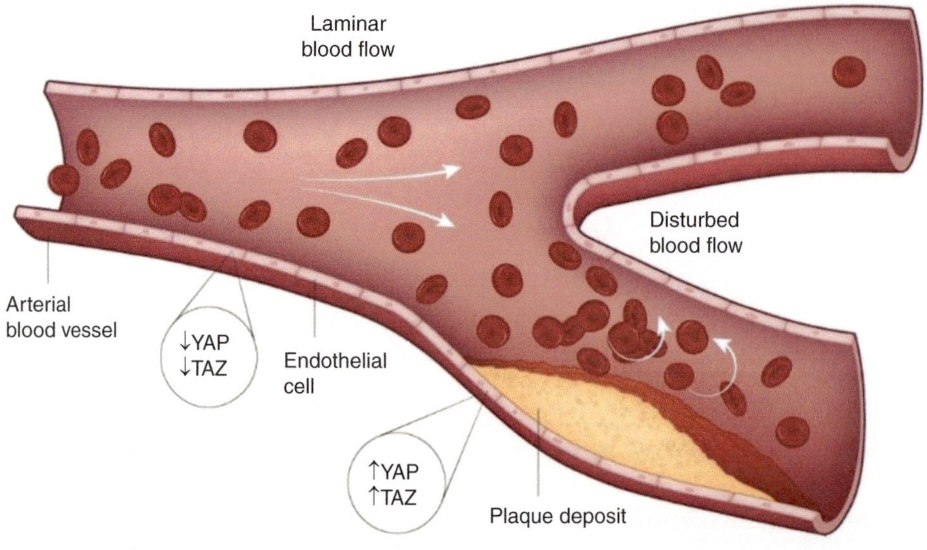

Fig. 35.2 Turbulent flow in CAS development. (Mehta and Tzima [17])

affect the CCAs is the anatomy of the arterial bifurcation. The hemodynamics of the blood flow through this channel with associated fluctuations of shear stress can predispose regions with lower flow velocity (i.e., the carotid bifurcation) to the development of atherosclerotic plaques. The hemodynamics of arterial flow at the carotid bifurcation can significantly increase the likelihood of atherosclerotic plaque, reducing vessel lumen diameter, and increasing risk of thrombotic or embolic event (Fig. 35.2).

Plaques form in part due to the inflammatory response (platelet deposition, smooth muscle cell proliferation, and slow accumulation of lipoproteins) involved in the repair process. The atherosclerotic plaques form due to several reasons, including elevated blood cholesterol, long-term damage from smoking on the intima of the vessel wall, chronically elevated blood glucose, and genetic predisposition (Chap. 27).

Presentation of CAS

Patients with carotid artery disease can present with or without neurological symptoms. Symptomatology and degree of stenosis are both considered when evaluating for surgical revascularization. Patients with symptomatic carotid artery disease may present with a myriad of neurological symptoms (Table 35.1) and may be revascularized at a lower degree of stenosis, whereas patients with asymptomatic carotid artery disease may be revascularized at a higher degree of stenosis.

Table 35.1 Common historical features to consider with CAS

Suggestive of symptomatic CAS	Commonly not associated with CAS
Amaurosis fugax-loss of vision in one eye	Dizziness/vertigo without loss of balance
Difficulty speaking or understanding	Syncope or near syncope
Loss of strength on contralateral side	Muscle tension headache
Numbness and sensory loss on contralateral side	Tinnitus
Facial droop	
Slurred speech	
Sudden severe headache	

Physical Examination

It is common to see referrals from providers for patients who have been found to have a *carotid bruit.* Bruits can be heard when there is turbulent blood flow that must flow around an atherosclerotic plaque (stenosis) within the vessel wall.

For best clinical practice, the patient should be evaluated with their head secured and slightly tilted back with the chin elevated. Stand or sit next to the patient on the right when auscultating the right ICA and ask them to look to their left. Repeat the same technique on the left (sit or stand to their left and have them look right). Stethoscope should be placed approximately 2–3 cm above the clavicle and patient asked to briefly hold their breath as they are expiring. Reposition the stethoscope 2–3 times moving caudally toward the level of the bifurcation on both sides [1].

The presence or absence of a carotid bruit is not diagnostic for whether the patient has significant carotid artery stenosis. Additionally, carotid artery bruits are most often found to be benign. Multiple studies have shown varying degrees of specificity and sensitivity, with a consistent trend showing a positive bruit to be more specific than sensitive.

Imaging/Diagnostic Testing

There are four main diagnostic tests that are used to evaluate the degree of stenosis within carotid arteries: Cerebral angiography, Carotid Duplex Ultrasound (DUS), Magnetic Resonance Angiography, and Computed Tomographic Angiography. Also, there are three main methods of measuring the degree of stenosis: **NASCET, ECST,** and **CC.**

The first method of measuring carotid artery stenosis, the **North American Symptomatic Carotid Endarterectomy Trial (NASCET)**, measures the residual lumen diameter at the most stenotic portion of the vessel and compares this with the lumen diameter in the normal ICA distal to the stenosis. This differs from the **European Carotid Surgery Trial (ECST)**, which measures the lumen diameter at the most stenotic portion and compares this with the estimated probable original diameter at the site of maximum stenosis (Fig. 35.3). Lastly, the third most common method to measure carotid artery stenosis is the **Common Carotid (CC)** method, which measures the residual lumen diameter at the most stenotic portion of the vessel and compares it to the lumen diameter in the proximal CCA.

Conventional Cerebral Angiography: Pros of this diagnostic modality include being able to evaluate the entire carotid artery system, while also showing information about atherosclerotic disease, plaque morphology, and collateral circulation as well. However, the downside to this diagnostic imaging, and the main reasons that it is rarely used, are that it is invasive, quite expensive, and places patients at a slightly increased risk of morbidity (due to CVA) and mortality.

Carotid Artery Duplex Ultrasound (US): This imaging modality (Fig. 35.4) utilizes B-Mode and Doppler US techniques to find focal increases in blood flow velocity, which can be indicative of carotid artery stenosis. It combines data from the peak systolic velocity (PSV), end-diastolic velocity (EDV), spectral configuration, and the carotid index (ICA PSV to CCA PSV ratio). This imaging modality has been shown to be highly specific or highly sensitive for detecting a residual lumen diameter of <1.5 mm (Table 35.2). The benefits of this imaging modality include that it is noninvasive, safe, and relatively inexpensive. The downside to this specific imaging

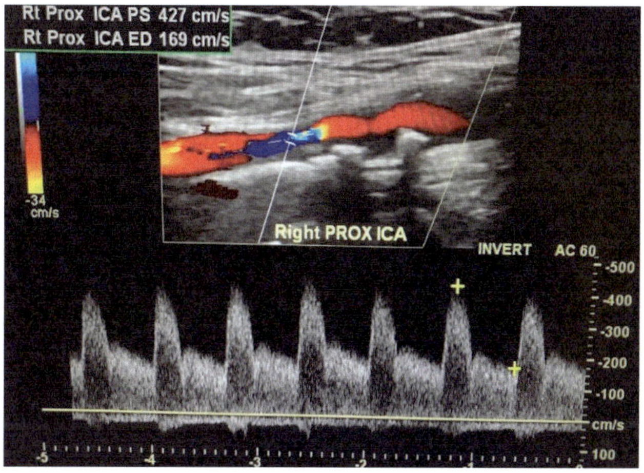

Fig. 35.4 Carotid duplex ultrasound with high grade stenosis of the proximal ICA (PS Peak Systolic, ED End Diastolic)

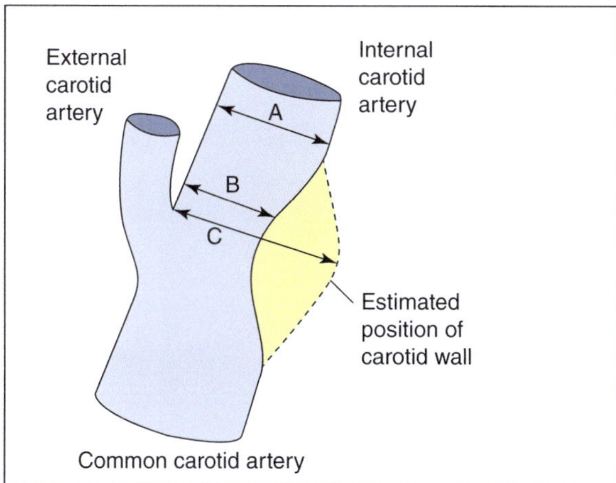

NASCET $\frac{A-B}{A}$ ECST $\frac{C-B}{C}$

NASCET	ECST
30	65
40	70
50	75
60	80
70	85
80	91
90	97

Approximate equivalent degrees of internal carotid artery stenosis used in ASCET and ESCT according to recent direct comparisons

Fig. 35.3 Assessing carotid stenosis severity. (Saxena et al. [18])

modality includes that near occlusions can be missed, the degree of stenosis can be overestimated, and the cervical portion of the ICA is best seen. The natural anatomic variances of patients make it difficult to obtain accurate results as well.

Magnetic Resonance Angiography: This diagnostic image shows a 3D image of the carotid bifurcation with good sensitivity for detecting high-grade stenosis, but less accurate for detecting moderate stenosis. Contraindications to potentially utilizing this modality are that MRA is more expensive, time-consuming, and less readily available. In addition, MRA is not a safe option for patients with significantly reduced kidney function.

Table 35.2 Duplex ultrasound evaluation for carotid severity—Atrium Health vascular laboratory standardization values

Stenosis	ICA PSV (cm/sec)	Plaque	ICA EDV (cm/sec)	ICA/CCA PSV ratio
Normal	<125	None	<40	<2.0
<50%	<125	<50% diameter reduction	<40	<2.0
50–69%	≥125–230	>50% diameter reduction	≥40–≤ 100	2.0–4.0
>70%	>230	>50% diameter reduction	>100	>4.0
Near occlusion	High, low, or undetectable	Visible	Variable	Variable
Occlusion	Undetectable	Visible, no detection	Not applicable	Not applicable

CCA Common Carotid, *ICA* Internal Carotid, *EDV* end diastolic velocity, *PSV* Peak systolic velocity, *PSV* ratio Carotid Index

Computed Tomography Angiography: This imaging modality shows an in-depth anatomic depiction of the lumen, adjacent soft tissues, and bony structures (Fig. 35.5). It can be particularly useful when the Carotid Duplex is not reliable. CTA is more readily available than MRA, but still expensive. Lastly, impaired renal function is a relative contraindication.

Management of Carotid Artery Stenosis

If the patient is asymptomatic and there is less than <70% ICA stenosis, conservative management is the best option. Optimal medical therapy includes aspirin 81 mg and statin therapy. Statin medications have been proven through many studies to be very beneficial at reducing atherosclerotic plaque buildup as well as stabilizing existing plaque. Atorvastatin and rosuvastatin are the most common as they have been shown to be the most efficacious as high-potency statins. Dual antiplatelet therapy may be recommended. Modifiable risk factors that are encouraged include smoking cessation, routine exercise, adequate blood pressure control, blood glucose control, and adherence to a medical regimen.

Surgical options for carotid revascularization include: TCAR (Trans Carotid Artery Revascularization), transfemoral carotid artery stenting, CEA (Carotid Endarterectomy), and carotid artery bypass

CEA: This surgery is an open surgical procedure where the carotid artery is opened, the plaque within the vessel is removed, and the artery is repaired.

TCAR: This surgery can be ideal for many high-risk surgical patients. Direct visualization of the diseased carotid and a reversal of flow away from the brain is established with a

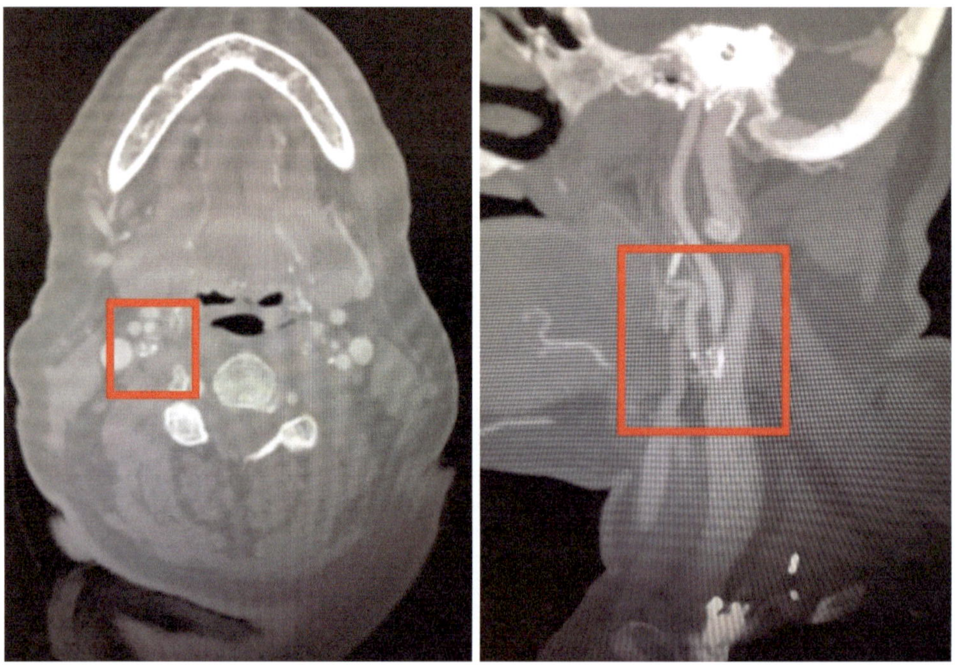

Fig. 35.5 CT angiography of the neck with 90% ICA stenosis (coronal and orbital views)

Table 35.3 Qualifying characteristics for TCAR

>75 years of age
HFrEF <35%
CAD with >75% stenosis
Abnormal stress testing
Severe pulmonary disease
Prior head and neck radiation
Prior CEA with restenosis
Surgically inaccessible lesion
Contralateral occlusion
Able to use clopidogrel for 60 days

small pump removing debris and reducing embolic potential. A filter is utilized, and the blood is removed from the carotid artery and returned to the femoral vein. Once this reversed flow is safely established, stenting of the carotid lesion is undertaken with a reduction in the risk of neurologic injury. There are several qualifying factors for patients (Table 35.3).

Surveillance

Doppler ultrasound imaging is traditionally used for postoperative surveillance after carotid revascularization to evaluate patency or recurrent disease. Restenosis can occur after revascularizations due to in-stent restenosis or thrombosis in TCAR, intimal hyperplasia, thrombosis, or recurrent atherosclerotic disease after CEA.

Clinical Pearls

- The presence or absence of a carotid bruit does not correlate with the severity of extracranial carotid disease
- Patients with risk factors, or known coronary, neurovascular, or peripheral arterial disease should be screened for carotid artery disease
- *Symptomatology in conjunction with the degree of stenosis* will determine the need for carotid revascularization
- TCAR may be a good surgical option for high-risk surgical patients meeting TCAR criteria
- Ultrasound surveillance is needed after carotid intervention to assess for restenosis.

Diseases of the Aorta

Pathophysiology involving the aorta is common, well-studied, and has a myriad of clinical presentations and management options. Aortic aneurysms and aortic dissections are two of the most common causes of sudden cardiovascular death. They develop due to hemodynamic stress on the specific layers of the vessel in conjunction with a plethora of biochemical and cellular processes, including atherosclerosis, genetic predisposition, and other contributory cardiovascular/connective tissue comorbidities. There has been much research in detecting these disease processes and standardizing treatments, including operative treatments, endovascular interventions, and medical management. The following section covers the anatomy and physiology, pathophysiology, diagnosis, physical exam, management, and varying treatment options for aortic aneurysms and aortic dissections.

Aneurysm

Anatomy & Physiology

The term aneurysm describes dilatation of any blood vessel greater than 1.5× increase in diameter compared with the expected normal diameter. Excluding intracranial vessels, arterial aneurysms are most prevalent in the infrarenal aorta [3]. Aortic aneurysms are commonly associated with concomitant aneurysms of the ascending aorta, thoracic aorta, iliac, femoral, or popliteal arteries.

Arterial walls are made up of three layers: Tunica intima, media, and adventitia. A true aneurysm involves dilation of all intact layers of the arterial wall due to remodeling of the extracellular matrix (ECM) (Fig. 35.6).

Pathology/Description

Aneurysmal degeneration of the aorta is a multifactorial, systemic process generally felt to be due to alterations in vascular wall biology leading to a loss of vascular structural proteins (namely collagen) and wall strength. Biomechanical forces, including stress across the arterial wall, are also felt to play a role [4]. As the aorta enlarges, turbulent flow develops within the aneurysm due to the flow dynamics and can lead to thrombus formation along the aortic wall [5]. This can lead to distal embolization.

Classification

The shape of aneurysms is defined as fusiform or saccular. A fusiform aneurysm is a ballooning on all sides of the aorta, whereas a saccular aneurysm is a focal enlargement that is one-sided. A false aneurysm (pseudoaneurysm) develops from arterial injury with subsequent hematoma formation and does not involve all 3 layers of the arterial wall (Fig. 35.7).

Aneurysms can occur throughout the entirety of the aorta. Location of aneurysms includes the aortic root, ascending aorta, aortic arch, thoracoabdominal aorta (Type I, II, III, IV), suprarenal aorta, juxta renal and infrarenal aorta. Abdominal aortic aneurysms (AAAs) are a leading cause of death in the United States [3]. AAA are classified based on anatomical location, shape, and size (Fig. 35.8).

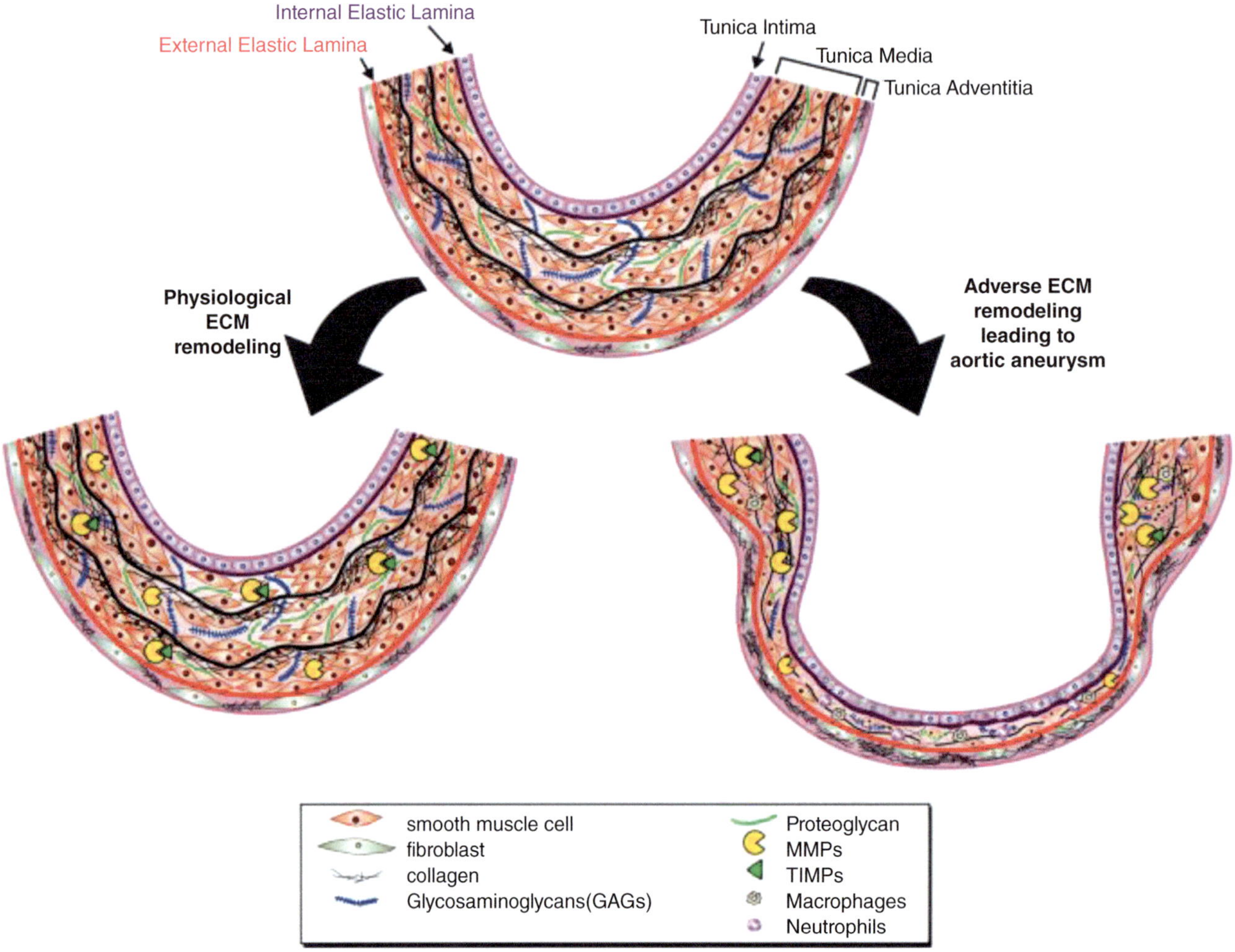

Fig. 35.6 Extracellular matrix, regional heterogeneity of the aorta, and aortic aneurysm. (Jana et al. [6])

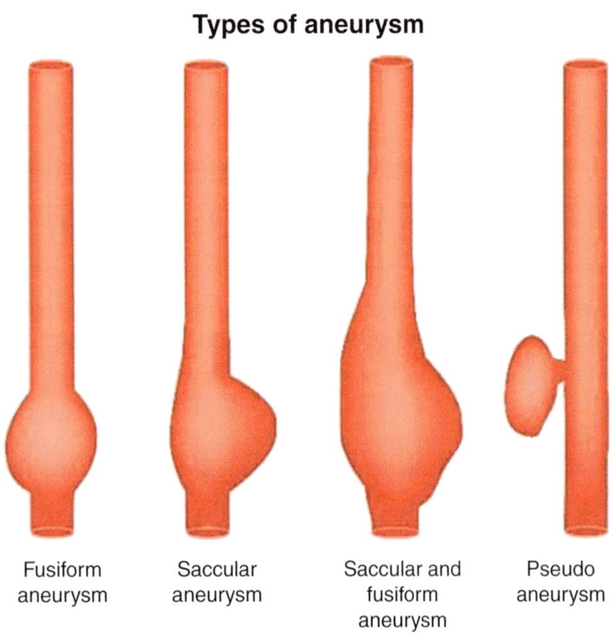

Fig. 35.7 The types of vascular aneurysms are shown, depicting their various forms

Depending on the location and size of the aneurysmal segment, the management and classification can vary. Aneurysm size is described by diameter and length, with diameter being the important risk factor for rupture (Table 35.4).

Risk Factors

Aortic aneurysms often occur in the setting of other concomitant diseases. Most AAAs are related to atherosclerotic *disease* (Table 35.5).

Incidence of AAA increases in males aged greater than 60 years and females aged greater than 70 years of age. Males are more likely to develop AAA than females. However, females are more likely to rupture at a smaller size than males [2]. Genetic conditions that are known to be associated with developing aortic aneurysms include **Ehlers–Danlos Syndrome (EDS)** and **Marfan's syndrome.** These conditions are more concerning in patients who present with aneurysms at a younger age. There is a high association between smoking and the development of an aneurysm.

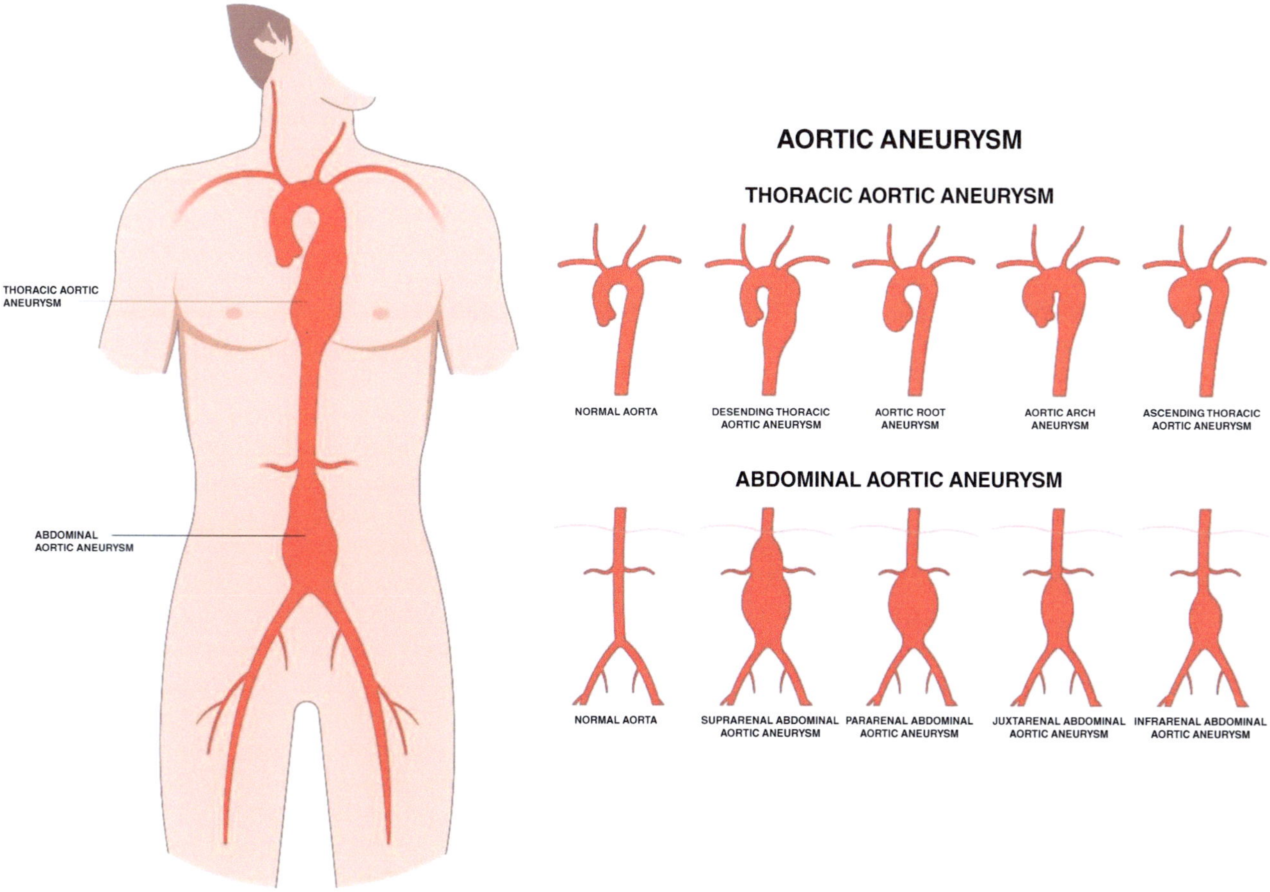

Fig. 35.8 Aortic aneurysm morphology and location

Table 35.4 Size and rupture risk [2]

Size of aneurysm	Annual risk of rupture
Small (3–3.9 cm)	No increased risk
Medium (4–4.9 cm);	1%
Large (5–5.9 cm)	5–10%
Very large (6–6.9 cm)	10–20%
Giant (7–7.9 cm)	20–40%
>8 cm	30–50%

Table 35.5 Risk factors for aneurysm development

Atherosclerotic disease	Any tobacco use
Family history	Male sex
Genetic predisposition	PAD/PVD
Autoimmune/inflammatory process	Remote aortic surgery
Infection	Hypertension
Age > 60 years	Caucasian race
Obesity	Trauma

Asymptomatic screening is recommended in patients with tobacco use.

Signs and Symptoms

AAAs are *commonly asymptomatic* and found incidentally during workup for other disease processes or on an age-related screening exam. Symptomatic patients can present with a wide array of symptoms. This may include abdominal, back, or flank pain. If there is evidence of a large AAA, the patient can present with obstructive symptoms such as Gastric Outlet Obstruction (GOO), nausea/vomiting, urinary symptoms due to obstruction of the ureters, and inferior vena cava compression and deep vein thrombosis (DVT). If an AAA has evidence of thrombus along the aortic wall, a patient may present with embolic changes (i.e., claudication, discoloration of toes and feet).

Physical Exam

When examining the vascular patient for a concern of aortic aneurysm, it is important to complete a *full* vascular exam. This includes a full abdominal examination, lower extremity and peripheral pulse examination, including palpation of the popliteal fossa for pulsatile masses, auscultation of carotid bruits, and cardiac auscultation. The provider must keep in mind the following list of physical exam findings as the patient may present with any of the following (Table 35.6). *Do not rely on a physical exam to diagnose a AAA since it is a difficult clinical diagnosis.* **Always check distal pulses** due to the risk of embolic disease and concomitant PAD.

Imaging

When working up a AAA, there are many different imaging modalities. Duplex ultrasound (DUS) is the modality of choice for screening and surveillance of AAA and lower extremity aneurysms [2]. This is also the cheapest and least invasive. It is not uncommon that an abdominal CT scan will be ordered for a patient during work up of abdominal pain revealing an incidental finding of AAA. Noncontrasted abdominal CT scans can help to identify AAAs but are not an ideal study for surgical planning. A CT angiography of the abdomen and pelvis is the most accurate modality for preoperative workup or concern for ruptured AAA. A CTA chest/abdomen/pelvis should be considered for any thoracic or thoracoabdominal aortic aneurysm. MRI of the lumbar spine can also help to identify AAA but are not ideal studies for AAA and are not appropriate for surgical planning (Fig. 35.9).

Management

Aortic aneurysms are managed medically with regular imaging surveillance until they reach the size criteria for surgical intervention. A goal of aneurysmal disease is early detection, surveillance, and elective repair to prevent complications of rupture, thrombosis, or embolism. The diagnosis and treatment will depend on the stability of the aneurysm [2]. Vascular surgery referral can be placed for any aortic aneurysm. Any incidence of ruptured aortic aneurysms requires emergent operative repair.

Medical management is indicated for stable aortic aneurysms of less than 5.5 cm in males and less than 5.0 cm in women. Modifiable risk factors in the medical management of aortic aneurysms include smoking cessation, management of hypertension, cholesterol, obesity, and atherosclerotic disease. Medical therapy includes antiplatelet therapy, statin drugs, and blood pressure management with a goal of normotension. Beta-blocker therapy is preferred as first line agent. Full anticoagulation is needed if thromboembolic disease distal to an aneurysm is identified with mural thrombus within the aneurysm. Avoid use of fluoroquinolones as they have been shown to increase the size of AAA and complications associated with rupture or dissection.

Once an aneurysm is diagnosed, DUS surveillance is obtained and is based on size and location (Table 35.7).

The timing of surgical intervention is often guided by the size of the aneurysm (Table 35.8).

Surgical intervention is then further defined based on endovascular repair versus open repair. EVAR is the most common repair but there are still cases in which open repair is preferred. Endovascular repair is defined as EVAR (endo-

Table 35.6 Physical findings consistent with AAA

Abdominal pulsatile mass	Enlarged popliteal pulse
Aortic bruit	Painful aortic palpation
Abdominal, inguinal, or flank pain	Embolic changes in lower extremity

Table 35.7 Aneurysm surveillance AAA

Aneurysm size	Duplex imaging frequency
<4.0 cm	Annually
4.0–5.0 cm	Every 6 months
>5.0	CTA

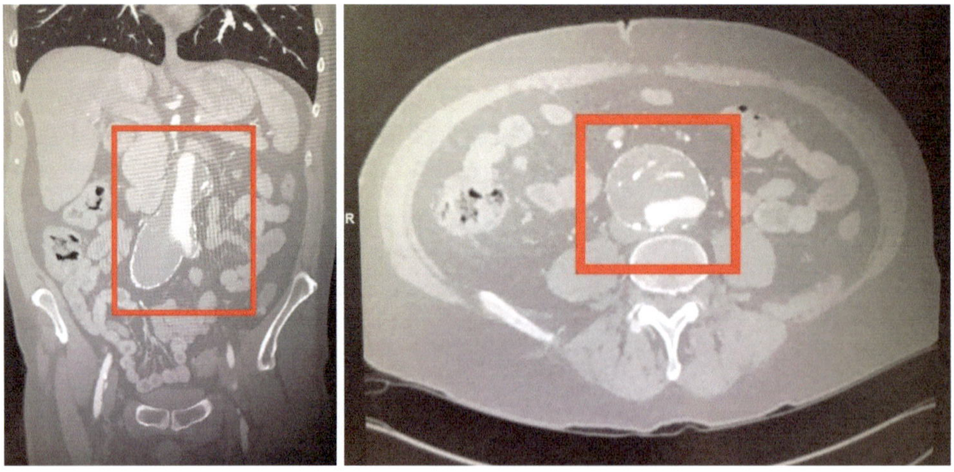

Fig. 35.9 Infrarenal AAA pre-EVAR with heavy thrombus (DARK) and atherosclerotic burden (calcification in wall of aorta) on CT imaging

vascular aortic repair), TEVAR (thoracic endovascular repair), and FEVAR (fenestrated endovascular aortic repair).

Open aortic repair is completed with aortic bypass grafting with either aortoiliac, aortobifemoral bypass graft, or straight aortic tube graft for patients without iliac artery involvement. Open repair may be indicated in younger patients who are otherwise healthy, patients with anatomy not conducive to EVAR, including short or angulated infrarenal aortic neck, and multiple branch vessels, increasing risk for endoleak. Patients with connective tissue disorders may be favored for open repair.

Endovascular aortic repair is completed via percutaneous or open arterial access. Straightforward EVAR can be completed with procedural sedation versus general sedation. Open access may be indicated in patients with concomitant peripheral arterial disease, small access vessels, or prior surgical interventions. Depending on the complexity of the repair, alternative access sites may also be indicated, including brachial artery or open axillary artery conduit. Repair is completed by placing a bifurcated endograft within the aorta, thereby excluding the aneurysm sac (Fig. 35.10). Prior to completion, a final angiogram is imaged to ensure no evidence of endoleak at the remainder of the case. Occasionally, assistive devices are used to aid with the seal zone, including fixation devices, coiling, or onyx glue, in patients with a short neck.

Open aortic repair is completed via midline or retroperitoneal incision (Fig. 35.11). The extent of repair is based on anatomical involvement of the iliac and femoral arteries or concomitant PAD. The incision is carried down to the abdominal cavity exposing the aorta. A retroperitoneal approach is performed with the patient in right lateral decubitus position through a left flank incision. The proximal and distal arteries are then clamped, repair is completed by replacing the aneurysmal segment with a synthetic graft, the aneurysm is then oversewn, and the abdomen is closed.

Table 35.8 Aneurysm size and indication for surgical intervention

Rapid growth 0.5 cm over 6 months
Ascending and abdominal >5.5 cm males, >5.0 cm females
Ascending and abdominal Marfan's > 5.0 cm male, 4.5 cm female
>4.5 cm ascending root if aortic valve disease involvement
Isolated aortic arch >5.5 cm
Popliteal >2.5 cm asymptomatic
Common iliac >3.5 cm asymptomatic

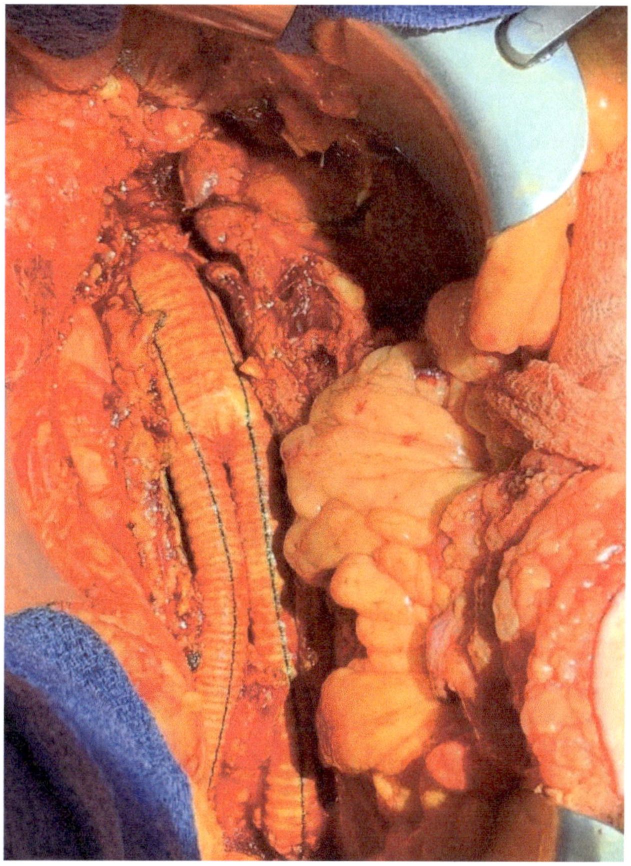

Fig. 35.11 Open aorto-bi-iliac bypass with Dacron graft

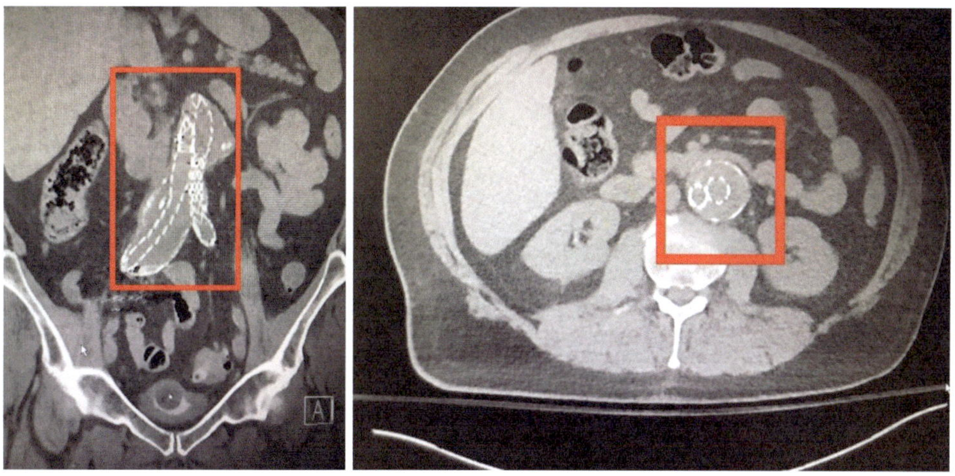

Fig. 35.10 EVAR treatment of AAA with exclusion of residual thrombus

Postoperative surveillance of EVAR of the infrarenal segment can be completed with aortic duplex in the vascular surgery clinic. An endoleak is defined as flow outside of the endograft and within the remaining AAA sac, risking continued aneurysm growth (Table 35.9).

Clinical Pearls

- Consider screening patients with risk factors for AAA given they are commonly asymptomatic.
- Fluroquinolones are contraindicated in patients with history of aortic aneurysm or dissection as there is an increased risk of aneurysm and dissection with this drug class.
- Consider TTE screening for ascending aortic aneurysm with new diagnosis of AAA and vice versa.
- Endocarditis prophylaxis should be recommended for any patient s/p aortic graft.
- There is risk for genetic inheritance of aneurysms, thus recommend family screening.

Table 35.9 Types of endoleaks (EL)

1 ab	Proximal (a) distal (b) graft attachment site leaks
2	Retrograde flow into the sac via aortic side branches (i.e., lumbar, mesenteric)
3	Defect in the graft either d/t fabric tear or disconnection of modular overlap
4	Graft wall porosity
5	Increase in maximum aneurysm diameter with no identifiable endoleak; endotension

Intervention is indicated for Types 1, 3 and 2 when EL sac with increasing aortic size

Aortic Dissection

Anatomy & Physiology

An aortic dissection is a tear within the layers of the aorta. The tear occurs within the intima, which causes a separation of the media, creating a new channel that is defined as the false lumen. The native channel is defined as the true lumen. Throughout the aortic dissection, there are many communications between the true and false lumen defined as fenestrations. The presence of an "intimal flap," representing the intimomedial septum between the true and false lumen, is the most characteristic pathology in acute aortic dissection [7] (Fig. 35.12). Aortic dissections are classified as acute versus chronic based onset timing and on the location of the entry tear. An acute aortic dissection is defined as the onset of symptoms within 2 weeks, subacute >14 days to 90 days, and chronic >90 days.

Historically, there were two classification systems: Debakey (1965) and Stanford (1970). The Debakey classification defines the intimal tear and the extent of aortic dissection. The standard Stanford classification describes only the tear and defines a type A as involving the proximal aorta or type B (TBAD), which is distal to the left subclavian artery [7] (Fig. 35.13).

DeBakey

- Type 1. Dissection originates in the ascending aorta, extending to descending and abdominal aorta

Type 2. Dissection originates and is confined to the ascending alone

Type 3. Dissection originates in the descending aorta

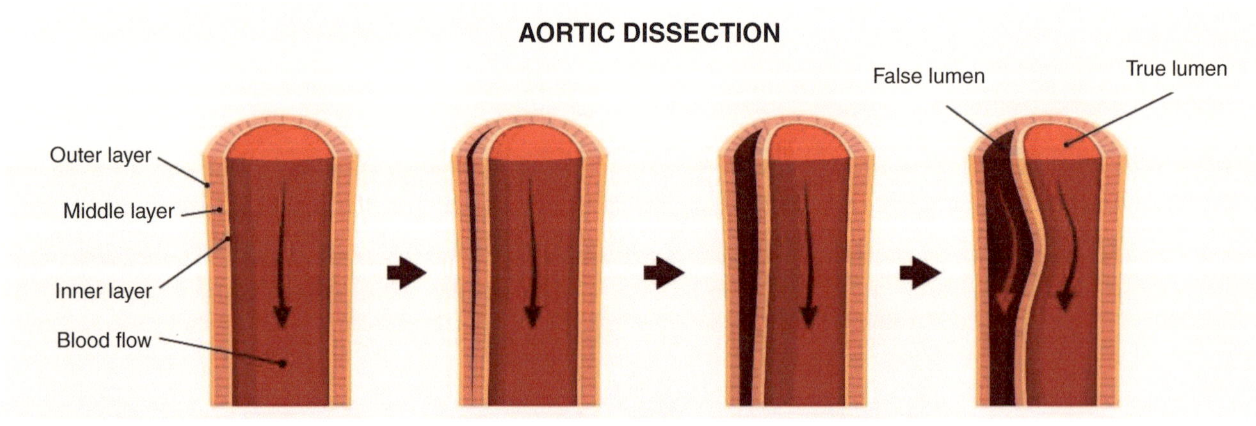

Fig. 35.12 Development and progression of aortic dissection

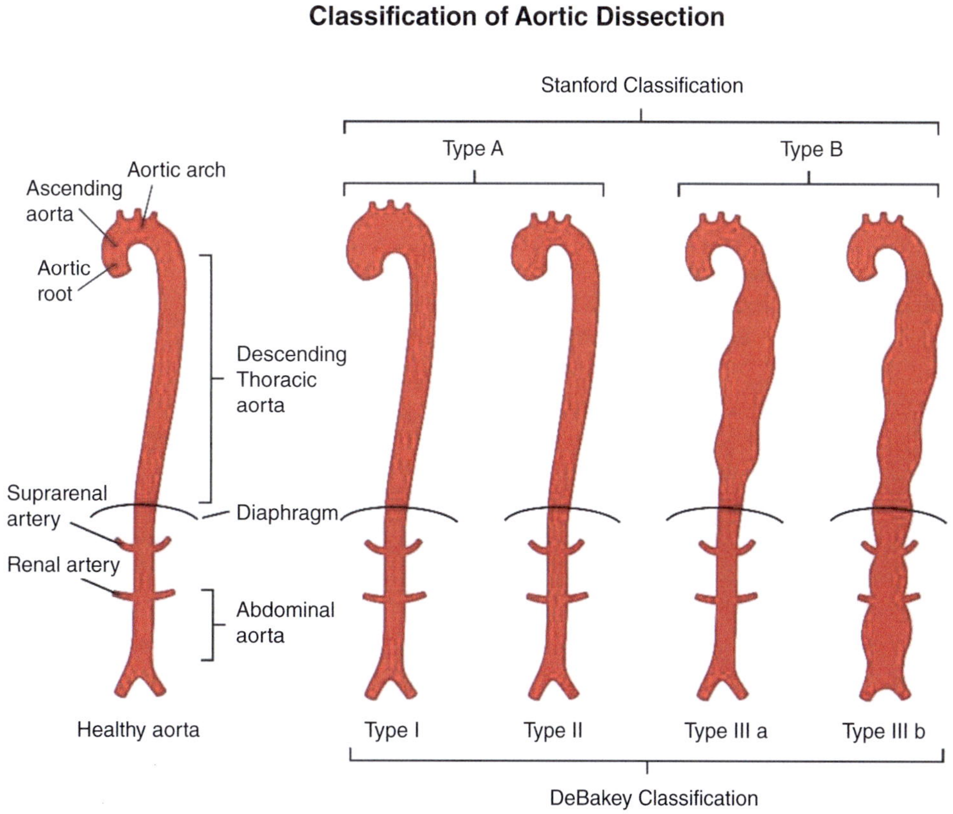

Fig. 35.13 Dissection classification: Stanford and Debakey

3a = supra-diaphragm
3b = below diaphragm

The newest classification system as defined by the Society for Vascular Surgery (SVS) in 2020 helps to overcome previous limitations and further develop more accurate communication when describing the complex aortic dissection patient. Within the new SVS classification scheme for aortic dissection, the distinction between **Type A** and **Type B** is predicated on entry tear location alone and defined in zones [8].

When discussing aortic syndromes, intramural hematoma (IMH) as well as the penetrating aortic ulcer (PAU) should also be included. IMH does not have a clear tear or communication as an aortic dissection but rather appears as hemorrhage within the aortic wall [8]. A PAU is defined as atherosclerotic plaque that penetrates the aortic wall. PAU rupture risk is directly associated with the ulcer depth [8].

Pathology/Description

The process of an aortic dissection is dynamic; therefore, it can occur anywhere along the aorta and present with an array of symptoms. The entry tear occurs within the intima and media layers of the aortic wall, creating an intimal flap in which blood rushes into the space both proximal and distal with multiple fenestrations between layers [7]. Rupture of the intima and media is the initial event in most cases of aortic dissection. The violation of the intimal surface results in the formation of a cleavage plane into the outer media and subsequent propagation for a varying distance in this plane, either antegrade or retrograde [7] (Fig. 35.12).

Aortic dissections are classified as complicated versus uncomplicated. Complicated dissections are defined by malperfusion of end organs, true lumen compression, aneurysmal degeneration, uncontrolled pain, or aortic rupture.

Risk Factors for Dissection (Table 35.10)

Physical Exam

The patient may present with a wide array of symptoms. The classic description is described as a ripping, tearing, sharp, "worst ever" anterior chest or back pain. There may be evidence of an anxious appearing patient with tachycardia and tachypnea. If there is a flow-limiting dissection, the patient can present with hypoperfusion symptoms and commonly abdominal pain. The medical provider should always obtain blood pressure readings in both upper extremities as the patient may present with loss of pulses to extremities, which could represent ischemia. Always complete a thorough cardiac exam and auscultate for a cardiac murmur. If the dissection involves the intracranial vessel, there could be evidence of neurologic changes presenting with stroke, Horner's syndrome, voice hoarseness, and spinal cord ischemia.

Imaging

When working up aortic dissections, consider the following imaging modalities. The gold standard imaging is a CT angiogram of the chest, abdomen, and pelvis. An acute dissection flap (Fig. 35.14) is thin in appearance compared with a chronic dissection, which will appear as a clearly defined dissection flap that usually is thicker and more dense [8]. IMH will appear as a hyperdensity within the aortic wall. PAU will appear as an atherosclerotic lesion with ulcer like projection within the aortic wall. A chest X-ray can reveal widening of the cardiac or aortic silhouette with widened mediastinum. A TTE or TEE can be used to evaluate for any evidence of cardiac tamponade or aortic insufficiency in the setting of a type A aortic dissection. A TTE should be ordered with diagnosis of acute aortic dissection. MR angiograms are not recommended. An EKG should always be obtained in the setting of acute Type A Aortic Dissection. Proximal dissection into a coronary artery (RCA) can create STEMI in addition to aortic dissection.

Table 35.10 Risk factors for dissection

Uncontrolled and sudden variation in blood pressure
Cocaine
Pregnancy
Genetic predisposition (Marfan, Ehlers–Danlos Syndrome (EDS), Loeys–Dietz syndrome (LD)
Blunt Force Trauma
Bicuspid aortic valve
Inflammatory conditions of Giant Cell Arteritis (GCA), Takayasu arteritis

Management

Prompt diagnosis and management are key; aortic dissections are associated with high morbidity and mortality. Type B aortic dissections are either managed medically or occasionally surgically. The cornerstone of medical therapy is the reduction of arterial blood pressure [7]. Acute aortic dissection patients will be admitted to the ICU for anti-impulse therapy and vasodilator therapy. Beta Blockade (labetalol or esmolol) is always initiated first, as vasodilators can cause a reflex tachycardia, which can worsen the dissection. Intravenous nicardipine is commonly used as a vasodilator. The goal is prompt control of heart rate and systolic blood pressure goal <120 mmHg or HR < 70 bpm.

Urgent surgical repair is indicated for acute type A aortic dissections because medical treatment is associated with 60% in-hospital death rate [7]. The anatomic goal is resection of the aortic intimal tear to eliminate the threat of rupture and to reconstruct the aortic wall layers. Type A dissection may require aortic valve repair/replacement, aortic root/aortic arch/hemiarch repair/replacement. Acute tamponade may develop with dissection into the pericardium. This is a surgical emergency, and pericardial tap should be avoided as this may worsen hemodynamic collapse and delay emergent surgical intervention.

In patients with uncomplicated type B dissection (TBAD), surgical therapy has not shown superiority over medical therapy [7]. Therefore, most TBAD are managed medically if uncomplicated. The goal of medical therapy is anti-impulse control, pain control, and evaluation for malperfusion or disease progression. TEVAR or surgical intervention may be warranted in TBAD with persistent/recurring pain, uncon-

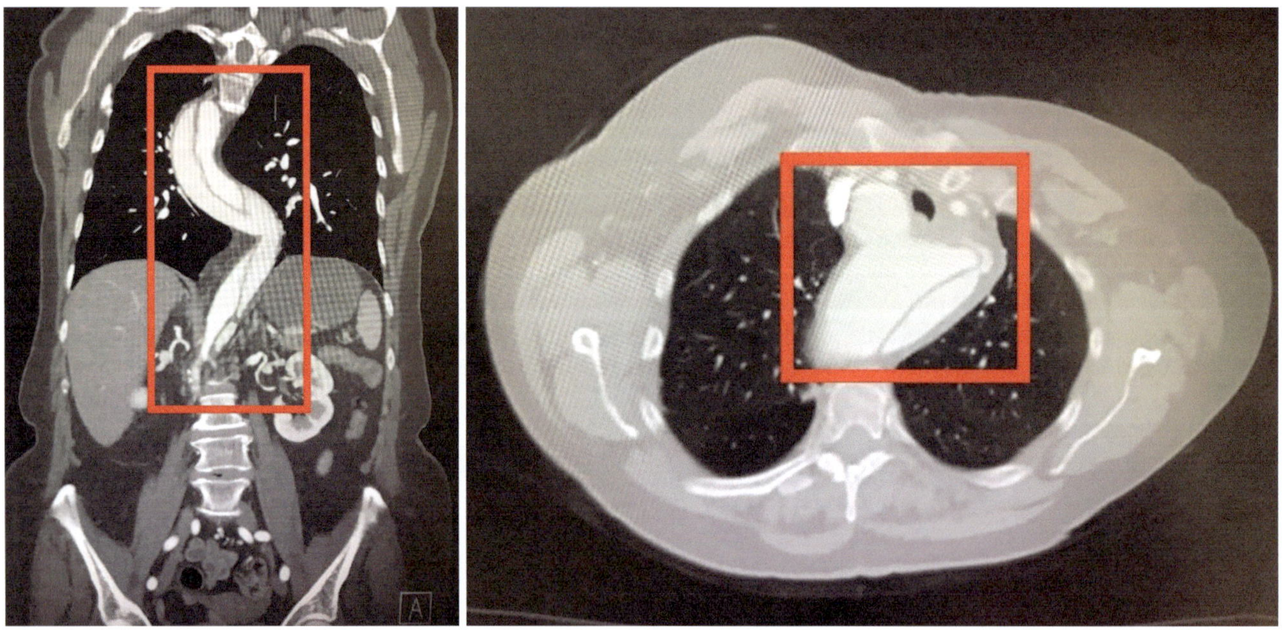

Fig. 35.14 CTA with acute thoracic aortic dissection

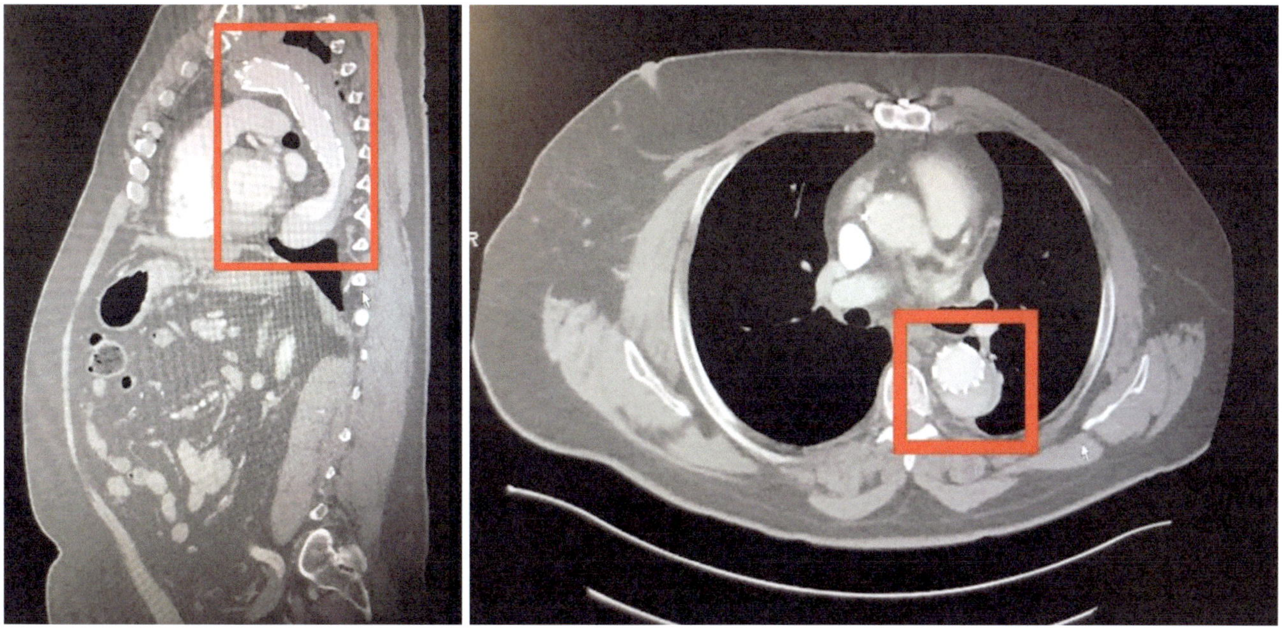

Fig. 35.15 TEVAR within true lumen excluding thrombus in false lumen

trolled hypertension despite medical therapies, advancing aortic expansion or any evidence of malperfusion. A TEVAR may be performed to prevent late complications and promote aortic remodeling as well. During this procedure, a stent graft is deployed in the true lumen to cover the entry tear with the goal of improving aortic perfusion and encouraging thrombosis of the false lumen (Fig. 35.15).

Surveillance

The principal late complication of aortic dissection is aneurysmal dilatation of the outer wall of the false lumen [7]. Regular follow-up with serial imaging for routine surveillance is recommended lifelong with a vascular surgery clinic. False lumen patency or thrombosis is an important predictor of regional luminal growth and reintervention rate [8]. In follow-up, the maximal aortic diameter is documented and followed over time. Patients with aortic dissection undergo at least annual surveillance with CT angiogram.

Clinical Pearls

- Patients diagnosed with aortic dissection should be referred to an aortic center when possible.
- Anti-impulse therapy is the mainstay of treatment for heart rate and blood pressure in patients with aortic dissection.
- A bicuspid aortic valve is associated with increased risk of aortic dissection and thoracic aortic aneurysm.
- Genetic referral for screening should be considered in patients with acute aortic dissections, especially in the younger population.

Peripheral Vascular Disease

In this section, we will review two of the most common peripheral vascular disease processes: peripheral arterial disease (PAD) and deep vein thrombosis (DVT). These can be progressive disease states with long-lasting effects if left untreated. It is important to recognize and diagnose PAD or DVT to prevent lifelong debilitation, reduced functional status, and quality of life or limb loss. First, we will review anatomy and pathophysiology, followed by physical exam findings, diagnostic imaging, and management. Surgical intervention may be indicated for patients with PAD who present with lifestyle-limiting symptoms, ischemic pain, or tissue loss. Patients with DVT may require surgical intervention to reduce long lasting impacts of post-thrombotic syndrome. For patients that do not require surgical intervention will require optimal medical therapy.

Peripheral Arterial Disease (PAD)

Anatomy

The body's circulatory system is made of an amazing network of vessels. Systemic arteries bring oxygenated blood flow from the heart to all the tissues and organs throughout the body, through tiny capillaries, and back to the heart via the venous system. The arterial system is continuous from the heart and structured to accommodate the high pressures of blood being ejected from the heart with each heartbeat. Arteries have three layers, the innermost being the intima, which is lined with endothelium. This single-celled layer is a continuous layer present throughout the arteries, capillaries, veins, heart valves, and endocardial surfaces. The intima secretes multiple factors that adjust vessel tone (vasodilation) and affect platelet aggregation and formation of thrombus. The middle layer, or media, of arteries is made of smooth muscles, elastin, and collagen, and it responds to signals along the intima. The outermost wall of arteries is the adventitia, made up of long fibrinous collagen chains, autonomic nerves, and vasa vasorum (perfuse external walls of larger vessels) (*see* Fig. 35.6).

When evaluating the total arterial anatomy (Fig. 35.16), it may be easiest to start from the heart, and follow the aortic arch into the brachiocephalic, common carotids, and subclavian arteries, and continue into the head/neck /chest. These arteries are also called the great vessels. From the subclavian arteries, the arm will further perfuse via the axillary, brachial, radial, and ulnar arteries into the palmar arch and smaller arteries of the hands. Blood flow continues to the descending aorta just left of the left subclavian artery, and follows the thoracic aorta through the chest, and past the diaphragm, where the abdominal aorta will lead you to the visceral segment. Here you will find the celiac, superior mesenteric, bilateral renal, and inferior mesenteric arteries that supply blood flow to structures and organs of the abdomen. Proceed distally, and you will reach the common iliac arteries, where the aorta bifurcates into smaller arteries of the pelvis and provides inflow to the bilateral lower extremities. The iliac arteries will bifurcate into internal and external iliac arteries, and then continue to the femoral arteries. The common femoral arteries will bifurcate into the profunda and superficial femoral arteries. The superficial femoral arteries will travel along the medial thighs posteriorly behind the knee, where the popliteal artery will lead to the tibioperoneal trunk, the peroneal artery, the posterior tibial artery, and the anterior tibial artery. These distal arteries will then perfuse the arteries of the foot (Fig. 35.17).

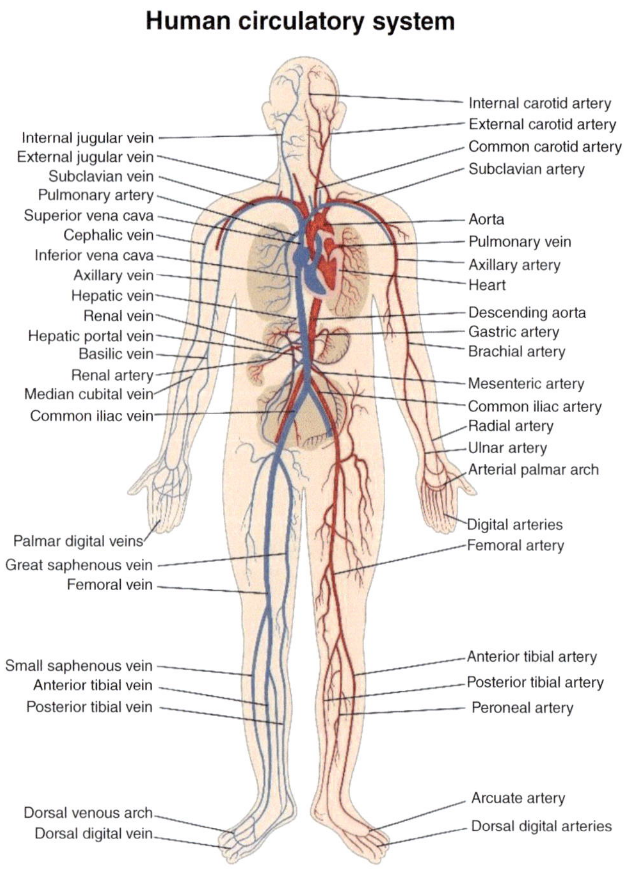

Fig. 35.16 Human Circulatory System

Physical Examination

A clinician's physical exam should be thorough to best evaluate for PAD, as well as to determine the potential need for intervention. Upon inspection, a clinician may appreciate muscle atrophy, hair loss, color changes (cyanosis or pallor), ischemic tissue changes, wounds, or decreased motor function of an area affected by arterial insufficiency. When palpating, the clinician may note cooler temperatures along the skin, which may correspond with the level of disease. The clinician should evaluate motion and sensation along the extremities, including hands, fingers, feet, and toes, where the most distal arteries may be compromised. A clinician should evaluate their patient for palpable pulses (brachial, radial, ulnar, femoral, popliteal, posterior tibial, and dorsalis pedis), their quality, and if there is variation in laterality.

Pulse may be qualified as: 0—Absent, 1—Diminished, 2—Normal, 3—Bounding

If pulses are nonpalpable, a clinician can further evaluate with a handheld Doppler while listening to the quality of arterial signals in the same anatomical locations—these may be described as triphasic, biphasic, monophasic, or absent arterial signals. In addition to auscultation via Doppler, a clinician may apply the bell of a stethoscope to evaluate for turbulent blood flow (i.e., bruit), which could indicate stenosis, fistula, and other vascular pathologies.

Pathology/Pathophysiology

Peripheral Arterial Disease (PAD) is a condition that is caused by atherosclerosis, which reduces tissue perfusion over time. Atherosclerosis is the pathophysiologic process of accumulation of lipids and fibrous materials between the layers of the arterial wall, reducing the diameter of the arterial lumen, thereby limiting arterial blood flow to tissue. This development of atherosclerosis over time leads to the formation of plaque, which can eventually thrombose or rupture, causing occlusion of distal vessels (Fig. 35.18). PAD affects the lower extremities more often than the upper; however, PAD may occur anywhere in the body and manifests through

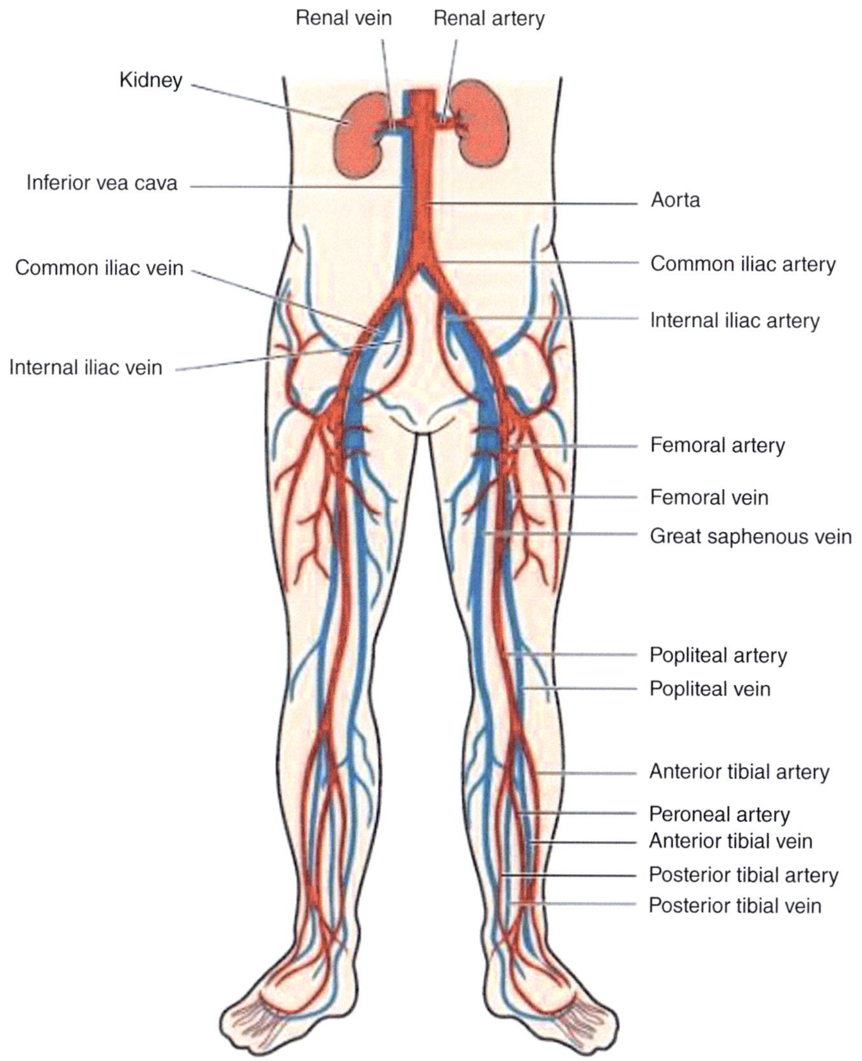

Fig. 35.17 Lower extremity vasculature

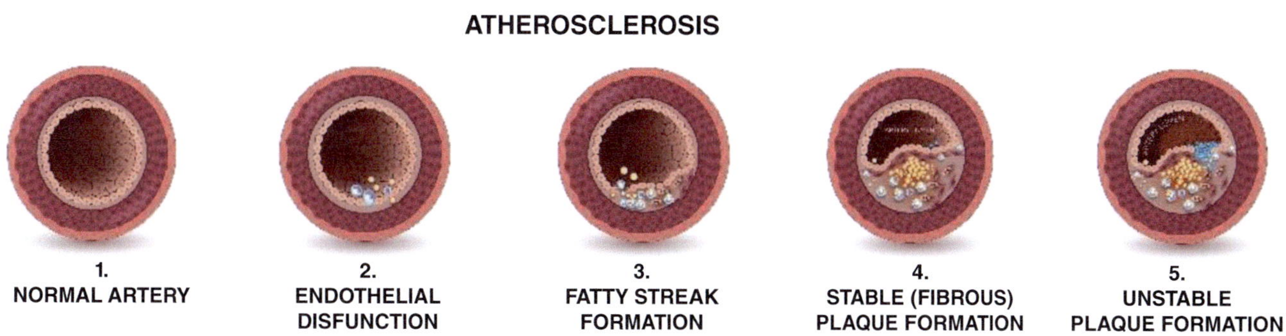

Fig. 35.18 PAD progression of arterial disease

varying degrees of symptoms based on the severity of the disease, as well as collateralized blood flow. PAD is a chronic and progressive disease in which the severity of symptoms will worsen with time if not appropriately managed. In its mildest form, patients may present with abnormal test results but without symptoms. In mild to moderate disease, patients may experience symptoms such as nonlimiting or limiting claudication. The Rutherford Classification System is the gold standard among most vascular practices within the United States to aid in classifying the severity of claudication (Fig. 35.19).

Patients who suffer from severe disease may develop tissue injury, nonhealing wounds, or ischemic pain. Patients who suffer from ruptured atherosclerotic plaque may present with acute limb ischemia and need to be revascularized quickly to minimize irreversible ischemic injury—please refer to the Rutherford classification of acute limb ischemia (Fig. 35.20).

Grade	Category	Clinical description
I	0	Asymptomatic; not hemodynamically correct
	1	Mild claudication
	2	Moderate claudication
	3	Severe claudication
II	4	Ischemic rest pain
	5	Minor tissue loss; non-healing ulcer, focal gangrene with diffuse pedal ischemia
III	6	Major tissue loss extending above transmetatarsal level; foot no longer salvageable

Fig. 35.19 The Rutherford classification system of claudication

Imaging/Diagnostic Testing

Ankle Brachial Index

Physiologic testing is used to establish the diagnosis of PAD. Depending on the specific type of testing, this can assist in defining the severity and extent of disease in patients with risk factors or suspicion for PAD. A cost-effective, easily available, and appropriate diagnostic tool to first evaluate a patient for PAD is by obtaining an Ankle Brachial Index (ABI). This simple and noninvasive test can determine the presence and extent of PAD. An ABI can be calculated on each leg by using the systolic blood pressure at the ankle, divided by the highest brachial systolic blood pressure (Fig. 35.21).

A normal ABI is > or = to 1 as the systolic blood pressure in the ankle is typically higher than in the arm. An ABI of < or = to 0.9 is diagnostic of the presence of PAD. An ABI of 0.4 to 0.9 is suggestive of a degree of arterial obstruction often associated with claudication. An ABI of less than 0.4 represents severe, multilevel disease that risks nonhealing ulcerations, ischemic rest pain, and pedal gangrene (Fig. 35.20). ABI results of >1.3 are falsely/artificially elevated, which signifies that the lower extremity ankle arteries are calcified and/or noncompressible. In this case, the values recorded are considered nondiagnostic. If the values are nondiagnostic, then the use of toe brachial indices (TBI) and toe pressures (TP) becomes even more valuable in predicting the ability to heal a current wound. TBIs are obtained by placing a pneumatic cuff on one of the toes (usually the great toe) (Table 35.11).

Grade	Category	Sensory loss	Motor deficit	Prognosis	Doppler signals	
					Arterial	Venous
I	Viable	None	None	No immediate threat	Audible	Audible
IIA	Marginally threatened	None or minimal (toes)	None	Salvageable if promptly treated	Inaudible*	Audible
IIB	Immediately threatened	More than toes	Mild/moderate	Salvageable if prompty revascularised	Inaudible	Audible
III	Irreversible	Perfound, anaesthetic	Perfound, paralysis (rigor*)	Major tissue loss amputadon. Permanent nerve damage inevitable	Inaudible	Inaudible

This is an identical replica of the table in the 1997 publication by Rutherford *et al.*,[2] with the exception of the asterisks (*).
* In the original 1997 classification it was stated that arterial Doppler sounds are never present in Stage IIA, and that rigor (mortis) is always present in Stage III. However, it is the opinion of the Writing Committee that exceptions to these rules do exist, and a slight modification of the Rutherforcd classification from 1997 may be appropriate in the future.

Fig. 35.20 Rutherford classification of acute limb ischemia

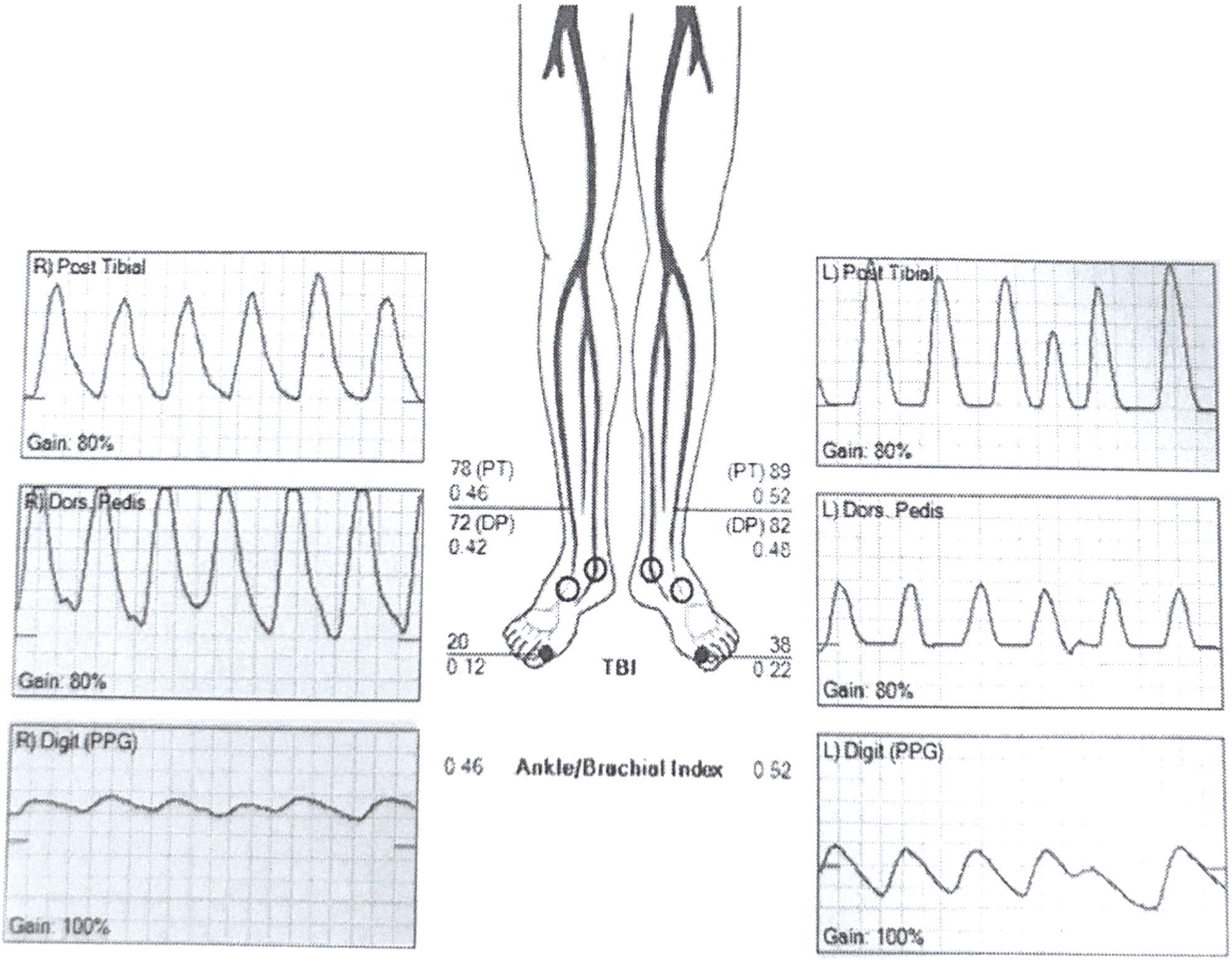

Fig. 35.21 Performance and interpretation of ABIHighest brachial systolic pressure was 169 mmHg. Right posterior tibial (PT) measured pressure of 78 mmHg and ABI of 0.46 suggestive of PAD. ABI of left extremity is also abnormal at 0.52. Toe pressures are significantly abnormal bilaterally suggestive of impaired wound healing

Table 35.11 Toe pressure utilization for nondiagnostic ABI> 1.3

Toe Brachial Index 0.7–0.8 normal
Toe pressure > 30 mmHg in diabetic favorable wound healing
Toe pressure > 50 mmHg nondiabetic favorable wound healing

Arterial Duplex Ultrasound

Arterial duplex ultrasound is considered the mainstay and often the initial noninvasive vascular imaging obtained when PAD is suspected. Duplex evaluation visualizes perfusion through the arteries in real time and measures peak systolic velocities (PSV) of arterial blood flow. Ratios are then determined from the change in PSV, which indicates a particular degree of stenosis.

Computed Tomography Angiography (CTA)

CT imaging uses contrast to obtain a large series of still images to better visualize and evaluate arterial blood flow. CTA can be used when considering an open operative approach or concern for inability to cannulate for endovascular intervention. CT evaluation requires intravenous contrast for adequate visualization of vessels; thus, consider the risk of contrast exposure in renal patients.

Management

Medical management and risk factor modification are crucial in maintaining vascular wellness, reducing complications and recurrent ischemic events, minimizing atherosclerotic progression, and achieving limb salvage. Medical therapies may include antiplatelet therapy, lipid-lowering agents (statins), and full anticoagulation when deemed appropriate. High-dose/high-potency statin therapy is recommended for all patients with atherosclerotic disease regardless of baseline LDL level. Hypertension impacts plaque formation; thus, adequate blood pressure management according to guidelines is important. Glucose management in diabetics is important for long-term vascular health, as well as minimizing the risk of lower extremity wounds. Tobacco cessation is important for overall cardiovascular health, as well as maintaining patency of prior vascular interventions. Lifestyle modification should also include regular exercise or implementing a regular walking program. Many patients can avoid (or at least delay) the need for endovascular or surgical intervention by adhering to a walking program and successfully modifying risk factors.

Currently, there is no definitive evidence for the efficacy of aspirin in patients with asymptomatic PAD. The guidelines vary in their treatment recommendations for patients with asymptomatic PAD. The American Heart Association/American College of Cardiology PAD guideline recommends antiplatelet therapy as reasonable if the ankle-brachial index is ≤0.90; the European Society of Cardiology guideline recommends against routine antiplatelet therapy in asymptomatic patients; and the Society for Vascular Surgery guideline provides no specific recommendations for this. Patients with symptomatic PAD should be treated with antithrombotic therapy to reduce cardiovascular risk. Single antiplatelet therapy with either aspirin or clopidogrel is recommended. Patients who undergo revascularization for PAD should be prescribed lifelong antithrombotic therapy. With respect to surgical revascularization, aspirin, clopidogrel, and rivaroxaban plus aspirin are all reasonable strategies [16].

Revascularization management and procedures of the lower extremities include a variety of endovascular and open surgical techniques. Age, risk factors, acute vs chronic disease, and a multitude of variables are considered in a patient's plan of care. Generally, the endovascular approach is preferred over an open surgery procedure. An endovascular approach consists of a surgeon evaluating and treating arterial blockages from within the lumen of an artery. After accessing the artery, an angiogram will be performed to visualize disease along the vessel, then interventions such as angioplasty, atherectomy, thrombectomy, drug-coated balloon angioplasty, stenting, and administration of medications (i.e., nitroglycerin, thrombolytics) may be performed (Figs. 35.22 and 35.23).

There are multiple open revascularization options depending on a patient's extent of disease. Some examples of open surgical revascularization are provided below:

- Aortobifemoral bypass—performed to treat aortoiliac occlusive disease or aneurysmal disease. A bypass is placed from the aorta to both femoral arteries.
- Iliofemoral bypass—used to treat iliofemoral occlusive disease. A bypass is placed from the iliac to femoral artery.

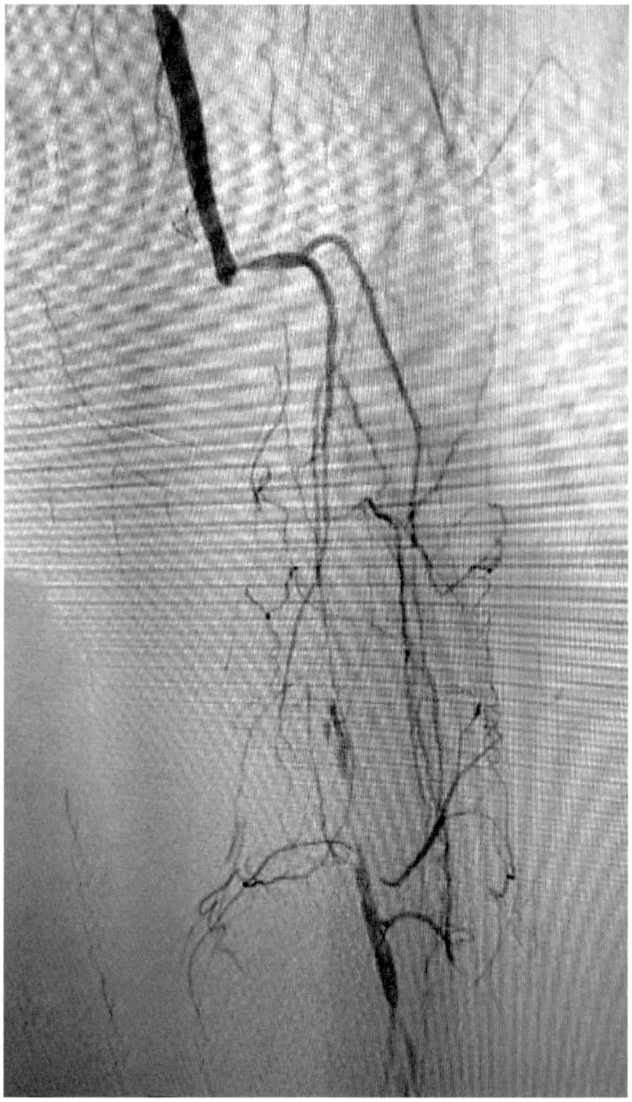

Fig. 35.22 Occluded superficial femoral artery (SFA)

- Axillofemoral bypass—extra-anatomic bypass performed axillary artery to the femoral artery. Lower patency rates long-term.

Revascularization may be performed using autologous vein harvest, synthetic material, or donor vessel.

Autogenous Vein conduit bypass—Generally are preferred over synthetic grafts.

Prosthetic conduit bypass—have an increased risk of needing graft explantation and infection.

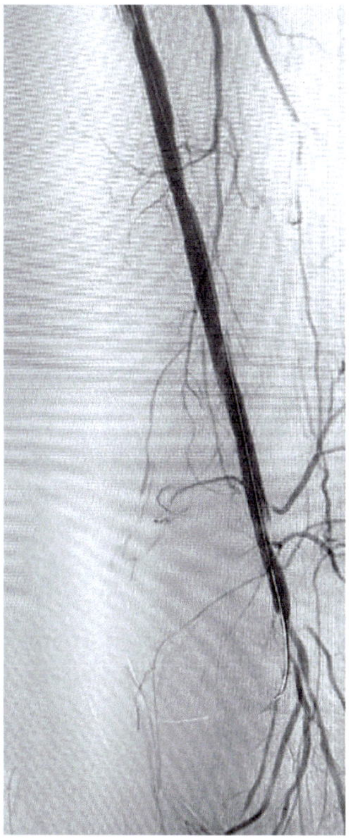

Fig. 35.23 SFA after percutaneous revascularization

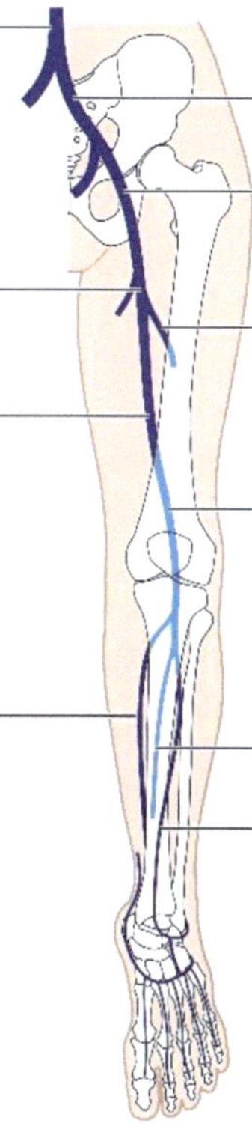

Fig. 35.24 Deep veins of lower extremity

Surveillance

Patients having undergone vascular intervention will need lifelong management and surveillance. This is often done with duplex ultrasound follow-up at least annually. CTA may be more appropriate for certain patients. Ankle and toe brachial index pressures are typically followed long-term for reassessment of trending patient's baseline arterial flow. At every follow-up, symptoms are evaluated in conjunction with testing results to determine the potential need for reintervention. It is important to maintain close follow-up as the patient will require lifelong medical therapy and potentially require repeat intervention.

Clinical Pearls

- Critical Limb Ischemia (CLI) is a classification of severe peripheral arterial disease. These patients suffer ischemic rest pain and/or tissue loss. If revascularization is unsuccessful, amputation may be needed.
- Patients with severe PAD, as evidenced by testing, may not require surgical intervention if asymptomatic, but warrant medical management.
- Patients with severe peripheral arterial disease should be considered for screening of disease in other vascular beds (neurovascular, coronary, carotid).
- After revascularization in patient with acute limb ischemia, evaluate for compartment syndrome, an acute process that leads to repeat occlusion of arterial perfusion and potential nerve damage.

Deep Vein Thrombosis

Anatomy & Physiology

Deep vein thrombosis (DVT) is when thrombus forms within a deep vein of the leg. Deep veins are identified as they have corresponding arterial vessels, whereas superficial veins do not (Fig. 35.24).

Superficial veins can be found in the subcutaneous tissues, while deep veins travel among muscles and bones below the fascia. Perforator veins drain superficial venous blood flow into the deep vein system. Veins differ from arteries in that they are a low-flow system, have a thin muscular wall, and blood is traveling against gravity. Veins have one-way valves, which prevent regurgitation of blood flow back down the leg while it travels back to the heart for recirculation. Skeletal muscle contraction of the lower extremities also aids in the propulsion of blood flow up through the low-flow venous system. DVTs are more common in the lower extremities due to the flow against gravity.

DVTs should be classified as either provoked or unprovoked, which guides management. Anatomical location of DVT also helps guide management, taking into consideration proximal or distal involvement in the extremities [9] (Table 35.12).

A myriad of other complications may arise from DVT, including post-thrombotic syndrome (PTS), venous insufficiency, venous wound development (venous stasis ulceration), and potential limb loss.

Post-thrombotic syndrome (PTS) occurs in 20–50% of patients with DVT, with 5% developing severe PTS [5]. Patients can develop chronic leg pain, itching, neuropathy, erythema, edema, ulcers, and limited activity tolerance (Table 35.13). PTS is managed with compression garments (usually 30–40 mmHg), wound care, and medical therapy (i.e., moisturizer, topical steroids, anti-inflammatories) [10].

Physical Exam

Patients with DVT may exhibit swelling, tenderness, erythema, firmness along the leg, as well as a positive Homan's sign. Patients with Homan's sign experience increased calf pain with dorsiflexion of the foot; however, this is a poor predictor of DVT.

Pathology/Description

DVTs can develop due to stasis of blood flow within the deep vein system, endothelial injury, or because of a hypercoagulable state, known as Virchow's Triad. DVTs occur in 300,000–600,000 people in the United States per year [13]. For common risk factors, see Table 35.14 below.

Symptoms will develop in the affected limb. Most patients will experience pain, swelling, warmth, erythema, hyperpigmentation, aching, throbbing, and limb heaviness. If patients experience chest pain, shortness of breath, tachypnea, tachycardia, or unexplained cough with DVT, they should be screened for pulmonary embolus [11] (Chap. 22).

Table 35.12 DVT location and risk

Proximal—Higher risk of PE and mortality	Distal—Lower risk
Iliac	Peroneal
Femoral	Posterior Tibial
Popliteal	Anterior Tibial

Table 35.13 Risk factors for post-thrombotic syndrome (PTS)

DVT above the knee
Recurrent DVT in the ipsilateral limb
Persistent symptoms beyond 1 month of therapy
Therapy noncompliance/subtherapeutic AC levels
Obesity
Residual thrombus

Imaging and Diagnosis

D-dimer can be tested, but it is not recommended given its low specificity. Diagnosis of DVT is obtained via visualization of the thrombus in the vein. Venous duplex for evaluation of DVT is the gold standard (Figs. 35.25 and 35.26); however, computed tomography venography (CTV) can also be obtained (Fig. 35.27). Interventional venogram can be diagnostic, as well as therapeutic. Patients who have unprovoked DVT should undergo a hypercoagulable workup. EKG, echocardiogram (to evaluate for right heart strain), CT angiography of the chest, or ventilation-perfusion (VQ) scan may be used to evaluate for pulmonary embolism.

Management

The aim of DVT management is to reduce the risk of thrombus propagation, embolization, relieve acute symptoms, and reduce the risk of lasting complications [14]. DVTs are managed with anticoagulation (AC). Intravenous options for this include systemic regular-dose unfractionated heparin in the acute setting. Therapeutic low molecular weight heparin (enoxaparin) or oral anticoagulation can be used in the acute, subacute, or chronic phase. Oral anticoagulants include direct-acting oral anticoagulants (DOACs) (Apixaban, dabigatran, edoxaban, rivaroxaban) or warfarin (vitamin k antagonists-VKA).

The CHEST Guidelines can help aid clinician decision-making based on DVT classification. CHEST recommends serial imaging (weekly venous ultrasound) for 2 weeks instead of anticoagulation in patients with isolated **distal DVT** of the leg without severe symptoms or risk factors for extension. Upon repeat imaging, AC is not recommended if no extension is seen, and is recommended if thrombus has propagated (even if remaining in the distal veins).

CHEST recommends AC for patients with isolated DVTs who are experiencing severe symptoms. Apixaban, dabigatran, edoxaban, or rivaroxaban over VKA is recommended in the first 3 months (treatment phase), and AC alone over inter-

Table 35.14 Risk factors for DVT

Family history/genetics	History of prior thrombotic event
Malignancy	Spinal cord injury/paralysis
African American race	Tobacco use
Oral contraceptives	Pregnancy (6 weeks postpartum)
Surgery within 3 months	Venous Catheters
Prolonged immobility-travel, cast	Hospitalization
Age > 40 yrs. and risk doubles with every 10 yrs.	Hypertension
Congestive heart failure	Sickle cell disease
Autoimmune disorders	Hypercoagulable states

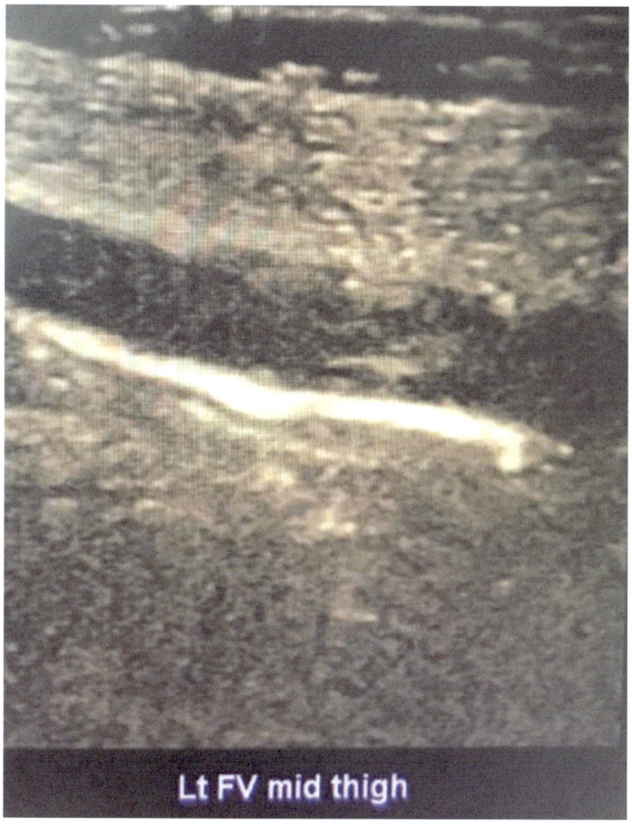

Fig. 35.25 Femoral vein imaging on venous duplex scan

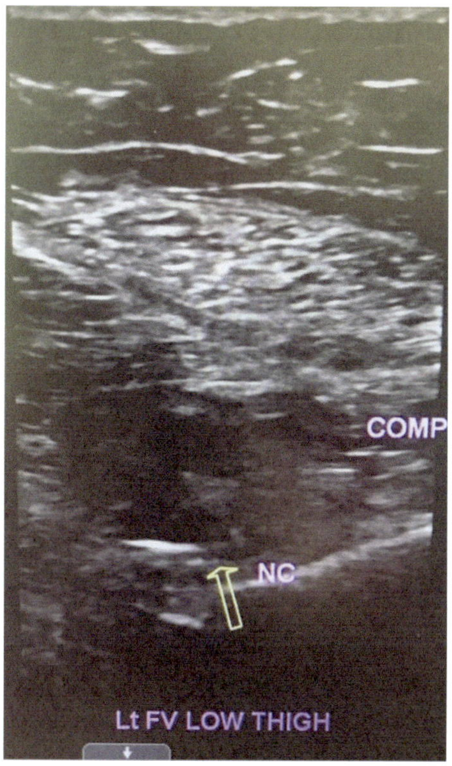

Fig. 35.26 Femoral vein that does not collapse with pressureThe lack of compression is suggestive of thrombus and DVT at the yellow arrow

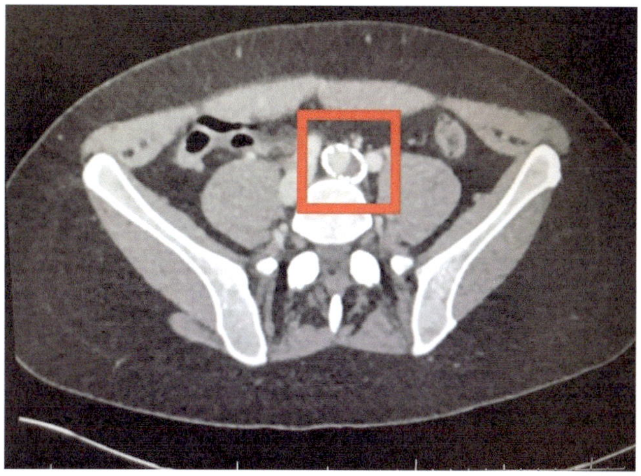

Fig. 35.27 CTV to evaluate IVC stented segmentDark thrombus formation is seen on the right side of the stented IVC segment

ventional therapies (thrombolytic, mechanical, or pharmacochemical) for acute DVTs. Oral Xa inhibitor (apixaban, edoxaban, rivaroxaban) over LMWH is recommended for initiation and treatment phases for patients with cancer. VKA (with INR target 2.5) is recommended for patients diagnosed with triple antiphospholipid syndrome.

The CHEST guidelines also provide recommendations on the duration of treatment. Patients with acute DVT without contraindication for AC should begin a treatment phase of 3 months of AC. At the completion of 3 months, patients should be assessed for extended therapy. Therapy should be extended for patients if the VTE was unprovoked or provoked by a persistent risk factor (prefer DOAC over VKA).

Surgical interventions for the management of DVT include thrombolysis, catheter-directed therapy, and thrombectomy. Thrombolysis, catheter-directed thrombolysis, and surgical thrombectomy are reserved for extensive proximal lower extremity DVT (ilio-femoral) for those with severe symptoms, threatened limb (phlegmasia), and with thrombus burden for <14 days [14] (see Table 35.15). For these patients, the benefit of more aggressive intervention may outweigh the associated risks [12]. The 2016 AC Forum and 2020 NICE recommend individual risk-to-benefit analysis for catheter-directed therapy (CDT), and that patients with iliofemoral DVT who have symptoms for <14 days, good functional status, life expectancy of 1+ years, and low risk for bleeding be considered for CDT [12].

Patients should undergo repeat venous ultrasound to evaluate DVT if symptoms worsen—this will evaluate for thrombus propagation. Swelling and leg heaviness may persist for those with extensive DVTs, despite surgical intervention and postintervention therapies. This can be alleviated by consistent use of compression garments, leg elevation, and regular exercise. Patients can begin wearing compression garments once a DVT is deemed stable and not propagating.

Table 35.15 Contraindication to thrombolysis and DVT [15]

Absolute	Relative
Recent intracranial Hemorrhage (ICH)	History of uncontrolled HTN
Severely uncontrolled HTN	Severe hypertension at presentation (SBP >180, DBP >110)
Cerebral vascular lesion-neoplasm	CPR > 10 minutes within last 3 weeks
Ischemic stroke within 3 months	Remote ischemic stroke
Possible aortic dissection	Dementia
Head trauma or facial trauma within 3 months	Pregnancy
Recent intracranial or spinal surgery	Major surgery within 3 weeks
Active bleeding (except menses)	Internal bleeding within 2–4 weeks
Streptokinase within 6 months	Active peptic ulcer disease
	Noncompressible vascular puncture

Compression garments help support venous structure and reduce venous stasis. There is no evidence that the use of graduated compression garments reduces the risk of DVT. Bed rest is not recommended after DVT diagnosis while starting anticoagulation therapy [14].

Clinical Pearls

- Aside from patients with asymptomatic distal DVT, patients without contraindication to AC should be treated for a minimum of 3–6 months with the option of extending the duration of therapy.
- When selecting AC, DOACs are preferred over VKA EXCEPT in patients with moderate-severe liver disease, or antiphospholipid syndrome [13].
- Oral Xa inhibitor (apixaban, edoxaban, rivaroxaban) over LMWH is recommended for initiation and treatment phases for patients with cancer.
- Clinicians should weigh the risk of bleeding when considering anticoagulation. Risk factors for major bleeding while taking AC include age > 65, alcohol use, liver failure, renal failure, anemia, antiplatelet therapy, cancer, reduced functional capacity, frequent falls, prior bleeding issues, prior stroke, and recent surgery [14].
- An inferior vena cava (IVC) filter may be placed in patients with acute proximal DVT of the leg who have a contraindication to AC.
- It is important to educate patients on modifiable risk factors to prevent new or recurrent thrombotic events. These risk factors include medication compliance, smoking cessation, heart-healthy diet, regular exercise, weight management, and surgical prophylaxis.
- Phlegmasia dolens is a rare and life-threatening complication of extensive, acute DVT. Surgical intervention due to arterial perfusion compromise and risk of limb loss may be needed.

References

1. Kass J, Krishnamohan P. Clinical overview: carotid artery stenosis. Elsevier; 2022. ClinicalKey. Accessed 14 Mar 2022.
2. Abdominal Aortic Aneurysm March 10, 2021. Elsevier BV. https://www-clinicalkey-com.ahecproxy.ncahec.net/#!/content/67-s2.0-7c5e261c-ea6f-4cab-aae7-cb8155587799.
3. Lawrence PF, Rigberg DA. Arterial aneurysms, epidemiology, and natural history. In: Rutherford's vascular surgery and endovascular therapy. Elsevier; 2019. p. 875–83. https://www-clinicalkey-com.ahecproxy.ncahec.net/#!/content/book/3-s2.0-B9780323427913000694?scrollTo=hl0000575.
4. Dalman R, Mell M. Overview of abdominal aortic aneurysm; 2022. https://www.uptodate.com/contents/overview-of-abdominal-aortic-aneurysm#!.
5. Schermerhorn M, Cronenwett JL. Arterial anuerysms: abdominal and iliac aneurysms. In: Rutherford vascular surgery. 6th ed. Elsevier; 2005.
6. Jana S, Hu M, Shen M, Kassiri Z. Extracellular matrix, regional heterogeneity of the aorta, and aortic aneurysm. Exp Mol Med. 2019;51:1–15.
7. Black J, Cambria RP. Aortic dissection: perspectives for the vascular/endovascular surgeon. In: Rutherford's vascular surgery. Elsevier; 2005. p. 1512–31.
8. Lombardi JV, Chad Hughes G, Appoo JJ, et al. Society for Vascular Surgery (SVS) and Society of Thoracic Surgeons (STS) reporting standards for type B aortic dissections. J Vasc Surg. 2020;71:723–47. https://www.jvascsurg.org/article/S0741-5214(19)32649-7/fulltext
9. Berger J, Davies M. Overview of lower extremity peripheral arterial disease. UpToDate. 2021. www.uptodate.com/contents/overview-of-lower-extremity-peripheral-artery-disease?source=history_widget#H16453723. Accessed 14 Mar 2022.
10. Douketis J. Overview of the venous system. 2021. https://www.merckmanuals.com/home/heart-and-blood-vessel-disorders/venous-disorders/overview-of-the-venous-system.
11. Kushner A, West P, Pillarisetty L. Virchow triad. 2021. https://www.ncbi.nlm.nih.gov/books/NBK539697/.
12. Lip GYH, et al. Overview of the treatment of lower extremity deep vein thrombosis. 2022. https://www.uptodate.com/contents/overview-of-the-treatment-of-lower-extremity-deep-vein-thrombosis-dvt.

13. Stevens SM, et al. Antithrombotic therapy for vte disease: second update of the chest guidelines and expert panel report. CHEST. 2021;160. https://journal.chestnet.org/article/S0012-3692(21)01507-5/fulltext?_ga=2.38742947.1844619104.1647184408-751823456.1647184408.
14. Ortel TL, et al. American society of hematology 2020 guidelines for management of thromboembolism: treatment of deep vein thrombosis and pulmonary embolism. Blood Adv. 2020;4:4693–738. https://ashpublications.org/bloodadvances/article/4/19/4693/463998/American-Society-of-Hematology-2020-guidelines-for.
15. Wilburn J, Shian B. Deep venous thrombosis and pulmonary embolism: current therapy. Am Fam Physician. 2017;95(5):295–302. https://www.aafp.org/afp/2017/0301/p295.html.
16. Hussain MA, Al-Omran M, Creager MA, Anand SS, Verma S, Bhatt DL. Antithrombotic therapy for peripheral artery disease: recent advances. J Am Coll Cardiol. 2018;71:2450–67.
17. Mehta V, Tzima E. A turbulent path to plaque formation. Nature. 2016;540:531–2. https://doi.org/10.1038/nature20489.
18. Saxena A, Ng EYK, Lim ST. Imaging modalities to diagnose carotid artery stenosis: progress and prospect. BioMed Eng OnLine. 2019;18:66. https://doi.org/10.1186/s12938-019-0685-7.

36 Vascular Emergencies

Annabella Olson and Tam T. T. Huynh

Introduction

Prompt recognition and treatment of vascular emergencies can save lives and limbs. The evaluation of patients presenting with a vascular emergency starts with a succinct history taking and physical examination, which usually leads to a working diagnosis. Vascular imaging studies can be acquired expeditiously to confirm the diagnosis. The delay in the diagnosis of a vascular emergency can result in increased morbidity and mortality. Vascular emergencies are broadly grouped into 2 clinical categories: (A) **clotting** or (B) **bleeding.** Acute vascular thrombosis (clotting) involves either the arterial or venous system. In these situations, systemic anticoagulation should be initiated and thrombectomy or declotting may be indicated, depending on the clinical situation. *Acute thrombosis of a major* ***artery*** *can lead to reduced distal perfusion and ischemia of the affected limb or end organ* (e.g., heart, brain, kidneys, intestine, etc.), and hence an *emergency revascularization intervention* is usually indicated in such cases. On the other hand, acute deep venous thrombosis (DVT) or pulmonary embolism (PE)are more common diagnoses but require surgical intervention *infrequently.* This chapter is intended to guide physician assistants and nurse practitioners in the evaluation and management of patients with common clinical conditions that require emergency or urgent vascular treatment. We aim to provide an overview of the basic principles in the diagnosis and management of the following common clinical problems: **acute limb ischemia (ALI), venothromboembolic disease (DVT and PE), hemodialysis access complications, and bleeding due to arterial pseudoaneurysms.** The management of aortic dissection and aneurysm rupture, vascular trauma, gastrointestinal bleeding, and mesenteric ischemia are outlined elsewhere in this textbook and hence, will not be discussed in this chapter.

Acute Limb Ischemia (ALI)

Incidence, Etiology, and Risk Factors

The incidence of **acute limb-threatening ischemia (ALI)** in the United States of America is estimated between 4 and 26 per 100,000 person-years. Over the last decades, the amputation rate related to ALI has decreased, currently at approximately 6–8%. ALI-related death rate has remained around 5–6%. ALI affects older patients (mean age around 70) and men slightly more than women. Most patients will have known risk factors, including *peripheral artery disease (PAD), heart disease, hypertension, diabetes, hyperlipidemia, tobacco smoking, and advanced age.* The common causes of ALI are (a) *embolic, (b) acute thrombosis of prior vascular interventions* (stent or bypass graft), and (c) *acute thrombosis of native arteries in patients with chronic PAD.* Left atrial thrombus formation related to **paroxysmal atrial fibrillation** is the <u>most common</u> source of cardiogenic emboli. Other less common causes of cardiogenic thrombus include post-myocardial left ventricle thrombus or valvular heart disease. Other rare sources of emboli come from the more proximal vasculature (plaque or aneurysm disease of the aorta). Less common causes of ALI include acute thrombosis of a popliteal artery aneurysm, arterial dissection, or trauma. ALI can also affect the upper extremity, but *much less* commonly. The management of ALI is similar for the upper and lower extremities. However, acute ischemia of the upper extremity is typically better *tolerated due to a larger network of natural collaterals stemming from the subclavian and axillary artery segments.*

Clinical Presentation

The clinical presentation of ALI can vary depending on the location of the blockage and the presence of collaterals. The

A. Olson · T. T. T. Huynh (✉)
Department Cardiovascular Surgery, Houston Methodist Hospital Houston, Houston, TX, USA
e-mail: tthuynh@houstonmethodist.org

S. Atallah, J. Dragoljevic (eds.), *Fundamentals of Surgery for Physician Assistants*,
https://doi.org/10.1007/978-3-032-21069-2_36

Rutherford classification of ALI (Table 36.1) is well accepted as a useful tool in determining the severity of ischemia and predicting prognosis. A useful mnemonic to remember regarding the symptoms and signs of ALI is the **6 "P"s: pain, pallor, pulselessness, paresthesia (numbness or tingling sensation), paralysis (motor weakness), and poikilothermia (in this context, means cold).** Typically, the patient presents with complaints of acute onset of pain, pale color (Fig. 36.1a), coldness, numbness, and weakness of the lower leg or foot, and is found to have absent pulses in the affected limb. The *skin is most sensitive (least tolerant) to ischemia,* followed by the nerves, and muscles (most tolerant). The **common peroneal nerve** is the *most commonly affected* nerve in the early stage of ALI, manifested as *reduced sensation in the webspace between first and second toe,* and *weak ankle dorsiflexion or foot drop.* The traditional teaching purports that skeletal muscles can generally tolerate **up to 6 hours** of **warm ischemia** before irreversible cell death occurs. *However, the clinical ischemic time is generally imprecise, and the tissue ischemic tolerance varies greatly, depending on the presence (or absence) of collaterals.* Limb **rigor mortis** can *set in within the hour in case of complete sudden severe ischemia with no collaterals.* On the other hand, some patients can have full recovery after revascularization despite prolonged period of ischemia due to presence of collateral flow.

Table 36.1 Categories of Acute Limb Ischemia

Category Prognosis Sensory Loss Motor Deficit				
I Viable No immediate None None threat				
Arterial Doppler Audible				
IIA Marginally threatened	Salvageable if promptly treated	Minimal	None	Often inaudible
IIB Immediately threatened	Salvageable if immediately revascularized	More than toes, rest pain	Mild/ moderate	Usually inaudible
III Irreversible	Major tissue loss, permanent nerve damage inevitable	Profound, anesthetic	Profound, paralysis, rigor	Inaudible

Adopted by the Society for Vascular Surgery Standards. Modified from Rutherford et al. [9]

Typical characteristics of ALI include a *sudden onset of pain* in the *lower part of the leg* (calf or foot/toe). **Ischemic pain at rest is indicative of severe ischemia**. Ischemic pain is typically in the foot/toes, constant, and *improved with dangling of the foot* (to allow better perfusion with gravity). **Claudication pain** (defined as pain in the leg muscles with walking or exercise, which is relieved with rest) usually indicates less severe ischemia. **Calf claudication** can be seen in patients with *occluded iliac, femoral, or popliteal arteries. Buttock/thigh* claudication usually means that the *occlusion is at the level of the* ***aortoiliac artery.*** Important factors that may help determine the diagnosis should be sought, including prior heart disease, history of arrhythmia, PAD, and PAD interventions (stenting, angioplasty, or bypass). For instance, a patient *without* prior PAD symptoms, presenting with new onset of atrial fibrillation and ALI, likely has an *embolic* occlusion. On the other hand, a different patient with a history of endovascular stenting of the iliac/femoral artery or iliac/femoral bypass surgery for chronic symptoms of PAD, but now presenting with ALI, likely has developed *acute thrombosis* of the stent or bypass graft. **Embolic occlusion** usually occurs *at bifurcation or branch points*, such as the common femoral artery bifurcation or the popliteal artery trifurcation/bifurcation. Typically, when the occlusion is at the level of the popliteal artery, a normal pulse can still be felt (above it) in the femoral (in the groin), **but pedal pulses are not likely palpable.**

On the other hand, if the clot or occlusion starts at the femoral artery bifurcation, *popliteal* and *pedal pulses* are *not palpable.* In this latter case scenario, the femoral pulse may or may not be palpable. On occasion, even if the clot is blocking the common femoral artery, one can still feel a transmitted pulse from the external iliac artery. An absent

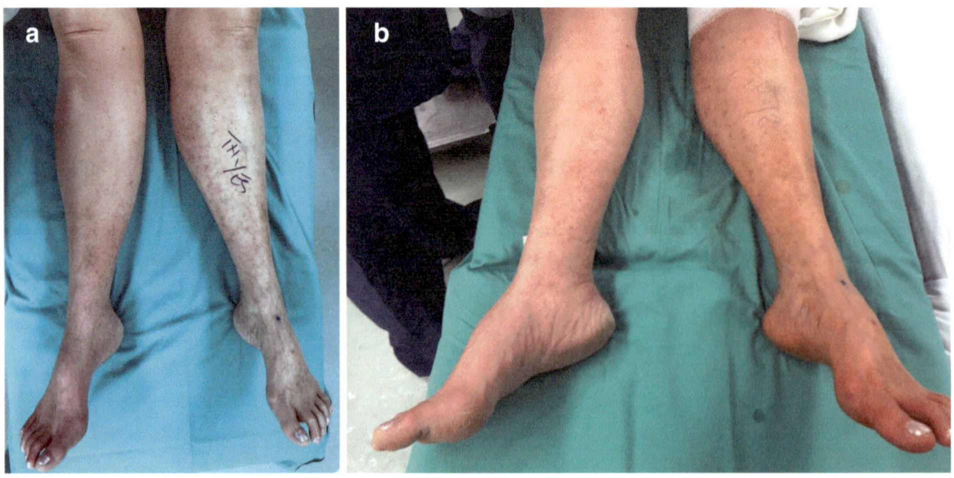

Fig. 36.1 Photographs of a patient who had acute limb-threatening ischemia of the left leg. (**a**) Before revascularization, note the pale color of the left leg compared to the normal right leg. (**b**) After successful revascularization, note the hyperemia of the left lower leg and foot after successful reperfusion

unilateral femoral pulse is usually diagnostic of *unilateral chronic iliac artery occlusion.* When bilateral femoral pulses are not palpable or absent, *it is diagnostic of either acute aortic occlusion or chronic aorto-iliac occlusive disease.* **Hand-held Doppler can detect flow when pulses are not palpable, and this test should be performed in this setting.** Normal arterial flow produces triphasic/biphasic (multiphasic) Doppler sounds. Monophasic sounds are heard when the pulse pressure is lower than normal, or when there is proximal occlusion.

Diagnostic Testing/Imaging

Standard laboratory testing, including complete blood cell count (CBC), basic metabolic panel (BMP), creatinine kinase level, prothrombin time/international normalized ratio (INR), baseline partial thromboplastin time (PTT), and type and screen, should be obtained. **An electrocardiogram (ECG) is obtained to assess for atrial fibrillation or other** types **of arrhythmia**. A significantly **elevated creatinine kinase** may indicate *muscle damage* and leakage. A **CT angiogram (CTA)** of the chest/abdomen/pelvis and bilateral leg run-off is generally diagnostic. **CTA run-off** is the imaging of choice for patients *with normal renal function and no iodine contrast allergy.* The CTA is usually readily available and takes less than 30 minutes to obtain and interpret. For patients with contraindications to getting CTA, an <u>**arterial**</u> duplex ultrasound of the affected leg can help confirm the diagnosis. **PA and advanced practitioners should note well: Bilateral lower extremity doppler to rule out DVT, <u>do not</u> assess *arterial* perfusion, and normal venous** Dopplers **of the lower extremity <u>have no bearing on arterial inflow</u>.**

Availability of a qualified vascular technologist is a limiting factor in getting duplex <u>***arterial***</u> ultrasound imaging. If neither imaging modality is readily available and the patient has immediately limb-threatening ischemia, *he or she can be taken directly to the hybrid operating room, or an interventional suite for diagnostic arteriogram, and endovascular intervention, or even directly to surgical revascularization as indicated.* For patients suspected of having cardiogenic embolization, a transthoracic 2D Echocardiogram with Doppler is indicated, but can be done *after* revascularization. Interestingly, the echocardiogram rarely shows evidence of thrombus even in patients with paroxysmal atrial fibrillation (possibly because the clot had embolized).

Management

Intravenous unfractionated **heparin** weight-based protocol is initiated as soon as possible once the diagnosis of ALI is made to stop clot propagation. In general, a loading dose of **80 units of heparin per kg is given as a bolus**, followed by an infusion rate of **18 units/kg/h**; the rate is titrated according to the **PTT or anti-Xa level**. *Currently, there is no role for intravenous systemic thrombolysis as it is not effective for ALI, and it is associated with a high risk of bleeding.* **Vascular surgeons** are a group of specialists formally trained and most often called on to provide the comprehensive management for patients with ALI. However, in some institutions, **interventional radiologists (IR)** and **interventional cardiologists** can also provide endovascular treatment. Up until the late 1990s, there were two treatment options for ALI.

First, conventional ***surgical thromboembolectomy*** with direct cut down and exposure of the involved arteries was preferred for patients with embolic occlusion or patients with more severe ischemia who would need <u>prompt</u> revascularization. **Second, *Catheter-directed thrombolysis (CDT)*** became a popular **option** in the late 1990s, as less invasive, with direct *infusion of low-dose TPA* (typically 1 mg/h) into the thrombosed vessels/stents/grafts. This therapy would typically require an overnight stay in the ICU for close monitoring and re-imaging with or without additional endovascular intervention, such as balloon angioplasty or stenting, or surgical revision. *CDT for ALI has been shown to be as effective as surgical revascularization regarding limb salvage rate, but it did require more subsequent interventions.* There are two main drawbacks to CDT: (a) longer period to reperfusion, generally from 8 to 24 hours, and (b) bleeding complications (at access sites and internal bleeding).

Fast forward to the late 2010s and early 2020s, with advances in catheter-based thrombus aspiration technology, **percutaneous thrombectomy** is now widely available, and *has been shown to be as effective as surgical thrombectomy in achieving prompt revascularization, without the added risk of bleeding associated with CDT.* The urgency of limb revascularization depends on the severity of ALI. **Surgical revascularization**, in the form of *open thrombectomy* and/or *bypass,* can be attempted *when endovascular intervention fails.* In general, revascularization can be done non-emergently for patients with ischemia that does *not* immediately threaten limb viability. **Rutherford I.** Revascularization should be done *as soon as possible* for patients with **Rutherford IIa** and *emergently* for **IIb.** For patients with severe ischemia in the **Rutherford III group**, with suspected irreversible tissue damage, particularly those with signs of rigor mortis, *revascularization is not recommended as it is likely futile.* This latter unfortunate group of patients is better served by having primary leg amputation.

<u>Frequent vascular assessment</u> is imperative after revascularization for ALI to detect post-intervention complications. Regular vascular checks should include assessment of the distal lower extremity/foot: presence of pain or numbness in the foot, color appearance, motor and sensory function of the foot and toes, and presence of palpable pulses or arterial Doppler signals. Comparison of symptoms and signs prior to and post-revascularization can be valuable. **Hyperemia** of

the lower leg and foot is typically a *good sign of reperfusion* after successful revascularization (Fig. 36.1b). This tends to be more marked in patients who had severe ischemia. Acute recurring thrombosis after revascularization can occur due to a variety of reasons, including technical failure.

Immediate re-intervention may be indicated for a select group of patients with recurring thrombosis. Bleeding complications are more frequent in these patients, particularly because they are anticoagulated during the procedure and/or need to remain on anticoagulation post-procedure. Bleeding can occur at the vascular access site (typically the common femoral artery) or in surgical wounds. **Compartment syndrome** is another concern after successful revascularization for ALI, *particularly in patients who sustained a severe and prolonged period of limb ischemia.* The onset of compartment syndrome after reperfusion can vary but is typically within a few hours after reperfusion. Increased compartmental pressures can cause pain in the calf and can lead to reduced arterial perfusion of the foot. Compartment pressures can be measured in the calf at the bedside to confirm diagnosis (compartment pressures greater than 30–40 mmHg). *Prophylactic 4-compartment calf fasciotomy immediately after revascularization procedure has been advocated for patients with severe and/or prolonged ischemia.* The fasciotomy wounds can be closed later when reperfusion swelling subsides. Following successful revascularization, there can be a **surge of potassium**, leaked from the muscle cells, into the bloodstream, acutely *causing acute hyperkalemia* in the initial postoperative period, and appropriate treatment should be planned.

Postoperatively, *long-term anticoagulation is indicated for patients with cardiogenic embolism.* **Direct oral anticoagulation (DOAC)** with **factor Xa inhibitors** (like Rivaroxaban and Apixaban) is commonly used for long-term anticoagulation. For patients with PAD, **antiplatelet therapy** (aspirin and/or clopidogrel) *is preferred*, with or without DOAC. Currently, there are no consensus regarding the benefit of long-term anticoagulation for PAD patients. Low-dose DOAC has been shown in some studies to be beneficial in PAD patients, but this must be weighed against risk of bleeding in elderly patients. Patients should follow up in the outpatient clinic, 2–3 weeks after discharge, for a wound check and review of the treatment plan. Patients with PAD will require long-term periodic surveillance. On the other hand, patients who had successful revascularization after a thromboembolic event, without underlying PAD, may not require long-term vascular surveillance.

Venothromboembolism (VTE)

The incidence of **venothromboembolism (VTE),** encompassing both **deep venous thrombosis (DVT)** and **pulmonary embolism (PE)** diagnoses, is estimated at around 100 persons per 100,000 per year in the USA. DVT and PE are one of the most common diagnoses of patients presenting to the emergency department. **Virchow's triad** describes the three primary factors that contribute to the development of thrombosis: **venous stasis, endothelial injury**, and **hypercoagulability.** Common clinical risk factors include advanced age, immobility, recent major surgery, cancer, obesity, dehydration, and hypercoagulable conditions. *DVT involves the lower extremity much more commonly than the upper extremity* (ratio ~ 20:1). The majority of PEs occur due to embolization *from a DVT in the lower extremity or pelvis.* However, it is not uncommon to find no evidence of DVT in patients presenting with PE.

A VTE is considered **"provoked"** when it is associated with a (a) recent event (like surgery) *or* (b) a reversible risk factor (immobility from illness or trauma). Conversely, an **"unprovoked"** VTE occurs without a clear identifiable risk factor. For patients with provoked VTE, current consensus guidelines recommend anticoagulation for 3–6 months. Unprovoked VTE may warrant further investigation to identify underlying causes or risk factors. Additional testing for hypercoagulable conditions, such as **Factor V Leiden deficiency** or underlying **malignancy** (*most cancers result in a hypercoagulable state*). Consultation with a hematologist is advisable for patients with unprovoked VTE. The VTE recurrence rate is higher in patients with unprovoked VTE. The duration of anticoagulation therapy is not well defined for patients with unprovoked VTE and can be longer (than 6 months) or at times indefinite.

Acute Lower Extremity DVT

Acute **leg swelling and pain** are the two main symptoms of DVT. Typically, swelling is in the calf when the thrombosis involves the femoral/popliteal or tibial veins. Swelling tends to be more severe and affects the entire leg (thigh and calf) when the thrombosis involves the common femoral and iliac veins. The classic **Homan sign** refers to *pain in the calf on forced dorsiflexion*. This sign is described in a past textbook as an indicator for presence of DVT *but has been shown to be neither specific nor sensitive*. Elevated levels of **D-dimer** in the blood are found in nearly all patients with acute lower extremity DVT. However, *high levels of D-dimer can also be found in conditions such as cancer and other acute illnesses.* It has been *suggested* that a normal D-dimer level can *rule out* the presence of DVT, but this has not been conclusively shown.

Currently, ***venous*** *duplex ultrasound* is the diagnostic test of choice to confirm the presence of extremity DVT. Typical sonographic signs of acute venous thrombosis are *noncompressibility* of the vein as the lumen is filled with hypoechoic mass (clots), *expansile vessel size* (due to accumulation of clots), and *lack of color-flow or absence of*

Doppler flow in complete vessel thrombosis. **CT venogram** of the pelvis and abdomen can be useful to show extension of thrombosis into the *iliac veins* (and *inferior vena cava*) in patients with severe leg swelling and suspected iliofemoral venous thrombosis. *Primary treatment for DVT remains systemic* ***therapeutic anticoagulation*** *to stop the propagation of the clot and reduce the risk of PE.*

Anticoagulation can be started as soon as possible if the patient's history and exam are highly suggestive of the diagnosis of DVT, while waiting for the confirmation on imaging. Ambulatory patients with mild symptoms can be treated in the outpatient setup and followed up in the clinic. **DOACs have become the mainstay of treatment for DVT.** The currently accepted treatment with DOAC consists of 2 weeks of higher loading dosing followed by a maintenance dose.

Patients with moderate to severe swelling *should be admitted to the hospital for further observation.* Some patients will show improved swelling with initiation of anticoagulation and leg elevation. However, if the extremity swelling is severe, does not improve, or worsens, mechanical thrombectomy can be considered. For patients in whom venous thrombectomy is considered, anticoagulation can be initiated with either intravenous unfractionated heparin or low molecular weight heparin, and hold initiation of DOAC until after the intervention. In general, a loading dose of 80 units of heparin per kg is given as a bolus, followed by an infusion rate of 18 units/kg/h, and followed by *titration of the infusion rate according to the PTT or anti-Xa level.*

Phlegmasia Cerulae or Alba Dolens

In its most severe form, iliofemoral DVT can lead to severe pain, swelling, and the development of compartment syndrome. The terms **phlegmasia *cerulae* dolens** and **phlegmasia *alba* dolens** refer to the pathognomonic findings of cyanotic appearance or blanching of the extremity, respectively, that occur in extensive DVT. The risk of venous gangrene and limb loss is increased in these patients, and urgent intervention is indicated. *Remarkable advances have been made in the mechanical thrombectomy device technology in the last decades.* **Image-guided percutaneous mechanical thrombectomy** of iliofemoral DVT can now effectively restore venous drainage, decrease tissue swelling, and promptly reduce calf compartment pressures in most cases, and *obviate the need for surgical thrombectomy or calf fasciotomy. Percutaneous mechanical thrombectomy* is minimally invasive and well tolerated by most patients with a low risk of embolization and access site complications. It is gaining popularity and is increasingly used as an adjunctive treatment of patients with iliofemoral DVT who manifest moderate to severe leg swelling.

Successful **venous thrombectomy** offers the benefit of more rapid resolution of leg swelling and potentially reduces the incidence of chronic venous insufficiency. Historically, catheter-directed thrombolysis and open surgical thrombectomy have been alternative treatment options for patients with severe, extensive extremity DVT, but these are now rarely used. In general, percutaneous mechanical thrombectomy can be done with local anesthesia and conscious sedation. However, patients frequently prefer general anesthesia or deeper sedation for comfort.

Venous access is gained with ultrasound guidance below the segment to be treated, typically the popliteal or tibial vein in the leg (and the basilic vein in the arm). Large bore sheaths (11–24 F) are required to accommodate the thrombectomy devices, but access site complications are rare. Patients can be started on DOAC soon after mechanical thrombectomy. *The total duration of anticoagulation remains the same,* ***at least 3 months*** *for provoked DVT, or greater for unprovoked DVT, regardless of whether the mechanical thrombectomy was performed.*

May-Thurner Syndrome (MTS)

The classic description of **May-Thurner Syndrome (MTS)** involves compression of the left common iliac vein between the right common iliac artery (anteriorly) and the lumbar spine (posteriorly). MTS is present in over 20% of the general population, even though *most are asymptomatic.* Compression of the iliac vein can be seen on CT venogram or following thrombectomy on selective contrast venography and on intravascular ultrasound (IVUS) imaging. Stenting of the compressed iliac vein segment is generally recommended to reduce the risk of recurring DVT. *Antiplatelet therapy with aspirin or clopidogrel is usually recommended* after venous stenting in addition to anticoagulation therapy.

Acute Pulmonary Embolism (PE)

In the United States, **Pulmonary Embolism (PE)** is the third *most common cause of cardiovascular death,* following coronary artery disease and stroke, with mortality rates for untreated acute PE reaching as high as 30%. The clinical presentation of PE spans over a spectrum—from asymptomatic patients, mild to severe symptoms, to sudden death. Common symptoms and signs include mild shortness of breath on exertion to dyspnea at rest, cough, pleuritic chest pain (pain on deep inspiration, a symptom of **pulmonary infarction**), hypotension, hypoxemia, tachycardia, and syncope. Risk factors for PE are as listed for DVT in the previous section. **CT pulmonary angiogram (CTPA)** is the gold standard and diagnostic test of choice. Emboli/clots are seen as filling defects obstructing the pulmonary vasculature, partially or completely. **Ventilation perfusion (V/Q) nuclear scan** is the alternate imaging modality for patients who have a contrast allergy or severe kidney disease. Ventilation-perfusion mismatch can predict PE probability. The original and simplified **pulmonary embolism severity index (PESI)** is a well-recognized risk stratification model. Currently, a com-

Table 36.2 Pulmonary Embolism (PE) Risk Stratification

Classification	Characteristics	Percentage of PEs	Estimated 30-Day Mortality
Intermediate (sub-massive) High-intermediate Risk	RV strain on CTA or echocardiogram **and** elevated troponin	5%	Up to 65%
Low-intermediate Risk	RV strain **or** elevated troponin	40%	5–25%
Low-Risk	No RV strain and normal troponin	55%	< 1%

Modified from the American Heart Association (AHA) and European Society of Cardiology (ESC) (Giri et al. [4], Konstantinides et al. [5])
RV right ventricular strain, *CTA* CT angiogram of pulmonary arteries

monly adopted PE risk classification stratifies risks into *low, intermediate* (also known as *submassive*), and *high* (*massive*). The intermediate risk (submassive) group can be further stratified as low-intermediate and high-intermediate-risk (Table 36.2). In its most severe form, a large **saddle PE** involves clots occluding *both main pulmonary arteries, which causes outflow obstruction of the right ventricle (RV), leading to acute pressure overload in the RV, pulmonary hypertension, and RV dilatation/strain and failure.* Signs of RV strain include elevated blood level of troponin (cardiac biomarker), RV/LV ratio greater than 1 on CTPA, dilated right atrium and RV on echocardiogram (*right heart strain*), and elevated pulmonary artery pressures.

Ambulatory patients with mild symptoms (low-risk PE) are prescribed *oral anticoagulation* or low molecular weight heparin and *do not require hospital admission.* In contrast, patients with intermediate and high-risk PE *should be admitted to the hospital for close observation. High-risk PE* patients presenting with syncope, hypoxia, tachycardia, and hypotension (< 90 mmHg) requiring vasopressor support are at significant risk for hemodynamic deterioration and death. **Urgent systemic thrombolysis** (10 mg IV as a bolus then 90 mg over 2 hours) *is indicated for high-risk PE patients who are in shock, unless they have contraindications to thrombolysis.* Absolute contraindications to thrombolysis include coagulopathy, severe thrombocytopenia, history of recent head trauma, stroke, and head or spine surgery.

Patients are monitored closely during and immediately after systemic thrombolysis for signs of bleeding (such as *intracranial hemorrhage*, which can occur in up to 2% of cases). Low-dose systemic thrombolysis treatment (50 mg IV or less) is as effective with a lower risk of intracranial hemorrhage. Historically, emergency surgical thromboembolectomy on cardiopulmonary bypass has been done for unstable high-risk PE patients, but these are now rarely performed emergently.

Image-guided catheter-based interventions have been shown to be beneficial for patients with high-intermediate and high-risk PE and have been adopted widely in the United States. Urgent intervention is indicated for high-risk PE patients to reduce the risk of deterioration. In hemodynamically stable patients with high-intermediate risk PE, the urgency is less, but in general, intervention should be done a priori. Systemic intravenous heparin should be started as soon as possible after the PE diagnosis is made while waiting for the intervention. **Percutaneous mechanical PE thrombectomy** *provides prompt, effective treatment and has become the intervention of choice for intermediate and high-risk (not in shock) PE patients.* Catheter aspiration thrombectomy technology continues to evolve, but currently still requires a large-bore sheath (~24 F) via the common femoral or internal jugular vein.

The risk of cardiac collapse upon induction of general anesthesia is very high in patients with severe RV dysfunction. Hence, *mechanical PE thrombectomy is best done under local anesthesia and conscious sedation.* In high-risk patients, **extracorporeal membrane oxygenation (ECMO)** should be readily available during mechanical PE thrombectomy, although it is rarely needed. The clinical improvement is often remarkable after successful PE mechanical thrombectomy, and patients typically are discharged home within a few days. **Catheter-directed thrombolysis (CDT)** is an effective alternative treatment option. The infusion catheter is placed inside the pulmonary arteries using fluoroscopic guidance, and a low dose of **tPA** (**tissue plasminogen activator**; 1 mg/h) is delivered continuously into the clots for 6–24 h. Patients are monitored closely in the ICU while receiving CDT. While the bleeding risk is lower with CDT when compared to systemic thrombolysis, it is not negligible. CDT may be more effective than aspiration thrombectomy for PEs that are in the peripheral/segmental location (versus central), but there has been no randomized direct comparison between the two techniques. DOAC therapy can be initiated soon after catheter-based interventions. The recommended total duration of anticoagulation is the same for all VTE (PE and DVT), at least 3–6 months if provoked, greater if unprovoked, regardless of whether the patient had an intervention.

Hemodialysis Access Complications

It is estimated that **808,000 people in the United States have end-stage renal disease (ESRD)**, and *over two-thirds of those people are on hemodialysis. Complications related to hemodialysis access account for a large portion of ESRD patients presenting to the emergency department.* A surgically made **Arteriovenous fistula** in the upper extremity is the preferred long-term access over an indwelling tunneled hemodialysis catheter, *because the former is more durable and associated with much lower infection rates.* The arteriovenous fistulas are created either using the patient's *autoge-*

nous cephalic or basilic veins or using *non-autogenous conduits* (most commonly synthetic **PTFE graft** and less commonly biologic graft (such as commercially available bovine carotid artery). Autogenous **arteriovenous fistulas (AVF)** are usually preferred in patients who have good caliber autogenous veins, as they have a better long-term primary patency rate, require fewer secondary interventions, and are associated with a lower risk of infection compared to synthetic **arteriovenous grafts (AVG).**

Bleeding Complications

Bleeding related to AVF/AVG ranges from minor bleeding from the needle punctures to massive, life-threatening bleeding due to ulcerated skin overlying the AVF/AVG. It is imperative to examine the bleeding site to assess the integrity of the skin. Minor bleeding from needle access sites on AVF and AVG can usually be stopped with *direct pressure on the bleeding site*. Direct pressure onto bleeding site of AVF/AVG *can be done by any person, including the patient.* Pressure dressings should be applied for reinforcement. When direct pressure fails to control the bleeding, the skin around the bleeding site can be approximated by placing a *purse-string or figure-of-eight 2–0 Silk or Nylon suture to stop the bleeding*. Application of a tourniquet proximal to the bleeding site can help reduce or stop the bleeding. On occasions, bedside control of the bleeding is tenuous, and emergency surgical exploration is indicated. When the bleeding is coming from an *ulcerated skin site on the AVF/AVG, it can be difficult to control and become life-threatening.* Ulceration of the skin typically happens due to repeated cannulations at the same spot that is associated with attenuated skin overlying a chronic aneurysmal segment of an AVF or a pseudoaneurysm segment of an AVG.

The presence of large skin ulceration usually requires urgent surgical revision of the access, even if the bleeding was temporarily stopped, as the risk of recurring brisk bleeding is imminent without definitive repair. Surgical revision and AVF salvage are usually possible, unless the skin defect is extensive and associated with a large underlying **AVF aneurysm**. AVF aneurysm excision and AVF ligation may be required in the latter case. On the other hand, salvage of AVG may or may not be possible depending on the presence of associated infection/contamination of the synthetic segment. Ligation of AVF/AVG may be required to stop life-threatening bleeding.

AVF/AVG Thrombosis

Acute thrombosis of AVF/AVG is not a true emergency, but *intervention is best done as soon as possible to restore the patency of the access.* In general, anticoagulation is not indicated for acute thrombosis of AVF/AVG unless there is associated extension of the acute thrombosis into the central veins. Acute thrombosis of AVF/AVG may or may not cause symptoms. Symptoms may include pain and swelling. *On physical exam, there is* ***loss of palpable thrill*** *and* ***audible bruit*** *in the outflow.* Confirmatory ultrasound duplex of the AVF/AVG is not necessary, but can provide helpful information regarding the outflow veins. ***Thrombectomy*** *of AVF/AVG can usually restore access patency, and the access can be used immediately for hemodialysis.* However, the development of outflow or central venous obstruction may limit long-term patency of AVF/AVG. Insertion of a new tunneled hemodialysis catheter may be necessary when thrombectomy and revision of thrombosed AVF/AVG fail to restore access patency. On occasions, temporary non-tunneled central venous catheter placement may be indicated for urgent hemodialysis for hyperkalemia or fluid overload prior to AVF/AVG thrombectomy.

Steal Syndrome Related to AV Access

Hemodialysis access **steal syndrome** occurs in approximately 1–5% patients with AVF/AVG and is probably the <u>most common</u> cause of **hand ischemia** overall. Hand ischemia due to steal spans over a spectrum. *Steal symptoms are usually insidious and include coldness, numbness, and pain in the hand and fingers in the arm with the AVF/AVG. Symptoms are usually worse during hemodialysis sessions or with arm exercise.* Signs of hand ischemia are cool/cold fingers, pale, decreased sensation to light touch, muscle weakness, and atrophy in the affected hand. Steal syndrome is complex, and a thorough evaluation and treatment are beyond the scope of this chapter. Mild symptoms that develop acutely after AVF/AVG creation may improve with time and adaptation. In contrast, the development of steal in chronic AVF/AVG will usually progress and require intervention. Ultrasound arterial and venous duplex of the affected extremity with the AVF/AVG will provide useful information, including inflow vs distal disease, reversal of flow from the hand, and access volume flows. Moderate to severe ischemia due to steal will require **access revision** to reverse distal ischemia while preserving AVF. ***Ligation*** *of AVF/AVG may be required to prevent loss of fingers or hand when revision is not possible or fails. Rarely,* acute severe limb-threatening ischemia can occur *immediately after creation of a new AVF/AVG*, and emergency access ligation is recommended to reverse the ischemia for limb salvage.

Post-catheterization and Post-operative Bleeding and Pseudoaneurysms; Groin and Retroperitoneal Hematomas

For decades, the **common femoral artery** was the *primary access site* for diagnostic angiograms and therapeutic interventions such as coronary artery stenting or peripheral artery interventions. Several percutaneous femoral artery *access* *closure devices* are now commercially available. These are intended to close the femoral artery access puncture and reduce the bedrest time after the procedure. Access site bleeding is an infrequent complication (iatrogenic injury) of arterial catheterization, occurring between 0.1% and 6% of catheterization procedures. ***Trans-radial artery catheterization*** is gaining popularity, as its use is associated with better patient tolerance and lower rates of complications than transfemoral access.

Nearly all bleeding that occurs acutely following arterial access can be controlled and stopped with direct manual pressure onto the bleeding access site. There are external devices such as a **"C-clamp"** or **"sandbag"** that can be applied to the bleeding access site to control and stop the bleeding. *Most groin hematomas are self- contained* and can be controlled with direct external compression. When the access site is a "high stick" above the inguinal ligament, in the **external iliac artery**, a *retroperitoneal hematoma* can form. *Most retroperitoneal hematomas are also self- contained by tissue tamponade. Most post-catheterization hematomas are small, asymptomatic, and resolve with time, and hence do not require intervention.*

Femoral Artery Pseudoaneurysms

Less than 1% of patients undergoing arterial catheterization may develop a **femoral artery pseudoaneurysm** (or also known as a **false aneurysm**), which is not an aneurysm, but rather, a defect (hole) in the vessel wall caused by the catheterization puncture, surrounded by a hematoma. Typically, the pseudoaneurysm presents as a *pulsatile "mass"* at the vascular access site that may or may not be painful or tender; the "mass" is the hematoma. The risk of pseudoaneurysm formation increases with the size of the sheath (sizes 4F- 24F) and the use of anticoagulation post- catheterization. *Ultrasound duplex imaging* is indicated to assess for the presence of a femoral artery pseudoaneurysm, particularly in an *expanding hematoma* or when the hematoma feels pulsatile. The classic finding of a pseudoaneurysm on duplex shows the *to and from* (ying/yang) flow pattern in the neck of the pseudoaneurysm. CT angiogram imaging can provide a more comprehensive anatomical assessment of the pseudoaneurysm and the extent of the hematoma. The pseudoaneurysm is seen as a sac or pocket of contained *contrast extravasation* in proximity to the iliac or femoral artery. Diagnosis of pseudoaneurysm as a sequelae of vessel catheterization does not require emergency intervention, unless it is causing a rapidly expanding hematoma, but does require close monitoring. Small pseudoaneurysms (less than 2 cm) may resolve spontaneously. Anticoagulation should be withheld to allow thrombosis of the pseudoaneurysm. Non-invasive bedside compression with or without ultrasound guidance has been used to promote thrombosis of pseudoaneurysm with mixed results. **Ultrasound-guided thrombin injection** (500–1000 IU) is effective and has become the *accepted treatment of choice for closing pseudoaneurysms caused by catheterization.* Contra-indications to thrombin injection treatment are the presence of infected hematoma and pseudoaneurysms associated with a large or short neck. Surgical repair is recommended for pseudoaneurysms that are not amenable to, or have failed thrombin injection, or are infected.

Chronic femoral artery pseudoaneurysms tend to grow over time. Untreated enlarging pseudoaneurysms can exert local compression on the adjacent femoral vein and nerve, although they rarely rupture. Surgical repair generally entails suturing the hole in the artery. When the hole is complex or large, repair may require a patch and, rarely a short interposition bypass graft.

Active Bleeding and Expanding Hematomas

On *rare* occasions, patients can develop hypotension and hemorrhagic shock due to *uncontained bleeding* in the groin or retroperitoneum after trans-femoral artery catheterization. **This presentation is a true vascular emergency**, requiring immediate fluid resuscitation (see below for details regarding management of arterial bleeding), blood replacement, and emergency vascular intervention. A rapid (STAT) CT angiogram of the abdomen and pelvis is useful to identify the exact location of the bleeding. In this setting, thrombin injection is usually not possible, particularly if the bleeding is in the retroperitoneum. In general, the common femoral artery and its bifurcation can be exposed via a groin incision. However, a retroperitoneal exposure is required if the external iliac artery is involved. Most of the time, the defect in the arterial wall can be repaired primarily (using sutures). A patch angioplasty or bypass graft may be required for more complex vessel wall defects. Endovascular placement of a covered stent-graft to cover the puncture hole/pseudoaneurysm has been used successfully and is an accepted alternative treatment option in patients with suitable anatomy.

Post-operative Arterial Bleeding

Bleeding complications following *any* type of surgery can be potentially life-threatening. Major postoperative arterial bleeding occurs rarely and is usually associated with the development of postoperative infection. Bleeding complications can happen in the early or late postoperative period. In the early postoperative period, the tissues at the operative site are friable and unorganized, and arterial bleeding will most likely be brisk and uncontained (free). In the later postoperative period (3 weeks after surgery or more), surrounding tissue tamponade can contain the bleeding and lead to the formation of a pseudoaneurysm/hematoma. Patients with arterial reconstruction or bypass are particularly at increased risk for postoperative bleeding. Catastrophic bleeding is often heralded by a **sentinel bleed**. Symptoms and signs vary depending on the anatomical location of the arterial bleeding. When assessing a patient with major hemorrhage, a quick initial survey is carried out, and includes noting the patient's vital signs, airway patency, and level of alertness. An initial focused history regarding the patient's symptoms and medical history and surgical treatment allows for the rapid formation of a differential diagnosis.

Bleeding into the chest or abdominal cavity can cause localized pressure or pain. The accumulation of extravasated blood in the abdomen can show as an expanding, tender mass. Large volume bleeding into the chest cavity can cause dyspnea due to compression of the lung. On the other hand, a large volume of blood can accumulate in the retroperitoneum before causing symptoms. Bleeding into an extremity is typically associated with swelling and pain.

The management of acute major arterial bleeding requires prompt diagnosis and simultaneous treatment. *Large-bore intravenous access is established, and rapid fluid and blood resuscitation is initiated. Mechanical maneuvers to apply a tamponade onto visible bleeding site.* **Uncross-matched O-NEGATIVE packed red blood cells (PRBCs)** can be transfused in patients who are in hemorrhagic shock while waiting for cross-matched blood to be administered as soon as it is available. **The patient's hemodynamic response to blood and fluid administration dictates the *rate and volume* of ongoing resuscitation**. Admission to the critical care unit should be requested for close monitoring.

Consultation with the respective surgical specialty is made. Multi-detector CT angiogram is the diagnostic imaging of choice for suspected hemorrhage and can be rapidly obtained within minutes. The high resolution of CT imaging and multiplanar reformatting of the axial images provide a high rate of diagnostic yield for localizing the bleeding (extravasation of contrast), or identifying a pseudoaneurysm, or vessel irregularity in proximity of the affected area. Furthermore, *CTA is useful in planning endovascular intervention or surgical treatment*. Selective angiography is rarely used for diagnosis, but rather is reserved for endovascular interventions. Endovascular interventions such as embolization of small pseudoaneurysms or placement of a covered stent-graft across a large bleeding vessel are generally effective in stopping the hemorrhage. Control of the infection source is usually necessary to prevent recurrence. Surgical debridement and healthy soft tissue coverage of the involved vessel are often required. Examples of soft tissue coverage include omental patch and pedicle muscle flaps. Excision of the infected synthetic graft may be indicated to eradicate the infection, and vascular reconstruction is usually required.

Summary

In summary, in this chapter, we have described the management of patients presenting with acute limb-threatening ischemia, venothromboembolic disease (DVT and PE), complications of hemodialysis access, and bleeding related to trans- femoral arterial catheterization and postoperative arterial pseudoaneurysms. We provided an overview of the common vascular emergencies *intended for the physician assistants and nurse practitioners*. The diagnosis of these conditions can usually be made promptly after a thorough focused history and physical examination. Diagnostic imaging can confirm the diagnosis and is useful in planning intervention. These challenging vascular emergencies are generally treated by vascular surgeons. However, depending on the organizational structure of the local institution, other specialties such as interventional radiology, interventional cardiology, interventional nephrology, or general surgery can be part of the multidisciplinary treating team providing treatment for these patients. In the *Appendix*, we include illustrative clinical vignettes of the common vascular emergencies.

Appendix: Clinical Vignettes

Case 1. Acute Limb Ischemia Due to Thromboembolism

A 54-year-old non-smoker woman with no prior medical history presented to the emergency department with acute right lower extremity ischemia, Rutherford IIB. This patient had symptoms and signs of right foot pain, mild numbness, and weakness (foot drop). Arterial duplex showed reduced flow in the right popliteal and tibial arteries (Fig. 36.2a–c). CTA showed embolic occlusion of the right popliteal artery (Fig. 36.3a, b). The patient was started on intravenous unfractionated heparin and taken urgently for revascularization. A combination of mechanical thrombectomy and catheter-directed thrombolysis of the popliteal and tibial arteries (Figs. 36.4) achieved good revascularization with return of palpable right pedal pulses. Fasciotomy was not required. The patient's right foot drop (peroneal nerve palsy) improved postoperatively. At one-year follow-up, the patient has remained free from reintervention on long-term low-dose apixaban. The source of embolization remains unclear with a negative cardiac work-up.

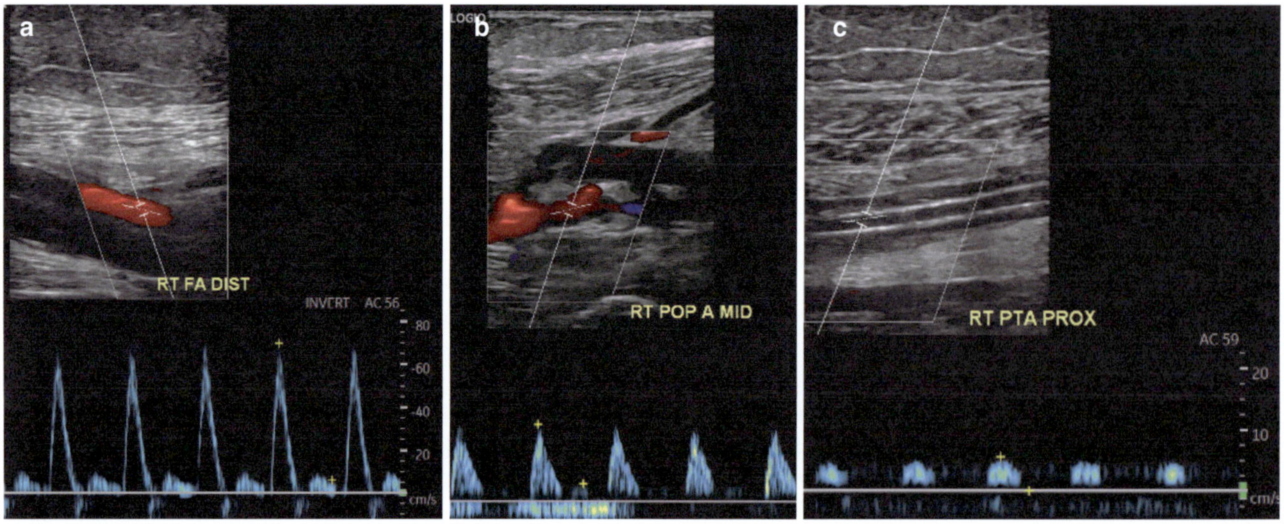

Fig. 36.2 Duplex ultrasound transverse images show: (**a**) Normal triphasic flow in the superficial femoral artery (FA). (**b**) Abnormal blunted flow in the nearly occluded right popliteal (pop) artery; thrombus is usually not well seen on ultrasound. (**c**) Monophasic flow in the reconstituted posterior tibial artery (PTA) distal to the occlusion with markedly reduced flow velocities

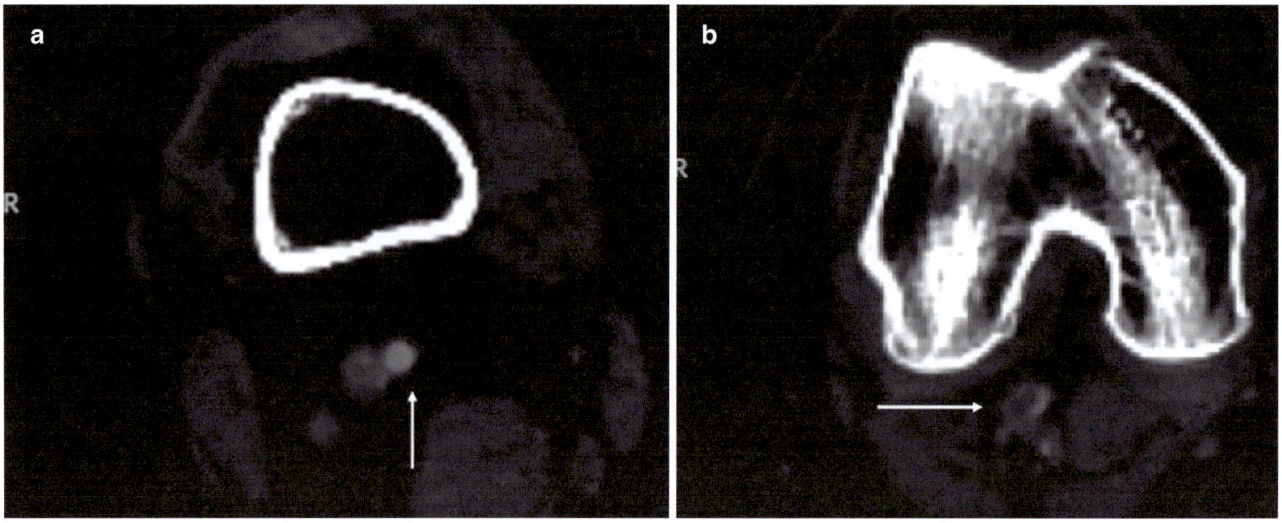

Fig. 36.3 Axial CTA images show: (**a**) Contrast in the distal normal superficial femoral artery (arrow); the femoral vein is seen adjacent to the artery. (**b**) Arrow points to the popliteal artery filled with thrombus; rim of contrast seen around the thrombus (dark grey) inside the lumen

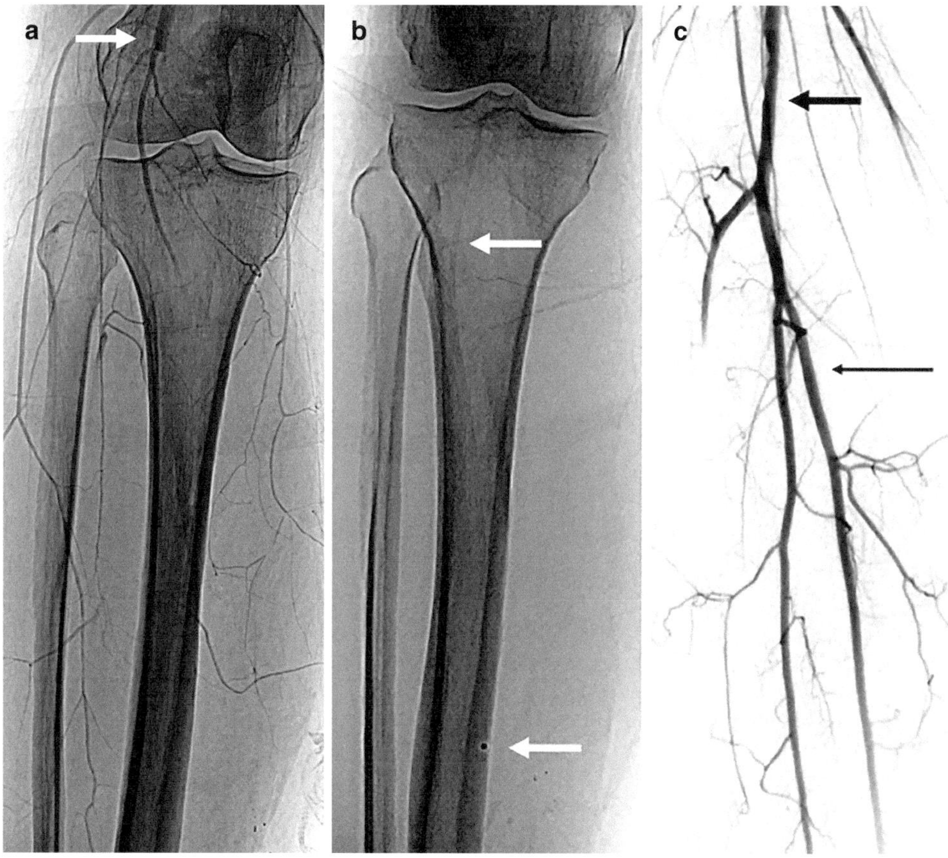

Fig. 36.4 Selective arteriogram, image-guided mechanical aspiration thrombectomy, and catheter-directed thrombolysis treatment. (**a**) Arrow points to the sharp cut-off of contrast filling in the above knee popliteal artery; a classic finding of an embolus. (**b**) After aspiration thrombectomy, a multi-side hole infusion catheter was placed inside the vessel with a radio-opaque tip (arrow points to black tip) for continuous catheter-directed thrombolysis. (**c**) Final digital subtraction image shows contrast filling the popliteal artery (short arrow), and all three tibial arteries (thin arrow)

Case 2. Acute Iliofemoral DVT

A 70-year-old woman on maintenance immunotherapy for stage 3 breast cancer treatment presented to the emergency department with an acute onset of severe swelling and pain in her left leg. On exam, the patient showed severe left leg swelling and discoloration of the thigh, calf, and foot, consistent with phlegmasia cerulea dolens (Fig. 36.5). Venous duplex showed extensive left femoral and popliteal DVT, including the common femoral vein (Fig. 36.6). CT venogram showed expansile thrombosis of the left external and common iliac veins (Fig. 36.7). Unfractionated intravenous heparin was initiated, and the patient underwent percutaneous image-guided iliofemoral mechanical DVT thrombectomy successfully (Fig. 36.8). Venogram and IVUS showed evidence of severe left common iliac vein compression, consistent with May-Thurner syndrome (Fig. 36.9a). Stenting of the left common iliac vein (Fig. 36.9b) was successful with prompt clinical improvement (Fig. 36.10). The patient was discharged the day after intervention on apixaban for 3 months for provoked DVT and compression stockings.

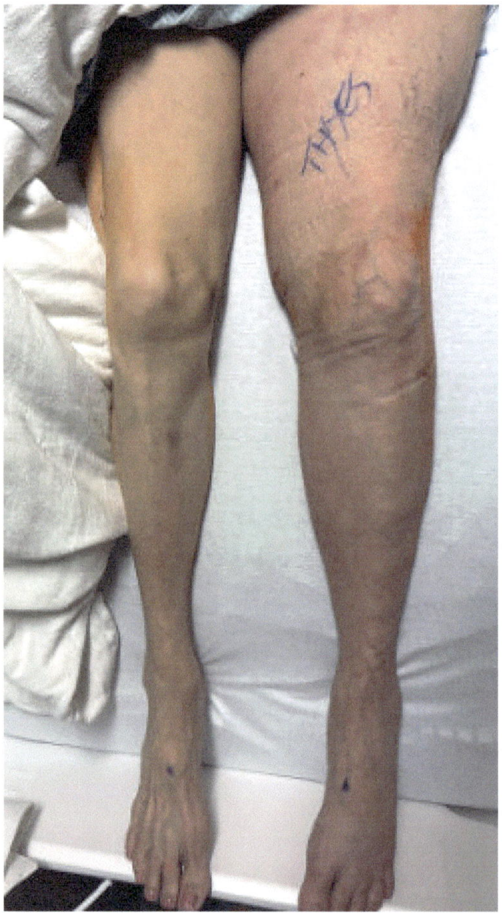

Fig. 36.5 Photograph of the patient on admission shows left leg swelling and discoloration, consistent with phlegmasia cerulea dolens

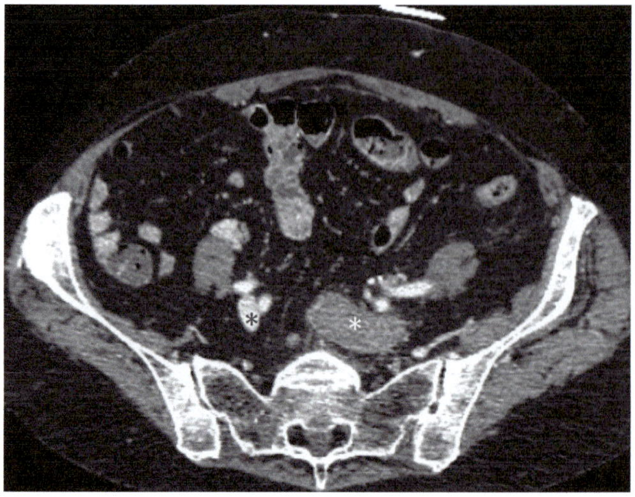

Fig. 36.7 CT Venogram axial image of the pelvis. The white asterisk shows a large expansile left common iliac vein with a large thrombus (white asterisk) and a patent right common iliac vein (black asterisk)

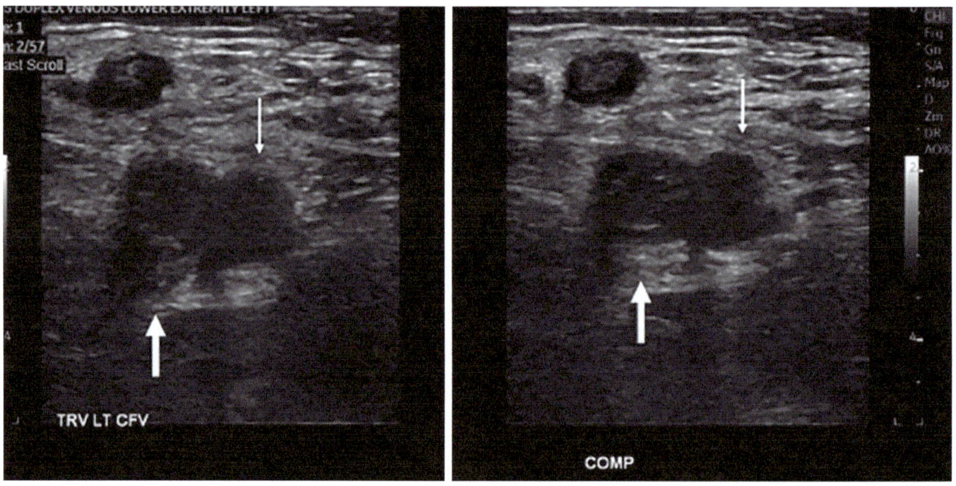

Fig. 36.6 Gray scale duplex ultrasound transverse images show incompressible left common femoral vein (comp: view seen during compression) filled with thrombus. Large arrow points to the common femoral vein (CFV) and thin arrows point to the common femoral artery

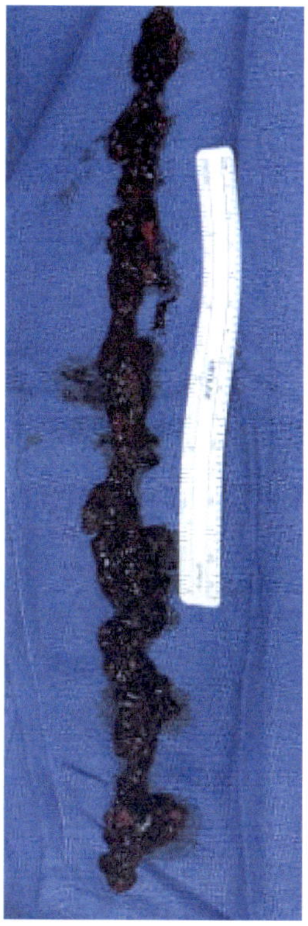

Fig. 36.8 Clots removed from left iliofemoral DVT using image-guided mechanical aspiration thrombectomy

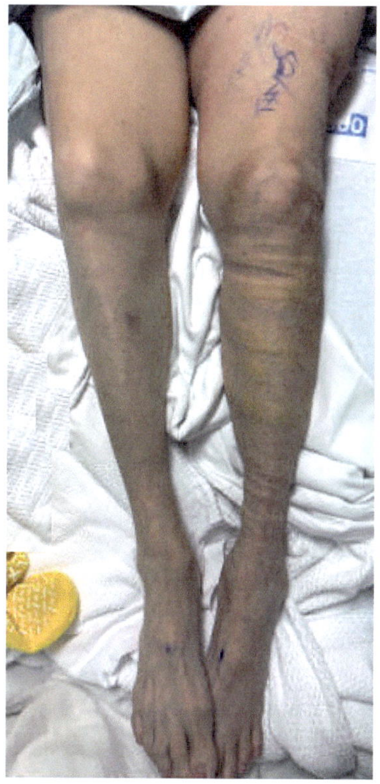

Fig. 36.10 Photograph of the patient after successful thrombectomy with much improved left leg swelling

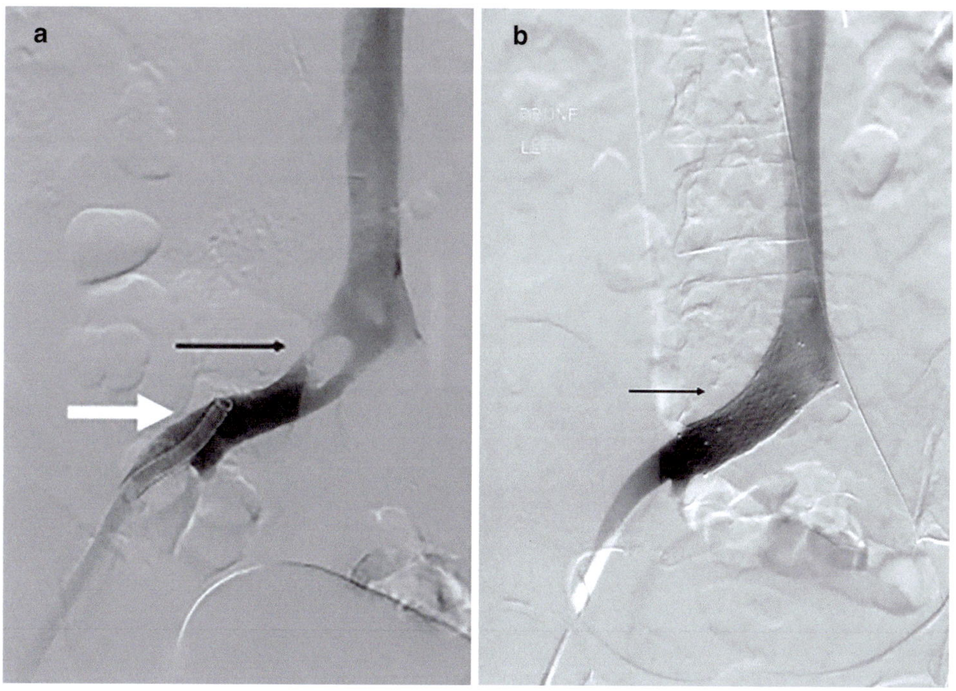

Fig. 36.9 Digital subtraction images (**a**) and (**b**) show focal severe stenosis/compression of the left common iliac vein (May-Thurner syndrome). The black arrow points to the left common iliac vein stenosis. White arrow indicates the position of the thrombectomy catheter inside the iliac vein

Case 3. Acute Pulmonary Embolism

A 70-year-old man with a history of chronic atrial fibrillation and hypertension presented to the emergency room with fatigue and dyspnea on exertion for several weeks. The patient had been on apixaban but missed several doses. CTPA showed bilateral multi-lobar pulmonary embolism and evidence of right heart strain (RV/LV ratio > 1.1; Fig. 36.11a–c). A large in-transit thrombus in the right atrium was demonstrated on CTPA and transthoracic echocardiogram (Fig. 36.12a, b). The patient underwent successful image-guided percutaneous mechanical aspiration thrombectomy, which removed the large in-transit clot in the right atrium (Fig. 36.13a), and clots in bilateral pulmonary arteries (Fig. 36.13b). The patient improved symptomatically and was discharged home 3 days after intervention on apixaban. Repeat echocardiogram showed resolution of RV strain and absence of clots in the right atrium.

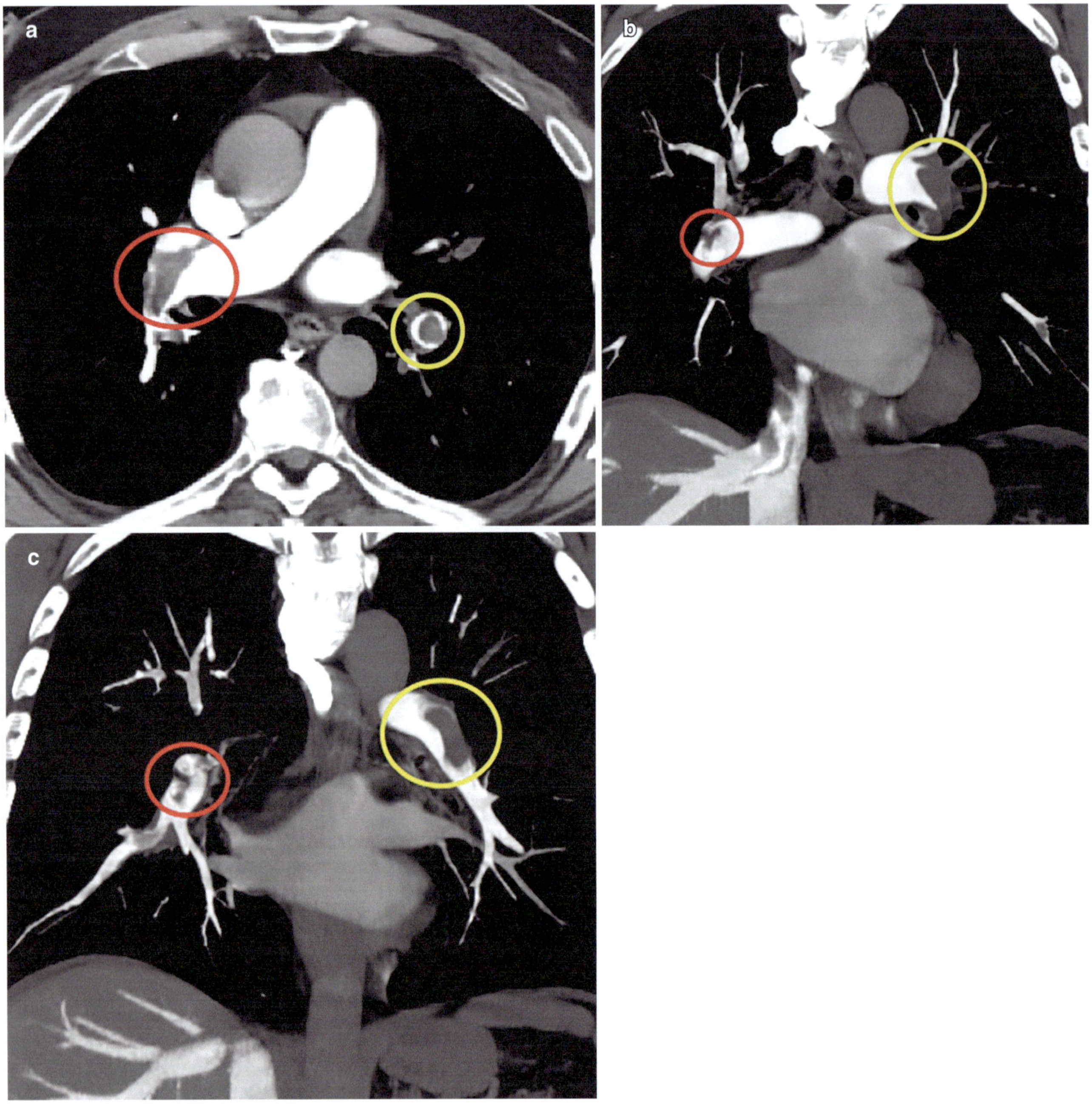

Fig. 36.11 CT of pulmonary arteries (CTPA) showed acute emboli (filling defects) in bilateral multi-lobar arteries (encircled) in axial (**a**) and sagittal (**b** and **c**) views

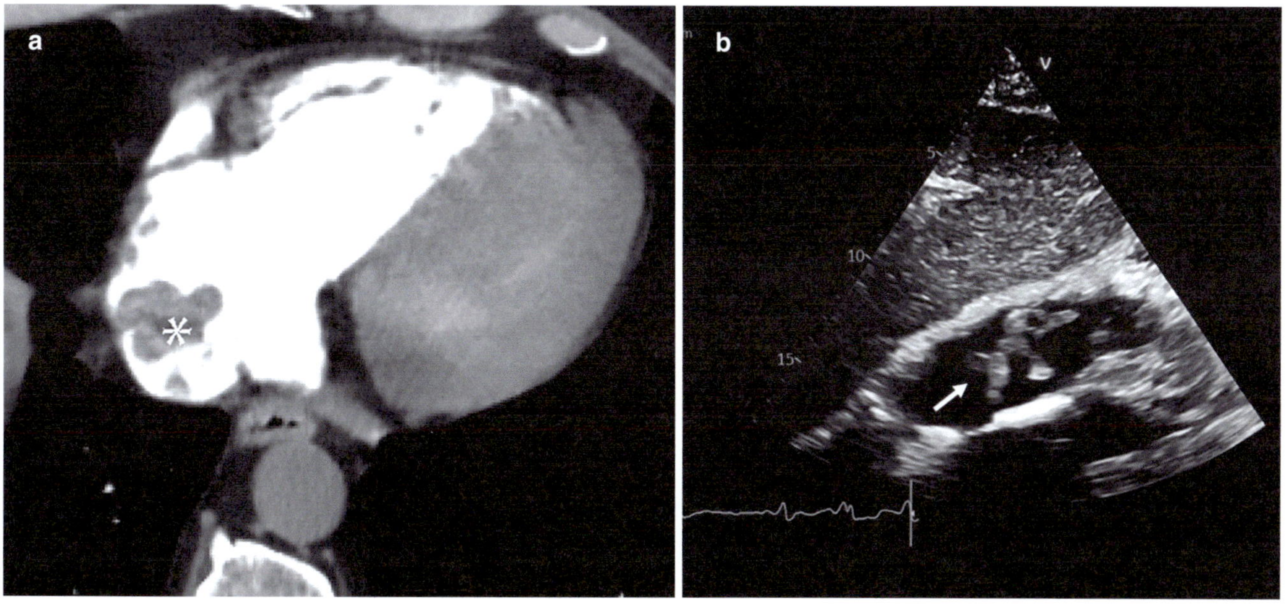

Fig. 36.12 Large in-transit thrombus seen on CTPA (**a**), marked with an asterisk, and transthoracic echocardiogram (**b**) indicated by the arrow

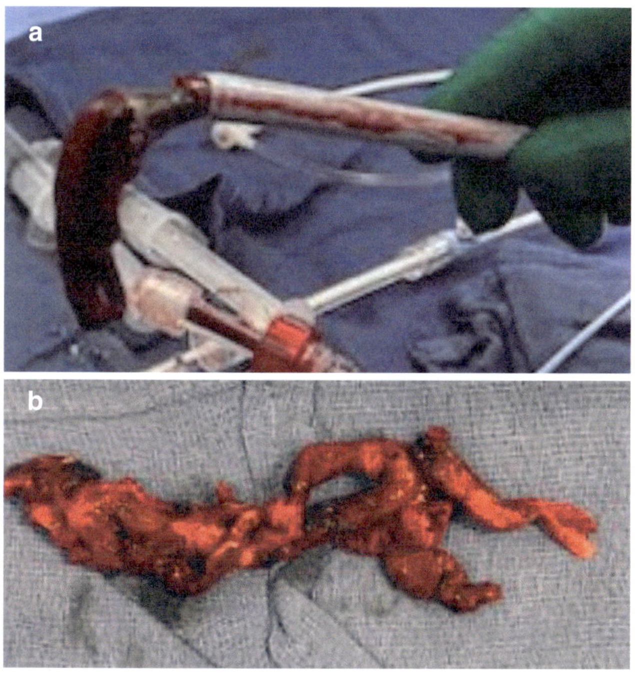

Fig. 36.13 Image-guided mechanical thrombectomy retrieved the large clot from the right atrium seen at end of the aspiration catheter (**a**), and large volume of clots from bilateral pulmonary arteries (**b**)

Case 4. Acute Bleeding Hemodialysis AV Fistula

A 69-year-old man with ESRD, diabetes, and peripheral artery disease presented to the emergency room with recurring AVF bleeding. The bleeding stopped with direct pressure. A large, ulcerated area can be seen involving an aneurysmal segment of the brachiocephalic AVF (Fig. 36.14a). The AVF was about 3–4 years old. Emergency AVF revision was successful, and the patient was able to continue to use the AVF immediately after revision surgery (Fig. 36.14b).

Case 5. Femoral Artery Pseudoaneurysm Post-catheterization

An 88-year-old man underwent staged bilateral antegrade transfemoral artery catheterization for popliteal intervention. This patient developed severe right flank pain and hypotension after right femoral artery access. The patient's blood pressure responded appropriately to 4 units of packed red blood cell transfusion. CTA imaging showed a larger right retroperitoneal hematoma and a pseudoaneurysm of the

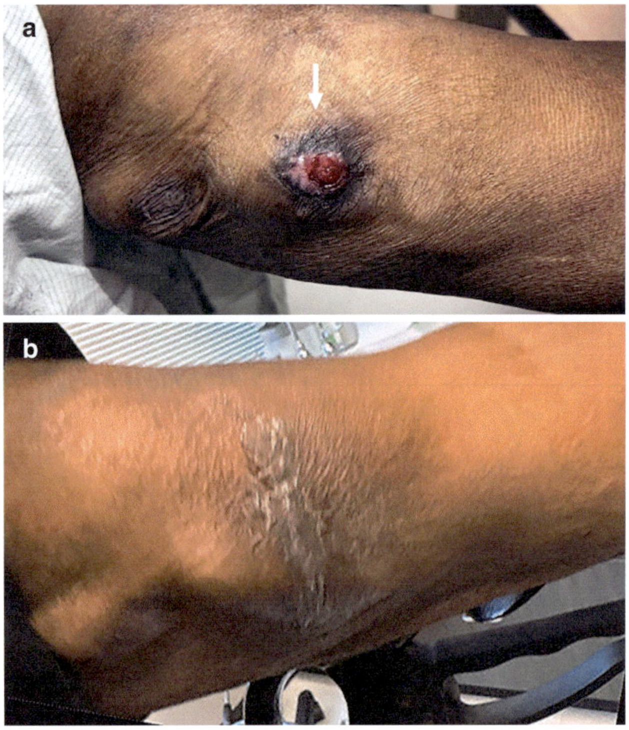

Fig. 36.14 (**a**) Photograph of the brachiocephalic AV fistula of a patient who had bled at home. Arrow points to an ulcerated aneurysmal segment of the outflow. (**b**) Photograph of the revised AVF 2 months post-operatively

proximal common femoral artery (Fig. 36.15a–d). Ultrasound-guided thrombin injection of the right common femoral artery performed at the bedside produced complete thrombosis of the pseudoaneurysm (Fig. 36.16a–c).

Case 6. Infected Femoral Artery Pseudoaneurysm After Femoral Endarterectomy and Bypass

A 65-year-old woman with a history of diabetes, hypertension, chronic kidney disease, and peripheral disease presented with acute right groin pain and swelling. The patient had multiple prior surgical and endovascular interventions for multilevel occlusive disease within the last 2 years. CTA showed a large complex bilobed pseudoaneurysm of the right common femoral artery (Fig. 36.17a–c). The patient was taken urgently to the operating room for repair of the large, expanding right common femoral artery pseudoaneurysm. A temporary occluding balloon was placed in the proximal right external iliac artery to mitigate a potential massive bleeding when exposing the large pseudoaneurysm (Fig. 36.18a). The previous common femoral artery patch was completely disrupted. The stented proximal *superficial femoral artery* (SFA) appeared occluded and was resected. The right profunda artery was reconstructed using an inter-

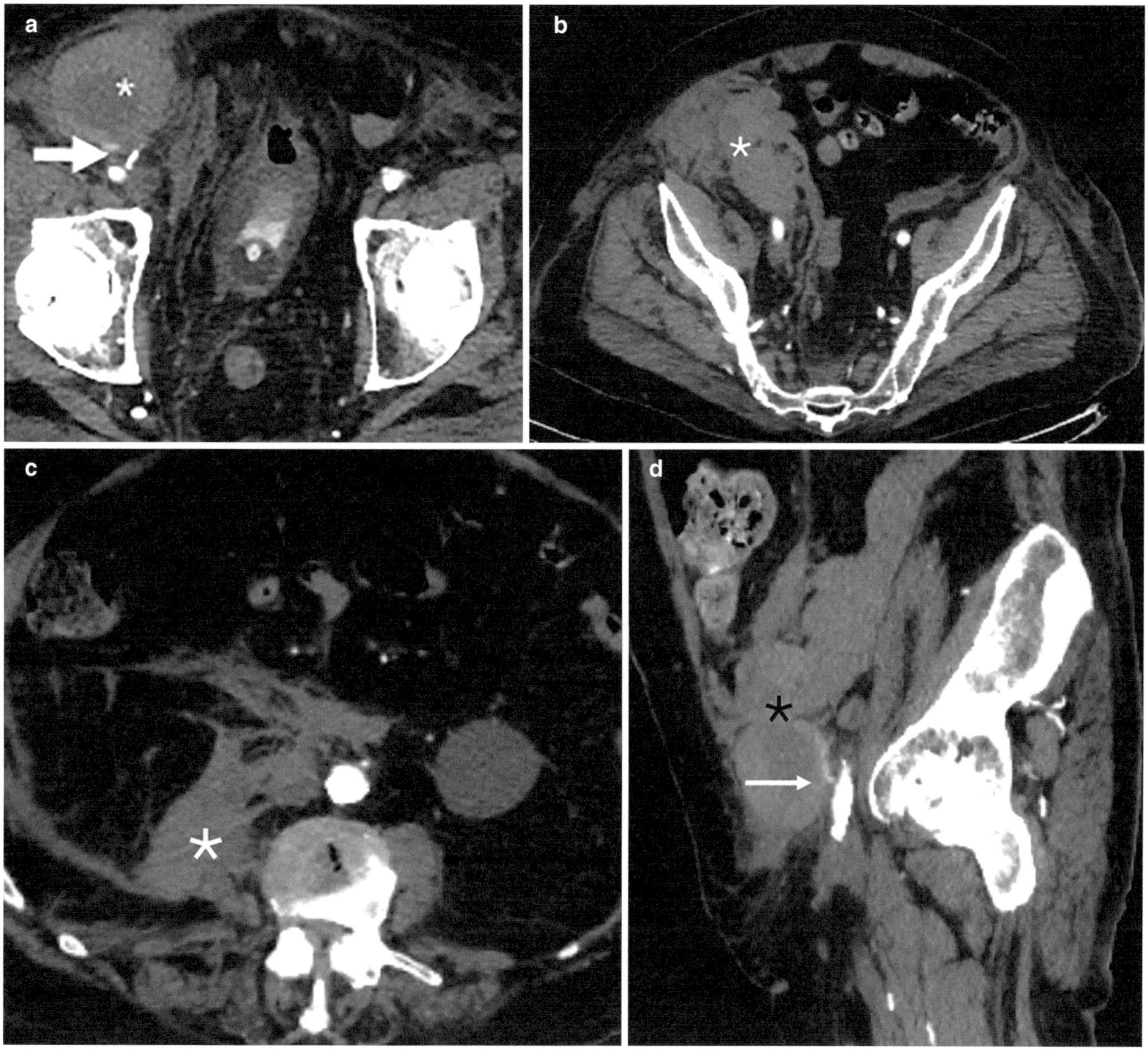

Fig. 36.15 CTA images show the large right groin hematoma extending into the retroperitoneum. (**a**) Axial image of the right groin hematoma (marked by the asterisk) and extravasation of contrast (arrow), indicating the presence of a pseudoaneurysm of the right common femoral artery. (**b**) Axial image of the hematoma extending into the right pelvis (asterisk). (**c**) Axial image of extension of the hematoma into the right retroperitoneum (asterisk). (**d**) Sagittal image of the large hematoma (asterisk) and a small pseudoaneurysm of the common femoral artery

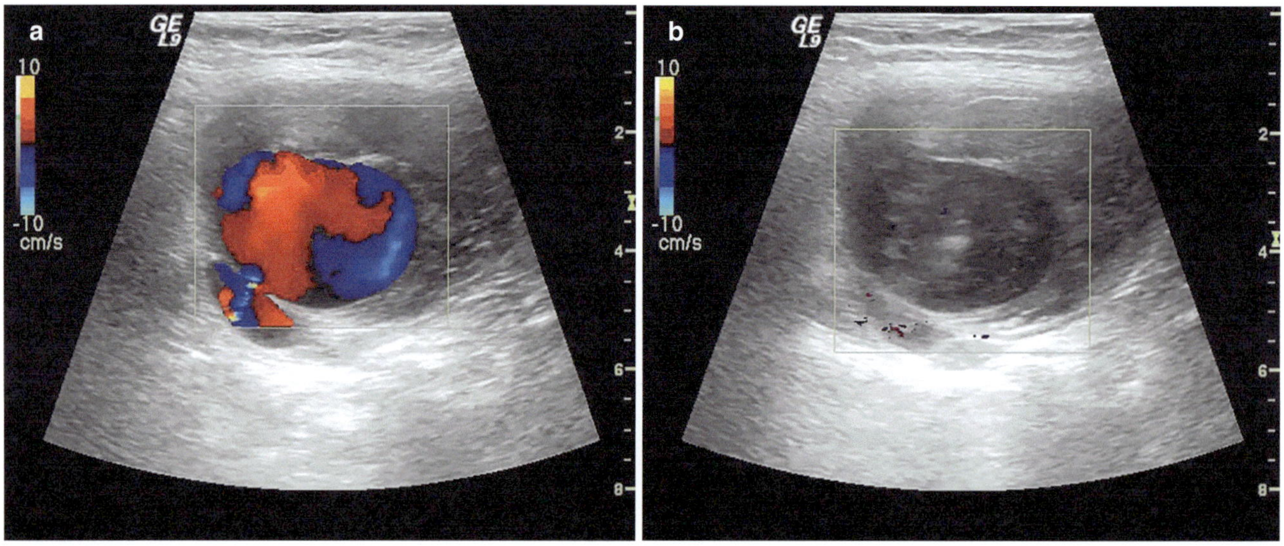

Fig. 36.16 Ultrasound-guided thrombin injection. (**a**) Colorflow transverse image shows the to-and-fro classic flow pattern of the common femoral artery pseudoaneurysm. (**b**) Complete cessation of flow indicating thrombosis of the pseudoaneurysm

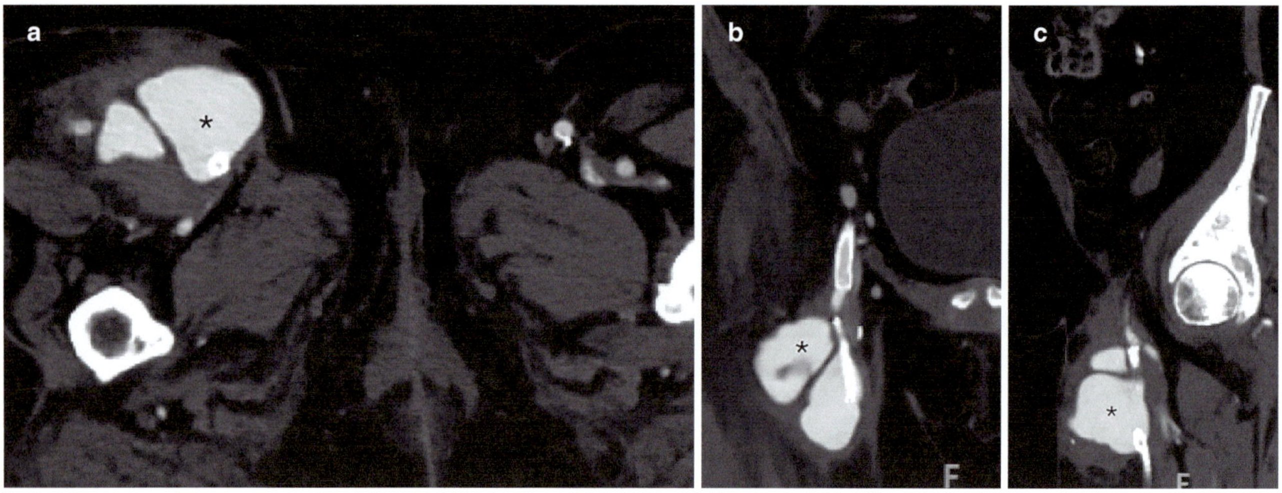

Fig. 36.17 CTA images show the large complex bilobed right common femoral artery pseudoaneurysm (asterisk) on (**a**) transverse (axial), (**b**) coronal, and (**c**) sagittal views

position cryopreserved arterial homograft; completion arteriogram showed satisfactory appearance (Fig. 36.18b). Reconstruction of the occluded superficial femoral artery was not possible, and this artery was ligated. Antibiotic beads were placed in the groin and subsequently rotated a pedicled sartorius muscle flap to cover the vascular structures. Intra-operative cultures from the deep tissues of the right groin grew multiple organisms, including coagulase-negative *Staphylococcus aureus* and *Pseudomonas*. The patient was maintained on long-term suppressive antimicrobial therapy.

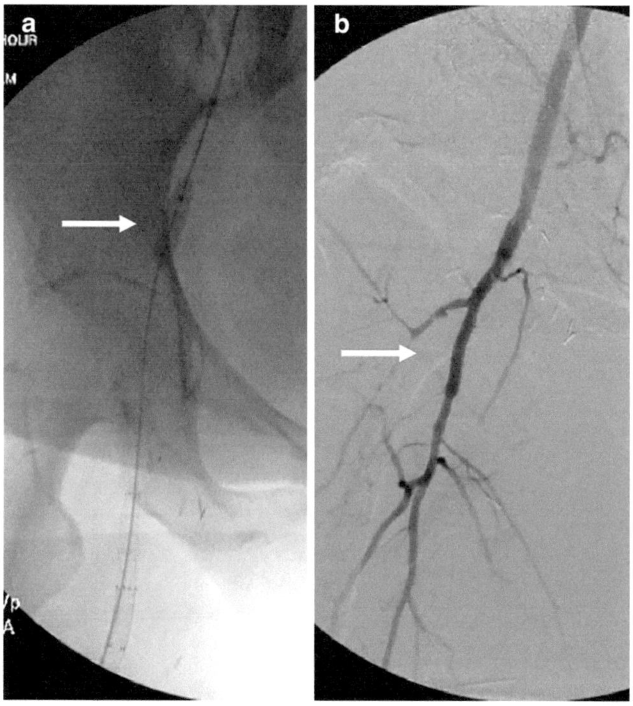

Fig. 36.18 Common femoral artery pseudoaneurysm repair and reconstruction (**a**) Radio—raphic image shows temporary occluding balloon in the right external iliac artery (arrow). (**b**) Digital subtraction image shows the right common femoral artery to profunda artery using an interposition cryopreserved femoral artery homograft (arrow)

Suggested Reading

1. BjorcK M, Earnshaw JJ, Acosta S, et al. European Society for Vascular Surgery 2020 clinical guidelines on the management of acute limb ischemia. Eur J Vasc Endovasc Surg. 2020;59:173–218.
2. Carlton WC, Franklin DP, Elmore JR, et al. Ultrasound-guided thrombin injection is a safe and durable treatment for femoral pseudoaneurysms. Vasc Surg. 2001;35:379–83.
3. Ferrer C, Cannizzaro GA, Borlizzi A, Caruso C, Giudice R. Acute ischemia of the upper and lower limbs: tailoring the treatment to the underlying etiology. Semin Vasc Surg. 2023;36(2):211–23. https://doi.org/10.1053/j.semvascsurg.2023.04.006.
4. Giri J, Sista AK, Weinberg I, et al. Interventional therapies for acute pulmonary embolism: status and principles for the development of novel evidence: a scientific statement from the AHA. Circulation. 2010;140(20):e773–801.
5. Konstantinides SV, Meyer G, Becattini C, et al. ESC Guidelines for the diagnosis and management of acute pulmonary embolism developed in collaboration with the European Respiratory Society (ERS): the task force for the diagnosis and management of acute pulmonary embolism of the European Society of Cardiology (ESC). Eur Heart J. 2019;41:543–603.
6. Moore WS, Lawrence PF, Oderich GS, editors. Moore's vascular and endovascular therapy surgery E-Book: a comprehensive review. Elsevier.
7. Padberg FT, Calligaro KD, Sidawy AN. Complications of arteriovenous hemodialysis access: recognition and management. J Vasc Surg. 2008;48(5S):55S–80S.
8. Roy P-M, Douillet D, Penaloza A. Contemporary management of acute pulmonary embolism. Trends Cardiovasc Med. 2022;32:259–68.
9. Rutherford RB, Baker JD, Ernst C, et al. Recommended standards for reports dealing with lower extremity ischemia. J Vasc Surg. 1997;26:517–38.
10. Sidawy A, Perler B, editors. Rutherford's vascular surgery and endovascular therapy. 10th ed. Elsevier; 2023.
11. Vedantham S, Goldhaber SZ, Julian JA, et al. Pharmacomechanical catheter-directed thrombolysis for deep-vein thrombosis. N Engl J Med. 2017;377:2240–52.
12. Veenstra EB, van der Laan MJ, Zeebregts CJ, et al. A systematic review and meta-analysis of endovascular and surgical revascularization techniques in acute limb threatenting ischemia. J Vasc Surg. 2020;71(2):654–68.
13. Vyas V, Sankari A, Goyal A. Acute pulmonary embolism. In: StatPearls; 2024. https://www.ncbi.nlm.nih.gov/books/NBK560551/.

Mesenteric Ischemia

37

Donna Bahroloomi, Ali Azizzadeh, and Heitham T. Hassoun

Introduction

Mesenteric ischemia occurs when blood flow to the gastrointestinal organs is insufficient to meet their oxygen and nutrient needs. This imbalance between oxygen supply and demand may result from either arterial or venous disease. The extent of ischemic injury depends on which vessels are affected and how well the body's natural collateral pathways can maintain blood flow to the affected areas. In milder cases, the injury may be limited to the mucosal layer, while more severe or prolonged ischemia can lead to full-thickness bowel infarction. While treatment techniques have evolved significantly, the most important determinant of patient outcomes remains the timeliness of diagnosis and intervention [1]. Delayed recognition of mesenteric ischemia can result in bowel infarction, sepsis, and death, with mortality rates for acute presentations reaching 60–80% [2]. This chapter reviews the fundamental principles of mesenteric ischemia, including vascular anatomy, pathophysiology, clinical presentation, diagnostic evaluation, and contemporary treatment strategies.

Anatomic Considerations

The mesenteric circulation consists of three main arterial branches from the abdominal aorta: the **celiac artery**, the **superior mesenteric artery (SMA)**, and the **inferior mesenteric artery (IMA)** (Fig. 37.1). These vessels supply the foregut, midgut, and hindgut, respectively, including the stomach, small intestine, colon, pancreas, and spleen. A rich network of collateral pathways connects the major mesenteric arteries, providing critical redundancy that helps protect the bowel from ischemia in the event of arterial narrowing or occlusion. For instance, in cases of chronic celiac artery obstruction, blood flow to the foregut can be maintained through retrograde perfusion via the pancreaticoduodenal arcades, which link branches of the SMA to the gastroduodenal and hepatic arteries. When either the SMA or the celiac artery remains patent, these collateral pathways are often sufficient to sustain adequate intestinal perfusion and prevent the onset of acute ischemia, even in the presence of significant disease in one vascular territory. This mechanism can effectively preserve blood supply to vital organs such as the liver, stomach, and pancreas despite celiac artery occlusion.

Similarly, the **arc of Riolan** and the **marginal artery of Drummond** form important connections between the superior and inferior mesenteric arteries, supporting continued perfusion of the colon when flow is compromised in either system. It is important to distinguish, however, between chronic and acute mesenteric disease. In chronic disease, collateral networks have time to develop and adapt to gradual changes in perfusion. In the acute setting, the sudden loss of blood flow does not allow sufficient time for collateral circulation to compensate, increasing the risk of intestinal ischemia and infarction.

Moreover, not all regions of the bowel benefit equally from these compensatory pathways. **Watershed zones** such as the *splenic flexure* and the *rectosigmoid junct*ion lie at the borders of major arterial territories and are particularly susceptible to low-flow states. The mid to distal small intestine, supplied by the terminal branches of the SMA, also has limited collateral input and is often the first area to suffer in acute ischemia. Understanding the structure and function of these collateral pathways is essential to recognizing patterns of injury in mesenteric ischemia and planning effective interventions. These principles are also important when evaluating patients with a history of prior abdominal surgery, aortic repair, or other vascular procedures that may have disrupted or compromised collateral blood flow.

D. Bahroloomi · A. Azizzadeh · H. T. Hassoun (✉)
Cedars-Sinai Medical Center, Los Angeles, CA, USA
e-mail: Heitham.Hassoun@cshs.org

S. Atallah, J. Dragoljevic (eds.), *Fundamentals of Surgery for Physician Assistants*,
https://doi.org/10.1007/978-3-032-21069-2_37

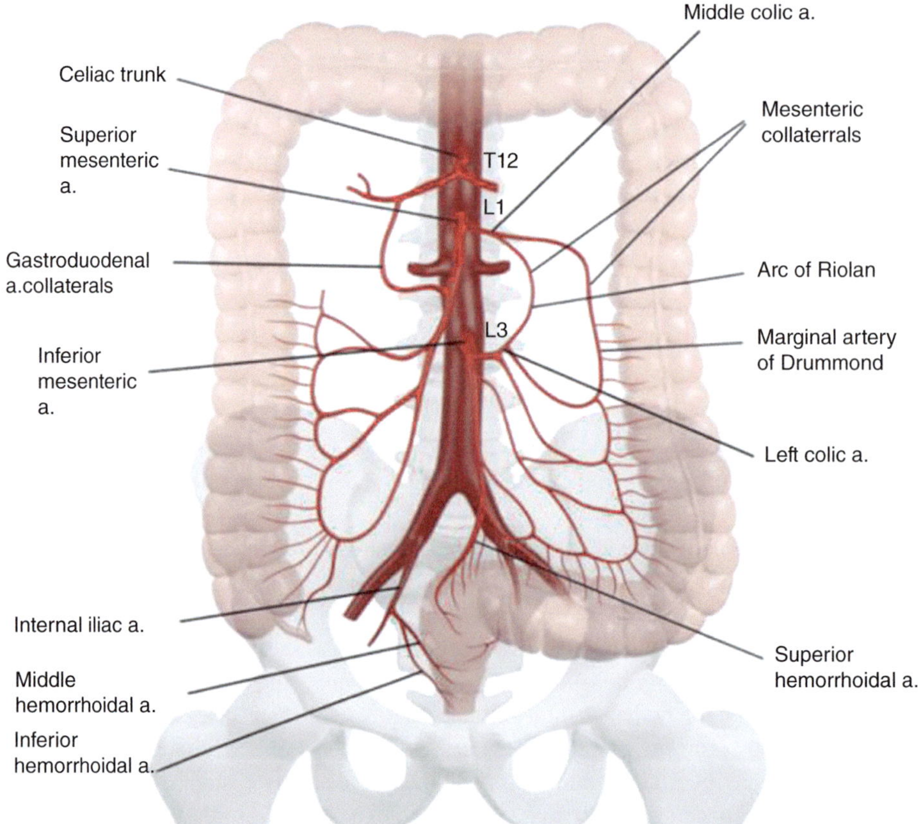

Fig. 37.1 Mesenteric vasculature [3]

Pathophysiology

Mesenteric ischemia is broadly categorized as acute or chronic, based on the duration of symptom onset. **Acute mesenteric ischemia (AMI)** is a vascular emergency most commonly caused by *arterial embolism, acute thrombosis of a preexisting atherosclerotic plaque, or nonocclusive low-flow states*. Without timely intervention, AMI can progress rapidly to bowel necrosis and systemic sepsis. **Chronic mesenteric ischemia (CMI)** develops gradually, most often due to *progressive atherosclerotic narrowing or occlusion* of the celiac, SMA, or IMA.

Mesenteric ischemia is also classified in terms of *four major categories* based on the underlying mechanism: **arterial embolism, arterial thrombosis, nonocclusive mesenteric ischemia (NOMI), and mesenteric venous thrombosis (MVT)**. Understanding these distinct etiologies is essential for timely diagnosis and effective treatment.

Chronic Mesenteric Ischemia

Chronic mesenteric ischemia is most often caused by progressive atherosclerotic narrowing at the origins of the celiac and SMA. The condition typically presents in older adults with cardiovascular risk factors such as smoking, hypertension, hyperlipidemia, end-stage renal disease (ESRD), and diabetes [1]. These patients often have widespread atherosclerotic disease affecting the coronary, cerebral, or peripheral arteries. Symptoms typically occur when two or more mesenteric vessels are affected, leading to postprandial pain, weight loss, and food avoidance. Collateral circulation between the mesenteric arteries is usually sufficient to prevent ischemia when at least one major vessel remains patent [4]. However, when all three vessels are compromised, symptoms are more likely.

While atherosclerosis is the primary cause, less common etiologies include vasculitides such as Lupus or Buerger disease, fibromuscular dysplasia, radiation injury, and certain drugs such as cocaine and ergot derivatives [1]. Although these conditions are less frequent, they should be considered in younger patients or those without traditional cardiovascular risk factors.

Acute Mesenteric Ischemia

Arterial Ischemia

Embolic Occlusion

Arterial embolism is the most frequent cause of acute mesenteric ischemia (AMI), and is responsible for 40–50% of cases

[5]. Emboli commonly originate from the heart and are associated with atrial fibrillation, recent myocardial infarction, dilated cardiomyopathy, structural defects, or infective endocarditis [1]. Less frequently, emboli may arise from ulcerated aortic plaques or thrombus within aneurysmal segments of the thoracic or abdominal aorta.

The SMA is a particularly vulnerable point of embolic occlusion due to its relatively large diameter and its straight angle of origin from the aorta, which allows emboli to bypass the proximal high-flow segment before becoming impacted at a branching point. As a result, the proximal jejunal branches are often spared, whereas the embolus obstructs flow to more distal branches supplying the jejunum, ileum, and portions of the right colon, including the cecum and ascending colon. In some cases, perfusion to the transverse colon may also be compromised, particularly if middle colic flow is interrupted. The pancreas and duodenum are typically spared due to robust collateralization from the celiac axis via the pancreaticoduodenal arcades. This segmental distribution of ischemia often results in patchy bowel infarction, with the mid to distal small intestine being particularly vulnerable.

Arterial Thrombus

Acute arterial thrombosis accounts for 20–35% of AMI cases and usually occurs in the setting of advanced atherosclerosis involving the mesenteric artery origins [6]. Patients often have preexisting symptoms of chronic mesenteric ischemia (CMI), such as postprandial abdominal pain or weight loss [7]. Thrombosis tends to affect the proximal SMA, often within 2 cm of its aortic origin, leading to extensive bowel involvement [8]. Given the more proximal location of arterial occlusion compared to embolism, thrombosis is associated with worse outcomes [8]. This is likely due to more proximal and extensive vessel occlusion and delayed diagnosis in patients with previously compensated chronic ischemia. Other contributing factors may include prothrombotic conditions such as antiphospholipid syndrome or malignancy [9]. Thrombosis may also result from extension of an aortic dissection into the mesenteric vessels and subsequent thrombosis of the false lumen [9].

Nonocclusive Mesenteric Ischemia

Nonocclusive mesenteric ischemia refers to intestinal ischemia that occurs without any arterial or venous obstruction. It accounts for approximately 5–15% of mesenteric ischemia cases and is most commonly seen in critically ill patients with reduced blood flow, such as those with cardiogenic or septic shock, severe heart failure, or prolonged low blood pressure during or after major cardiac or abdominal surgery [10]. The underlying mechanism involves intense constriction of the splanchnic circulation, triggered by systemic low blood pressure and heightened sympathetic nervous system activity [10]. This results in diversion of blood away from the intestines to preserve perfusion of vital organs. In individuals with underlying atherosclerosis of the mesenteric vessels, the ability to compensate through vasodilation is impaired, which further worsens intestinal ischemia. Other risk factors for NOMI include advanced age, hypovolemia, use of systemic vasoconstrictors or vasoactive agents, aortic insufficiency, cardiopulmonary bypass, major abdominal or cardiovascular surgery, abdominal compartment syndrome, and liver failure [1]. NOMI is also increasingly observed in patients receiving dialysis, where episodes of low blood pressure during treatment are a major precipitating factor [11]. Additional contributing factors include advanced age, long duration of dialysis, diabetes, and the use of medications such as erythropoietin, which may increase blood thickness. Preventing significant drops in blood pressure during dialysis is essential for reducing the risk of this condition in vulnerable patients.

Mesenteric Venous Thrombosis

Mesenteric venous thrombosis (MVT) accounts for 5–15% of all mesenteric ischemia cases and usually involves the superior mesenteric vein [12]. It may extend to the portal, splenic, or inferior mesenteric veins [12]. Unlike arterial ischemia, MVT typically presents with a more *gradual onset* of symptoms and carries a better prognosis when recognized early [12]. MVT is classified as either *primary, or idiopathic, or secondary to an identifiable underlying condition.* Secondary causes include local inflammation such as pancreatitis, diverticulitis, or inflammatory bowel disease; direct vascular injury from abdominal trauma or surgery; and venous stasis related to obesity or increased intra-abdominal pressure. Inherited or acquired hypercoagulable states are also common contributors and include conditions such as factor V Leiden mutation, antithrombin III deficiency, protein C or S deficiency, antiphospholipid antibody syndrome, and myeloproliferative disorders [13]. Most patients with MVT respond well to systemic anticoagulation and treatment of the underlying cause [14]. Surgical intervention is rarely required unless there is evidence of bowel infarction or perforation.

Diagnosis

Clinical Presentation

Acute mesenteric ischemia presents with the *sudden onset* of severe abdominal pain, classically described as being out of proportion to physical examination findings. The pain is typically diffuse, constant, and may occur without focal tenderness in the early stages [15]. As the disease progresses, peritoneal signs such as guarding, rebound tenderness, and rigidity may develop, indicating transmural bowel infarction [15]. Associated symptoms may include nausea, vomiting, diarrhea, or hematochezia, although these are not always present. In advanced cases, systemic signs such as hypotension, altered mental status, and signs of sepsis may occur. Laboratory findings are nonspecific but may reveal leukocytosis, elevated serum lactate, high anion gap metabolic acidosis, and elevated D-dimer [15, 16]. These findings reflect tissue hypoperfusion, but are not diagnostic and should not be relied upon alone for diagnosis. The nonspecific nature of early symptoms and laboratory data often leads to diagnostic delays. Early diagnosis requires a high index of clinical suspicion, especially in patients with atrial fibrillation, recent myocardial infarction, heart failure, or known atherosclerotic disease, all of which increase the risk of mesenteric embolism or thrombosis.

Chronic mesenteric ischemia, by contrast, presents in a more insidious manner and is typically seen in older adults with generalized atherosclerosis. The hallmark symptom is postprandial abdominal pain, which usually begins 30 to 60 minutes after eating and may persist for several hours [17, 18]. This pain is often described as dull, crampy, and epigastric, and it tends to occur consistently with food intake. As a result, patients may develop food aversion and significant unintended weight loss [17, 18]. Additional symptoms may include early satiety, nausea, bloating, or diarrhea. On physical examination, findings are often minimal, although an abdominal bruit may be present in some cases. With prolonged symptoms, patients may often appear cachectic, malnourished, and significantly underweight. Because symptoms overlap with other gastrointestinal disorders, including peptic ulcer disease, gallbladder dysfunction, or irritable bowel syndrome, diagnosis is frequently delayed. A thorough clinical history in conjunction with appropriate vascular imaging is essential for timely recognition and to prevent progression to acute mesenteric ischemia due to arterial thrombosis.

Imaging

Imaging plays a central role in diagnosing mesenteric ischemia and guiding treatment. The most commonly used noninvasive imaging tests include **duplex ultrasound (DUS), computed tomography angiography (CTA), and magnetic resonance angiography (MRA)**. *The choice of study depends on the urgency of the presentation, patient stability, and any prior vascular interventions.*

DUS is often used as an initial screening tool in patients with suspected chronic mesenteric ischemia. It measures blood flow velocities and resistance patterns in the celiac, superior mesenteric, and sometimes the inferior mesenteric arteries [19]. Specific velocity thresholds can help estimate the degree of arterial narrowing. In recent literature, the peak systolic velocity (PSV) in the SMA of greater than 275 cm/s, or a PSV of greater than 200 cm/s in the celiac trunk has been described as a reliable indicator of 70% or greater angiographic stenosis [20]. In patients with suspected median arcuate ligament syndrome, DUS during respiration can demonstrate dynamic compression of the celiac artery [21]. These measurements are accurate in native arteries, but after stenting, velocities can remain elevated even without significant narrowing [20]. For this reason, a baseline study soon after revascularization is recommended for future comparison. Despite the useful information obtained by DUS, not all patients with elevated velocities have symptoms or require repeat treatment, so results must always be interpreted alongside the clinical picture.

Computed tomography angiography is the preferred imaging test for both acute and chronic mesenteric ischemia. It provides high-resolution images quickly and allows direct visualization of the arteries, veins, and bowel. In acute cases, CTA can show findings such as bowel wall thickening, submucosal edema, pneumatosis, portal venous gas, or ascites [23]. It can also identify emboli (Fig. 37.2), thrombosis, dissections, or aneurysms. In mesenteric venous thrombosis, CTA may reveal dilated veins, filling defects, or thrombus, often seen as a "target sign" in the superior mesenteric vein [23]. A standard protocol includes both arterial and venous phases to improve detection and characterization. CTA is also useful for evaluating bypass grafts and stents. However, heavy calcification near vessel origins can make it harder to

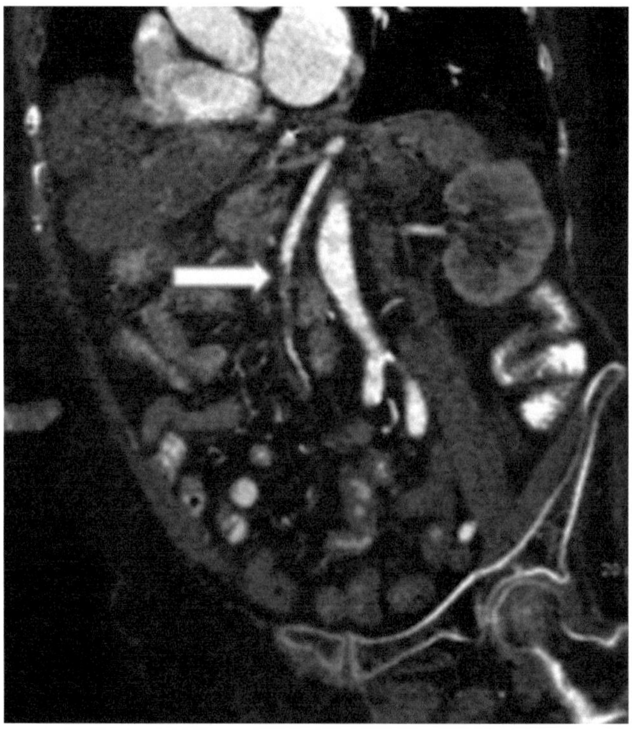

Fig. 37.2 CTA image of SMA thrombus from embolic source [22]

distinguish contrast from plaque. Reviewing noncontrast images and adjusting window settings helps improve accuracy. While CTA does involve radiation and iodinated contrast, its diagnostic value often outweighs these risks in the setting of ruling out acute mesenteric ischemia.

Magnetic resonance angiography (MRA) is an alternative when CTA is contraindicated, such as in patients with contrast allergy or severe kidney disease [24]. MRA can visualize the main mesenteric arteries and veins, but its resolution is lower than CTA, and it may not show smaller vessels or calcified plaque as clearly. It is also less accurate for assessing in-stent restenosis [24]. As a result, MRA is typically reserved for selected patients, while CTA remains the first-line imaging choice in most cases.

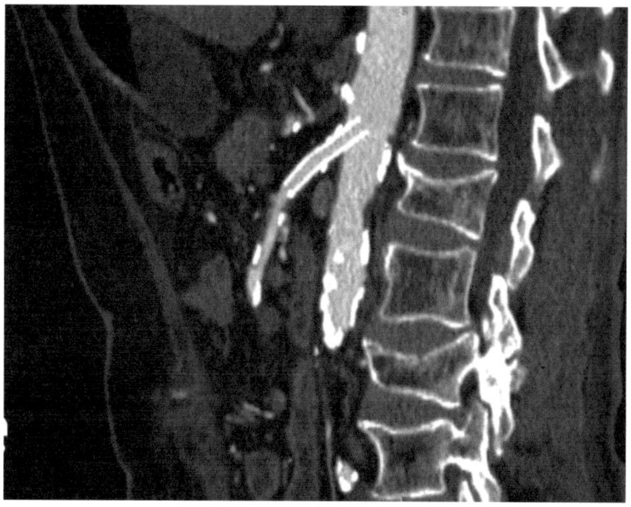

Fig. 37.3 Patent SMA stent placed for chronic mesenteric ischemia [27]

Treatment

The management of mesenteric ischemia depends on the underlying cause, the severity of bowel injury, and the overall clinical status of the patient. Broadly, treatment strategies are tailored to four major subtypes: acute arterial mesenteric ischemia (either embolic or thrombotic), chronic mesenteric ischemia, nonocclusive mesenteric ischemia (NOMI), and mesenteric venous thrombosis (MVT). Across all forms, early recognition, supportive medical care, and timely revascularization or anticoagulation are central to improving outcomes.

Chronic Mesenteric Ischemia

Patients with chronic mesenteric ischemia benefit from aggressive medical optimization. Preventive measures such as risk factor modification are critical in slowing the progression of atherosclerosis. High-intensity statin therapy has been shown to reduce cardiovascular events, mortality, and overall vascular complications in other arterial beds, and its use is reasonable in patients with mesenteric vascular disease [25]. For patients with known or suspected inherited thrombophilias, screening and appropriate anticoagulation should be considered.

Patients with chronic mesenteric ischemia often have significant malnutrition due to longstanding postprandial pain and reduced oral intake [17]. Preoperative nutritional assessment, including serum albumin, prealbumin, transferrin, and inflammatory markers such as C-reactive protein, should guide the need for nutritional supplementation. In severely malnourished patients, initiation of enteral or parenteral nutrition before revascularization may improve outcomes [26].

The treatment of chronic mesenteric ischemia has shifted toward less invasive approaches in recent years [26]. Endovascular revascularization with balloon angioplasty and stenting (Fig. 37.3) has become the preferred first-line therapy in most centers due to its lower morbidity, shorter recovery time, and favorable long-term patency in appropriately selected patients [26, 28]. This approach is particularly beneficial in patients with limited comorbid disease, single-vessel involvement, or moderate symptoms [28]. Following endovascular stenting for mesenteric revascularization, dual antiplatelet therapy is commonly employed. At many institutions, a clopidogrel loading dose of 300 milligrams is administered after the procedure, followed by 1 to 3 months of clopidogrel in addition to lifelong aspirin and statin therapy, unless contraindicated [1].

Surgical revascularization remains an option in patients with extensive disease, long-segment occlusions, failed prior endovascular interventions, or those with contraindications to endovascular therapy. Open surgical revascularization for chronic mesenteric ischemia typically involves antegrade or retrograde bypass (Fig. 37.4) from the aorta or common iliac artery to the affected mesenteric vessels, most commonly the superior mesenteric and celiac arteries [30]. Conduits may include prosthetic grafts or autologous vein, with inflow taken from the supraceliac or infrarenal aorta depending on patient anatomy and extent of disease. It can also involve transaortic endarterectomy or patch angioplasty [31]. Although more invasive than endovascular approaches, open bypass offers durable long-term patency and is often preferred in younger patients, those with extensive calcification, or when endovascular treatment has failed.

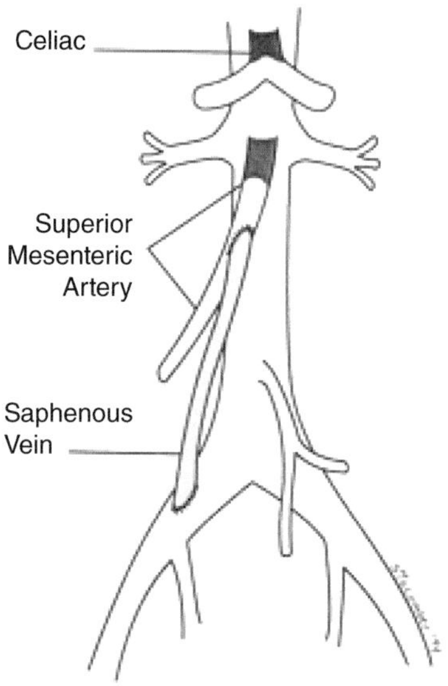

Fig. 37.4 Superior mesenteric artery bypass with saphenous vein conduit [29]

Acute Mesenteric Ischemia

The first step in the medical management of acute mesenteric ischemia is rapid hemodynamic stabilization and supportive care, initiated immediately upon suspicion of the diagnosis. Patients typically present with varying degrees of hypovolemia, electrolyte disturbances, and metabolic acidosis due to fluid losses, third spacing, and ongoing intestinal ischemia. Aggressive intravenous fluid resuscitation is essential to restore adequate organ perfusion and urine output, correct acid–base imbalances, and support cardiac output [32]. Broad-spectrum intravenous antibiotics should be administered early to prevent or treat sepsis, particularly given the risk of bacterial translocation through a compromised intestinal mucosa [32]. Empiric coverage should include gram-negative and anaerobic organisms [32]. Nasogastric decompression is often used to reduce intestinal distension and minimize further compromise of mesenteric perfusion. Concurrently, anticoagulation with intravenous unfractionated heparin is generally initiated in the absence of contraindications, as it may limit thrombus propagation and reduce the risk of additional vascular events [1]. These measures are not curative but are critical in optimizing the patient's physiological status prior to surgical or endovascular intervention and may improve overall outcomes.

Patients with acute mesenteric ischemia due to arterial embolism or thrombosis require urgent intervention. In cases with signs of peritonitis or suspected bowel necrosis, emergent laparotomy is indicated to assess bowel viability and perform revascularization [33]. Embolic occlusions typically occur distally in the SMA, often sparing the proximal jejunum and transverse colon due to preserved flow in the middle colic and ileocolic branches. Thrombotic occlusions, by contrast, usually involve the proximal origin of the SMA and result in more extensive bowel injury.

Open surgical options include embolectomy, thrombectomy, bypass grafting, or endarterectomy [34]. After restoring flow, intraoperative reassessment of the bowel is crucial, as segments previously thought to be nonviable may recover following reperfusion [34]. A wide range of adjuncts can aid in this decision, including Doppler ultrasound, visual inspection of bowel color and peristalsis, vessel palpation, and use of fluorescence or oximetric technologies [1]. Intraoperative angiography may also be helpful to confirm technical success. Most patients should undergo a planned second-look laparotomy within 24 hours to reassess bowel viability and determine whether further resection is necessary [35]. If resection is performed at the initial operation, bowel ends are stapled and left in discontinuity until the second procedure [1].

Endovascular therapy may be considered in patients with localized disease, significant comorbidities, previous abdominal operations, or poor nutritional status [35]. In selected cases with early diagnosis and no evidence of infarction, percutaneous revascularization with angioplasty and stenting has shown promising outcomes [35]. However, many patients with acute mesenteric ischemia ultimately require open exploration due to the frequency of associated bowel injury.

Nonocclusive Mesenteric Ischemia

NOMI is a distinct clinical entity that typically arises in the setting of low cardiac output, hypoperfusion, or vasospastic response following cardiac surgery or critical illness. Management focuses on correcting the underlying circulatory insufficiency. Efforts should be made to improve cardiac output, optimize volume status, and discontinue vasoconstrictive agents whenever possible [1].

Selective mesenteric angiography is the gold standard for diagnosis and can be used for therapeutic intervention [36]. Intra-arterial infusion of vasodilators such as papaverine or prostaglandin E1 may improve blood flow [36]. Studies have also demonstrated efficacy with intravenous or intra-arterial prostacyclin analogs, such as iloprost, particularly in models of cardiac tamponade or other severe low-flow states. Angioplasty and stenting are less commonly required but may be considered in patients with coexisting fixed stenoses contributing to the ischemia [37].

Mesenteric Venous Thrombosis

The primary treatment for acute or subacute mesenteric venous thrombosis is the prompt initiation of systemic anticoagulation [12].This approach improves survival, reduces the risk of recurrence, and may allow for complete resolution without the need for surgery [38]. In patients with signs of bowel infarction, peritonitis, or gastrointestinal hemorrhage, exploratory laparotomy is indicated to resect nonviable bowel [38]. Resection should be conservative, and a second-look laparotomy is often scheduled 24 hours later to reassess and avoid unnecessary removal of viable bowel [1].

Long-term anticoagulation is generally recommended in all patients with MVT. In those with identifiable thrombophilias or prior thrombotic events, lifelong anticoagulation with vitamin K antagonists is advised [12]. Transition from heparin to oral therapy can be initiated once bowel function has returned and there is no evidence of ongoing bleeding [1].

Conclusion

Mesenteric ischemia represents a spectrum of vascular disorders with high morbidity and mortality if not promptly diagnosed and treated. A thorough understanding of the varied presentations and etiologies is essential for timely intervention. While advances in endovascular and surgical techniques have expanded therapeutic options, successful management still relies on a tailored, multidisciplinary approach.

References

1. Rutherford RB, Cronenwett JL, Johnston KW. Rutherford's vascular surgery and endovascular therapy. 8th ed. Elsevier; 2014.
2. Kassahun WT, Schulz T, Richter O, Hauss J. Unchanged high mortality rates from acute occlusive intestinal ischemia: six year review. Langenbeck's Arch Surg. 2008;393(2):163–71. https://doi.org/10.1007/s00423-007-0263-5.
3. Revzin MV, Pellerito JS, Nezami N, Moshiri M. The radiologist's guide to duplex ultrasound assessment of chronic mesenteric ischemia. Abdom Radiol. 2020;45(10):2960–79. https://doi.org/10.1007/s00261-019-02165-2.
4. Upchurch GR, Henke PK. Clinical scenarios in vascular surgery. Lippincott Williams & Wilkins; 2005.
5. Bradbury AW, Brittenden J, McBride K, Ruckley CV. Mesenteric ischaemia: a multidisciplinary approach. J Br Surg. 1995;82(11):1446–59.
6. Mansour MA. Management of acute mesenteric ischemia. Arch Surg. 1999;134(3):328–30.
7. Jaster A, Choudhery S, Ahn R, et al. Anatomic and radiologic review of chronic mesenteric ischemia and its treatment. Clin Imaging. 2016;40(5):961–9. https://doi.org/10.1016/j.clinimag.2016.04.003.
8. Schoots IG, Koffeman GI, Legemate DA, Levi M, Van Gulik TM. Systematic review of survival after acute mesenteric ischaemia according to disease aetiology. J Br Surg. 2004;91(1):17–27.
9. Acosta S, Ögren M, Sternby NH, Bergqvist D, Björck M. Clinical implications for the management of acute thromboembolic occlusion of the superior mesenteric artery: autopsy findings in 213 patients. Ann Surg. 2005;241(3):516–22.
10. Acosta S. Epidemiology of mesenteric vascular disease: clinical implications. In: Seminars in vascular surgery, vol. 23. Elsevier; 2010. p. 4–8. Accessed 1 Aug 2025. https://www.sciencedirect.com/science/article/pii/S0895796709000854.
11. Quiroga B, Verde E, Abad S, et al. Detection of patients at high risk for non-occlusive mesenteric ischemia in hemodialysis. J Surg Res. 2013;180(1):51–5.
12. Kumar S, Sarr MG, Kamath PS. Mesenteric venous thrombosis. N Engl J Med. 2001;345(23):1683–8. https://doi.org/10.1056/NEJMra010076.
13. Acosta S, Alhadad A, Svensson P, Ekberg O. Epidemiology, risk and prognostic factors in mesenteric venous thrombosis. Br J Surg. 2008;95(10):1245–51. https://doi.org/10.1002/bjs.6319.
14. Hmoud B, Singal AK, Kamath PS. Mesenteric venous thrombosis. J Clin Exp Hepatol. 2014;4(3):257–63. https://doi.org/10.1016/j.jceh.2014.03.052.
15. Oldenburg WA, Lau LL, Rodenberg TJ, Edmonds HJ, Burger CD. Acute mesenteric ischemia: a clinical review. Arch Intern Med. 2004;164(10):1054–62. https://doi.org/10.1001/archinte.164.10.1054.
16. Challenges in diagnosing mesenteric ischemia - PMC. Accessed 1 Aug 2025. https://pmc.ncbi.nlm.nih.gov/articles/PMC3602491/.
17. White CJ. Chronic mesenteric ischemia: diagnosis and management. Prog Cardiovasc Dis. 2011;54(1):36–40. https://doi.org/10.1016/j.pcad.2011.04.005.
18. Moawad J, Gewertz BL. CHRONIC MESENTERIC ISCHEMIA: clinical presentation and diagnosis. Surg Clin. 1997;77(2):357–69. https://doi.org/10.1016/S0039-6109(05)70554-5.
19. Mitchell EL, Moneta GL. Mesenteric duplex scanning. Perspect Vasc Surg Endovasc Ther. 2006;18(2):175–83. https://doi.org/10.1177/1531003506291885.
20. Moneta GL, Yeager RA, Dalman R, Antonovic R, Hall LD, Porter JM. Duplex ultrasound criteria for diagnosis of splanchnic artery stenosis or occlusion. J Vasc Surg. 1991;14(4):511–20. https://doi.org/10.1016/0741-5214(91)90245-P.
21. Goodall R, Langridge B, Onida S, Ellis M, Lane T, Davies AH. Median arcuate ligament syndrome. J Vasc Surg. 2020;71(6):2170–6. https://doi.org/10.1016/j.jvs.2019.11.012.
22. Bala M, Kashuk J, Moore EE, et al. Acute mesenteric ischemia: guidelines of the World Society of Emergency Surgery. World J Emerg Surg. 2017;12(1):38. https://doi.org/10.1186/s13017-017-0150-5.
23. Menke J. Diagnostic accuracy of multidetector CT in acute mesenteric ischemia: systematic review and meta-analysis. Radiology. 2010;256(1):93–101. https://doi.org/10.1148/radiol.10091938.
24. Shih MCP, Hagspiel KD. CTA and MRA in mesenteric ischemia: part 1, role in diagnosis and differential diagnosis. Am J Roentgenol. 2007;188(2):452–61. https://doi.org/10.2214/AJR.05.1167.
25. Chou R, Dana T, Blazina I, Daeges M, Jeanne TL. Statins for prevention of cardiovascular disease in adults: evidence report and systematic review for the US Preventive Services Task Force. JAMA. 2016;316(19):2008–24. https://doi.org/10.1001/jama.2015.15629.
26. Terlouw LG, Moelker A, Abrahamsen J, et al. European guidelines on chronic mesenteric ischaemia – joint United European Gastroenterology, European Association for Gastroenterology, Endoscopy and Nutrition, European Society of Gastrointestinal and Abdominal Radiology, Netherlands Association of Hepatogastroenterologists, Hellenic Society of Gastroenterology, cardiovascular and interventional radiological Society of Europe, and Dutch Mesenteric Ischemia Study group clinical guidelines on the diagnosis and treatment of patients with chronic mesenteric

ischaemia. United Eur Gastroenterol J. 2020;8(4):371–95. https://doi.org/10.1177/2050640620916681.
27. Karkos CD, Mitka MA, Asaloumidis N, Sotiriadis S, Giagtzidis IT, Papazoglou KO. Laparotomy and jejunal arterial access for retrograde superior mesenteric artery stenting as a bailout option after failed percutaneous approach. Cardiovasc Intervent Radiol. 2019;42(11):1658–9. https://doi.org/10.1007/s00270-019-02271-0.
28. Kougias P, Sayed HFE, Zhou W, Lin PH. Management of chronic mesenteric ischemia. The role of endovascular therapy. J Endovasc Ther. 2007;14(3):395–405. https://doi.org/10.1583/07-2102.1.
29. McMillan WD, McCarthy WJ, Bresticker MR, et al. Mesenteric artery bypass: objective patency determination. J Vasc Surg. 1995;21(5):729–41.
30. Atkins MD, Kwolek CJ, LaMuraglia GM, Brewster DC, Chung TK, Cambria RP. Surgical revascularization versus endovascular therapy for chronic mesenteric ischemia: a comparative experience. J Vasc Surg. 2007;45(6):1162–71. https://doi.org/10.1016/j.jvs.2007.01.067.
31. Alahdab F, Arwani R, Pasha AK, et al. A systematic review and meta-analysis of endovascular versus open surgical revascularization for chronic mesenteric ischemia. J Vasc Surg. 2018;67(5):1598–605. https://doi.org/10.1016/j.jvs.2017.12.046.
32. Jamieson WG, Pliagus G, Marchuk S, et al. Effect of antibiotic and fluid resuscitation upon survival time in experimental intestinal ischemia. Surg Gynecol Obstet. 1988;167(2):103–8.
33. Wyers MC. Acute mesenteric ischemia: diagnostic approach and surgical treatment. Semin Vasc Surg. 2010;23(1):9–20. https://doi.org/10.1053/j.semvascsurg.2009.12.002.
34. Duran M, Pohl E, Grabitz K, Schelzig H, Sagban TA, Simon F. The importance of open emergency surgery in the treatment of acute mesenteric ischemia. World J Emerg Surg. 2015;10(1):45. https://doi.org/10.1186/s13017-015-0041-6.
35. Zhao Y, Yin H, Yao C, et al. Management of acute mesenteric ischemia: a critical review and treatment algorithm. Vasc Endovasc Surg. 2016;50(3):183–92. https://doi.org/10.1177/1538574416639151.
36. Mitsuyoshi A, Obama K, Shinkura N, Ito T, Zaima M. Survival in nonocclusive mesenteric ischemia: early diagnosis by multidetector row computed tomography and early treatment with continuous intravenous high-dose prostaglandin E: 1. Ann Surg. 2007;246(2):229–35.
37. Kang H, Manasia A, Rajamani S, et al. Intravenous iloprost increases mesenteric blood flow in experimental acute nonocclusive mesenteric ischemia. Crit Care Med. 2002;30(11):2528–34.
38. Acosta S, Ögren M, Sternby NH, Bergqvist D, Björck M. Mesenteric venous thrombosis with transmural intestinal infarction: a population-based study. J Vasc Surg. 2005;41(1):59–63.

Abdominal Imaging: Radiologic Findings of Common General Surgical Conditions and Best Imaging Studies for Common Clinical Scenarios

38

Landon Fike, Kathleen Donais, Lisa M. Truett, and Katherine Frederick-Dyer

Introduction

Welcome to the Dark Side: Diagnostic Radiology. Radiology can seem overwhelming with the sheer number of studies and diagnoses. The good news is you don't need to become a radiology expert. This chapter will equip you with the essential skills and knowledge to navigate imaging as a PA or NP. We will cover the most common imaging modalities, key diagnoses, and how to choose the correct study for a variety of clinical scenarios.

Imaging Modalities

Imaging Interpretation Basics

Think of each radiological study as a map leading to a diagnosis. To get to the diagnosis, you need to be able to recognize the common landmarks (the anatomy), follow your directions (your approach), and recognize the signposts that tell you when you are close (radiological signs).

Anatomy

Over 600 muscles, 206 bones, plus numerous ligaments, arteries, and nerves. No problem, right? For now, we will focus on recognizing *how* certain things look on different studies. The specific anatomy will come with study and practice. Resources like Radiopaedia.org, e-Anatomy (with free and paid options), or an image search for "Normal CT abdomen anatomy labeled" will be helpful along the way. Common structures will be highlighted with each modality.

Approach

Your approach is your search pattern or checklist for reviewing a study, ensuring nothing critical is missed. While the non-radiologist is not responsible for incidental findings (diagnoses unrelated to the current clinical situation that may require additional work-up or follow-up), having a systematic approach will help avoid missing major issues. Your approach should align with the clinical question and the type of study.

Signs

You need go-to signs to help guide you toward a diagnosis—warning flags to tell you something is wrong, even if you cannot see the actual problem. Here are three:

- **Air**: Air belongs in the lungs and gastrointestinal (GI) tract. If found elsewhere (e.g., under the diaphragm), consider causes like perforation (Fig. 38.1) or recent surgery. Context is essential. "Lung windows" on CT may help make air more conspicuous (Fig. 38.2) (discussed later in the Computed Tomography section).
- **Fluid**: Fluid normally resides in vessels, the gallbladder, urinary bladder, and the GI tract. Small amounts of pelvic free fluid in pre-menopausal women may be normal from ovulation. Excess fluid in the abdomen could indicate ascites, abscess, bleed, or perforation. History and imaging can help distinguish between these.
- **Fat Stranding**: Inflammation causes dilation and leakiness of blood vessels, making affected areas appear hazy on imaging. Normally, fat appears dark on radiographs/CT. With inflammation (from trauma, infection, etc.), fat appears brighter and hazier due to the increased fluid in the tissue fluid (Fig. 38.2) (fluid is brighter or "more dense" than fat on radiographs/CT).

L. Fike · K. Donais · L. M. Truett · K. Frederick-Dyer (✉)
Vanderbilt University Medical Center, Nashville, TN, USA
e-mail: landon.fike.1@vumc.org; kathleen.donais@vumc.org; lisa.m.truett@vumc.org; kate.f-dyer@vumc.org

S. Atallah, J. Dragoljevic (eds.), *Fundamentals of Surgery for Physician Assistants*,
https://doi.org/10.1007/978-3-032-21069-2_38

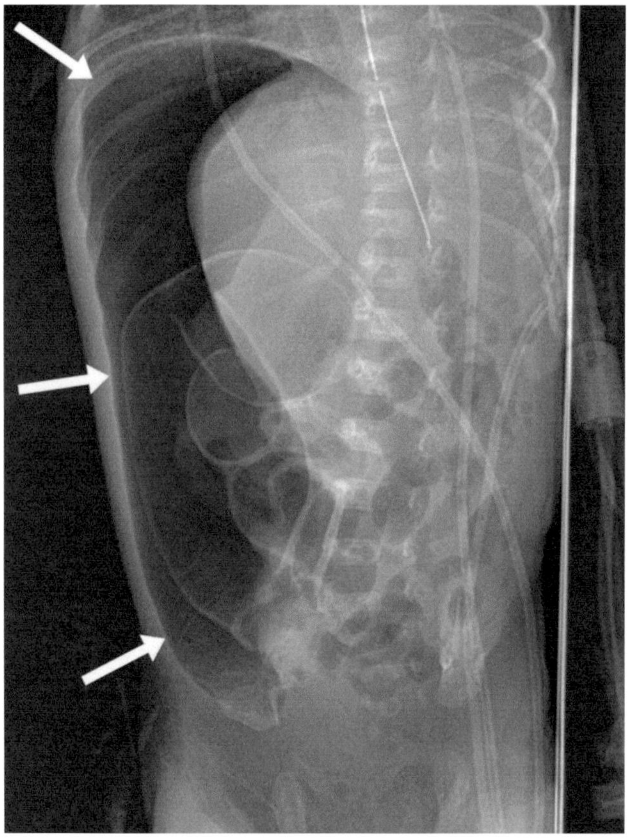

Fig. 38.1 Left lateral decubitus radiograph demonstrating a large amount of free air (white arrows)

Radiographs and Fluoroscopy

Radiographs (X-rays) and fluoroscopy work by shining X-rays (higher frequency photons than visible light) through the body, with denser materials stopping more X-rays and appearing whiter (bones are white). Typically, brightness on X-rays follows: Metal > Barium Contrast > Bone > Iodinated Contrast > Soft tissue > Water > Fat > Air. Fluoroscopy functions similarly but adds real-time imaging with different angles (projections), often with color-inverted images by convention (bones appear dark).

Radiographs are often the first choice for imaging since they are quick, portable, and inexpensive. As 2D images, they provide a basic screening test for obvious issues. If you find something, great! If not, it doesn't necessarily rule out a problem. For example, radiographs are useful for detecting post-surgical perforations because you might see free air, but they are not ideal for cholecystitis because you probably won't be able to see the gallbladder or gallstones. You can enhance the utility of radiographs by requesting specific views depending on the clinical question. For example, a lot of free air may be inconspicuous on a supine radiograph (since the air will layer along the anterior abdomen), but if you change the patient's position, you can make the air collect under the diaphragm (upright radiograph) or along the patient's flank (lateral decubitus radiograph).

Fluoroscopy is often used in the acute setting to evaluate for leak or in the outpatient setting to define pre-surgical

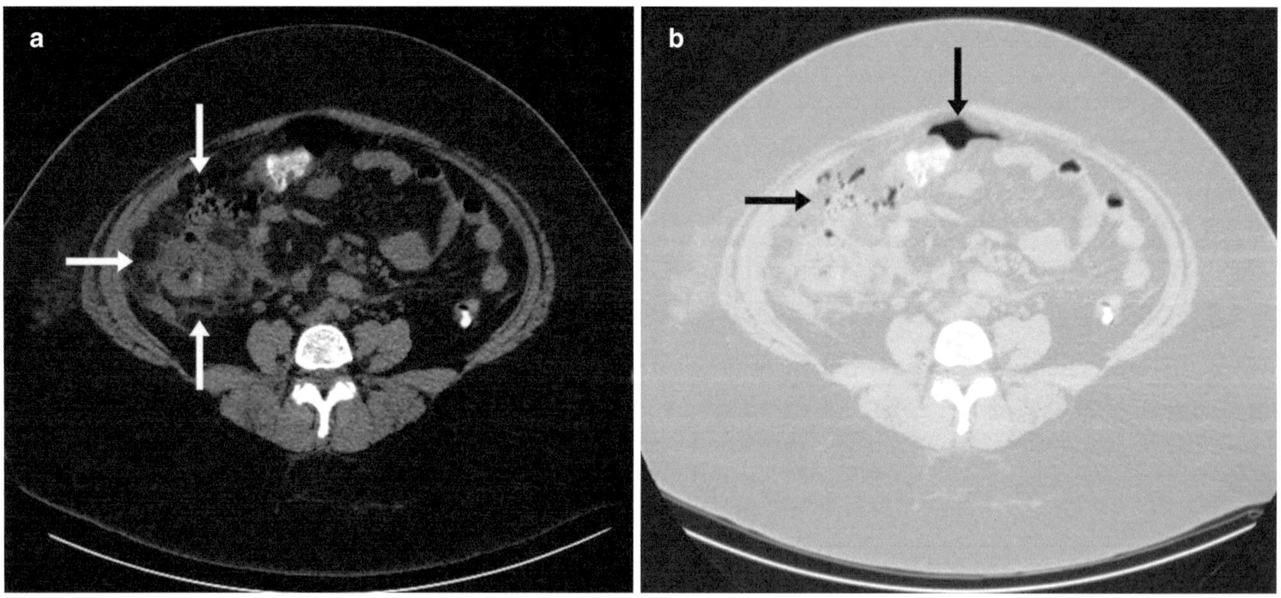

Fig. 38.2 (**a**) Axial non-contrasted CT image with soft-tissue window demonstrating right lower quadrant fat stranding and trace free fluid in the region marked by white arrows. (**b**) The same axial CT image with lung windows highlighting the presence of free air (black arrows) raising concern for bowel perforation

Table 38.1 Considerations for using Barium, Diatrizoate, and Iohexol as oral/rectal contrast agents

Contrast type	Barium	High Osmolarity Iodinated Contrast - example: Diatrizoate (Gastrografin)	Low Osmolarity Iodinated Contrast - example: Iohexol (Omnipaque)
Benefits	Brightest (densest) PO/PR contrast, shows more detail on fluoroscopy and radiography No iodine, less allergy risk	Water-soluble Inexpensive No significant CT artifact if diluted with water appropriately	Water-soluble Safest option for PO in patients with aspiration risk No significant CT artifact if diluted with water appropriately
Risks	Not water-soluble Problematic if aspirated Causes significant streak artifact on CT (due to high density)	Can cause chemical pneumonitis if aspirated Contains iodine, allergy risk Hypertonic, can cause fluid to be drawn into lumen, avoid use in dehydrated patients Subjectively the worst tasting PO contrast	More expensive Contains iodine, allergy risk

anatomy. If there is clinical concern for an esophageal, gastric, urinary bladder, or anastomotic leak, ordering fluoroscopy can help demonstrate the exact location of the leak.

There are several different types of by mouth or per rectum contrast that can be administered (Table 38.1). Barium is a very dense substance and can help to define the anatomy of gastrointestinal structures as well as assess physiologic parameters such as motility. However, Barium should not be administered when there is a suspected leak. Instead, water-soluble Iodinated contrasts, such as Diatrizoate (trade name Gastrografin) or Iohexol (Omnipaque) should be utilized if there is a leak as they can be reabsorbed by the body if they leak out from a perforation. Please note that Diatrizoate (Gastrografin) should not be administered PO if the patient is at risk for aspiration as it can cause pneumonitis if aspirated because of its high osmolarity. Administration per gastrostomy tube could be considered in this setting. Also, patients should be asked about allergies to iodinated contrast agents prior to administration of water-soluble agents.

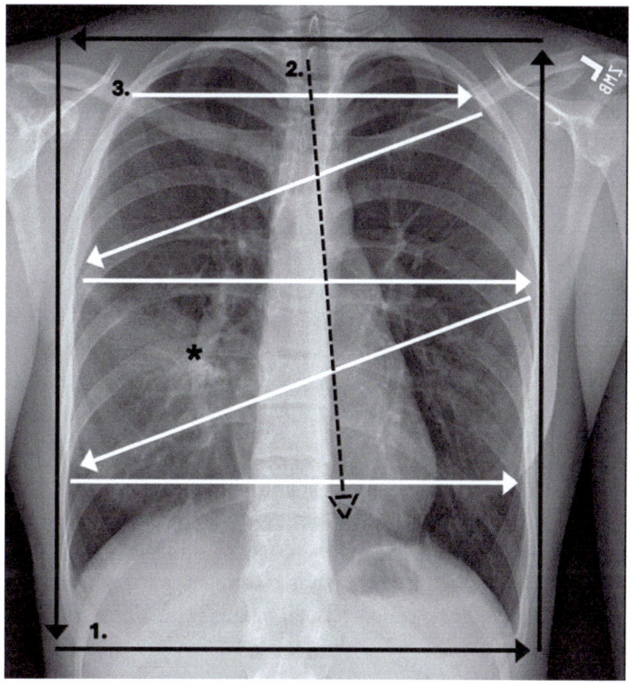

Fig. 38.3 Frontal chest radiograph demonstrating a simple approach. Examine the chest wall by starting at 1. and following the solid black arrows. Next, examine the mediastinum and spine by starting at 2. and following the dashed black arrow. Lastly, examine the lungs side-to-side starting from the top at 3. and following the white arrows. The patient's right middle lobe pneumonia is marked by the black asterisk

Basic Approach

Focus on structure outlines and hidden free air. Always consider positioning to guide your search for air. Start by assessing hardware, lines, and tubes, then examine the radiographs systematically to avoid missing key areas. For excellent and light reading to help build your approach and skills to radiographs, see Felson's textbook referenced at the end of the chapter.

- Chest (Fig. 38.3): Upper abdomen (free air?), soft tissues, bones, mediastinum/heart, lungs
- Abdomen/pelvis (Fig. 38.4): Chest/film edges, diaphragm, bowel gas, organ areas (liver, spleen, kidneys, pelvis), bones

Computed Tomography (CT)/CTA

CT uses the same x-rays as radiographs/fluoroscopy but rotates around the patient to create a 3D image data set, which can be reformatted in various ways. Typically, radiologists review an exam using axial reformats—slices oriented horizontally through the patient's body, but images can be reformatted coronally (vertical slides from anterior to posterior), sagittally (vertical slices from side to side), or obliquely (Fig. 38.5). Brightness on CT follows the same pattern: **Metal > Bone > Iodinated Contrast > Most soft tissues > Water > Fat > Air**. In fact, each tissue has a relatively specific brightness on CT (called Hounsfield Units or HU) that can help identify it; for example, simple fluids are 0–20 HU, so if you see a fluid brighter than this, you should con-

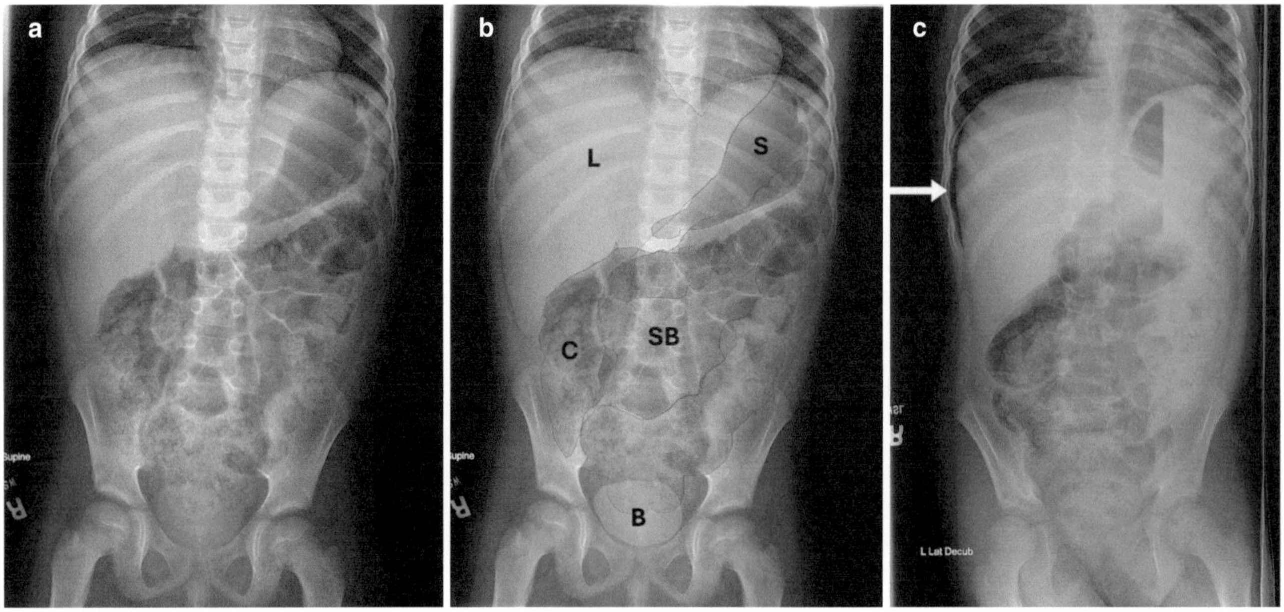

Fig. 38.4 (**a**) Supine frontal abdominal radiograph showing subtle free air, (**b**) The same image with anatomy labeled including the liver (L), stomach (S), colon/large bowel (C), small bowel (SB), bladder (B), (**c**) The same patient in the left lateral decubitus position showing trace pneumoperitoneum collecting along the right flank (white arrow)

sider a more complicated fluid, such as blood, abscess, or bowel contents.

CT provides detailed anatomy of organs, viscera, and small pockets of free air that cannot be seen on radiographs. The downside: CTs are not portable and are typically less available compared to radiographs. Furthermore, there is increased radiation exposure and increased cost relative to radiography, and if you are utilizing IV iodinated contrast, you will need to consider additional risks such as allergic reactions and, in patients with poor renal function, injury to the kidneys (Table 38.2).

CTA (CT angiography) is a CT scan that is specifically protocolled to evaluate blood vessels, cardiac structures, and potential bleeds or thrombus/emboli. They often have thinner slices and are timed with IV contrast administration to optimize assessment of these structures, usually a non-contrast phase, a phase where the contrast timing is optimized for assessment of the arteries, and a phase where the contrast timing is optimized for assessment of the veins. Additionally, they are often reformatted as MIP or Maximal Intensity Projections, whereby a "thicker" image is created by taking the brightest pixel from several sequential images (Fig. 38.6).

Approach

The significantly higher amount of detail means there is a lot to see—or miss. Generally, having an organ/organ system-based approach will help keep you from missing an obvious abnormality. Two things deserve specific imaging for abdominal surgery: running the bowel and CT windows.

Running the bowel: start at the anus and follow the large bowel to the cecum. Then, start at the esophagus and follow through the stomach and duodenum. After this, divide the small bowel in regions (scroll all the way through looking at the left flank, mid abdomen, right flank). If you see evidence of obstruction, then back up and take your time following the loops to find the area where the caliber abruptly changes, called the transition point. Coronal and Sagittal reformats are often helpful for following the bowel and localizing an obstruction. Please see later section discussing "Ileus and Obstruction" for more information.

CT windows: these settings help highlight different tissues by changing the brightness and darkness. A bone window is better for bones because they may be too bright on other sequences. Lung windows are not only good for evaluating the lungs. They are extremely helpful for examining the abdomen for free air. Always review a CT with lung windows to look for free air in the abdomen (Fig. 38.5).

Ultrasound

Ultrasound can be more challenging for the non-radiologist reviewer because anatomic detail and orientation may be less clear. Ultrasound works by sending high-frequency sound waves into the patient and "listening" for the reflections—which means it does not use radiation. The more sound is reflected, the brighter an area will be on ultrasound. Simple fluid, such as a cyst or seroma, is not reflective and will allow sound to pass through, making it appear dark (Fig. 38.7).

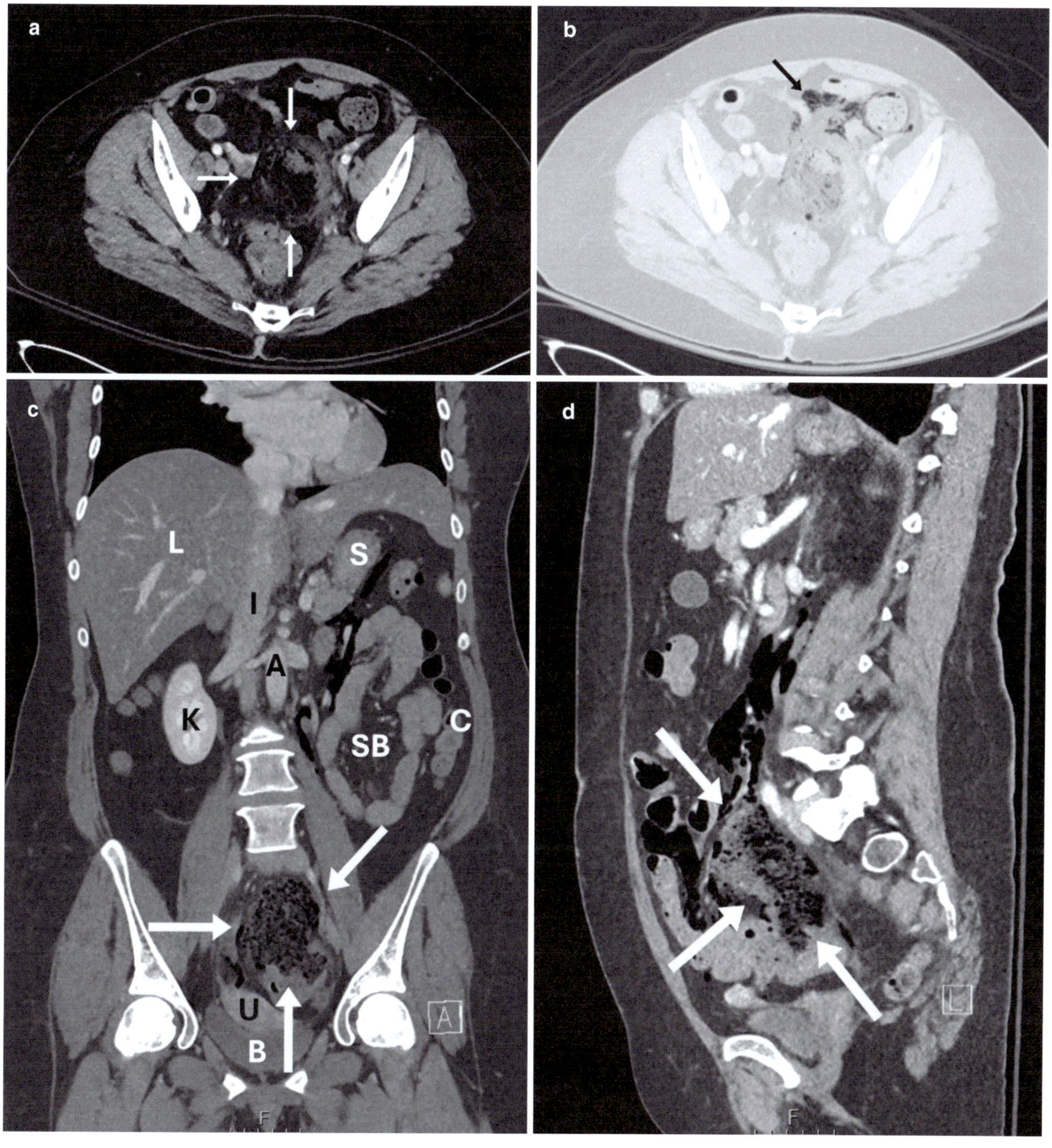

Fig. 38.5 (**a**) Axial contrast-enhanced CT image through the pelvis showing an area of fat stranding (white arrows), (**b**) The same image on lung window highlighting the free air (black arrow) concerning for perforation that was difficult to notice on panel a, (**c**) Coronal reformat of the sigmoid perforation with normal anatomy labeled including liver (L), stomach (S), kidney (K), IVC (I), aorta (A), colon (C), small bowel (SB), uterus (U), and bladder (B), (**d**) Sagittal reformat of the same area

Table 38.2 Selected CT and MRI IV contrast considerations (Reference ACR Manual on Contrast Media 2024)

Modality	CT	MRI
Typical contrast agent	Iodinated contrast media (ICM) (modern agents are low osmolar)	Gadolinium based contrast media (GBCM)
Risk of acute adverse event (allergic or physiologic)	~0.2–0.7%	~0.15%
Risk of serious acute reaction	~0.04%	~0.006%
Greatest risk factor for Allergic Reaction	Prior allergic reaction to ICM	Prior allergic reaction to GBCM
Risk in patients with poor renal function	Contrast-induced nephropathy (risk increases with worsening renal function)	Nephrogenic Systemic Fibrosis (risk is very low and possibly nonexistent with group II agents, but continued caution is advised)
Risk in pregnancy (FDA category)	Pregnancy Category B—probably low risk but no well controlled studies	Pregnancy Category C—recommend avoiding unless benefits outweigh risks
Breastfeeding	<0.01% excreted and absorbed by infant's gut. No requirement to stop breastfeeding.	<0.0004% estimated excreted and absorbed by infant's gut. No requirement to stop breastfeeding

Please refer to the ACR Manual on Contrast Media and your own institution's protocols for premedication strategies for patients with history of contrast allergy needing IV contrast. Your local radiologist may be able to offer alternative exam recommendations depending on the clinical scenario.

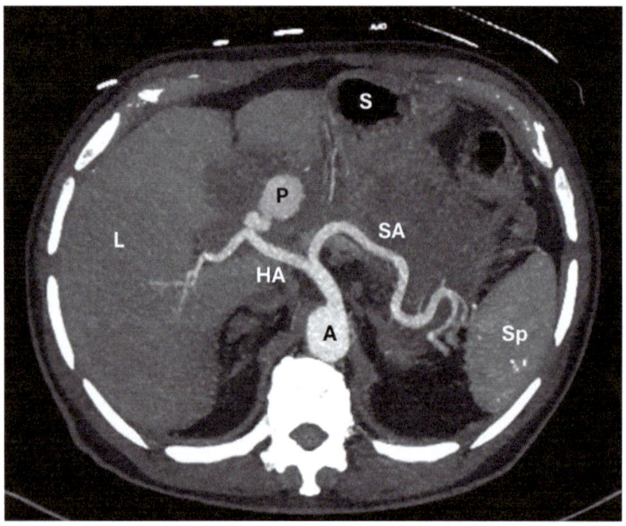

Fig. 38.6 Axial CT image in arterial phase with maximal intensity projection (MIP) demonstrating a large pseudoaneurysm (P) arising from the common hepatic artery (HA). Additional anatomy labeled including liver (L), spleen (Sp), stomach (S), aorta (A), and splenic artery (SA)

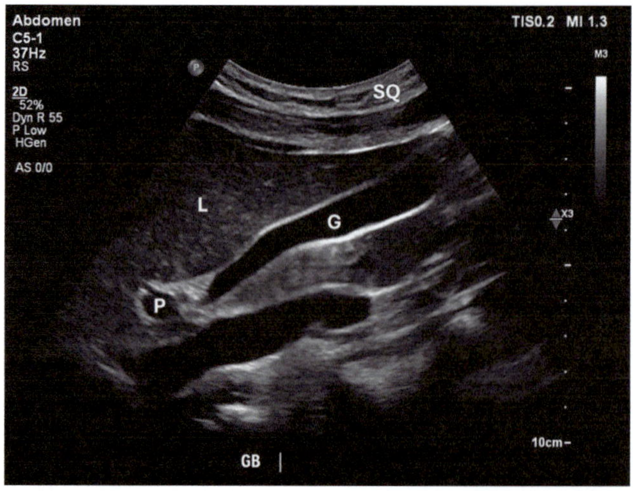

Fig. 38.7 Grayscale ultrasound image through the long-axis of a normal gallbladder (G). The fluid within the gallbladder appears dark, the liver (L) less dark, and the subcutaneous fat (SQ) and other interfaces brighter. Portal vein (P)

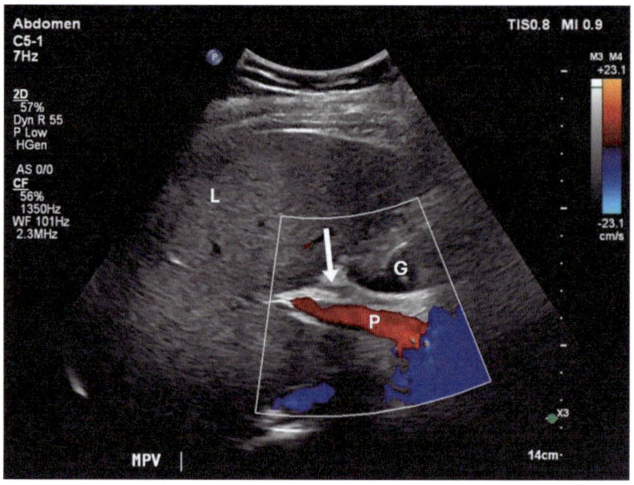

Fig. 38.8 Ultrasound with color doppler showing patency and normal directional flow of the main portal vein (P). Liver (L), gallbladder (G), common hepatic duct (white arrow)

Bone is very reflective, and the closer surface of the bone will show up as bright white. However, because it is so reflective, no soundwaves will pass through, and you will see a dark "shadow" behind the surface of the bone. Gas will also reflect a lot of sound and show a bright interface with a dark shadow making it impossible to image through normal lung. In fact, gel must be applied to a patient to remove the air between the patient and the ultrasound probe for the ultrasound probe to work! We can add Doppler assessment to ultrasounds, allowing us to visualize flow within an area and even evaluate the speed blood is flowing in a vessel (Fig. 38.8).

When reviewing an ultrasound, the images will often be labeled to tell you what the sonographer is showing you—

this is key to getting oriented. The ability to perform targeted real-time imaging with assessment of blood flow makes ultrasound an incredibly useful tool for specific questions. Some applications include looking for blood clots, superficial fluid collections, and assessing solid organs. Limitations arise from the inability to visualize beyond gas/bone, so ultrasound is typically not useful for looking at the brain (outside of infants), lungs, or gas-filled bowel.

It is important to note that ultrasound is often essential in the work-up of pelvic pain in females because of its superior soft tissue discrimination abilities. In addition to transabdominal evaluation, specially designed transvaginal ultrasound probes are available to facilitate highly detailed evaluation of the uterus and ovaries.

Magnetic Resonance Imaging (MRI)/MRCP

Like CT and ultrasound, MRI allows 3D assessment of anatomy. MRI uses powerful magnets, radiofrequency, and the properties of hydrogen atoms in different tissues to create images without radiation. Changing imaging parameters creates different sequences that can highlight or subtract different tissue signals. This allows for sequences that highlight fluid and blood or suppress unwanted signals like fat. Two basic sequences are T1 and T2. On T1, fluid is dark and fat is bright. On T2, fluid is bright (think H2O) and fat is somewhat bright. If you are looking for inflammation and abscess, look for a bright collection on T2 that is dark on T1 (Fig. 38.9). MRCP (Magnetic Resonance Cholangiopancreatography) is a specific type of MRI which is often used as a non-invasive alternative to ERCP (Endoscopic Retrograde Cholangiopancreatography) to evaluate the bile ducts, gallbladder, pancreas, and pancreatic duct. It can be useful to detect biliary stones and strictures.

The utility of MRI comes from using multiple types of images to better characterize specific abnormalities. The cons of MRI compared with CT include longer imaging time (30 mins to a couple hours), decreased availability of MRI, and higher cost.

When reviewing an MRI, start with your T1 and T2 sequences and take an organ-by-organ approach like for CT. You can use some of the more complicated sequences to help further evaluate abnormalities that you find, although the description of more advanced sequences is beyond the scope of this text.

MRI evaluation can also be performed with intravenous contrast, although it is important to note that MRI contrast utilizes gadolinium (a rare earth metal) instead of iodine. MRIs are typically performed both with and without IV contrast when contrast is utilized so that the non-contrast sequences are obtained as well as the with contrast sequences for a more complete characterization of the patient's pathology. The risk of allergic reaction with MRI contrast is less than the risk with CT contrast. Gadolinium contrast (especially older Type I contrast agents) should be used with caution in patients with poor renal function due to the risk of nephrogenic systemic fibrosis (Table 38.2).

Nuclear Medicine

In nuclear medicine, instead of shining x-rays through a patient, we are giving the patient a radioactive pharmaceutical—a tracer—that localizes to an organ and/or physiologic/pathologic process and creates x-rays through radioactive

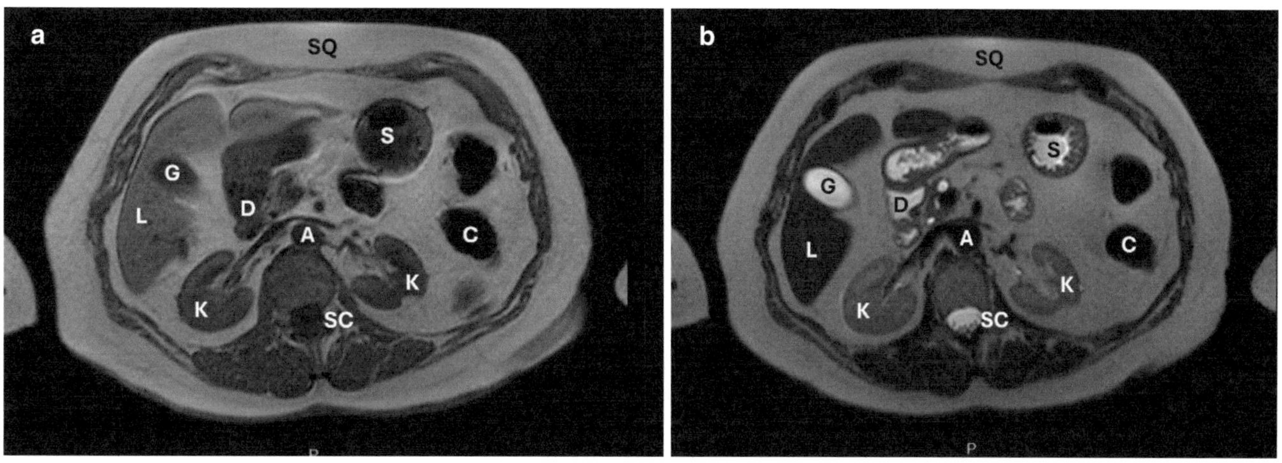

Fig. 38.9 (**a**) Axial T1-weighted MR image through the abdomen showing bright subcutaneous fat (SQ) and typical appearances of the liver (L), gallbladder (G), duodenum (D), kidney (K), aorta (A), stomach (S), colon (C), and spinal canal (SC), (**b**) Axial T2-weighted image at the same level showing that a key difference is that fluid is bright on the T2 sequence as seen in the gallbladder, GI tract, and CSF (labels identical to (**a**))

decay that our detectors outside of the patient will convert into an image. The patient (or more specifically the radiopharmaceutical inside the patient) are the source instead of our x-ray machines. Each radiopharmaceutical used will have different properties that allow it to highlight different tissues or tissue functions. For example, some are excreted into the biliary system, some stay in the blood, and some go to the bones.

We can use these properties to tell us about the function of different organs/tissues. Each study has a specific utility. A HIDA (hepatobiliary iminodiacetic acid) scan can assess gallbladder function in cases of questionable cholecystitis (Fig. 38.10), a bone scan can evaluate for osteomyelitis (Fig. 38.11), and a tagged RBC scan is an extremely sensitive method to evaluate for an occult slow intermittent GI bleed. PET (Positron Emission Tomography) scans can help identify malignancy and follow it over time (Fig. 38.12).

The approach to each of these will be study specific. Areas that take up the radiopharmaceutical for that study will show up as brighter or darker than the surrounding tissue depending on the study. The general question will be: is the tracer where it is expected to be and going where it is expected to go? Numbers may be provided for functional assessment and normal values/interpretation can be looked up for each study.

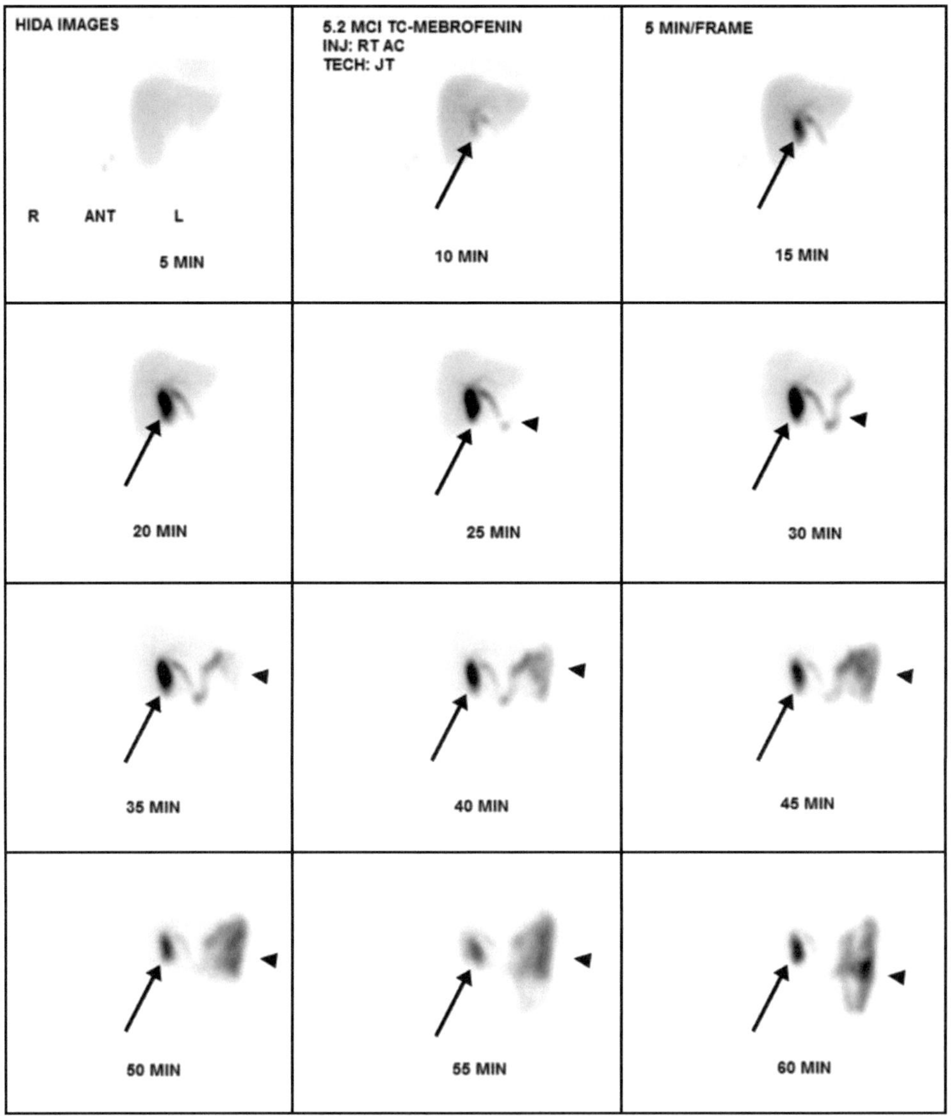

Fig. 38.10 Normal nuclear medicine HIDA scan showing the radiopharmaceutical entering the gallbladder (black arrows) by 10 min and the small bowel (black arrowheads) by 25 min

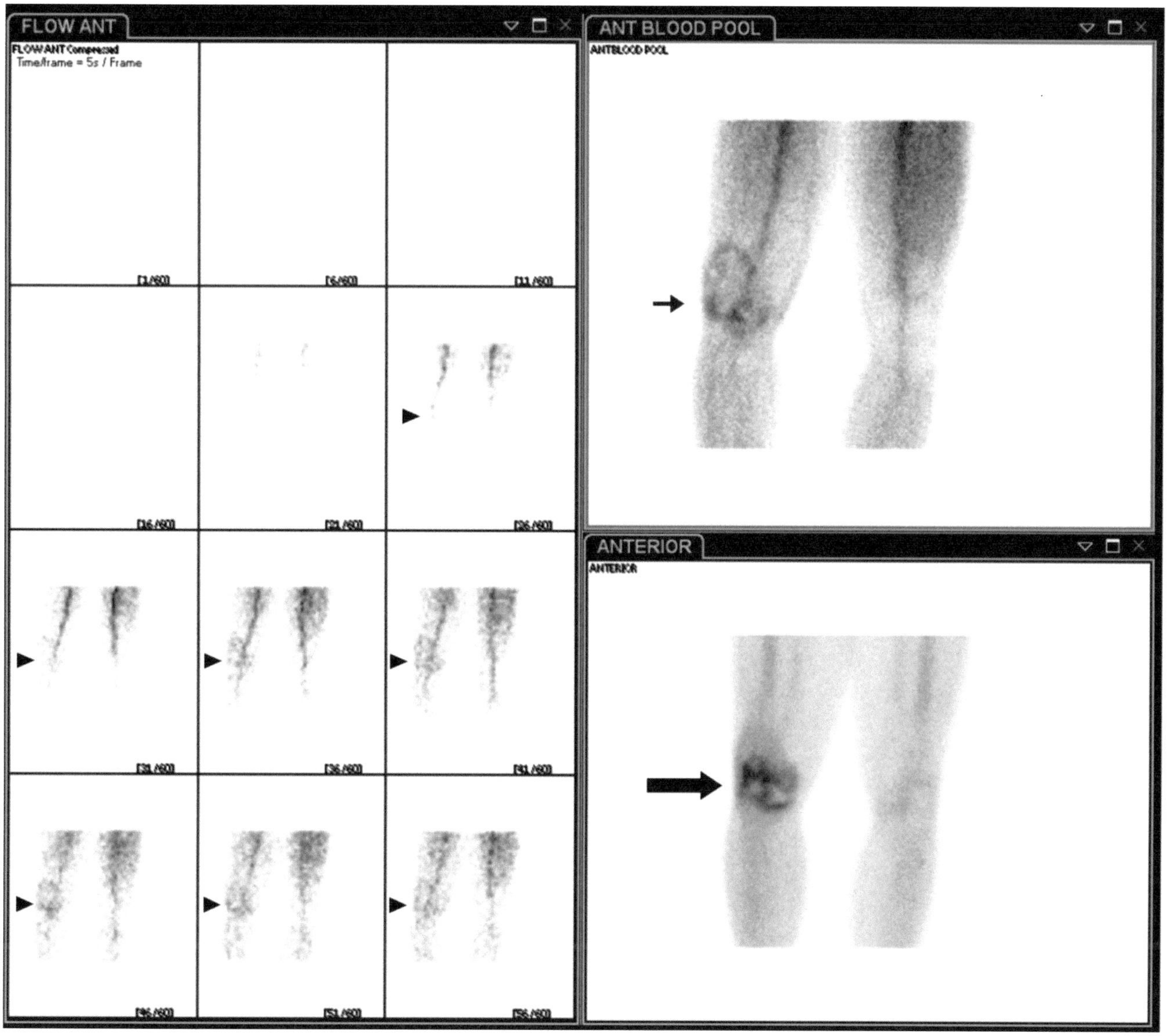

Fig. 38.11 Three-phase nuclear medicine bone scan consistent with acute osteomyelitis. The left panels show the dynamic angiographic images showing increased flow to the right knee (arrow heads). The upper right blood pool image shows increased soft tissue uptake/hyperemia of the right knee (small black arrow). The delayed image in the bottom right panel shows increased bone uptake of the radiopharmaceutical (larger black arrow)

Special Populations

Pediatric Patients

Ionizing radiation effects in radiation biology are considered deterministic (related to dose, such as skin burns) or stochastic (related to random chance, such as risk of developing cancer later in life). Growing children are more sensitive to radiation than adults. Therefore, more caution is used when considering what type of imaging to obtain in children. For acute abdominal pain in children, for example, the workup will often begin with ultrasound and radiographs. CT is reserved for cases when initial studies are negative or inconclusive, as might be the case if there is high clinical suspicion for acute appendicitis but both radiographs and ultrasound are negative or equivocal.

MRI has the benefit of no ionizing radiation exposure; however, it is unreasonable to expect small children to hold still for the long duration of an MRI. Faster sequences are often used in children at the expense of some resolution. If an MRI is needed in a young child, it is often necessary to perform the study under anesthesia, which must factor into the risk-benefit analysis when choosing your imaging.

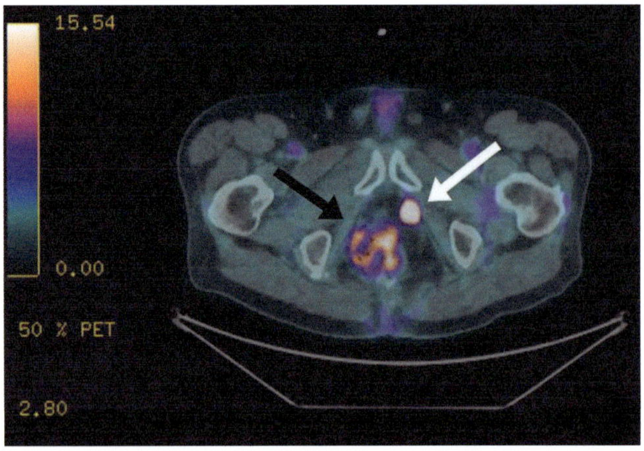

Fig. 38.12 FDG (Fluorodeoxyglucose) PET scan showing a very avid left pelvic lymph node (white arrow) concerning for metastatic disease. The activity within the adjacent rectum (black arrow) may represent normal gastrointestinal activity

Pregnant Patients

Imaging in pregnant patients follows a similar thought process to imaging children. The fetus is even more susceptible to radiation than infants, and that risk increases with earlier gestational age. The risks and benefits for each situation and gestational age must be considered; for example, a CT chest, abdomen, and pelvis in a pregnant patient after a high-speed car accident will often be worth the risk. Specific safety considerations in pregnancy in the Table 38.3 below.

If available, MRI may be an appropriate alternative to CT in many clinical scenarios. According to the American College of Radiology Manual on MR Safety 2024, "The vast majority of data today has failed to show that exposure to MR has deleterious effects on the developing fetus." However, MRI gadolinium contrast should be avoided (pregnancy category C).

Table 38.3 Summary of suspected in utero induced deterministic radiation effects[a]

Menstrual or gestational age	Conception age	<50 mGy (<5 rad)	50–100 mGy (5–10 rad)	>100 mGy (>10 rad)
0–2 weeks (0–14 days)	Prior to conception	None	None	None
3rd and 4th weeks (15–28 days)	1st–2nd weeks (1–14 days)	None	Probably none	Possible spontaneous abortion.
5th–10th weeks (29–70 days)	3rd–8th weeks (15–56 days)	None	Potential effects are scientifically uncertain and probably too subtle to be clinically detectable	Possible malformations increasing in likelihood as dose increases
11th–17th weeks (71–119 days)	9th–15th weeks (57–105 days)	None	Potential effects are scientifically uncertain and probably too subtle to be clinically detectable	Risk of diminished IQ or of mental retardation, increasing in frequency and severity with increasing dose
18th–27th weeks (120–189 days)	16th–25th weeks (106–175 days)	None	None	IQ deficits not detectable at diagnostic doses
>27 weeks (>189 days)	>25 weeks (>175 days)	None	None	None applicable to diagnostic medicine

[a]Stochastic risks are suspected, but data are not consistent. For exposure to a newborn child, the lifetime attributable risk of developing cancer is estimated to be 0.4% per 10 mGy (1 rad) dose to the baby. The potential risks in utero for the second and third trimesters and part of the first trimester may be comparable, but the uncertainties in this estimate are considerable

Reproduced with permission from the ACR-SPR Practice Parameter for Imaging Pregnant or Potentially Pregnant Patients With Ionizing Radiation (Revised 2023)

IQ intelligence quotient, *ACR* American College of Radiology, *SPR* Society for Pediatric Radiology

Common Conditions

Lines/Tubes

Evaluation of lines and tubes is critically important and often accomplished with radiographs. Misplacement of a tube can cause issues with proper function or can even lead to significant patient harm—imagine putting tube feeds directly into the lungs! See Table 38.4 and Fig. 38.13 for common lines and tubes and associated complications (Fig. 38.14).

Table 38.4 Common lines and tubes and selected common complications

Device	Appropriate position	Common complications
Endotracheal tube	Mid-thoracic Trachea (Landmarks: clavicles and carina)	Mainstem intubation: tube within the right or left main bronchi leading to collapse of the non-ventilated lung Cuff overinflation: balloon cuff on tube overexpands the trachea. Can lead to tracheal injury/necrosis and later stenosis
Central venous catheter/port Peripherally inserted central catheters (PICC)	Lower SVC/superior cavoatrial junction (landmark: Two vertebral bodies below the carina) Upper extremity approach: Lower lower SVC/superior cavoatrial Junction Lower extremity approach: Intrahepatic intrahepatic IVC or inferior cavoatrial junction (landmark: where the heart meets the diaphragm)	Pneumothorax Vascular perforation Arterial placement: will follow artery towards aorta. Can verify with blood gas. Other misplacement: may end up in non-ideal vein (internal jugular/subclavian/azygos) which may increase the risk of clot, perforation, or malfunction Deep placement: Tip at distal right atrium or right ventricle increases risk of arrhythmia
Feeding tube	Generally, should pass below the diaphragm If attempting post-pyloric placement, should curve toward the patient's right side past midline. Higher confidence if it starts to take a downward turn after crossing midline If there is a sidehole, this should be within the stomach	Too high (pharynx or esophagus): increased aspiration risk Malposition in airways Malposition and perforation into other structures (peritoneum, pleura, brain stem)
Surgical tube	Variable positions depending on goal. If there are sideholes, these should be internal to the patient	Kinking, displacement, malposition
Pulmonary artery (Swan-Ganz) catheter	Proximal right or left pulmonary artery	Too peripheral (extending beyond the hila) leads to risk of pulmonary artery perforation/ischemia

Post-operative Problems

Anastomotic Leak and Bowel and Bladder Perforation

Brief Description

Bowel perforation occurs when a breach in the bowel wall allows bowel contents (including gas, enzymes, and bacteria-filled material) to escape into the free abdomen. This can cause peritonitis, sepsis, and abscess formation. Causes include trauma, ischemia, peptic ulcer disease, or post-surgical complications. Free air and fluid are often seen in these cases.

Similarly, bladder perforation occurs when a disruption in the bladder allows urine to escape into the abdomen. Both bowel and bladder perforations can be intraperitoneal or extraperitoneal.

Anastomotic leak results from a breakdown of the connection between two surgically connected or repaired parts of an organ, generally parts of the GI and/or genitourinary (GU) tract.

Best Imaging Study

- Bowel perforation and anastomotic leak:
  - Initial screening: radiography to look for free air (increase yield by adding upright or decubitus views) (Figs. 38.1 and 38.4).
  - Most sensitive test: CT with IV contrast (provides best anatomic evaluation and identifies small leaks of fluid and air) (Figs. 38.2 and 38.5).
  - Alternatives: Fluoroscopy or CT with oral contrast to identify site of active leak. CT can be performed immediately after fluoroscopy if fluoroscopy evaluation is positive or equivocal to provide better anatomic assessment and help confirm or exclude a possible leak. Water soluble contrast (rather than Barium) should be administered in the setting of a suspected leak (Table 38.1).
- Bladder perforation and GU anastomotic leak:
  - Upper collecting system: CT urogram—CT performed with and without IV contrast with additional 8–10 min delayed CT to visualize excreted contrast in the upper collecting system and bladder.
  - Bladder: CT or fluoroscopic cystogram—CT or fluoroscopic imaging performed before and after contrast administered to bladder via foley catheter.
  - Urethra: Fluoroscopy (retrograde urethrogram)—contrast administered via small catheter to distal (usually male) urethra with visualization under fluoroscopy. Can also be performed bedside with multiple radiographs in patients unable to travel to the radiology department for exam.

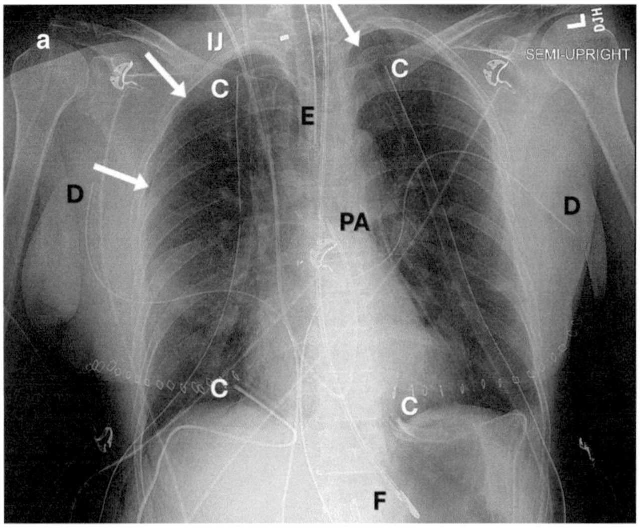

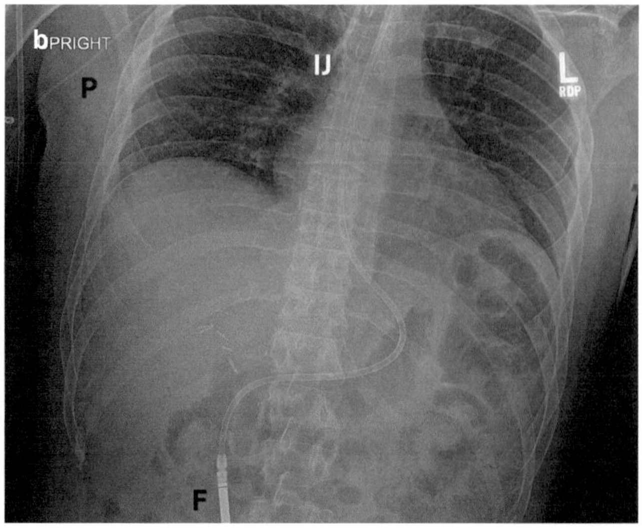

Fig. 38.13 (**a**) Semi-upright frontal chest radiograph. This complicated chest radiograph shows normal placement of multiple tubes, including right internal jugular central venous catheter (IJ), PA catheter (PA), endotracheal tube (E), feeding tube (F), and multiple surgical drains (D) and chest tubes (C). Bilateral pneumothoraces also present (white arrows), (**b**) Frontal abdominal radiograph showing a post-pyloric feeding tube (F) which has crossed mid-line and is coursing into the descending duodenum. Right PICC (P) and central venous catheter (IJ) are partially visualized

  - Voiding cystourethrogram—contrast administered to bladder via Foley, which is then removed and patient voiding into a urinal observed with fluoroscopy.
- Fluoroscopy can be tailored for clinical questions. For example, in patients with altered anatomy such as ileal conduit, contrast can be instilled directly into the conduit; it can also be instilled into percutaneous nephrostomy tubes.

Classic Imaging Findings

Leaked contents: fluid and gas from bowel (Fig. 38.15) and mainly fluid from GU anastomosis (Fig. 38.16). It can be challenging to distinguish anastomotic leak from normal post-surgical changes, which may include small amounts of air and fluid depending on how recently the surgery was performed. However, using clues such as worsening over time and proximity to the actual anastomosis can help. Giving contrast that will traverse the anastomosis (PO or per tube for bowel, IV or per tube for GU) can help demonstrate active anastomotic leak and confirm the diagnosis (Fig. 38.17).

Bleed

Brief Description

Ongoing bleeding from vessels/organs involved in the surgery as well as structures that may have been unintentionally involved.

Best Imaging Study

CTA of the relevant body region. Hematomas can be identified on non-angiographic CT but findings may be non-specific and may prompt more definitive assessment with CTA.

Classic Imaging Findings

- Fluid collection: distinguished from simple fluid by higher density (>20 Hounsfield units) and sometimes heterogeneity reflecting clot formation and layering blood products.
- Active extravasation (Fig. 38.18): on a classic CTA with non-con, arterial, and venous phases, active bleeding is identified by contrast appearing up outside of a blood vessel on arterial phase images that is not seen on non-

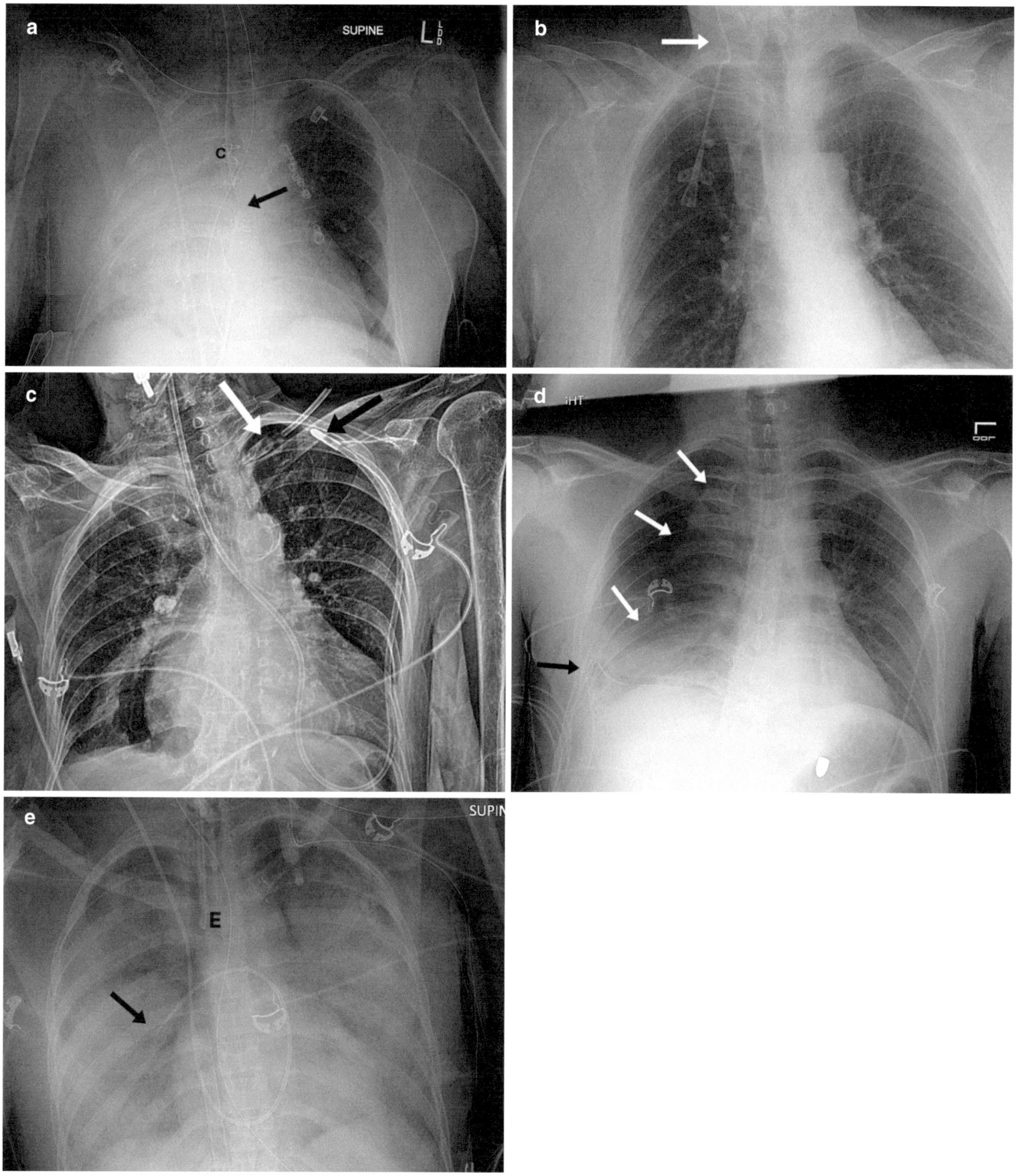

Fig. 38.14 (**a**) Frontal chest radiograph showing the endotracheal tube (C) in the left mainstem bronchus (black arrow) which resulted in complete atelectasis of the right lung, (**b**) Right central venous catheter within the right internal jugular vein (white arrow), (**c**) Frontal chest radiograph with a significantly malpositioned feeding tube coursing down the trachea, left mainstem bronchus, lung parenchyma, and puncturing through the pleura with tip at the lung apex (black arrow) adjacent to the small pneumothorax (white arrow) caused by the placement, (**d**) Frontal chest radiograph showing a kinked right chest tube (black arrow) preventing adequate treatment of the patient's large pneumothorax and pleural effusion (hydropneumothorax) (white arrows), (**e**) Frontal chest radiograph showing a pulmonary arterial catheter in a slightly too-peripheral position (black arrow) placing the patient at risk of pulmonary artery injury and infarct. A good rule of thumb is not extending more than 3 cm beyond the midline. Endotracheal tube (E)

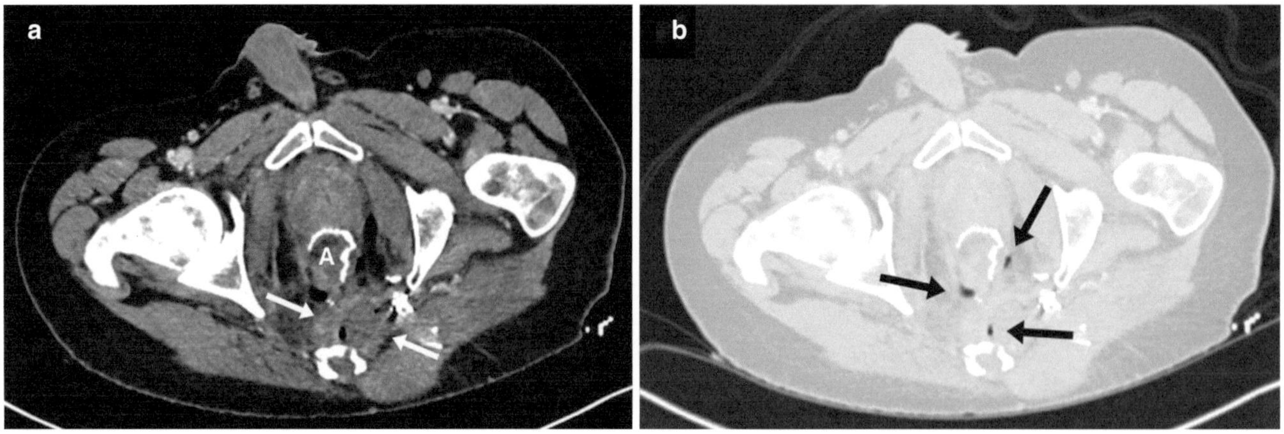

Fig. 38.15 (**a**) Contrast-enhanced axial CT image at the level of a post-surgical anastomosis (A) showing an adjacent fluid collection (white arrows) concerning for anastomotic leak. (**b**) The same image on lung window highlighting the adjacent free air (black arrows) further raising suspicion for anastomotic leak

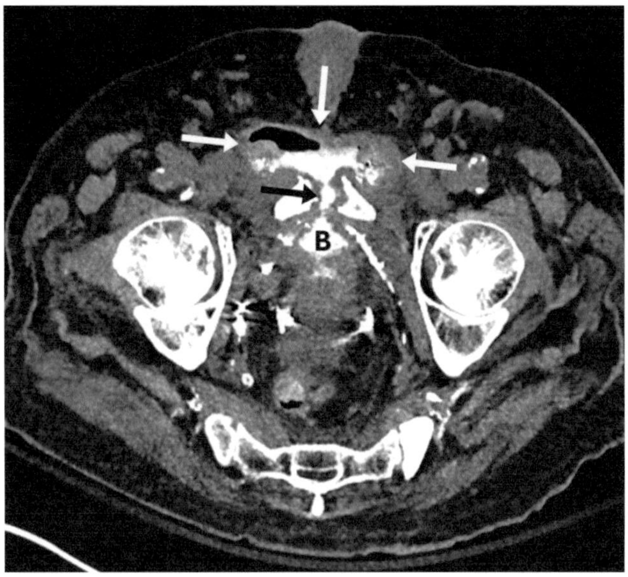

Fig. 38.16 Axial CT cystogram showing bladder (B) contrast communicating along a fistula (black arrow) through the pubic symphysis into a focal collection anteriorly (white arrows)

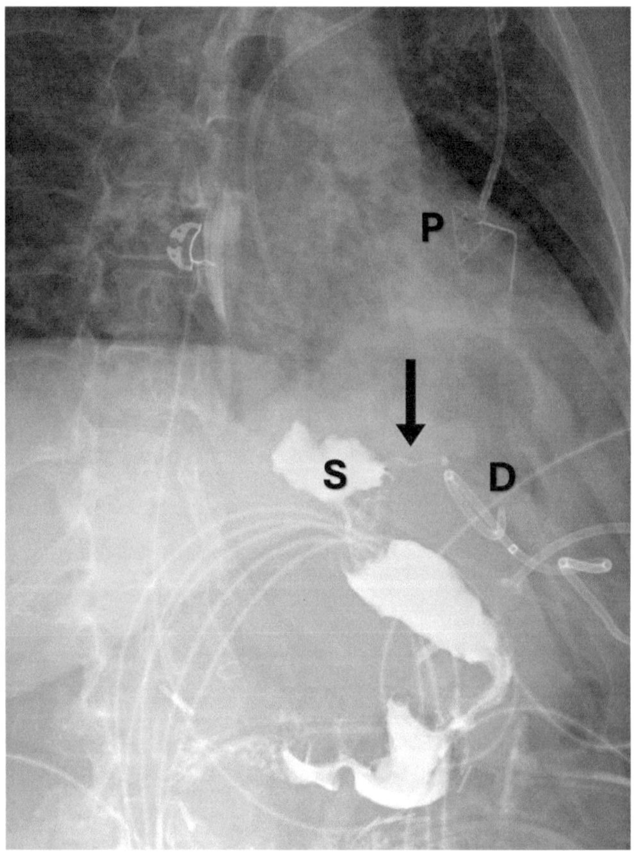

Fig. 38.17 Frontal fluoroscopic image showing a thin area of extraluminal contrast (black arrow) localizing the site of the patient's gastric leak/perforation. Stomach (S), surgical drain (D), chest port (P)

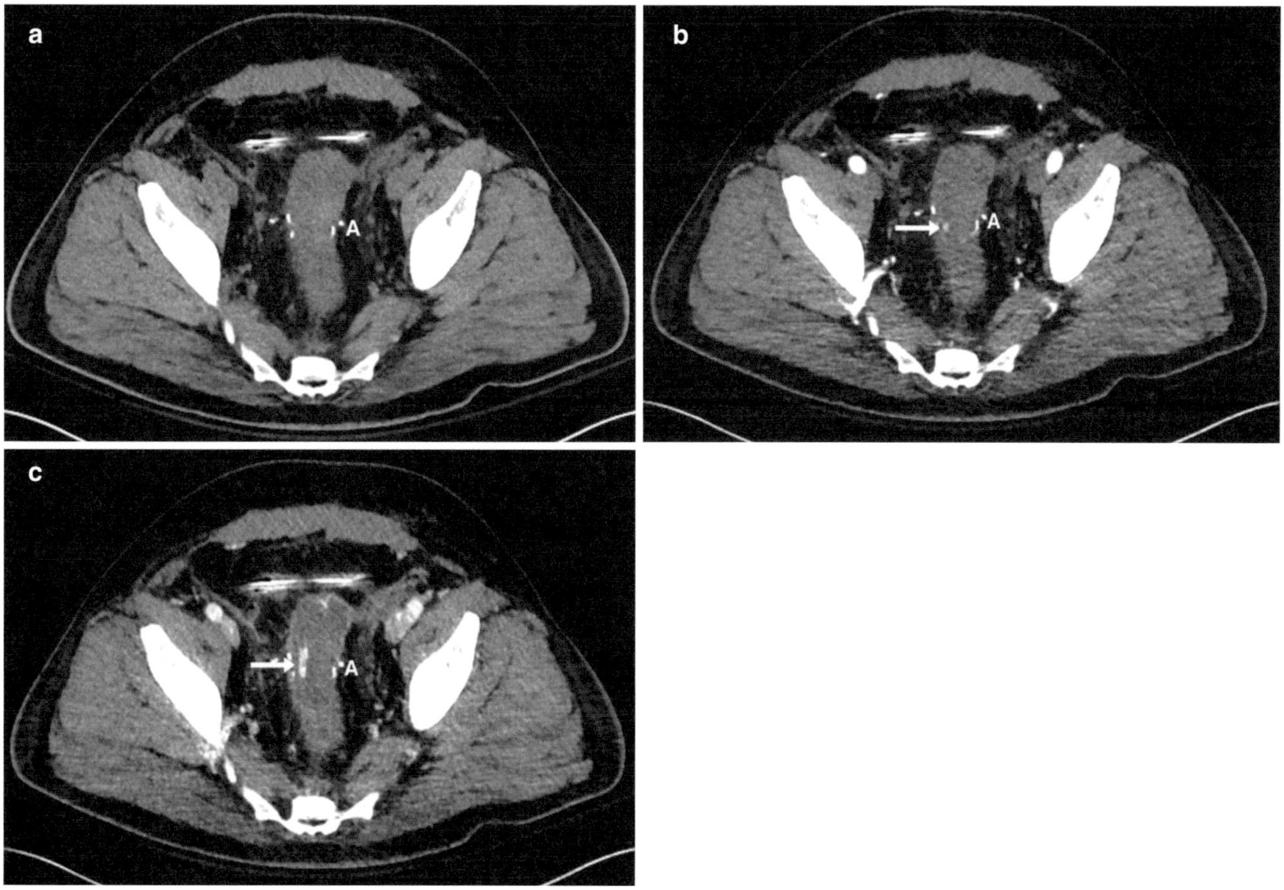

Fig. 38.18 (**a**) Non-contrasted axial CT angiography image through the pelvis at an area of anastomosis (A) in the sigmoid colon, (**b**) Arterial phase at the same level demonstrates a focus of contrast not seen on the non-contrasted image raising the possibility of acute bleed, (**c**) Venous phase image showing accumulation of contrast at this area confirming the suspicion of acute bleed/active extravasation

con images, with accumulation and pooling on venous phase. Some bleeds may only show up on the venous phase or not at all if the bleeding is very slow or intermittent.

Phlegmon, Abscess, and Seroma

Brief Description

A seroma is a non-inflamed fluid collection after surgery. Infection after surgery may start as unorganized infected tissue known as a phlegmon. When an area of infection becomes walled off with fluid internally, it is called an abscess. Abscesses are always a differential consideration for fluid collections in post-operative patients—though less likely in the first hours after surgery.

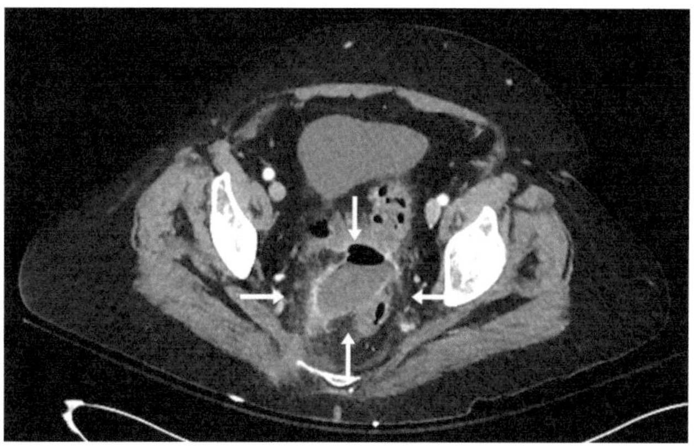

Fig. 38.19 Contrast-enhanced axial CT image through the pelvis showing a large fluid and gas collection (white arrows) with surrounding fat stranding concerning for abscess

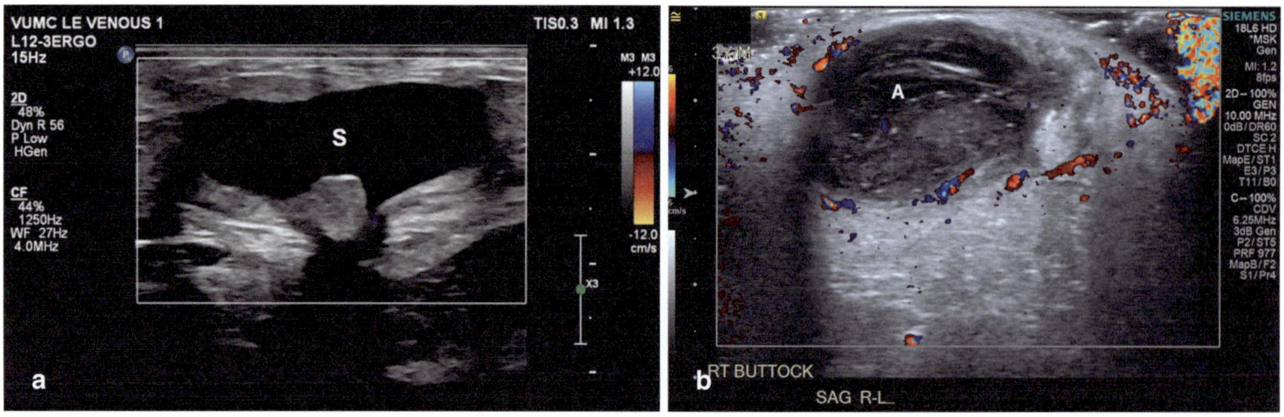

Fig. 38.20 (**a**) Color doppler image of a post-operative seroma (S). The important features in this image are the lack of both internal and peripheral vascularity, the simple appearance of the fluid, and the normal appearance of the adjacent soft tissue, (**b**) Color doppler image of an abscess (A). Contrasted from the seroma, this collection has significant peripheral vascularity (hyperemia), a brighter appearance of the surrounding fat (edema), and complex internal fluid

Best Imaging Study

- Intra-abdominal infection: CT abdomen and pelvis with contrast (Fig. 38.19).
- Superficial infections/wound infections: Targeted US (Fig. 38.20) for superficial drainable collections, but CT may be needed to exclude involvement of deeper structures.

Classic Imaging Findings

- Fat stranding: as discussed, this is our body's general response to inflammation including infection. If a simple collection is identified with no surrounding fat stranding, then a non-infected seroma may be more likely than abscess although sometimes difficult to distinguish. An infection will tend to cause increasing haziness/stranding over time whereas uninfected post-surgical changes should improve over time, so correlation with prior studies will be helpful.
- Abscess: well-defined collection of fluid with an enhancing rim (gets brighter with IV contrast) and surrounding fat stranding.

Ileus Versus Bowel Obstruction

Brief Description

Ileus is stunning of the bowel, leading to poor motility and bowel dilation. It occurs for various reasons and is common in the acute post-operative setting. Bowel obstruction is a mechanical issue where the bowel is unable to move contents beyond a certain point, resulting in upstream distention and downstream decompression. Obstruction and several of its many causes are described in the Bowel Obstruction section. Compared to ileus, obstruction is less common post-operatively, compared to ileus but should be suspected in any patient with abdominal pain and a history of abdominal surgery.

Best Imaging Study

Abdominal radiographs are often the best screening tool for post-surgical patients with abdominal pain, followed by CT of the abdomen and pelvis with IV contrast to localize the obstruction and assess for complications like ischemia or rupture. Small bowel follow-through (serial abdominal radiographs performed pre and post PO administration of water-soluble contrast) may help to differentiate ileus from partial or complete bowel obstruction.

Classic Imaging Findings

Radiographs may show dilated bowel loops, but often cannot definitively differentiate between ileus and obstruction. Signs favoring obstruction include localized dilation and absence of gas in the pelvis. On CT, a "transition point" where the bowel caliber changes from dilated to narrow suggests obstruction. Additional important findings include pneumatosis (air dissecting in the wall of the bowel), free air, or portal venous gas, which indicate ischemia or perforation complicating an obstruction. Please see Bowel Obstruction and Bowel Ischemia sections later in this chapter for more information (FIg. 38.21).

Wound Dehiscence

Brief Description

Breakdown of a surgical wound with partial or complete opening of the wound that may occur at the deep or superficial level.

Best Imaging Study

Superficial or complete wound dehiscence is usually diagnosed clinically. For deeper dehiscence or complications, CT with contrast is best for evaluating the extent and any associated

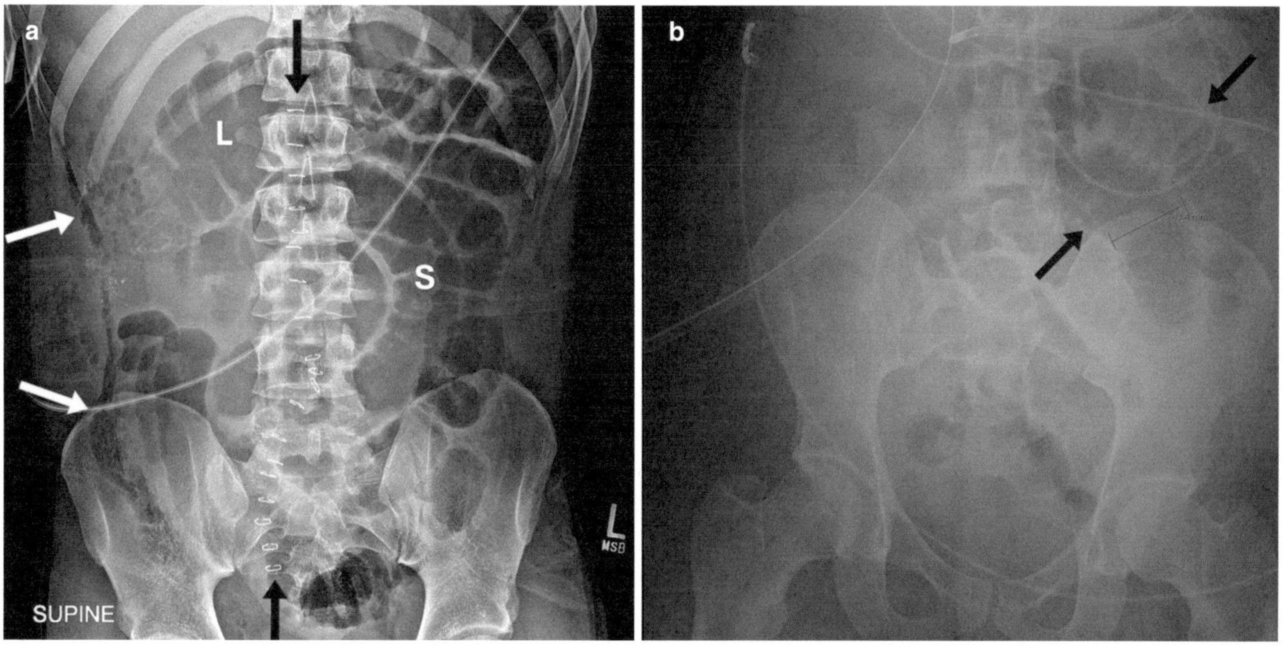

Fig. 38.21 (**a**) Supine frontal abdominal radiograph in the acute post-operative setting with skin staples (black arrows) and soft tissue air along the right flank (white arrows). There is diffuse dilation of both large (L) and small bowel (S) loops consistent with ileus. (**b**) Supine frontal abdominal radiograph showing a more focal dilated loop of small bowel (black arrows) which is more suspicious for obstruction

abscess or infection. Ultrasound may be used to evaluate associated abscesses but is often limited by gas in the soft tissues.

Classic Imaging Findings
Look for areas of widening along the incision with soft tissue gas, fat stranding, and surrounding inflammatory changes (Fig. 38.22). Stranding should decrease over time after trauma or surgery; persistent or worsening stranding may indicate an underlying infection.

Inflammatory and Infectious Conditions

The longer body contents (bile, GI contents, urine) stay in one place, the more inflammation will occur and the greater the risk of infection. Therefore, a common starting point among the inflammatory and infectious conditions described in this section is obstruction and stasis. Stasis leads to distension and inflammation. Infection can follow. The combination of distension, inflammation, and infection can cause ischemia of the wall of the associated organ which can ultimately lead to necrosis or perforation.

Appendicitis

Brief Description
Inflammation of the appendix, often due to obstruction, leading to distention, infection, and possible perforation.

Best Imaging Study
CT abdomen and pelvis with contrast is the best initial imaging choice in most cases because it can detect complications

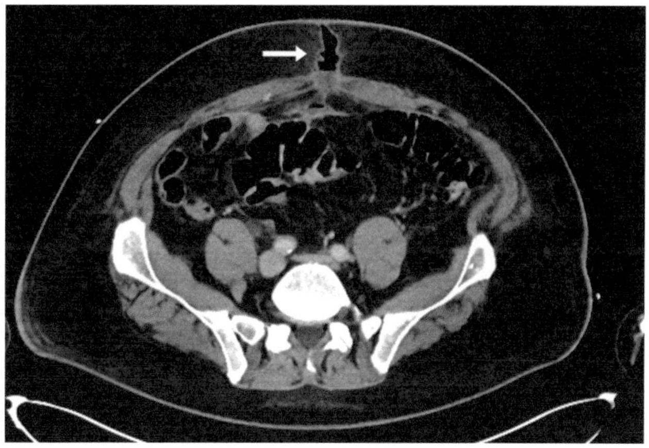

Fig. 38.22 Axial contrast-enhanced CT demonstrating an area of wound dehiscence (white arrow) along the prior midline surgical incision

of appendicitis and alternative diagnoses. Ultrasound or MRI should be considered as alternatives, especially in pediatric or pregnant patients.

Classic Imaging Findings
Distended appendix (>6 mm), adjacent fat stranding, and occasionally free fluid or gas (suggesting perforation) (Fig. 38.23). An appendicolith (stone) may also be seen. Ultrasound findings include a non-compressible appendix and echogenic fat (Fig. 38.24). MRI shows fat stranding as bright T2 signal surrounding the dilated appendix (Fig. 38.25).

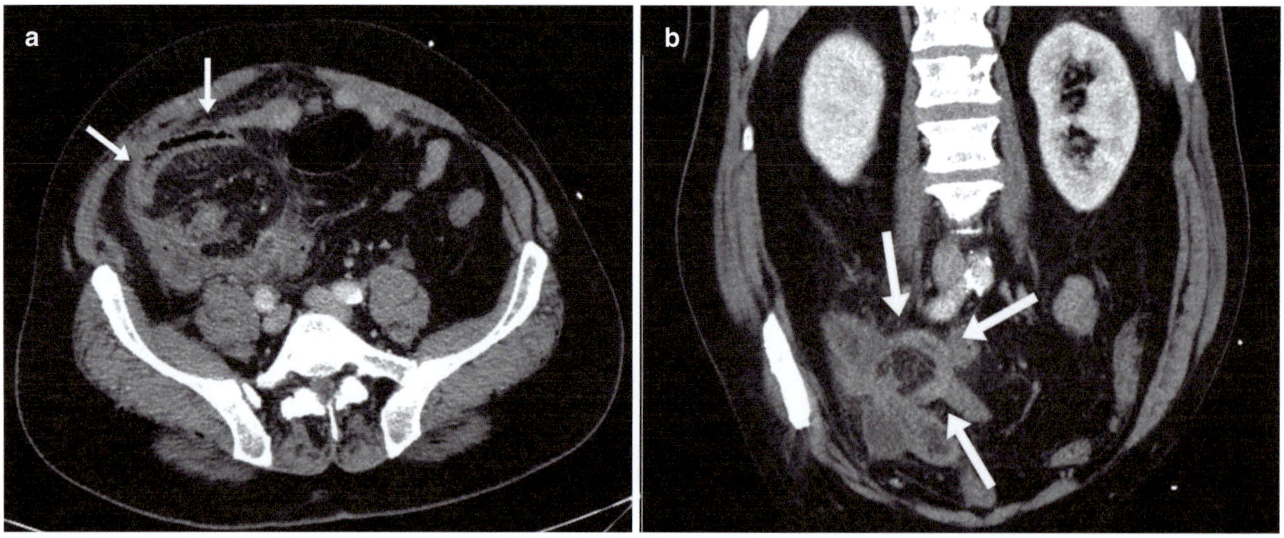

Fig. 38.23 (**a**) Acute appendicitis: contrast-enhanced axial CT image through lower abdomen/upper pelvis showing significant fat stranding in the right lower quadrant adjacent to a dilated appendix with wall-thickening (white arrows), (**b**) Coronal CT image in the same patient showing the inflamed appendix (white arrows)

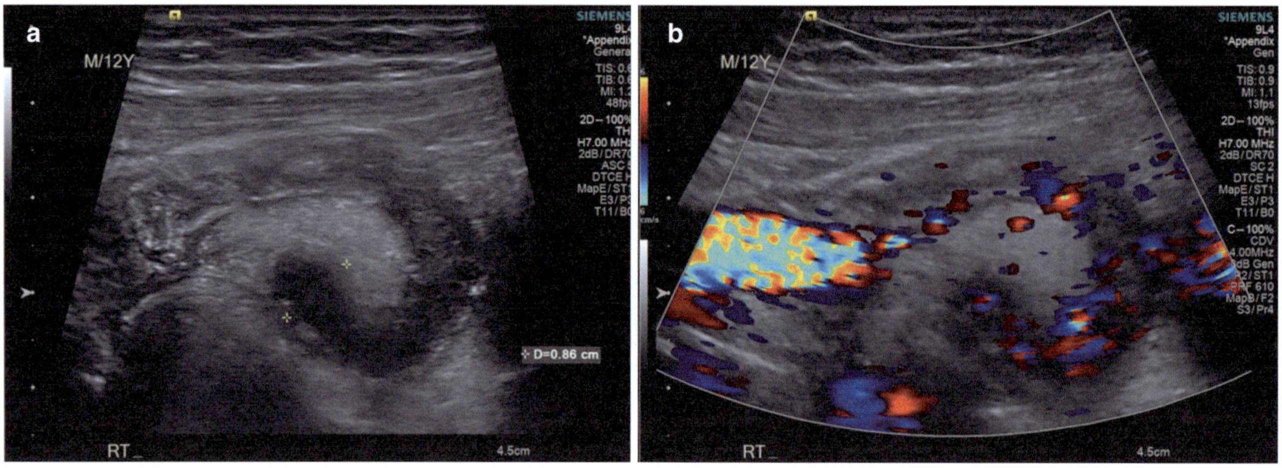

Fig. 38.24 (**a**) Grayscale ultrasound in the right lower quadrant showing a dilated appendix with wall thickening and brightness (edema) of the surrounding fat consistent with acute appendicitis, (**b**) Color doppler at the same area showing increased vascularity of the wall (hyperemia) further supporting the diagnosis

Cholecystitis/Choledocholithiasis

Brief Description

Cholecystitis often results from a stone blocking gallbladder outflow, leading to distention and inflammation. Acalculous (no stone) cholecystitis can occur but typically is seen in critically ill patients. Choledocholithiasis involves stones obstructing the common bile duct, which may progress to ascending cholangitis (inflammation of the biliary tree).

Best Imaging Study

Right upper quadrant ultrasound is the best initial test for suspected biliary issues. This is because the gallbladder is usually well-visualized with ultrasound and ultrasound is more sensitive for detection of gallstones since the stones are often fluid density on CT and obscured by the surrounding bile. If findings are equivocal, follow-up imaging may include MRCP, CT, or HIDA scan.

Classic Imaging Findings

- **Cholecystitis**: Gallbladder distention (>4 cm width), wall thickening (>3 mm), stones, fat stranding, and pain during ultrasound exam (especially pain as the sonographer presses on the patient with the gallbladder in the field of view—the sonographic Murphy's sign) (Fig. 38.26). Complications include gas in the wall or perforation. On HIDA scan, non-visualization of the gallbladder after 4 h indicates that the cystic duct going to the gallbladder is obstructed and is diagnostic of acute

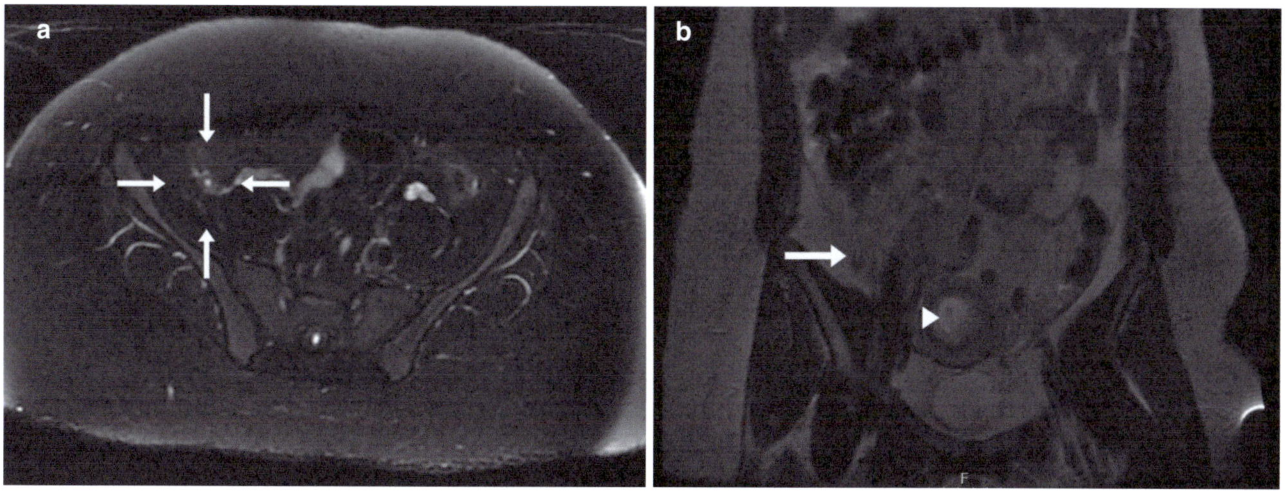

Fig. 38.25 (**a**) Axial T2 fat-saturated image through the upper pelvis in a pregnant patient showing increased T2 signal surrounding a dilated appendix (white arrows), (**b**) coronal T2-weighted image partially showing the dilated appendix (white arrow) as well as the first-trimester gestational sac and embryo (white arrowhead)

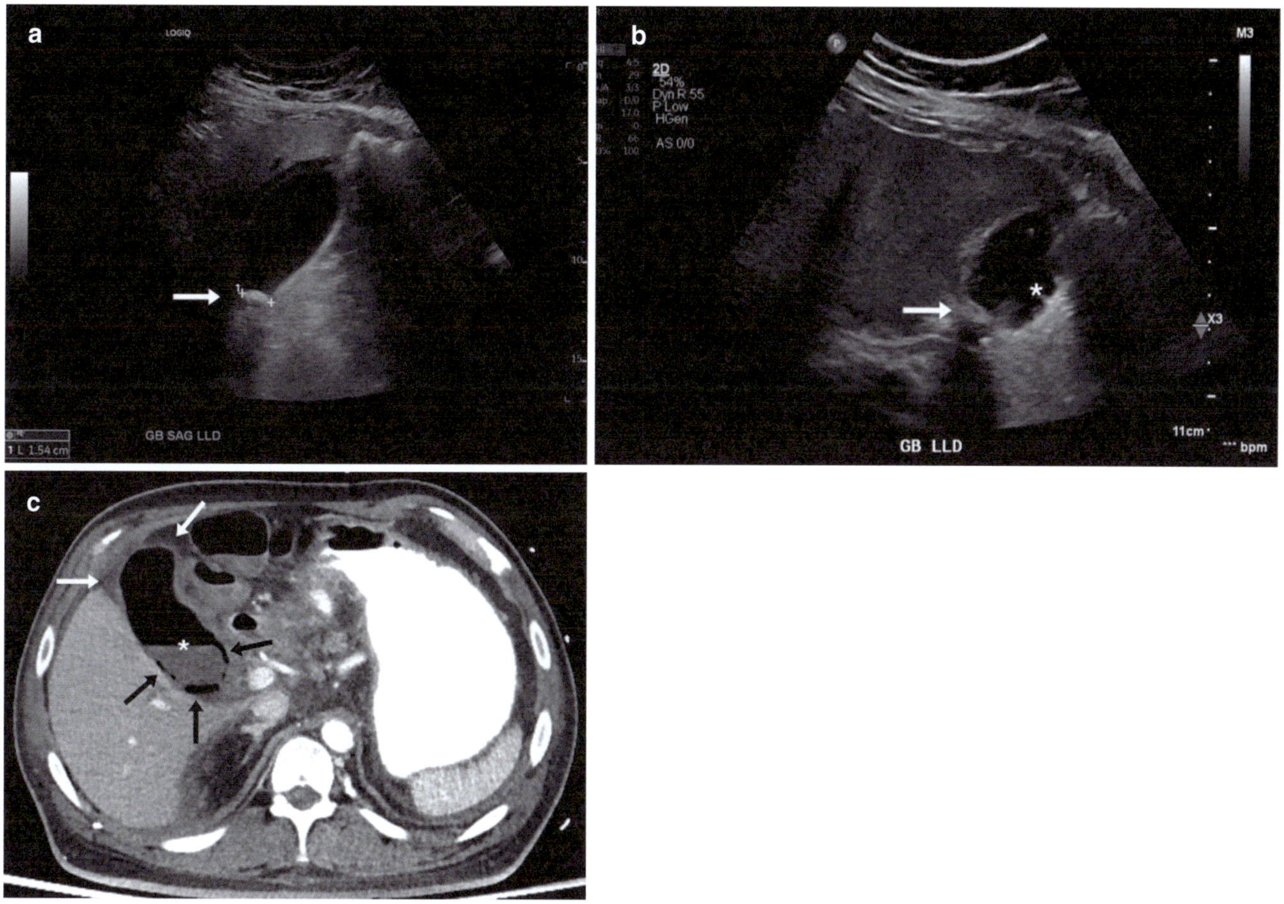

Fig. 38.26 (**a**) Grayscale ultrasound of the gallbladder showing a large stone (white arrow) near the gallbladder neck, gallbladder distension, and wall-thickening in a patient with acute cholecystitis, (**b**) Grayscale ultrasound in a different patient showing gallbladder perforation (asterisk) in the setting of distension, wall thickening, and a shadowing stone near the neck (white arrow), (**c**) Axial contrast enhanced CT showing emphysematous cholecystitis with wall thickening and adjacent fat stranding (white arrows), air-fluid level highlighting intraluminal air and fluid (asterisk), and intramural (inside the wall) gas (black arrows)

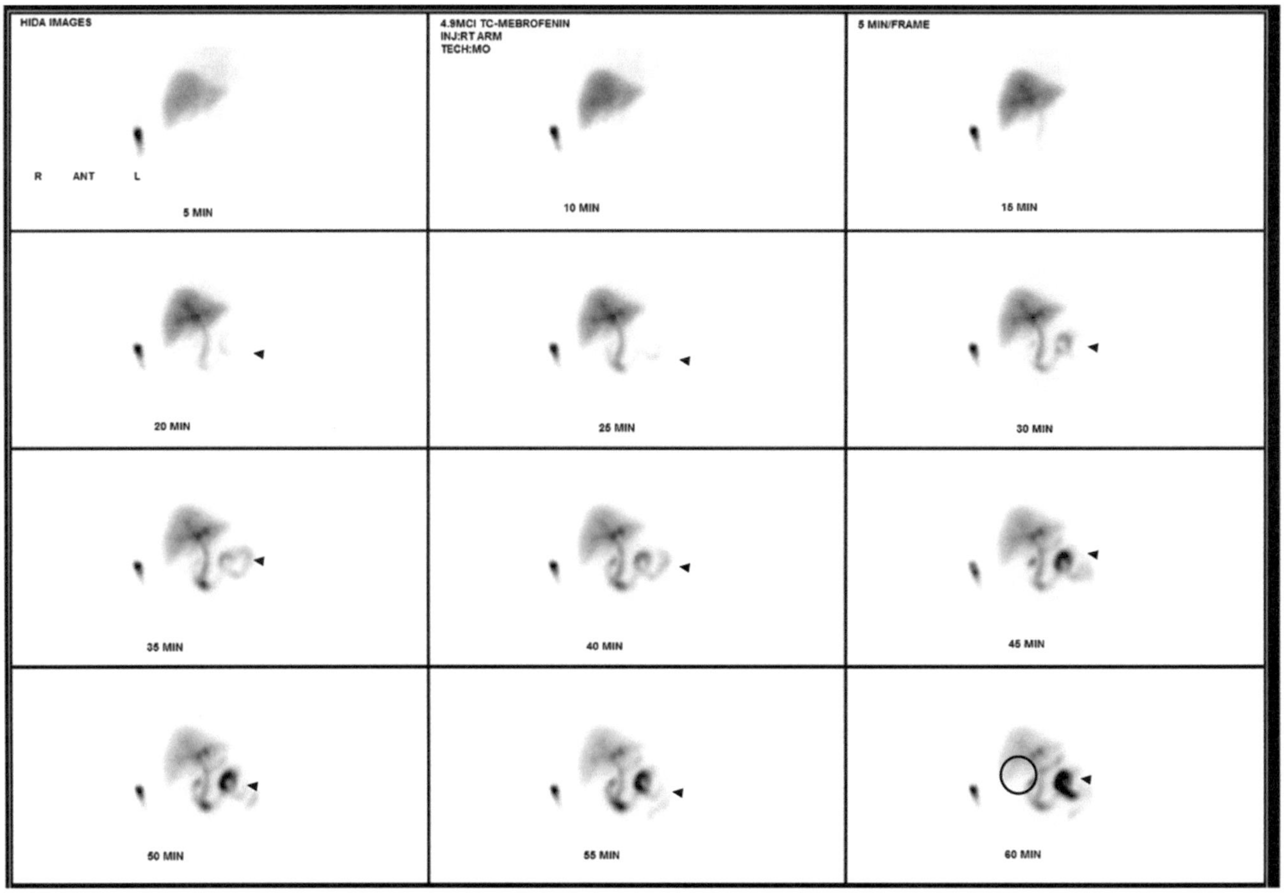

Fig. 38.27 Nuclear medicine HIDA scan consistent with acute cholecystitis. The radiopharmaceutical can be seen passing from the common bile duct into the small bowel (black arrowheads) by 20 min. The gallbladder is never filled with the radiopharmaceutical suggesting obstruction of the cystic duct as expected in acute cholecystitis (black circle on final image showing the empty gallbladder fossa)

cholecystitis (Fig. 38.27). Fat stranding or increased T2 signal on MRI can be seen around an inflamed gallbladder (Fig. 38.28).

- **Choledocholithiasis**: Common bile duct distention (>6 mm) may help indicate an obstruction, although the common bile duct is often dilated but still normal in older patients or post-cholecystectomy patients. Stones may be visible on CT if they are calcified but are often visible on MRCP, with T2 dark stones against T2 bright bile (Fig. 38.29).

Diverticulitis

Brief Description

Diverticulosis refers to the presence of outpouchings in the bowel wall, common in older adults. Diverticulitis occurs when one of these outpouchings becomes obstructed and inflamed, leading to infection and perforation.

Best Imaging Study

CT abdomen and pelvis with IV contrast

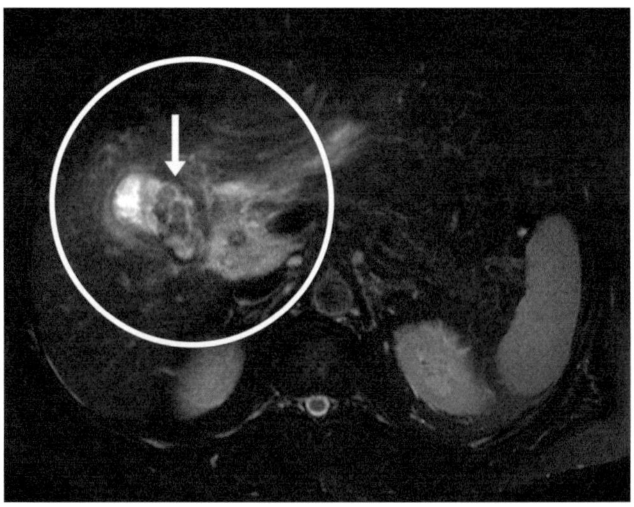

Fig. 38.28 Axial T2 fat-saturated image in the abdomen showing a significant amount of hazy increased T2 signal around the gallbladder (region in white circle) and right upper quadrant. The bright T2 fluid signal is the MRI equivalent of fat stranding. Multiple low signal gallstones (white arrow) are also seen within the distended gallbladder with wall thickening consistent with acute cholecystitis

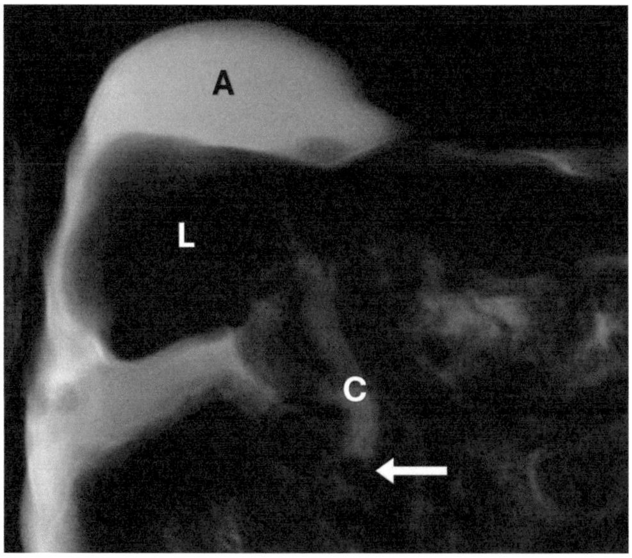

Fig. 38.29 Coronal MRCP image showing a large obstructing low-signal stone (white arrow) in the common bile duct (C) with associated ductal dilation. Cirrhotic liver (L) and ascites (A)

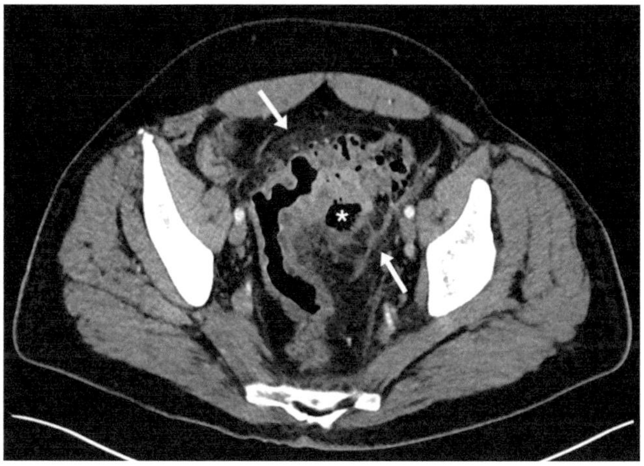

Fig. 38.30 Axial contrast-enhanced CT through the pelvis showing a segment of sigmoid colon (white arrows) with wall-thickening, diverticuli, and surrounding fat stranding consistent with acute diverticulitis. Small focus of adjacent free air (white asterisk) consistent with perforation

Classic Imaging Findings

Diverticulitis is characterized by the presence of diverticula, adjacent fat stranding, and bowel wall thickening (Fig. 38.30). Inflammation should be somewhat centered around diverticula as colitis may be a differential consideration with more diffuse bowel inflammation and wall thickening. Microperforation may manifest as small gas locules outside of the bowel, while more severe complications include abscesses, fistulas, and blood clots.

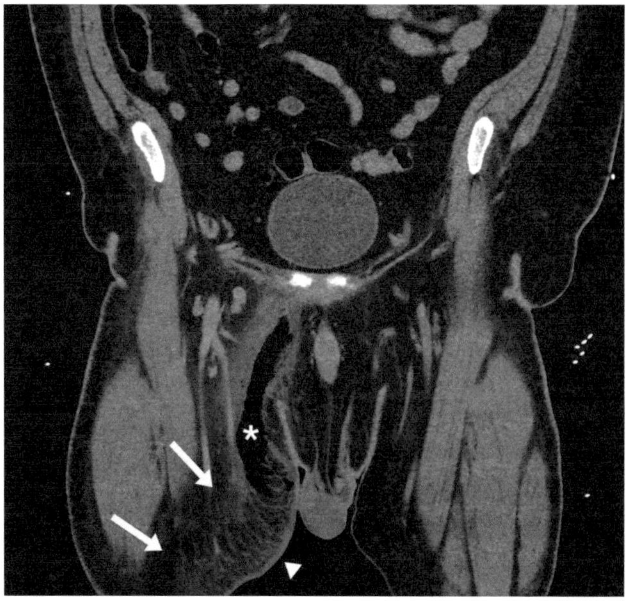

Fig. 38.31 Coronal CT image showing fat stranding of the right medial thigh (white arrows), gas tracking along the fascia (asterisk), and skin thickening (white arrowhead) highly concerning for necrotizing fasciitis in a patient without recent surgery

Necrotizing Fasciitis

Brief Description

A rapidly spreading soft tissue infection involving the subcutaneous tissue and fascia, leading to extensive tissue damage.

Best Imaging Study

Necrotizing fasciitis is primarily a clinical diagnosis. CT with contrast may help in equivocal cases to assess for gas or assist with surgical planning (Fig. 38.31). MRI can also be helpful, but it is not suitable for unstable patients.

Classic Imaging Findings

Deep soft tissue gas is highly concerning, especially without clinical explanation such as recent surgery or penetrating injury. Fascial thickening, fat stranding on CT, or T2 bright edema on MRI may also be present. Non-enhancing areas suggest necrosis.

Pyelonephritis and Nephrolithiasis

Brief Description

Common causes of flank pain. The kidneys can form stones for many reasons and those stones can travel down the ureter and result in pain and obstruction. Pyelonephritis is an infection of the kidney.

Best Imaging Study

In cases where stones are suspected, non-con CT will be sufficient. In cases of suspected complicated infection, CT with contrast will be helpful. Renal ultrasound can be used in pregnant patients although further evaluation with CT or MRI (if available) may be needed. If CT is needed, informed consent should be obtained, and radiation dose should be optimized. Radiographs are sometimes used to follow known stone disease.

Classic Imaging Findings

Renal stones are radiopaque similar to bones and can be found all along the urinary tract from renal calyces to urethra. When they become lodged in the ureter, they cause obstruction that results in hydronephrosis (dilation of the fluid filled renal pelvis and renal calyces) and hydroureter (dilatation of the ureter).

Pyelonephritis is often suspected clinically but can be seen on contrast enhanced CT as a relative darker appearance of a focal portion of the kidney (focal pyelonephritis) (Fig. 38.32). This is because the swelling and edema from the infection makes it more difficult for the contrast to enhance the involved portion of the kidney. Complications such as renal abscess can also be demonstrated. Pyonephritis is a combination of pyelonephritis and urinary obstruction and is a surgical emergency that requires urgent decompression to avoid severe sepsis.

Fistulas

Brief Description

A fistula is a connection between two different structures of the body. These can occur in a variety of locations, such as between organs (for example cholecystoduodenal fistula between the gallbladder and duodenum or a vesicovaginal fistula between the bladder and vagina) and between the skin and an organ (e.g., an enterocutaneous (EC) fistula between the intestine and the skin). They can be congenital, such as a congenital tracheoesophageal fistula, or created intentionally, as in the case of an arteriovenous fistula for dialysis. Often, fistulas are complications related to surgery or an infectious process. These often present clinically as specific fluid (urine, bile, blood, lymph, or stool) or air excreting from the wrong structure or from a wound.

Best Imaging Study

The best imaging depends on the suspected fistula. For example, a cholecystoduodenal fistula is generally best seen with CT rather than ultrasound because of the presence of bowel gas, which will degrade ultrasound imaging. If a patient has had a recent abdominal surgery and has a wound with ongoing drainage (especially of feculent material), an EC fistula should be considered and can potentially be demonstrated with CT with PO contrast. Administering contrast into a chronically draining wound under fluoroscopic visualization (a fistulogram) can also be considered to help

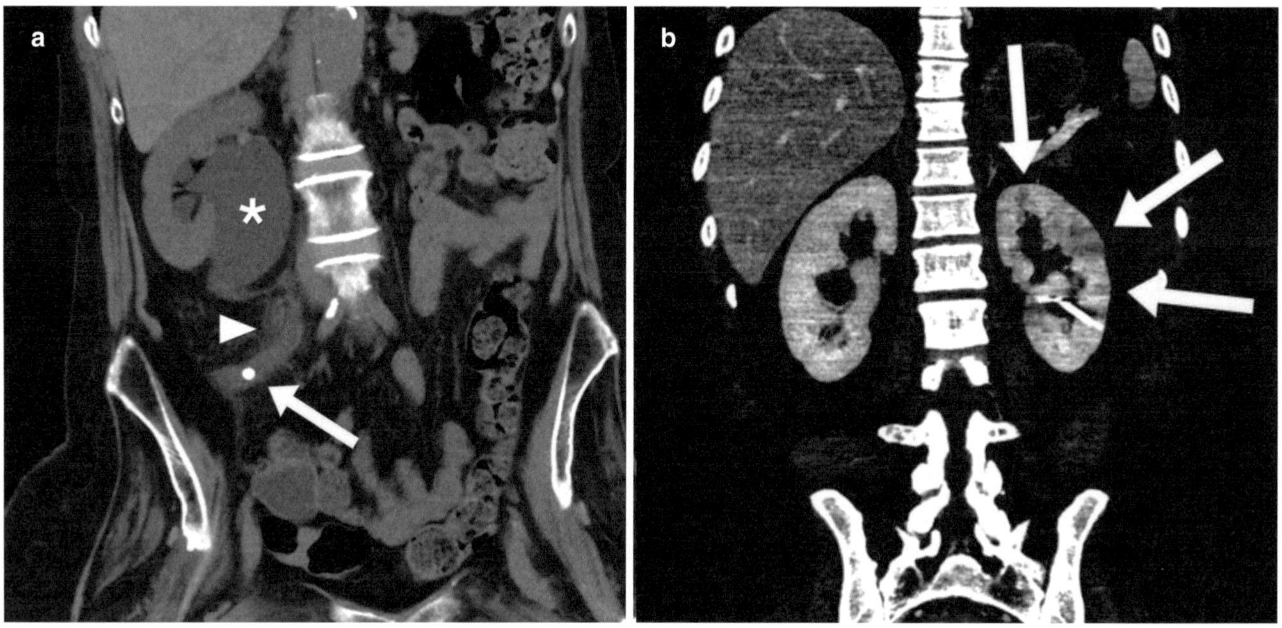

Fig. 38.32 (**a**) Coronal CT through the abdomen and pelvis showing a right mid-ureteral stone (white arrow) with significant upstream hydronephrosis (asterisk) and ureteral dilation. Fat stranding adjacent to the ureter (white arrowhead) is common and likely reflects inflammation from the adjacent stone and stasis, (**b**) Coronal contrast-enhanced CT showing a striated pattern of enhancement in the left kidney with multiple hypo-enhancing cortical areas (white arrows) consistent with acute pyelonephritis

differentiate an EC fistula from a non-healing wound. MRI may be helpful for evaluation of fistulas involving complex soft tissue structures such as the anal sphincter. A rectovaginal fistula (between the rectum and vagina) can be seen with the use of contrast within the rectum while a vesicovaginal fistula can be demonstrated by administering contrast into the bladder.

Classic Imaging Findings

It is important to understand the patient's history when you are evaluating for a fistula so you know where to look. The classic imaging findings are a tract between two structures and air, fluid, or contrast that should not be in one of these structures (Fig. 38.33).

For example, if you suspect a fistula in the gallbladder related to stones, you may see pneumobilia (gas in the gallbladder or biliary tree). However, context is essential since pneumobilia would be a normal finding for a patient who has had recent instrumentation of their biliary tree.

For an EC fistula, you may see a soft tissue tract from the bowel directly connecting to the skin or bowel loops abutting the skin surface on CT. To demonstrate communication and exclude other possibilities such as scaring or phelgmon, fistulogram or CT with PO contrast can demonstrate a true connection between the skin and bowel lumen.

Inflammatory Bowel Disease

Brief Description

Autoimmune inflammation of the bowel, manifesting as ulcerative colitis (continuous inflammation starting at the rectum) or Crohn's disease (segmental inflammation that can be transmural and affect any part of the GI tract, commonly the terminal ileum).

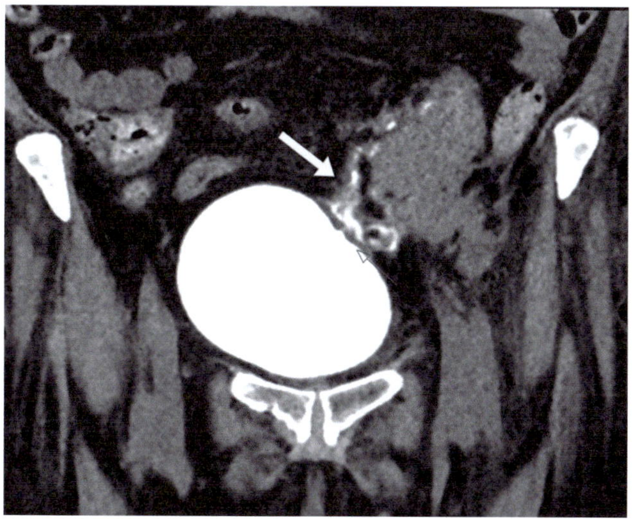

Fig. 38.33 Coronal CT cystogram showing contrast tracking from the bladder toward the sigmoid colon concerning for colovesical fistula (white arrow)

Best Imaging Study

CT or MR enterography with "negative" (fluid density) oral contrast and positive (bright) IV contrast is preferred to evaluate the bowel wall and complications like fistulas. Fluid density PO contrast allows for better evaluation of the bowel mucosa by not obscuring vascular enhancement, often present in active inflammation. MR enterography is not necessarily a better exam as it can be more susceptible to artifacts, but it does avoid radiation exposure to these patients who tend to need multiple exams to evaluate their disease progression and are typically younger and more susceptible to radiation stochastic effects such as malignancy. CT abdomen/pelvis with IV contrast is an alternative, especially in the acute setting and in patients who cannot tolerate PO.

Classic Imaging Findings

- **Crohn's Disease** (Fig. 38.34a): Segmental bowel involvement with mural hyperenhancement, strictures, fistulas, and abscess formation. Associated complications include bowel obstruction and ischemia.
- **Ulcerative Colitis** (Fig. 38.34b): Continuous mucosal hyperenhancement with submucosal edema, starting from the rectum. Severe cases may develop toxic megacolon (colonic dilation >8 cm) with risk of perforation.

Obstructive

Bowel Obstructions—(See Above for Discussion of Postoperative Ileus Versus Obstruction)

Bowel obstruction is a mechanical issue, where something like a mass, scar tissue (such as adhesions), bowel entrapment (such as within a hernia), and/or bowel twisting leads to an inability of the bowel to move contents beyond a certain point, resulting in upstream distention and downstream decompression (Fig. 38.35).

Volvulus

Brief Description

A volvulus occurs when the bowel twists on itself and its blood supply, leading to obstruction and ischemia. Closed loop means that there are two transition points and enteric contents trapped between those two transition points cannot be decompressed with vomiting. Common types include sigmoid and cecal volvulus.

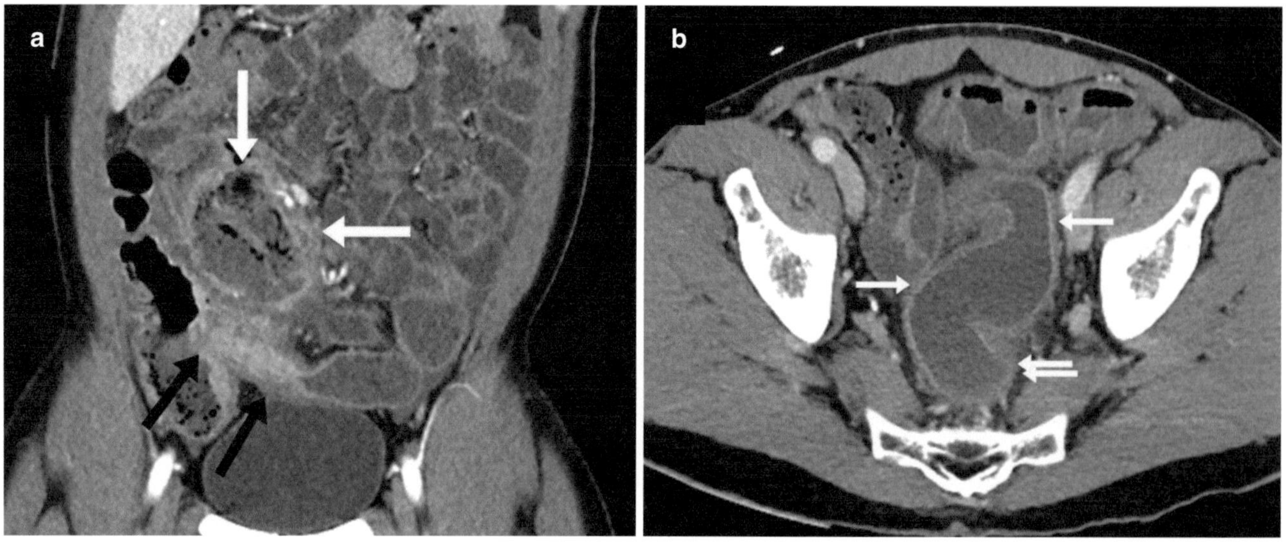

Fig. 38.34 (**a**) Coronal contrast-enhanced CT enterography image showing significant wall thickening of the terminal ileum (black arrows) and mucosal hyperenhancement consistent with Crohn disease. Area of ill-defined fluid and gas (white arrows) above the terminal ileum concerning for developing abscess, (**b**) Axial CT image through the pelvis showing mild wall thickening and lack of folds (featureless) of the rectum/sigmoid colon (white arrows) with mucosal hyperenhancement which may be seen in ulcerative colitis

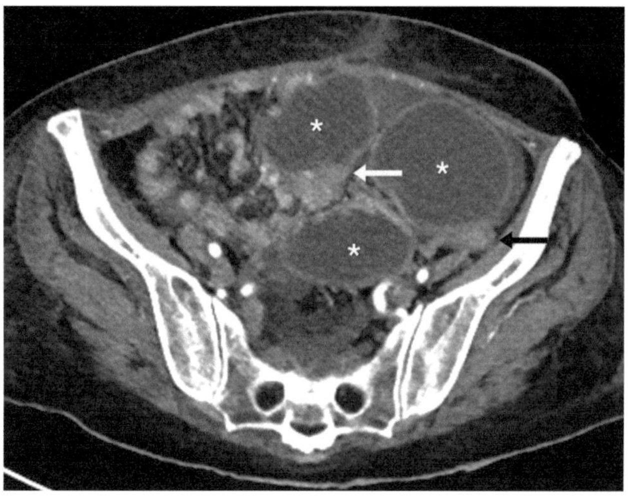

Fig. 38.35 Axial contrast-enhanced CT through the lower pelvis showing dilated small bowel loops (asterisks), decompressed colon (black arrow), and a transition point (white arrow) consistent with small bowel obstruction

Best Imaging Study

CT abdomen and pelvis with IV contrast is the preferred imaging. Abdominal radiographs may also help identify the volvulus.

Classic Imaging Findings

- **Sigmoid Volvulus** (Fig. 38.36): "Coffee bean sign" on radiographs, with the bowel distended and gas-filled, tapering into the pelvis. On CT, the "whirl sign" indicates twisting of mesenteric vessels.
- **Cecal Volvulus** (Fig. 38.37): The cecum appears distended and may shift abnormally into the left upper quadrant, with decompression of distal colon.

Hernias

Brief Description

A hernia occurs when an organ or tissue moves beyond its anatomic containment. In the abdomen, hernias most commonly occur at weak points where other structures naturally pass through, such as the inguinal canal or umbilicus. These are called external hernias. Internal hernias occur when bowel moves into pockets within the abdomen, such as congenital spaces or those created post-surgically. Herniated bowel can become trapped (incarcerated), and if blood supply is compromised, ischemia and bowel death can occur (strangulation).

Best Imaging Study

If a patient presents with a lump and a hernia is suspected, an ultrasound (US), or CT abdomen and/or pelvis is usually appropriate. For patients with acute abdominal pain or suspected complications of a known hernia, CT abdomen and pelvis with IV contrast is the best test (Fig. 38.38). Small bowel follow-through may be useful in equivocal cases, especially in cases of obstruction.

Classic Imaging Findings

- **General:** The hernia neck refers to the defect through which the contents pass, while the hernia sac refers to the contents beyond the normal boundaries, often containing fat or bowel.

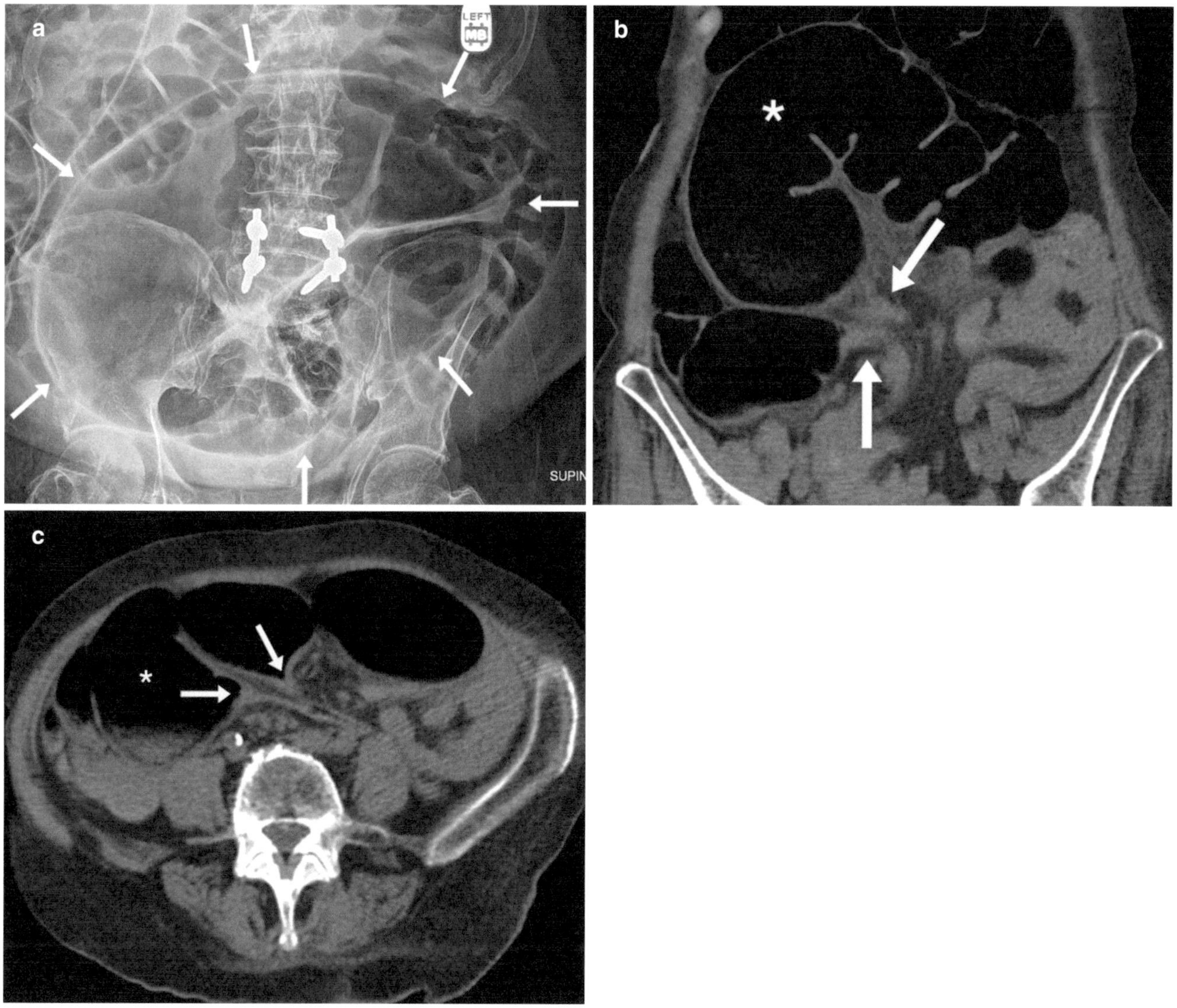

Fig. 38.36 (**a**) Frontal abdominal radiograph of sigmoid volvulus showing the classic coffee-bean sign with a significantly dilated loop of sigmoid colon arising from the pelvis (white arrows), (**b**) Coronal CT image showing the dilated sigmoid colon (asterisk) and two adjacent transition points (white arrows) which is the classic finding of a closed-loop obstruction, (**c**) Axial CT image through the pelvis again demonstrating the dilated sigmoid colon (asterisk) and two adjacent areas of abrupt tapering (white arrows) consistent with closed loop obstruction

- **Ultrasound:** May visualize the hernia neck and sac. Pressure or Valsalva maneuver can demonstrate the contents moving in and out, indicating that the hernia is not incarcerated. Look for signs of inflammation such as increased echogenicity, free fluid, or altered vascularity.
- **CT:** Can visualize the hernia neck and sac contents and is better at assessing complications such as strangulation and obstruction. Findings include upstream obstruction, adjacent fat stranding, poor wall enhancement, and possible perforation. Note that CT is unable to access for dynamic findings such as hernia reducibility to exclude incarceration.

Intussusception

Brief Description

Intussusception is the telescoping of a segment of bowel into a distal segment, often starting at a "lead point" such as a tumor, post-surgical scar, enlarged lymph node, or abnormal bowel (e.g., in Celiac disease). This process can lead to obstruction, ischemia, and perforation. It is much more common in children and may resolve spontaneously or be treated with air/hydrostatic enema. In adults, treatment usually requires surgery.

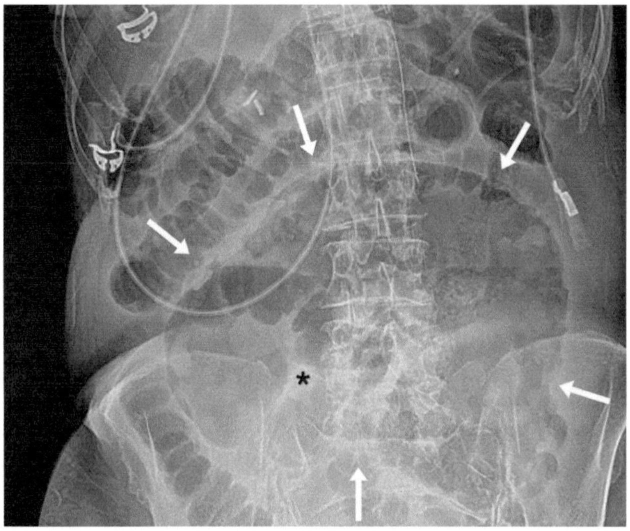

Fig. 38.37 Frontal abdominal radiograph showing a markedly dilated loop of large bowel (white arrows) centered on the right lower quadrant (black asterisk) concerning for cecal volvulus

Best Imaging Study

For adults with abdominal pain, a CT abdomen and pelvis with IV contrast is appropriate (Fig. 38.39). In children, abdominal radiographs are typically followed by ultrasound (Fig. 38.40), which is the best imaging modality. Fluoroscopic-guided air enema or ultrasound-guided hydrostatic enema may be both diagnostic and therapeutic in pediatric cases (Fig. 38.41).

Classic Imaging Findings

- **General:** Bowel-in-bowel appearance with alternating layers of bowel wall and mesenteric fat, sometimes containing lymph nodes. Longer segments (>4 cm) are more concerning due to increased difficulty with reduction and risk of complications.
- **CT:** Alternating layers of bowel wall and mesenteric fat. CT is better for visualizing complications like obstruction or perforation.

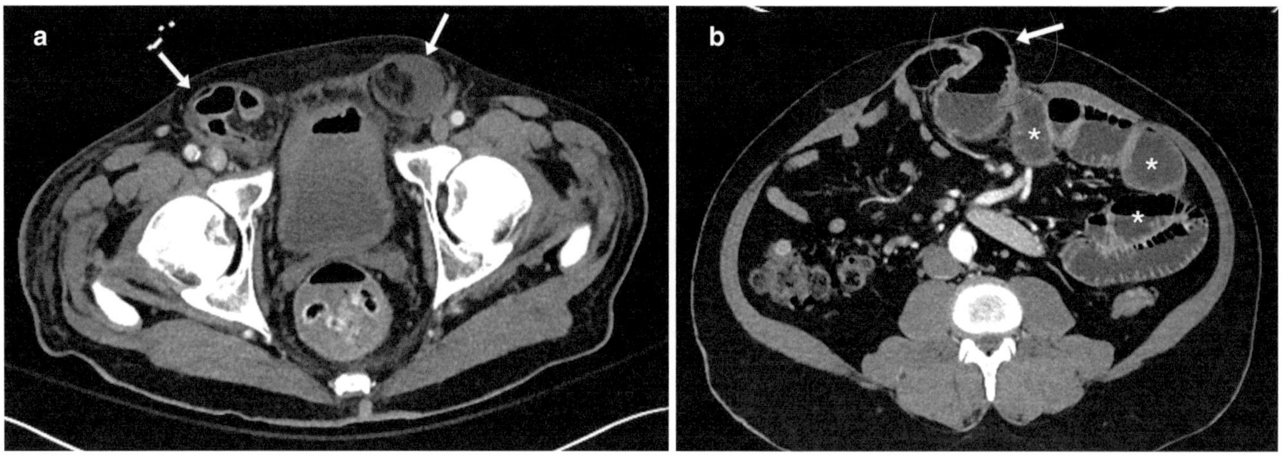

Fig. 38.38 (**a**) Axial contrast enhanced CT through the pelvis showing bilateral inguinal hernias (white arrows) containing bowel on the right and fluid/fat on the left, (**b**) Axial contrast-enhanced CT through the mid-abdomen showing a peri-umbilical hernia (white arrow) and upstream dilation of the small bowel (asterisks) consistent with small bowel obstruction from an incarcerated hernia

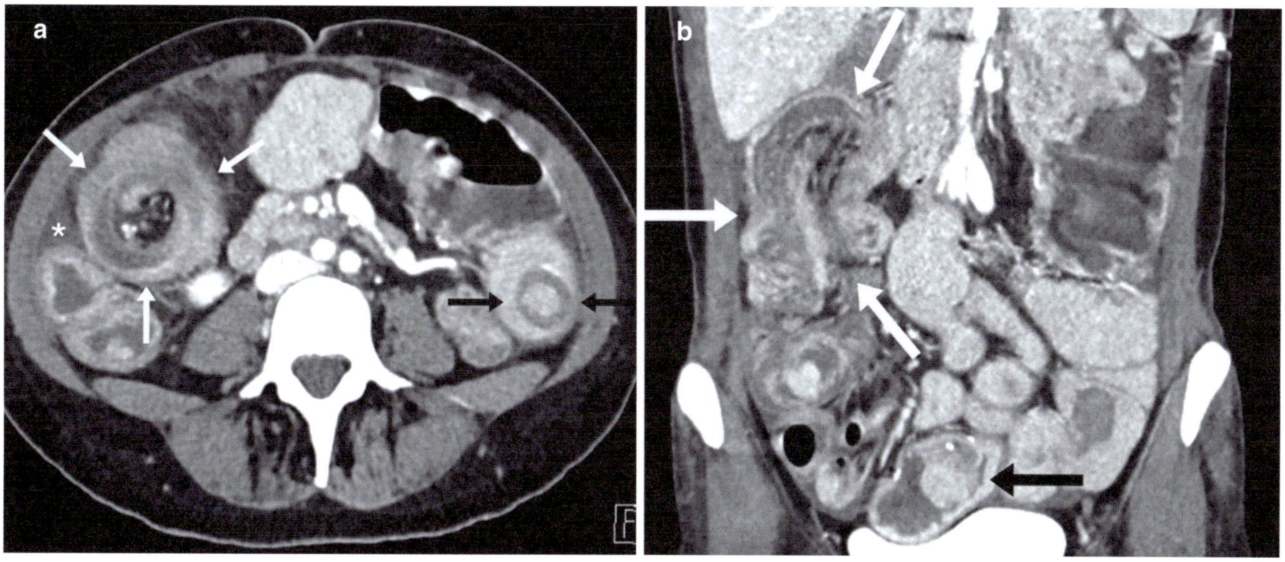

Fig. 38.39 (**a**) Axial contrast-enhanced CT through the lower abdomen showing an ileocolic intussusception in the right lower quadrant (white arrows) with adjacent free fluid (asterisk) as well as fluid within the intussusception which are worrisome signs. Incidental small bowel-small bowel intussusception in the left lower quadrant (black arrows), (**b**) Coronal image of the same patient showing the ileocolic (white arrows) and small bowel (black arrow) intussusceptions

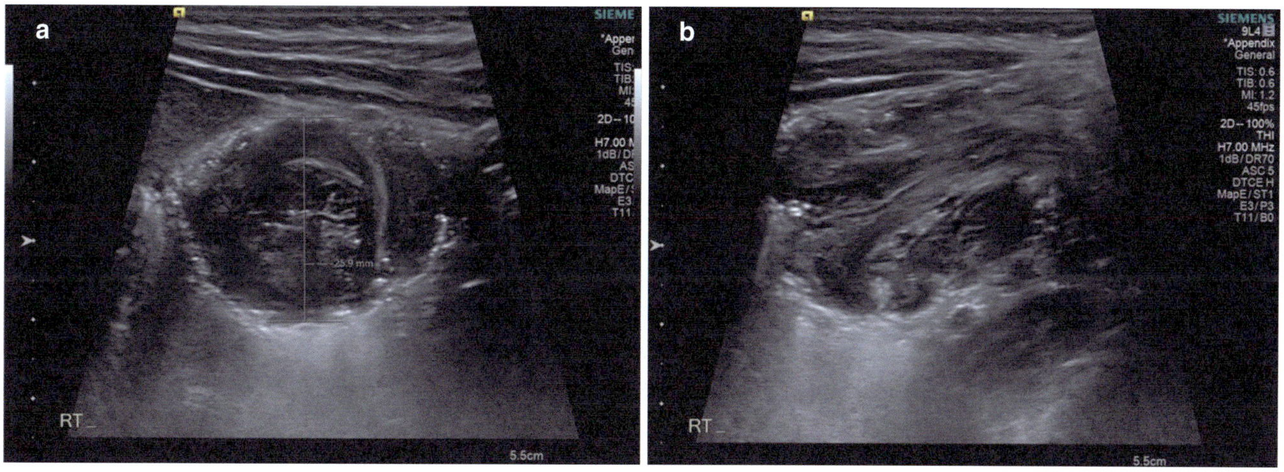

Fig. 38.40 (**a**) Grayscale ultrasound in the right hemi-abdomen showing a transverse image of an ileocolic intussusception with alternating layers of bright and dark bowel wall and fat, (**b**) Sagittal ultrasound image of the same ileocolic intussusception better capturing the bowel being pulled into itself

- **Ultrasound:** Hypoechoic and echogenic layers of bowel wall with intervening mesenteric fat. Doppler may show mesenteric blood vessels between bowel loops.

Trauma

Full discussion of trauma is outside the scope of this test. Some of the more commonly encountered traumatic injuries are listed below.

Solid Organ Injury

Brief Description

The liver and spleen are the most common organs injured in trauma although any organ is at risk, including the kidneys and pancreas. Blunt force, rib fracture, or gunshot wounds (Fig. 38.42) can lead to disruption of the associated organs with possible hemorrhage.

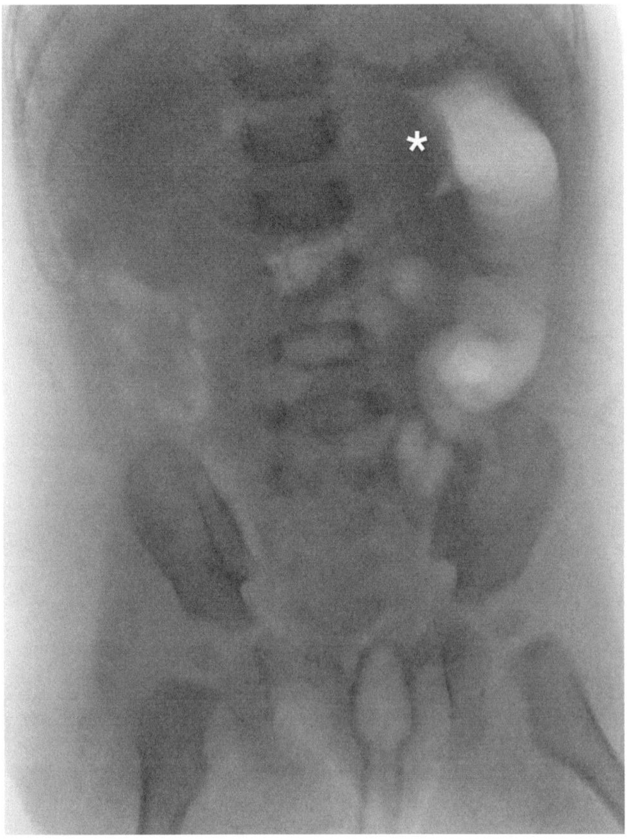

Fig. 38.41 Fluoroscopic radiograph (bone is dark, air is bright), showing the intussusception as a soft tissue thickening (asterisk) within the colon immediately adjacent to the air being instilled during the enema

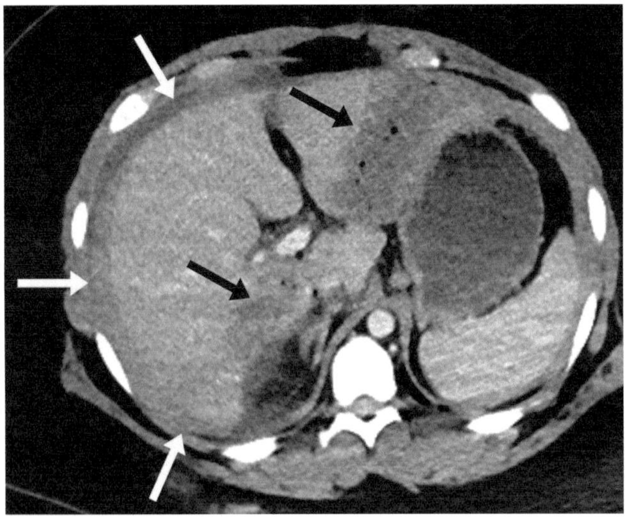

Fig. 38.42 Axial contrast-enhanced CT through the upper abdomen showing a low attenuating tract (black arrows) with air locules through the liver from recent gunshot wound. High attenuation fluid around the liver (white arrows) which is brightest near the tract is concerning for acute bleeding

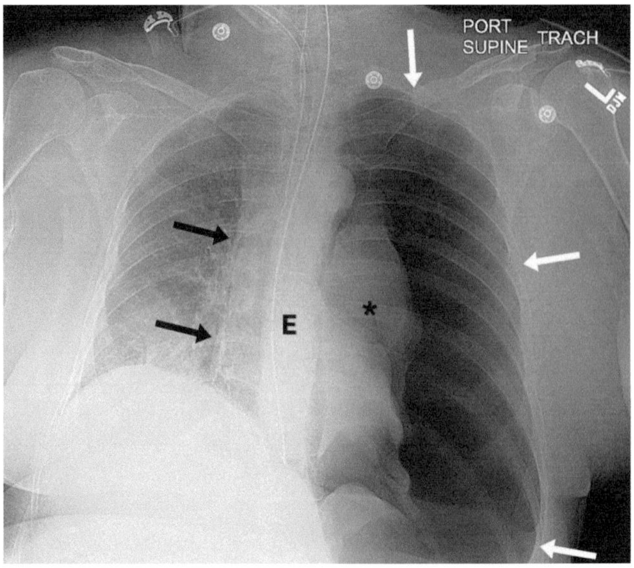

Fig. 38.43 Frontal chest radiograph showing a very large left pneumothorax (white arrows), left lung collapse (asterisk), and rightward mediastinal shift (black arrows along right mediastinum) consistent with tension pneumothorax. Incidentally, the enteric suction tube (E) is too high within the esophagus and would need to be advanced until the sidehole (adjacent to the E label) is within the stomach

Classic Imaging Findings

Disrupted normal parenchyma from its blood supply will not enhance. This means it will show up darker than the adjacent parenchyma. Active extravasation may be present with a small amount of bright contrast or denser than simple fluid blood near the site of bleeding. Large volumes of high attenuation fluid (>20 HU) in a trauma patient are highly concerning for hemoperitoneum. The American Association for the Surgery of Trauma (AAST) has developed grading systems for solid organ injuries including injuries of the liver, spleen, and kidneys with I being the mildest injury and V being the most severe (for example a shattered spleen).

Pneumothorax

Brief Description

"Popped lung." Air inside the pleural cavity lining the lung. Common after trauma but can also occur spontaneously or be iatrogenic. If large enough, it is possible for the pneumothorax to put pressure on the heart, mediastinal vessels, and diaphragm. This is called a tension pneumothorax (Fig. 38.43).

Best Imaging Study

Chest radiographs are the best first test. Supine radiographs can be insensitive for a small pneumothorax. Obtaining upright or decubitus radiographs increases the sensitivity.

CT will reveal trace amounts of air but evaluation with radiographs is usually sufficient in post-surgical or outpatient cases.

Classic Imaging Findings

Look for a "white pleural line" representing the edge of the lung. Lung vascular markings should not extend beyond the line. Beware outline of the ribs and scapula as well as artifacts from patient bedding and skin folds. Air should rise to the highest point—the lung apices on upright views. Tension pneumothorax may be suspected if there is shift of the heart away from the pneumothorax and/or depression or inversion of the diaphragm.

Vascular

Acute Mesenteric Ischemia and Bowel Ischemia

Brief Description

Acute mesenteric ischemia is like a stroke, but of the gut. Decreased blood flow can arise from a variety of causes, including arterial/venous clot and obstruction. Other causes of bowel ischemia include closed-loop obstruction, strangulated hernia, and severe hypotension.

Best Imaging Study

Beyond a standard CT abdomen and pelvis with IV contrast, when acute mesenteric ischemia is suspected, the best test is a CTA of the abdomen and pelvis. Catheter angiography is recommended for definitive evaluation and treatment.

Classic Imaging Findings

Some specific findings will vary based on the etiology: clot within the associated blood vessels (Fig. 38.44), injury from trauma, bowel obstruction. Early findings of bowel ischemia can include wall thickening and fat stranding. As ischemia progresses, the injury can lead to associated ileus/dilation without obstruction, lack of enhancement of the associated bowel loop, and pneumatosis. Pneumatosis is air within the bowel wall, which is sometimes difficult to separate from normal gas inside the bowel lumen. Normal intraluminal gas should accumulate at whichever side is "up". On a CT, this will be the anterior aspect of the bowel because the patient is supine. Pneumatosis may be seen within the wall regardless of patient positioning. You may be able to see portal venous gas collecting in the adjacent mesenteric veins and eventually traveling to the liver in the portal venous system—look for fine branching gas in the periphery of the liver on lung windows.

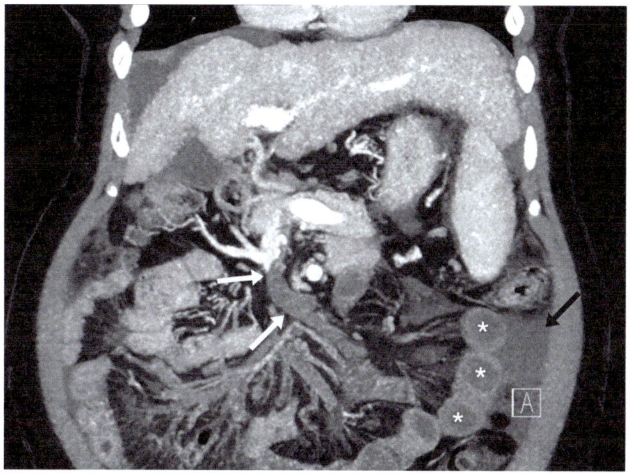

Fig. 38.44 Coronal contrast-enhanced MIP image of the abdomen showing complete occlusion of the SMV (white arrows). This leads to congestion of the associated bowel which can be seen in the left lower quadrant bowel (asterisk) which has wall thickening, hypo-enhancement, and adjacent free fluid (black arrow)

GI Bleed

Brief Description

The findings of active extravasation have been previously discussed—accumulation of IV contrast on more delayed sequences. Clinically significant bleeding will generally be evaluated by direct endoscopic visualization. If not visualized but the patient continues to lose blood, the source may be in the small intestine.

Best Imaging Study

CTA abdomen and pelvis without and with IV contrast often appropriate. Multiphase CT enterography where the patient ingests negative contrast (low density to help better evaluate the bowel) wall can be helpful. Interventional arteriography can also be used for both diagnostic evaluation and treatment. In cases where a source of GI bleeding remains obscured, a very sensitive tool is nuclear medicine GI bleeding scintigraphy often using labeled red blood cells (Fig. 38.45).

Classic Imaging Findings

Whether by CTA (Fig. 38.18) or nuclear medicine, look for accumulation of contrast or radioactivity within the lumen of the GI tract. Over time, the blood should progress along the GI tract which will be more evident with delayed imaging as on a nuclear medicine study (Fig. 38.45).

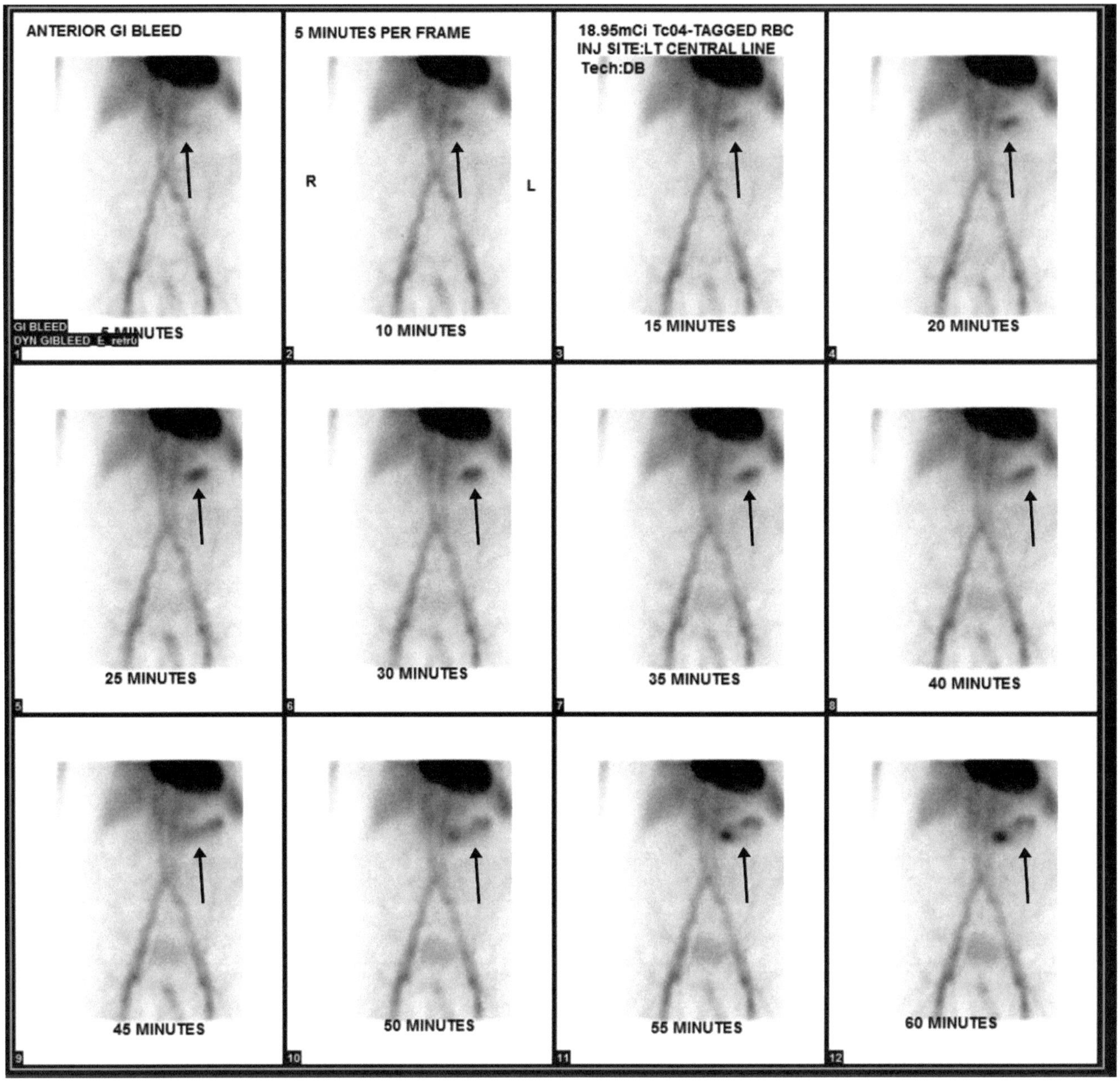

Fig. 38.45 Nuclear medicine GI Bleeding study using tagged red blood cells. The radiopharmaceutical can be seen on 5-min image in the left upper quadrant (black arrows) and gradually accumulates over the course of the study confirming the presence of active GI bleeding

Abdominal Aortic Aneurysm (AAA)

Brief Description

Dilation of the abdominal aorta, most often related to atherosclerotic disease.

Best Imaging Study

If symptomatic, then CTA (Fig. 38.46). US is usually sufficient for screening high risk patients although noncontrast CT can also be considered, especially in patient with a known aneurysm needing follow-up for growth.

Classic Imaging Findings

Aorta >1.5 times the normal diameter. Generally, >3 cm in the infrarenal aorta. Risk of rupture increases with diameter. CTA can also visualize other complications such as dissection and assess stent grafts for endoleak.

Miscellaneous

Neoplasia

Discussion of the myriad types and imaging findings of cancer is beyond the scope of this text, but the most important thing to be aware of is that the radiologists and technologists can tailor the imaging protocols of CT and MRI to the specific type of cancer suspected or being followed. Providing these clinical details on the exam request is extremely helpful as it allows the radiologists to optimize an exam for the patient.

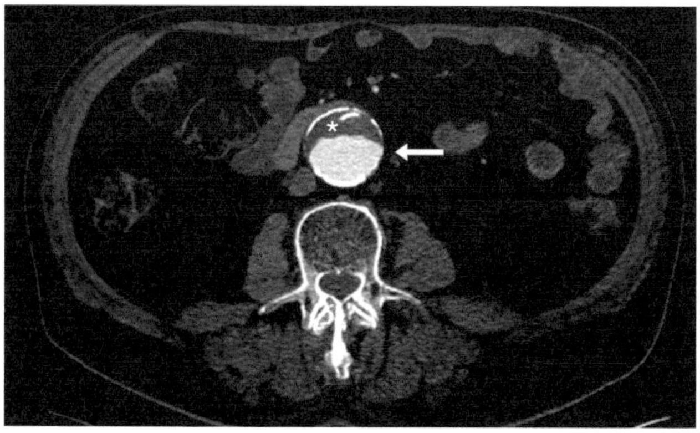

Fig. 38.46 Axial arterial-phase CTA image through the infrarenal aorta showing an abdominal aortic aneurysm (white arrow) with eccentric thrombus/plaque (asterisk)

Foreign Body

Brief Description

Can result from accidental or intentional ingestion, penetrating injury, or iatrogenic causes.

Best Imaging Study

Radiography can be used to screen for metallic foreign bodies (Fig. 38.47a), such as ingested batteries or ballistics. Retained surgical sponges often include radiopaque fibers to make them visible on radiographs (Fig. 38.47b). Glass is typically radiopaque, though usually the density is closer to bone making it more difficult to visualize on radiographs.

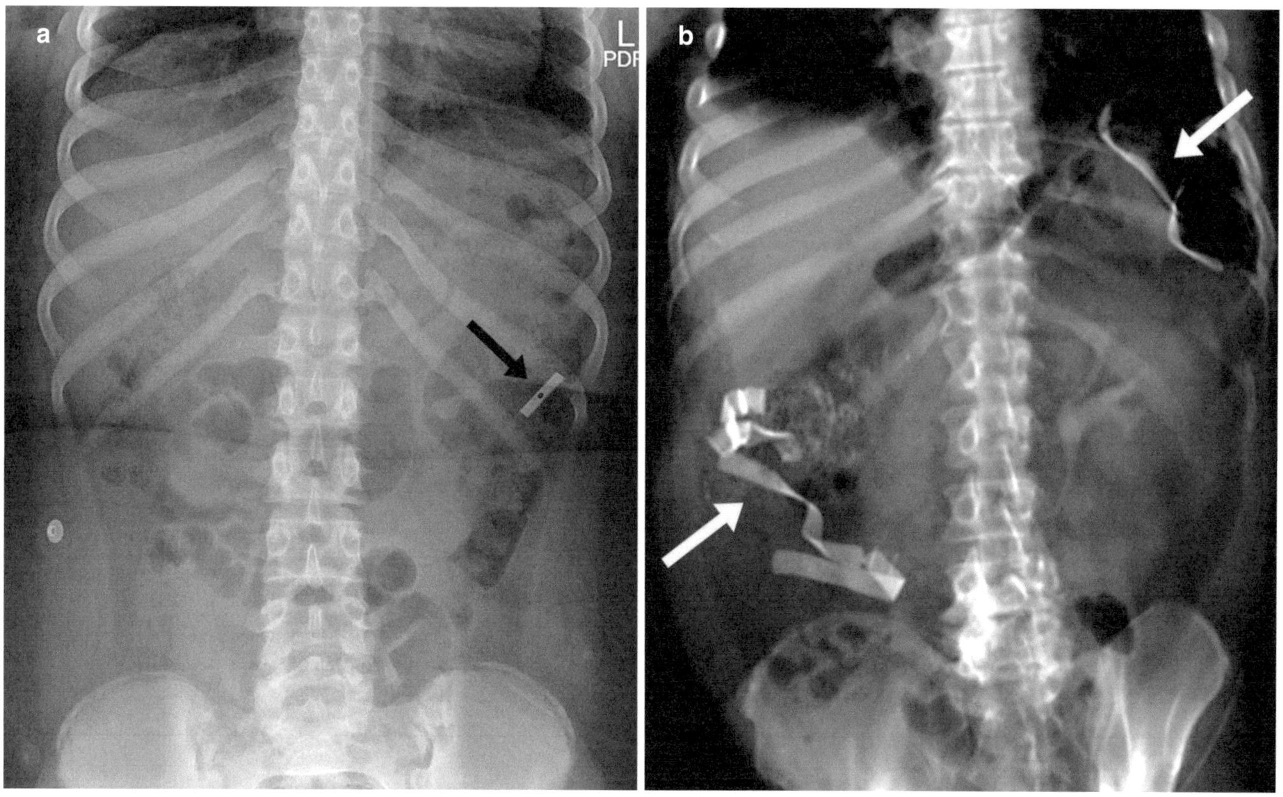

Fig. 38.47 (**a**) Abdominal radiograph showing an ingested razor blade (black arrow) in the left upper quadrant, (**b**) Frontal abdominal radiograph showing retained surgical sponges in the right lower quadrant and left upper quadrant (white arrows)

CT can help clarify cases of suspected ingestion or complications not seen on radiographs. Wood (such as splinters) is isodense and typical not visible on radiographs or CT but may be visible on targeted ultrasound or MRI.

Classic Imaging Findings

Non-metallic foreign bodies are often not visible on radiographs. Sharp objects, multiple magnets, and button batteries are the most dangerous ingested foreign bodies and most crucial to identify. Retained surgical sponges will have a looped appearance.

Choosing Wisely

It is an overwhelming task to remember all the available tests and what specific factors will change the best test to choose. Fortunately, the ACR (American College of Radiology) has published and useful tool called the Appropriateness Criteria® which is an evidence-based guide to what tests are appropriate or inappropriate for a given clinical situation. We have provided a summary of many of the clinical scenarios discussed in this chapter and the preferred radiologic test in the following Quick Reference Table (Table 38.5):

Table 38.5 Quick reference table

Indication	Best test	Caveats/distinctions
Anastomotic leak, GI	CT with IV contrast Radiography and fluoroscopy may be useful alternatives	CT provides best anatomic evaluation and identifies small leaks of fluid and air
Anastomotic leak, GU	Upper collecting system: CT urogram Bladder: Cystogram (CT or fluoroscopy) Urethra: Fluoroscopy (retrograde urethrogram)	No air in normal GU tract so less utility to start with radiographs
Bleed	CTA	Active extravasation: CTA with non-con, arterial, and venous phases
Abscess	CT abdomen and pelvis with contrast	Superficial infections/wound infections may be visible with targeted US
Ileus and bowel obstruction	Abdominal radiographs	CT abdomen and pelvis with contrast can assess for obstruction, ischemia, or abscess
Wound dehiscence	Clinically	CT with contrast for deeper dehiscence or complications
Appendicitis	CT abdomen and pelvis with contrast	US or MRI can be considered in pediatric or pregnant patients
Cholecystitis/Choledocholithiasis	Right upper quadrant US	If findings are equivocal, follow up imaging may include MRCP, CT, or HIDA scan
Diverticulitis	CT abdomen and pelvis with IV contrast	Microperforation may manifest small gas locules, while larger compilations include abscesses, fistulas, or blood clots
Nephrolithiasis	Non-contrast CT sufficient in most cases	CT with contrast for suspected complicated infection. Renal US can be used to screen for hydronephrosis in pregnant patients
Necrotizing fasciitis	Primarily clinical diagnosis	CT with contrast may help in equivocal cases to assess for gas or assist with surgical planning. MRI can be helpful in stable patients
Inflammatory bowel disease	CT or MR enterography (with IV contrast and negative oral contrast) to evaluate the bowel wall and complications	CT abdomen/pelvis with IV contrast is an alternative
Volvulus	CT abdomen and pelvis with IV contrast	Abdominal radiographs or fluoroscopic enema may also help identify the volvulus
Hernia	US for screening; CT for complications	
Intussusception	CT in adults; Radiographs then US in children	
Perforation	CT; upright/decubitus radiographs to screen	
Soid organ injury	CT with contrast	In trauma, often includes chest, abdomen, and pelvis
Pneumothorax	Chest radiographs	Uprights or decubitus radiographs increase the sensitivity

(continued)

Table 38.5 (continued)

Indication	Best test	Caveats/distinctions
Acute mesenteric ischemia	CTA abdomen and pelvis with contrast	CT of the abdomen and pelvis may help initially with work-up of abdominal pain
GI bleed	CTA abdomen and pelvis without and with IV contrast Nuclear medicine tagged RBC scan for slow intermittent GI bleed	CT enterography can help better evaluate the bowel wall Interventional arteriography can also be used as both imaging and treatment
Abdominal aortic aneurysm	CT with contrast if symptomatic	US for screening in high-risk patients
Neoplasia	CT and MRI with tailored imaging protocols	Provide adequate clinical detail in the order
Foreign body	Screen with radiographs (multiple views can be helpful)	CT can help clarify cases of suspected ingestion or complications not seen on radiographs Some foreign bodies are not visible on radiographs or CT and US or MRI may be needed
Pelvic Pain in female patients	Pelvic US	CT abdomen and pelvis or MRI pelvis may be need if US is inconclusive

Conclusion

This chapter provides PA and NPs the essential skills and knowledge to efficiently and safely navigate imaging. We have reviewed imaging interpretation basics, common imaging modalities, key diagnosis, and how to choose the correct study for a variety of clinical scenarios. The recommendations in this chapter have been put together as a reference for providers to use to enhance quality of care and contribute to the most efficacious use of radiology.

References and Suggested Readings

ACR Appropriateness Criteria. https://www.acr.org/Clinical-Resources/ACR-Appropriateness-Criteria. Reference for determining the best imaging study for a multitude of clinical scenarios.

American College of Radiology. ACR Manual on Contrast Media. Revised 2024. https://www.acr.org/-/media/acr/files/clinical-resources/contrast_media.pdf.

America College of Radiology. ACR Manual on MRI Safety. Revised 2024. Available at: https://www.acr.org/-/media/ACR/Files/Radiology-Safety/MR-Safety/Manual-on-MR-Safety.pdf.

American College of Radiology. ACR–SPR practice parameter for imaging pregnant or potentially pregnant patients with ionizing radiation. Revised 2023. Available at: https://www.acr.org/-/media/acr/files/practice-parameters/pregnant-pts.pdf.

e-Anatomy. The anatomy of imaging. https://www.imaios.com/en/e--anatomy. Excellent online reference atlas for imaging anatomy. Subscription service.

Goodman LR. Felson's principles of chest roentgenology, a programmed text: a programmed text. 5th ed. Elsevier; 2021.

Radiopaedia. https://radiopaedia.org/?lang=us. Free online radiology reference.

The American Association for the Surgery of Trauma—Injury Scoring Scales. Accessed 2024. https://www.aast.org/resources-detail/injury-scoring-scale. Reference for specific injury classifications in trauma.

Interventional Radiology: Core Applications in General and Vascular Surgery

39

B. Bobby Chiong

Introduction

PA school goes by fast, and you often just have 27 or 28 months to learn everything in medicine and surgery, which is not adequate. Most students spend substantial time on core rotations—surgery, medicine, obstetrics, gynecology, family medicine, and pediatrics. Many clinical rotations take place in low-acuity centers, and most curricula and PA programs do not provide students with information about important ancillary service lines. Perhaps one of the most important service lines, especially in (but not limited to) the hospital setting, is the field known as ***interventional radiology*** (IR). *Surgeons work hand in hand with IR physicians*, and it is at least important that PAs, both in training and in practice, are aware of the value and service of IR. Although exposure to IR in PA school is limited, this is a specialty that allows advanced practitioners considerable autonomy, and is a niche specialty worth exploring for the practicing PA who desires to perform and assist with IR procedures.

What *is* interventional radiology and what do these physicians do exactly? This is generally a difficult thing to explain, but let's try and make it simple. In the beginning, there were doctors. If you needed surgery, you went to the barber (yes, surgeons actually started out as *barbers*). Fast forward a millennium and now physicians have become increasingly specialized in their scope and nature of practice.

With the discovery that high-energy photons (X-rays) could be used to take pictures of bones, the field of radiology was born. Fast forward today, where radiologists who *do procedures* predicated upon X-ray information are called ***interventional radiologists*** (you will often hear this abbreviated to **IR**). Many of these procedures are carried out in highly sophisticated IR-suites inside of hospitals facilities (Fig. 39.1a, b).

B. B. Chiong (✉)
SBH Health System, Department of Interventional Radiology,
Bronx, NY, USA

S. Atallah, J. Dragoljevic (eds.), *Fundamentals of Surgery for Physician Assistants*,
https://doi.org/10.1007/978-3-032-21069-2_39

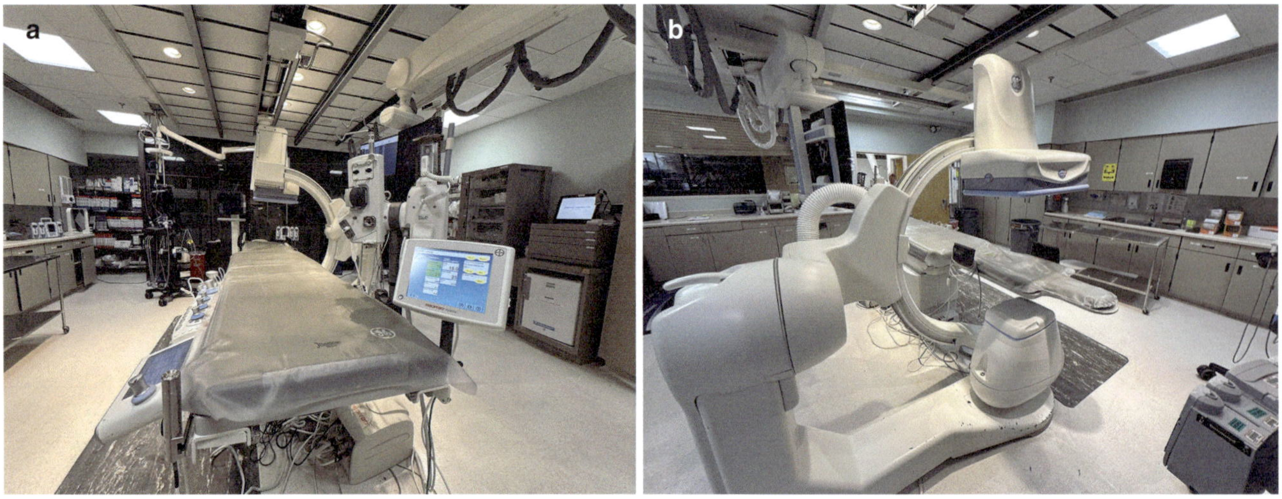

Fig. 39.1 (**a**) An IR suite is shown. It is a complex, and highly sophisticated theater that allows for precision instrumentation under radiographic guidance with or without intravenous contrast, depending on the nature of the procedure. IR specialists work hand in hand with patients who are being managed on a surgical service in many cases. (**b**) View of the fluoroscopy machine that can provide "live" or continuous imaging, which can be helpful in certain interventions

Training to Become and Interventional Radiologist

IR physicians follow a long road. Traditionally, after 4 years of college and 4 years of medical school, an internal medicine internship training was required. After this, 4 years of radiology residency, then 1 year of interventional radiology fellowship are necessary, making post-graduate training 5 years in duration. At the time of this writing, this is no longer the way that most interventional radiologists are trained. Now, the training is a direct pathway out of medical school. Similar to the way that radiation oncology is now a separate training and a separate specialty from diagnostic radiology, there is an undercurrent of discussion about interventional radiology breaking off completely from diagnostic radiology. IR physicians think differently, work differently, and possess a different mindset and approach. The main difference in the specialties is that diagnostic radiologists don't typically *treat* patients, while IR physicians *do*, by providing therapeutic intervention.

The Role of IR in Clinical Medicine

So, what exactly is it that IR docs do? There is a wide variation in the scope of practice, and a *general* distribution of IR uses by specialty in the United States is shown in Fig. 39.2. Basically, IR is performing a procedure under **imaging guidance** (Table 39.1). Every IR center is different, and different interventional radiologists in the same practice may not all cover the same procedures.

Let's focus on the basics. The three most common procedures interventional radiologists perform are:

- **Image Guided Biopsy**
- **Image Guided Drainage (such as of abscess or fluid collection)**
- **Image Guided Vascular Access**

Biopsies would seem to me the most obvious purview of interventional radiology. Most suspicious findings in the body show up on medical imaging such as computed tomography (CT), ultrasound (US), or magnetic resonance imaging (MRI). If you need to biopsy a lesion not easily accessible so as, for example, to obtain histologic confirmation of malignancy, you can always check with IR to see if an adequate tissue sample can be obtained under image guidance. There are other pertinent examples of when IR can be helpful. For example, if a kidney or liver is failing, an image-guided biopsy of those solid organs can be informative to the clinical team. Under imaging guidance, with or without sedation (but almost always with local anesthesia), the interventional radiologist can perform a biopsy using a specialized needle with a biopsy chamber to get a **core** biopsy for diagnosis. Importantly, *a core tissue biopsy preserves **histological architecture**,* which is especially important in telling the difference between *pre*-cancer (carcinoma in situ) and *invasive* cancer.

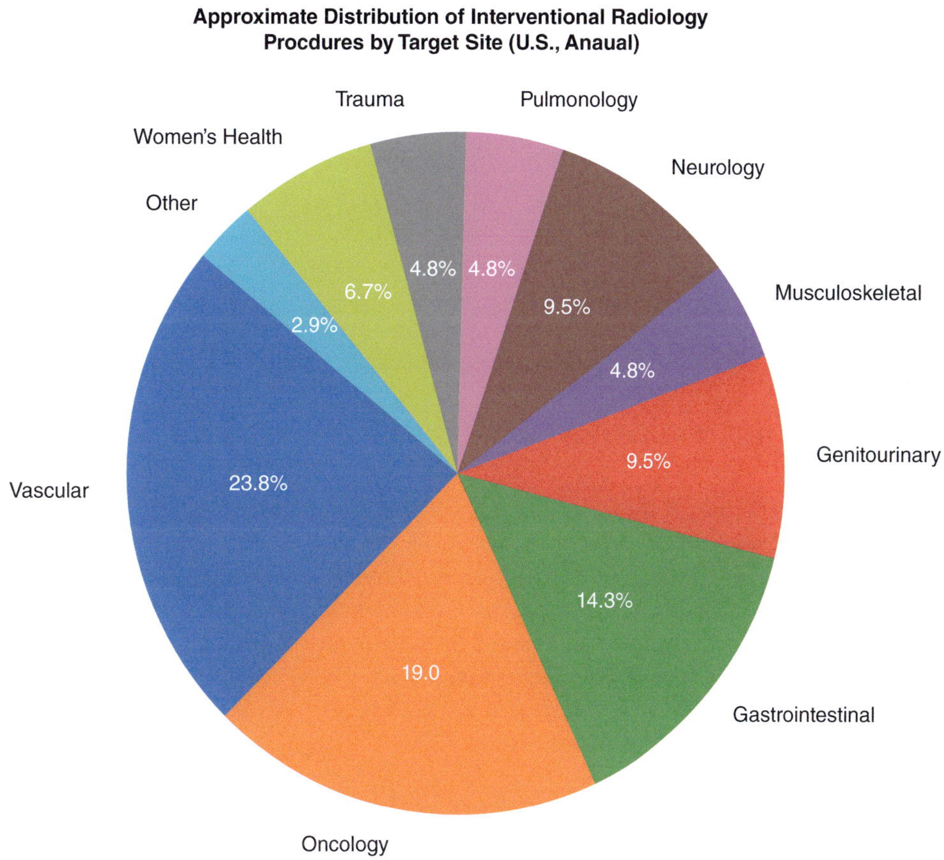

Fig. 39.2 The approximate distribution of IR procedures by target site (organ) is shown

Table 39.1 Uses of interventional radiology in modern medicine

Clinical specialty	Procedure	Indication/use	Description
Vascular	Angioplasty and stenting	Atherosclerotic vascular disease, peripheral artery disease	Balloon dilation and stent placement to open narrowed blood vessels
Vascular	Embolization	Aneurysms, bleeding, tumors	Intentional occlusion of blood vessels to stop bleeding or cut blood supply to tumors
Vascular	Thrombolysis/thrombectomy	Acute DVT, PE, arterial thrombosis	Dissolution or mechanical removal of blood clots
Oncology	Transarterial chemoembolization (TACE)	Hepatocellular carcinoma, metastatic liver tumors	Direct delivery of chemotherapy into tumor vasculature followed by embolization
Oncology	Radioembolization (Y-90 therapy)	Liver tumors (HCC, metastases)	Delivery of radioactive particles to tumors via hepatic artery
Oncology	Percutaneous tumor ablation	Renal, liver, lung tumors	Destruction of tumor cells using heat (RFA, microwave), cold (cryoablation), or other techniques
Gastrointestinal	Percutaneous gastrostomy tube	Feeding access in patients unable to eat orally	Image-guided placement of a feeding tube directly into the stomach
Gastrointestinal	Biliary drainage and stenting	Biliary obstruction from stones or tumors	Decompression of the biliary tree via internal/external drainage or stent placement
Genitourinary	Nephrostomy and ureteral stenting	Urinary obstruction due to stones, tumors	Image-guided drainage or bypass of the urinary tract.
Genitourinary	Varicocele embolization	Varicoceles causing infertility or pain	Non-surgical treatment by embolizing dilated testicular veins
Musculoskeletal	Vertebroplasty/kyphoplasty	Osteoporotic vertebral compression fractures	Injection of bone cement into fractured vertebra to relieve pain and stabilize spine
Neurology	Cerebral angiography and coiling	Aneurysms, AVMs, stroke	Vascular imaging and minimally invasive treatment of brain aneurysms and vascular malformations
Neurology	Mechanical thrombectomy	Acute ischemic stroke	Catheter-based removal of clots from cerebral arteries
Pulmonology	Pulmonary angiography	Pulmonary embolism diagnosis and management	Imaging of pulmonary arteries; may assist in catheter-directed thrombolysis
Pulmonology	Bronchial artery embolization	Hemoptysis	Control of bleeding from bronchial arteries
Infectious disease	Abscess drainage	Intra-abdominal, pelvic, or soft tissue abscesses	Percutaneous drainage of infected fluid collections under image guidance
Trauma	Angiographic embolization	Solid organ injury (liver, spleen, kidney)	Control of internal bleeding without surgery
Women's health	Uterine fibroid embolization (UFE)	Symptomatic uterine fibroids	Minimally invasive alternative to hysterectomy for fibroid treatment
Women's health	Fallopian tube recanalization	Infertility due to tubal blockage	Image-guided reopening of blocked fallopian tubes

Thermal Ablative Procedures

To take it a step further, if there is a malignancy that needs treatment, and if you can get a needle there to take the biopsy, it's not that much difference in skill to get a needle there for *thermal ablation*. **Thermal ablation** is an alternative to resection surgery, where instead of cutting out the tumor, you can cook it with microwaves or freeze the lesion (the latter is known as **cryoablation**). Of course, there's a deep level of nuance to this, but this is the 30,000 ft overview.

The Seldinger Technique

Perhaps you've heard of the ***Seldinger Technique?*** Before Sven Ivar Seldinger and his landmark paper in 1953, if you wanted a central line, you had to cut through the skin (that is, perform a *surgical cut-down*), find the vein, and directly insert the line you wanted into the vessel.

Seldinger figured out that you could use a much thinner needle for the first puncture, then use a *guidewire* (that closely resembles a modern-day guitar string), then dilate your way up to using whatever catheter you need over the guidewire. *This general concept, commonly referred to as the* ***Seldinger Technique****, is something that now forms the basis of most vascular access and drainage procedures for the interventional radiologist. Of course, all of this is done under X-ray-based image guidance—such as CT-imaging, or fluoroscopy.*

Vascular Access Procedures

To expand on vascular access, there are many ways to get medications into veins. If you are new to the field of medicine, surgery, and anesthesia, you will soon learn that *vascular access, whether short-term or long-term is a lifeline*. Let me try and briefly list the different types of venous access. First, there are the ***peripheral*** **intravenous lines**, the thing we generally first think of when we talk about "getting an IV." These access IVs are generally only a few cm in length, and are placed into a superficial vein that is just below the skin, which can be felt and/or seen. Next, we have ***midlines,*** which are so-called because they bridge the gap between peripheral IV (PIV) lines and **PICCs** (peripherally inserted central catheters).

Midlines are generally placed in the upper arm, sometimes forearm, and are generally 10–20 cm in length. Midlines are introduced into an anatomically *named* vein—like the *brachial, basilic,* or *cephalic vein.* The crucial difference between a midline and a PICC is that for a midline, *the tip ends outside the central venous system,* no further than the axillary vein outside (distal to) where the first rib and clavicle cross. A few centimeters more proximally, the axillary vein becomes the *subclavian vein*, which is considered part of the *central venous system.*

Functionally, midlines will remain useful for a longer time than a PIV because they go into larger diameter veins with improved blood flow that will be *less likely to clot.* PICCs will remain useful the longest of all, up to 18 months at some centers, while others may not impose a time limit, and PICCs are kept in place for as long as they are functional. Again, PICCs have a long life because the blood in the central veins moves much faster than in the extremities (think of water flowing in a small stream versus a large river as an analogy). Blood in the veins of the arms and legs often is not move at all, and is quite sluggish.

Special Considerations for Patients with Kidney Failure

In general, a PICC should be avoided if the patient is on dialysis for chronic kidney disease or if the GFR is less than 45. Having a PICC for too long makes it difficult to make an AV fistula for dialysis. If your patient requires long-term vascular access, ask IR to place a **tunneled central** line (aka Hickman, Broviac, Groshong) rather than a PICC.

Tunneled Vascular Access Lines

This brings us to the concept of *tunneling a line.* Most commonly, tunneled lines will be for vascular access, usually for hemodialysis access. A ***non*****-tunneled central line** will enter through the skin with a relatively short course between the skin and the vein. This short distance makes the presence of a central line a relatively high risk for bacteremia. *Tunneling means that the line will travel for a distance of about 5–10 cm under the skin before going into the vein.* Don't think about it too hard, but this *tunneling protects against skin flora and outside pathogens from getting into the bloodstream*. While a *non-tunneled central line should only stay in for a few days*, a tunneled central line can stay in for a much longer period of time, even years in some cases.

Venous Access Ports

One step further and IR specialists can implant a **venous access port**. This means that we tunnel the central line, and this line connects to a port that goes *under* the skin that can be accessed by a special kind of needle. Typically, these ports are going to be placed for patients requiring *systemic chemotherapy*. Because many kinds of chemotherapy are too caustic to be placed into a peripheral vein, they need to go to the fast-flowing central veins. Instead of placing a central line every time, it's easier to place a port and then access the port for chemotherapy, using a special needle. When not in use, there are no lines or tubes "sticking out of the body"; but the port is easily palpable and often visible just beneath the dermis. Nowadays, both (general/vascular) surgeons and IR physicians are trained to place central venous access ports, and this may vary by institution, availability, and preference.

Drainage Procedures

When an interventional radiologist carries out a drainage procedure, it essentially combines the skillset of IR-biopsy and the skillset for IR-vascular access. If there is a pocket of fluid that requires drainage (e.g., abscess, ascites, pleural effusion, pericardial effusion, etc.), ultrasound and/or CT-body imaging can be used to position the needle toward the target fluid collection. Then, if needed, the Seldinger technique can be used to place a drainage catheter. These techniques can also be used to drain a blocked system, such as *nephrostomy tubes* for hydronephrosis, suprapubic catheters for bladder outlet obstruction, cholecystostomy tubes for cholecystitis, biliary drains for bile duct obstruction, and more. Rarely, if there is a need for long-term drainage, sometimes a tunneled drain can be placed, typically for malignant ascites or pleural effusion in a hospice patient (e.g., PleurX® catheter, Aspira® catheter).

Similar to drainage procedures in the IR technique, if a *feeding tube* is required to deliver feeds into the alimentary tract (stomach or jejunum), some interventional radiologists will place *gastrostomy* and *gastrojejunostomy* tubes. Jejunostomy tubes are also possible, but much more challenging.

Vascular Interventional Radiology

Interventional Radiologists were the doctors who performed many of the first cardiac catheterization cases, placing catheters into coronary arteries to treat myocardial infarction. This has since been taken over almost completely by cardiology. IR doctors still, however, treat many conditions within the vascular system—including placement of inferior vena cava (IVC) filters, and even the TIPS procedure (see later).

Most arterial interventions will be to improve *arterial flow,* to reestablish distal extremity perfusion or to treat claudication using a combination of balloons and stents to increase blood flow (IR techniques that are beyond the scope of this introductory chapter). Interventional radiologists can also use embolic material such as tiny particles or platinum **coils**, to reduce blood flow—to stop bleeding—and this is a "go-to" to treat several important diseases, the ones most relevant in the field of general surgery are:

- **Diverticular Bleeding**
- **Gastric/Peptic Ulcer Bleeding**

Here, the first line therapeutic treatment is *not* surgical intervention, but rather interventional radiology for image-guided embolization of the bleeding vessel. This is a very important point. *Surgery is a last resort* for diverticular bleeding and peptic ulcer bleeding. Due to the high success rate of IR for controlling GI bleeding, nowadays it is rare for surgeons to operate on patients due to these reasons, as IR has proven extremely effective, and is not nearly as invasive as an operation.

IR Applications in Trauma Surgery and Special Conditions

Trauma embolization is still mostly done by interventional radiologists, such as for *traumatic solid organ (esp., liver and spleen) laceration* and *post-traumatic pelvic bleeding.* As stated, gastrointestinal bleeding is often treated with interventional radiology with similar techniques (using coil embolization).

In terms of non-trauma arterial embolization, a common target organ is the uterus. IR can successfully treat abnormal uterine bleeding, usually from fibroids, although there are other uterine pathologies that can be effectively treated as well. Prostate embolization is becoming a more common method to reduce the volume of the prostate gland as an alternative to prostatectomy. Hemorrhoid embolization is becoming more common, although the standard is operative except in special circumstances, such as anorectal variceal bleeding in high-operative-risk patients with portal hypertension and Child's C liver cirrhosis.

IR techniques can be used to embolize joints (knees and shoulders) to reduce inflammation and treat pain. Certain cancers can also be targeted for therapy using IR ablative techniques. For example, hepatocellular carcinoma can be controlled and volume reduced using advanced IR technology.

IR and the Portal Venous System

If you didn't know, there are actually *two venous systems in our body:* the **systemic** venous system and a separate one, known as the **portal** venous system. The portal veins are *very important clinically* as they can lead to intestinal bleeding, especially **esophageal variceal bleeding** from portal *hypertension.* **Portal hypertension** can be an extremely serious and in some instances life-threatening condition, and *is most commonly attributed to liver cirrhosis.*

For portal vein disease, portal veins are not easy to get to—for a surgeon, or for an interventional radiologist. The portal vein *proper* is the main supplier of blood to the liver, supplying most of the liver (in normal physiology) *with about three times more flow than it gets from the heart through the hepatic artery.* The portal vein is (usually) supplied by the *splenic vein* and *superior mesenteric vein* and not blood directly pumped by the heart. To oversimplify things, nutrition from the gut needs to be processed by the liver, so the blood brings nutrients from the gut into the liver for processing. *When the liver is damaged in hepatic cirrhosis, the pressure in the portal venous system increases, and many pathologies can ensue.* Esophageal and gastric variceal bleeding from portal hypertension is one of the most important, clinically relevant conditions that results from portal hypertension

Transjugular Intrahepatic Portosystemic Shunt (TIPS)

Portal venous hypertension and its sequelae (especially esophageal variceal bleeding) is one of the most serious complications related to *liver cirrhosis,* which can be a life-threatening condition. TIPS is a treatment for portal venous hypertension and it is performed by IR. In short, this is a way to access the portal vein system by entering the internal jugular vein and placing a needle through the liver parenchyma into the portal vein system. The tract is then dilated and a stent is placed to *shunt blood from the* ***portal system*** *into the* ***hepatic vein (systemic venous system)****.*

TIPS combines a lot of skills that don't exist outside of IR. There are other methods to access the portal venous system, typically for bleeding associated with portal hypertension. One can access it by a direct stick through the liver, through the spleen, and sometimes even through superficial varices. These techniques are beyond the scope of this introductory chapter.

Endoscopic Therapies for Surgical Conditions

40

Abdul Mohammed and Mariam Naveed

Introduction

Endoscopy has revolutionized the management of many surgical conditions by offering minimally invasive alternatives that reduce morbidity, accelerate recovery, and improve patient outcomes. This chapter explores how advancements in endoscopic techniques have redefined the management of various conditions, highlighting their indications, benefits, limitations, and clinical applications.

Historically, many of these conditions required open or laparoscopic surgery. While effective, such procedures often involve significant risks, including prolonged recovery times, higher complication rates, and increased healthcare costs. With the advent of advanced endoscopic tools and techniques, addressing these conditions with similar or superior outcomes is possible while avoiding the risks associated with traditional surgery. This shift is particularly valuable for patients who are poor surgical candidates due to comorbidities, advanced age, or other risk factors.

Endoscopic therapies (Fig. 40.1) offer several advantages: reduced procedural time, lower risk of infection, shorter hospital stays, and quicker return to normal activities. In addition, the continuous evolution of endoscopic technology and techniques has broadened the range of conditions that can be treated endoscopically, contributing to a paradigm shift in surgical management.

This chapter aims to provide a practical overview of endoscopic interventions, focusing on their indications, techniques, and outcomes. Topics include the endoscopic management of surgical complications, emergencies, and conditions traditionally treated with surgery but now amenable to endoscopic therapy. This chapter will address applications in motility disorders, GERD, obesity, neoplasia, strictures, and pancreaticobiliary disease. By understanding these evolving approaches, healthcare professionals can better support interdisciplinary teams, enhance patient care, and contribute to advancing minimally invasive surgical practices.

A. Mohammed
Advanced Endoscopy Fellow, Center for Interventional Endoscopy, Advent Health Orlando, Orlando, FL, USA

M. Naveed (✉)
Gastroenterology and Hepatology Fellowship, AdventHealth Medical Group Gastroenterology Altamonte Springs, Altamonte Springs, FL, USA
e-mail: Mariam.Naveed.MD@AdventHealth.com

S. Atallah, J. Dragoljevic (eds.), *Fundamentals of Surgery for Physician Assistants*, https://doi.org/10.1007/978-3-032-21069-2_40

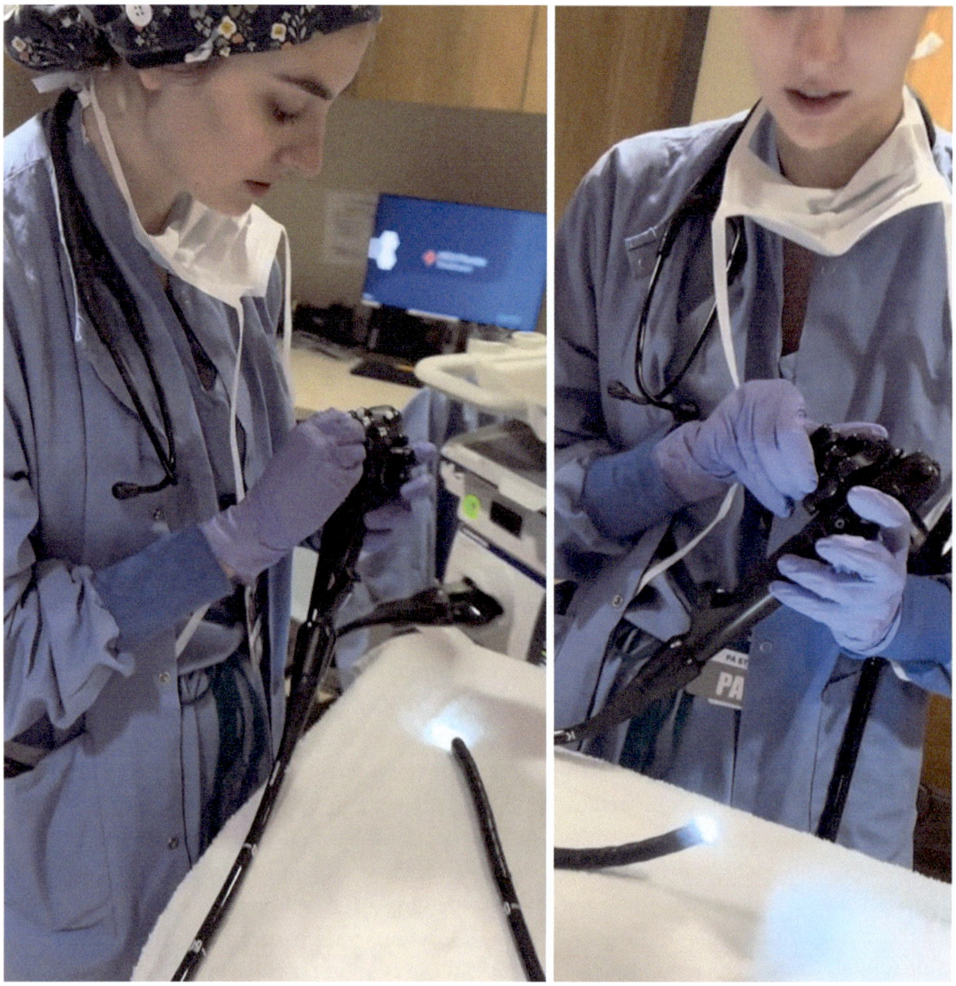

Fig. 40.1 A physician assistant student learns to use an endoscope in a dry lab setting. This device is used to evaluate the entire colon (*colonoscopy*) and the foregut (*esophagogastroduodenoscopy,* almost always abbreviated EGD). *This is the main instrument used by practicing gastroenterologists.* The device consists of a flexible fiberoptic shaft that transmits light along its length and allows visualization of structures at the tip of the scope. This video image is then displayed on an LCD monitor in real-time. The tip orientation and direction is controlled by the proceduralist via two rotating wheels (as depicted here). Endoscopes allow for suction, insufflation, and high-quality visualization of target anatomy within the alimentary tract. Additionally, they have channels used to transmit tiny forceps, snares, and sophisticated instrumentation, which allow target lesions to be biopsied or removed (e.g., polypectomy). There are multiple other applications of endoscopy, many of which are delineated in this chapter. It is important to understand that surgeons often work closely with gastroenterologists, and a multidisciplinary approach to problems of the alimentary tract is taken under a variety of scenarios

Applications of Third Space Endoscopy

Esophageal Per-Oral Endoscopic Myotomy

Per-oral endoscopic myotomy (POEM) was first described in humans by Inoue et al. in 2008 in Japan [1]. This novel minimally invasive technique was developed as a primary treatment of achalasia. While a surgical Heller's myotomy requires laparoscopy and dissection of the esophagogastric junction (EGJ), POEM offers a less invasive alternative. Peroral endoscopic myotomy (POEM) is a safe and effective treatment for classic (straight type) achalasia. However, its efficacy in patients with sigmoid-type achalasia, characterized by high lower esophageal sphincter (LES) pressure and morphological changes such as esophageal dilation, acute angulation, and rotation, was initially controversial. Originally indicated solely for classic achalasia, POEM is now increasingly recognized as an effective option for more complex cases, including sigmoid-type achalasia and patients who have failed previous treatments such as laparoscopic Heller's myotomy. The indications for POEM have expanded to include non-achalasia motility spastic motility disorders (e.g., distal esophageal spasm, hypercontractile esophagus) and esophagogastric junction outflow obstruction. The

POEM technique integrates principles of natural orifice transluminal endoscopic surgery (NOTES) and endoscopic submucosal dissection (ESD). It involves creating a submucosal tunnel using a forward-viewing endoscope, followed by a selective myotomy of the circular muscle fibers with a dissection knife. The myotomy typically extends at least 6 cm in the esophagus and continues approximately 2 cm below the squamocolumnar junction into the gastric cardia.

Prospective studies report a clinical success rate exceeding 90%. POEM offers superior outcomes compared to Heller's myotomy in type III achalasia, while demonstrating comparable efficacy in types I and II [2]. Despite its proven effectiveness, the widespread adoption of POEM has been limited by concerns over post-procedure gastroesophageal reflux. A systematic review and meta-analysis reported abnormal acid exposure in 39% of patients following POEM, compared to 16.8% after surgical myotomy. Similarly, the incidence of esophagitis was significantly higher post-POEM (29.4%) than after surgical myotomy (7.6%) [3].

Gastric Per-Oral Endoscopic Myotomy

Gastric POEM (G-POEM) is an extension of esophageal POEM, designed to access and treat the pyloric sphincter via submucosal tunneling and pyloromyotomy [4]. The pyloric sphincter plays a key role in regulating gastric emptying. Abnormal pyloric resting tone and impaired coordination of pyloric contractions and relaxations can disrupt gastric emptying and contribute to the development of gastroparesis. G-POEM is considered safe and effective when performed by experienced endoscopists. Among patients with medically refractory gastroparesis, clinical success rates reach approximately 61% at 1 year [5], with the highest success observed in diabetic gastroparesis. Compared to surgical pyloromyotomy, G-POEM offers similar symptom control with fewer postprocedural complications and shorter hospital stays. Adverse events, such as delayed bleeding, pain, or pre-pyloric ulceration, occur in 5.1–6.8% of cases [6]. In contrast, the Heineke-Mikulicz pyloroplasty, a surgical approach involving longitudinal incision and transverse closure of the pylorus, is associated with a 6.8% morbidity rate. Complications include leaks, jejunostomy, and even subtotal gastrectomy [7].

Zenker's Per-Oral Endoscopic Myotomy

Zenker's diverticulum (ZD), also known as hypopharyngeal diverticulum, is an acquired pouching of the mucosa and submucosa at the posterior wall of the pharyngoesophageal junction. It typically presents with dysphagia, regurgitation, coughing, aspiration, and weight loss. Symptomatic patients benefit from treatment regardless of the diverticulum size. Surgical approaches, such as transcervical surgery involving pharyngeal pouch excision, were used as early as 1886. Due to the need for a large neck incision, high morbidity rates, and prolonged recovery times, there has been a shift in the management of ZD towards minimally invasive techniques. Flexible endoscopic septotomy (FES) has emerged as a safe and effective alternative to surgery, demonstrating a 90% clinical response rate. However, recurrence rates range from 11% to 32%, likely due to incomplete cricopharyngeal myotomy and technical limitations in septal division [8]. Zenker's peroral endoscopic myotomy (Z-POEM) was introduced as an alternative to FES, allowing submucosal access to the diverticular septum via a mucosal incision. Once the septum is isolated, a full-thickness myotomy is performed, followed by closure of the initial mucosal incision to restore luminal integrity. Comparative analysis demonstrated that Z-POEM and FES have similar procedural times and recurrence rates, though Z-POEM may be associated with higher clinical success rates at follow up [8].

Endoscopic Management of GERD

Gastroesophageal reflux disease (GERD) is the pathological reflux of gastric contents into the esophagus, leading to symptoms such as heartburn and regurgitation. GERD affects approximately 2–5% of the Westen population [9]. Initial management focuses on dietary and lifestyle modification. For patients with refractory or severe symptoms, maximal acid suppressive therapy is recommended. Surgical fundoplication remains the gold-standard treatment for those who fail medical therapy or cannot tolerate long-term acid suppression.

Transoral Incisionless Fundoplication

Transoral Incisionless Fundoplication (TIF) is a minimally invasive technique that reconstructs the gastroesophageal flap valve, similar to a partial fundoplication. It creates a 2–4 cm, 270° wrap of the gastric fundus around the lower esophagus.

TIF is indicated for symptomatic GERD patients who:

- Have persistent symptoms despite maximal acid suppressive therapy.
- Present with LA Grade A or B esophagitis.
- Have a small (<2 cm) hiatal hernia.
- Are not candidates for surgery or prefer to avoid long-term medical therapy.

Contraindications include:

- Hiatal hernia >2 cm.
- Hill Grade III or higher.
- Before esophageal surgery.
- LA grade C or D esophagitis.
- Presence of Barrett's esophagus.

As with surgical fundoplication, all patients should undergo endoscopy, esophageal manometry, and esophageal pH monitoring before the procedure. The procedure is performed under general anesthesia using the EsophyX endoscopic suturing device (EndoGastric Solutions, Redmond, WA, USA) in combination with a gastroscope. It typically requires two operators—one for the EsophyX device and one for the endoscope. The endoscope, equipped with the EsophyX device, is advanced and retroflexed to provide a clear view of the gastroesophageal (GE) junction. Using a helical retractor, gastric tissue is drawn into the device, allowing for the creation of full-thickness plications. This process is repeated sequentially by rotating the endoscope. The goal is to achieve a 2–4 cm serosa-to-serosa full-thickness approximation, covering approximately 270°. This reconstructs the flap valve and results in effacement of the GE junction at its base and the lower esophagus, re-establishing the flap valve and reducing reflux.

TIF is associated with significant improvements in both short-term and long-term outcomes compared to medical therapy. At 6 months, 97% of patients who underwent TIF showed clinical improvement, compared to only 50% in the proton pump inhibitor (PPI) group [10]. TIF also leads to notable improvements in GERD-related quality of life and significantly reduces distal esophageal acid exposure at 6 months compared to PPItherapy [11]. These benefits appear to be sustained at 36 months, with many patients able to reduce their PPI use by half or discontinue it entirely [12]. However, long-term efficacy data beyond this point are still limited. The rate of major adverse events is low (2–5%) and includes complications such as perforation, bleeding, infection, pneumothorax, and mediastinal abscesses.

Stretta Procedure

The Stretta procedure (Mederi Therapeutics, Greenwich, CT, USA) uses radiofrequency (RF) energy to remodel the lower esophageal sphincter (LES) and the gastric cardia. The proposed mechanism is that ablation promotes connective tissue deposition within the LES and decreases transient lower esophageal sphincter relaxations (tLESRs). Increased tLESRs are considered the primary pathogenic mechanism in pathologic acid reflux [13].

The Stretta procedure involves:

- Positioning the Stretta catheter at the squamocolumnar junction
- Infusing cold water through the device
- Inflating a balloon
- Deploying needle electrodes into the LES musculature
- Delivering controlled RF energy to the muscularis propria

Over 30 clinical trials and four systematic reviews have assessed Stretta's efficacy. Long-term data are encouraging: at 10 years, 72% of patients reported normalized GERD-health-related quality of life (GERD-HRQL) scores, and 60% had reduced their PPI use by at least 50% [14].

Endoscopic Bariatric Therapies

The prevalence of obesity in the United States has risen to 35% [15] and is a major contributor to the development of numerous comorbid conditions, including increased cardiovascular mortality. Obesity and its related complications account for approximately 21% of annual healthcare expenditures in the USA. Total body weight loss (TBWL) has been shown to reduce obesity-related mortality and morbidity by altering neuroendocrine signaling, gut microbiota, gut motility, and autonomic regulation. While bariatric surgery is highly effective, it carries significant risks. Lifestyle and pharmacologic interventions are safer but often yield modest and non-durable results. Endoscopic bariatric therapies (EBTs) have emerged as a minimally invasive solution to bridge this "care gap" in obesity treatment.

Gastric EBTs

Intragastric Balloons (IGB)

Intragastric balloons (IGB) are space-occupying, volume-restricting devices used to manage obesity. They promote satiety by stimulating gastric mechanoreceptors, which activate vagal pathways to the brain, trigger satiety, and delay gastric emptying. Several IGBs are Food and Drug Administration (FDA)-approved—The Orbera IGB (Apollo Endosurgery, Austin, TX), previously known as the BioEnterics Intragastric Balloon (Allergan, Irvine, CA); the Spatz3 adjustable balloon system (Spatz Medical, Great Neck, NY); and the Obalon IGB (Obalon Therapeutics, Inc., Carlsbad, CA). The balloons are approved for use for 6 months. Compared to lifestyle modifications alone, IGBs are associated with 2–3 times greater weight loss at 6 months [16–19].

Device	Balloon	Volume/material	TBWL	Adverse event
Orbera IGB (Apollo Endosurgery, Austin, TX)	Elastic spherical single silicone balloon	400–700 ml of saline	10.2% +/− 6.6% at 6 months	10%
Spatz3 adjustable balloon system (Spatz Medical, Great Neck, NY)	Elastic adjustable single silicone balloon	400–500 ml of saline and 1% methylene blue (adjustable to 850 ml)	14.9% +/− 7.2% at 6 months	5.3%
Obalon IGB (Obalon Therapeutics, Inc., Carlsbad, CA	Ingestible capsule with a collapsed balloon that is released in the stomach[a]	250 ml of nitrogen mix gas	6.6% +/− 5.1% at 6 months	0.5%

TBWL total body weight loss
[a]Up to 3 balloons can be swallowed over 6–8 weeks

A meta-analysis by Abu Dayyeh et al. reported low rates of serious adverse events associated with IGB, including perforation (0.1%), migration (1.4%), bowel obstruction (0.3%), and gastric ulcer (2%) [20].

Gastric Volume Reduction Procedures

Several endoscopic gastric volume reduction procedures are available to manage obesity, including Endoscopic Sleeve Gastroplasty (ESG), POSE 2.0, Endomina, and Endozip. Among these, ESG is the most widely adopted and utilized technique.

Introduced in 2013, ESG is a minimally invasive, transoral procedure designed to reduce gastric volume by creating a sleeve-like configuration, similar in concept to laparoscopic gastric gastrectomy (LSG), but without surgical resection. It is performed using a cap-based flexible endoscopic suturing system (Overstich, Apollo Endosurgery), which places full-thickness sutures along the greater curvature of the stomach to achieve gastric retraction and volume reduction. Unlike LSG, ESG preserves the gastric fundus. The procedure aims to reduce both the volume and length of the stomach, resulting in approximately 70% reduction in functional gastric capacity and a 30% decrease in gastric length. Contraindications to ESG include a family history of gastric cancer, the presence of premalignant gastric lesions, gastric anomalies that preclude safe intervention (e.g., large hiatal hernia, PUD), pregnancy, or breastfeeding. ESG has demonstrated sustained effectiveness, with studies showing an average total body weight loss (TBWL) of 16% at 12 months and 16–17% at 18–24 months. The pooled adverse event rate is low, at 2.3% [16, 17]. Long-term data also support its durability, with one study reporting 15.9% TBWL at 5-year follow-up [18]. A large multicenter randomized controlled trial compared ESG with a medically supervised diet and lifestyle modification regimen in patients with a BMI of 30–40. The ESG group not only achieved significantly greater weight loss but also showed improvements in metabolic syndrome, hypertension, GERD symptoms, type 2 diabetes mellitus, and overall improved quality of life at 24 months [19].

Aspiration Therapy

Aspiration therapy is a novel endoscopic bariatric procedure that enables partial removal of ingested food through a modified percutaneous gastrostomy tube. The A-Tube (Aspire Bariatrics, King of Prussia, PA) is placed using the same technique as a standard percutaneous gastrostomy tube. Once in place, the Aspire Assist device (Aspire Bariatrics) is connected to the external port, allowing for gastric irrigation and aspiration of approximately one-third of stomach contents after meals. This approach is effective, achieving a 14.2% TBWL at 12 months, compared to 4.9% TBWL with lifestyle intervention alone [21].

Small Bowel Endoscopic Bariatric Therapies

Small bowel endoscopic bariatric therapies (EBTs) function similarly to malabsorptive bariatric surgeries. The small intestine plays a key role in insulin regulation through incretin hormones and is involved in mucosal maladaptation in response to caloric overexposure. By bypassing portions of the proximal small bowel and redirecting nutrients to distal segments, these therapies enhance the glucose-lowering effects of GLP-1 and may also influence intestinal permeability.

EndoBarrier

The EndoBarrier (GI Dynamics, Lexington, MA) is a 65 cm impermeable duodenal-jejunal liner placed over a guidewire under endoscopic and fluoroscopic guidance. It creates a mechanical barrier to proximal nutrient absorption, redirecting nutrients to the distal small intestine. The EndoBarrier has been shown to produce a 35.3% TBWL at 12 months and significant improvements in HbA1c levels [20].

Duodenal Mucosal Resurfacing (DMR)

Duodenal mucosal resurfacing (DMR) is an endoscopic procedure using hydrothermal ablation to remodel the duodenal lining (Fractyl Health, Inc., Lexington, MA, USA). Given the duodenum's easy endoscopic accessibility, the procedure involves advancing specially designed balloon catheters over a guidewire through the endoscope. Saline is injected to lift the mucosa and protect the outer layers of the duodenum. Circumferential hydrothermal ablation of the duodenal mucosa is then performed, followed by natural mucosal regeneration. This process is believed to reset glucose homeostasis by modulating enteroendocrine cell function in the duodenum. In addition to promoting weight loss, DMR has demonstrated sustained improvements in fasting plasma glucose, HbA1c, insulin resistance, and transaminase levels at 24 weeks—effects that were sustained at 12 months [22].

Endoscopic Revision of Surgical Bypass

In patients who undergo Roux-en-Y gastric bypass (RYGB) for weight loss, 10 years after RYGB, patients regain on average 20–30% of the weight they initially lost, with approximately one-third reverting to their pre-surgical weight. There are several reasons for this—behavioral, medical, and anatomic factors. Dilation of the gastrojejunal anastomosis (GJA) is an anatomic factor that causes weight gain. Transoral outlet reduction (TORe) is an endoscopic procedure developed to reduce the size of the GJA. TORe suturing is performed with the Overstitch device (Apollo EndoSurgery). Before suturing, argon plasma coagulation (APC) is applied to the gastric side of the GJA. The Overstitch device is then used to perform single purse-string, interrupted, double purse-string, or running suture patterns. Reinforcement suturing can be performed in the distal pouch. Patients experience approximately 8.4% TWL at 1 year with significant improvement in obesity-related comorbidities [23]. Significant weight loss is maintained at 3 years and 5 years after TORe [24, 25]. The serious AE rate of TORe at 5 years was 3.9%, with most being intraprocedural and device-related. Compared with surgical revision, endoscopic revision of the GJA is associated with significantly fewer total and serious AEs and similar long-term weight loss [26].

Percutaneous Endoscopic Colostomy

Percutaneous Endoscopic Colostomy (PEC) is a minimally invasive endoscopic technique that affixes the colon to the abdominal wall for therapeutic access. It serves as a conduit for decompression, irrigation, or stabilization of the colon, especially in patients who are poor candidates for surgical intervention. Clinical indications include recurrent colonic pseudo-obstruction, sigmoid volvulus, chronic refractory constipation, and neurogenic bowel in high-risk surgical patients. Contraindications include bowel obstruction, ischemia, sepsis, and inadequate transillumination. Although effective, PEC carries a notable risk of serious complications, including infection, tube migration, perforation, abdominal wall bleeding, and, in some rare cases, death.

The following outlines a typical procedural approach to percutaneous endoscopic colostomy (PEC) placement for the management of sigmoid volvulus in a patient deemed a poor candidate for surgery:

1. The colonoscope is advanced beyond the volvulus and then withdrawn to the proximal limb.
2. The colon is insufflated to closely approximate the colonic wall to the abdominal wall.
3. Transillumination uses a high-intensity light source, and the colonoscope tip is angled toward the abdominal wall.
4. The finger indentation test is used to confirm appropriate positioning—indentation from an external finger creates a visible tenting effect internally.
5. Once the site is selected, the area is sterilized and anesthetized locally.
6. A small skin incision is made, and a trocar is used to access the colon under direct endoscopic visualization.
7. A guidewire is passed through the trocar and snared intraluminally.
8. The colonoscope is then withdrawn along with the wire and snare.
9. A percutaneous gastrostomy tube is affixed to the wire and pulled through the abdominal wall using the Ponsky pull technique. The proper placement is confirmed by reinserting the colonoscope.

Endoscopic Management of Early GI Neoplasia

Endoscopic Resection Techniques

Endoscopic resection techniques have become a cornerstone in treating premalignant and early-stage malignant gastrointestinal (GI) neoplasms. The techniques offer curative resection (R0) with negative histologic margins while avoiding the higher morbidity, mortality, and cost of traditional surgical approaches.

The main resection methods include:

- Endoscopic submucosal dissection (ESD)
- Endoscopic mucosal resection (EMR)
- Endoscopic full-thickness resection (EFTR)

Each technique aims to achieve complete tumor removal while minimizing procedural risks such as bleeding or perforation. EMR is technically less demanding and suitable for smaller lesions, where en-bloc resection is possible. EMR typically requires piecemeal resection for larger lesions, which limits accurate assessment of lateral margins.

ESD enables *en-bloc* resection (i.e., removal of the growth in a single piece) regardless of lesion size and allows precise histological assessment of lateral and deep margins (Fig. 40.2). It is the preferred approach for lesions with features suggestive of submucosal invasion. These features include non-granular morphology, depression, ulceration, converging mucosal folds, firmness on palpation with biopsy forceps, fixation to the underlying bowel wall, and non-lifting sign [27]. EFTR is reserved for select lesions where standard resection methods are insufficient, offering the advantage of full-thickness excision in an endoscopic setting. Together, these techniques provide safe and effective alternatives to surgery for carefully selected GI lesions, advancing curative intent while minimizing patient burden.

Endoscopic Mucosal Resection

With EMR, a submucosal lifting agent is injected to create a submucosal cushion that elevates the lesion away from the muscularis propria, enabling safe and curative resection. Various injections are available to provide a sustained lift and enhance the distinction between abnormal and normal mucosa. A dynamic injection technique—combining simultaneous injection and directional manipulation—is critical for optimal visualization. Resection is then performed using a stiff snare or a banding cap. Electrocautery use depends on lesion size, morphology, location, and endoscopist preference. En-bloc resection is preferred for smaller lesions; for larger lesions, careful piecemeal resection is effective and associated with a low risk of recurrence [28]. Resection margins are often ablated with snare tip soft coagulation or argon plasma coagulation (APC). A variation of this technique, underwater EMR, involves immersing the lesion in water, allowing the mucosal lesion to float away from deeper layers, and facilitating resection without a submucosal lifting agent [29].

Endoscopic Submucosal Dissection

ESD, first described in 1988, enables precise delineation of lesion margins. Marking dots are placed approximately 5 mm outside the tumor margin, followed by a submucosal injection cushion to create a lifting cushion. An initial incision is made with an endoscopic knife—chosen based on endoscopist preference—and extended along the marked perimeter. The submucosal plane is dissected parallel to the lesion, close to the mucosal surface and away from the muscularis propria. Submucosal bleeding vessels are cauterized during dissection to minimize immediate and delayed bleeding. The key advantage of ESD is its ability to achieve en-bloc resection and facilitate curative (R0) outcomes.

Endoscopic Full Thickness Resection

Endoscopic full-thickness resection allows for better histologic evaluation of resection tissue, as it removes all layers of the gastrointestinal wall. The resection device is an over-the-scope clip system (Ovesco Endoscopy AG, Tübingen, Germany) that comprises a cap that is mounted on the endoscope, a snare that is affixed on the outside of the scope with a sleeve, and a mounted clip. First, the clip is deployed to grasp the tissue, and then the snare is closed around the lesion to cut the tissue. The lesion that can be resected is restricted by the cap size. Indications for endoscopic full-thickness resection include lesions <30 mm, particularly non-lifting or those involving diverticulum.

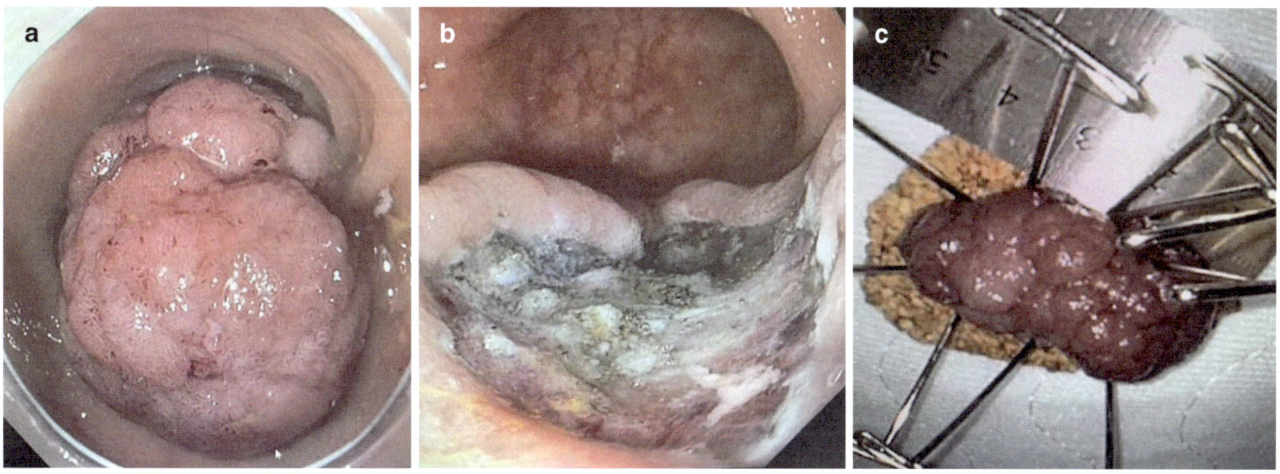

Fig. 40.2 A bulky polypoid lesion of the colon is removed using ESD. (**a**) endoscopic view prior to resection; note the considerable size of the neoplasm as it occupies nearly the entire lumen. (**b**) The base of the colon wall post-excision. (**c**) The *en bloc* resected specimen is pinned out, prior to final pathologic assessment. ESD is a very important procedure because it allows patients to have pre-cancerous growths removed without resorting to surgery, which is considerably more invasive and comes at a higher risk to patients. ESD requires highly specialized training and is typically only performed by interventional endoscopists

Clinical Applications by GI Cancer Type

Esophageal Squamous Cell Neoplasia

Endoscopic resection is an appropriate treatment for selected patients with esophageal squamous cell dysplasia or early, well-differentiated, nonulcerated squamous cell carcinoma without clear signs of submucosal invasion. Both EMR and ESD can be considered, although ESD is preferred for lesions larger than 15 mm [30]. Long-term outcomes of ESD compared with esophagectomy remain uncertain—especially for lesions with superficial submucosal invasion (SM1), which carry a higher risk of lymph node metastasis. However, because esophagectomy is associated with high morbidity, ESD is often favored for patients with significant comorbidities or elevated surgical risk. Notably, endoscopic resection has not been shown to increase the risk of complications in patients who later undergo definitive surgery [31].

Early-Stage Gastric Adenocarcinoma (GAC)

Endoscopic resection is a safe and effective treatment for selected patients with early-stage gastric adenocarcinoma. The choice between ESD and EMR depends on factors such as tumor differentiation (well/moderate vs. poor), morphology (ulcerated vs. nonulcerated), cancer subtype (intestinal vs. diffuse), and lesion size.

For well-differentiated, nonulcerated, intestinal-type GACs measuring <20 mm, either EMR or ESR may be used. However, ESD is preferred for lesions >20 mm [30]. Surgical resection is recommended for any poorly differentiated lesion, regardless of size. Following endoscopic resection, additional surgery may be indicated if the pathology report shows lymphovascular invasion, deeper submucosal invasion (SM2 or deeper), and positive deep margins [32].

Colorectal Neoplasia

Endoscopic resection is widely used in the treatment of colorectal neoplasia. For lesions larger than 20 mm, both EMR and ESD are viable options. Hot-EMR is associated with lower recurrence rates, whereas cold-EMR has fewer adverse events but a higher rate of residual neoplasia [33, 34].

ESD is preferred for lesions with low to moderate risk of submucosal invasion, particularly when en-bloc resection is needed. Surgery is reserved for lesions with suspected or confirmed deep submucosal invasion [28].

Stricture Management

Endoscopic Management of Post-transplant Biliary Strictures

Biliary strictures are a common complication following liver transplantation and are often associated with elevated liver enzymes, recurrent cholangitis, and potential graft failure [35]. While surgical repair is an option, it is associated with significant morbidity and is generally avoided when less invasive approaches are available.

Endoscopic retrograde cholangiopancreatography (ERCP) is the preferred method for managing post-transplant biliary strictures. The procedure is performed with a side-viewing endoscope to access the ampulla of Vater. A sphincterotome is used to deeply cannulate the ampulla, and contrast dye is injected to visualize the biliary anatomy under fluoroscopy.

Once the stricture is identified, a guidewire is passed through the narrow segment, and either plastic or metal stents are deployed across the stricture to allow biliary drainage. ERCP is favored over percutaneous transhepatic biliary drainage (PTBD), as PTBD often requires multiple drains for multi-lobar strictures, carries a higher risk for dislodgement, and is more challenging for patients to manage [36].

Endoscopic Management of Crohn's Disease Strictures

Up to 5–24% of patients with Crohn's disease develop a stricturing phenotype. Strictures may be either inflammatory or fibrotic [37]. Inflammatory strictures are more amenable to endoscopic therapy, including balloon dilation.

Endoscopic balloon dilation is typically performed using a controlled radial expansion (CRE) balloon. Graded dilation in a stepwise fashion up to 18–20 mm is recommended for optimal effectiveness. The endoscope and the CRE balloon with an integrated guidewire are positioned at one end of the stricture. The CRE balloon is advanced across the narrowed segment. The balloon is then inflated to the desired diameter. When available, dilation can also be performed under fluoroscopic guidance.

Following dilation, the site is inspected for tearing, bleeding, and perforation, and to assess the proximal small bowel.

Balloon dilation is most effective for short strictures (<5 cm), whether primary or post-surgical anastomotic strictures. In cases of longer strictures (>5 cm) or multiple strictures, success rates decrease, and surgical intervention may be more appropriate [38]. The presence of prestenotic dilation often indicates long-standing disease or high-grade stenosis and predicts a poor response to balloon dilation.

Endoscopic electroincision is an emerging technique for managing Crohn's strictures, especially in patients who have not responded to balloon dilation. There are two main approaches:

1. Stricturotomy—Incision alone is used to widen the stenotic lumen.
2. Stricturoplasty—Incision is followed by the placement of endoscopic clips to hold the lumen open, functioning similarly to a surgical stricturoplasty.

The procedure is performed using electrocautery-equipped needle knives to incise the stricture and progressively enlarge the lumen carefully. Clips may be placed at the incision margin to serve as spacers. Early studies suggest that endoscopic electroincision may be more effective than balloon dilation in select patients, particularly those with prior treatment failure [39].

Therapeutic EUS & Interventional Drainage

EUS Gallbladder Drainage (EUS-GBD)

Endoscopic ultrasound-guided gallbladder drainage (EUD-GBD) is an emerging, minimally invasive alternative for managing gallbladder disease in patients who are poor surgical candidates. It is particularly useful when the major papilla cannot be accessed via ERCP, such as in patients with an indwelling metal biliary stent that obstructs the cystic duct or those with a large gallstone burden.

In EUS-GBD, a connection is created between the gallbladder and the gastrointestinal tract, typically the stomach or duodenum. Using an echoendoscope (an endoscope equipped with ultrasound capabilities), the endoscopist visualizes the gallbladder and surrounding structures. A needle is then advanced through the gastric or duodenal wall into the gallbladder under ultrasound guidance. A lumen-apposing metal stent (LAMS) is deployed to form a channel that allows bile to drain directly into the gastrointestinal tract. EUS-GBD has demonstrated comparable efficacy and safety to both transpapillary drainage and percutaneous transhepatic biliary drainage (PTBD). However, it should be avoided in specific patient populations, including liver transplant candidates, patients with gallbladder perforation, emphysematous cholecystitis, and those who may undergo cholecystectomy in the future. In contrast, transpapillary drainage via ERCP is preferred in patients with ascites, malignant infiltration of the gallbladder, severe coagulopathy, and limited access to EUS-GBD due to lack of operator expertise or equipment [40].

Endoscopic Drainage of Pancreatic Fluid Collection and Necrosectomy

Pancreatic fluid collections (PFCs) can develop following acute or chronic pancreatitis, pancreatic trauma, or pancreatic surgery. In the early stages of pancreatitis, acute peri-PFCs, which are typically sterile, rarely become infected and resolve spontaneously. However, approximately 20% of individuals with acute pancreatitis will develop necrosis. Over 2–4 weeks, these collections may mature into either pseudocysts or walled-off necrosis (WON). When these collections become symptomatic or infected, endoscopic drainage has increasingly replaced surgical and percutaneous approaches for symptomatic sterile or infected pseudocysts and WON [41].

Transmural drainage of PFCs involves using an echoendoscope to identify the fluid collection and create a tract through the gastric or duodenal wall. The tract is then dilated, and one or more stents are placed to facilitate drainage. Historically, plastic stents were used; however, lumen-apposing metal stents (LAMS) are now preferred because they lead to rapid drainage, reduced risk of stent occlusion, and allow repeat access to the collection for endoscopic necrosectomy if needed. In cases of walled-off necrosis, patients may require multiple debridement sessions, typically performed every 48 to 72 hours, until all necrotic material is removed [42].

EUS-Guided Gastroenterostomy

Gastric outlet obstruction (GOO), whether from benign or malignant causes, results in impaired passage of gastric contents from the stomach into the jejunum. Gastroduodenal and pancreatic cancers are the most common causes of malignant GOO, while peptic ulcer disease remains the most frequent benign etiology.

Endoscopic placement of self-expanding metal stents (SEMS) is a durable alternative to surgical gastrojejunostomy (GJ) for the palliation of unresectable malignancies. Using an echoendoscope, the endoscopist identifies a loop of distal jejunum adjacent to the stomach. A tract is created between the two lumens, and a stent is deployed to bridge the defect, allowing gastric contents to bypass the obstruction.

Compared to surgery, SEMS placement is associated with a shorter time to resumption of oral intake and reduced hospital stay. However, studies show no significant difference in overall efficacy, major adverse event rates, or postoperative mortality between SEMS and surgical GJ. Surgical GJ is generally preferred in patients with a life expectancy greater than 6 months due to lower reintervention rates, as SEMS are prone to obstruction or migration over time. Contraindications to EUS-GE include inadequate access to the target jejunal loop, perigastric varices, large volume ascites, peritoneal carcinomatosis, and bowel obstruction distal to the intended bypass site [43].

Endoscopic Management of Bile Leaks

Bile leaks are a common complication of hepatobiliary surgery, particularly after laparoscopic cholecystectomy. A biliary leak may be asymptomatic but can also lead to life-threatening biliary peritonitis. Surgical management in the immediate postoperative period is not ideal and carries significant morbidity.

ERCP plays a critical role in diagnosing and treating symptomatic bile leaks. The goal of endoscopic therapy is to promote healing by reducing the pressure gradient across the sphincter of Oddi, thereby enhancing bile flow into the duodenum [44].

During ERCP, selective cannulation of the common bile duct is performed, followed by contrast injection to identify the leakage site. The leaks appear as contrast extravasation outside the biliary tree on fluoroscopy.

The Strasberg classification is commonly used to categorize bile duct injuries after cholecystectomy:

- Major injuries involve complete or partial involvement of the CBD, common hepatic duct, or major segmental ducts at the porta hepatis.
- Minor injuries include leaks from the cystic duct, subvesical duct of Luschka, or gallbladder fossa).

Once the leak is localized, a guidewire is advanced and positioned proximally to the site of the leakage. Transpapillary plastic stents are then placed over the guidewire to facilitate preferential bile drainage and support leak resolution.

Future Directions

Access to a wide range of endotherapy therapies allows the modern endoscopist to go beyond diagnosis and engage in a broad spectrum of therapeutic interventions. This progress is blurring the lines between endoscopy and traditional surgery.

One example is concomitant transoral incisionless fundoplication (cTIF), which combines laparoscopic hiatal hernia repair with endoscopic TIF in a single session. This hybrid approach illustrates the expanding role of endoscopy in areas once dominated by surgery.

Advances in technology and the pursuit of less invasive approaches have also led to the growth of the endobariatrics field. New techniques such as duodenal electroporation and the incisionless, sutureless magnet anastomosis system are being developed and have the potential to transform metabolic and bariatric surgery.

Looking ahead, the next frontier in therapeutic endoscopy lies in integrating artificial Intelligence (AI) and robotic endoscopy. Currently, AI is primarily applied in pattern recognition and the identification of high-risk lesions. Robotic platforms are being designed to enhance the precision and performance of complex therapeutic procedures, although the pace of advances in mechanical and electrical engineering still limits progress. Combining AI with robotic endoscopy could support clinical decision-making, semi-automated device movements and enable more complex maneuvers. However, these innovations must be backed by robust clinical trials and supported by structured, rigorous training to ensure safe and effective implementation.

References

1. Inoue H, Minami H, Kobayashi Y, et al. Peroral endoscopic myotomy (POEM) for esophageal achalasia. Endoscopy. 2010;42(4):265–71. https://doi.org/10.1055/s-0029-1244080.
2. Rohof WO, Salvador R, Annese V, et al. Outcomes of treatment for achalasia depend on manometric subtype. Gastroenterology. 2013;144(4):718–25; quiz e13–14. https://doi.org/10.1053/j.gastro.2012.12.027.
3. Repici A, Fuccio L, Maselli R, et al. GERD after per-oral endoscopic myotomy as compared with Heller's myotomy with fundoplication: a systematic review with meta-analysis. Gastrointest Endosc. 2018;87(4):934–943.e18. https://doi.org/10.1016/j.gie.2017.10.022.
4. Kawai M, Peretta S, Burckhardt O, Dallemagne B, Marescaux J, Tanigawa N. Endoscopic pyloromyotomy: a new concept of minimally invasive surgery for pyloric stenosis. Endoscopy. 2012;44(2):169–73. https://doi.org/10.1055/s-0031-1291475.
5. Kamal F, Khan MA, Lee-Smith W, et al. Systematic review with meta-analysis: one-year outcomes of gastric peroral endoscopic myotomy for refractory gastroparesis. Aliment Pharmacol Ther. 2022;55(2):168–77. https://doi.org/10.1111/apt.16725.
6. Yan J, Tan Y, Zhou B, Zhang S, Wang X, Liu D. Gastric per-oral endoscopic myotomy (G-POEM) is a promising treatment for refractory gastroparesis: a systematic review and meta-analysis. Rev Esp Enferm Dig. 2020;112(3):219–28. https://doi.org/10.17235/reed.2020.6559/2019.
7. Shada AL, Dunst CM, Pescarus R, et al. Laparoscopic pyloroplasty is a safe and effective first-line surgical therapy for refractory gastroparesis. Surg Endosc. 2016;30(4):1326–32. https://doi.org/10.1007/s00464-015-4385-5.
8. Singh S, Chandan S, Bapaye J, et al. Peroral endoscopic myotomy (Z-POEM) versus flexible endoscopic septotomy (FES) for treat-

ment of Zenker's diverticulum: does either make the cut? A systematic review and meta-analysis of outcomes. Ann Gastroenterol. 2025;38(1):20–7. https://doi.org/10.20524/aog.2024.0934.
9. Savarino E, Marabotto E, Bodini G, et al. Epidemiology and natural history of gastroesophageal reflux disease. Minerva Gastroenterol Dietol. 2017;63(3):175–83. https://doi.org/10.23736/S1121-421X.17.02383-2.
10. Trad KS, Barnes WE, Simoni G, et al. Transoral incisionless fundoplication effective in eliminating GERD symptoms in partial responders to proton pump inhibitor therapy at 6 months: the TEMPO randomized clinical trial. Surg Innov. 2015;22(1):26–40. https://doi.org/10.1177/1553350614526788.
11. Witteman BPL, Conchillo JM, Rinsma NF, et al. Randomized controlled trial of transoral incisionless fundoplication vs. proton pump inhibitors for treatment of gastroesophageal reflux disease. Am J Gastroenterol. 2015;110(4):531–42. https://doi.org/10.1038/ajg.2015.28.
12. Testoni PA, Testoni S, Mazzoleni G, Vailati C, Passaretti S. Long-term efficacy of transoral incisionless fundoplication with Esophyx (Tif 2.0) and factors affecting outcomes in GERD patients followed for up to 6 years: a prospective single-center study. Surg Endosc. 2015;29(9):2770–80. https://doi.org/10.1007/s00464-014-4008-6.
13. Sandhu DS, Fass R. Stretta therapy in the management of gastroesophageal reflux disease (GERD). Ann Esophagus. 2019;2. https://doi.org/10.21037/aoe.2019.01.01.
14. Noar M, Squires P, Noar E, Lee M. Long-term maintenance effect of radiofrequency energy delivery for refractory GERD: a decade later. Surg Endosc. 2014;28(8):2323–33. https://doi.org/10.1007/s00464-014-3461-6.
15. Ogden CL, Carroll MD, Kit BK, Flegal KM. Prevalence of childhood and adult obesity in the United States, 2011-2012. JAMA. 2014;311(8):806–14. https://doi.org/10.1001/jama.2014.732.
16. de Miranda Neto AA, de Moura DTH, Ribeiro IB, et al. Efficacy and safety of endoscopic sleeve gastroplasty at mid term in the management of overweight and obese patients: a systematic review and meta-analysis. Obes Surg. 2020;30(5):1971–87. https://doi.org/10.1007/s11695-020-04449-9.
17. Hedjoudje A, Abu Dayyeh BK, Cheskin LJ, et al. Efficacy and safety of endoscopic sleeve gastroplasty: a systematic review and meta-analysis. Clin Gastroenterol Hepatol. 2020;18(5):1043–1053.e4. https://doi.org/10.1016/j.cgh.2019.08.022.
18. Sharaiha RZ, Hajifathalian K, Kumar R, et al. Five-year outcomes of endoscopic sleeve gastroplasty for the treatment of obesity. Clin Gastroenterol Hepatol. 2021;19(5):1051–1057.e2. https://doi.org/10.1016/j.cgh.2020.09.055.
19. Dayyeh BKA, Bazerbachi F, Vargas EJ, et al. Endoscopic sleeve gastroplasty for treatment of class 1 and 2 obesity (MERIT): a prospective, multicentre, randomised trial. Lancet. 2022;400(10350):441–51. https://doi.org/10.1016/S0140-6736(22)01280-6.
20. ASGE Bariatric Endoscopy Task Force and ASGE Technology Committee, Abu Dayyeh BK, Kumar N, et al. ASGE Bariatric Endoscopy Task Force systematic review and meta-analysis assessing the ASGE PIVI thresholds for adopting endoscopic bariatric therapies. Gastrointest Endosc. 2015;82(3):425–438.e5. https://doi.org/10.1016/j.gie.2015.03.1964.
21. Thompson CC, Abu Dayyeh BK, Kushner R, et al. Percutaneous gastrostomy device for the treatment of class II and class III obesity: results of a randomized controlled trial. Am J Gastroenterol. 2017;112(3):447–57. https://doi.org/10.1038/ajg.2016.500.
22. van Baar ACG, Holleman F, Crenier L, et al. Endoscopic duodenal mucosal resurfacing for the treatment of type 2 diabetes mellitus: one year results from the first international, open-label, prospective, multicentre study. Gut. 2020;69(2):295–303. https://doi.org/10.1136/gutjnl-2019-318349.
23. Jirapinyo P, Kröner PT, Thompson CC. Purse-string transoral outlet reduction (TORe) is effective at inducing weight loss and improvement in metabolic comorbidities after Roux-en-Y gastric bypass. Endoscopy. 2018;50(4):371–7. https://doi.org/10.1055/s-0043-122380.
24. Kumar N, Thompson CC. Transoral outlet reduction for weight regain after gastric bypass: long-term follow-up. Gastrointest Endosc. 2016;83(4):776–9. https://doi.org/10.1016/j.gie.2015.08.039.
25. Jirapinyo P, Kumar N, AlSamman MA, Thompson CC. Five-year outcomes of transoral outlet reduction for the treatment of weight regain after Roux-en-Y gastric bypass. Gastrointest Endosc. 2020;91(5):1067–73. https://doi.org/10.1016/j.gie.2019.11.044.
26. Dolan RD, Jirapinyo P, Thompson CC. Endoscopic versus surgical gastrojejunal revision for weight regain in Roux-en-Y gastric bypass patients: 5-year safety and efficacy comparison. Gastrointest Endosc. 2021;94(5):945–50. https://doi.org/10.1016/j.gie.2021.06.009.
27. Bilal M, Pohl H. Updates in colon endoscopic mucosal resection. Clin Gastroenterol Hepatol. 2024;22(12):2388–91. https://doi.org/10.1016/j.cgh.2024.07.022.
28. Kaltenbach T, Anderson JC, Burke CA, et al. Endoscopic removal of colorectal lesions: recommendations by the US Multi-Society Task Force on Colorectal Cancer. Am J Gastroenterol. 2020;115(3):435–64. https://doi.org/10.14309/ajg.0000000000000555.
29. Thiruvengadam SS, Fung BM, Barakat MT, Tabibian JH. Endoscopic mucosal resection: best practices for gastrointestinal endoscopists. Gastroenterol Hepatol. 2022;18(3):133–44.
30. ASGE standards of practice committee, Forbes N, Elhanafi SE, et al. American Society for Gastrointestinal Endoscopy guideline on endoscopic submucosal dissection for the management of early esophageal and gastric cancers: summary and recommendations. Gastrointest Endosc. 2023;98(3):271–84. https://doi.org/10.1016/j.gie.2023.03.015.
31. Takeuchi M, Suda K, Hamamoto Y, et al. Technical feasibility and oncologic safety of diagnostic endoscopic resection for superficial esophageal cancer. Gastrointest Endosc. 2018;88(3):456–65. https://doi.org/10.1016/j.gie.2018.04.2361.
32. Zhao B, Zhang J, Zhang J, et al. Risk factors associated with lymph node metastasis for early gastric cancer patients who underwent non-curative endoscopic resection: a systematic review and meta-analysis. J Gastrointest Surg. 2019;23(7):1318–28. https://doi.org/10.1007/s11605-018-3924-5.
33. Steinbrück I, Ebigbo A, Kuellmer A, et al. Cold versus hot snare endoscopic resection of large nonpedunculated colorectal polyps: randomized controlled German CHRONICLE trial. Gastroenterology. 2024;167(4):764–77. https://doi.org/10.1053/j.gastro.2024.05.013.
34. O'Sullivan T, Cronin O, van Hattem WA, et al. Cold versus hot snare endoscopic mucosal resection for large (≥15 mm) flat non-pedunculated colorectal polyps: a randomised controlled trial. Gut. 2024;73(11):1823–30. https://doi.org/10.1136/gutjnl-2024-332807.
35. Kohli DR, Desai MV, Kennedy KF, Pandya P, Sharma P. Patients with post-transplant biliary strictures have significantly higher rates of liver transplant failure and rejection: a nationwide inpatient analysis. J Gastroenterol Hepatol. 2021;36(7):2008–14. https://doi.org/10.1111/jgh.15388.
36. Kohli DR, Amateau SK, Desai M, et al. American Society for Gastrointestinal Endoscopy guideline on management of post-liver transplant biliary strictures: summary and recommendations. Gastrointest Endosc. 2023;97(4):607–14. https://doi.org/10.1016/j.gie.2022.10.007.
37. Thia KT, Sandborn WJ, Harmsen WS, Zinsmeister AR, Loftus EV. Risk factors associated with progression to intestinal com-

plications of Crohn's disease in a population-based cohort. Gastroenterology. 2010;139(4):1147–55. https://doi.org/10.1053/j.gastro.2010.06.070.
38. Lan N, Shen B. Multiple primary Crohn's disease-associated strictures had poor response to endoscopic balloon dilation: 748. Am J Gastroenterol. 2018;113:S421.
39. Shen B, Kochhar G, Navaneethan U, et al. Practical guidelines on endoscopic treatment for Crohn's disease strictures: a consensus statement from the Global Interventional Inflammatory Bowel Disease Group. Lancet Gastroenterol Hepatol. 2020;5(4):393–405. https://doi.org/10.1016/S2468-1253(19)30366-8.
40. ASGE Standards of Practice Committee, Pawa S, Marya NB, et al. American Society for Gastrointestinal Endoscopy guideline on the role of therapeutic EUS in the management of biliary tract disorders: summary and recommendations. Gastrointest Endosc. 2024;100(6):967–79. https://doi.org/10.1016/j.gie.2024.03.027.
41. Working Group IAP/APA Acute Pancreatitis Guidelines. IAP/APA evidence-based guidelines for the management of acute pancreatitis. Pancreatology. 2013;13(4 Suppl 2):e1–15. https://doi.org/10.1016/j.pan.2013.07.063.
42. ASGE Standards of Practice Committee, Muthusamy VR, Chandrasekhara V, et al. The role of endoscopy in the diagnosis and treatment of inflammatory pancreatic fluid collections. Gastrointest Endosc. 2016;83(3):481–8. https://doi.org/10.1016/j.gie.2015.11.027.
43. ASGE Standards of Practice Committee, Jue TL, Storm AC, et al. ASGE guideline on the role of endoscopy in the management of benign and malignant gastroduodenal obstruction. Gastrointest Endosc. 2021;93(2):309–322.e4. https://doi.org/10.1016/j.gie.2020.07.063.
44. Huang CS, Lichtenstein DR. Postcholecystectomy bile leak: what is the optimal treatment? Gastrointest Endosc. 2005;61(2):276–8. https://doi.org/10.1016/s0016-5107(04)02799-3.

Acute Care Surgery for the Pregnant Patient

41

Goran Augustin

Acute Appendicitis

Incidence

The rate of AA during pregnancy is in the range of 1/1000—1/4167 pregnancies. The highest incidence is in Taiwan—1/181 and varies significantly between countries, and even between regions and hospitals within the same country. In the USA (2002–2015), there was a 5% average annual decrease in AA rates, with a steep decline in overall AA appendicitis and AA rates after 2011. Pregnancy is a protective factor for AA, with rates lower than in the general population. The highest incidence is during the second trimester and then early puerperium. AA during pregnancy, especially in advanced pregnancy and at term, may be underestimated. Mild attacks could be interpreted as the ordinary discomforts of pregnancy, and the severe cases in the puerperium were probably regarded as types of puerperal sepsis.

Risk Factors

The most attributed risk factors for AA in pregnancy include age <30 years, multiple pregnancies, African-American and Hispanic women, nonobese, attacks of AA before pregnancy, and (pregnancy-induced) constipation. Pregnant women during the antepartum period were 35% less likely to be diagnosed with AA than during the time outside pregnancy, with the lowest risk reported during the third trimester.

G. Augustin (✉)
University Hospital Centre Zagreb, Zagreb, Croatia

School of Medicine University of Zagreb, Zagreb, Croatia

Clinical Presentation

During the first 6 months of pregnancy, symptoms and signs of AA are the same as in nonpregnant women. Still, diagnostic difficulties remain due to (1) blunting/masking of symptoms and signs (abdominal distension, intra-abdominal organ dislocation, diminished tissue response to inflammation), (2) possible changes in appendiceal location as pregnancy advances, and (3) nausea, vomiting, and abdominal pain of normal pregnancy, especially in the first trimester.

Constant RLQ pain is the most common symptom. The most challenging interpretation of abdominal pain is immediately before, during, and immediately after labor. With uterine contractions before labor, AA is likely when severe abdominal pain remains between contractions or persists after delivery. Approximately 50–70% have a low-grade fever, similar to the general population. There is no single and reliable sign for the diagnosis of AA in pregnancy. Some classic signs of AA, such as Rovsing's or Psoas's sign, have no diagnostic value for AA in pregnancy. Rebound tenderness is the most common sign.

Diagnosis

Clinical examination is inaccurate, resulting in negative appendectomy in more than a third of patients. One reason is the broader differential diagnosis compared to the general population. Additional conditions include threatened abortion, placental abruption, chorioamnionitis, pelvic inflammatory disease, fibroid degeneration, ectopic pregnancy, (pre) eclampsia, round ligament syndrome/pain, preterm labor, metritis, and ovarian vein syndrome.

Leukocytosis is not diagnostic due to the physiologic rise in pregnancy. Only if previous values during the same pregnancy were normal should it raise suspicion. Neutrophil

S. Atallah, J. Dragoljevic (eds.), *Fundamentals of Surgery for Physician Assistants*,
https://doi.org/10.1007/978-3-032-21069-2_41

granulocytosis with a left shift implies acute bacterial infection. Without the left shift, granulocytosis >80% is suggestive of AA. CRP starts to increase within 8–12 h. All perforated AA have high levels of CRP. The CRP-to-albumin ratio (CAR) is significantly higher in patients with AA than in those under acute abdominal observation or in healthy pregnant women. The lymphocyte-to-CRP ratio (LCR) is significantly lower in patients with AA than in healthy pregnant women. Elevated procalcitonin confirms bacterial infection and, in combination with the clinical presentation of AA, is highly diagnostic, though expensive.

Clinical-laboratory-imaging scoring systems have been developed to more accurately diagnose AA in the nonpregnant population. These include the Alvarado Score, Appendicitis Inflammatory Response Score, Tzanakis Score, RIPASA, and ATMOS.

Despite suggestive laboratory findings and scoring systems, transabdominal ultrasound in pregnant patients with RLQ pain is mandatory. The sensitivity in the first, second, and third trimesters of pregnancy is 69%, 63%, and 51%, respectively. The corresponding figures for specificity are 85%, 85%, and 65%. After an indeterminate US, abdominal MRI or CT, when MRI is unavailable, is recommended.

Treatment

Surgical treatment is recommended for complicated AA, but also for uncomplicated cases. Laparoscopic access results in shorter hospital stay, earlier ambulation, and less pain without adverse outcomes on the fetus or delivery. An open approach, by gridiron incision, is an alternative, especially in the advanced third trimester when laparoscopic space and manipulation are limited due to an enlarged gravid uterus.

Conservative management in pregnancy is increasing and is used only for uncomplicated AA, defined by MRI. In Korea, 25% of pregnancies affected by uncomplicated AA are treated conservatively, compared to 63% in China and 65% (until 2016) in the USA. The first conservative strategy is definitive antibiotic treatment. Still, no consensus exists on the route, type, or duration of antibiotic therapy (3–10 days). The second strategy is to use antibiotics to localize abscesses and evacuate them percutaneously. The last strategy used for complicated AA during active labor is when delivery is imminent; surgery may be delayed for a short time until the placenta is delivered. Otherwise, immediate appendectomy is advised if prolonged labor is anticipated.

Maternal and Fetal Outcome

The severity of AA and duration of symptoms increase maternal morbidity (intra-abdominal abscess formation, conversion to laparotomy or pneumonia), as in the general population. Maternal mortality is almost nil. The severity and longer duration of AA increase the preterm labor or spontaneous abortion rate. AA during the third trimester could increase the Cesarean section rate.

Acute Cholecystitis

Incidence

Acute biliary disease is the second most common indication for surgery in pregnancy. The incidence in pregnancy is 0.05–0.3%. Asymptomatic gallstones occur in 2.5–10% of pregnant patients and 12% in the early puerperium versus 1.3% in nonpregnant controls. Approximately 60–69% of pregnant women with gallstones are asymptomatic, while acute cholecystitis (AC) occurs in 1/1000–1/10,000. Approximately 40% of pregnant patients with symptomatic cholelithiasis require cholecystectomy during pregnancy, and 1% with gallbladder disease underwent cholecystectomy in the first postpartum year. Cholelithiasis is the cause of cholecystitis in over 90% of cases.

The incidence of acute biliary conditions during pregnancy, listed in descending order, includes biliary colic and AC (62.7–86.3%), biliary acute pancreatitis (AP) (3–25.4%), choledocholithiasis (6.8–7.0%), and acute cholangitis (2.6–5%).

Risk Factors

Risk factors for acute cholecystitis include advanced age, multiparity (interrelated with age), oral contraceptive use, (gestational) diabetes mellitus, and obesity.

In pregnancy, progesterone levels increase and remain high during the second and third trimesters, leading to smooth muscle relaxation, *gallbladder dilatation, and stasis.* A similar mechanism is found with diabetes mellitus, resulting in impaired gallbladder emptying. As a result, at term, new sludge or stones were found in 30% and 2% of the women, respectively; however, postpartum ultrasonography revealed their disappearance in 61% and 28%, respectively, suggesting that the findings are transient. The number of pregnancies does affect this, and the prevalence increases from 1.3% in nulliparous women to 12.2% in multiparous women.

Clinical Presentation

Presentation during pregnancy is the same as in nonpregnant patients. Acute biliary pain usually begins as right upper quadrant or mid-epigastric pain that may increase in severity. The pain may radiate to the interscapular area, the angle of the right scapula, or the right shoulder. It may be precipitated by a fatty or large meal following a fasting period. Nausea and vomiting are found in half of the patients. Many patients will have a history of known gallbladder stones, colic attacks, and fatty food intolerance. The increasing severity of colicky pain, fever, or chills (rigors) usually implies an underlying complication, i.e., acute cholecystitis, acute pancreatitis, or cholangitis. Common bile duct (CBD) stones should be excluded if jaundice persists.

With acute cholecystitis, direct abdominal tenderness in the upper right quadrant is always present because even an enlarged uterus cannot cover the gallbladder. Murphy's sign (cessation of inspiration during palpation of the inflamed gallbladder) may be elicited less frequently in pregnant patients and indicates AC. Abdominal muscle rigidity is present with gallbladder perforation and biliary peritonitis. Fever and tachycardia are variably present. Vomiting and dyspepsia can mimic peptic ulcers. If itching is present, liver disease should be excluded, and biliary obstruction should be considered when jaundice is found.

Diagnosis

Many diseases present with pain in the upper right abdominal quadrant (Table 41.1).

Granulocytosis (left shift) indicates a bacterial infection. C-reactive protein (CRP) is elevated, and bacterial infection is expected with values >40 mg/L. Serum bilirubin and transaminases may be elevated, as in nonpregnant women. Serum alkaline phosphatase is less helpful because it's value doubles due to estrogen even during normal pregnancy. Serum amylase levels are elevated transiently in up to 33%.

Table 41.1 Differential diagnosis of right upper quadrant pain in pregnancy [1]

Jaundice[a]	No jaundice
Common bile duct stones	Diaphragmatic myocardial infarction
Hepatitis	Acute appendicitis
Intrahepatic cholestasis	Pancreatitis
Preeclampsia-eclampsia	Symptomatic/perforated peptic ulcer
HELLP syndrome	Pyelonephritis/nephrolithiasis
Acute fatty liver in pregnancy	Radiculopathy
Hepatic malignancy	Herpes zoster (Shingles)
Cholangitis	Perihepatitis (Fitz-Hugh-Curtis sy.)
Choledochal cyst	Rib fracture/Costal margin pain
Hepatic vascular engorgement	Pleural effusion
Hepatic hematoma	Lower lobe pneumonia
	Colon cancer (hepatic flexure)

[a]Jaundice in these conditions is not obligatory

The accuracy of transabdominal ultrasonography (US) in diagnosing gallbladder disease in pregnancy is 95–98%. US criteria for AC include gallbladder calculi, gallbladder wall thickening (>3 mm), pericholecystic fluid, and sonographic Murphy's sign (focal tenderness under the US transducer positioned over the gallbladder). CBD obstruction should be ruled out, as it alters the therapeutic approach. The following US findings are highly suggestive: CBD >7 mm in diameter, dilatation of intra- and extrahepatic ducts, and gallbladder calculi smaller than the cystic duct diameter.

Magnetic resonance cholangiopancreatography (MRCP) helps differentiate CBD stones from intrahepatic cholestasis of pregnancy, as their clinical and biochemical presentations overlap. MRCP is indicated when dilatation of intrahepatic and extrahepatic ducts is present on the transabdominal US.

Treatment

A decade ago, conservative therapy with antibiotics was the recommended treatment. Traditional "bridge" therapy was to delay the cholecystectomy until the second trimester, when the spontaneous abortion rate after cholecystectomy is the lowest.

Today, laparoscopic cholecystectomy is indicated for AC or related complications. Recurrence rates after nonoperative treatment are trimester-dependent—92% when the initial presentation is in the first trimester, 64% in the second trimester, and 44% in the third trimester. The average number of relapses during pregnancy is between two and six. Laparoscopic cholecystectomy can be performed in all trimesters. It is technically demanding due to the limited space in the advanced third trimester. Therefore, if AC occurs in the near term, it can be managed conservatively. The clinical condition of the patient dictates when a postpartum cholecystectomy will be performed.

Prognosis

Cholecystectomy has significantly lower maternal complication rates compared to conservative treatment (4.3% versus 16.5%).

Nonoperative management is associated with a significantly higher rate of labor induction and preterm delivery requiring neonatal intensive care, as well as a higher fetal death rate and spontaneous abortion rate compared to cholecystectomy. Cesarean section (CS) rate with conservative treatment is significantly higher (35%) than with cholecystectomy.

Acute Pancreatitis

Incidence

The incidence varies more than in the general population (England, Denmark, and the United States: 4.8–24.2/100,000), ranging from 1/1000 to 1/12,000 pregnancies, and rarely progresses to the necrotizing form. It is more common in East Asian countries, including China, where AP in pregnancy accounts for 4.25% of all AP [20] or 1/441 pregnancies. Mild disease may be underreported because women experiencing mild abdominal pain attribute it to the "normal" state of pregnancy.

Risk Factors

Women are becoming pregnant at a more advanced age, and the incidence of AP in the general population increases with age. AP is more prevalent in advanced pregnancy. The trimester distribution varies from 19–28% in the first, 21–33% in the second, 43–78% in the third, and 2–38% in the puerperium. The severe AP (SAP) proportion also increases with gestational age (first, second, third, at 0%, 11.1%, and 88.9%, respectively). The trimester distribution is consistent with (1) a lithogenic effect of estrogen, (2) physiological insulin resistance in the advanced pregnancy, (3) a progressive physiologic increase in serum cholesterol and triglyceride concentrations, with peak levels reached at term, in response to elevated estrogen levels, (4) compression of the uterus on the biliary tree, pancreatic vessels and pancreas itself, and (5) rise in intra-abdominal pressure with a prolonged second stage of labor.

Clinical Presentation

Clinical presentation is the same as in nonpregnant patients. The symptomatology of primary hyperparathyroidism (PHPT)-induced AP starts after 20 weeks of gestation, similar to other, more frequent causes of AP (gallstones, hypertriglyceridemia). However, adenoma PTH secretion is probably completely independent.

Diagnosis

As in nonpregnant patients, laboratory findings require at least a three-fold elevation in serum amylase and lipase levels. No enzyme assay has a predictive role in determining the severity or etiology of AP in pregnancy. HTG-induced AP is triggered when TG levels exceed 1000 mg/dL (10 mmol/L). Mild to moderate elevations in TGs (2–10 mmol/L) are extremely common in the early phase of AP of any cause. Serum calcium levels should be obtained in pregnant women with persistent nausea, vomiting, and abdominal pain, especially when AP is suspected. Primary hyperparathyroidism is the cause when elevated calcium and elevated or normal intact PTH levels are found. Serum CRP at 48 h is the best available laboratory marker of AP severity.

Transabdominal US is the initial diagnostic imaging of choice. However, the sensitivity in the general population for detecting CBD stones is 20–38%. The US can reveal focal accumulations >2–3 cm and pancreatic pseudocysts (accuracy of 54%). An additional role of the US is the estimation of fetal growth and development.

Magnetic resonance imaging (MRI) is indicated if transabdominal US is nondiagnostic. MRPC allows the detection of rare and complex pathologies, such as intrahepatic biliary stones, Mirizzi syndrome, and choledochal cysts. MRCP also obviates the need for intraoperative cholangiography. It accurately detects pancreatic pathology, including pancreatic pseudocysts and fluid collections in surrounding areas.

During emergent exploration, the diagnosis and even the cause of AP can be found. Intraperitoneal fluid can be milky and lipemic. Similarly, emergent CS reveals a placenta covered with milky fluid (Fig. 41.1), contributing to the diagnosis of hyperlipidemic AP.

Treatment

Treatment has two aspects. The first is the treatment of the AP itself, and the second is the elimination of its cause. The initial management of AP during pregnancy is similar to management in nonpregnant patients—fluid restoration, oxygen, analgesics, antiemetics, and monitoring of vital signs. Adequate IV fluid administration corrects the volume deficit, which is monitored by maternal vital signs. Fetal monitoring is mandatory with maternal left tilt after 24 weeks of gestation to avoid inferior vena cava obstruction.

Prophylactic use of antibiotics is controversial, and the choice of antibiotics in pregnancy is challenging. Antibiotics have no role in treating mild acute pancreatitis (MAP). Imipenem is the antibiotic of choice in the general population with necrotizing AP. Still, dose adjustment in pregnancy (FDA category C) should be considered even though the optimal dose has not been established. Metronidazole did not show teratogenic risk (FDA category B). Quinolones (FDA category C) are alternatives to first-line antibiotic therapy.

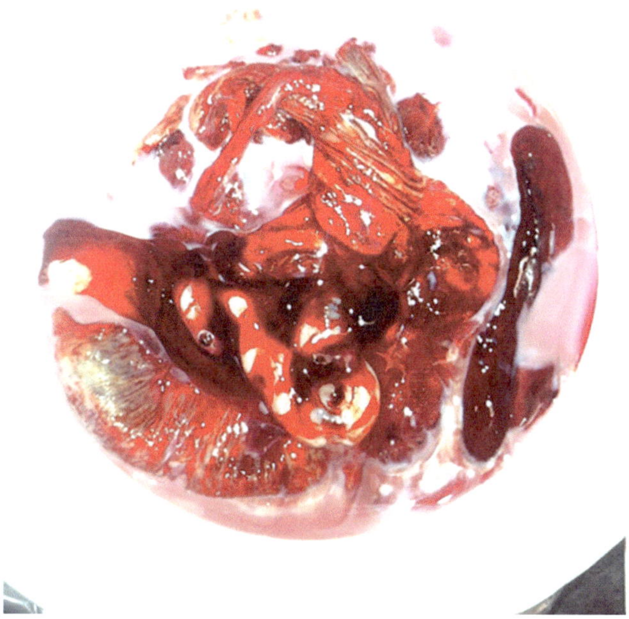

Fig. 41.1 Placenta covered with milky fluid suggestive of severely increased serum lipid levels. (Reproduced from Ref. [205] under the CC Attribution License)

Continuous renal replacement therapy (CRRT), continuous venovenous hemofiltration (CVVH), or hemoperfusion (HP) can prevent sepsis by removing excess circulating inflammatory mediators and improve survival in AP. However, they are rarely used in pregnancy, primarily for hypertriglyceridemic AP. Lipid-lowering diet or lipid-lowering medications (fibrates or statins) are also used for hypertriglyceridemic AP.

When treated conservatively, MAP usually resolves within 7 days. The severe course occurs in 10% of patients and should be managed in an intensive care unit (ICU).

Surgical treatment includes intervention for local (biliary tract disease, pancreatic pseudocysts) or distant (PHPT—parathyroidectomy) causes/complications of the AP. Surgery for necrotizing AP in pregnancy should be delayed as long as possible. Indications for surgery are pancreatic necrosis and infection (3–4 weeks after the onset of symptoms), large intra-abdominal exudates, or clinical deterioration.

Percutaneous, endoscopic, or minimally invasive surgical techniques are widely used. Decompression and percutaneous drainage avoid or delay surgery in most patients with SAP and pancreatic abscesses. Necrosectomy should be performed as late as possible, and if CS is indicated, it is made through median laparotomy.

Therapeutic delivery is indicated for AP resistant to conservative or surgical treatment. An additional beneficial effect of therapeutic delivery is that medications contraindicated during pregnancy can be used after delivery. The mode of delivery is determined by obstetric factors. Stimulating fetal lung maturation with corticosteroids in the critical period for delivery is essential. The most common indications for therapeutic delivery include hyperlipidemias/dyslipidemias, preeclampsia/eclampsia, acute fatty liver of pregnancy, and HELLP syndrome.

Prognosis

Maternal mortality during the 20 years before the millennium in Japan was 7.5%, without a maternal death since 1985. Recent maternal mortality is <1%. It depends on AP severity, AP etiology, gestational trimester, maternal age, and maternal comorbidities. Non-gallstone AP had worse maternal and fetal outcomes compared to simple gallstone AP. The recent perinatal mortality is 0.57–4.7%, and preterm labor is 19%. The fetal outcome depends on the trimester, AP severity, AP etiology, and maternal organ failure.

Intestinal Obstruction

Incidence

Incidence varies widely, from 1/1500 to 1/66,431, depending on the population analyzed. Common causes are postoperative adhesions, volvulus, and intussusception. Intra-abdominal adhesions cause 60–77% of intestinal obstructions in pregnancy. Intestinal volvulus accounts for 25% in pregnant patients, compared with only 3–5% in nonpregnant patients. In comparison, incarcerated groin hernias are the second most common cause of intestinal obstruction in the general population; however, hernias in pregnancy account for less than 5% of obstructions. The incidence of intussusception is similar in pregnant and nonpregnant women (5–6%).

Clinical Presentation

Intestinal obstruction presents with a wide range of obstructive symptoms and signs that depend on the location, degree, rate of progression, intestinal perforation, and underlying malignancy. Classic symptoms are abdominal pain, nausea, and vomiting with abdominal distension and lack of flatus. All colicky pain in pregnancy is not necessarily uterine, and premature labor can complicate intestinal obstruction and vice versa.

The average duration from symptom onset to hospital admission ranges from 48 to 84 h. Once admitted, an average of 48–60 h passes before definitive surgery. An average delay of 4 days remains a significant factor in high morbidity and mortality in the pregnant population.

Diagnosis

Differential diagnosis includes constipation (common in pregnancy), irritable bowel syndrome, and postpartum acute colonic pseudo-obstruction.

The first imaging modality of choice is a plain abdominal X-ray. Air-fluid levels are diagnostic and define the level of obstruction. X-ray accurately distinguishes between cecal and sigmoid volvulus, which is important because sigmoid volvulus can be treated nonoperatively.

Transabdominal US is diagnostic for intussusception only. The classic features include "target", "doughnut", or "crescent-in-doughnut" signs on a transverse view and the "pseudokidney" sign in the longitudinal view.

Abdominal MRI or CT can define the location and cause of intestinal obstruction. The cause and location of obstruction are important for diagnosing and determining the type of abdominal access.

Treatment

Initial conservative measures can be therapeutic, alleviate symptoms, and minimize the complications of intestinal obstruction, especially with small bowel obstruction. Nasogastric tube insertion can be therapeutic for adhesive small bowel obstruction. However, it is not indicated in patients after Roux-Y gastric bypass, as it can lead to bowel perforation at several sites (narrow gastrojejunostomy, blind loop of the Roux limb, etc.) with a false sense of decompression. Due to third-space loss, IV hydration with at least 2.5 L/day of crystalloids should be administered immediately. Urinary output, best determined by urine catheterization, reflects hydration status. If peristalsis is present or begins, prokinetics could be administered. Metoclopramide and pyridostigmine are safe in pregnancy, while other groups of medications should be used if clearly needed.

Sigmoid volvulus can be treated by colonoscopic detorsion and decompression. However, the success rate is lower in the (advanced) third trimester because the enlarged gravid uterus prevents detorsion.

Operative treatment is indicated if conservative treatment fails, when signs of peritonitis are present, or when complete obstruction is detected on imaging. Laparoscopy would be the best option, but it can be challenging to complete due to a distended bowel and distorted anatomy from an enlarged gravid uterus. Most operations are done through midline laparotomy, except for local approaches to incarcerated abdominal wall hernias. The negative side of laparotomy, especially in advanced pregnancy, is that uterine contractions and abdominal wall contractions can result in abdominal wall dehiscence or postdelivery hernia.

Prognosis

The prognosis depends on the state of the bowel. Maternal prognosis is excellent after resection for ischemic bowel or without bowel resection. Bowel ischemia or peritonitis leads to higher rates of spontaneous abortion and preterm labor. The diagnostic process is shorter in the puerperium because clinicians are not reluctant to use ionizing imaging.

Symptomatic Abdominal Wall Hernia

Incidence

A reported incidence of inguinal hernia is 1/1000–1/3000, with 50% to 75% occurring in multiparas. The predominant side was right (86%). The incidence of incarcerated/strangulated groin hernias in pregnancy is at least 10 times lower than in the general population. First, patients with a hernia planning pregnancy undergo an operation before or after pregnancy, lowering the incidence in future pregnancies. The growing uterus blocks the entrance of intra-abdominal contents into the hernia sack.

Risk Factors

The risk factors are the same as in the general population (family history, collagen diseases, smoking, renal failure, chronic lung disease, diabetes mellitus, steroid use, malignancy, malnutrition, cirrhosis, ascites, and obesity). Epigastric and umbilical hernias are the most common types after pregnancy.

Clinical Presentation

A reducible lump that enlarges during the Valsalva maneuver (sharp increase in intra-abdominal pressure) is diagnostic. An incarcerated hernia does not demonstrate an expansile cough impulse but is painful on palpation. Palpation of hernia content differentiates a solid structure (greater omentum or uterine fibroid) from the intestine (gas sounds on pressure, which can be pushed back, shrinking the hernia). The Valsalva maneuver is completed with forceful exhalation with a closed glottis so that no air exits through the mouth or nose (strenuous coughing, straining during a bowel movement, or lifting a heavy weight).

Severe abdominal pain with nausea and sometimes vomiting occurs with incarceration. Bowel incarceration results in severe vomiting, sometimes with the absence of stool and flatus. Fever develops if perforation due to distension or strangulation occurs. Redness of the overlying skin follows due to the spread of infection through the abdominal wall.

Diagnosis

Differential diagnosis is essential only for an inguinal hernia. Conditions with similar presentation include inguinal/round ligament endometriosis, hydrocele of the canal of Nuck, myoma of the round ligament, and two conditions found only during pregnancy—round ligament stretch/pain and round ligament varicosities (RLV). The distinction between a groin hernia and RLV is difficult because both present with a lump in the groin. When the lump is painful RLV has thrombosed. Both swellings disappear when lying down (because these veins lack valves) and reappear when standing, provoked by increased intra-abdominal pressure during coughing or the Valsalva maneuver. RLVs also transmit cough impulses because increased abdominal pressure leads to vein distension. Associated lower limb or labial varicosities suggest RLV. Thrombosed RLV, which are irreducible, mimic an incarcerated inguinal hernia.

Clinical examination is usually diagnostic, and no additional diagnostic workup is generally needed. Transabdominal ultrasound confirms the hernia or excludes RLV in the groin. If the clinical presentation in a patient with a hernia is atypical, an abdominal MRI or CT scan can exclude other causes of obstruction.

Treatment

Asymptomatic, reducible hernias can safely be managed nonoperatively until postpartum. Indications for emergent operation are incarcerated hernias or hernias with spontaneous skin rupture. Skin rupture develops in umbilical or incisional hernias with a gravid uterus as the hernia content. Semi-elective operation is indicated in severely painful hernias or hernias with skin necrosis from compression of the gravid uterus in the hernia sac. It occurs in advanced pregnancy, and the operation should be delayed as much as possible to deliver (near) term babies. In such situations, combined hernioplasty and CS are performed. With inguinal, umbilical, or inferior median laparotomies, both procedures are done through a single incision. Still, unsolved issues are the use of prosthetic materials during pregnancy and the role of the abdominal binder in the early postoperative period during pregnancy. The ideal timing for hernioplasty is after the last pregnancy, because every pregnancy increases the risk of primary hernia or hernia recurrence.

Prognosis

Due to the small number of patients undergoing treatment, many factors remain unknown. Maternal outcome is excellent, even with strangulation and bowel gangrene. Hernia recurrence is low. Fetal outcome is excellent, except for maternal bowel gangrene, which can lead to fetal death or preterm birth.

Maternal Abdominal Trauma

Incidence

Emergency department visits due to maternal trauma occur in 3–7% of pregnancies. Hospital admission is needed in 0.3–0.9%, with significant variations even within the country. Blunt trauma is the most common type, accounting for 69% of the total cases, whereas penetrating trauma accounts for only 1.5%. The most common cause is MVA, followed by falls, interpersonal violence, and burns.

Risk Factors

Risk factors are presented in Table 41.2.

Clinical Presentation

Blunt Abdominal Trauma

Blunt trauma, not sustained from a known motor vehicle accident or other explainable sudden event, mandates examination for signs of prior trauma due to physical abuse and

Table 41.2 Risk factors for maternal trauma during pregnancy [1]

Maternal factors	External factors
Age < 25 years	Low socioeconomic status
African-American/Hispanic race	Work outside the home
Illicit drugs/alcohol/smoking	Medicaid insurance
Domestic violence	Traffic/transportation law/regulations
Noncompliance with proper seatbelt use	The severity of a court sentence
Epilepsy or other seizures	
Overweight and obesity	
Primiparas	

violence. The entire body should be examined for hidden injuries under clothes, makeup, jewelry, or wigs. Injuries range from cuts, bruises, and black eyes to miscarriage, bony injuries, splenic and liver trauma, partial loss of hearing or vision, and scars from burns or knife wounds. *Soft tissue wounds, cuts, and bruises in different stages of healing should always alert the clinician to the possibility of physical abuse.*

Abdominal pain is the most common symptom. It can be localized or generalized depending on the severity of abdominal trauma. It is challenging to determine abdominal distension and free fluid in advanced pregnancy due to an enlarged gravid uterus.

Penetrating Abdominal Trauma

Penetrating abdominal trauma results in a more straightforward diagnosis of abdominal injury. The path of a stab or a gunshot wound should be estimated. Exit wounds from gunshot wounds are essential to reconstruct the path of a missile.

Diagnosis

In the pregnant population, the diagnostic process is more complex because of the potential injuries to the mother, the fetus, and the uteroplacental unit.

Laboratory Findings

- Base deficit (BD) > −6 has a probability of ≥95% for the absence of intra-abdominal bleeding.
- BD ≤ −6 and increased heart rate indicate a markedly enhanced risk for intra-abdominal bleeding.

A decrease in hemoglobin indicates bleeding. A hemoglobin fall of 20–30 g/L is significant, and a search for its cause is mandatory. Significant loss occurs with fractures of long bones, pelvis, or a contained retroperitoneal hematoma.

Diagnostic Imaging

Hemodynamic stability directs diagnostic algorithm. In hemodynamically unstable patients without severe trauma other than abdominal trauma, emergent exploratory laparotomy without diagnostic workup is indicated. Stable patients undergo transabdominal ultrasound to check maternal abdominal injuries and fetal status. If several organ systems are injured, abdominal CT better defines the location, type, and severity of every organ injured.

Obstetric Conditions

Cardiotocography is mandatory for patients with abdominal trauma. The algorithm for the management of the pregnant woman after blunt abdominal trauma is presented in Fig. 41.2.

Placental abruption is difficult to predict based on the severity of trauma. The seatbelt sign during pregnancy increases the risk of traumatic placental abruption and, to a lesser degree, fetal head injury and uterine rupture. Placental abruption presents as vaginal bleeding, abdominal cramps, uterine tenderness, amniotic fluid leakage, and maternal hypovolemia out of proportion to visible bleeding. Only 35% of clinically significant placental abruptions had vaginal bleeding. The remaining hematomas are confined to the uterus and do not manifest as vaginal bleeding. Up to 2 L of blood can accumulate in the uterus, which can cause maternal shock.

Fetal-maternal hemorrhage (FMH) or transplacental hemorrhage is a physiological transplacental passage of low fetal blood volume (fetal cells) into the maternal circulation. Therefore, it remains clinically insignificant and undetected. Severe FMH is a fetal blood loss >30 ml. Detection of fetal cells in the maternal bloodstream is necessary for confirmation. The tests used for confirmation are the Kleihauer–Betke test, the Rosette test, and the most precise test, a flow cytometry, using monoclonal antibodies directed against fetal hemoglobin. Positive results mandate treatment (see section "Hospital Management").

Treatment

Prehospital Management

Prehospital management is the initial key to maternal and fetal survival. Pregnancy is a criterion for transport to a trauma center that can provide obstetrical care whenever possible, as long-term monitoring is usually required. The criteria for the transfer to level I trauma centers, according to Advanced Trauma Life Support (ATLS) guidelines, are (the last four are added for pregnant patients):

- Glasgow Coma Score <14
- Respiratory rate <10/min or >29/min
- Systolic blood pressure <90 mmHg
- Revised Trauma Score <11
- Anatomy or mechanism of injury
- *Pulse >110 bpm*
- *Chest pain*
- *Loss of consciousness*
- *Third trimester*

The decision to intubate in the field is mainly unaffected by pregnancy.

Avoiding supine hypotension syndrome (uterocaval compression) prevents decreased cardiac output, which leads to prolonged resuscitation and increased acidosis and vasopres-

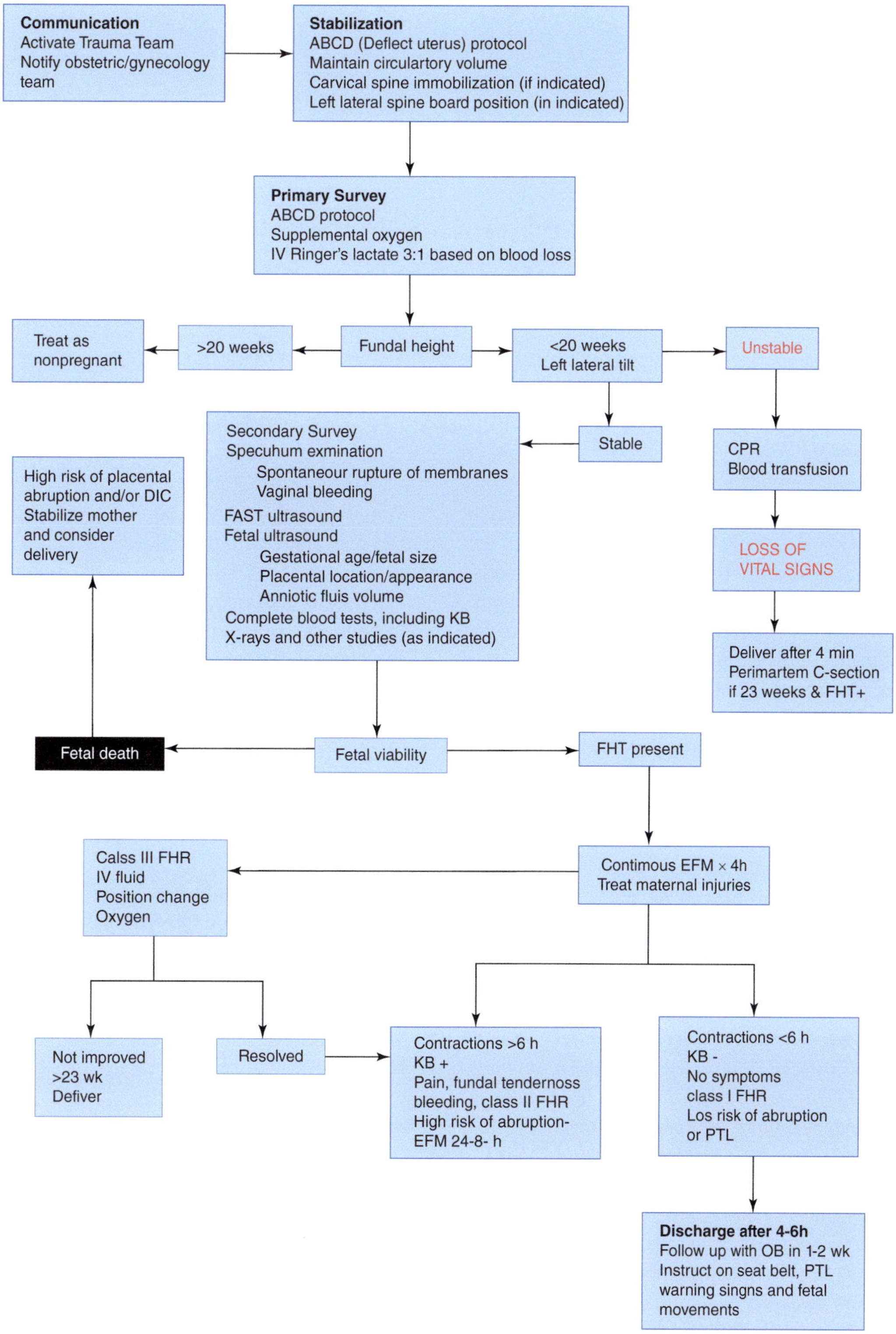

Fig. 41.2 Algorithm for the management of the pregnant woman after blunt (abdominal) trauma. KB Kleihauer-Betke test, FHT fetal heart tones, EFM electronic fetal monitoring, PTL preterm labor. (Modified from Refs. [281–283]; Augustin [1])

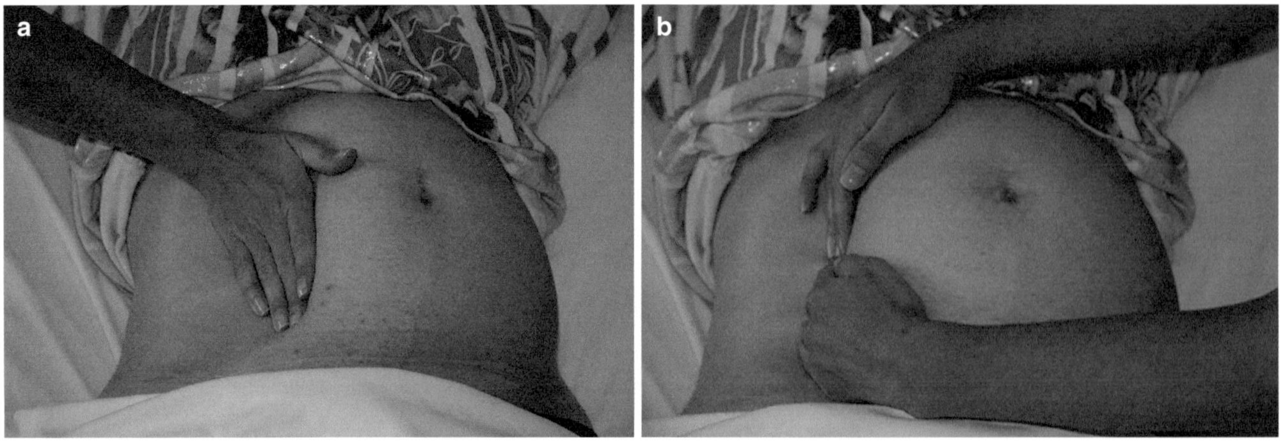

Fig. 41.3 Left lateral uterine displacement using (**a**) 1-handed technique and (**b**) 2-handed technique. (Reproduced with permission from Ref. [45])

sor requirements. Beyond 20 weeks of gestation, the patient is placed on a backboard with a 15° angle to the left. For less than 24 weeks, 1-handed (Fig. 41.3a) and 2-handed (Fig. 41.3b) manual left lateral displacement techniques might be sufficient. The increased breathing effort in the advanced pregnancy indicates a transport in a 30° reversed Trendelenburg position. A left lateral tilt can be utilized even with a suspected spinal fracture.

Femoral IV access should be avoided because potential uterocaval compression alters the distribution of medications or fluids. Oxygen supplementation by nasal cannula or face mask should be routine. If prehospital transfusion is required, O-negative blood should be used whenever possible.

Hospital Management

The volume of fetal blood loss after trauma is 5–40 ml. As little as 1 ml of Rh + blood can sensitize 70% of Rh-women [190,195]. *Therefore, all Rh-negative mothers with abdominal trauma should receive a prophylactic dose (300 μg) of Rh immune globulin*. It should be administered within 72 h of trauma. The same applies to positive FMH.

Wounds should be cleaned and debrided. *Tetanus toxoid* should be given if the last booster was 10 years ago or if vaccination history is unknown. If the previous immunization was >10 years ago, tetanus immune globulin should be given. The tetanus toxoid dose is 5 IU intramuscularly (IM), while tetanus immune globulin prophylaxis dosing is 250 or 500 IU IM (in the opposite extremity to tetanus toxoid) [100]. Pregnancy has no immunosuppressive effect on the mother's response to tetanus toxoid.

Nonoperative management in penetrating abdominal trauma may apply with the following criteria:

- The fetus is deceased
- The entrance wound is below the level of the fundus
- The bullet is radiographically shown to be in the uterus
- Maternal evaluation is reassuring
- Hematuria or rectal bleeding are absent

The algorithm for stabbing abdominal wounds is presented in Fig. 41.4.

Emergency CS in viable pregnancies (>24 weeks) is indicated if:

- Maternal resuscitation fails/cardiac arrest
- The uterus interferes with the examination and repair of maternal injuries
- A viable fetus suspected of having direct injury
- Maternal shock
- Possible exsanguinations from any cause
- Irreparable uterine injury
- Fetal distress in a viable fetus
- Unstable thoracolumbar spine injury
- Amniotic fluid embolism

Perimortem CS should only be considered when:

- Uterine size exceeds the umbilicus or gestation ˃24 weeks
- Evidence of fetal heart activity (Doppler or M-mode US)
- Unsuccessful maternal CPR 4–5 min (up to 15 min if fetal vital signs persist)

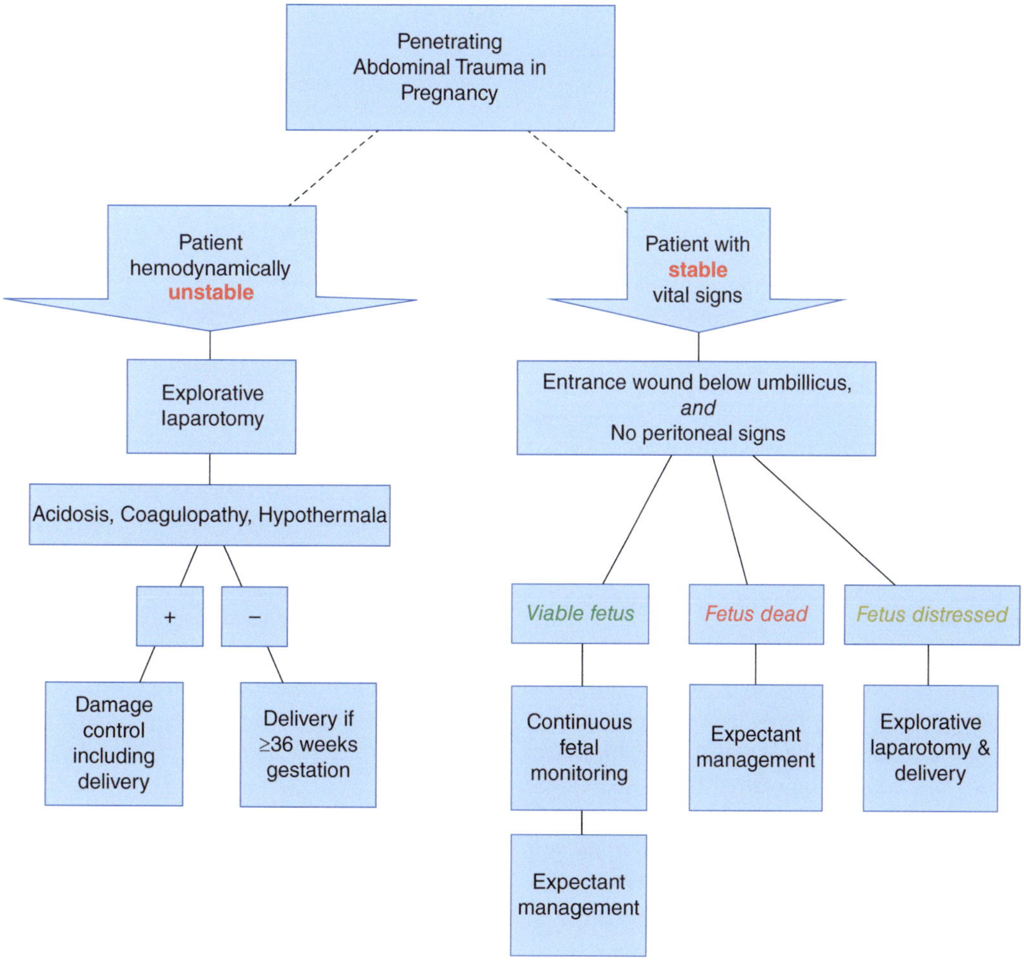

Fig. 41.4 Treatment algorithm for penetrating maternal abdominal trauma in pregnancy. (Reproduced from Ref. under the CC Attribution License)

Splenic Emergencies

Incidence

Less than 100 cases of spontaneous splenic ruptures in pregnancy have been published. Of the reported cases, 60% occurred in the third trimester [18]. Similarly, fewer than 100 cases of traumatic splenic rupture in pregnancy are recorded. Most cases result from road traffic accidents, rarely after bicycle falls, domestic violence, or even coitus. Traumatic splenic rupture occurs in the third trimester in half of patients. Seventy-five ruptured and nine unruptured SAA (splenic artery aneurysm) cases were published. The mean age was 31.1 ± 5.2 years, of which 64.4% were multiparous and 54.8% presented in their third trimester. Thirty-two cases of primary splenic pregnancy were reported worldwide, 28 in the English literature until 2021.

Classification and Etiopathogenesis

Two types of etiology include spontaneous or traumatic rupture. Some spontaneous cases are likely from minor trauma (coughing, sneezing, vomiting) that the patient does not recall. Criteria for spontaneous rupture include:

- No history of trauma
- No systemic disease that can affect the spleen
- No evidence of perisplenic adhesions to suggest previous trauma
- Splenic parenchyma, vasculature, and capsule are normal macroscopically and histologically
- Lack of viral infections related to the spleen

Predisposing factors for spontaneous splenic rupture include:

- Local lesions as points of weakness
- The increase of capsular tension due to splenic enlargement (>200 g) in the second half of pregnancy
- Hypervolemic state
- Diminished peritoneal cavity volume
- Compression by the abdominal musculature
- Increased intra-abdominal pressure

Primary splenic pregnancy can be the cause of spontaneous splenic bleeding. The spleen is favorable for implantation because it is a flat organ with abundant blood flow and is easily reached by the fertilized ovum. However, the spleen does not allow placental attachment, leading to rupture with massive hemoperitoneum.

The third common cause of splenic rupture is rupture of the SAA.

Clinical Presentation

In traumatic cases, splenic rupture may become manifest immediately after trauma or may be delayed and only recognized following a latent period. The classic triad of epigastric pain, tenderness, and Kehr's sign after blunt abdominal trauma is characteristic of a ruptured spleen. *Kehr's sign* represents diaphragmatic irritation with referred pain to the left shoulder tip region. It is almost pathognomonic when present with blunt abdominal trauma. Blood from any cause in the left subphrenic space causes Kehr's sign. The pain worsens with coughing, deep breathing, and movement. Dyspnea results from blood loss into the intra-abdominal cavity and from diaphragmatic compression. In advanced pregnancy, the enlarged gravid uterus does not give rise to Ballance's sign (dullness to percussion in the left flank or left upper abdominal quadrant and shifting dullness to percussion in the right flank). The dullness in the left flank is due to coagulated blood, and the shifting dullness on the right in altering position is due to fluid blood. The pain can become generalized in later stages, with distention and rigidity. Eventually, more than half of patients develop hemorrhagic shock.

Diagnosis

Differential diagnoses according to the cause and trimester of organ rupture are presented in Table 41.3.

The initial imaging method is transabdominal US or abdominal CT, depending on the severity of the trauma. The transabdominal US can also evaluate the viability of the fetus. Free fluid localization depends on the severity of the bleeding. Free fluid in the upper abdomen or left upper quadrant should raise suspicion of splenic rupture. Doppler US can detect SAA. If SAA is suspected in a hemodynamically stable patient, angiography can detect the cause and is also therapeutic, with embolization or stenting of the SAA. Abdominal CT is rarely performed for isolated blunt abdominal trauma, especially in hemodynamically stable patients. It is mainly used in polytrauma patients with evidence of injury to several systems. An exploratory laparotomy is done in hemodynamically unstable patients when the cause of bleeding is unknown preoperatively.

Table 41.3 Differential diagnosis of splenic rupture during pregnancy [1]

Traumatic	Spontaneous			
	First trimester	*Second trimester*	*Third trimester*	*Puerperium*
Liver rupture	Ruptured ectopic pregnancy		Placental abruption	Postpartum pain
Uterine rupture			Uterine rupture	Uterine rupture
Renal rupture			Acute pancreatitis	Acute pancreatitis
			Renal artery rupture	Postpartum bleeding

Treatment

Nonoperative management (NOM) with close hemodynamic monitoring has been advocated in well-selected cases, most of which are traumatic in origin. There are no criteria or guidelines for pregnant patients, but criteria from the general population can be used:

- Hemodynamic stability
- Absence of peritoneal signs
- Absence of other abdominal injuries requiring surgery

Splenic artery angiography followed by embolization has an 85% success rate in the general population. In several cases during pregnancy, the treatment was successful via radial artery catheterization. For primary splenic pregnancy, immediate post-embolization angiography evaluates the procedural success. The entire pathologic vascularity should disappear. Adjuvant treatment consists of a single IM dose of methotrexate 50 mg/m^2. After 10–14 days, transabdominal US confirms infarct formation and the avascular cystic splenic lesion reduction.

Surgery is indicated in hemodynamically unstable patients or when NOM or splenic embolization fails. If CS is required, a midline vertical incision is recommended to facilitate access and visualization. The obstetrician often sees the patient first with a pelvic pathology diagnosis. Therefore, the standard incision is a lower midline or Pfannenstiel incision. In spontaneous rupture of the normal spleen, 75% resulted in splenectomy, but through an inadequate incision. Some patients needed extensions, and some required a new incision due to insufficient exposure from the original incision.

Splenectomy or partial splenectomy, if possible, is indicated. For primary splenic pregnancies, intragestational sac feticide instillation is indicated without splenectomy. Feticide solutions include methotrexate (1 mg/kg) and potassium chloride.

Prognosis

Until 2011, the maternal mortality from a spontaneous splenic rupture in pregnancy was 14.3% and is declining further.

Maternal hemodynamic decompensation leads to an acute decrease in uteroplacental perfusion, resulting in "fetal distress" and, ultimately, fetal demise. Therefore, early diagnosis and intervention before hemorrhagic shock lowers the fetal mortality rate.

Hepatic Emergencies

Spontaneous Hepatic Rupture

Incidence

The subcapsular hepatic hematoma formation with capsular rupture in pregnancies varies from 1/30,863 to 1/250,000 deliveries. Hepatic rupture in patients with HELLP syndrome is 0.4–1.8%. Less than 500 cases have been reported. Most patients with HELLP syndrome present during the third trimester or early postpartum.

Etiopathogenesis

The condition is common in preexisting pre-eclampsia or even more common in HELLP syndrome. HELLP syndrome consists of hemolysis, elevated liver function tests, and low platelet counts. Initial vasospasms are due to increased concentration and sensitivity to circulating vasopressors during pregnancy. This leads to increased Ca^{2+} concentration, vasoconstriction, and reduced blood perfusion. This is followed by endothelial damage, creating a proinflammatory and procoagulant state with platelet aggregation and the subsequent formation of microvascular thrombi and fibrin deposition. The result is ischemia, necrosis, and ultimately, liver rupture.

Clinical Presentation

The clinical presentation ranges from mild symptoms to sudden hemodynamic instability. Most patients with HELLP syndrome present with upper abdominal pain, hemodynamic instability, and a distended abdomen. Additional symptoms include vomiting and shoulder pain (*Kehr's sign*), resulting from blood irritating the diaphragm. Patients can present with one or more symptoms.

Diagnosis

Several conditions can cause SLR during pregnancy, but the most common cause is HELLP syndrome (Table 41.4).

Previously, the diagnosis was made during emergency laparotomy. Today, half of patients undergo diagnostic imaging, while the other half, due to initial hemodynamic instability, are emergently explored; this exploration is also diagnostic, as hepatic rupture is diagnosed intraoperatively.

The diagnostic protocol is dictated by maternal hemodynamic status. As a FAST procedure, the transabdominal US is sufficient in hemodynamically unstable patients. It shows abundant free intra-abdominal fluid. In hemodynamically stable patients, abdominal CT with IV contrast shows a subcapsular liver hematoma or liver rupture with free intra-abdominal fluid.

Complete blood count, potassium, sodium, BUN, creatinine, serum glucose, bilirubin, AST, ALT, ALP, and amylase values are mandatory. Depending on its volume, hemoglobin values will be lower even with a subcapsular hematoma.

Treatment

Treatment is dictated by maternal hemodynamic stability. Initially or after FAST, emergency laparotomy is performed in hemodynamically unstable patients. Control of bleeding is the primary aim, achieved primarily through liver packing. In severe ruptures, the control of bleeding can be done only with liver resection. In the most severe cases with destruction of both liver lobes, liver transplantation is the only option. In stable patients, percutaneous embolization of hepatic arteries or branches is minimally invasive and efficient. In all cases, Factor VIIa should be administered. Patients with unruptured, subcapsular hematoma can be initially managed conservatively with serial transabdominal US and close monitoring in the ICU.

Most pregnancies were completed by CS. The rate of CS has increased over the decades due to the earlier use and more accurate diagnostic modalities while the fetus was still

Table 41.4 Underlying causes of spontaneous hepatic rupture during pregnancy [1]

Hemangioma/metastasis/hepatoma
Infections (malaria, syphilis, amoebic abscess)
Hepatic tuberculosis
Hepatic sarcoidosis
Peliosis hepatis
Splanchnic artery aneurysms
Cocaine use
Anabolic steroid therapy
Systemic amyloidosis

alive. In viable fetuses (gestational week 26), CS should be done during emergency laparotomy. Continuation of pregnancy is possible in stable patients with subcapsular hematoma or after successful percutaneous hepatic artery embolization. This decision should be made in consultation with a gynecologist.

Prognosis

After 1990, maternal and fetal mortality were 33.7% and 18.8%, respectively. Almost all cases of maternal mortality were the result of the initial presentation of hemodynamic instability. Patients after percutaneous hepatic artery embolization have better maternal survival because these patients were also initially hemodynamically stable.

Hepatic Trauma

Incidence

Isolated liver trauma in pregnancy is extremely rare. The most common cause is blunt abdominal trauma from motor vehicle accidents. Another cause is cardiopulmonary resuscitation (CPR) during pregnancy. Liver lacerations after CPR in pregnancy are significantly higher than in the general population (0.6–2.1%).

Etiopathogenesis

HELLP syndrome is a risk factor for liver laceration or rupture, even with minor trauma. Another risk factor is CPR. An enlarged gravid uterus during pregnancy and early puerperium lessens free intra-abdominal space, increasing intra-abdominal pressure, and resulting in a physiologic compression of the liver capsule. Also, increased intravascular volume and hepatic congestion increase hepatic susceptibility to rupture.

Clinical Presentation

Presentation depends on the severity of liver trauma and associated injuries, especially in motor vehicle or motorcycle accidents. Presentation is the same as with spontaneous liver rupture (see section "Clinical Presentation").

Diagnosis

Diagnostic workup is the same as with spontaneous liver rupture (see section "Diagnosis").

Treatment

Management is the same as with spontaneous liver rupture (see section "Treatment").

Prognosis

Maternal survival after liver laceration from CPR is 50%. It depends on the severity of the bleeding, the diagnostic delay, and the underlying cause that necessitated CPR. The prognosis after a blunt abdominal trauma-induced liver injury is excellent.

Reference

1. Augustin G. Acute abdomen during pregnancy. 3rd ed. Springer; 2023.

Cardiac Surgery

42

Sandra A. Hyder and Anthony L. Estrera

Introduction

From vessel occlusions and anatomic anomalies to valvular diseases, the aim of cardiovascular surgical interventions is to restore adequate oxygenation to the brain and vital organs. Through advances in medical technology, surgical interventions include open sternotomy approaches, minimally invasive techniques, and endovascular methods. Regardless of the procedure, a working understanding of anatomy and the pathophysiology behind the original disease state is imperative in understanding perioperative management.

Surgical Techniques

Coronary Artery Bypass Graft

The surgical approach to severe coronary artery disease should be explored when percutaneous coronary intervention (PCI) is inappropriate or when the advantages of coronary artery bypass graft (CABG) surgery outweigh those of PCI [1]. The conventional method for CABG involves a median sternotomy incision, myocardial preservation via cardioplegic arrest, and the utilization of a cardiopulmonary bypass (CPB) machine. Alternative approaches include "off-pump" CABG, in which revascularization occurs without CPB; minimally invasive direct coronary artery bypass, which facilitates vessel bypass through a small incision in the left and/or right thorax, thereby, removing the necessity for CPB; robotic or complete endoscopic coronary artery bypass, employing robotics for vessel dissection and grafting via small ports, with or without CPB through femoral cannulation; and transmyocardial revascularization, which utilizes CO2 or holmium-YAG lasers to create channels in the myocardium to enhance perfusion, executed through a left thoracotomy in patients deemed to have inoperable coronary artery disease in areas of viable myocardium.

Numerous factors influence the selection of the graft conduit, which is essential for the surgical success of coronary blockage bypass. This decision impacts patient outcomes, including survival, independence from myocardial infarction, symptoms, and reinterventions [2]. The primary benefit of arterial grafts is their increased long-term patency in comparison to saphenous vein grafts (SVGs). Consequently, arterial grafts are more appropriate for younger patients (those with a life expectancy of more than 10 years) as they surpass the benefits of SVGs. Conversely, the technique of arterial grafting is more time-consuming and difficult, which is why venous grafting is the preferred option for patients with a higher operative risk and in emergencies [2].

The saphenous vein is generally retrieved endoscopically. However, it may also be harvested by open techniques, which may result in pain, edema, and prolonged wound healing [3]. When employing the saphenous vein graft as a conduit, it is important to excise the valves or invert the vessel to prevent blood flow restriction. The vein is subsequently sutured to the aorta at one end, while the opposite end is attached to the coronary artery distal to the obstruction. The internal mammary arteries extend from the subclavian artery to both the right and left sides of the chest wall, rendering them suitable candidates for bypass grafting procedures. The left internal mammary artery is predominantly employed to circumvent blockages in the left descending artery, whereas the right internal mammary artery is utilized for bypassing occlusions in the right coronary artery [4]. The artery undergoes minimal manipulation as the surgeon meticulously dissects its distal end from the chest wall and positions it into the coronary artery beyond the site of occlusion. This mitigates the likelihood of arterial vasospasms occurring.

S. A. Hyder (✉)
Department of Graduate Studies, Cizik School of Nursing at UTHealth Houston, Houston, TX, USA
e-mail: sandra.a.hyder@uth.tmc.edu

A. L. Estrera
Department of Cardiothoracic and Vascular Surgery, McGovern Medical School at UTHealth Houston, Houston, TX, USA

S. Atallah, J. Dragoljevic (eds.), *Fundamentals of Surgery for Physician Assistants*,
https://doi.org/10.1007/978-3-032-21069-2_42

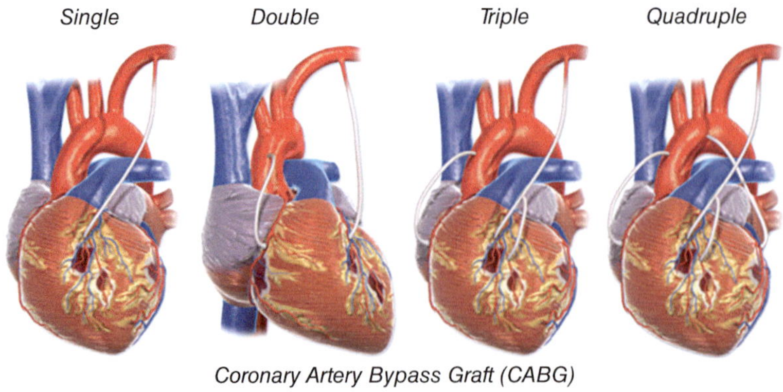

Fig. 42.1 Coronary artery bypass grafting (CABG) [26]

The procedure for harvesting the radial artery from the nondominant arm is accomplished through either an open or endoscopic technique. Before initiating the harvesting process, Allen's test, Doppler evaluation, pulse oximetry, perfusion index, or a combination of these assessments is performed to determine whether the ulnar artery is providing adequate perfusion to the hand. Given the susceptibility of the radial artery to spasm, the administration of intravenous nitroglycerin or diltiazem may be warranted [5] (Fig. 42.1).

Upon completion of the bypass grafts, the surgeon inserts chest tubes into the mediastinal and pleural spaces to facilitate the drainage of any accumulated blood or fluid. Pacer wires are affixed to the anterior surface of the right ventricle and/or atrium, with the opposite end passed through the chest wall to postoperative arrhythmias, if necessary [6].

Valvular Surgery

The primary role of the four heart valves is to ensure unidirectional flow of blood through the body by opening and closing sufficiently, allowing forward flow and preventing backflow in the heart. Failure to perform this function by one or more valves can lead to significant health implications for patients and may necessitate surgery. Surgical interventions can occur as isolated valvular treatment or in combination with other interventions, such as CABG, or other therapies. Like coronary artery bypass surgery, surgical approaches to valvular repair include sternotomy (open approach), minimally invasive surgery (robotic-assisted), and transcatheter procedures. Method and type (tissue vs. mechanical valve) of repair is dependent on the type and severity of valvular disease, with consideration of the patient's overall health condition and comorbidities. Patients requiring valvular surgery may have valve repair or replacement. Although repairing a native valve is preferred over replacement, given its reduction of postoperative complications, valve replacement may be required for severe and symptomatic conditions, such as aortic stenosis/regurgitation, mitral stenosis/regurgitation, tricuspid stenosis/regurgitation, and valvular endocarditis [1, 7].

Aortic valve surgeries using a complete median sternotomy incision also include CPB. The conventional treatment for aortic stenosis is aortic valve replacement using either a tissue or mechanical valve, the latter necessitating lifetime anticoagulant therapy. The Ross method involves utilizing the patient's pulmonary valve to replace the aortic root, followed by the replacement of the pulmonary valve with a homograft. This approach is suitable for individuals under 50 years of age who wish to avoid anticoagulation [1]. For patients requiring simultaneous ascending aortic replacement, the Bentall procedure may be performed with a valved conduit (Fig. 42.2). Aortic valve repair, using the reapproximation of valve leaflet segments to enhance leaflet coaptation, has demonstrated efficacy in younger patients with aortic regurgitation. Alternatively, aortic valve-sparing root replacement is viable in individuals with severe conditions if sufficient remodeling of the root can be achieved. Following these surgeries, meticulous attention must be paid to hemodynamics and electrocardiography, due to the necessity of reimplanting the coronary ostia buttons.

In patients with moderate-to-severe mitral stenosis, percutaneous balloon mitral commissurotomy is the preferred technique when echocardiographic assessment indicates acceptable valve morphology or in cases where CPB should be avoided [1, 8]. Mitral repair can be achieved using annuloplasty rings, leaflet repairs, and chordae transfers. Mitral valve replacement is warranted in cases of calcified or fibrotic valvular leaflets associated with mitral stenosis when repair is impracticable, or in instances of papillary muscle rupture in patients with mitral regurgitation. Similar to mechanical aortic valves, mechanical mitral valves necessitate lifelong anticoagulation, but the requirement for anticoagulation in bioprosthetic mitral valves remains a topic of discussion among clinicians [9]. In patients with paroxysmal or persistent atrial fibrillation, a concurrent procedure utilizing radiofrequency, cryoablation, or high-frequency ultrasound to establish transmural ablation lines should be considered.

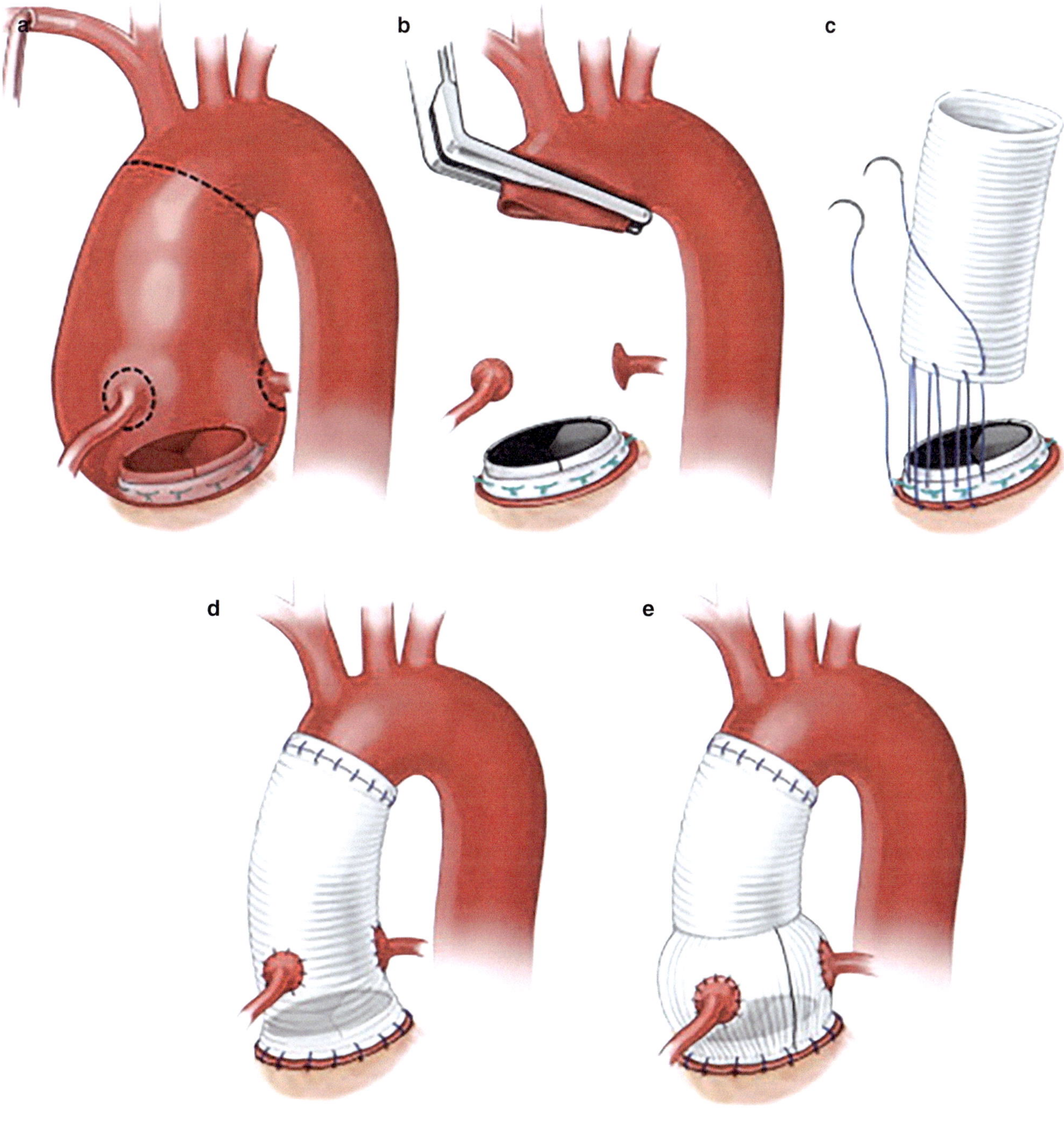

Fig. 42.2 The Completion Bentall Procedure [27]. (Reproduced with permission)

Like aortic and mitral valve conditions, the tricuspid valve can be repaired via annuloplasty with a ring or suture technique in patients with functional tricuspid regurgitation. However, when leaflet shrinkage and poor coaptation exclude successful elimination of tricuspid regurgitation through annuloplasty, tricuspid valve replacement is required. With close proximity to the coronary sinus and conduction system, there is a high risk of developing atrioventricular heart block postoperatively, and the placement of epicardial pacing wires is required [1, 10].

While this chapter focuses on the most common indications for open cardiac surgery, other conditions, such as left ventricular aneurysm, ventricular septal rupture, hypertrophic obstructive cardiomyopathy, aortic dissections, thoracic aortic aneurysms, and pericardial diseases, are also important considerations. The indications for surgical intervention in these conditions are beyond the scope of this discussion. However, they share similar risks and postoperative complications to those addressed in this chapter.

Intraoperative Considerations

Cardiopulmonary Bypass

The CPB circuit, referred to as the "heart-lung" machine, diverts venous blood from the patient, filters and oxygenates it and, subsequently, returns the blood to the arterial system through venous and arterial cannulas, oxygenators, heat exchangers, and pumps, thereby ensuring the perfusion of vital organs during cardiac arrest [11]. Utilizing CPB enables surgeons to conduct heart surgery while preserving oxygenation and perfusion across the body. Central or arterial cannulation is performed to deliver oxygenated blood from the circuit to the patient. Single- and dual-stage venous cannulation is utilized to extract deoxygenated blood from the patient to the CPB circuit. The CPB circuit administers cardioplegia and recovers blood lost during surgery, thereby minimizing the necessity for blood transfusions.

While CPB has enabled the implementation of modern cardiac surgical techniques that were previously impossible, it is essential to recognize that CPB induces a systemic inflammatory response characterized by leukocyte activation and endothelial cell dysfunction. The secretion of pro-inflammatory cytokines, nitric oxide, and reactive oxygen species contributes to oxidative stress, elevating postoperative morbidity and mortality [11]. Vasoplegic syndrome may occur due to an inflammatory response during CPB. It is marked by significant hypotension, resulting from low systemic vascular resistance that is unresponsive to volume expansion or catecholamines, attributable to the dysregulation of the vasodilator and vasoconstrictor functions of smooth muscle cells [12]. Platelet dysfunction and the depletion of clotting factors from the CPB circuit might result in coagulopathy and bleeding issues during and after surgery. Blood transfusion may increase the risk of hemolysis and infection as complications associated with the procedure. Neurologic problems related to CPB include stroke, emboli, hypoperfusion, and abnormalities in cerebral blood flow. Moreover, changes in vascular perfusion may result in acute renal damage and electrolyte abnormalities in individuals undergoing CPB.

Complications Following Cardiac Surgery

A comprehensive preoperative assessment is essential in identifying potential risks and preventing postoperative complications. By thoroughly evaluating a patient's medical history, current health status, and any other relevant factors, healthcare providers can optimize surgical outcomes. Despite meticulous preparation and planning, unforeseen challenges may still arise during or after surgery, highlighting the importance of continued vigilance and adaptability in patient care. While not comprehensive, listed below are several of the most prevalent complications that may arise following surgery.

Postpericardiotomy Syndrome

Postpericardiotomy syndrome is a prevalent complication after cardiac surgery and is included in the postcardiac injury syndromes, along with Dressler's syndrome and posttraumatic pericarditis. Postpericardiotomy syndrome affects up to 30% of patients and, generally, presents as pleuritic chest pain and fever occurring days or up to 6 months following cardiac or pericardial injury [13]. It is caused by an immune response impacting the pericardium, epicardium, and pleural cavity.

The emphasis for treatment is early recognition and treatment to reduce complications and relieve symptoms. Anti-inflammatory medications, such as ibuprofen, indomethacin, and salicylic acid, have been proven to reduce symptoms and shorten illness duration [13]. Colchicine, given within the initial 3 days post-surgery, has been shown to diminish inflammation. However, it does not affect effusion volume or the onset of cardiac tamponade and was linked to a significant incidence of gastrointestinal adverse events [14, 15].

Pericardial Effusion

Postoperative pericardial effusion is common after cardiac surgery, usually presenting as small and asymptomatic, and affects up to 84% of patients [16]. Effusions typically peak around the postoperative day 10 and resolve without intervention. However, in some cases, they can persist or worsen, potentially leading to life-threatening cardiac tamponades.

Tamponade

Cardiac tamponade, which is a life-threatening accumulation of blood or fluid in the pericardial space that impacts cardiac output, is a risk associated with cardiac surgery. Clinical manifestations are dictated by the rate of fluid accumulation. To alleviate this issue, mediastinal and pericardial chest tubes are inserted postoperatively and can be manipulated to prevent or remove clots (Fig. 42.3). Inducing negative pressure through milking, tapping, and stripping are chest tube maneuvers that can assist in clot elimination; however, insufficient data exists to endorse one way over another [17, 18]. Currently, there is no standardized approach to postoperative chest tube management, as prac-

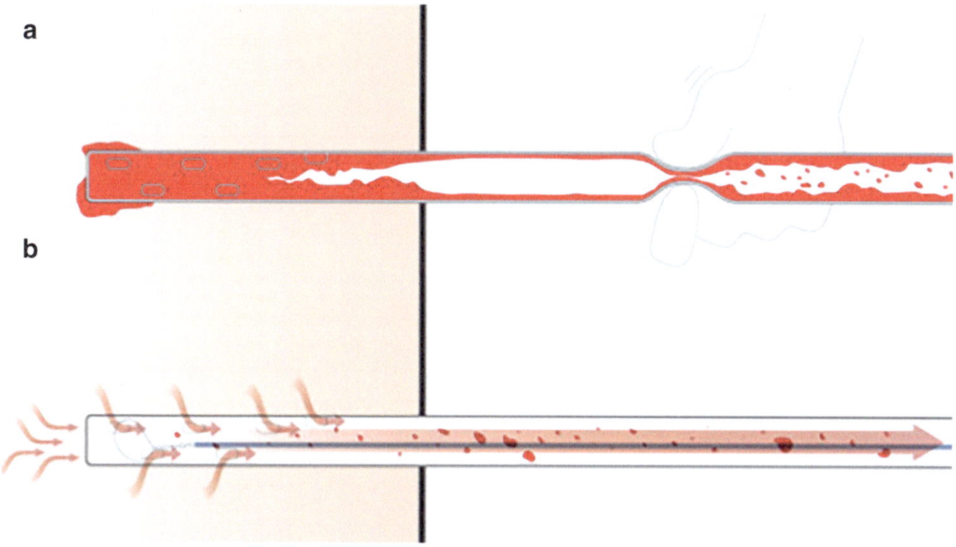

Fig. 42.3 Active clearance of chest tube [28]

tices vary depending on surgeon preference and institutional guidelines. Routine monitoring of chest tubes typically involves daily chest X-rays to assess the position and function of the tube, evaluation for tidaling or air leaks, and measurement of drainage output. Surgical reintervention may be necessary if the drainage exceeds 200 cc per hour for 4 consecutive hours, even after addressing coagulopathy with appropriate blood products [19].

Conversely, an abrupt reduction in chest tube drainage with hemodynamic instability can suggest tamponade. When cardiac tamponade is suspected, a point-of-care ultrasound or echocardiogram should be ordered but a clinical diagnosis can be made by noting signs of cardiogenic shock, such as low cardiac output, increased filling pressures, pulsus paradoxus, and tachycardia [20].

Pleural Effusion

Pleural effusions are another common postoperative complication, occurring in approximately 90 percent of patients following cardiac surgery. Most occur in the first 7 days, resolve naturally, and are due to the inflammatory response postprocedure. Large and clinically significant effusions can occur due to underlying pericarditis, pleural inflammation, and postcardiac injury syndrome [21]. The management of postoperative pleural effusions is dictated by their location, size, and associated symptoms.

Symptomatic effusions refractory to diuresis necessitates further workup by assessing volume status, ruling out hemothorax, infectious processes (i.e. pneumonia or empyema), and pulmonary embolism. Infectious processes can be evaluated by obtaining a complete blood count, erythrocyte sedimentation rate, and C-reactive protein. A significant drop in hemoglobin and hematocrit may indicate a hemothorax, while an elevated brain natriuretic peptide can indicate heart failure [21].

Point-of-care ultrasound, CT scan, or chest x-ray can be used to evaluate effusion size and determine if diagnostic or therapeutic thoracentesis is warranted. Pleural fluid analysis will assist in determining further management strategies. In cases of suspected empyema or hemothorax, chest tube or catheter drainage may be preferred.

Vasoplegic Syndrome

The inflammatory response to prolonged CPB, the use of angiotensin-converting enzyme inhibitors, or diuretics prior to surgery can result in uncontrolled peripheral vasodilation, which can lead to severe arterial hypotension. Inflammatory mediators release an excessive amount of nitric oxide, which can deplete calcium stores and affect vascular tone for up to 72 h following surgery [22]. Vasoplegic syndrome is characterized by hypotension that is resistant to volume resuscitation and low systemic vascular resistance with normal or increased cardiac output.

Catecholamine therapies, specifically norepinephrine, are the initial treatment for Vasoplegic syndrome. Vasopressin, methylene blue, hydroxocobalamin, angiotensin II, and Vitamin C are alternative non-catecholamine treatments that can address vasoplegia [22] (Fig. 42.4).

Dysrhythmias

Arrhythmias frequently occur as complications following cardiac surgery, with atrial tachyarrhythmias, especially atrial fibrillation, being the most common postoperative cardiac rhythm abnormalities. Although infrequent, ventricular

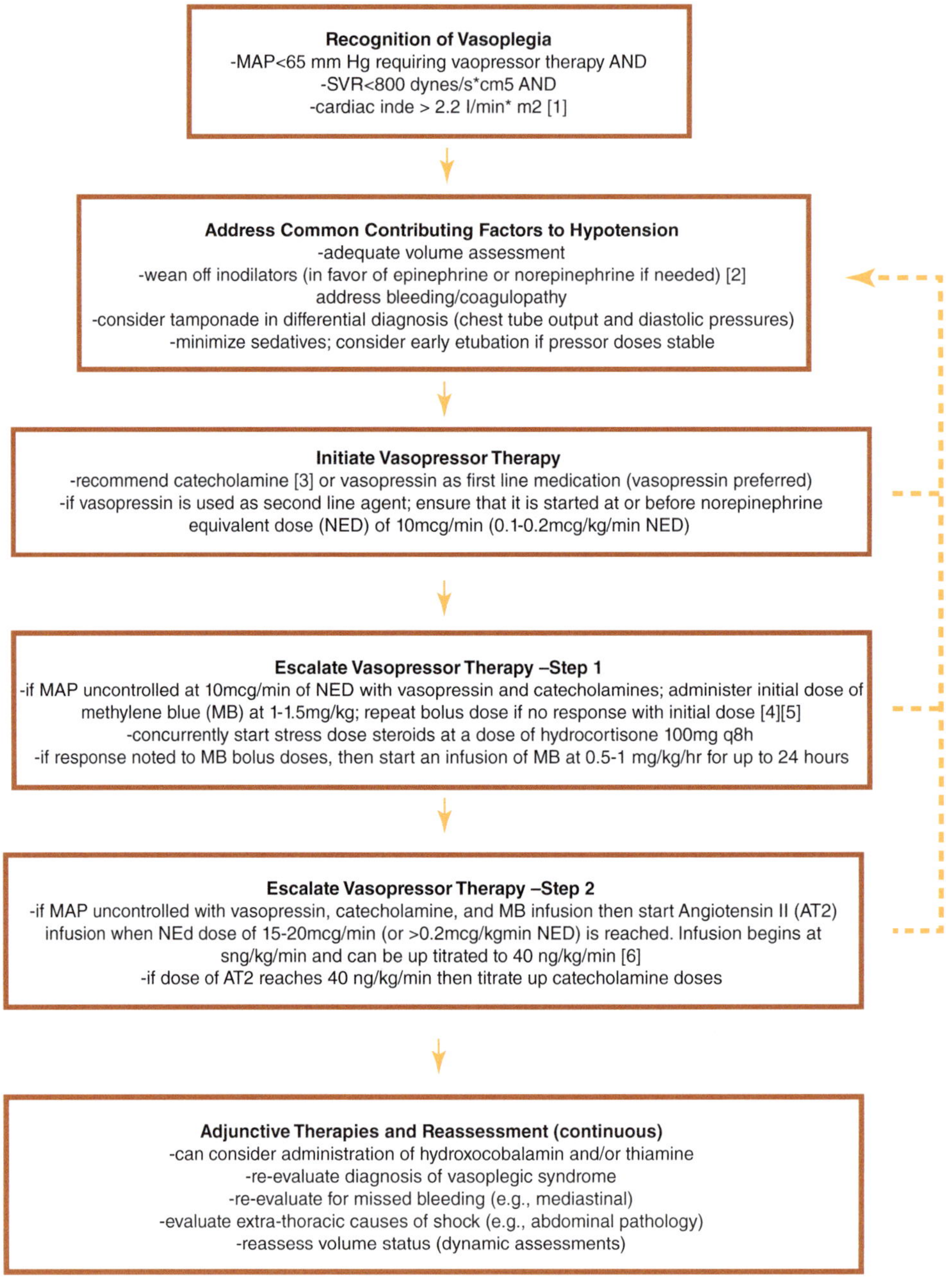
Recognition of Vasoplegia
-MAP<65 mm Hg requiring vaopressor therapy AND
-SVR<800 dynes/s*cm5 AND
-cardiac inde > 2.2 l/min* m2 [1]
Address Common Contributing Factors to Hypotension
-adequate volume assessment
-wean off inodilators (in favor of epinephrine or norepinephrine if needed) [2]
address bleeding/coagulopathy
-consider tamponade in differential diagnosis (chest tube output and diastolic pressures)
-minimize sedatives; consider early etubation if pressor doses stable
Initiate Vasopressor Therapy
-recommend catecholamine [3] or vasopressin as first line medication (vasopressin preferred)
-if vasopressin is used as second line agent; ensure that it is started at or before norepinephrine equivalent dose (NED) of 10mcg/min (0.1-0.2mcg/kg/min NED)
Escalate Vasopressor Therapy –Step 1
-if MAP uncontrolled at 10mcg/min of NED with vasopressin and catecholamines; administer initial dose of methylene blue (MB) at 1-1.5mg/kg; repeat bolus dose if no response with initial dose [4][5]
-concurrently start stress dose steroids at a dose of hydrocortisone 100mg q8h
-if response noted to MB bolus doses, then start an infusion of MB at 0.5-1 mg/kg/hr for up to 24 hours
Escalate Vasopressor Therapy –Step 2
-if MAP uncontrolled with vasopressin, catecholamine, and MB infusion then start Angiotensin II (AT2) infusion when NEd dose of 15-20mcg/min (or >0.2mcg/kgmin NED) is reached. Infusion begins at sng/kg/min and can be up titrated to 40 ng/kg/min [6]
-if dose of AT2 reaches 40 ng/kg/min then titrate up catecholamine doses
Adjunctive Therapies and Reassessment (continuous)
-can consider administration of hydroxocobalamin and/or thiamine
-re-evaluate diagnosis of vasoplegic syndrome
-re-evaluate for missed bleeding (e.g., mediastinal)
-evaluate extra-thoracic causes of shock (e.g., abdominal pathology)
-reassess volume status (dynamic assessments)

Fig. 42.4 *Vasoplegia syndrome algorithm.* Norepinephrine is recommended as the first-line catecholamine agent, with the recognition that cardiogenic shock and vasoplegia can occur simultaneously [29]

arrhythmias and bradyarrhythmia may also manifest. Factors such as duration, ventricular response rate, underlying heart function, and preexisting comorbidities influence the clinical impact and presentation, thereby, determining the urgency and type of treatment required [23].

As a result of surgical trauma, including cannulation, acute atrial enlargement, and ischemia, up to 40% of patients undergoing CABG and 50% of those undergoing valvular surgery develop atrial fibrillation. Atrial fibrillation typically reaches its peak by the third postoperative day and may resolve spontaneously within 24 hours. Atrial fibrillation lasting more than 48 hours increases the likelihood of stroke. Patients displaying symptoms of chronic atrial fibrillation should be evaluated for electrical or pharmacologic cardioversion. Class IA, IC, or II antiarrhythmics serve as pharmacological agents [23]. Ventricular and brady arrhythmias can occur from ischemia or infarction and evaluation of coronary artery patency, specifically post-CABG, should be prioritized.

Chylothorax

Chylothorax refers to the accumulation of chyle in the pleural cavity, resulting from the disruption of the thoracic duct, responsible for transporting chyle from the intestines to the circulatory system. The thoracic duct begins at the cisterna chyli, located in the retroperitoneum near the second lumbar vertebra, and ends at the junction of the left subclavian and jugular veins [24]. Surgical interventions adjacent to the thoracic duct are the principal cause of traumatic chylothorax, as they may unintentionally injure the duct or its branches [25].

In postsurgical patients, chylothorax may initially present as a pleural effusion detected on serial chest imaging or as continuous pleural fluid drainage from the chest tube. The initial step in diagnosing chylothorax involves pleural fluid analysis.

Fluid analysis includes the assessment of triglyceride and cholesterol levels, in addition to routine serum tests, including white blood cell count with differential, glucose, lactic dehydrogenase, total protein, cytology, and microbiologic smear and culture [24]. These tests assist in differentiating chylothorax from other conditions.

Key diagnostic findings for chylothorax include:

- Triglycerides: >110 mg/dL or higher than serum triglycerides.
- Proteins: >20 g/L.
- Cholesterol: <200 mg/dL.
- White blood cell count: >1000 cells/μL, with >80% lymphocytes.

The management of postoperative chylothorax focuses on alleviating respiratory symptoms and preventing further chyle accumulation. Treatment focuses on addressing the underlying cause, with conservative management as the primary approach. Conservation management targeting chylous reduction involves a low-fat diet administered orally for 5–7 days, followed by escalation to total parenteral nutrition for patients who cannot tolerate oral intake or exhibit high chylous output for an additional 5–7 days [25]. Adjunctive pharmacologic agents include octreotide to reduce lymphatic output through somatostatin receptors and diuretics to decrease the size of the effusion. For patients presenting with persistent output exceeding 100 ml/kg/day for 5 days, surgical interventions, such as thoracic duct ligation, pleurodesis, or lymphatic duct embolization, may be considered [24].

It is imperative to promptly diagnose and administer staged treatment for chylothorax to mitigate its substantial systemic effects and facilitate recovery in postoperative patients. Before advancing to interventional or surgical interventions, conservative measures must be fully implemented.

Conclusion

Cardiac surgery performed with CPB involves risks and potential postoperative complications. Perioperative monitoring necessitates continuous telemetry and invasive hemodynamic evaluations to promptly identify potential adverse events, including unexplained hypotension, tachycardia, or pulmonary edema, which may signify postoperative cardiac dysfunction. A multidisciplinary approach is crucial for managing postoperative complications, and an emphasis on comprehensive care improves outcomes and patient safety. Clinical expertise is crucial for identifying complications, administering timely interventions, and overseeing adverse events.

Disclosure Dr. Estrera is on the advisory board of Artivion and a consultant for WL Gore and Terumo Aortic. The other authors have no conflicts of interest.

Funding No funding was obtained for this study.

References

1. Bojar RM. Manual of perioperative care in adult cardiac surgery. 5th ed. Wiley-Blackwell; 2011. ISBN: 978-1-444-34824-8
2. Cuminetti G, Gelsomino S, Curello S, Lorusso R, Maessen JG, Hoorntje JC. Contemporary use of arterial and venous conduits in coronary artery bypass grafting: anatomical, functional and clinical aspects. Neth Heart J. 2017;25(1):4–13. https://doi.org/10.1007/s12471-016-0919-2.
3. Altshuler P, Nahirniak P, Welle NJ. Saphenous vein grafts. In: StatPearls [Internet]. Treasure Island (FL): StatPearls Publishing; 2024.
4. Shahoud JS, Kerndt CC, Burns B. Anatomy, thorax, internal mammary (internal thoracic) arteries. In: StatPearls [Internet]. Treasure Island (FL): StatPearls Publishing; 2024.
5. Curtis E, Fernandez R, Lee A. The effect of vasodilatory medications on radial artery spasm in patients undergoing transradial coronary artery procedures: a systematic review. JBI Database System Rev Implement Rep. 2017;15(7):1952–67.
6. Waqanivavalagi SWFR. Temporary pacing following cardiac surgery - a reference guide for surgical teams. J Cardiothorac Surg. 2024;19(1):115. https://doi.org/10.1186/s13019-024-02619-9.
7. Mick SL, Keshavamurthy S, Gillinov AM. Mitral valve repair versus replacement. Ann Cardiothorac Surg. 2015;4(3):230–7.
8. Brown KN, Ahmed I, Kanmanthareddy A. Catheter management of mitral stenosis. In: StatPearls [Internet]. Treasure Island (FL): StatPearls Publishing; 2024.
9. Carlin S, Eikelboom J. Advances in anticoagulation: patients with bioprosthetic heart valves. Cardiovasc Res. 2022;118(3):e26–8.
10. Bazire B, Algalarrondo V, Dreyfus J. Permanent pacemaker implantation after tricuspid valve surgery. JACC Case Rep. 2023;13:101805.
11. Ismail A, Semien G, Sharma S, Collier SA, Miskolczi SY. Cardiopulmonary bypass. In: StatPearls [Internet]. Treasure Island (FL): StatPearls Publishing; 2024.
12. Ferreira LO, Vasconcelos VW, Lima JS, Neto JRV, da Costa GE, Esteves JC, et al. Biochemical changes in cardiopulmonary bypass in cardiac surgery: new insights. J Pers Med. 2023;13(10):1506.
13. Lehto J, Kiviniemi T. Postpericardiotomy syndrome after cardiac surgery. Ann Med. 2020;52(6):243–64.
14. Meurin P, Lelay-Kubas S, Pierre B, Pereira H, Pavy B, Iliou MC, et al. Colchicine for post-operative pericardial effusion:

preliminary results of the POPE-2 study. J Am Coll Cardiol. 2015;66(10):1198–9.
15. European Society of Cardiology. The 2015 ESC guidelines on the diagnosis and management of pericardial diseases. Eur Heart J. 2015;36(42):2873–85. https://doi.org/10.1093/eurheartj/ehv479.
16. Khan NK, Järvelä KM, Loisa EL, Sutinen JA, Laurikka JO, Khan JA. Incidence, presentation and risk factors of late postoperative pericardial effusions requiring invasive treatment after cardiac surgery. Interact Cardiovasc Thorac Surg. 2017;24(6):835–40.
17. Tabaie AS, Rasoul A, Bahador B, Shariar M, Tabaei SS4. The effect of negative pressure applied on chest tubes in the amount of pleural effusions in postcoronary artery bypass grafting patients. Res Cardiovasc Med. 2018;7(1):10–4. https://doi.org/10.4103/rcm.rcm_20_17.
18. Wallen M, Morrison A, Gillies D, O'Riordan E, Bridge C, Stoddart F. Mediastinal chest drain clearance for cardiac surgery. Cochrane Database Syst Rev. 2004;2002(4):CD003042.
19. Merkle A, Cindass R. Care of a chest tube. In: StatPearls [internet]. Treasure Island (FL): StatPearls Publishing; 2024.
20. Kearns MJ, Walley KR. Tamponade: hemodynamic and echocardiographic diagnosis. Chest. 2018;153(5):1266–75.
21. Heffner JE. Etiology, clinical presentation, and diagnosis of chylothorax. UpToDate. 2025. https://www.uptodate.com/contents/etiology-clinical-presentation-and-diagnosis-of-chylothorax?topicRef=6703&source=see_link.
22. Heyman HM, Serrano RA. Vasoplegic syndrome and noncatecholamine therapies. In: StatPearls [internet]. Treasure Island (FL): StatPearls Publishing; 2024.
23. Peretto G, Durante A, Limite LR, Cianflone D. Postoperative arrhythmias after cardiac surgery: incidence, risk factors, and therapeutic management. Cardiol Res Pract. 2014;2014:615987.
24. Heffner JE. Evaluation and management of pleural effusions following cardiac surgery. UpToDate. 2025. https://www.uptodate.com/contents/evaluation-and-management-of-pleural-effusions-following-cardiac-surgery/print.
25. Ahmed MA Sr. Post-operative Chylothorax in children undergoing congenital heart surgery. Cureus. 2021;13(3):e13811.
26. Blaus B. Coronary artery bypass graft. Wiki J Med. 2014;1(2) https://doi.org/10.15347/wjm/2014.010.
27. Malekan R, Spielvogel D, Saunders PC, Lansman SL, Griepp RB. The completion Bentall procedure. Ann Thorac Surg. 2011;92(1):362–3.
28. Vistarini N, Gabrysz-Forget F, Beaulieu Y, Perrault LP. Tamponade relief by active clearance of chest tubes. Ann Thorac Surg. 2016;101(3):1159–63.
29. Rizvi G. April. Vasoplegic syndrome after cardiovascular surgery - a clinical practice guideline: PCCM Lecture Series. Houston; Memorial Hermann Hospital; 2024.

Preoperative Care of the Thoracic Surgery Patient

43

Brittney J. Roberts and Steven D. Miller

Introduction

Thoracic surgery is a broad topic that goes beyond the confines of this chapter. For a more detailed review of thoracic surgery, consider studying a dedicated thoracic surgery text. The purpose of this chapter is to review common problems and conditions related to general thoracic surgery that can be encountered by a wide variety of clinicians who are not thoracic surgeons. Clinicians practicing in ambulatory care, emergency medicine, and critical care often encounter issues that require a basic fund of knowledge in thoracic surgery. In this chapter, we will cover common disease processes such as pneumothorax, hemothorax, rib fractures, pneumomediastinum, lung abscess & empyema, chest tube management, malignant pleural effusion, anterior mediastinal mass, lung cancer, and esophageal perforations. Common pearls include respective etiology, clinical presentation, diagnosis, and treatment of said diseases.

Pneumothorax

Introduction

Pneumothorax is the presence of air in the pleural space originating from the tracheobronchial tree. This is usually the result of a defect on the lung surface (e.g., ruptured bullae) or damage to the chest wall (e.g., trauma).

Air within the pleural space means there is a loss of normal negative pressure, which impedes lung expansion.

B. J. Roberts (✉) · S. D. Miller
Department of Thoracic Surgery, Oklahoma Heart Hospital, Oklahoma City, OK, USA
e-mail: sdmiller@okheart.com

Types

Pneumothoraces can be divided into two types: traumatic or spontaneous. Traumatic pneumothorax results from blunt or penetrating trauma. Spontaneous pneumothoraces are typically related to underlying lung disease that produces the formation of bullae, which trap air and can develop enough tension to rupture.

A tension pneumothorax occurs when enough air is present in the pleural space to cause respiratory and hemodynamic compromise. The pneumothorax causes a shift of the mediastinum with compressive atelectasis and impeded venous return to the heart. Tension pneumothorax can occur with either a traumatic or spontaneous pneumothorax. Treatment requires prompt decompression of the pleural space either with chest tube insertion or needle decompression of the pleural space. Needle decompression should be performed in the second or third intercostal space at the midclavicular line. Chest tubes should be placed in the fifth intercostal space of the mid-axillary line within the borders of the triangle of safety (latissimus dorsi, pectoralis major, and nipple line significant for the fifth intercostal space) [9].

Providers who practice emergency medicine should be comfortable with chest tube insertion, pleural catheter insertion, and needle decompression because of the need to manage tension pneumothorax promptly.

Clinical Presentation

Patients with spontaneous pneumothorax will often present with the sudden onset of chest pain and dyspnea. Patients presenting with spontaneous pneumothorax are often young males with a tall, thin body habitus and a smoking history. Older patients tend to have a history of asthma or COPD.

S. Atallah, J. Dragoljevic (eds.), *Fundamentals of Surgery for Physician Assistants*,
https://doi.org/10.1007/978-3-032-21069-2_43

Diagnosis and Treatment

A chest x-ray will confirm the diagnosis. For a very small pneumothorax (<2 cm collapse on x-ray) with minimal symptoms and no signs of respiratory compromise—observation and repeat chest x-ray in a few hours is a reasonable option for initial management. If the pneumothorax remains stable and asymptomatic, conservative management is a consideration if the patient has the means for reliable follow-up.

If the pneumothorax is larger (>2 cm collapse on x-ray) or produces symptoms of room air hypoxia or decreased tolerance of mild activity, then chest tube or pleural catheter insertion is indicated. Resolution of the pneumothorax and the absence of an air leak within 24–48 h are indications for removal.

When there is a persistent air leak or failure of the lung to completely re-expand, surgical management with VATS (Video Assisted Thoracoscopy) or thoracotomy is indicated for wedge resection of bullae, which are commonly seen at the apex of the lung. Mechanical pleurodesis, consisting of abrasion of the parietal pleura, is often performed at the time of surgery as well.

In the case of recurrent spontaneous pneumothorax, either on the same side or contralateral, surgery is indicated immediately upon presentation. A chest tube can be inserted to temporize the patient prior to surgery. The occurrence of spontaneous pneumothorax places the patient at increased risk for occurrence on the contralateral side.

Hemothorax

Introduction

Hemothorax is a medical condition in which blood enters the pleural cavity either via traumatic or non-traumatic causes.

Etiology

Hemothoraces can be caused by blunt trauma from falls, motor vehicle accidents, and sports injuries. Penetrating trauma, such as gunshot wounds or stab wounds, can cause Hemothoraces. There are also iatrogenic causes associated with procedures, including central line placement, thoracentesis, and lung biopsy.

Non-traumatic causes include pneumonia, lung cancer, pulmonary embolism, and coagulation disorders, which require anticoagulation, leading to the risk of bleeding into the pleural cavity.

Clinical Presentation

Depending on the severity of the bleeding into the pleural cavity, patients may experience worsening shortness of breath due to compression of the lung parenchyma, pleuritic chest pain with deep breathing, tachycardia and hypotension with abrupt blood loss, and cough secondary to alveolar collapse.

Diagnosis and Treatment

Chest radiology will show a dependent white out, depending on whether the imaging is portable or upright. It will also show a blunted costophrenic angle of the affected side.

Computed tomography scans can help determine the consistency of the fluid, the severity of bleeding, and possible vascular injuries.

Ultrasound can be used in an emergency to confirm pleural fluid accumulation.

Treatment is determined by the extent of the bleeding and the patient's condition. Assessing airway and breathing are essential, resuscitating volume with intravenous fluids, and then potentially placing a chest tube if the fluid accumulation seems to be greater than 300 mls of fluid and patient deteriorates. Chest tube placement is to drain blood, relieve pressure, and allow re-expansion of the lung. You should perform a Chest x ray post procedure to confirm appropriate tube placement.

Surgical intervention with open thoracotomy or video-assisted thoracoscopy may be indicated in the event of massive bleeding >1500 mls or continuous bleeding post chest tube placement. Supportive care with assessment of anemia and appropriate blood transfusions, continuous monitoring of vital signs and respiratory function, and pain control.

Rib Fractures

Introduction and Etiology

Rib fractures are simply defined as a break in one or more of the ribs. They are the most common result of blunt force trauma, such as motor vehicle accidents or falls. Penetrating traumas such as gunshot wounds and stab wounds may also result in rib fractures. Iatrogenic causes of rib fractures include surgical procedures that involve applying stress on ribs with retractors, chest tube insertions, and thoracenteses. Non-traumatic causes include pathological fractures secondary to insidious cancers, osteoporosis, or osteogenesis imperfecta. Chronic coughing secondary to diseases like COPD and bronchitis can contribute to rib fractures.

Pathophysiology

Rib fractures are classified as displaced or non-displaced. Displaced fractures result in the misalignment of the bone fragments. Non-displaced rib fractures maintain their alignment and therefore pose less risk. Displaced rib fractures can injure adjacent structures such as the pleura, lung, vasculature, and nerves, which can lead to pneumothorax, hemothorax, and nerve injury.

Clinical Presentation

Patients with rib fractures tend to present with sharp localized pain to the chest wall that is worse with movement, breathing, and coughing. Cough and dyspnea may be present depending on vascular and parenchymal compromise. Crepitus may be palpated over the injured area.

Diagnosis and Treatment

Chest x-ray is the first modality of choice and will define larger rib fractures, but some rib fractures are very subtle and can be difficult to detect on x-ray.

CT of the chest can further define the extent of rib fractures and associated injuries of the lungs and vasculature.

Single fractures and non-displaced fractures can be managed conservatively with reasonable follow-up. Severe rib fractures with 3 or more displaced fractures in multiple places (flail chest) are associated with vascular injury and may require surgical fixation. Elderly females with 3 or more rib fractures should be admitted and monitored closely with serial chest x-rays for respiratory compromise due to high mortality in this demographic.

If a significant pneumothorax or hemothorax develops secondary to rib fractures, chest tube thoracostomy may be necessary.

Pneumomediastinum

Introduction

Pneumomediastinum is a medical condition that occurs when air from within the airway, lungs, and esophagus leaks and migrates into the mediastinal space.

Types

Primary or spontaneous pneumomediastinum tends to occur in healthy individuals with no identifiable cause. Some risk factors for spontaneous occurrence include smoking or tobacco use, and other inhalation exposures, including marijuana, methamphetamine, and cocaine. [4].

Secondary pneumomediastinum occurs secondary to trauma. There are several different forms of trauma-related pneumomediastinum, including trauma within the lung parenchyma, iatrogenic trauma, and blunt trauma [4].

Iatrogenic causes should also be considered. Certain medical interventions, like positive pressure ventilation, endotracheal intubation, or esophageal instrumentation, can also introduce air into the mediastinum [4].

Clinical Presentation and Physical Exam

Patient presentation can be variable due to the cause and the extent of air accumulation. Most common symptoms include:

- Dyspnea or shortness of breath from pressure on the airways.
- Chest pain, sharp, localized, and worse with deep breaths.
- Coughing may be encountered if there is bronchial involvement.
- Dysphagia or difficulty swallowing due to esophageal involvement.

A clinician may encounter physical exam findings such as crepitus, which is palpable subcutaneous emphysema that can be felt on the chest wall or neck, tachycardia, hypotension, and decreased breath sounds signifying pulmonary involvement [4].

Secondary pneumomediastinum is rare, but generally presents in the young, tall male population with low body mass index. This is thought to be due to the lack of fibrotic tissue in the younger population, which allows for easier air extravasation.

Pathophysiology

Spontaneous pneumomediastinum develops secondary to increased intra-alveolar pressure, which results in alveolar rupture, then air dissects into peribronchial and perivascular sheaths. Excessive vomiting, coughing, physical exertion, or valsalva maneuvers can increase intra-alveolar pressure. Respiratory diseases such as COPD and asthma cause bronchoconstriction and predispose patients to the airway due to increased baseline alveolar pressures [6].

Secondary pneumomediastinum is typically caused by trauma to the trachea or esophagus. Blunt trauma, such as motor vehicle accidents and penetrating trauma, such as a stab wound or impalement, can result in tracheal or esophageal injury, resulting in air extravasation to the mediastinum.

Iatrogenic pneumomediastinum is usually traumatic in nature and is usually associated with endoscopy procedures, endotracheal intubation, or central line placement [6].

Diagnosis and Treatment

Pneumomediastinum is initially evaluated with a chest x-ray, which can show subcutaneous emphysema and usually a translucent line around the mediastinal space. Computed tomography shows a more detailed view and is highly sensitive for detecting air in the mediastinum. CT can help identify sources of air entry. Of note, CT findings of posterior mediastinal air, air in all mediastinal compartments, and concurrent hemothorax are associated with increased mortality. This type of finding should be relayed to the trauma surgeon on call [7].

Treatment depends on the extent of the air extravasation and the underlying pathology. Conservative management with observation, bowel rest (if esophagus involved), and pain management is reasonable in the setting of spontaneous pneumomediastinum without underlying disease.

Surgical intervention is rare, but can be a necessary intervention in the setting of rupture of the esophagus or tracheobronchial tree, or with overwhelming signs of persistent shortness of breath or signs of mediastinal tension.

Lung Abscess and Empyema

Introduction

Lung abscess is the liquefactive necrosis of lung parenchyma resulting from infection, most commonly bacterial.

Empyema thoracis, or more commonly, empyema, is a collection of purulent fluid in the pleural space.

Etiology

Lung abscesses are often the result of aspiration. Alcoholics, those with swallowing dysfunction from chronic neurologic or esophageal motility disorders, and any condition that inhibits the reflexive protection of the airway are at risk for aspiration and the subsequent development of pneumonia and lung abscess.

Empyema is most often seen as a complication of pneumonia in which an abscess or multiple abscesses form in the lung and rupture into the pleural space. Empyema can result from any condition that introduces an infectious process into the pleural space, such as trauma, infection involving an adjacent structure, such as the liver or kidney, or a complication of surgery. Patients who are at risk for the development of empyema include diabetics, those who are immunosuppressed, alcoholics, and those with preexisting pulmonary disease.

Clinical Presentation

Lung Abscess and Empyema present with similar symptoms, including a productive cough (sometimes foul-smelling sputum if bacterial), fever, pleuritic chest pain with deep breathing, and shortness of breath. Hemoptysis may be encountered with cavitary lesions associated with lung abscesses. Physical exam findings of dullness to percussion or decreased breath sounds of the affected side can be a telltale sign of empyema.

Diagnosis

Chest radiography can disclose localized opacity, which is often associated with pulmonary abscesses. Unilateral pleural effusion is often encountered when dealing with infection of the pleural space or empyema.

For more detailed visualization, computed tomography can differentiate between pulmonary abscesses and empyema.

Sputum cultures can determine the infectious organism associated with pulmonary abscess cases.

Procedures, such as thoracentesis, utilize either ultrasound or CT guidance and may be used to obtain and evaluate pleural fluid for cell counts, culture, and biochemical analysis to confirm empyema. Light's criteria are utilized to determine if pleural fluid is exudative. Exudative fluid is associated with an empyema diagnosis.

Treatment

Treatment for lung abscess consists of broad-spectrum antibiotics, chest physiotherapy, and postural drainage. Most lung abscesses resolve without surgical management.

Typically, empyema has three stages. First, an exudative parapneumonic effusion, which is often free-flowing and at this stage amenable to management with thoracentesis or a chest tube. The next stage is the fibrinopurulent stage, in which fibrous septae develop within the fluid collection. Imaging often refers to a multiloculated pleural effusion at this stage. Finally, the organizing stage in which scarring of the pleura develops and a rind of fibrinous material develops on the visceral pleural surface of the lung. This rind prevents the lung from completely expanding. At the fibrinopurulent stage and organizing stage, surgical drainage and decortication of the lung is required to drain the purulent fluid and to allow the lung to re-expand. At the earlier fibrinopurulent stage, empyema can be managed with VATS or intrapleural lytic therapy. At the organizing stage thoracotomy with decortication is usually required for adequate treatment.

Chest Tube Management

Many common surgical conditions in the thorax are treated with chest tubes (tube thoracostomy). Most thoracic surgical procedures result in the placement of chest tubes for postoperative care. A basic understanding of chest tubes is a must when considering thoracic surgical problems.

The first thing that must be known about a chest tube is its location. Chest tubes can be placed in the pleural space, mediastinum, or pericardial space. Chest tubes serve two purposes; to evacuate air or fluid from the space (the pleural space, mediastinum, or pericardial space).

Management of chest tubes and the decision to remove them are based on the presence of a bronchopleural fistula (commonly referred to as an air leak) or the volume of fluid (blood, pleural fluid, chyle, etc.) drained. The chest tube drainage system consists of three chambers. First is the suction chamber. Next is the collection chamber, which collects fluid from the pleural space. Finally, the water seal chamber allows the one-way passage of air from the pleural space.

When asked to cough or produce a Valsalva maneuver, bubbles will appear in the fluid in the water seal chamber. Bubbling of the water seal chamber indicates the presence of a bronchopleural fistula. Removal of the tube with a bronchopleural fistula will result in a recurrent pneumothorax.

Volume of fluid in a 24-h period is also a determinant for safe removal of a chest tube. Typically, for most conditions, removal is warranted with an output less than 200–250 ml over a 24-h period.

When removing a chest tube, ensure that the patient does not aspirate air into the pleural space through the insertion site by asking the patient to hold their breath or to take a deep breath and exhale as the tube is being removed.

When a chest tube is removed, an occlusive dressing should be placed over the insertion site for at least 24 h. After this, it is safe to assume the pleura has sealed, and aspiration of air into the pleural space through the insertion site is not likely.

Malignant Pleural Effusion

Introduction

Malignant pleural effusion is the development of a pleural fluid collection due to cancer. These effusions are exudative. Breast and lung cancer are often the primary site of origin in malignant pleural effusions. Malignant pleural effusions are incurable, reflect advanced disease, and reduce quality of life. The average life expectancy of patients with malignant pleural effusion is 3–12 months.

Clinical Presentation

The clinical presentation depends on the amount of fluid accumulated, the severity of the underlying disease, and the patient's overall health. Shortness of breath is the most common symptom secondary to lung compression. Other symptoms include: pleuritic chest pain, fatigue, weakness, unintentional weight loss, and persistent cough due to alveolar Compression.

Clinicians may notice decreased breath sounds or dullness to percussion on the affected side. In the event of advanced disease or more rapid fluid accumulation, patients can experience hypoxemia, confusion, and severe respiratory distress.

Diagnosis and Treatment

Initial treatment often consists of simple drainage via thoracentesis. Commonly, malignant effusions recur quickly after thoracentesis. Diagnosis of malignant pleural effusion is based on the presence of malignant cells in the pleural space, seen on either analysis of pleural fluid or by pleural biopsy via video-assisted thoracoscopy (VATS).

Treatment of malignant pleural effusion is palliative and seeks to relieve dyspnea, which can be debilitating. Thoracentesis is the most common modality for diagnosis and initial management of malignant pleural effusions. It can be performed in a variety of settings and by several medical and surgical specialties. A common finding with malignant pleural effusions is the development of trapped lung. Trapped lung results when fibrinous exudate or tumor prevents complete reexpansion of the lung following drainage. A trapped lung limits the effectiveness of thoracentesis.

Another disadvantage to thoracentesis is the rapid recurrence of the effusion following drainage. Surgery is reserved for more difficult cases, either in the diagnosis of a refractory pleural effusion or the inability to relieve dyspnea durably by thoracentesis. VATS provides the ability to obtain pleural fluid and pleural biopsy, as well as mechanical or chemical pleurodesis with sclerosing agents such as talc or doxycycline. At the same time, an indwelling pleural catheter can be inserted for longer-term management of malignant pleural effusion at home. Indwelling pleural catheters can be inserted without thoracoscopy as well.

Disadvantages to indwelling pleural catheters are most notably infectious complications at the insertion site or in the pleural space. Aggressive surgical approaches such as pleurectomy or decortication are not favored with malignant pleural effusion and are associated with significant risk of complications such as persistent bronchopleural fistula and bleeding.

Anterior Mediastinal Mass

Introduction

The anterior mediastinum is the portion of the mediastinum located anterior to the heart and great vessels, posterior to the sternum, and bounded laterally by the pleural spaces.

Mediastinal masses in general are usually benign. However, anterior mediastinal abnormalities on imaging are to be taken seriously, as more than half of anterior mediastinal masses are malignant. The mediastinum contains the thymus, which plays a vital role in the development of the immune system in early life. By adulthood, the thymus involutes and is replaced by fat.

Pathophysiology

Masses of the anterior mediastinum typically involve one of the 4 T's: Thymoma, teratoma (germ cell tumors), thyroid, and "terrible" lymphoma. Thymomas make up 1% of adult malignancies, but are the most common mediastinal mass in adults. It is commonly associated with myasthenia gravis. Thymomas as a group consist along a spectrum of biologic behavior from indolent, slow-growing tumors, the classic thymoma, to very aggressive and fortunately rare thymic carcinomas. Diagnosis and treatment in most cases is surgical resection via median sternotomy, with adjuvant therapy reserved for capsular or gross invasion of adjacent structures.

According to the National Cancer Institute Dictionary of Cancer Terms germ cell tumors form from cells that develop into sperm or eggs. Commonly, germ cell tumors involve the testes or ovaries but account for about 15% of anterior mediastinal masses and are the most common extragonadal germ cell tumor. The location in the anterior mediastinum is owed to failure of primitive germ cells to migrate during embryonic development. Benign teratoma is the most common germ cell tumor and consists of cells originating from at least two germ cell layers.

Immature teratomas contain fetal or neuroendocrine tissue. Immature teratomas are malignant and carry a poor prognosis. Testicular germ cell tumors are the most common cancer in young adult men. They are classified as seminoma, non-seminoma (yolk sac, embryonal carcinoma, and choriocarcinoma, immature teratoma), and mixed. Ovarian germ cell tumors include germinoma, dysgerminoma (yolk sac, embryonal carcinoma, choriocarcinoma, immature teratoma), and mixed. Serum markers are important in the diagnosis and differentiation of germ cell tumors. Alpha-fetoprotein and beta-human chorionic gonadotropin levels are often but not always elevated with germ cell tumors.

Germ cell tumors are most often seen in younger patients presenting with anterior mediastinal masses. Most of the time, the diagnosis can be made with clinical exam, imaging findings, and serum markers. Seldom do these patients require biopsy of their mediastinal mass.

Diagnosis and Treatment

An enlarged cervical thyroid gland (goiter) extending directly into the mediastinum can produce an anterior mediastinal mass. Substernal goiter is defined as having more than 50% of its volume below the thoracic inlet. Substernal goiters can cause dyspnea and dysphagia due to mass effect on the trachea and esophagus. Imaging with CT scanning usually demonstrates continuity between the cervical thyroid and substernal portion with a heterogenous appearance to the mass with deviation of the trachea, esophagus or aortic arch and great vessels by mass effect.

Treatment involves resection in symptomatic cases and can usually be resected through a cervical incision. Primary mediastinal lymphomas are a small fraction of lymphomas involving the mediastinum. Usually, lymphomas with mediastinal involvement show disease in other sites besides the mediastinum. For those involving the mediastinum as a primary, the majority are Hodgkin lymphoma, with a small minority being non-Hodgkin lymphoma. The diagnosis of lymphoma involves obtaining larger volumes of tissue than are obtainable with CT-guided or other needle biopsy. Flow cytometry is used to diagnose a monoclonal cell population, which is diagnostic of most lymphomas (the exception being Hodgkin lymphoma, which is diagnosed by the presence of Reed-Sternberg cells on staining). This requires a larger specimen, which is sent fresh in media such as RPMI solution as well as in formalin for routine pathologic exam. Surgical biopsy in many of these cases can be accomplished with anterior mediastinotomy through the second intercostal space on either the right or left, or a cervical incision. The ideal surgical approach is determined by imaging findings (CT scan).

Lung Cancer

Introduction

Lung cancer remains the leading cause of cancer death in the USA. The best results in terms of overall survival, in non-small cell lung cancer (the most common type of bronchogenic carcinoma), are seen with complete anatomic resection of the primary tumor and mediastinal lymph node dissection. Most patients are not surgical candidates at the time of diagnosis due to metastatic disease or physiologic compromise (most commonly due to COPD). Smoking remains the leading risk factor associated with the development of lung Cancer. Others include: environmental exposures (second-hand smoke, radon gas, asbestos, and air pollution, previous lung diseases (COPD and pulmonary fibrosis), and genetic predispositions.

Classification

Lung cancer can be classified into two different groups: *non-small cell carcinomas (NSCLC)* and *small cell carcinomas (SCC)*. Non-small cell carcinomas encompass adenocarcinomas, squamous cell carcinomas, and large cell carcinomas. Adenocarcinomas are the most commonly occurring lung cancer, predominantly in non-smoking females and located peripherally in the lung parenchyma. Squamous cell carcinomas are found in smokers and are located more centrally in the lung parenchyma. Large cell carcinomas are uncommon and have a poorer prognosis. 85% of lung cancer cases are of the NSCLC type. Small cell carcinomas are known for their rapid growth and quick metastasis. Smoking is a risk factor of SCC. Small cell carcinomas represent 15% of lung cancer cases.

Screening

Low-dose screening CT scanning of patients at high risk for lung cancer has been shown to reduce mortality from lung cancer (NEJM reference). The early development of primary lung cancers is most often asymptomatic, and early detection of lung cancers at lower clinical stages, where they can be completely resected, greatly improves survival. The United States Preventive Services Task Force currently recommends annual low-dose screening CT for adults aged 50–80 years with a 20-pack-year history of smoking who currently smoke or have quit smoking in the last 15 years. Screening should be discontinued once a patient has not smoked for 15 years or develops a health problem that substantially limits life expectancy or the ability to undergo curative lung surgery.

Clinical Presentation

Symptomatology in patients with lung cancer includes: a persistent cough, hemoptysis, dyspnea (due to pleural effusion or tumor invasion of surrounding structures), chest pain, unintentional weight loss, and fatigue.

Diagnosis and Treatment

Initial studies include a chest x-ray which can detect a solid white mass in the lung parenchyma. CT scans are more sensitive for evaluating and detecting lung masses and provide more information for staging. Bronchoscopy with biopsy is used for central lesions. CT-guided biopsy may be used if the lesions are peripheral or if the clinician is unable to obtain bronchoscopically. Endobronchial ultrasound (EBUS) is used to biopsy associated mediastinal lymph nodes for staging purposes.

Staging is used to determine the extent of treatment. The TNM classification system is utilized. T = tumor and represents the size of the tumor, N = node and represents the nodal involvement, and M = metastasis and shows the presence of metastasis.

NSCLC, if detected in the early stages, can be resected with a wedge resection, lobectomy, or pneumonectomy +/− radiation therapy. Adjuvant or neoadjuvant chemotherapy may be considered with stage 3 disease. Immunotherapy may be an option in more advanced disease, and multidisciplinary care should be established [3].

SCC is usually detected too late due to its rapid growth. Chemotherapy +/− radiation therapy may be considered. Multidisciplinary care should be established with oncology, social work, and palliative care.

Esophageal Perforations

Introduction

Esophageal rupture or perforation is a critical condition in which a tear is formed in the esophagus, leading to extravasation of gastric contents into the mediastinum. It is important for clinicians to understand the anatomy of the esophagus to further aid in the care of these patients.

Anatomy of the Esophagus

The esophagus is made up of 3 layers (mucosa, submucosa, and muscularis propria). It does not have a serosal layer, making it more vulnerable to rupture.

Esophageal Sphincters

- Upper esophageal sphincter (UES)—Starts at the crico-pharyngeal muscle. It is located about 15 centimeters from the incisors. It is the most common site for iatrogenic perforation, likely secondary to endotracheal intubation and foreign body aspiration. The sphincter prevents air swallowing and is contracted at rest. It is innervated by the recurrent laryngeal nerve. Failure of the sphincter to relax after a CVA can result in aspiration. The normal pressure of the UES during rest is 50–70 mmhg and during swallowing is 15 mmhg. (The Operative).
- Lower Esophageal Sphincter (LES)—It is not a true sphincter. LES works indirectly through the inner circular muscle layer. It is located 40 cm from the incisors. Its mechanism of action is to prevent reflux based on its high resting tone. The sphincter only relaxes with swallowing and gastric distention. The normal pressure of LES during rest is 10–20 mmhg and during swallowing is 0 mmhg. (The Operative).

Esophageal Perforation: Etiology

Spontaneous rupture is the most common form of non-iatrogenic perforations (15% of all esophageal perforations. The rupture results from a sudden increase in intra-esophageal pressure, combined with negative intrathoracic pressure. It usually occurs in a longitudinal fashion on the left side and varies in size [5].

Boerhaave's Syndrome is a form of spontaneous rupture that affects the distal third of the esophagus and results in a full-thickness or transmural tear [2]. Patients with a history of recent intractable vomiting or retching and alcoholism are most commonly affected. Symptomatology includes Mackler's triad with severe thoracic pain, vomiting, and subcutaneous emphysema [10]. Other signs of advanced disease include: fever, dyspnea, and signs of mediastinitis. It is diagnosed with a CT scan and extravasation of gastric contents into the mediastinum. This is a medical emergency and requires urgent surgical intervention due to the risk of mediastinitis and sepsis [11].

Mallory Weiss tear is a less serious form of spontaneous rupture that affects the superficial mucosa of the gastroesophageal junction. It is usually a result of uncontrolled vomiting or retching. It is more commonly associated with symptoms of hematemesis and abdominal pain. Patients usually do not experience the severe chest pain and signs of mediastinitis exhibited by patients with Boerhaave's. Mallory-Weiss tears are diagnosed under direct visualization with an endoscopy. CT scans can be used to evaluate for other associated injuries, but it is not the primary method for diagnosing these tears. Treatment is usually conservative and the lesion heals spontaneously. There are instances where an endoscopic procedure is utilized if there is excess bleeding.

Traumatic ruptures are rare and usually secondary to penetrating or blunt forces such as gunshot wounds or stab wounds. Iatrogenic injuries with endoscopic procedures, esophageal dilation, endotracheal intubation and surgical interventions are the most common [1].

Foreign body impaction can result in esophageal rupture and most commonly occurs in the distal third of the esophagus. It is more common in patients with a history of esophageal stricture (i.e., peptic stricture, achalasia), esophageal obstruction (i.e., neoplasm), or inflammatory/infectious processes (i.e., esophagitis or mediastinitis that can weaken the wall of the esophagus). Foreign body impactions can be complicated by pressure necrosis, leading to wall ischemia in the affected segment and resulting in necrosis with subsequent perforations [5].

Esophageal Perforation: Clinical Presentation

The clinical signs and symptoms of esophageal perforations include acute chest pain or abdominal pain. Other symptoms include shortness of breath, fever, and tachycardia due to gastric contents leaking into the pleural space and mediastinum, subcutaneous emphysema, and crepitus. Some patients may experience pain with swallowing or difficulty swallowing. Oftentimes, symptoms are associated with intractable vomiting or retching. Some patients may experience epigastric pain that radiates to the left shoulder and this symptom lends to an abdominal component.

Advanced disease leading to mediastinitis will present with fever, tachycardia, hypotension, tachypnea, cyanosis, and shock. All of which are poor prognostic indicators.

Esophageal Perforation

Diagnosis and Treatment

Diagnosis

Early and accurate diagnosis is vital for successful management.

X-ray will show air that has escaped from the ruptured esophagus (i.e., free air under the diaphragm) +/− pleural effusion.

CT scan is the gold standard for diagnosis. Imaging can show the site and severity of the perforation and associated injuries.

Contrast esophagography with water or barium can show extravasation from the esophagus and can determine the location and degree of perforation. Although barium swallows are more accurate and specific, there is concern for barium-induced chemical mediastinitis. In lieu of this, water contrast studies are favored [5].

Treatment

Treatment depends on the severity of the esophageal tear and the stability of the patient. There are nonoperative and operative forms of management. Nonoperative management is for the patient population with mild symptoms or minimal signs of sepsis, or those diagnoses that go undetected [8].

For unstable patients with multiple symptoms and underlying comorbidities, conservative management is recommended. ICU admission with hemodynamic monitoring, volume resuscitation, and stabilization are key. Bowel rest is imperative in the event of a transmural tear, as consumption of gastric contents in the wrong compartments will further lead to sepsis. Consider total parenteral nutrition. Broad-spectrum antibiotics should be started after two blood cultures have been obtained. Consider IV proton pump inhibitors. Depending on the degree of the tear, a surgical evaluation may be necessary.

Surgical intervention within 24 h of perforation can be treated with debridement of contaminated tissues with primary repair of the defect with a vascularized tissue (pedicle flap of serratus anterior, latissimus dorsi, or diaphragm). Perforations with extensive leakage of fluid and tissue necrosis should undergo emergent stenting, debridement, and drainage. If a patient is at high risk for the above interventions, in the case of friable tissue or pre-existing esophageal disease such as an inoperable malignancy, patients can undergo an esophagogostomy and feeding gastrostomy/jejunostomy.

The patient should only resume oral feedings once stable, and the integrity of the esophagus has been confirmed via contrast esophagography. If there is any evidence of leakage, the patient should not resume feedings. The surgical team should be consulted. [5].

The multi-disciplinary team should consist of a general surgeon, radiologist, intensivist, thoracic surgeon, expert endoscopist, dietician, speech therapist, respiratory therapy, intensive care nursing, rehabilitation, and case management involving resources for therapy after discharge [11].

References

1. Norton-Gregory AA, Kulkarni NM, O'Connor SD, Budovec JJ, Zorn AP, Desouches SL. CT esophagography for evaluation of esophageal perforation. Radiographics. 2021 Mar;41(2):447–61.
2. Teh E, Edwards J, Duffy J, Beggs D. Boerhaave's syndrome: a review of management and outcome. Interact Cardiovasc Thorac Surg. 2007;6(5):640–3. https://doi.org/10.1510/icvts.2007.151936.
3. Guo Q, Liu L, Chen Z, Fan Y, Zhou Y, Yuan Z, Zhang W. Current treatments for non-small cell lung cancer. Front Oncol. 2022;12:945102. https://doi.org/10.3389/fonc.2022.945102.
4. Iteen AJ. Pneumomediastinum. In: StatPearls [Internet]. U.S. National Library of Medicine; 2023. www.ncbi.nlm.nih.gov/books/NBK557440/.
5. Kassem MM, Wallen JM. Esophageal perforation and tears. [Updated 2023 Aug 7]. In: StatPearls [Internet]. Treasure Island (FL): StatPearls Publishing; 2024. Available from: https://www.ncbi.nlm.nih.gov/books/NBK532298/.
6. Kouritas VK, et al. Pneumomediastinum. J Thorac Dis. 2015;7(Suppl 1):S44–9. https://doi.org/10.3978/j.issn.2072-1439.2015.01.11.
7. Lee WS, Chong VE, Victorino GP. Computed tomographic findings and mortality in patients with pneumomediastinum from blunt trauma. JAMA Surg. 2015;150(8):757–62. https://doi.org/10.1001/jamasurg.2015.1138.
8. Mubang RN, Sigmon DF, Stawicki SP. Esophageal trauma [Updated 2023 Jul 25]. In: StatPearls [Internet]. Treasure Island (FL): StatPearls Publishing; 2024. Available from: https://www.ncbi.nlm.nih.gov/books/NBK470161/.
9. "Pneumothorax." TeachMeSurgery. teachmesurgery.com/cardiothoracic-surgery/pleural/pneumothorax/.
10. Turner AR, Collier SA, Turner SD. Boerhaave Syndrome. [Updated 2023 Dec 4]. In: StatPearls [Internet]. Treasure Island (FL): StatPearls Publishing; 2024. Available from: https://www.ncbi.nlm.nih.gov/books/NBK430808/.
11. Wang J, Wang D, Chen J. Diagnostic challenge and surgical management of Boerhaave's syndrome: a case series. J Med Case Rep. 2021;15:553. https://doi.org/10.1186/s13256-021-03080-1.

Urology

44

Jelena Dragoljevic and Hannah Chelliah

Introduction

Urology is a medical and surgical specialty that focuses on the diagnosis, treatment, and management of disorders affecting the urinary tract and male reproductive system. This chapter will explore some of the most frequently encountered urological conditions that require surgical or emergent intervention.

Benign Prostatic Hyperplasia

Etiology

Benign prostatic hyperplasia (BPH) is a condition characterized by prostate gland enlargement, which may result in *lower urinary tract symptoms* (LUTS). Proliferation of stromal and epithelial cells of the *prostatic transition zone,* which directly surrounds the urethra (Fig. 44.1), leads to urethral compression and *bladder outlet obstruction*. While the etiology is not entirely clear and is likely multifactorial, the androgen dihydrotestosterone (DHT) has been associated with the growth of prostatic stromal and epithelial cells [1], contributing to BPH.

Prostate Gland Anatomy

The prostate gland is divided into five lobes: anterior, posterior, lateral (left and right), and median lobe (Fig. 44.1). The two lateral lobes comprise the bulk of the prostate gland and are associated with BPH symptoms. The median lobe of the prostate is located between the urethra and the two ejaculatory ducts. *Enlargement of the median lobe tends to cause more significant BPH symptoms* due to protrusion into the bladder and closure of the bladder outlet. The clinical significance lies in the fact that patients with median lobe enlargement may be more resistant to medical therapy and may require surgical intervention more frequently.

Clinical Presentation

Classic obstructive symptoms of BPH include straining to void, incomplete emptying, weak urinary stream, hesitancy, intermittency, and post-void dribbling. In response to bladder outlet obstruction, the *detrusor muscle* (which is the main muscle of the bladder wall) becomes overactive in order to overcome the resistance and empty the bladder of stored urine. This results in irritative urinary symptoms consisting primarily of frequency, urgency, and nocturia. *BPH with LUTS* is a term frequently used to describe these obstructive and irritative symptoms, though the term LUTS is not necessarily specific to BPH.

Diagnosis

The *International Prostate Symptom Score (IPSS)* is a validated questionnaire frequently used to help diagnose BPH and, more importantly, to assess a patient's response to treatment.

Uroflowmetry is a diagnostic test that primarily measures a patient's urine flow rate. Ideally, the maximum flow rate (*Qmax*) should be *>15 mL/s*. To ensure an accurate Qmax measurement, voided volume should be greater than 150 mL. A low Qmax may indicate any type of obstruction in the urinary tract *or* a weak detrusor muscle. Thus, a low Qmax is not exclusive to BPH.

A *bladder scan* is an ultrasound of the bladder that aids in the diagnosis of BPH by assessing *post-void residual* (PVR)

J. Dragoljevic (✉)
Telemed2U, Roseville, CA, USA

H. Chelliah
Reproductive Endocrinology, Brown Fertility, Orlando, FL, USA

S. Atallah, J. Dragoljevic (eds.), *Fundamentals of Surgery for Physician Assistants*,
https://doi.org/10.1007/978-3-032-21069-2_44

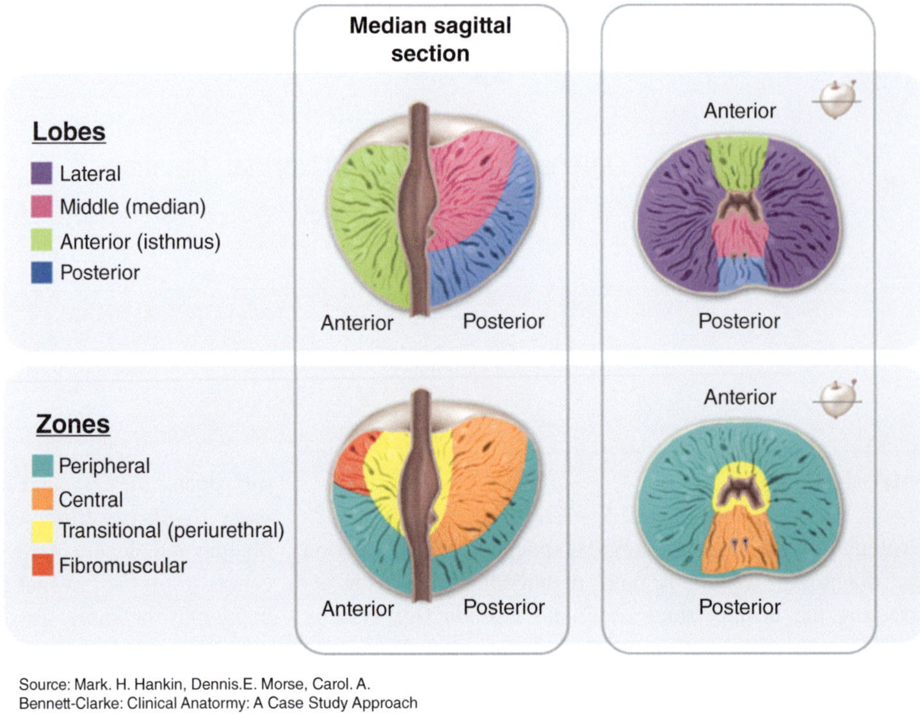

Fig. 44.1 Prostate gland anatomy. The prostate gland can be divided into five anatomical lobes: left lateral, right lateral, median, anterior, and posterior. The lateral and median lobes are most frequently referenced in clinical practice and on cystoscopic examination. The prostate gland can also be divided into histologically distinct zones. The anterior fibromuscular stroma is non-glandular, while the glandular zones include the central, peripheral, and transitional zones

volume. *PVR <50 mL suggests adequate bladder emptying.* PVR >200 mL indicates urinary retention, which is also nonspecific and can be seen in many conditions aside from BPH. Catheterization is required if PVR >400 mL *or* in the case of acute urinary retention with abdominopelvic distension and discomfort. If severe urinary retention is discovered on a bladder scan, the next step in the workup is a renal ultrasound to rule out the development of subsequent hydronephrosis.

Cystoscopy and transrectal ultrasound of the prostate (TRUS*)* are two diagnostic procedures that are often performed together, as the final step in the workup. Cystoscopy allows for direct visualization of any narrowing or compression of the urethra at the prostatic level. This procedure also reveals which lobes of the prostate are contributing to the obstruction, which is an important factor when considering eligibility for certain surgical interventions. Additionally, secondary effects of BPH, such as *trabeculation* (bladder wall thickening) resulting from retention and increased bladder pressure, can be visualized on cystoscopy. It is important to note that cystoscopy can simultaneously rule out other causes of a patient's urinary symptoms, such as urethral strictures, bladder stones, and malignancy. TRUS is used to assess the size and shape of the prostate. Prostate measurements and prostate volume are determined, which aid in diagnosis and treatment planning.

Treatment

Medical Treatment

Alpha-blockers are the mainstay of treatment for BPH/LUTS. They work by relaxing the smooth muscle of the prostate and the bladder neck. More specifically, they block alpha-1 adrenergic receptors to oppose the effects of the sympathetic nervous system, resulting in decreased smooth muscle contraction. Medications in this class include tamsulosin, silodosin, alfuzosin, doxazosin, and terazosin. The most common side effects are orthostatic hypotension, dizziness, headaches, retrograde ejaculation, and erectile dysfunction. *Tamsulosin and silodosin are known to have a greater incidence of retrograde ejaculation*, and patients who develop this side effect should be switched to one of the nonselective alpha-blockers (alfuzosin, doxazosin, or terazosin).

5-Alpha reductase inhibitors work by shrinking the prostate gland. This is accomplished by blocking the enzyme 5-alpha reductase, which normally converts testosterone into dihydrotestosterone (DHT). Medications in this class include finasteride and dutasteride. Side effects of 5-alpha reductase inhibitors are primarily sexual and may include retrograde ejaculation, decreased libido, and erectile dysfunction.

Key points to keep in mind regarding 5-alpha reductase inhibitors:

- They falsely lower serum PSA values by about 50% after 3–6 months of use [2]. In practice, this means that for patients on 5-alpha reductase inhibitors, one must *double their reported PSA* in order to get the *true*, corrected PSA value.
- It may take between 3 and 6 months for these medications to shrink the prostate and thus to have a noticeable effect on the patient's symptoms.

PDE-5 inhibitors are typically used for the treatment of erectile dysfunction; however, tadalafil has also been FDA-approved for the treatment of BPH/LUTS. The mechanism of action is inhibition of phosphodiesterase type 5, resulting in increased cyclic GMP and relaxation of the smooth muscles of the prostate and bladder neck. Tadalafil is particularly beneficial for patients with both ED and BPH/LUTS, and the usual dosage for this indication is 5 mg once daily. The most common side effects are headaches, flushing, dizziness, dyspepsia, nasal congestion, and myalgia. *PDE-5 inhibitor use with nitrates is contraindicated due to the risk of severe hypotension.*

Surgical Treatment

Surgical treatment for BPH is indicated when a patient fails to respond to maximum medical therapy. Additional indications include development of refractory urinary retention, hydronephrosis, renal insufficiency, recurrent or persistent gross hematuria, recurrent UTIs, and recurrent bladder stones [3].

One of the most important considerations with surgical intervention for BPH is impact on sexual function. BPH procedures can cause erectile and ejaculatory dysfunction to varying degrees, which are often *irreversible*. Given the sensitivity of this issue and impact on quality of life, it is essential to counsel patients on the risk of *permanent* sexual adverse effects when discussing treatment options. The following is a review of several of the most common surgical interventions currently used for BPH.

Minimally Invasive

Prostatic Urethral Lift (Urolift)

Prostatic urethral lift is a minimally invasive, tissue-sparing procedure in which small implants are permanently placed into the prostate to *retract* the obstructing prostate tissue and relieve compression on the urethra. Suitable candidates for a Urolift are those with a *prostate volume 30–80 cc* and *the absence of an obstructive median lobe*. Additionally, this procedure may be ideal for those who are concerned about preserving sexual function, as it has minimal effect on erectile and ejaculatory function. Patients do not usually require catheterization post-procedure. Improvement in urinary symptoms can be seen within 1–2 weeks.

Water Vapor Thermal Therapy (Rezum)

Water vapor thermal therapy is a minimally invasive procedure that essentially uses steam to ablate the obstructive prostate tissue, as opposed to mechanically retracting it with Urolift. Ideal prostate volume for Rezum is similarly *30–80 cc*. This is another procedure that may be a good option for those wishing to preserve sexual function. Patients do require catheterization for about 3–4 days after the Rezum procedure. Improvement in urinary symptoms after Rezum can be seen after about a month, as it takes some time for the destroyed tissue to be resorbed.

Conventional Surgical Therapy

Transurethral Resection of the Prostate (TURP)

TURP is the most commonly performed surgical procedure for BPH and has historically been considered the gold standard treatment, although some newer procedures are becoming increasingly favored. TURP removes obstructive prostate tissue using electrocautery. During the procedure, a resectoscope is inserted into the urethra to visualize the prostate. Excess prostatic tissue is removed with an electric loop and then flushed into the bladder. Patients with a prostate volume of *<80 cc* are most suitable. Catheterization for about 3–5 days is standard post-procedure to prevent urinary retention secondary to the passage of tissue or blood clots. Recovery time following a TURP can take up to 4–6 weeks, although many patients will see improvement in urination within a few days following removal of the catheter. *The most common long-term complication of TURP is damage to the internal urethral sphincter resulting in retrograde ejaculation, with a risk of up to 70–90%* [4].

Robotic Waterjet Treatment (Aquablation)

Aquablation is performed via the AquaBeam® Robotic System, which utilizes a robotically controlled, heat-free water jet to resect portions of the prostate contributing to obstruction/LUTS. It is most appropriate for patients with prostate volume of *30–80 cc*. Prior to the procedure, a transrectal ultrasound (TRUS) is used to map out the specific regions of the prostate to be targeted. During the surgery, both a cystoscope and TRUS provide real-time imaging to ensure accurate visualization. Once the treatment plan is confirmed, the robotic water jet precisely resects the designated tissue, minimizing the risk of damage to surrounding structures. Post-procedure, a catheter is typically left in place for 3–5 days to facilitate the passage of any remaining tissue or blood clots. Most patients can resume normal activities within 1–2 weeks, with full recovery expected in 3–4 weeks. *Due to its precision, Aquablation carries a lower risk—approximately 10%—of retrograde ejaculation compared to traditional procedures* [5].

Holmium Laser Enucleation of the Prostate (HoLEP)

Holmium laser enucleation of the prostate is a minimally invasive procedure that uses pulses of a laser beam to resect and vaporize prostate tissue surrounding the urethra. The holmium laser, inserted via a resectoscope, separates the prostate core from its capsule. The detached tissue is then pushed into the bladder, where it is cut into smaller pieces, or *morcellated,* for easier evacuation. Laser enucleation is beneficial in that it can be offered to patients with significantly enlarged prostate glands *greater than 100 cc*. Catheterization for about 1–2 days is typical post-procedure. The expected recovery time is typically 4–8 weeks. *Prevalence of retrograde ejaculation following laser enucleation is between 70% and 80%* [6].

Simple Prostatectomy

A simple prostatectomy involves resection of the *core* of the prostate via open surgery, laparoscopic surgery, or laparoscopic surgery with robotic assistance. This procedure is not to be confused with a *radical* prostatectomy, which involves the removal of the *entire prostate gland*, seminal vesicles, vas deferens, and occasionally surrounding pelvic lymph nodes. Simple prostatectomy is ideal for patients with significantly enlarged prostate glands measuring *>100 cc* or those with severe urinary retention/obstruction. This procedure is not often performed, as it has a higher risk of complications and a longer recovery time compared to the above-mentioned procedures. When performed, it is most often done using a robot-assisted approach. In this procedure, the prostate core is excised while the outer capsule is preserved. A urinary catheter is placed, and drainage tubes may be inserted through abdominopelvic incisions into the surgical site. Drains are usually removed within 1–2 days, while the catheter remains in place for 7–10 days. Complete recovery typically takes 6–8 weeks. The risk of retrograde ejaculation is significant. However, several studies have suggested that urethral-sparing simple prostatectomy via minimally invasive robotic approach has preserved antegrade ejaculation in about 80% of patients [7].

Urolithiasis

Etiology

Urolithiasis (a.k.a., *'kidney stones'*) is characterized by hard, crystalline deposits made up of minerals and salts that develop when certain substances in the urine become highly concentrated. There are several types of calculi. Dehydration or low urine volume are significant risk factors for all types. Calcium stones, *the most common type*, are made of calcium oxalate or calcium phosphate. They are associated with hyperparathyroidism, hypercalciuria, hyperoxaluria, hypomagnesemia, and hypocitraturia. Dietary factors contributing to calcium stones include high intake of oxalate-rich foods, sodium, and animal protein. *Low dietary calcium intake is a risk factor for calcium stones*, as it results in increased absorption of oxalate due to a lack of calcium to bind to it in the digestive tract. Moderate calcium intake is recommended to reduce the risk of calcium stones. Struvite stones are usually caused by urinary tract infections, more specifically by Gram-negative, urease-producing organisms such as *Pseudomonas, Proteus, and Klebsiella.* These organisms break urea into ammonia, resulting in more alkaline urine and promoting the formation of struvite crystals. Uric acid stones are associated with persistently low urine pH, high dietary intake of purines (fish, legumes, red meat), metabolic disorders such as gout, type 2 diabetes, metabolic syndrome, and obesity. Cystine stones, the least common type, are caused by the inherited disorder cystinuria, which leads to excessive excretion of the amino acid cystine in the urine.

Clinical Presentation

Clinical presentation of urinary tract calculi may vary depending on multiple factors, including the location and size of the stone. Microscopic or gross hematuria is a common finding. Kidney stones are often asymptomatic and may incidentally be discovered on imaging. Symptoms may not develop until the stone causes infection or obstruction, either at the level of the kidney, ureteropelvic junction (UPJ), ureter, or ureterovesical junction (UVJ). Patients may present with *sudden, colicky unilateral flank pain radiating to the lower abdomen and groin*, hematuria, nausea, vomiting, and changes in urination (dysuria, frequency, urgency). Classically, ureteral stone patients tend to be *writhing* in pain. Signs of concomitant infection include fever, chills, malaise, and malodorous urine. Physical exam may reveal CVA tenderness.

Diagnosis

Patients with acute renal colic or suspected urolithiasis should be evaluated with urinalysis and urine culture if indicated, laboratory studies including CBC to assess for leukocytosis and creatinine to assess kidney function, as well as imaging studies. Initial imaging with ultrasonography may be used to assess for obstruction and hydronephrosis, although ultrasound cannot easily detect ureteral stones or kidney stones <5 mm in diameter. Non-contrast CT abdomen/pelvis is the gold-standard imaging modality. X-ray of the kidneys, ureters, and bladder (KUB) can detect radiopaque stones (calcium, struvite, and cysteine), but not radiolucent stones (uric acid). The primary advantage of KUB is monitoring stone growth over time and determining whether a stone is amenable to extracorporeal shockwave lithotripsy *(see below)*. Therefore, for urology follow-up and management purposes, it is recommended to order KUB as an adjunct to non-contrast CT abdomen/pelvis. For patients with evidence of long-standing obstruction or hydronephrosis, a nuclear renal scan should be ordered to evaluate kidney function.

Treatment

Medical Management

Urinary tract stones that are asymptomatic, nonobstructive, or <5 mm in size can be managed conservatively. Approximately 90% of stones <5 mm will pass spontaneously [8]. Conservative management comprises *pain control (esp. with the anti-inflammatory medication ketorolac), anti-emetics*, and *medical expulsive therapy (MET)* for <10 mm, distal ureteral stones. MET involves the use of alpha-blockers, such as tamsulosin, to relax the muscles in the ureter and help the ureteral stone pass spontaneously. Duration of MET is between 2 and 6 weeks. Patients should be encouraged to drink plenty of fluids and, if possible, strain the urine to collect the stone for analysis. This can decrease the need for repeat imaging. If it is unclear whether the stone has passed, repeat imaging with renal ultrasound (US) and KUB is preferred to assess for stone progression and hydronephrosis. While every attempt should be made to minimize radiation exposure, non-contrast CT body imaging may need to be repeated if the US and/or KUB are inconclusive regarding stone passage or in the case of a radiolucent stone. Ureteral stones that have not passed within 4–6 weeks are unlikely to pass spontaneously, and surgical intervention is often indicated.

Surgical Management

If non-emergent surgical intervention is warranted, definitive treatment for stones may involve extracorporeal shockwave lithotripsy (ESWL), ureteroscopy (URS), percutaneous nephrolithotomy (PCNL), and rarely open or laparoscopic approaches.

Extracorporeal shockwave lithotripsy is a non-invasive procedure that uses shock waves to break stones down into smaller fragments that can be passed spontaneously. ESWL is only indicated for radiopaque stones, as it relies on fluoroscopy (continuous X-ray imaging) to visualize and target the stones. ESWL is primarily used for *proximal ureteral* or *non-lower pole renal stones <2 cm in diameter.* Although lower-pole renal stones can successfully be fragmented with ESWL, they are less likely to pass due to the gravity-dependent position of the lower calyces. ESWL may still be offered for smaller lower-pole stones <1 cm in diameter. Additional factors that may rule out ESWL as a treatment option include cases involving *distal ureteral stones, dense stones resistant to ESWL (cystine), obesity, use of anticoagulant therapy, pregnancy, or active urinary tract infection* [9]. Repeat imaging with KUB and renal ultrasound is performed to evaluate for adequate stone fragmentation, and multiple ESWL treatments are sometimes needed in order to clear stones completely. Ureteral stent placement during ESWL may be considered depending on stone characteristics or the presence of anatomic abnormalities, although current guidelines discourage routine stent placement during ESWL [10].

Ureteroscopy is a minimally invasive procedure in which a flexible ureteroscope is passed through the urethra and bladder and up to the ureter/kidney to locate the stone. Stones can then be removed via a stone extraction basket, or they can be fragmented with holmium laser lithotripsy and allowed to pass spontaneously. Ureteroscopy can be used for *any* renal or ureteral stones <2 cm in diameter. URS is preferred over ESWL for *mid-ureteral and distal-ureteral stones, lower-pole renal stones <2 cm, and dense stones resistant to shock waves.* Ureteral stents are almost always placed after ureteroscopy to ensure adequate urine drainage and passage of smaller stone fragments. *Post-operative KUB and renal ultrasound* are performed to assess for residual stones and hydronephrosis. If the patient is stone-free, the ureteral stent is typically removed in the clinic within 1–2 weeks. Ureteroscopy is contraindicated in the case of *active urinary tract infection.*

Percutaneous nephrolithotomy (PCNL) is a more invasive procedure that involves placement of a nephrostomy tube percutaneously through the flank and into the kidney to establish access to the renal collecting system (Fig. 44.2). In clinical practice, the term *percutaneous nephrostomy* is often shortened to "*perc-neph.*" This procedure is usually performed by interventional radiology (IR) prior to the PCNL. A plastic access sheath is left in place to safely allow for instruments (nephroscope, lithotripters, stone retrieval devices, etc.) to be passed through. PCNL is indicated for *stones >2 cm in diameter, staghorn stones, stones in patients with CKD, and for patients that have failed or have contra-*

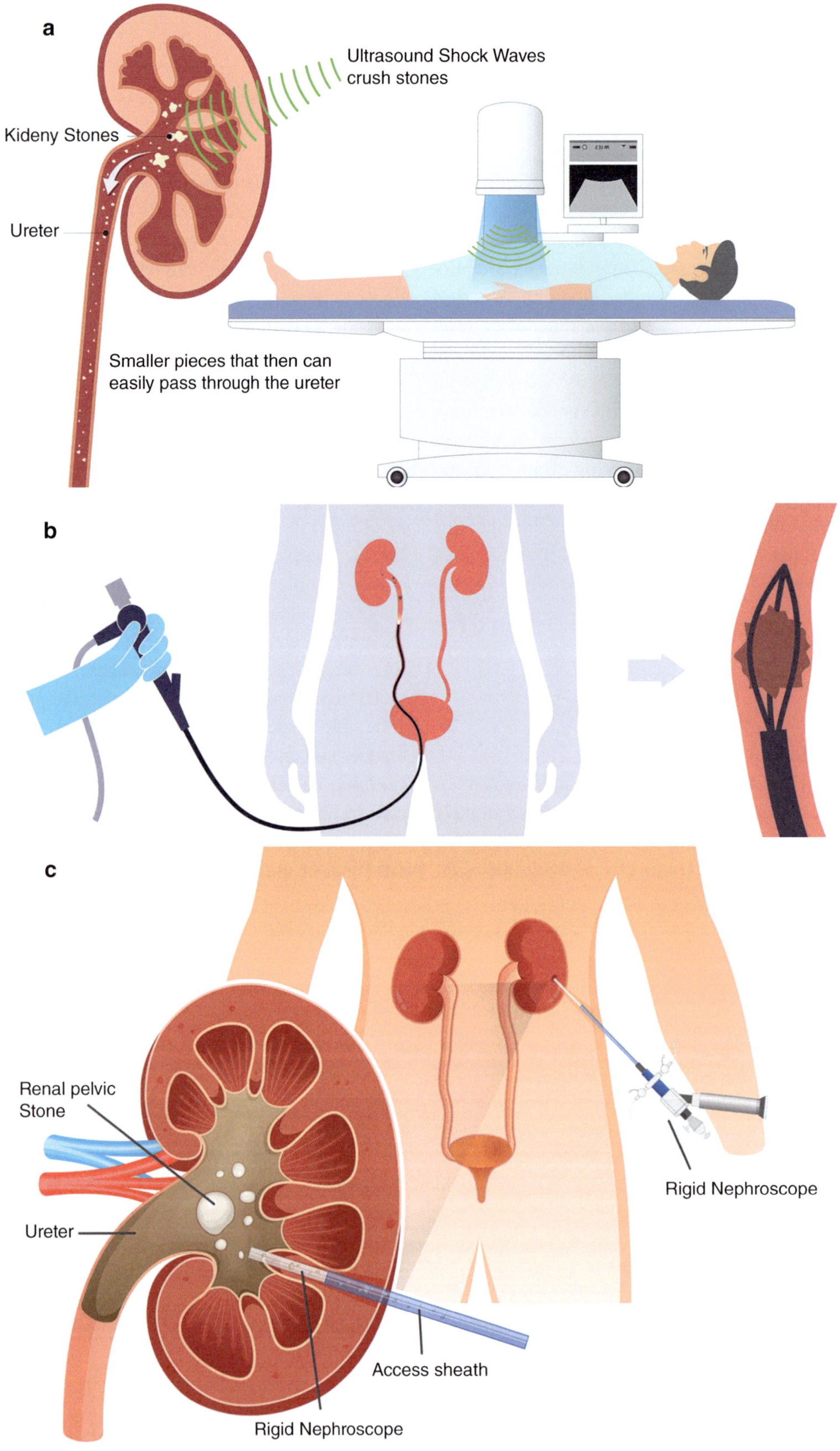

Fig. 44.2 (**a**) Extracorporeal shockwave lithotripsy. (**b**) Ureteroscopy. (**c**) Percutaneous nephrolithotomy

indications to URS or ESWL [11]. At the end of the procedure, patients are often left with both an indwelling nephrostomy tube and a ureteral stent to promote passage of any remaining stone fragments and to ensure adequate urine drainage during the healing process. Repeat imaging with *antegrade nephrostogram* is performed post-operatively to confirm ureteral patency and assess residual stone burden/need for repeat PCNL. The nephrostomy tube is removed prior to hospital discharge or within a few days. Ureteral stents are removed in the clinic within 1–2 weeks following discharge. Contraindications to PCNL include *pregnancy, coagulopathy, use of anticoagulant therapy, pregnancy, and active urinary tract infection* [12].

Robotic, laparoscopic, or open surgical treatment of kidney stones is very rarely needed—the main indications are *non-functioning kidneys* with stones, presence of *anatomic abnormalities (ureteral stricture, UPJ obstruction)* complicating stone removal, and for *ectopic kidneys* with stones [13]. Nephrectomy or partial nephrectomy may be performed for non-functioning kidneys with stones, particularly when associated with persistent pain, bleeding, or recurrent infections. Kidney stones in the presence of concomitant UPJ obstruction may require surgical reconstruction with pyeloplasty, in which the obstructed segment of the ureter is removed, and the unobstructed segment is reconnected to the renal pelvis.

Emergent Management

Obstructive uropathy secondary to calculi requires urgent or emergent decompression in the presence of *infection (urosepsis), immunosuppression, acute decline in renal function (elevated creatinine), solitary kidney, bilateral obstruction, uremia, and hyperkalemia* [14]. Decompression of the urinary tract simply means relieving the pressure caused by the obstruction and allowing urine to flow freely again. Decompression entails temporary urinary diversion via placement of a double J ureteral stent *or* percutaneous nephrostomy. Ureteral stents are flexible, hollow tubes that are endoscopically placed in the ureter to allow for temporary relief of obstruction. Percutaneous nephrostomy, as mentioned above, is often performed by interventional radiology and allows for urine to drain into a nephrostomy bag, essentially bypassing the obstruction. There is a lack of consensus in the literature regarding which method of decompression is preferred, however there appears to be no significant difference in outcomes between the two [15]. Both of these procedures are frequently performed on an urgent/emergent basis while a patient is hospitalized, in which case the patient follows up as an outpatient for scheduling of definitive treatment of the stone (ESWL, URS, PCNL) and eventual removal of the stent or nephrostomy tube. Complications of obstructive uropathy include *infectious* complications (UTI, pyelonephritis, abscess formation, urosepsis), as well as *permanent and severe kidney damage* (chronic hydronephrosis leading to renal failure, chronic kidney disease, renal scarring, and atrophy).

Urologic Oncology

Testicular Cancer

Although testicular cancer is a relatively rare malignancy, it is the *most common cancer in young men aged 15–34* [16]. Risk factors include *undescended testicles (cryptorchidism)*, previous history of testicular cancer, family history, Caucasian race, infertility, and certain genetic conditions (Klinefelter syndrome) [17]. Testicular cancer most often originates in germ cells and is classified into *seminoma* and *non-seminoma* based on the type of germ cells involved. *Seminomas are the more common type*, accounting for just over half of germ cell tumors. Compared to non-seminomas, seminomas are slower-growing, less aggressive, more radiation-sensitive, and overall have a better prognosis.

The most common presentation of testicular cancer is a *painless lump or swelling in the testicle.* Additional symptoms may include testicular pain/discomfort, dull ache in the lower abdomen or lower back, and a general sense of heaviness in the scrotum. Diagnosis relies on physical examination, laboratory tests, and imaging. Key tumor markers for testicular cancer are alpha-fetoprotein (AFP), beta-human chorionic gonadotropin (beta-hCG), and lactate dehydrogenase (LDH). Non-seminomas are characterized by *elevated AFP*, often *significantly* elevated hCG, and elevated LDH. On the other hand, *seminomas do NOT produce AFP,* so they are characterized by *normal AFP, mildly* elevated hCG, and elevated LDH [18]. Scrotal ultrasound is the first-line imaging study, which helps to distinguish solid tumors from benign fluid-filled cysts. CT chest/abdomen/pelvis is the primary imaging modality used for staging.

Definitive diagnosis and treatment for testicular cancer is *radical inguinal orchiectomy* with possible retroperitoneal lymph node dissection, with or without chemotherapy and/or radiation. Testicular cancer has an excellent prognosis when detected early, with a five-year survival rate of 95% for all types of testicular cancer [16].

Bladder Cancer

The *most common type of bladder cancer* is urothelial carcinoma, also known as transitional cell carcinoma (TCC). The most significant risk factor, accounting for about half of all bladder cancers, is tobacco smoking. Additional risk factors include chronic bladder infections or inflammation, family history, previous pelvic radiation, age >65, male sex, and occupational exposure (aromatic amines, dyes, and pesticides) [19]. The hallmark clinical presentation of TCC is *painless gross hematuria*. Patients may also present with irritative voiding symptoms (frequency, urgency, nocturia, dysuria) and/or obstructive symptoms (straining, intermittency, weak stream).

Workup consists of diagnostic tests, including laboratory tests (CBC, CMP), urine tests (urine cytology, Fluorescence In Situ Hybridization/FISH (UroVysion® Kit), cystoscopy, and CT urogram. Treatment for bladder tumors depends on the stage, grade (Fig. 44.3), and location of the tumor, as well as the patient's age and overall health. Surgery is the primary treatment.

The majority of bladder cancers are *non-muscle invasive* (carcinoma in situ, Ta, T1) and are treated with transurethral resection of bladder tumor (TURBT), which is both diagnostic and therapeutic. For intermediate and high-grade non-muscle invasive bladder cancer, TURBT is followed by intravesical immunotherapy (bCG) or intravesical chemotherapy (mitomycin C) to reduce the risk of recurrence.

Treatment for *muscle-invasive* bladder cancer (T2, T3, T4) may involve a combination of surgery, chemotherapy, and sometimes radiation. Main approaches to surgical treatment are partial or radical cystectomy, ideally with cisplatin-based neoadjuvant chemotherapy. Chemoradiation is an option for patients who are ineligible for cystectomy. Urinary diversion procedures, such as ileal conduit or neobladder, are required after radical cystectomy.

The standard of care for advanced or metastatic bladder cancer is chemotherapy. Immunotherapy (checkpoint inhibitors) and targeted therapy have also emerged as key treatments, particularly for patients who cannot tolerate chemotherapy. The prognosis for bladder cancer varies depending on many factors. The five-year survival rates for bladder cancer are 96% for non-muscle invasive, 71% for muscle-invasive, and 39% for metastatic cases [20].

Prostate Cancer

Prostate cancer is the most common cancer diagnosed in men, and the second-leading cause of cancer-related deaths in men. About 80–85% of all prostate cancers are diagnosed in the local or regional stages. The 5-year, 10-year, and 15-year survival rates for localized and regional prostate cancer are >99%, 98%, and 95%, respectively [21]. Well-established risk factors for prostate cancer include older age, African American race, a family history of prostate cancer, mutations in BRCA 1 and BRCA 2 genes, and Lynch syndrome [22]. Prostate cancer typically develops in the *peripheral zone* of the prostate gland.

Early prostate cancer is often asymptomatic, although early symptoms may include hematuria, hematospermia, and changes in urination. Advanced prostate cancer can present with fatigue, weight loss, erectile dysfunction, bone pain related to osseous metastases, and neuropathy related to spinal cord compression. Most of the time, prostate cancer is detected through prostate-specific antigen (PSA) screening prior to the development of symptoms.

A serum PSA level of *<4 ng/mL* is generally considered *normal*. A serum PSA level between 4 and 10 ng/mL is considered borderline and is associated with a 25% likelihood of prostate cancer. When the PSA level exceeds 10 ng/mL, the probability of having prostate cancer rises to over 50% [23]. While PSA is a valuable screening test for prostate cancer, it does not determine whether a prostate cancer is clinically significant or requires treatment. Screening guidelines have significantly differed between the United States Preventive Services Task Force (USPSTF) and the American Urological Association (AUA). However, both organizations aim to optimize the detection of clinically significant prostate cancer while minimizing unnecessary biopsy and overtreatment for clinically insignificant cancers. The AUA currently recommends initiating PSA screening between ages 45 and 50 for patients without risk factors, and this recommendation is

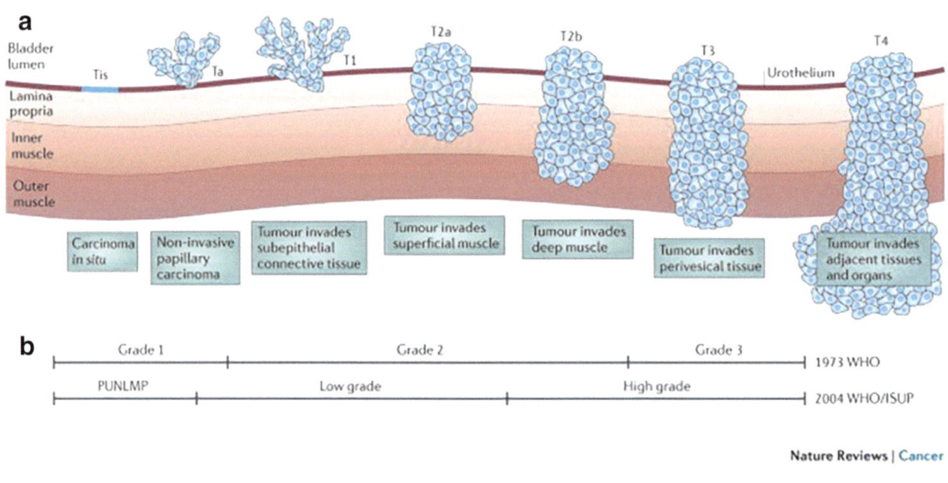

Fig. 44.3 Bladder cancer grading and staging. Staging of bladder TCC uses the TNM system. As depicted, CIS, Ta, and T1 are non-muscle invasive, while T2, T3, and T4 are muscle-invasive

most frequently followed in the urology community. For patients with specific risk factors (Black race, germline mutations, or strong family history), the AUA recommends offering PSA screening beginning at 40–45 [24].

Elevated PSA can be caused by conditions unrelated to prostate cancer, including BPH, prostatitis, recent ejaculation, or prostate manipulation (recent DRE, catheterization, cystoscopy, prostate biopsy). Aside from BPH, these factors can cause a transient elevation in PSA that may normalize upon retesting. For this reason, *the initial step in evaluating a newly elevated PSA is to repeat the test before moving forward with additional, potentially invasive workup.* A digital rectal exam is recommended mainly to establish the risk of clinically significant cancer. MRI of the prostate is the primary diagnostic imaging modality, which provides a PI-RADS score to classify the likelihood of prostate cancer and aid in the decision-making process. For patients with suspicious lesions identified on MRI, the next step in evaluation is a targeted, MRI/TRUS fusion-guided biopsy of the lesion, along with systematic biopsy to ensure uniform sampling of the entire prostate. In cases where no lesions are visible on MRI but the patient has a high risk of clinically significant cancer, a systematic TRUS biopsy is advised. The decision to proceed with a biopsy is complex and multifactorial. Urinary biomarker tests such as *myProstateScore* can be utilized to predict the likelihood of high-grade prostate cancer, helping patients and healthcare providers in making informed decisions about undergoing a biopsy. A prostate biopsy determines the cancer's grade, which is reported using the Gleason score, ranging from 6 to 10. The TNM classification system is used for staging. The most accurate imaging modality for staging is the PSMA PET scan, although CT abdomen/pelvis combined with a bone scan is acceptable in certain cases.

Treatment of prostate cancer depends on many factors, including the stage of disease, patient's age and overall health, the effect of treatment on quality of life, and patient preferences. The intricacies of individualized treatment are beyond the scope of this introductory chapter; however, general treatment options to be aware of include:

- Active surveillance or watchful waiting may be an option for low-risk, low-volume, slow-growing cancers, particularly for older patients with limited life expectancy.
- Some localized, low-risk lesions may be treated with focal ablation (cryoablation, radiofrequency ablation, or high-intensity focused ultrasound (HIFU) ablation). *Focal ablation minimizes damage to surrounding, healthy tissue and may help to preserve sexual and urinary function.*
- Radiation may involve either external beam radiation therapy (EBRT) versus radioactive seeds (brachytherapy) that are implanted into the prostate gland. *Radiation can adversely impact bowel, bladder, and sexual function to varying degrees.*
- Androgen deprivation therapy (leuprolide) may be utilized alongside radiation to improve outcomes. *Most common side effects include hot flashes, decreased libido, testicular atrophy, headache, and generalized pain.*
- Surgical treatment involves radical prostatectomy with possible lymph node dissection, which is typically reserved for younger, healthier patients. *The primary adverse effects patients must be aware of are temporary or permanent erectile dysfunction and urinary incontinence.*
- Treatment of metastatic prostate cancer focuses on androgen deprivation therapy, chemotherapy, and newer treatments such as immunotherapy and targeted therapy.

Urologic Emergencies

Priapism

Priapism is characterized by a prolonged (>4 h) erection that is not associated with sexual arousal. Priapism can be *ischemic* (low-flow) or *non-ischemic* (high-flow). *Ischemic priapism is more common and is a medical emergency.* It is distinguished by a *painful*, prolonged erection caused by dysfunction in venous outflow. Causes of ischemic priapism include *sickle cell disease, malignancy, medications, and illicit drugs (amphetamines).* Medication-induced priapism can be caused by antipsychotics (clozapine), phenothiazines (chlorpromazine), antidepressants (trazodone), erectile dysfunction medications (PDE-5 inhibitors, intracavernosal papaverine, alprostadil), antihypertensives (prazosin), and anticoagulants (heparin, coumadin) [25]. Initial treatment of ischemic priapism centers on draining the excess blood from the corpora via *aspiration, with or without normal saline irrigation.* The next step in treatment is *intracavernosal phenylephrine* (diluted in normal saline) injection, which results in contraction of cavernous smooth muscle and facilitates venous outflow and detumescence. Phenylephrine injection can be repeated every 5 min, up to three times total. Failure of medical therapy necessitates surgical intervention, which involves the creation of a shunt to allow for blood to drain from the corpora cavernosa. *If not treated promptly, priapism can lead to penile fibrosis, nerve damage, chronic pain, and potentially permanent erectile dysfunction.*

In contrast, non-ischemic priapism is characterized by a *painless, partial erection* and is caused by unregulated arterial blood flow into the penis, most often due to penile or pelvic trauma. Initial treatment of non-ischemic priapism is observation, as the condition is not a medical emergency and may resolve spontaneously. If conservative management fails, arterial embolization is the treatment of choice.

Testicular Torsion

Testicular torsion is a medical emergency characterized by twisting of the spermatic cord around the testicle, resulting in testicular ischemia. Torsion can occur spontaneously, and the precise etiology is not always known, however several factors that may increase the risk include *bell-clapper deformity* (Fig. 44.4), *varicocele, undescended testicle, trauma, and strenuous physical activity* [26]. Testicular torsion occurs most commonly in adolescent boys between 12 and 18 years of age. Patients classically present with a *sudden onset of severe, unilateral scrotal pain associated with nausea and vomiting*. A physical exam may reveal redness or swelling of the scrotum. *Absence of the cremasteric reflex*, in which stroking of the inner thigh does *not* cause the testicle to rise, can be a sign of testicular torsion but is not specific. If blood flow is not restored promptly (*within 6 h*), the risk of testicular necrosis and the need for orchiectomy significantly increase. Treatment for testicular torsion is immediate surgical detorsion and orchidopexy, in which the testicle is untwisted and permanently fixed to the walls of the scrotum. Manual detorsion, in which the testicle is rotated laterally in an "open-book maneuver", can sometimes be successful if done by an experienced provider. *However, surgery is still required and is the only definitive treatment to prevent future torsion. (See Pediatric Surgical Emergencies chapter for further details.)*

Paraphimosis

Paraphimosis is a urologic emergency that occurs when the foreskin becomes trapped in a retracted position. This results in a tight band of constricting tissue that obstructs venous and lymphatic drainage, leading to edema of the glans penis. Contributing factors include poor hygiene, infection, or genital trauma. Paraphimosis can also occur *iatrogenically*, due to failure to replace the retracted foreskin over the glans following physical exam, placement of a catheter, or urology procedure. Treatment of paraphimosis centers on *decreasing edema* (mechanical compression, ice, or mannitol-soaked gauze) followed by *manual reduction.* Due to severe pain, a dorsal penile nerve block is commonly performed prior. If manual reduction is unsuccessful, surgical intervention via the *dorsal slit* of the foreskin is indicated to allow for easier reduction. *Failure to treat promptly may result in ischemia and necrosis of the distal penis.*

Fournier's Gangrene

Fournier's gangrene is a rapidly progressing, life-threatening necrotizing fasciitis of the genitals or perineum. It is classified as a polymicrobial infection caused by both aerobic (*E. coli, Klebsiella, Proteus*) and anaerobic (*Bacteroides, Clostridium*) bacteria [27]. Fournier's gangrene is primaril y caused by pathogens entering the body through colorectal, urogenital, or cutaneous routes. Risk factors include *diabetes mellitus*, immunosuppression, obesity, chronic alcohol abuse, tobacco use, peripheral vascular disease, and hypertension. Patients may initially present with constitutional symptoms (fever, malaise), *tenderness and pain of the genital/perineal area*, genital edema, erythema, and warmth of the affected area. As the infection progresses, patients may develop more severe pain, and clinical signs may include *reddish-purple skin discoloration, formation of bullae, crepitus on palpation, and foul-smelling discharge.* The formation of gangrene and symptoms of systemic toxicity (hypotension, tachycardia, altered mental status, and septic shock) occur at the final stage. *Early recognition* and *aggressive management with broad-spectrum IV antibiotics and emergent surgical debridement are critical for establishing*

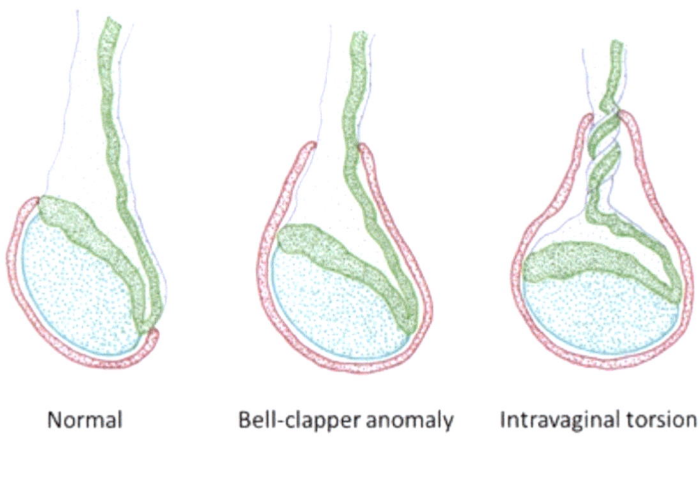

Fig. 44.4 Anatomy of the normal testis, bell clapper deformity, and testicular torsion. In a normal testis, the tunica vaginalis is securely attached to the epididymis, whereas in a bell clapper deformity, this attachment is abnormally high anatomically. This leads to a horizontal lie of the testicle and allows the testicle to freely rotate, increasing the risk of testicular torsion

overall source control and for patient survival, as this is a life-threatening condition. Empiric antibiotics involve triple therapy to cover gram-positive, gram-negative, and anaerobic organisms. The take-home message here is that *Fournier's gangrene is a surgical emergency.*

References

1. Goldenberg L, So A, Fleshner N, Rendon R, Drachenberg D, Elhilali M. The role of 5-alpha reductase inhibitors in prostate pathophysiology: is there an additional advantage to inhibition of type 1 isoenzyme? Can Urol Assoc J. 2009;3(3 Suppl 2):S109–14. https://doi.org/10.5489/cuaj.1114.
2. Adhyam M, Gupta AK. A review on the clinical utility of PSA in cancer prostate. Indian J Surg Oncol. 2012;3(2):120–9. https://doi.org/10.1007/s13193-012-0142-6. Epub 2012 Mar 3
3. Macey MR, Raynor MC. Medical and surgical treatment modalities for lower urinary tract symptoms in the male patient secondary to benign prostatic hyperplasia: a review. Semin Intervent Radiol. 2016;33(3):217–23. https://doi.org/10.1055/s-0036-1586142.
4. Liao J, Zhang X, Chen M, Li D, Tan X, Gu J, Hu S, Chen X. Transurethral resection of the prostate with preservation of the bladder neck decreases postoperative retrograde ejaculation. Wideochir Inne Tech Maloinwazyjne. 2019;14(1):96–101. https://doi.org/10.5114/wiitm.2018.79536. Epub 2018 Nov 14
5. Plante M, Gilling P, Barber N, Bidair M, Anderson P, Sutton M, Aho T, Kramolowsky E, Thomas A, Cowan B, Kaufman RP Jr, Trainer A, Arther A, Badlani G, Desai M, Doumanian L, Te AE, DeGuenther M, Roehrborn C. Symptom relief and anejaculation after aquablation or transurethral resection of the prostate: subgroup analysis from a blinded randomized trial. BJU Int. 2019;123(4):651–60. https://doi.org/10.1111/bju.14426. Epub 2018 Jul 26
6. Placer J, Salvador C, Planas J, Trilla E, Lorente D, Celma A, López MÁ, Morote J. Effects of holmium laser enucleation of the prostate on sexual function. J Endourol. 2015;29(3):332–9. https://doi.org/10.1089/end.2014.0502. Epub 2014 Oct 21
7. Bearelly P, Avellino GJ. The role of benign prostatic hyperplasia treatments in ejaculatory dysfunction. Fertil Steril. 2021;116(3):611–7. https://doi.org/10.1016/j.fertnstert.2021.07.1199.
8. Leslie SW, Sajjad H, Murphy PB. Renal Calculi, Nephrolithiasis. 2024. In: StatPearls [Internet]. Treasure Island (FL): StatPearls Publishing; 2025.
9. Manzoor H, Leslie SW, Saikali SW. Extracorporeal Shockwave Lithotripsy. 2024. In: StatPearls [Internet]. Treasure Island (FL): StatPearls Publishing; 2025.
10. Khanna A, Monga M, Gao T, Yerram N, Sun A, Schold J, et al. PD08-06 ureteral stent placement during shockwave lithotripsy: characterizing guideline discordant practice. J Urol [Internet]. 2018 [cited 2025 Apr 11];199(4S):e163–4. Available from: https://doi.org/10.1016/j.juro.2018.02.452.
11. Sabler IM, Katafigiotis I, Gofrit ON, Duvdevani M. Present indications and techniques of percutaneous nephrolithotomy: what the future holds? Asian J Urol. 2018;5(4):287–94. https://doi.org/10.1016/j.ajur.2018.08.004. Epub 2018 Sep 6
12. Paneque T, Richey J, Abdelrazek A, Morgan K, Fitz-Gerald J, Swinney S, Connelly ZM, Khater N. Current advances in pain regimens for percutaneous nephrolithotomy A comprehensive review. Can Urol Assoc J. 2023;17(11):E388–94. https://doi.org/10.5489/cuaj.8333.
13. Bhojani N, Lingeman JE. In: OMICS Publishing Group, editor. Is there still a need for open/laparoscopic surgery for urinary stones? [Internet]. Clinical Practice; 2012. p. 509–14. https://doi.org/10.2217/cpr.12.47.
14. Mourmouris P, Chiras T, Papatsoris AG. Obstructive uropathy: from etiopathology to therapy. World J Nephrol Urol [Online]. 2014;3.1:1–6. Web. 11 Apr. 2025
15. Zul Khairul Azwadi I, Norhayati MN, Abdullah MS. Percutaneous nephrostomy versus retrograde ureteral stenting for acute upper obstructive uropathy: a systematic review and meta-analysis. Sci Rep. 2021;11(1):6613. https://doi.org/10.1038/s41598-021-86136-y.
16. Gaddam SJ, Bicer F, Chesnut GT. Testicular cancer. 2023. In: StatPearls [Internet]. Treasure Island (FL): StatPearls Publishing; 2025.
17. Testicular cancer risk factors: risks for testicular cancer. In: Testicular Cancer Risk Factors | Risks For Testicular Cancer | American Cancer Society. https://www.cancer.org/cancer/types/testicular-cancer/causes-risks-prevention/risk-factors.html. Accessed 11 Apr 2025.
18. Testicular cancer tumor markers. In: Johns Hopkins Medicine. https://www.hopkinsmedicine.org/health/conditions-and-diseases/testicular-cancer/testicular-cancer-tumor-markers. Accessed 11 Apr 2025
19. Shadab R, Nerli RB, Bidi SR, Ghagane SC. Risk factors for bladder cancer: results of a survey of hospital patients. J Cancer Allied Spec. 2023;9(1):485. https://doi.org/10.37029/jcas.v9i1.485.
20. Cancer of the urinary bladder. In: Cancer Stat Facts: Bladder Cancer. https://seer.cancer.gov/statfacts/html/urinb.html. Accessed 11 Apr 2025.
21. SEER [Internet]. Cancer of the Prostate - Cancer Stat Facts; [cited 2025 Apr 30]. Available from: https://seer.cancer.gov/statfacts/html/prost.html
22. Giri VN, Beebe-Dimmer JL. Familial prostate cancer. Semin Oncol. 2016;43(5):560–5. https://doi.org/10.1053/j.seminoncol.2016.08.001. Epub 2016 Aug 18
23. David MK, Leslie SW. Prostate-specific antigen. 2024. In: StatPearls [Internet]. Treasure Island (FL): StatPearls Publishing; 2025.
24. Wei JT, Barocas D, Carlsson S, et al. Early detection of prostate cancer: AUA/SUO guideline part I: prostate cancer screening. J Urol. 2023;210(1):45–53.
25. Schifano N, Capogrosso P, Boeri L, et al. Medications mostly associated with priapism events: assessment of the 2015–2020 Food and Drug Administration (FDA) pharmacovigilance database entries. Int J Impot Res. 2024;36:50–4. https://doi.org/10.1038/s41443-022-00583-3.
26. Keays M, Rosenberg H. Testicular torsion. CMAJ. 2019;191(28):E792. https://doi.org/10.1503/cmaj.190158.
27. Leslie SW, Foreman J. Fournier gangrene. 2025. In: StatPearls [Internet]. Treasure Island (FL): StatPearls Publishing; 2025.

Pediatric Surgery

45

Susana Fortich, Sarah L. Mims, and Ravi S. Radhakrishnan

Introduction

Pediatric surgery is a specialty that covers a wide range of surgical conditions, beginning with the prenatal period and continuing through young adulthood. This varied patient population commits pediatric surgeons to deal not only with different pathophysiologies but also conditions covering all major organ systems. This chapter includes some of the most common pediatric conditions treated by pediatric surgeons, as well as important pre- and postoperative management considerations for the allied health professional.

Head and Neck Lesions

Thyroglossal Duct Cyst

The thyroid gland develops as it descends into the neck. During this migration, the middle portion of the gland remains connected to the foramen cecum at the tongue's base via the thyroglossal duct. This duct typically atrophies by the tenth week of gestation, but incomplete obliteration can lead to the formation of thyroglossal duct cysts [1]. Although found anywhere between the hyoid bone and the thyroid gland, the cysts' most common location is closer to the hyoid bone. It typically appears as a small midline mass, although it can also be seen just lateral to the midline [1]. It might also become inflamed and enlarged, occasionally draining. Active infections should be treated with antibiotics before considering surgical intervention [2]. When performed, the Sistrunk procedure is the gold standard operation for thyroglossal duct cysts [3]. Postoperatively, the area should be monitored for increased swelling and postoperative hematoma formation, given the extent of dissection. The risk of recurrence is 40–50% if the entire cyst and hyoid bone are not removed.

Branchial Cleft Remnants

Branchial cleft remnants present as lateral neck masses. These remnants result from the failure of embryological structures in the head and neck to regress. The location of the remnant typically dictates not only its origin but also the required surgical intervention. Clinical presentations of these remnants include mucinous drainage from a fistula or sinus tract, as well as localized infection of a cystic mass [4]. First branchial cleft remnants manifest as fistulas or masses at the front or back of the ear or in the upper neck near the mandible. An ENT specialist may need to be involved in excising these remnants, as they may traverse through the parotid gland. Second branchial cleft remnants, the most common type, appear along the anterior border of the sternocleidomastoid muscle in its upper third. Third branchial cleft remnants typically lack a fistula or sinus tract and present as a cyst or mass near the suprasternal notch, which can descend into the mediastinum. Complete excision of the sinus tract, fistula, or mass is crucial to reduce recurrence risk [4].

Diaphragmatic Conditions

Congenital Diaphragmatic Hernia

Congenital diaphragmatic hernia (CDH) is a rare birth defect characterized by incomplete closure of the diaphragm and herniation of fetal abdominal organs into the chest that results in pulmonary hypoplasia, postnatal pul-

S. Fortich
Department of Surgery, University of Texas Medical Branch, Galveston, TX, USA

S. L. Mims · R. S. Radhakrishnan (✉)
Division of Pediatric Surgery, Department of Surgery, University of Texas Medical Branch, Galveston, TX, USA
e-mail: rsradhak@utmb.edu

S. Atallah, J. Dragoljevic (eds.), *Fundamentals of Surgery for Physician Assistants*,
https://doi.org/10.1007/978-3-032-21069-2_45

monary hypertension owing to vascular remodeling, and cardiac dysfunction. This condition is usually diagnosed prenatally on ultrasound. Defects can be detected as early as 15 weeks of gestation. The overall incidence of CDH is 1 in 2000–5000 live births, with left-sided defects being more common. Low- and middle-income regions have a mortality ranging from 40% to 100%. This is associated directly with the severity of cardiopulmonary pathophysiology [5]. Predictors like the lung-to-head circumference ratio (LHR) of less than 1.4, along with the position of the liver, are strong indicators of poorer prognosis and survival [6], along with the need for ECMO. Fetal MRI is currently being utilized at some centers to assess fetal lung volume, providing an observed versus expected lung volume that can aid in counseling prenatally.

Clinical Presentation: Infants with known CDH should be delivered in hospitals equipped to provide advanced neonatal care. Initially, the patient may remain stable during what is known as the "honeymoon period," but after several hours, decompensation will begin. Symptoms include respiratory distress with retractions, grunting, dyspnea, and cyanosis. Bowel sounds may be auscultated over the chest, along with diminished breath sounds. Mediastinal shift is also common and may displace heart sounds. Chest radiography will show bowel loops in the thoracic cavity.

The mortality rate in CDH is linked to the severity of pulmonary hypoplasia and pulmonary hypertension. Due to the presence of bowel in the thoracic cavity and mediastinal shift, neither lung can develop properly, resulting in both hypoplasia and pulmonary hypertension. Current treatment focuses on respiratory support and managing the often-refractory pulmonary hypertension.

Patients should be intubated immediately after delivery and an orogastric tube placed to suction for gastric decompression. Practitioners should take care to avoid excess mean airway pressure, which can lead to barotrauma and compromise venous return to the heart. Gentle ventilation with permissive hypercapnia has resulted in improved survival [7] with the goal of pH greater than 7.2. Inhaled nitric oxide can be utilized for its pulmonary vasodilation effects. Medications such as sildenafil, a phosphodiesterase 5 inhibitor, or Flolan, a prostaglandin, can be used as an adjunct therapy for the management of pulmonary hypertension. Once the patient has stabilized, infants not requiring utilization of ECMO can undergo surgical repair of the defect. The exact timing of repair remains controversial, but it can be performed within the first 24 h after birth in many cases. The preferred approach for open repair is through a subcostal incision with reduction of viscera into the abdominal cavity and repair of the defect. While thoracoscopic repair of CDH has gained popularity in recent years, there is little research available on long-term outcomes and benefits. Infants requiring ECMO need a delay in repair, which is often performed while weaning off ECMO or even after decannulation. In patients repaired on ECMO, the major consideration is postoperative bleeding due to the use of anticoagulation.

Long-term considerations for patients born with CDH can vary and depend on multiple factors, such as the severity of the disease and the need for ECMO support at any time during their hospitalization. Some children may develop chronic respiratory dysfunction and pulmonary hypertension, as well as developmental delays, seizures, and hearing loss. Additionally, children are at risk for gastroesophageal reflux, chest wall deformities, and chronic lung diseases such as asthma and scoliosis. All children born with CDH should undergo brain imaging prior to discharge to establish their baseline status, as well as hearing assessment screening.

Respiratory System Conditions

Congenital Pulmonary Airway Malformation

Congenital Pulmonary Airway Malformations (CPAM) are multicystic lesions, whether microcystic or macrocystic, that replace normal lung tissue. These lesions are connected to the tracheobronchial tree and fed via the pulmonary blood supply. There is a risk of malignancy during the patient's lifetime, which is why resection is recommended [8]. The Stocker classification is used to differentiate between the various subtypes of CPAM. Type 1 lesions are the most common, accounting for approximately 75% of cases. These lesions consist of a small number of larger cysts, usually measuring 2–10 cm. Type 2 lesions comprise numerous smaller cysts, typically less than 1 cm in size. Type 3 lesions are rare and present with mediastinal shift and hydrops, exhibiting a poor prognosis despite the small size of the cysts, which are typically only a few millimeters in diameter.

CPAMs are often diagnosed prenatally via ultrasound and may undergo changes throughout the pregnancy. Many lesions will show some degree of regression, especially in the third trimester, although some may continue to grow during the pregnancy. Expectant management is used in cases where the size is stable and not causing other symptoms in the fetus. In cases with large lesions or in patients with hydrops, a single course of betamethasone has been shown to promote regression or size reduction, as well as resolve hydrops when present [9].

Upon delivery, all patients with known CPAM should be evaluated with chest radiographs. These may not always reveal the lesion, but they can rule out mediastinal shift and air trapping. Most infants are asymptomatic at birth and do not require emergent intervention. Close follow-up with further imaging closer to the time of surgical intervention is recommended.

Resection is recommended based on the risk of malignancy and the increased risk of infection in the affected lobe. Most surgeons perform surgery within the first year of life either via open thoracotomy or utilizing a thoracoscopic technique. After surgery, the patient will continue to develop new alveolar units, and overall lung capacity should not be affected.

Pulmonary Sequestration

Bronchopulmonary sequestration (BPS) differentiates itself from CPAM as there is no connection to the tracheobronchial tree, and the lesion is fed via an aberrant systemic artery. There are two types of BPS, intralobar and extralobar, which are differentiated by their location within the pleura. An intralobar sequestration is contained within normal lung parenchyma, while extralobar sequestration is encased by its own pleura. As there is no connection to the tracheobronchial tree, these cysts do not enlarge or cause pneumothoracies. The aberrant blood supply to these lesions can cause left to right shunting in infants, which can increase their risk for high output heart failure.

BPS, like CPAM, can be seen on prenatal imaging, and these patients are also at risk for hydrops as well as pleural effusions. Initial workup is similar, including chest radiographs and ultrasound with Doppler to evaluate for the arterial blood supply. Tomography and MRI can also be utilized for better anatomy delineation and surgical planning, but are typically not needed emergently.

Alimentary Tract Conditions

Esophageal Atresia and Tracheoesophageal Fistula

Esophageal atresia (EA) is a congenital disruption in esophageal development leading to discontinuity of the esophagus with proximal esophageal obstruction. EA may be seen with or without a tracheoesophageal fistula (TEF), which is a pathologic communication between the esophagus and trachea. The incidence of EA/TEF is 1 out of 1500–5000 live births [10]. There are five anatomical variants of EA/TEF that may be present with the Type C lesion (EA with distal TEF), seen most commonly.

Presentation after delivery often involves excessive salivation, coughing, or choking during feeds. Placement of an orogastric tube should be attempted; coiling at the thoracic inlet is a defining characteristic of EA with or without TEF. Neonates with Type C EA/TEF, where there is proximal EA with distal TEF, may present with acute gastric distention that can compromise respiratory status, potentially leading to respiratory failure. These neonates may require emergent gastric decompression, with continuous suction on the replogle tube, to support respiratory function. Initial imaging may show an absence of distal bowel gas, raising suspicion for pure EA (Type A), or it may show the presence of distal bowel gas indicative of TEF. Patients also benefit from elevation of the head of the bed and prone positioning to help prevent aspiration. Intubation and positive airway pressure should be avoided, as air could cross the TEF into the GI tract, causing severe gastric distention. Worsening gastric distention may then deteriorate respiratory status and complicate ventilation.

Surgical Considerations and Approach: All patients with TEF/EA should undergo a full VACTERL workup prior to surgery. A cardiac ECHO is of utmost importance prior to any surgical procedure. Patients should ideally undergo rigid bronchoscopy at the beginning of the procedure. This allows for the evaluation of tracheomalacia as well as the identification of the location of the fistula. Once bronchoscopy is completed, the patient should be intubated past the fistula if possible. Definitive treatment involves surgical repair, with the approach depending on the type of anomaly. For Type A–D (non-H-type), a right extra-pleural thoracotomy with primary repair is performed, while Type E (H-type) requires a right cervical approach due to its typical location near the thoracic inlet. General measures include separating the trachea and esophagus, ligating the fistula, and performing a primary anastomosis for atresia. In cases of long-gap atresia (greater than two vertebral bodies), management may involve placing a temporary gastrostomy tube and delaying repair for 2–3 months to allow esophageal growth. Internal or external traction may also be used to reapproximate the gap until delayed repair is feasible. If these measures fail, intestinal interposition or gastric transposition may be necessary. Long-gap esophageal atresia is the most common indication for esophageal replacement in pediatric patients, with caustic stricture being the second most common [11].

Long-term Outcomes: Mortality and morbidity with TEF and EA are linked to the concomitant anomalies associated with the disease process. These anomalies included cardiac, renal anomalies, and chromosomal disorders. Common complications from surgery include esophageal dysmotility, esophageal reflux, anastomotic leak, stricture, and tracheomalacia.

Hypertrophic Pyloric Stenosis

Hypertrophic pyloric stenosis (HPS) is a disease seen typically between 2 and 8 weeks of age. The incidence ranges from 1 in 300–900 live births, with boys affected more often than girls. Firstborn males have the highest risk. Hypertrophy of the circular muscle of the pylorus causes a gastric outlet obstruction, which progressively worsens. The typical presentation is a progressive worsening of nonbilious emesis over days to weeks that becomes projectile in nature as symptoms progress. Previously, students and practitioners were taught to palpate the pyloric "olive." Although it is pathognomonic for HPS, the "olive" is typically only palpable in severely lethargic infants or those under anesthesia.

Infants suspected of having HPS typically undergo ultrasound evaluation. On ultrasound, a pyloric muscle thickness greater than 3–4 mm and a length exceeding 14–18 mm, along with the inability of gastric contents to pass through the pylorus, is diagnostic for HPS. While ultrasound has become the preferred method for most institutions, an upper GI contrast study remains the gold standard diagnostic test. Once confirmed with ultrasound or upper GI series, preoperative resuscitation is the primary consideration.

Infants experiencing pyloric stenosis often present with electrolyte abnormalities, mainly metabolic alkalosis, which must be corrected prior to operative intervention. With progressive emesis, patients present with a loss of hydrochloric acid, which leads to hypokalemia, hypochloremia, and dehydration. In response, carbon dioxide and water are converted into hydrogen and bicarbonate ions; the final metabolic disturbance is a hypochloremic hypokalemic metabolic alkalosis. This requires aggressive IV fluids to increase urine output and restore acid–base balance. Infants should initially receive a bolus of 20 cc/kg of normal saline and then further resuscitation based on urine output and lab values.

To proceed with surgery, serum bicarbonate and chloride levels must be normalized. If left uncorrected, once the patient is under anesthesia, they risk postoperative apnea due to decreased respiratory drive from low carbon dioxide levels. HPS itself is not a surgical emergency, and lab correction is the primary concern. Depending on your institution, bicarbonate and chloride lab values should be normalized to less than 30 mEq/L and greater than 95 mEq/L, respectively.

The surgical approach involves a pyloromyotomy (Ramstedt procedure) by which the surgeon incises the thickened pyloric musculature to relieve the pyloric channel obstruction, which can be performed open or laparoscopically. Complications of the pyloromyotomy include full-thickness mucosal perforation or inadequate pyloromyotomy. Postoperatively, feeding is begun within 6 h of surgery. Small-volume emesis is common postoperatively and is usually self-limited. If emesis persists beyond 7–14 days, an upper GI series may be necessary to evaluate for incomplete pyloromyotomy.

Intestinal Atresia

Intestinal atresia presents as the failure of the intestinal lumen to be in complete continuity. This can include complete separation of the intestinal segments as well as obstructive intestinal webs. Intestinal atresia presents with obstructive bowel symptoms, including vomiting and abdominal distention.

Duodenal atresia is caused by failure of the duodenum to recanalize during development. Concern for duodenal atresia can be seen on prenatal imaging as an enlarged stomach bubble or double bubble with an enlarged stomach and the first portion of the duodenum. Duodenal atresia is associated with several other conditions and prenatal findings, including prematurity, trisomy 21, intestinal malrotation, biliary atresia, as well as maternal polyhydramnios [12]. Postnatal imaging reveals the classic double bubble sign, especially if obtained prior to gastric decompression. Surgery for duodenal atresia is typically not emergent due to the ability to adequately decompress the obstruction via an orogastric tube. Surgical treatment is done with a duodenoduodenostomy.

Jejunal-ileal atresia is the most common type of intestinal atresia. It is believed to be the result of intra-uterine vascular compromise, leading to the intestine closing off as a protective measure. Infants typically present with obstructive symptoms, including bilious emesis and progressive abdominal distension as the proximal intestine fills with air and bowel contents. Radiographs show large, distended bowel loops with no air in the rectum. During surgical repair, the primary goal is to achieve bowel continuity while also preserving as much bowel length as possible, since infants with jejunal-ileal atresia are at risk of short gut syndrome. Similar to the repair of duodenal atresia, the distal intestine should be assessed for additional atretic segments, which can occur in 10–15% of these patients' cases.

Intestinal Malrotation and Midgut Volvulus

During normal embryologic development, the midgut undergoes a series of rotations and fixations to achieve normal anatomic positioning within the abdominal cavity. By the sixth week of gestation, the midgut elongates and herniates into the umbilical cord, initiating a 270-degree counterclockwise rotation around the superior mesenteric artery (SMA). This rotation involves both the duodenojejunal and cecocolic loops and progresses through three key stages: initial bowel herniation and rotation (week 6), return of the midgut into the abdominal cavity (week 10), and mesenteric fixation. Fixation of the mesentery ensures stability and prevents abnormal movement or rotation of the gut. Intestinal malrotation arises when this normal process is disrupted, leading to incomplete or improper rotation and fixation of the midgut. Despite the generally constant positions of the pylorus and splenic flexure, malrotation can result in abnormal positioning of other intestinal structures and the formation of

Ladd's bands—fibrous attachments that may obstruct the duodenum [13].

Clinical presentation could range from chronic abdominal pain, esophageal reflux, poor feeding tolerance, or be completely asymptomatic to extremis with signs of shock, requiring aggressive resuscitation as well as prompt surgical intervention due to midgut volvulus. Midgut volvulus is a surgical emergency, as there will be progressive intestinal ischemia with worsening acidosis despite resuscitation attempts.

The diagnosis of intestinal malrotation typically involves imaging studies, with an upper gastrointestinal (GI) series being the gold standard in stable patients. In malrotation, the duodenum fails to cross the midline and is displaced to the right of the abdomen. Ultrasound may reveal abnormal vascular anatomy, such as the superior mesenteric vein (SMV) positioned to the left or anterior to the superior mesenteric artery (SMA). In cases of volvulus, characteristic findings include the "bird's beak" sign, indicating abrupt narrowing of the bowel, a mesenteric "whirl" sign caused by twisting of the mesentery, and a "double-bubble" appearance. If the patient is unstable, imaging is deferred, and immediate surgical intervention is required.

Surgical correction of intestinal malrotation is done by performing the Ladd's procedure. This surgery involves lysing all of Ladd's bands, straightening the duodenum, widening the mesentery, and appendectomy. Postoperatively, patients often experience prolonged ileus, which can take up to a week or more for bowel function to return. Patients who presented with midgut volvulus, requiring extensive resection, may develop short bowel syndrome.

Necrotizing Enterocolitis

Necrotizing enterocolitis (NEC) is primarily a disease of neonates and is the most common gastrointestinal surgical emergency in this population. The most significant risk factor for NEC is prematurity. NEC usually occurs within the first few days of life, coinciding with the start of enteral feeding. Infants receiving formula are also at an increased risk for NEC compared to those who are breastfed. The recent increase in the use of donor breast milk for infants with unavailable maternal breast milk has helped reduce the incidence of NEC.

The presentation of NEC can vary from patient to patient. Patients may exhibit acute distention, abdominal tenderness, and abdominal wall cellulitis, along with occult blood in the stool. Other less specific signs include temperature instability and increased episodes of apnea or bradycardia. As NEC worsens, sepsis, coagulopathy, and subsequent shock become evident. Pneumatosis intestinalis is a pathognomonic radiological finding in NEC, but patients may also present with portal venous gas, fixed loops of intestine, or free air. The modified Bell's staging criteria are utilized to classify the severity of NEC and help drive medical and surgical intervention.

Initial management of NEC consists of gastric decompression, resuscitation with IV fluids, and broad-spectrum antibiotics. Although the majority of NEC cases can be managed medically, surgical intervention is necessary in some cases. Absolute indication for surgery remains free air on plain radiographs. Relative indications for surgery included clinical deterioration despite medical management, persistent acidosis, and a fixed loop of intestine on radiography. Depending on weight at the time of the NEC episode, initial surgical intervention may involve peritoneal drain placement vs. laparotomy. Although not always a definitive therapy, peritoneal drain placement can improve abdominal distention and ventilation and, in patients less than 1 kg, may be sufficient. It is also believed to prevent further progression of sepsis, allowing time for medical management to take effect. While not definitive in most cases, some infants respond very positively to drain placement and do not require further surgical intervention. If no improvement is seen within 24–72 h after drain placement, exploratory laparotomy is indicated for more definitive surgery. If the infant is larger at the time of surgery (typically over 1 kg), exploratory laparotomy utilizing damage control principles is the preferred procedure, aiming to resect all nonviable intestines while preserving maximum intestinal length [14].

Following both medical and surgical treatment of NEC, patients are at risk for intestinal strictures. Patients with episodes of NEC should have a contrast enema approximately 6 weeks post-NEC. This procedure evaluates the colon for strictures, which are most commonly found at the splenic flexure but can occur anywhere in the colon. Despite advancements in medical and surgical care, NEC remains the leading cause of short gut syndrome, and the mortality rate for surgical NEC varies from 10% to 50%.

Hirschsprung Disease

This disease is characterized by an absence of ganglion cells in the myenteric (Auerbach) and submucosal (Meissner) plexus in the distal colon/rectum [15]. It occurs in 1 in 5000 live births, with boys being affected four times more than girls, with an increased risk in the presence of the disease in the family history. Of these patients, 3–5% have Down syndrome.

Aganglionosis begins at the anorectal or dentate line. In approximately 80% of cases, the transition to normal colon occurs in the rectosigmoid colon [15], 17% in the splenic or transverse colon, and 8% in the small intestine (involving the entire colon). The area between the dilated and contracted segments is referred to as the transition zone. Here, ganglion cells begin to appear, but in reduced numbers.

Most infants (>90%) present with abdominal distention and bilious vomiting, along with failure to pass meconium within the first 24 h of life. Those with undiagnosed Hirschsprung disease may present later in life with a persistent history of abdominal distention and constipation. Enterocolitis is the leading cause of death in patients with untreated Hirschsprung disease and can manifest with diarrhea alternating with periods of constipation, as well as symptoms such as abdominal distention, fever, hematochezia, peritonitis, shock, and potential death.

The initial diagnostic imaging study in a newborn is a contrast enema, with a subsequent rectal biopsy proximal to the dentate line serving as the gold standard. Absent ganglia, hypertrophied nerve trunks, and robust immunostaining for acetylcholinesterase are the histopathologic criteria. Calretinin immunostaining has now become a standard adjunct histologic study for the diagnosis of Hirschsprung disease. Once confirmed, the primary treatment is a pull-through procedure, which involves bringing the normally innervated bowel down to the anus while preserving normal sphincter function. In some cases, a colostomy may be necessary in cases of severe enterocolitis, perforation, malnutrition, or massively dilated proximal bowel.

Postoperatively, daily or weekly dilations are typically required for a few weeks. Normal temporary changes include increased stool frequency, perineal excoriation, streaks of blood in the stool, crying with defecation, and fecal soiling, all of which are very common and resolve with close postoperative follow-up.

Anorectal Malformation

Anorectal malformations are common anomalies observed in neonates. The reported incidence ranges between 1:3300 and 1:5000 live births. They vary in severity from mild anal stenosis to complete caudal regression [16]. The most common anorectal defect is an imperforate anus with a fistula between the distal colon and bulbar urethra in boys or the vestibule of the introitus in girls.

An anatomic classification of anorectal anomalies is based on the fistula present in the rectum. Boys can have recto-perineal, recto-bulbar urethra, recto-prostatic urethra, or recto-bladder neck fistulas or no fistula. Girls can have recto-perineal or recto-vestibular fistulas, no fistula, or a cloacal anomaly. In the past, these defects were classified as low, intermediate, or high in relationship to the levator ani musculature, but modern terminology uses the anatomic classification.

Rectal atresia, a rare anomaly associated with trisomy 21, is characterized by the lumen of the rectum being completely or partially interrupted, with the upper rectum being dilated and the lower rectum consisting of a small anal canal. A cloaca is defined as a defect in which the rectum, vagina, and urethra all fuse to form a single common channel that empties into the perineum. The severity of this lesion is characterized by the length of the common channel, with 3 cm being the cutoff between short and long defects. On physical exam, a single orifice in the perineum indicates a cloaca, which occurs only in females. Anorectal malformations often coexist with other lesions, and the VACTERL association must be considered during evaluation.

A newborn with a perineal or vestibular fistula may undergo a primary single-stage repair without colostomy. For anal stenosis, where the anal opening is normally positioned, serial dilation alone is usually sufficient. Dilations are performed daily, with gradual size increases over time. If the anal opening is anterior to the external sphincter (i.e., rectoperineal fistula), with a small distance between the opening and the center of the external sphincter, and the perineal body remains intact, a cut-back anoplasty or limited posterior sagittal anorectoplasty is indicated to restore the anal opening to its normal position within the center of the sphincter muscles, including reconstruction of the perineal body. The posterior sagittal anorectoplasty is the procedure of choice for the vast majority of anorectal malformations, with total urogenital mobilization added for cloacal anomalies.

Complications of anorectal malformations are related to their associated anomalies. Social fecal continence is the primary goal concerning the correction of the defect. Prognostic factors for continence include the level of the rectum and whether the sacrum is normal. In general, postoperative outcomes of social continence range from 75% to 99% and are related to how proximal the fistula is in relation to the sphincter mechanism. A bowel management program that combines oral stool softeners and laxatives, along with close outpatient follow-up, is essential to reduce the frequency of soiling and to enhance the quality of life for these patients.

Intussusception

Intussusception refers to the telescoping of the intestine into itself. While it can occur anywhere in the intestine, it is most commonly observed in the ileocolic region, where the distal ileum telescopes into the cecum with the ileocecal valve or mesenteric lymph nodes serving as the lead point [17]. Intussusception is often linked to a recent episode of gastroenteritis, but it may also occur following recent upper respiratory infections or the administration of the rotavirus vaccine. Typically, there is no identifiable anatomic lead point in younger children, and the condition is usually considered idiopathic. In older children, however, there is a higher incidence of a pathological lead point, most commonly a Meckel's diverticulum or a tumor, which necessitates further investigation and workup.

The presentation of intussusception includes severe, intermittent abdominal pain, typically occurring in children aged 3 months to 3 years. The incidence after the age of 2 years is less than 25%. Patients often bring their legs up to their abdomen during pain episodes. They may also experience vomiting and the passage of bloody, mucoid stools (currant jelly), along with a palpable abdominal mass, typically located in the right lower abdomen. The workup for intussusception includes an abdominal ultrasound, which can reveal the characteristic "target sign" of the intussuscepted intestine [17]. Following ultrasound findings consistent with intussusception, reduction via an enema using water-soluble contrast or air is the recommended therapy of choice.

Contraindications for air enema reduction include peritonitis, hemodynamic instability, and small bowel intussusception. Pediatric surgery should always be readily available for all patients undergoing enema reduction due to the risk of perforation. Enema reduction is successful in approximately 80% of cases, and if an attempt is unsuccessful, additional attempts can be made after a few hours with a high rate of success. Recurrence of intussusception is about 10% and typically occurs within the first 24 h after reduction. Patients with successful reduction may be discharged after a brief monitoring period in the emergency room, without needing admission. In cases where radiological intervention fails or is contraindicated, surgical intervention can be used to reduce the intussusception. This may be performed through either an open or laparoscopic approach, with reduction occurring in a retrograde manner. Bowel viability should be assessed once reduction is complete, and the bowel should be examined for any lead point. Rarely, bowel resection is necessary if the intussusception cannot be reduced, if the bowel is found to be non-viable, or to remove any lead point identified during visualization.

Hepatopancreaticobiliary Conditions

Extrahepatic Biliary Atresia

Biliary atresia (BA) is a rare disease in neonates that is characterized by the inflammatory obliteration of the extrahepatic bile ducts. There is marked variation in the incidence of BA, ranging from about 1 in 5–10,000 live births in Asia to about 1 in 15–20,000 in mainland Europe, England and Wales, and North America. It may be associated with other congenital malformations, such as splenic abnormalities (e.g., asplenia and polysplenia), absence of the inferior vena cava (IVC), cardiac anomalies, heterotaxy syndromes, and intestinal malrotation [18]. The exact mechanisms of BA are unknown, and the disease is progressive.

The disease is classified based on the level of the most proximal biliary obstruction. Type 1 BA has patency to the level of the common bile duct (CBD); type 2 has patency to the level of the common hepatic duct; and type 3, which accounts for more than 90% of cases, involves the left and right hepatic ducts at the level of the porta hepatis. This classification aids in differentiating between correctable BA and other types. Correctable BA requires that patent hepatic ducts exist to the porta hepatis.

Infants typically present shortly after birth with jaundice, pale stools, and dark urine. Advanced disease may present with failure to thrive, hepatomegaly, and ascites due to liver cirrhosis. If jaundice persists beyond 14 days of life in a term infant, an evaluation for liver disease should be initiated. This evaluation includes determining direct or conjugated bilirubin levels, which will be elevated (>2.0 mg/dL) in cases of liver disease. Other exclusionary studies include serologic testing for toxoplasmosis, rubella, cytomegalovirus, herpes (TORCH), and hepatitis B and C infections, as well as α1-antitrypsin deficiency and cystic fibrosis. Additionally, metabolic disorders such as galactosemia and tyrosinemia, along with endocrine abnormalities, must also be ruled out.

The gallbladder may be atrophic or absent, and intrahepatic ducts may also be notably absent on ultrasound evaluation. Hepatobiliary iminodiacetic acid (HIDA) scintigraphy, magnetic resonance cholangiopancreatography (MRCP), and endoscopic retrograde cholangiopancreatography (ERCP) are utilized with varying success. The timing of Kasai portoenterostomy has been shown to influence postoperative outcomes. Liver biopsy aids in supporting the diagnosis of BA. Optimal timing for the operation is typically before 60 days of life, where the 2-year survival rate with the native liver is approximately 60%. If the operative intervention is performed after 90 days of life, this number drops to about 40%.

Once a diagnosis is suspected, operative exploration with intraoperative cholangiography is indicated; the absence of contrast drainage into the duodenum confirms the diagnosis. If BA is confirmed, the surgical procedure of choice is hepatoportoenterostomy (Kasai procedure). Antibiotics are also continued postoperatively due to the high risk of cholangitis (45–60%), which arises from the ease with which intestinal bacteria can ascend and colonize the bile ducts. Unfortunately, if the Kasai procedure fails to reestablish bile flow and liver failure or cirrhosis develops, liver transplantation becomes necessary.

Even with an initially successful Kasai hepatoportoenterostomy, BA may continue to progress in more than 70% of infants who undergo the procedure. The rate at which the disease progresses, as evidenced by cirrhosis and portal hypertension, is variable but may be expedited by recurrent cholangitis. However, it is estimated that 80% of those who have successfully undergone a Kasai procedure can live up to 10 years before requiring liver transplantation. Among those infants who undergo transplantation, outcomes are generally positive, with 10-year graft survival and overall patient survival rates of 73% and 86%, respectively.

Choledochal Cyst

Choledochal cysts (CC) are cystic dilations of the CBD. CCs occur more frequently in Asian versus Western populations, with an incidence of 1 in 13,000 versus 1 in 150,000 people [19], respectively, and it has a female-to-male ratio of 3–4:1. These cysts are classified based on their location, and their frequency varies. The Todani classification classifies CCs as follows: type I CCs (50–80%) are congenital cystic dilations of the CBD, type II (2%) cysts are congenital diverticulum of the extrahepatic biliary tree with a narrow neck, type III (1.4–4.5%) cysts are congenital choledochoceles with dilation of the intraduodenal portion of the CBD, type IV (15–35%) involves both intrahepatic and extrahepatic bile ducts, and type V, or Caroli's disease (20%), is confined to the intrahepatic ducts only [19]. Choledochal cysts can be associated with various congenital anomalies, including duodenal and colonic atresia, imperforate anus, pancreatic arteriovenous malformation, and pancreatic divisum. Additionally, choledochal cysts are considered premalignant lesions.

The pathogenesis of choledochal cysts is largely unknown; however, pancreaticobiliary malunion, where the pancreatic duct and CBD join with a long common channel (>6 mm) before entering the duodenum, is observed in many cases.

The classic triad of jaundice, a palpable right upper quadrant mass, and abdominal pain is present in less than 20% of patients, although 85% show at least two of these symptoms. Infants typically present with obstructive jaundice and an abdominal mass, while older children may experience chronic intermittent pain, fever, and jaundice. Complications such as cholangitis and pancreatitis can occur, as well as bile peritonitis secondary to cyst rupture. Abdominal ultrasound reveals a cystic, enlarged ductal structure that is distinct from the gallbladder. A HIDA scan may show initially absent filling of the cyst, followed by delayed uptake and emptying into the duodenum. MRCP can further clarify the entire biliary system and the pancreatic head. Prompt surgical excision of the cysts, combined with Roux-en-Y hepaticojejunostomy, is recommended. Postoperative anastomotic strictures are common complications and likely result from chronic intrahepatic cholelithiasis and recurrent cholangitis.

Abdominal Wall Defects

Abdominal wall defects occur during normal fetal development when the midgut herniates outward through the abdominal wall at the umbilical ring. By the 11th week of gestation, the midgut that has herniated outward returns to the abdominal cavity and undergoes rotation, fixation, and closure of the umbilical ring. If this process fails to occur, it results in anterior abdominal wall defects, which are generally classified as either an omphalocele or gastroschisis, depending on the location of the defect, as well as an anomaly of intestinal rotation.

Omphalocele is a central defect occurring through the umbilical cord, typically larger than 4 cm and covered by a membranous sac. It is frequently associated with chromosomal anomalies like trisomy 13, 15, 18, and syndromes like Beckwith-Wiedemann [20]. Management depends on defect size, with small defects managed with primary closure, while larger defects may require staged closure, prosthetic patches, or the "paint and wait" method for epithelialization.

Gastroschisis is a congenital malformation characterized by visceral herniation, usually through a right-sided abdominal wall defect, to an intact umbilical cord and not covered by a membrane [21], leading to intestinal thickening and inflammation. It is rarely associated with anomalies except for intestinal atresia (15%). Immediate postnatal management includes placing the infant in a bowel bag to prevent fluid loss. Reduction of the abdominal contents may be done primarily or gradually via a ringed silo. Sutureless closure has gained popularity, reducing the need for general anesthesia. Gastroschisis patients face prolonged ileus, an increased risk of NEC (20%), and require extended NICU stays for feeding advancement.

Hernias

Hernia repair is one of the most frequently performed surgical procedures in pediatric surgery. The most common types of hernias encountered in pediatric patients are inguinal and umbilical hernias. Inguinal hernias require repair of the defect when detected, while umbilical hernias may close on their own.

Inguinal hernias require surgical repair, as they do not close spontaneously. They are congenital in nature, resulting from failure of the processus vaginalis to close [22]. The incidence is 3–5% in term infants and higher (9–11%) in premature infants, with right-sided hernias being most common [22]. Boys are six times more likely to be affected than girls. Diagnosis is clinical, with imaging rarely needed unless testicular torsion or epididymitis is suspected. The primary concern is incarceration and strangulation, which should be discussed with parents. While early repair is typically recommended, premature infants may have delayed surgery due to anesthesia risks. If a hernia is incarcerated, reduction is attempted first, followed by delayed surgery after 24–48 h to allow edema resolution. An incarcerated or strangulated hernia is a surgical emergency. Surgical options include open repair or laparoscopic closure, with higher recurrence rates occurring in laparoscopic repairs and higher rates of testicular complications occurring in open repairs.

Umbilical hernias often close spontaneously, with around 80% resolving by age 5. If a hernia persists beyond age 4–5, closure is unlikely, and repair is considered. Earlier intervention is recommended for defects larger than 2 cm or if the defect leads to poor cosmesis. Incarceration is rare, but parents should be educated on warning signs.

Pediatric Solid Tumors

While solid tumors detected at early stages of the disease tend to respond well, those diagnosed at advanced stages remain challenging to cure, despite multiple therapeutic options available. The latest discoveries in cancer biology and ongoing clinical trials are expected to have the greatest impact on children with advanced disease.

Neuroblastoma

Neuroblastoma is the most common extracranial solid tumor in infants and children, representing 8–10% of pediatric cancers and 15% of cancer-related deaths. The median age at diagnosis is 22 months, with 30% of cases occurring within the first year of life. This malignant tumor originates from neural crest cells and primarily affects the sympathetic nervous system, most commonly occurring in the abdomen (65%), followed by the chest, neck, and pelvis [23].

Clinically, neuroblastoma often presents as a painless abdominal mass, which is typically detected when parents notice a firm, non-tender swelling. Thoracic tumors are usually discovered incidentally on chest radiographs obtained for unrelated respiratory symptoms. Pelvic masses may cause constipation or bladder dysfunction due to compression effects, while neck tumors can lead to Horner syndrome in about 15% of cases. When the tumor extends into the spinal canal, patients may develop neurological deficits that can rapidly progress to paralysis. Bone marrow involvement can result in anemia, bruising, bone pain, and pathologic fractures. Metastatic disease may manifest as periorbital swelling and proptosis (raccoon eyes) or as blue subcutaneous nodules, also known as blueberry muffin syndrome. Some cases present with paraneoplastic syndromes, including intractable diarrhea due to vasoactive intestinal peptide secretion (VIP), encephalomyelitis, neuropathy, or opsoclonus-myoclonus syndrome, which is characterized by rapid eye movements and involuntary limb spasms.

The genetic profile of neuroblastoma influences prognosis. Whole chromosome gains, leading to hyperdiploidy, are associated with better outcomes, whereas segmental chromosomal aberrations, including *MYCN* amplification and deletions of chromosome 1p36 and 11q, correlate with more aggressive disease. *MYCN* amplification, present in 25% of cases, is found in 30–40% of advanced-stage tumors but only in 5% of localized or stage 4S cases. Deletion of 1p36 occurs in approximately 70% of MYCN-amplified, high-risk neuroblastomas and is linked to poor prognosis. Deletions of chromosome 11q, seen in 15–22% of cases, also indicate unfavorable outcomes, while whole chromosome 17 gain is associated with better survival rates.

Diagnosis relies on measuring urinary catecholamines and their metabolites, such as dopamine, vanillylmandelic acid, and homovanillic acid. Elevated serum levels of lactate dehydrogenase, ferritin, and neuron-specific enolase serve as nonspecific tumor biomarkers. Imaging plays a crucial role, with CT scans often revealing characteristic tumor calcifications. MRI is useful for assessing spinal cord involvement, while ^{131}I-metaiodobenzylguanidine (MIBG) scanning helps detect metastases and monitor treatment response. Histologically, neuroblastoma is characterized by small, round blue cells with poor differentiation. Fluorescent in situ hybridization (FISH) is used to assess chromosomal abnormalities, including *MYCN* amplification. Tumors are classified based on neuroblastic differentiation, mitosis-karyorrhexis index, and Schwann cell presence. The Children's Oncology Group stratifies patients into low-, intermediate-, or high-risk categories based on age at diagnosis, tumor stage, histopathology, DNA index, and *MYCN* amplification status [23].

Treatment strategies depend on risk classification. Localized tumors are managed with surgical resection, while high-risk cases require multimodal therapy. Induction chemotherapy typically includes cyclophosphamide, doxorubicin, cisplatin, carboplatin, etoposide, and vincristine. However, high-risk neuroblastomas frequently develop resistance, often necessitating autologous hematopoietic stem cell transplantation. Anti-GD2 immunotherapy has become a standard component of treatment for high-risk patients. Near-complete surgical resection improves local control and is particularly effective when combined with chemotherapy, radiation, and immunotherapy.

For early-stage disease (stages 1 and 2B), primary surgical resection is the standard approach. In advanced stages (3 and 4), an initial biopsy is performed for tumor biology assessment before initiating chemotherapy. While aggressive surgical resection for metastatic stage 4 neuroblastoma remains a subject of debate in Europe, it continues to be standard practice in the United States. Infants with stage 4S disease typically do not require surgical resection due to the high rate of spontaneous tumor regression. Radiation therapy is often used in high-risk cases for local and metastatic control, but is contraindicated in intraspinal tumors due to risks of vertebral damage, growth arrest, and scoliosis. However, it may be necessary for palliative management in cases of pain, hepatomegaly with respiratory compromise, or acute neurological symptoms from spinal cord compression.

Over the past few decades, outcomes for neuroblastoma patients have significantly improved, with 5-year survival rates increasing from 52% to 74%. While 50–60% of high-risk cases relapse after standard therapy, survival rates in low-risk patients now exceed 90%.

Wilms Tumor

Wilms tumor (WT), also known as nephroblastoma, is an embryonal renal neoplasm that accounts for 85% of pediatric renal tumors and 5.9% of all childhood malignancies. Approximately 75% of cases are diagnosed in children under the age of five, with bilateral involvement occurring in 13%. Several syndromes predispose to WT, including Beckwith-Wiedemann syndrome, Li-Fraumeni syndrome, Denys-Drash syndrome, and neurofibromatosis. Additionally, 10% of WT cases occur in children with congenital anomalies collectively referred to as WAGR syndrome, which includes aniridia, hemihypertrophy, genitourinary malformations, and intellectual disability [24].

WT arises due to mutations in tumor suppressor genes located on chromosome 11. The WT1 gene at 11p13 plays a crucial role in kidney and genitourinary tract development, and its mutation increases the risk of WT as well as genitourinary abnormalities such as cryptorchidism and hypospadias. Aniridia is present in 1.1% of WT cases, and when associated with WT1 deletions, the risk of tumor development rises to 40%. Mutations in the WT2 locus at 11p15 are linked to Beckwith-Wiedemann syndrome, with affected individuals carrying a 4–10% risk of developing WT, particularly if they also have hemihypertrophy.

Most cases of WT are detected incidentally during a physical examination when an abdominal mass is palpated by a caregiver or physician. Other presenting symptoms include vague abdominal discomfort and hematuria, which may indicate tumor invasion into the collecting system or ureter. Hypertension is observed in 25% of cases due to disturbances in the renin-angiotensin system. Less commonly, patients present with varicocele, hepatomegaly due to hepatic vein obstruction, ascites, or congestive heart failure.

Imaging plays a crucial role in diagnosis, with ultrasound often identifying tumor thrombus in the renal vein or inferior vena cava. CT scans help differentiate WT from other renal or adrenal tumors and assess regional adenopathy, contralateral kidney involvement, and distant metastases, with lung metastases present in 8% of cases at diagnosis.

Histologically, WT is classified based on the presence or absence of anaplasia. Favorable histology includes the classic triphasic composition of blastemal, stromal, and epithelial elements. Tumors with predominant epithelial differentiation are often diagnosed at an earlier stage and have a less aggressive course, whereas blastemal-predominant tumors tend to present with advanced disease. Unfavorable histology, defined by anaplasia, clear cell sarcoma, or rhabdoid tumor components, is associated with higher recurrence rates and chemoresistance. Nephrogenic rests, precursor lesions found in 25–40% of kidneys with WT, do not necessarily progress to malignancy but can undergo differentiation and spontaneous regression.

Staging systems for WT differ based on treatment approach. The International Society of Pediatric Oncology (SIOP) system evaluates tumor stage after preoperative chemotherapy, relying on imaging to assess metastatic spread before surgical resection. In contrast, the National Wilms Tumor Study Group (NWTSG) system determines tumor stage at the time of initial surgery and stratifies patients before chemotherapy. This approach allows for stage-based therapy, reducing unnecessary chemotherapy exposure in lower-risk patients.

Management of WT consists of surgery and chemotherapy, with radical nephrectomy and lymph node sampling serving as the standard treatment. Complete tumor resection with negative margins is critical, as intraoperative tumor spillage results in upstaging. In cases of vascular invasion extending into the inferior vena cava, tumors are classified as stage III and managed accordingly. Sampling of hilar, paraaortic, and paracaval lymph nodes is essential for accurate staging. Nephron-sparing surgery is reserved for patients with bilateral WT or a solitary kidney and may be facilitated by preoperative chemotherapy to reduce tumor burden. Partial nephrectomy is considered in select cases with bilateral disease or a localized pole-confined tumor with no evidence of vascular or collecting system involvement, and preserved renal function.

Chemotherapy regimens are determined by tumor stage and histologic classification. According to NWTSG guidelines, vincristine and dactinomycin form the bases of treatment, with doxorubicin or radiation therapy added in higher stage or unfavorable histology cases. The SIOP approach advocates preoperative chemotherapy to improve resectability and long-term survival. Prognosis varies based on stage and histology, with survival rates exceeding 95% for stages I and II with favorable histology. In contrast, unfavorable histology is associated with poorer outcomes, with 4-year survival rates of 70% for stage II, 56% for stage III, and 17% for stage IV.

Liver Tumors

Primary liver tumors in children are rare but are malignant in about 60% of cases. The most common are hepatoblastoma (80% of malignant liver tumors) and hepatocellular carcinoma (HCC). Hepatoblastoma typically occurs in children under five, with peak incidence at 3 years, while HCC is more common in older children and adolescents. Syndromes such as familial adenomatous polyposis and Beckwith-Wiedemann [25] increase hepatoblastoma risk, while HCC is associated with hepatitis B and C, tyrosinemia, and metabolic disorders.

Hepatoblastoma usually presents as a painless abdominal mass, while HCC may also show signs of cirrhosis, jaundice, and splenomegaly. Both tumors can metastasize, with lung and bone involvement common in HCC. Diagnosis involves ultrasound, CT, and MRI, with AFP levels elevated in most hepatoblastoma cases.

Histologically, hepatoblastoma can be epithelial (fetal or embryonal) or mixed with mesenchymal elements. HCC consists of large, pleomorphic hepatocyte-like cells and often has multifocal nodular growth. The PRETEXT system, developed by the International Childhood Liver Tumor Strategy Group (SIOPEL), classifies hepatoblastoma based on tumor-free liver segments noted preoperatively and additional risk factors, guiding treatment decisions.

Surgery is the main treatment, with segmentectomy or lobectomy for PRE-Treatment EXTent of disease (PRETEXT) I and II tumors. Liver transplantation is an option for unresectable tumors. Neoadjuvant chemotherapy (cisplatin, 5-fluorouracil, and vincristine) can decrease tumor size for better resection outcomes. Stage I tumors with pure fetal histology may not require chemotherapy, while others typically do. HCC has poorer survival rates with surgery alone, though early liver transplantation may improve outcomes. Chemoembolization and targeted chemotherapy are used in refractory cases. Resectable hepatoblastoma has an 85–90% long-term survival rate, with similar success for liver transplantation in unresectable cases.

Teratoma

Teratomas are typically benign tumors containing tissue from multiple embryonic germ layers. They can occur anywhere along the midline, most commonly in sacrococcygeal, mediastinal, retroperitoneal, and gonadal regions [26]. Teratomas may be solid, cystic, or mixed and are classified as mature or immature, with immature types carrying a potential risk of malignancy. They are more frequent in females (80%) and show an age-related distribution, with extragonadal tumors in neonates and young children and gonadal tumors in adolescents.

Sacrococcygeal Teratomas (SCTs)

SCTs account for 60% of all teratomas and can be detected in utero via ultrasound. Large tumors may cause complications such as polyhydramnios, fetal hydrops, and high-output heart failure due to vascular steal syndrome. Symptoms can include neurological deficits like paralysis or bladder dysfunction. Diagnosis is often clinical, but imaging (ultrasound, CT, and MRI) helps assess intra-abdominal involvement. Elevated AFP or β-hCG levels may indicate malignant components [26].

Surgical resection is the primary treatment and should be performed early to prevent complications like hemorrhage or rupture. The approach depends on tumor location: a posterior approach for most cases, combined abdominal and posterior approaches for extensive intra-abdominal involvement, and laparotomy or laparoscopy for entirely intra-abdominal tumors. Preservation and reconstruction of the anorectal complex is critical for continence.

Prognosis depends on age at diagnosis, with poorer outcomes for those identified before 30 weeks of gestation or after 2 months postnatally. AFP levels should be monitored every 3 months for 3–4 years to detect recurrence, which may require reexcision.

References

1. Gioacchini FM, Alicandri-Ciufelli M, Kaleci S, Magliulo G, Presutti L, Re M. Clinical presentation and treatment outcomes of thyroglossal duct cysts: a systematic review. Int J Oral Maxillofac Surg. 2015;44(1):119–26. https://doi.org/10.1016/j.ijom.2014.07.007.
2. Simon LM, Magit AE. Impact of incision and drainage of infected thyroglossal duct cyst on recurrence after Sistrunk procedure. Arch Otolaryngol Head Neck Surg. 2012;138(1):20–4. https://doi.org/10.1001/archoto.2011.225.
3. Lin ST, Tseng FY, Hsu CJ, Yeh TH, Chen YS. Thyroglossal duct cyst: a comparison between children and adults. Am J Otolaryngol. 2008;29(2):83–7. https://doi.org/10.1016/j.amjoto.2007.02.003.
4. Adams A, Mankad K, Offiah C, Childs L. Branchial cleft anomalies: a pictorial review of embryological development and spectrum of imaging findings. Insights Imaging. 2016;7(1):69–76. https://doi.org/10.1007/s13244-015-0454-5.
5. Zani A, Chung WK, Deprest J, et al. Congenital diaphragmatic hernia. Nat Rev Dis Primer. 2022;8(1):1–20. https://doi.org/10.1038/s41572-022-00362-w.
6. Jani J, Nicolaides KH, Keller RL, et al. Observed to expected lung area to head circumference ratio in the prediction of survival in fetuses with isolated diaphragmatic hernia. Ultrasound Obstet Gynecol. 2007;30(1):67–71. https://doi.org/10.1002/uog.4052.

7. Guidry CA, Hranjec T, Rodgers BM, Kane B, McGahren ED. Permissive hypercapnia in the management of congenital diaphragmatic hernia: our institutional experience. J Am Coll Surg. 2012;214(4):640–7. https://doi.org/10.1016/j.jamcollsurg.2011.12.036.
8. Breckenfelder C, Dawson-Gore CC, Galambos C, Corkum KS, Partrick D, Derderian SC. Congenital pulmonary airway malformation associated with papillary adenocarcinoma. Ann Thorac Surg Short Rep. 2024;2(3):400–3. https://doi.org/10.1016/j.atssr.2024.04.010.
9. Derderian SC, Coleman AM, Jeanty C, et al. Favorable outcomes in high-risk congenital pulmonary airway malformations treated with multiple courses of maternal betamethasone. J Pediatr Surg. 2015;50(4):515–8. https://doi.org/10.1016/j.jpedsurg.2014.08.019.
10. Mohammed S, Hamilton TE. Advances in complex congenital tracheoesophageal anomalies. Clin Perinatol. 2022;49(4):927–41. https://doi.org/10.1016/j.clp.2022.07.003.
11. Krishnan U. Eosinophilic esophagitis in esophageal atresia. Front Pediatr. 2019;7:497. https://doi.org/10.3389/fped.2019.00497.
12. Mirza B, Sheikh A. Multiple associated anomalies in patients of duodenal atresia: a case series. J Neonatal Surg. 2012;1(2):23.
13. Karlslätt KS, Husberg B, Ullberg U, Nordenskjöld A, Wester T. Intestinal malrotation in children: clinical presentation and outcomes. Eur J Pediatr Surg. 2023;34:228–35. https://doi.org/10.1055/s-0043-1764239.
14. Bellodas Sanchez J, Kadrofske M. Necrotizing enterocolitis. Neurogastroenterol Motil. 2019;31(3):e13569. https://doi.org/10.1111/nmo.13569.
15. Tjaden NEB, Trainor PA. The developmental etiology and pathogenesis of Hirschsprung disease. Transl Res. 2013;162(1):1–15. https://doi.org/10.1016/j.trsl.2013.03.001.
16. Turowski C, Dingemann J, Gillick J. Delayed diagnosis of imperforate anus: an unacceptable morbidity. Pediatr Surg Int. 2010;26(11):1083–6. https://doi.org/10.1007/s00383-010-2691-5.
17. Marsicovetere P, Ivatury SJ, White B, Holubar SD. Intestinal intussusception: etiology, diagnosis, and treatment. Clin Colon Rectal Surg. 2017;30(1):30–9. https://doi.org/10.1055/s-0036-1593429.
18. Lakshminarayanan B, Davenport M. Biliary atresia: a comprehensive review. J Autoimmun. 2016;73:1–9. https://doi.org/10.1016/j.jaut.2016.06.005.
19. Brown ZJ, Baghdadi A, Kamel I, Labiner HE, Hewitt DB, Pawlik TM. Diagnosis and management of choledochal cysts. HPB. 2023;25(1):14–25. https://doi.org/10.1016/j.hpb.2022.09.010.
20. Verla MA, Style CC, Olutoye OO. Prenatal diagnosis and management of omphalocele. Semin Pediatr Surg. 2019;28(2):84–8. https://doi.org/10.1053/j.sempedsurg.2019.04.007.
21. Bhat V, Moront M, Bhandari V. Gastroschisis: a state-of-the-art review. Children. 2020;7(12):302. https://doi.org/10.3390/children7120302.
22. Brandt ML. Pediatric hernias. Surg Clin North Am. 2008;88(1):27–43. https://doi.org/10.1016/j.suc.2007.11.006.
23. Park JR, Eggert A, Caron H. Neuroblastoma: biology, prognosis, and treatment. Hematol Oncol Clin North Am. 2010;24(1):65–86. https://doi.org/10.1016/j.hoc.2009.11.011.
24. Spreafico F, Fernandez CV, Brok J, et al. Wilms tumour. Nat Rev Dis Primer. 2021;7(1):1–21. https://doi.org/10.1038/s41572-021-00308-8.
25. Sharma D, Subbarao G, Saxena R. Hepatoblastoma. Semin Diagn Pathol. 2017;34(2):192–200. https://doi.org/10.1053/j.semdp.2016.12.015.
26. Barksdale EMJ, Obokhare I. Teratomas in infants and children. Curr Opin Pediatr. 2009;21(3):344. https://doi.org/10.1097/MOP.0b013e32832b41ee.

Orthopedic Surgery

46

Craig P. Eberson, Mary Lou, Joseph Moschella, Pooja Thyvalappil, and Julia Gillette

Introduction

Orthopedic surgery is the surgical subspecialty dedicated to the prevention, diagnosis, and treatment of musculoskeletal injuries and pathologies in patients of all age groups. The specialty is tremendously versatile, utilizing surgical and nonsurgical means to strengthen, shape, or repair elements of the musculoskeletal system in order to support and protect human locomotion and function. The spectrum of practice is vast, with subspecialized areas in hand and upper extremity, shoulder and elbow, foot and ankle, adult reconstruction, spine, sports medicine, pediatrics, trauma, and oncology [1]. Orthopedics is currently the most common surgical subspecialty among practicing physician assistants (PAs), comprising 11% of the workforce [2]. Since their first incorporation into the field in 1967, physician assistants (PAs) have played critical roles in the daily practice of orthopedics, participating in both outpatient and inpatient care of patients. Frequently cited clinical activities included first-assisting in surgeries, soft tissue injections, preoperative history-taking and physical exam, and patient education [3].

The purpose of this chapter is to serve as an overview of essential terminology and concepts in orthopedics that are critical for the practicing PA. We will aim to define and clarify the orthopedic language, review the key points of history-taking and physical exam when approaching musculoskeletal injuries in the inpatient and outpatient setting, and discuss treatment strategies for common orthopedic pathologies. This chapter is by no means a comprehensive review of orthopedics; it is a Herculean task to cover the breadth of orthopedics in a book; therefore, this chapter is, at best, a mere tip of the iceberg that is orthopedic surgery. However, we hope that this chapter can function as a point of reference for the specialized language and practice of orthopedics and offer a starting point for further reading.

The Orthopedic History and Physical Exam

A thorough history and physical exam are crucial to proper diagnosis and management of presenting injuries or pathologies. This central tenet is as important in orthopedic surgery as it is in all other medical specialties. However, in comparison to other specialties, the orthopedic interview and physical exam are more specific and problem-based. Priorities in the orthopedic assessment will thus vary depending on the patient's condition and the setting of the initial encounter. A 15-year-old presenting to the outpatient clinic for 2 months of ankle pain and a 63-year-old presenting to the emergency department (ED) after a fall from a ladder will likely be asked different sets of questions given the distinct contexts of both visits.

When assessing a patient in the ED, acuity of the chief concern is an initial question that can guide the remainder of the interview. Acute traumatic injuries should first be triaged to identify patients that may need emergent or urgent surgery. Emergent injuries are those that require surgery within 6 h of patient encounter and include open fractures (when fractured bone breaks through soft tissue and skin and is exposed to the external environment), traumatic amputations (loss of an extremity or digit), septic joints (infection within a joint space), compartment syndrome (increased pressure within a muscle compartment), and vascular-compromised limbs (limbs with occluded blood flow). Urgent surgeries require operation within 24–48 h, and include pelvis and acetabulum fractures, long bone (femur, tibia, and humerus) fractures, poly-traumatic injuries (multiple fractures), and unstable spine fractures. While the orthopedic service is often consulted for these patients after initial stabilization in the ED, providers should keep the components of a primary

C. P. Eberson (✉) · M. Lou · J. Moschella · P. Thyvalappil
J. Gillette
Department of Orthopaedic Surgery, Brown University, Warren Alpert Medical School, Providence, RI, USA

S. Atallah, J. Dragoljevic (eds.), *Fundamentals of Surgery for Physician Assistants*, https://doi.org/10.1007/978-3-032-21069-2_46

trauma assessment (airway, breathing, circulation, disability, and exposure) and the patient's general appearance (sick or not sick) and mental status (alert, oriented, or conscious) in mind when walking into the room to see the patient for the first time [4].

After ensuring stability of the patient in the ED, the interview can then be guided by the acuity of the chief concern. For acute injuries, additional information should be gathered on timing and mechanism. Understanding the "when," "where," and "how" of the injury can offer insights into the precise anatomical structures that were compromised. If similar episodes have happened before, ask patients how they were treated previously and in what ways the current presentation is similar or different. For chronic injuries, details on whether the severity of the chief concern has waxed or waned over time can help gauge whether the injury is from repetitive stress or has been exacerbated by a recent provocation. In addition, if the injury had been worked up before, obtaining the records and results of the tests and imaging that were previously done is helpful for comparison and to avoid unnecessary repeat testing. For both acute and chronic injuries, asking the patient to describe the quality of pain (e.g., burning, sharp, stabbing, and intermittent), radiation, and associated numbness or weakness also provides pertinent information to narrow the differential. Additional helpful questions asked include aggravating or alleviating factors or positioning, severity at presentation compared to time of injury, and baseline functional status. The patient's past medical history should also be verified with what may already be written in the electronic medical record (EMR). Components of the past medical history that are particularly relevant in orthopedic surgery include surgical/orthopedic history, diagnosis of connective tissue disorder, diagnosis of bone disease (e.g., osteoporosis, osteomalacia, Paget's disease), an increased bleeding risk (e.g., taking anticoagulant medications, coagulative disorder), an increased thromboembolic risk (e.g., prior history of distal venous thrombosis (DVT), pulmonary embolism (PE), antiphospholipid syndrome, taking an anticontraceptive), diabetes, or immunocompromised state (on immunomodulatory drugs, undergoing radiation or chemotherapy). Diet, occupation, exercise/baseline activity level, smoking history, and alcohol habits are also pertinent aspects of the patient's history as they inform the patient's general health status as well [5–11]. The above information pieces together the key background information needed to formulate a differential that can then be further refined with a physical exam, imaging, and labs.

Assessing a patient in the outpatient clinic/office follows similar guidelines as seeing a patient in the ED. However, with the delay of care from the time of injury to the time of the appointment, patients presenting to the office are more likely to have a chronic chief concern rather than acute traumatic injuries [12, 13]. A small fraction of patients may still present with more urgent injuries, upon which it will be important to assess whether it is something that can be taken care of in the office or if the patient should be sent to the nearest ED for treatment. However, the same questions are relevant for a thorough medical interview.

Physical exam of the patient can be broadly organized into five steps: inspection, palpation, range of motion, neurovascular assessment, and specialized tests [10, 11, 14]. General practice is to examine from the joint above to the joint below the site of injury, with the noninjured side assessed first as a point of reference if possible. Painful components of the physical exam should be performed last to prevent lingering pain from interfering with subsequent parts of the exam and also optimize patient comfort [10, 11, 15]. Inspection should examine for any obvious deformity along with any skin changes, erythema, open wounds, scarring, or rash. Systematic palpation should assess for swelling, tenderness, or warmth around the site of injury. Abnormalities around osseous and soft tissue landmarks should be noted and clinically correlated with the patient's history to confirm a diagnosis. Range of motion will vary depending on patient age, sex, and baseline mobility and activity; thus, comparing to the contralateral side is critical to assess the degree of restriction. Both active (patient independently moves the extremity) and passive (provider moves the extremity for the patient) ranges should be assessed, as differences can point to distinct pathologies. Any rigidity, spasticity, locking, clicking, or crepitus upon movement should also be noted. Neurovascular examination should focus on strength, sensation, pulses, and capillary refill. Pulses that cannot be palpated by hand should be followed up with a Doppler examination. Recognition of neurovascular compromise is especially important as delays in treatment can result in long-term functional deficits, amputation, or mortality [16]. One example is compartment syndrome, which is an orthopedic emergency that can occur after acute trauma due to increased pressure build-up within the muscle fascia. The classic presentation of compartment syndrome is remembered with the "5 Ps": pain, pulselessness, paresthesia, paralysis, and pallor. Suspicion of compartment syndrome should warrant immediate measurement of intracompartmental pressure to confirm diagnosis and prepare for surgical decompression [17, 18]. For patients presenting with symptoms concerning for spinal stenosis or radiculopathy, assessment of reflexes is also informative of spinal levels affected [11, 19, 20]. Further specialized testing can then be used to ascertain the findings of the prior physical exam parts and patient history. Some frequently used special tests and their corresponding pathologies are described in Table 46.1 [11, 14, 21–27]. It should be noted that results of special tests should be clinically correlated with patient history and imaging, as different maneuvers also have distinct sensitivity (rate of true positives) and specificity (rate of true negatives).

Table 46.1 Common physical exam tests in orthopedics

	Test	Indicative pathology	Description
Hand and forearm	Tinel's sign of the median nerve	Carpal tunnel syndrome	Patient has forearm supinated; examiner taps on wrist at the region of the median nerve. Positive if patient reports tingling along distribution of median nerve (1st through 3rd digits)
	Phalen's test (Fig. 46.1a)	Carpal tunnel syndrome	Patient places hands back-to-back with wrists fully in flexion for 60 s. Positive if patient reports numbness or tingling along distribution of median nerve (1st through 3rd digits)
	Finkelstein test (Fig. 46.1b)	de Quervain tenosynovitis	Patient stabilizes forearm in neutral rotation on table with clenched fist with thumb inside. Examiner moves wrist toward the ulnar side. Positive if patient experiences symptom exacerbation
	Wrist hyperflexion, abduction of the thumb (WHAT) test	de Quervain tenosynovitis	Patient hyperflexes wrist with thumb extended and abducted. Examiner applies resistance against thumb abduction. Positive if patient experiences symptom exacerbation
	Grind test	1st carpometacarpal (CMC) osteoarthritis	Patient holds hand in neutral position. Examiner applies axial compression along the thumb metacarpal and rotates the thumb base. Positive if pain is reproduced along the CMC joint
Elbow	Tinel's sign of the ulnar nerve	Cubital tunnel syndrome	Patient slightly flexes elbow. Examiner identifies the groove between the olecranon and medial epicondyle and taps the region. Positive if tingling elicited along distribution of ulnar nerve (4th–5th digits)
	Valgus stress test	Ulnar collateral ligament (UCL) tear	Patient flexes elbow to 90° with forearm supinated. Examiner applies force to the arm medially and the forearm laterally to stress UCL. Positive if pain or laxity is observed
	Hook test (Fig. 46.2)	Distal biceps rupture	Patient actively flexes elbow to 90° with forearm supinated. Examiner attempts to hook finger under biceps tendon from the lateral side. Positive if examiner can hook finger 1 cm underneath tendon and pull it forward
Shoulder	Shoulder apprehension test	Anterior shoulder instability	Patient lies supine. Examiner passively abducts and externally rotates arm. Positive if any apprehension is felt
	Neer sign	Subacromial impingement	Patient pronates forearm and internally rotates arm. Examiner stabilizes scapula and slowly flexes arm. Positive if pain is reproduced
	"Empty can" test	Supraspinatus tear	Patient flexes arm to 90° and 60° of horizontal abduction, with full internal rotation (as if emptying a can). Examiner applies downward force that patient resists. Positive if patient has pain or weakness
	External rotation test	Infraspinatus tear	Patient flexes elbow to 90° with arms by the side and externally rotates arm 45° against examiner's resistance. Positive if patient has pain or weakness
Spine	Spurling's test	Cervical radiculopathy	Patient seated with neck rotated and laterally flexed to one side. Examiner applies downward pressure on head. Positive if pain is reproduced
	Lhermitte's sign	Cervical myelopathy	Patient flexes neck to touch chin to chest. Positive if a "pins and needles" sensation is elicited from the head down the neck
	Hoffman's sign	Cervical myelopathy	Examiner flicks the fingernail of the patient's middle finger. Positive if involuntarily flexes thumb and index finger
	Straight leg raise test	Sciatica	Patient supine with knee extended. Examiner passively flexes the hip. Positive if patient has low back pain or shooting pain down the back of the buttocks
Knee	Lachman test (Fig. 46.3)	Anterior collateral ligament (ACL) tear	Patient supine with knee flexed to 30°. Examiner stabilizes thigh with one hand while other hand pull tibia forward. Positive if tibia able to be translated anteriorly
	Posterior drawer test	Posterior collateral ligament (PCL) tear	Patient spine with knee flexed to 90°. Examiner sits on foot and pushes tibia posteriorly. Positive is tibia translates posteriorly
	Valgus stress test	Medial collateral ligament (MCL) tear	Patient supine with knee slightly flexed. Examiner pushes thigh medially and moves ankles laterally. Positive if laxity present in medial knee
	Varus stress test	Lateral collateral ligament (LCL) tear	Patient supine with knee slightly flexed. Examiner pushes thigh laterally and moves ankles medially. Positive if laxity present in lateral knee
	Thessaly test	Meniscus tear	Patient stands on affected extremity and flexes knee to 20°. Patient pivots around the knee and body while keeping knee flexed. Positive if pain along joint line or locking in the knee is elicited
Foot and ankle	Thompson test	Achilles tendon rupture	Patient lies prone with feet hanging off the table. Examiner squeezes calf. Positive if foot does not plantar flex
Pediatric	Galeazzi test (Fig. 46.4)	Leg length discrepancy, hip dislocation	Patient lies supine and flexes hip and knees such that feet are flat on the table and ankles touch the buttocks. Positive if there is an inequality in height of the knees

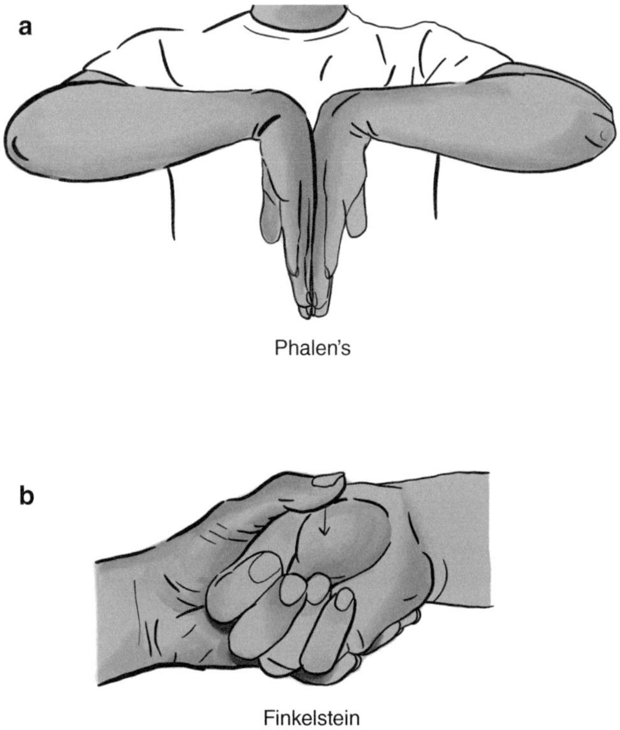

Fig. 46.1 Illustration of Phalen's test for carpal tunnel syndrome and Finkelstein test for De Quervain's tenosynovitis

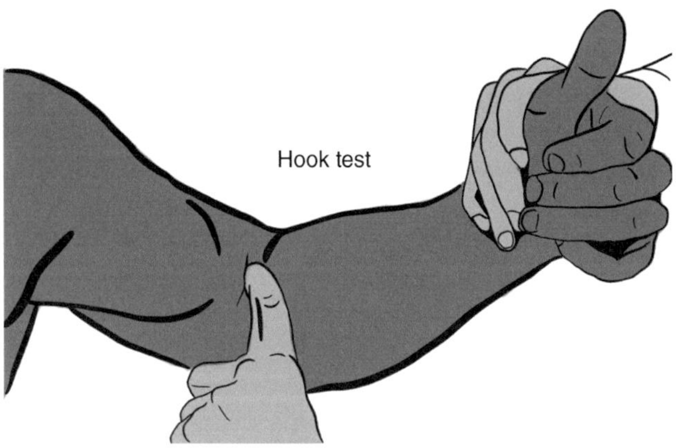

Fig. 46.2 Illustration of the Hook test for distal biceps rupture

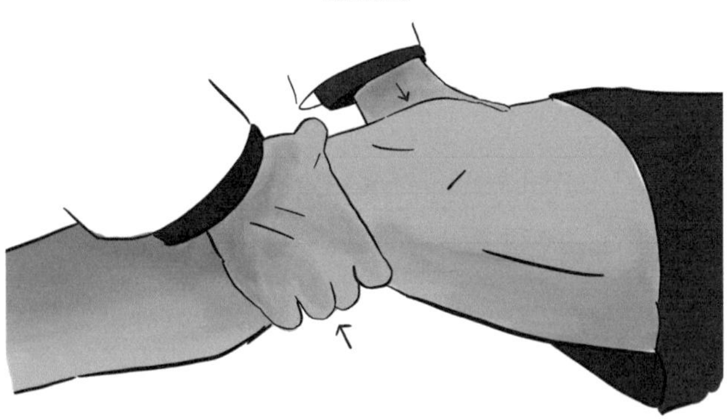

Fig. 46.3 Illustration of the Lachman's test for anterior cruciate ligament tears

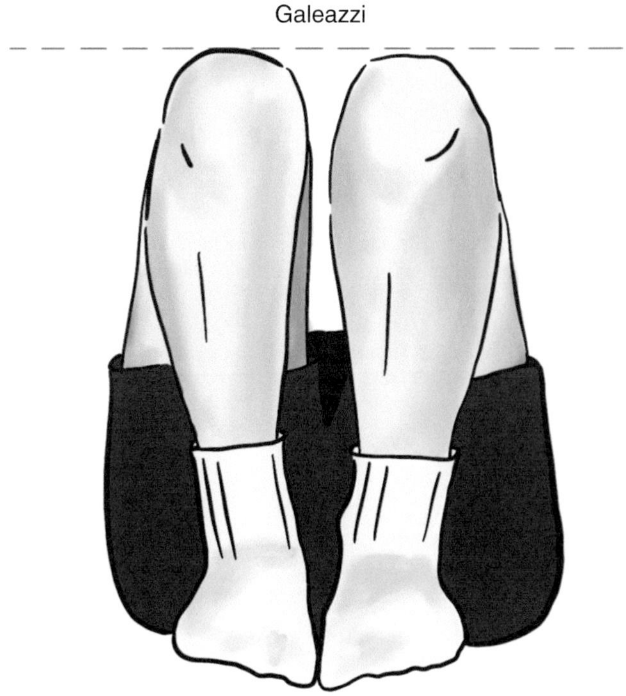

Fig. 46.4 Illustration of the Galeazzi test for leg length discrepancy and hip dislocation in pediatric patients

Essentials of Musculoskeletal Imaging

Radiographs (x-rays) are the primary imaging modality in orthopedics. This imaging technique captures a two-dimensional image by passing x-ray beams through the body to strike an image receptor behind the patient. Bone appears white (radiopaque), soft tissue is gray, and air is black (radiolucent); with this contrast, bony pathologies are easily visualized, thereby making radiographs the most common primary imaging modality to assess fractures. Radiographs are also relatively inexpensive compared to other imaging modalities and can be performed rapidly at the bedside, allowing for increased flexibility and rapid assessment of acute trauma. However, radiographs are unable to provide adequate visualization of soft tissues, and while minimal in quantity, still expose the patient to radiation [28–30]. Thus, special considerations of the radiation risks should be taken when ordering radiographs for pregnant patients or infants, and other imaging modalities that do not require radiation may be considered initially for these patient groups when possible [29–31]. As radiographs are only able to capture a two-dimensional image, it is thus important to always obtain at least two different views of the anatomic region of interest in order to appreciate the full extent of injury. For most injuries, these views are the anteroposterior (AP) and lateral [28]. Specific views can also be obtained for improved visualization of different anatomic regions, such as the scapular outlet ("Y") and axillary views of the shoulder, oblique and flexion-extension views of the spine, the oblique view of the elbow, Judet views of the pelvis, sunrise view of the knee, and Mortise view of the ankle [28, 32, 33].

Computed tomography (CT) is an imaging modality that allows for three-dimensional visualization of anatomic structures by performing cross-sectional x-rays at regular intervals. As in radiographs, bony structures are white (hyperdense), soft tissues are gray, and air and fluid are dark (hypodense). The additional dimension improves visualization of structures such as complex fractures, trabecular bone, and tumors, which aid in surgical planning. However, CT scans, by nature of the three-dimensional reconstruction, tend to have increased artifact, and also come with the risk of increased radiation exposure [34].

Magnetic resonance imaging (MRI) can also be used for three-dimensional imaging and is the best imaging modality for soft tissues such as ligaments, tendons, cartilage, and nerves. Contrast can be injected intravenously to identify herniated discs and into joints to identify tendon tears. Each MRI scan includes multiple variations of the image, called pulse sequences (e.g., T1 and T2), which help emphasize abnormalities in different tissue types. On T1, fat appears bright (hyperintense) and cortical bone, tendons, and ligaments appear dark (hypointense). On T2, fluids are hyperintense, with fat remaining relatively hyperintense as well; bone, tendons, and ligaments also remain relatively hypointense. T2 thus is useful for assessment of edema, joints, and marrow abnormalities [35, 36]. MRI is also the most sensitive imaging study for osteomyelitis, as it can detect bone marrow edema and early inflammatory changes [37, 38]. Despite its many uses, MRI is far more expensive than plain radiographs and CT, and is the most time-consuming and expensive to obtain out of the three modalities. The narrow tube and set-up of the machine is also not always tolerated by patients; young children who are unable to remain still require procedural sedation for the MRI to be performed, and adults with claustrophobia can have difficulty tolerating the study as well. Patients with implants such as pacemakers, hearing aids, artificial implants, and neurostimulation systems also cannot obtain MRIs as the implanted devices can have a projectile effect, malfunction, or cause burns. Detailed screening of patient history prior to MRI study is thus needed to ensure patient safety [39].

Ultrasound can also be used in orthopedics, with utility in identifying tendon tears, deep vein thrombosis, developmental hip dysplasia in infants, and foreign bodies. Notably, it does not emit ionizing radiation and can be safely used on patients with implanted devices, thereby circumventing the contraindications for radiographs, CT, and MRI. Unlike these three modalities, ultrasound provides a "live image" that can be interpreted during the scan. Thus, ultrasound can also be used for procedures such as intra-articular injections. It is also the cheapest imaging modality, and, with the advent of point of care ultrasound (POCUS), is easily portable for rapid assessment of injuries at the bedside. However, as sound waves cannot penetrate bone, bony structures cause artifact and shadowing in scans, leading to poor image resolution. Deep structures are also difficult to visualize as sound waves weaken the farther they travel [28, 34].

Common Orthopedic Conditions

Overview of Terminology

Orthopedic conditions can be broadly classified as traumatic and nontraumatic depending on the mechanism and acuity of the injury. Traumatic injuries are those that are caused by an external force and have a sudden onset and severity, and include fractures, sprains, dislocations, and tears. Other conditions are termed nontraumatic.

Of the traumatic conditions, fractures can further be subclassified as open or closed; open fractures warrant emergent treatment due to the increased risk of infection and osteomyelitis. Classification systems for fractures provide a framework for standardizing injury description and guide treatment. Open fractures are frequently described with the Gustilo-Anderson classification. Type I open fractures have a wound less than 1 cm and are clean, and Type II has a laceration greater than 1 cm without extensive soft tissue damage. Type IIIa fractures have adequate soft tissue coverage despite large soft tissue laceration; Type IIIb fractures have extensive soft tissue injury with exposed bone and extensive stripping of the periosteum; and Type IIIc fractures are large open wounds with associated arterial injury [40]. In children, where the growth plate is still present, fractures that involve the growth plate can be classified with the Salter-Harris system. Salter I fractures are within the growth plate, Salter II extend from the growth plate to the metaphysis (shaft of the bone), Salter III extend from the growth plate into the epiphysis (ends of the bone), Salter IV pass through metaphysis, growth plate, and epiphysis, and Salter V is the most severe, in which there is a comminution or crush injury on the growth plate (Fig. 46.5) [41].

Most orthopedic conditions are named based on the anatomic region that is compromised and a suffix describing the type of injury. For example, inflammation of the tendon is termed "tendinitis," inflammation of a bursa (fluid sacs that cushion the joints) is "bursitis," and inflammation of the tenosynovium is "tenosynovitis." The suffix "-opathy" is also commonly seen and means "diseased," while "-osis" is a long-term diseased structure. Thus, it can be seen that tendinitis is a type of tendinopathy, as tendonitis is an ill tendon that is inflamed, and tendinopathy, for a long time, becomes tendinosis [42].

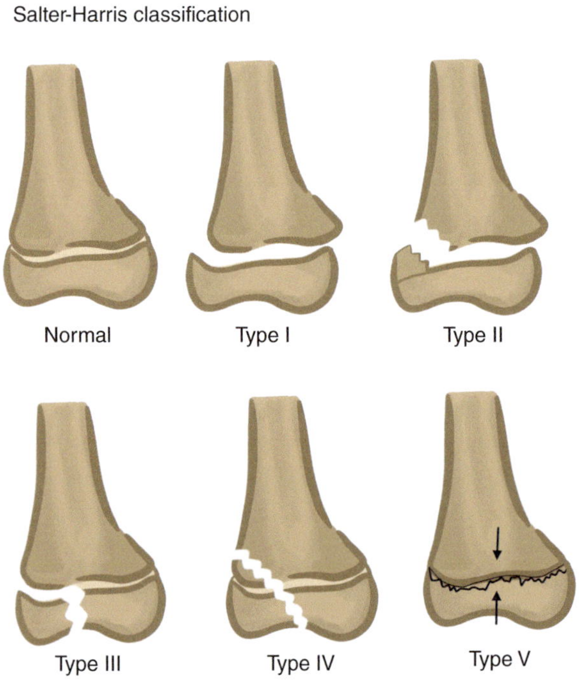

Fig. 46.5 Illustration of the Salter-Harris classification system for fractures that involve the growth plate

Procedures are similarly named. Common suffixes seen in orthopedic procedures include "-plasty" (to reshape or mold), "-ectomy" (to remove), "-otomy" (to cut or incise), "-scopy" (to view), "-desis" (to fuse or stabilize), and "-centesis" (to puncture). Thus, arthroscopy is a procedure involving a "view of the joint," usually with a camera inside the joint space. Arthroplasty is a "reshaping of the joint," or colloquially a joint replacement where some or all of a major joint is replaced [43].

Finally, open reduction internal fixation (ORIF) is a common abbreviation that is used to describe the process of open surgery to reduce a fracture, followed by stabilization with hardware such as plates, screws, and rods.

In the context of this terminology, the following sections will review common orthopedic conditions, briefly reviewing relevant anatomy, clinical features, and treatment strategies for each one.

Hand and Upper Extremity

The human hand consists of 27 bones: 8 carpals (scaphoid, lunate, triquetrum, pisiform, trapezium, trapezoid, capitate, hamate), 5 metacarpals (first through fifth), and 14 phalanges (five proximal, four intermediate, five distal) (Fig. 46.6). It is innervated by branches of the median, ulnar, and radial nerves, and receives blood supply from the ulnar and radial arteries that branch from the brachial artery. Rich blood supply is maintained in the hand with an anastomosis of the dorsal carpal branches of radial and ulnar arteries, creating the dorsal carpal arch [44].

The forearm consists of two bones: radius and ulna, which are connected via an interosseous membrane (Fig. 46.7a). Muscles of the forearm function for wrist and hand movements, with tendons that extend down into the hand (Fig. 46.7b). The median, radial, and ulnar nerves also innervate the muscles of the forearm. The median nerve and ulnar nerves divide up the muscles for wrist flexion, with the median nerve innervating all muscles in the anterior compartment other than the flexor carpi ulnaris and the ulnar portion of the flexor digitorum profundus. The radial nerve innervates the muscles of the posterior compartment. Blood supply is also from the ulnar and radial arteries [45].

Traumatic conditions of the hand and forearm and their respective treatment are listed in Table 46.2. Nontraumatic conditions and treatment strategies are described in Table 46.3.

Shoulder

The shoulder is a complex structure and is the most mobile joint in the body. It is formed by the junction of the clavicle, scapula, and humerus, and is supported by the rotator cuff muscles (supraspinatus, infraspinatus, teres minor, and subscapularis). The deltoid, pectoralis major and minor, and latissimus dorsi also aid in arm mobility. The various branches of the brachial plexus innervate these muscles, and the blood supply comes from the brachial, subclavian, and axillary arteries (Fig. 46.8) [59].

Due to the high degree of mobility inherent in the shoulder, the most common pathologies of the joint involve instability (subluxation and dislocation). The young, athletic population is particularly susceptible to instability events. A vast majority of instability is in the anterior direction, which can be the result of both traumatic and atraumatic injuries. Posterior instability is much rarer as it is usually caused by high-energy trauma, such as motor vehicle accidents, seizures, or electrocution [60]. Traumatic instability tends to be unilateral and unidirectional with labral injury, while atraumatic tends to be bilateral with hyperlaxity. Physical exam of an unstable shoulder will test positive for shoulder apprehension, and special emphasis should be made when gathering the history to ascertain if this is a recurrent instability or a first-time dislocation. Nonsurgical treatment of shoulder instability can involve a sling for immobilization and physical therapy, while surgical treatment entails open or arthroscopic repair of the unstable structures [61].

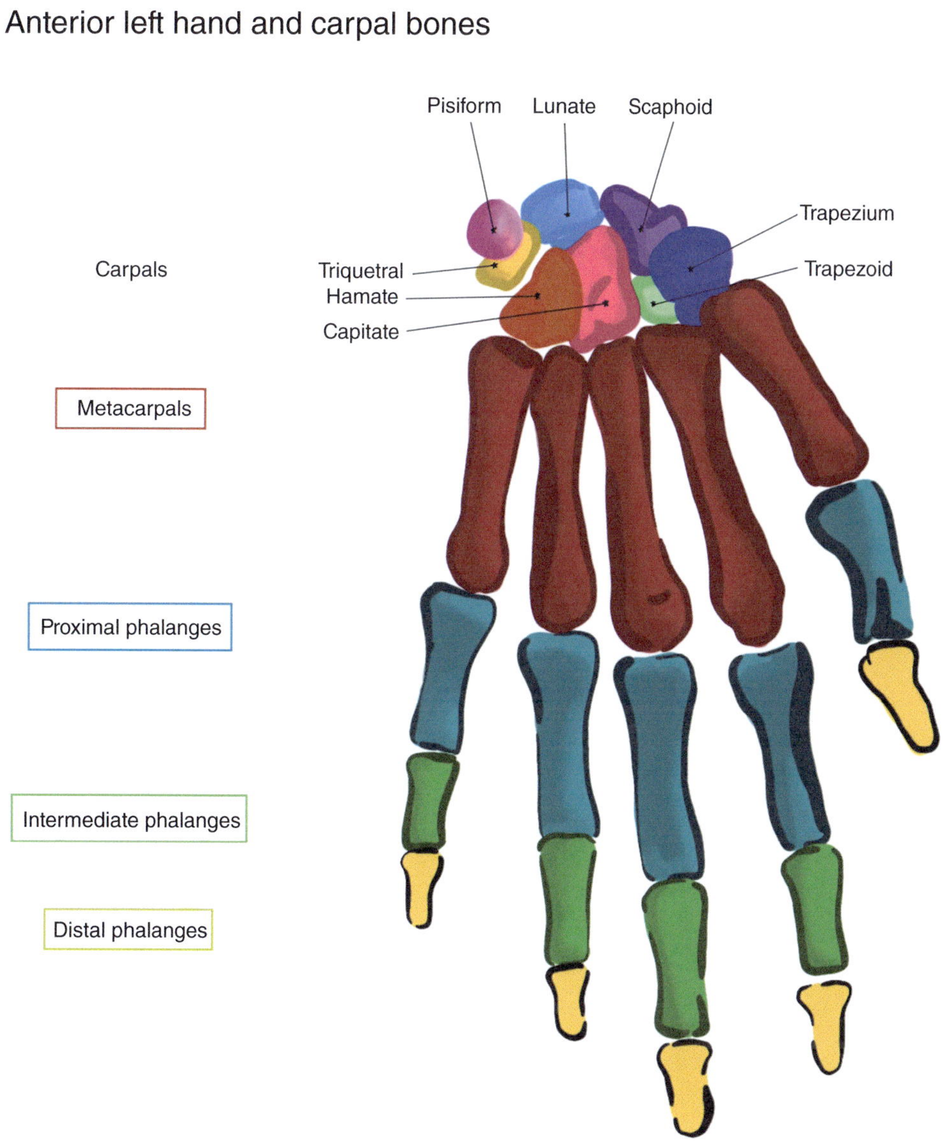

Fig. 46.6 Illustration of the bones of the hand (carpals, metacarpals, and phalanges)

Spine

The spine is comprised of 33 vertebrae, separated into 7 cervical, 12 thoracic, 5 lumbar, 5 sacral, and 1 coccygeal. Each individual vertebra is separated by intervertebral discs, which are cartilaginous structures that act as cushions for the spine. Common orthopedic spine conditions include low back pain and scoliosis [62].

Low back pain affects 10–30% of adults annually in the United States and is one of the chief concerns of patients reporting to the orthopedic surgery office. Etiologies of back pain include muscular strain, trauma, osteoarthritis, spinal stenosis, disc herniation, or malignancy [63]. The multivariable causes of low back pain thus warrant a very thorough history and physical exam in order to determine a diagnosis. Conservative treatment is frequently pursued first with medications such as nonsteroidal anti-inflammatory drugs (NSAIDs) and skeletal muscle relaxants. If symptoms do not resolve, then surgical intervention is utilized, such as surgical decompression for spinal stenosis [63].

Scoliosis is a spinal deformity defined as lateral curvature of the spine of at least 10°. It is mostly identified in pediatric patients but can be diagnosed in all ages. Most cases are idiopathic, but neurological conditions such as cerebral palsy and congenital syndromes like Marfan and neurofibromatosis can cause scoliosis [64]. For younger patients, nonsurgical treatment is initially pursued if possible, and the curvature of the spine is routinely monitored. Surgical treatment is indicated if the curve exceeds 45–50°, as increased curvature can compromise pulmonary function [65].

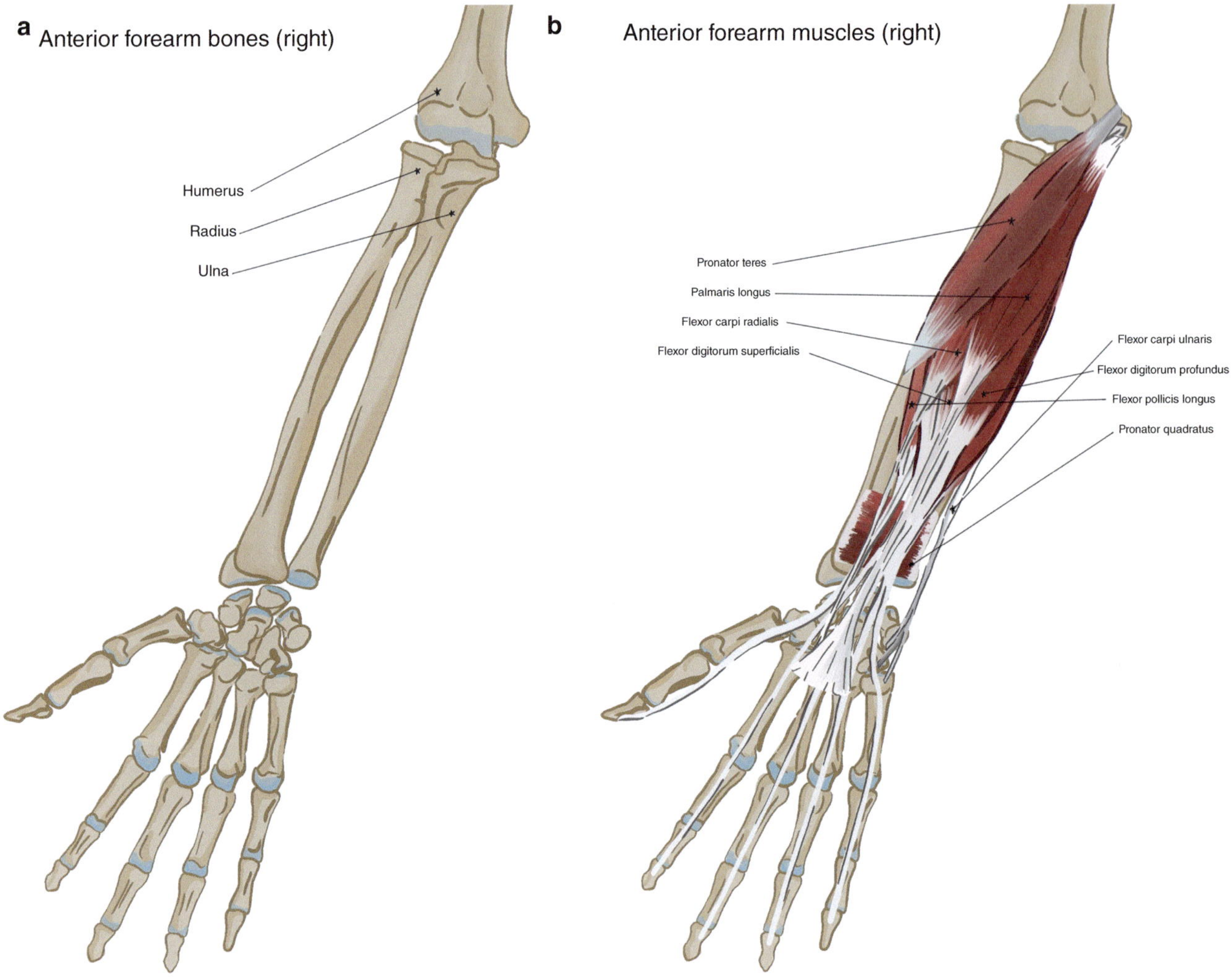

Fig. 46.7 Illustration of the forearm and hand bones and muscles of the forearm

Table 46.2 Traumatic conditions of the hand and forearm

	Epidemiology	Etiology	Clinical features	Nonsurgical treatment	Surgical treatment
Scaphoid fracture [46, 47]	The most common carpal fracture. Mostly seen in adult patients	A result of fall onto an outstretched hand	Pain and swelling around the base of the thumb and anatomic snuffbox on the radial side of the wrist	For nondisplaced fractures within the distal third of the bone, immobilize with long arm or short arm cast for at least 6 weeks. Can also be immobilized with a thumb spica	Insertion of screws or K-wires to stabilize broken scaphoid. In some cases, ORIF with bone grafting
Distal radius fracture [48]	Very common, mostly seen in pediatric and elderly patients	Trauma to the forearm commonly occurs when falling onto an outstretched hand	Distal upper extremity pain, radiographic evaluation	Short-arm cast immobilization. Pediatric patients can tolerate more angulation than adults	ORIF
Metacarpal fracture [49, 50]	Third most common fracture in contact-sport athletes and manual laborers	Direct trauma, such as direct blows to the dorsum of the hand	Swelling, loss of knuckle height, digit malrotation, and digit crossing over. Confirm with radiographs	Stable fractures with minimal displacement call for nonoperative treatment	Percutaneous wires, intramedullary fixation, or ORIF

(continued)

Table 46.2 (continued)

	Epidemiology	Etiology	Clinical features	Nonsurgical treatment	Surgical treatment
Phalanx fracture [51, 52]	Second most common fracture in children. Very common in adults as well	Sports injuries, blunt trauma	Pain, swelling, deformity, decreased range of motion, and/or instability around the injury site	A splint, worn for 3–4 weeks	Internal fixation using plates, screws, or K-wires
Supracondylar humerus fracture [53]	Most common fracture seen in children, relatively uncommon in adults	Fall on outstretched hand	Inability to lift the arm due to pain, using unaffected arm to hold onto the elbow of the injured arm. Confirm with a radiograph	If minimally displaced, can use a long arm cast and sling	Percutaneous pinning, ORIF

Table 46.3 Nontraumatic conditions of the hand and forearm

	Epidemiology	Etiology	Clinical features	Nonsurgical treatment	Surgical treatment
Carpal tunnel syndrome [54, 55]	1–3 per 1000 adults in the United States	Compression of the median nerve at the carpal tunnel	Wrist pain, numbness, and tingling along distribution of the median nerve. Positive Tinel's and Phalen's. Can confirm with EMG	Wrist bracing, corticosteroid injection, hand therapy	Carpal tunnel release
Trigger finger [56]	2% of general population in the United States	Inflammation and hypertrophy of the retinacular sheath restricts motion of flexor tendon	Finger locked in flexion, requires other hand to straighten	Splinting, corticosteroid injection	Trigger finger release
De Quervain's Tenosynovitis [57]	More common in women than in men. Adults aged 40–50 years old	Abductor pollicis longus and extensor pollicis brevis tendons entrapped against tendon sheath, causing inflammation	Positive Finkelstein or WHAT test	Corticosteroid injection	Release of the first dorsal compartment tendon sheath
Cubital tunnel syndrome [58]	1.8% of the general population in the United States	Compression of the ulnar nerve in the cubital tunnel	Numbness and tingling along distribution of ulnar nerve. Positive Tinel's sign at the elbow	Elbow splinting at night, NSAIDs	Cubital tunnel release

Hip and Thigh

The hip is a ball and socket joint where the femur articulates with the acetabulum in the pelvis. As a major joint for weight-bearing, the hip has many reinforcing structures, including the acetabular labrum and iliofemoral ligament. Flexion muscles include the psoas major and iliacus, extension includes gluteus maximus and the hamstrings (semimembranosus, biceps femoris, and semitendinosus), lateral rotation includes the obturators and quadratus femoris, and medial rotation includes the gluteus medius and minimus. Adduction is accomplished by the adductors (longus, brevis, and magnus) along with the gracilis and pectineus, while abduction is performed by the gluteus medius and minimus [66].

Traumatic injuries of the hip are high-energy, often from events like motor vehicle accidents. Initial treatment thus focuses on preliminary stabilization prior to surgical fixation. Proximal femur fractures have similar etiologies as pelvic fractures and also require stabilization before emergent surgery, usually with traction pins and weights. Surgical intervention is ORIF with plates in the pelvis and rods in the femur. If the femoral head or neck is fractured, then hemiarthroplasty to replace it will need to be done to avoid the possibility of avascular necrosis that otherwise may occur [67].

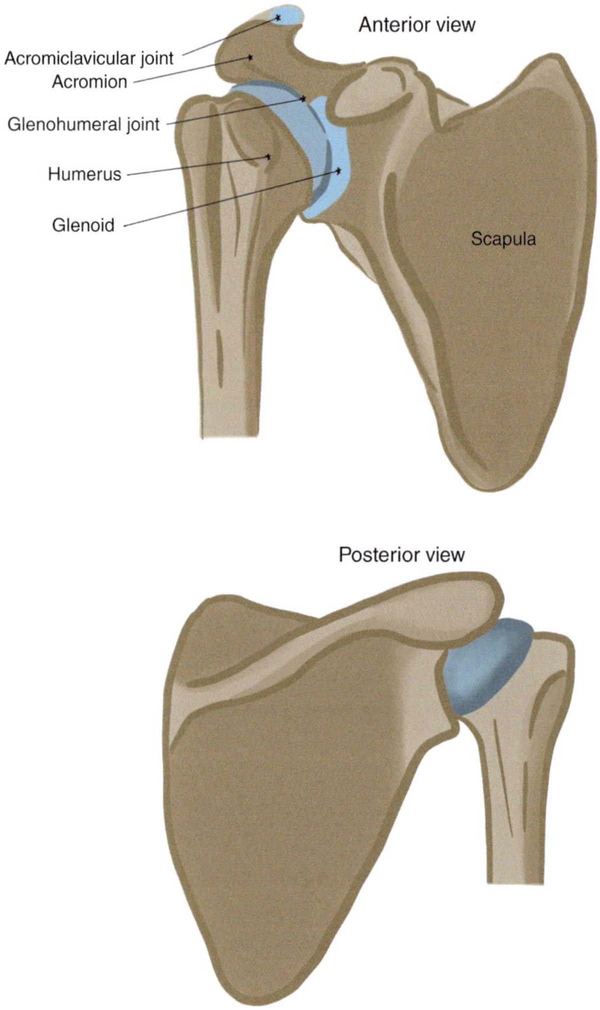

Fig. 46.8 Illustration

For nontraumatic hip conditions, osteoarthritis (OA) is one of the most common and debilitating, as the loss of articular cartilage and inflammatory bony changes cause pain that significantly affects mobility. Some causes of hip OA include avascular necrosis, history of trauma, developmental hip dysplasia, and idiopathic degenerative disease. The average OA patient is 50–70-years old with hip pain that slowly develops and worsens over time [68, 69]. Pain and stiffness typically are most apparent in the morning and after sitting for an extended period of time. Hip arthritis can be diagnosed by only clinical presentation, but imaging can be helpful for confirmation and tracking, with radiographs showing decreased joint space and osteophytes. Treatment plans involve nonoperative, nonpharmacologic treatment as first-line choices. These include low-impact exercise programs that focus on strengthening and stretching muscles around the hip, such as yoga, cycling, and swimming. For early and mild arthritis, physical therapy is recommended for similar reasons. Pharmacological therapy includes acetaminophen, corticosteroid injections, and NSAIDs for pain relief. For patients with persistent pain and progressive disease, surgical intervention with total hip arthroplasty (THA) is recommended, with studies demonstrating great success and outcomes even 10 years after the operation [68].

Femoroacetabular impingement (FAI) is another nontraumatic hip injury that presents with pain from abnormal contact of the proximal femur and acetabulum, leading to soft tissue damage such as labral tears and hip arthritis. There are two types: cam impingement and pincer impingement [70]. Cam impingement is more commonly seen in males; this impingement involves the edge of the femoral head or femoral neck and the hip when flexed. In an AP radiograph, a bony prominence can be seen on the femoral head [71]. Pincer impingement occurs when the acetabulum covers too much of the femoral head. Impingement presents with a gradual onset of hip pain, especially provoked by hip flexion and internal rotation. Physical exam should assess gait and hip range of motion. The FADIR test (hip flexion, adduction, and internal rotation) can be applied to assess for labral tears. A similar test, the FABER (hip flexion, abduction, and external rotation), can be used to assess for sacroiliac joint pathologies, particularly in cases of anterior hip or groin pain [72].

Any hip snapping, clicking, popping, and catching on exam can also point toward FAI as a diagnosis [72]. Nonoperative treatment, such as physical therapy and medication, should be initiated before surgery is considered. If nonoperative treatment fails, operative treatment can involve hip arthroscopy with bone shaving from the femoral neck, labral debridement, labral repair, or acetabular osteotomy [73].

Knee

The knee is a hinge joint that is critical to daily mobility, formed by the articulation of the femur, tibia, and patella (Fig. 46.9). It is stabilized by the quadriceps (rectus femoris, vastus lateralis, vastus intermedius, and vastus medialis), intra-articular ligaments (anterior cruciate ligament—ACL, posterior cruciate ligament—PCL), and extracapsular ligaments (lateral collateral ligament—LCL, medial collateral ligament—MCL). It is also supported by multiple bursae (prepatellar, suprapatellar, anserine, popliteus, etc.), small sacs that surround the joint and reduce friction between the numerous parts.

Traumatic impact to the knee can also cause tearing of the stabilizing ligaments and meniscus, along with fractures. MCL injuries generally occur due to a direct blow to the lateral aspect of the knee and present as a temporary valgus deformity. These are mostly treated using hinged knee bracing and physical therapy, with surgery recommended mainly when there is concurrent knee dislocation and instability

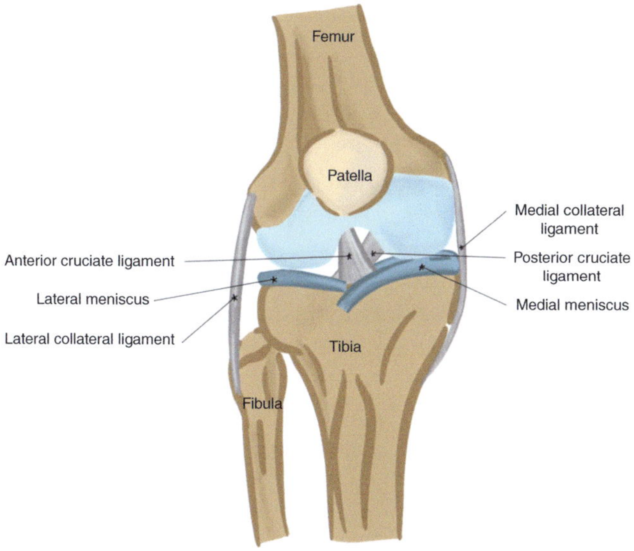

Fig. 46.9 Illustration of the bone, ligament, and meniscus anatomy of the knee joint

[74]. ACL tears are the most common ligamentous injury and usually arise from a pivoting injury where the tibia translates anteriorly while the knee is in valgus and flexed [75]. Treatment depends on associated injuries, age, functionality, and knee use of the individual patient. Surgical management is mostly done in the younger, more active population to optimize mobility. In the older population, physical therapy for strengthening is preferred, as the lack of an ACL does not completely hinder ambulation. For ACL repair, graft replacement is usually necessary; options are autograft, bone-tendon-bone, or allograft, with the optimal graft choice dependent on the patient's case. Treatment should prioritize early restoration of extension, flexion, and strengthening. If grafting is used, 6–12 months are necessary for the patient to fully be able to return to activity. The damage to the articular cartilage determines whether there will be eventual existence of osteoarthritis in the affected joint later on [74]. PCL and LCL injuries are rare compared to MCL or ACL tears, and are occasionally treated with a graft and surgical operation [76]. Stability to the knee is also provided by the meniscus, which is a relatively avascular structure that aids in shock absorption and improves knee articulation. Tears in the meniscus can cause joint line tenderness, swelling, clicking, and locking. Management is usually surgical, with arthroscopic repair or debridement [77].

Ligament and meniscus tears also have a high association with tibial plateau fractures, which are common in pediatric patients, young adults, and elderly patients [78]. Diagnosis of these fractures can be confirmed on plain radiographs, with CT scans supplemented to rule out neurovascular injury and MRI added to evaluate the need for concomitant MCL or ACL tears. Nonoperative treatment is suitable for minimally displaced fractures with no ligament injuries. Patients can be placed in a hinged knee brace, with non-weight-bearing restrictions for 6–8 weeks. Operative management is used for fractures with significant articular step-off, condylar widening, and ligamentous instability. Surgical management involves ORIF. Postoperatively, a hinged knee brace is used, with the patient instructed to be non-weight-bearing for 6 weeks, partial weight-bearing for the following 6 weeks, and then weight-bearing as tolerated. In some cases, external fixation or total knee arthroplasty may be required [79].

Nontraumatic knee injuries are commonly from overuse and include pathologies such as patellofemoral syndrome ("runner's knee"), pes anserine bursitis, and iliotibial band syndrome. Management of these conditions is usually conservative and involves some combination of activity modification, ice, and NSAID use. Corticosteroid injections have also been shown to provide symptom relief [80–82]. In addition, the knee is also a major joint affected by OA, with similar screening and treatment strategies as hip OA. Patients with persistent arthritic symptoms despite nonsurgical treatment can be surgically managed with total knee arthroplasty [68, 83].

Foot and Ankle

The foot is comprised of 26 bones: 7 tarsals, 5 metatarsals, and 14 phalanges. The complex anatomy helps to support the rest of the body. The foot is divided into forefoot (metatarsals and phalanges), midfoot (navicular, cuboid, and middle, medial, and lateral cuneiforms), and hindfoot (talus and calcaneus); articulation of the forefoot and midfoot is called the Lisfranc joint, and the junction between the hindfoot and midfoot is called the Chopart joint. Muscles and tendons in the foot function to maintain stability and allow for coordinated movement when walking [84].

In terms of traumatic injuries, ankle sprains are extremely common and can affect patients of all populations, arising often from a stretch of the anterior talofibular ligament (ATFL) or the calcaneofibular ligament (CFL) after rolling the foot. Rest, ice compression, and elevation are first-line for treatment of ankle sprains, with gradual resumption of daily activities encouraged to avoid stiffness from immobilization [84]. Trauma or repeated stress can also lead to foot bone dislocations and fractures. A Lisfranc injury is a frequently missed and misdiagnosed injury in the foot, which can come from high-energy or low-energy mechanisms, and can range from sprains to dislocations and fractures. Low-energy injuries are caused by lesions in the ligaments, bones, and soft tissues in the structures between the forefoot and midfoot, thereby leading to gradual dislocation of the tarsometatarsal Lisfranc joint (between the medial cuneiform and second metatarsal base). Over time, the lesions can cause biomechanical changes in the arch of the foot, thereby yielding abnormal weight distribution and causing severe pain that can affect gait. On the more severe end of the Lisfranc injury spectrum, a Lisfranc fracture, most commonly the result of high-energy trauma such as falls from a distance or a motorcycle accident, includes fracture of the metatarsal base along with ligament compromise [85]. Patients with Lisfranc injuries often present with midfoot pain that is worse when weight-bearing. Lisfranc injury should be expected if the patient with midfoot pain has persistent pain for at least 5 days, swelling, and a slightly altered gait. Nonsurgical management includes reduction, immobilization (boost or cast), and aggressive elevation. Surgical management is indicated if the Lisfranc joint becomes unstable, compartment syndrome is found in the foot, there is persistent malalignment of the tarsometatarsal joint despite nonsurgical management, or the fracture is open [86].

Of the nontraumatic injuries of the foot and ankle, plantar fasciitis is the most common, occurring in nearly 10% of the general population. This condition has a degenerative etiology, resulting from repetitive strain causing micro-tears in the plantar fascia over a period of time. Patients thus present with progressive pain in the heel that is sharp and worse with the first steps in the morning or extended standing. Ambulation and activity tend to help with the pain, and the pain is reproduced with passive dorsiflexion of the foot and toes. Plantar fasciitis is a clinical diagnosis, and so no imaging is needed. First-line treatment is rest from the painful activities and a night splint, along with ice and NSAIDs for pain. If these conservative measures do not help, then more invasive techniques such as injections can be used. If the pain continues to persist despite nonsurgical treatments, surgery can be recommended. Surgery should be approached with caution in plantar fasciitis, as it does not guarantee a successful outcome as the fasciitis can still return later on [87].

Basics of Fracture Immobilization

Casts and splints are two techniques for joint immobilization that stabilize fractures to permit healing. The rigid materials also allow for molding to reduce the fracture. Casts are wrapped circumferentially to immobilize a given joint, offering greater stability and rigidity. Meanwhile, splints do not circumferentially cover the joint, leaving space for edema. Thus, splints are more commonly used for acute injuries to leave space for swelling, while casts are used for unstable fractures and injuries that cannot be managed with splinting.

There are a variety of casts that can be wrapped depending on the body part they are to support. As general practice, fiberglass should be dipped in cold water before wrapping, and bony prominences should be padded with cotton before layering on the cast material. In the lower extremity, a below-knee (short-leg) cast wraps from the base of the toes up to the proximal tibia. The ankle should be in a neutral position for this cast, and so when applied, the knee should be in flexion. For the above-knee (long-leg) cast, the fiberglass extends from the toes to the distal femur. Knee should be flexed at 5–20° and extra padding should be applied around the patella for comfort. For lower extremity casts, the toes should be kept free. In the upper extremity, short arm casts extend from the palm to below the elbow, while long arm casts go above the elbow. The thumb and MCP joints should be free, and the distal part of the cast should not go past the proximal palmar crease [88].

Similar to casts, there are also many variations for splints depending on the joint it is attempting to immobilize. Table 46.4 provides a list of different types of splints along with their indications and general structure. Because they do not circumferentially wrap, and therefore are easily removable, splints are often a temporizing measure for patients'

Table 46.4 Splints, their indications, and structure, with illustrations of upper body splints of the arm, forearm, and hand in Fig. 46.10 and lower body splints of the ankle and thigh in Fig. 46.11

Splint type	Indications	Structure
Sugar-tong splint	Distal radius and ulna fractures	Splint from palm to above elbow. Splint material goes from volar surface of palm down the forearm, around the elbow and then along the dorsal surface of the forearm
Coaptation splint	Humerus fractures	Splint the arm from shoulder to elbow. Splint material goes from axilla around the elbow up the arm toward the acromioclavicular joint
Volar/dorsal forearm splint	Wrist sprain, acute carpal bone fracture (excluding scaphoid and trapezium), childhood buckle fractures of the distal radius	Splint material extending from palmar crease to the mid-forearm on both the volar/palmar and dorsal sides
Ulnar gutter splint	Fractures of the 4th and 5th metacarpal	Splint material folded longitudinally to wrap around ulna and 4th and 5th phalanges. Extend from the fingers to the mid-forearm
Thumb spica splint	Scaphoid and trapezium fractures. Stable thumb fractures.	Splint material from palm to the mid-forearm, wrapped around the base of the thumb and folded along the radial side
Posterior slab splint (ankle)	Nondisplaced malleolar fractures, acute foot fractures, and severe sprains	Splint material from plantar surface of metatarsal heads extends posteriorly to the fibular head
Posterior slab splint (thigh)	Injuries to the knee and leg (proximal tibia, distal femoral fractures)	Splint extends from mid-thigh to ankle, wrapped posteriorly around the leg

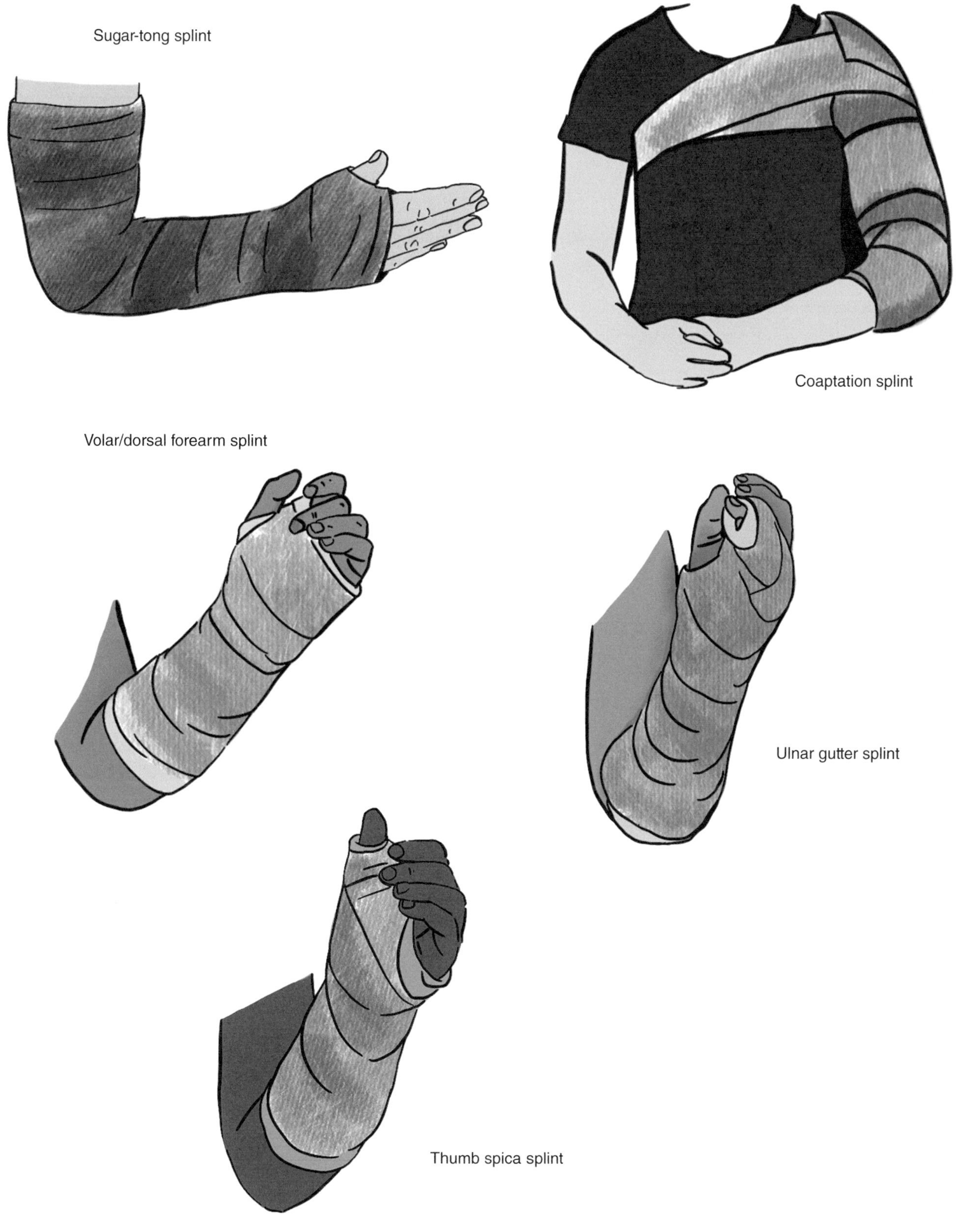

Fig. 46.10 Illustration of various types of upper body splints

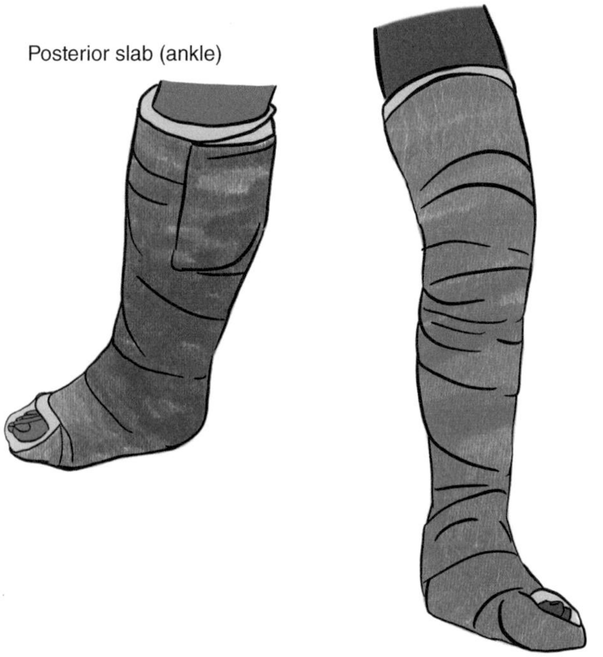

Fig. 46.11 Illustration of the posterior slab splint of the ankle and the posterior slab splint of the thigh

fractures until they can get treated in the operating room with an open reduction. As general practice for splints, when wrapping with plaster, warmer water decreases molding time, but overly hot water can burn the patient's skin, so either ensure that the patient has enough protective layers of padding before applying the plaster or check the water temperature before dipping the wrapping plaster [89, 90].

While splints and casts are incredibly useful, they also have their complications. Increased external pressure can cause pressure necrosis and, in casts that are wrapped too tight, can even cause compartment syndrome. Thus, care must be taken to ensure that a well-fitting but safe cast or splint is applied.

Conclusion

In this chapter, we reviewed the basics of assessing a new orthopedic patient in the ED and the office, including the key components of the interview and physical exam that are relevant when forming a differential and treatment plan for an orthopedic injury. Benefits and costs of imaging modalities, and a rapid overview of common orthopedic conditions was also presented. Finally, we discussed the basics of fracture immobilization and casting and splinting techniques.

References

1. Gehrig LMB. Orthopedic surgery. Am J Surg. 2011;202(3):364–8. https://doi.org/10.1016/j.amjsurg.2011.06.007.
2. Statistical Profile of Board Certified Physician Assistants ANNUAL REPORT National Commission on Certification of Physician Assistants. Published online May 3, 2024. Accessed 3 Oct 2024. https://www.nccpa.net/wp-content/uploads/2024/05/2023-Statistical-Profile-of-Board-Certified-PAs5_3_24.pdf.
3. Larson EH, Coerver DA, Wick KH, Ballweg RA. Physician assistants in orthopedic practice. A national study. J Allied Health. 2011;40(4):174–80.
4. Best practices in the management of orthopaedic trauma. ACS Committee on Trauma. Published online 2015.
5. Lin S, Alepuz A, Tritsch T, Schwartz G. Deep vein thrombosis prophylaxis in orthopedic surgery. Cureus. 2024;16(2):e53726. https://doi.org/10.7759/cureus.53726.
6. Lan P, Chen X, Fang Z, Zhang J, Liu S, Liu Y. Effects of comorbidities on pain and function after total hip arthroplasty. Front Surg. 2022;9:829303. https://doi.org/10.3389/fsurg.2022.829303.
7. Castano-Betancourt MC, Fruschein Annichino R, De Azevedo E, Souza Munhoz M, Gomes Machado E, Lipay MV, Marchi E. Identification of high-risk groups for complication after arthroplasty: predictive value of patient's related risk factors. J Orthop Surg Res. 2018;13(1):328. https://doi.org/10.1186/s13018-018-1036-2.
8. Santos C, Gabriel AT, Quaresma C, Nunes IL. Risk factors, symptoms, and prevalence of lower limb work-related musculoskeletal disorders among orthopedic surgeons. Int J Ind Ergon. 2024;101:103597. https://doi.org/10.1016/j.ergon.2024.103597.
9. Greenstein AS, Gorczyca JT. Orthopedic surgery and the geriatric patient. Clin Geriatr Med. 2019;35(1):65–92. https://doi.org/10.1016/j.cger.2018.08.007.
10. Hippensteel KJ, Brophy R, Smith MV, Wright RW. A comprehensive review of physical examination tests of the cervical spine, scapula, and rotator cuff. J Am Acad Orthop Surg. 2019;27(11):385–94. https://doi.org/10.5435/JAAOS-D-17-00090.
11. Payares-Lizano M, Pino C. Pediatric orthopedic examination. Pediatr Clin N Am. 2020;67(1):1–21. https://doi.org/10.1016/j.pcl.2019.09.004.
12. Babayoff O, Shehory O, Geller S, Shitrit-Niselbaum C, Weiss-Meilik A, Sprecher E. Improving hospital outpatient clinics appointment schedules by prediction models. J Med Syst. 2022;47(1):5. https://doi.org/10.1007/s10916-022-01902-3.
13. MacKechnie MC, Nadeau M, Deering E, Thaller J, MacKechnie MA. Orthopaedic walk-in clinics: a model to lessen the burden on emergency departments during the COVID-19 pandemic. J Orthop. 2020;20:293–6. https://doi.org/10.1016/j.jor.2020.05.014.
14. Cleland J, Koppenhaver S, Su J, Netter F. Netter's orthopaedic clinical examination: an evidence-based approach. 4th ed. Elsevier; 2022.
15. Koetter P, Gallo R, Kasmire KE. Assessing the necessity for the "joint above and below" radiography approach for lower-extremity long bone fractures in children. Pediatr Emerg Care. 2022;38(1):e316–20. https://doi.org/10.1097/PEC.0000000000002274.
16. Faraz A, Qureshi AI, Noah H Khan M, et al. Documentation of neurovascular assessment in fracture patients in a tertiary care hospital: a retrospective review. Ann Med Surg (Lond). 2022;79:103935. https://doi.org/10.1016/j.amsu.2022.103935.
17. Raza H, Mahapatra A. Acute compartment syndrome in orthopedics: causes, diagnosis, and management. Adv Orthop. 2015;2015:543412. https://doi.org/10.1155/2015/543412.

18. Torlincasi AM, Lopez RA, Waseem M. Acute compartment syndrome. In: StatPearls. StatPearls Publishing; 2024. Accessed 6 Oct 2024. http://www.ncbi.nlm.nih.gov/books/NBK448124/.
19. Shahrokhi M, Asuncion RMD. Neurologic exam. In: StatPearls [Internet]. StatPearls Publishing; 2023. Accessed 6 Oct 2024. https://www.ncbi.nlm.nih.gov/books/NBK557589/.
20. Gracy JA. Orthopedics for physician assistant and nurse practitioner students: an introductory guide. Springer International Publishing; 2022. https://doi.org/10.1007/978-3-031-04406-9.
21. Larkins LW, Baker RT, Baker JG. Physical examination of the ankle: a review of the original orthopedic special test description and scientific validity of common tests for ankle examination. Arch Rehabil Res Clin Transl. 2020;2(3):100072. https://doi.org/10.1016/j.arrct.2020.100072.
22. Hippensteel KJ, Brophy R, Smith MV, Wright RW. Comprehensive review of provocative and instability physical examination tests of the shoulder. J Am Acad Orthop Surg. 2019;27(11):395–404. https://doi.org/10.5435/JAAOS-D-17-00637.
23. Kuschner SH, Ebramzadeh E, Johnson D, Brien WW, Sherman R. Tinel's sign and Phalen's test in carpal tunnel syndrome. Orthopedics. 1992;15(11):1297–302. https://doi.org/10.3928/0147-7447-19921101-08.
24. Dawson C, Mudgal CS. Staged description of the Finkelstein test. J Hand Surg Am. 2010;35(9):1513–5. https://doi.org/10.1016/j.jhsa.2010.05.022.
25. Model Z, Liu AY, Kang L, Wolfe SW, Burket JC, Lee SK. Evaluation of physical examination tests for thumb basal joint osteoarthritis. Hand (N Y). 2016;11(1):108–12. https://doi.org/10.1177/1558944715616951.
26. Erickson BJ, Romeo AA. The ulnar collateral ligament injury: evaluation and treatment. J Bone Joint Surg. 2017;99(1):76–86. https://doi.org/10.2106/JBJS.16.01277.
27. Teoli D, Rocha Cabrero F, Smith T, Ghassemzadeh S. Lhermitte sign. In: StatPearls. StatPearls Publishing; 2024. Accessed 6 Oct 2024. http://www.ncbi.nlm.nih.gov/books/NBK493237/.
28. Hodler J, Kubik-Huch RA, Von Schulthess GK, editors. Musculoskeletal diseases 2021–2024: diagnostic imaging. Springer International Publishing; 2021. https://doi.org/10.1007/978-3-030-71281-5.
29. Yoon I, Slesinger TL. Radiation exposure in pregnancy. In: StatPearls. StatPearls Publishing; 2024. Accessed 6 Oct 2024. http://www.ncbi.nlm.nih.gov/books/NBK551690/.
30. Schlacter JA, Roussos D, Masrouha K, et al. Effect of a protocol to reduce radiographic imaging in pediatric patients with suspected fractures. J Pediatr Orthop. 2023;43(1):61–4. https://doi.org/10.1097/BPO.0000000000002262.
31. Rajaraman P, Simpson J, Neta G, et al. Early life exposure to diagnostic radiation and ultrasound scans and risk of childhood cancer: case-control study. BMJ. 2011;342:d472. https://doi.org/10.1136/bmj.d472.
32. Goud A, Segal D, Hedayati P, Pan JJ, Weissman BN. Radiographic evaluation of the shoulder. Eur J Radiol. 2008;68(1):2–15. https://doi.org/10.1016/j.ejrad.2008.02.023.
33. Min W, Sanders R. The use of the mortise view of the ankle to determine hindfoot alignment: technique tip. Foot Ankle Int. 2010;31(9):823–7. https://doi.org/10.3113/FAI.2010.0823.
34. Carrino JA, Ibad H, Lin Y, et al. CT in musculoskeletal imaging: still helpful and for what? Skeletal Radiol. 2024;53(9):1711–25. https://doi.org/10.1007/s00256-024-04737-w.
35. Hartley KG, Damon BM, Patterson GT, Long JH, Holt GE. MRI techniques: a review and update for the orthopaedic surgeon. J Am Acad Orthop Surg. 2012;20(12):775–87. https://doi.org/10.5435/JAAOS-20-12-775.
36. Hong A, Liu JN, Gowd AK, Dhawan A, Amin NH. Reliability and accuracy of MRI in orthopedics: a survey of its use and perceived limitations. Clin Med Insights Arthritis Musculoskelet Disord. 2019;12:1179544119872972. https://doi.org/10.1177/1179544119872972.
37. Dobaria DG, Cohen HL. Osteomyelitis imaging. In: StatPearls [Internet]. StatPearls Publishing; 2023. Accessed 7 Oct 2024. https://www.ncbi.nlm.nih.gov/books/NBK594242/.
38. Jha Y, Chaudhary K. Diagnosis and treatment modalities for osteomyelitis. Cureus. 2022;14(10):e30713. Published online October 26, 2022. https://doi.org/10.7759/cureus.30713.
39. Ghadimi M, Sapra A. Magnetic resonance imaging contraindications. In: StatPearls. StatPearls Publishing; 2024. Accessed 7 Oct 2024. http://www.ncbi.nlm.nih.gov/books/NBK551669/.
40. Kim PH, Leopold SS. Gustilo-Anderson classification. Clin Orthop Relat Res. 2012;470(11):3270–4. https://doi.org/10.1007/s11999-012-2376-6.
41. Levine RH, Thomas A, Nezwek TA, Waseem M. Salter-Harris fracture. In: StatPearls [Internet]. StatPearls Publishing; 2023. Accessed 7 Oct 2024. https://www.ncbi.nlm.nih.gov/books/NBK430688/.
42. Bass E. Tendinopathy: why the difference between tendinitis and tendinosis matters. IJTMB. 2012;5(1):14–7. https://doi.org/10.3822/ijtmb.v5i1.153.
43. Banay GL. An introduction to medical terminology I. Greek and Latin derivations. Bull Med Libr Assoc. 1948;36(1):1–27.
44. Arias DG, Black AC, Varacallo M. Anatomy, shoulder and upper limb, hand bones. In: StatPearls. StatPearls Publishing; 2024. Accessed 7 Oct 2024. http://www.ncbi.nlm.nih.gov/books/NBK547684/.
45. Patel M, Varacallo M. Anatomy, shoulder and upper limb, forearm bones. In: StatPearls. StatPearls Publishing; 2024. Accessed 7 Oct 2024. http://www.ncbi.nlm.nih.gov/books/NBK545260/.
46. Fowler JR, Hughes TB. Scaphoid fractures. Clin Sports Med. 2015;34(1):37–50. https://doi.org/10.1016/j.csm.2014.09.011.
47. Sabbagh MD, Morsy M, Moran SL. Diagnosis and management of acute scaphoid fractures. Hand Clin. 2019;35(3):259–69. https://doi.org/10.1016/j.hcl.2019.03.002.
48. Corsino CB, Reeves RA, Sieg RN. Distal radius fractures. In: StatPearls [Internet]. StatPearls Publishing; 2023. Accessed 7 Oct 2024. https://www.ncbi.nlm.nih.gov/books/NBK536916/.
49. Fatima A, Ahmed O, Ahmed M, Beg MSA, Batool A, Siddiqui MM. Metacarpal fractures, management techniques, and outcomes in our center. Cureus. 2021;13(9):e17828. Published online September 8, 2021. https://doi.org/10.7759/cureus.17828.
50. Werntz RL, Varacallo M. Metacarpal fracture. In: StatPearls [Internet]. StatPearls Publishing; 2023. Accessed 7 Oct 2024. https://www.ncbi.nlm.nih.gov/books/NBK551532/.
51. McDaniel DJ, Rehman UH. Phalanx fractures of the hand. In: StatPearls. StatPearls Publishing; 2024. Accessed 7 Oct 2024. http://www.ncbi.nlm.nih.gov/books/NBK557625/.
52. Kremer L, Frank J, Lustenberger T, Marzi I, Sander AL. Epidemiology and treatment of phalangeal fractures: conservative treatment is the predominant therapeutic concept. Eur J Trauma Emerg Surg. 2022;48(1):567–71. https://doi.org/10.1007/s00068-020-01397-y.
53. Supracondylar humerus fractures - StatPearls - NCBI Bookshelf. Accessed 7 Oct 2024. https://www.ncbi.nlm.nih.gov/books/NBK560933/.
54. Joshi A, Patel K, Mohamed A, et al. Carpal tunnel syndrome: pathophysiology and comprehensive guidelines for clinical evaluation and treatment. Cureus. 2022;14(7):e27053. Published online July 20, 2022. https://doi.org/10.7759/cureus.27053.

55. Sevy JO, Sina RE, Varacallo M. Carpal tunnel syndrome. In: StatPearls. StatPearls Publishing; 2024. Accessed 7 Oct 2024. http://www.ncbi.nlm.nih.gov/books/NBK448179/.
56. Makkouk AH, Oetgen ME, Swigart CR, Dodds SD. Trigger finger: etiology, evaluation, and treatment. Curr Rev Musculoskelet Med. 2008;1(2):92–6. https://doi.org/10.1007/s12178-007-9012-1.
57. Satteson E, Tannan SC. De Quervain tenosynovitis. In: StatPearls. StatPearls Publishing; 2024. Accessed 7 Oct 2024. http://www.ncbi.nlm.nih.gov/books/NBK442005/.
58. Anderson D, Woods B, Abubakar T, et al. A comprehensive review of cubital tunnel syndrome. Orthop Rev (Pavia). 2022;14(3):38239. https://doi.org/10.52965/001c.38239.
59. Hyland S, Charlick M, Varacallo M. Anatomy, shoulder and upper limb, clavicle. In: StatPearls. StatPearls Publishing; 2024. Accessed 7 Oct 2024. http://www.ncbi.nlm.nih.gov/books/NBK525990/.
60. Doehrmann R, Frush TJ. Posterior shoulder instability. In: StatPearls. StatPearls Publishing; 2024. Accessed 7 Oct 2024. http://www.ncbi.nlm.nih.gov/books/NBK557648/.
61. Varacallo M, Musto MA, Mair SD. Anterior shoulder instability. In: StatPearls. StatPearls Publishing; 2024. Accessed 7 Oct 2024. http://www.ncbi.nlm.nih.gov/books/NBK538234/.
62. DeSai C, Reddy V, Agarwal A. Anatomy, back, vertebral column. In: StatPearls [Internet]. StatPearls Publishing; 2023. Accessed 7 Oct 2024. https://www.ncbi.nlm.nih.gov/books/NBK525969/.
63. Urits I, Burshtein A, Sharma M, et al. Low back pain, a comprehensive review: pathophysiology, diagnosis, and treatment. Curr Pain Headache Rep. 2019;23(3):23. https://doi.org/10.1007/s11916-019-0757-1.
64. Janicki JA, Alman B. Scoliosis: review of diagnosis and treatment. Paediatr Child Health. 2007;12(9):771–6. https://doi.org/10.1093/pch/12.9.771.
65. Maruyama T, Takeshita K. Surgical treatment of scoliosis: a review of techniques currently applied. Scoliosis. 2008;3(1):6. https://doi.org/10.1186/1748-7161-3-6.
66. Gold M, Munjal A, Varacallo M. Anatomy, bony pelvis and lower limb, hip joint. In: StatPearls. StatPearls Publishing; 2024. Accessed 7 Oct 2024. http://www.ncbi.nlm.nih.gov/books/NBK470555/.
67. Tullington JE, Blecker N. Pelvic trauma. In: StatPearls [Internet]. StatPearls Publishing; 2023. Accessed 7 Oct 2024. https://www.ncbi.nlm.nih.gov/books/NBK556070/.
68. Katz JN, Arant KR, Loeser RF. Diagnosis and treatment of hip and knee osteoarthritis: a review. JAMA. 2021;325(6):568. https://doi.org/10.1001/jama.2020.22171.
69. Lespasio MJ, Sultan AA, Piuzzi NS, et al. Hip osteoarthritis: a primer. Perm J. 2018;22:17–084. https://doi.org/10.7812/TPP/17-084.
70. O'Rourke RJ, El Bitar Y. Femoroacetabular impingement. In: StatPearls. StatPearls Publishing; 2024. Accessed 7 Oct 2024. http://www.ncbi.nlm.nih.gov/books/NBK547699/.
71. Trigg SD, Schroeder JD, Hulsopple C. Femoroacetabular impingement syndrome. Curr Sports Med Rep. 2020;19(9):360–6. https://doi.org/10.1249/JSR.0000000000000748.
72. Fortier LM, Popovsky D, Durci MM, Norwood H, Sherman WF, Kaye AD. An updated review of femoroacetabular impingement syndrome. Orthop Rev. 2022;14(3):37513. https://doi.org/10.52965/001c.37513.
73. Harris JD, Erickson BJ, Bush-Joseph CA, Nho SJ. Treatment of femoroacetabular impingement: a systematic review. Curr Rev Musculoskelet Med. 2013;6(3):207–18. https://doi.org/10.1007/s12178-013-9172-0.
74. LaBella CR, Hennrikus W, Hewett TE, et al. Anterior cruciate ligament injuries: diagnosis, treatment, and prevention. Pediatrics. 2014;133(5):e1437–50. https://doi.org/10.1542/peds.2014-0623.
75. Evans J, Mabrouk A, Nielson JL. Anterior cruciate ligament knee injury. In: StatPearls. StatPearls Publishing; 2024. Accessed 7 Oct 2024. http://www.ncbi.nlm.nih.gov/books/NBK499848/.
76. Lundblad M, Hägglund M, Thomeé C, et al. Epidemiological data on LCL and PCL injuries over 17 seasons in men's professional soccer: the UEFA elite club injury study. OAJSM. 2020;11:105–12. https://doi.org/10.2147/OAJSM.S237997.
77. Bhan K. Meniscal tears: current understanding, diagnosis, and management. Cureus. 2020;12(6):e8590. Published online June 13, 2020. https://doi.org/10.7759/cureus.8590.
78. Malik S, Herron T, Mabrouk A, Rosenberg N. Tibial plateau fractures. In: StatPearls [Internet]. StatPearls Publishing; 2023. Accessed 7 Oct 2024. https://www.ncbi.nlm.nih.gov/books/NBK470593/.
79. Prat-Fabregat S, Camacho-Carrasco P. Treatment strategy for tibial plateau fractures: an update. EFORT Open Rev. 2016;1(5):225–32. https://doi.org/10.1302/2058-5241.1.000031.
80. Hadeed A, Tapscott DC. Iliotibial band friction syndrome. In: StatPearls. StatPearls Publishing; 2024. Accessed 7 Oct 2024. http://www.ncbi.nlm.nih.gov/books/NBK542185/.
81. Bump JM, Lewis L. Patellofemoral syndrome. In: StatPearls. StatPearls Publishing; 2024. Accessed 7 Oct 2024. http://www.ncbi.nlm.nih.gov/books/NBK557657/.
82. Mohseni M, Mabrouk A, Li DD, Graham C. Pes anserine bursitis. In: StatPearls. StatPearls Publishing; 2024. Accessed 7 Oct 2024. http://www.ncbi.nlm.nih.gov/books/NBK532941/.
83. Hsu H, Siwiec RM. Knee osteoarthritis. In: StatPearls. StatPearls Publishing; 2024. Accessed 7 Oct 2024. http://www.ncbi.nlm.nih.gov/books/NBK507884/.
84. Melanson SW, Shuman VL. Acute ankle sprain. In: StatPearls. StatPearls Publishing; 2024. Accessed 7 Oct 2024. http://www.ncbi.nlm.nih.gov/books/NBK459212/.
85. Chen J, Sagoo N, Panchbhavi VK. The Lisfranc injury: a literature review of anatomy, etiology, evaluation, and management. Foot Ankle Spec. 2021;14(5):458–67. https://doi.org/10.1177/1938640020950133.
86. Buchanan BK, Iii CJD. Lisfranc dislocation. In: StatPearls [Internet]. StatPearls Publishing; 2023. Accessed 7 Oct 2024. https://www.ncbi.nlm.nih.gov/books/NBK448147/.
87. Buchanan BK, Sina RE, Kushner D. Plantar Fasciitis. In: StatPearls. StatPearls Publishing; 2024. Accessed 7 Oct 2024. http://www.ncbi.nlm.nih.gov/books/NBK431073/.
88. Egol KA, Koval KJ, Zuckerman JD. Handbook of fractures. 6th ed. Wolters Kluwer; 2020.
89. Althoff AD, Reeves RA. Splinting. In: StatPearls. StatPearls Publishing; 2024. Accessed October 7, 2024. http://www.ncbi.nlm.nih.gov/books/NBK557673/.
90. Boyd AS, Benjamin HJ, Asplund C. Splints and casts: indications and methods. Am Fam Physician. 2009;80(5):491–9.

Otolaryngology

47

Vincent Pretorius

Introduction

This chapter provides an overview of frequently encountered ear-nose-throat (ENT) conditions. It provides a foundational understanding of their key features, potential complications, and management strategies.

Upper Airway Obstruction—The Stridulous Patient

It can be very easy to feel overwhelmed when dealing with airway emergencies. It is important to try to remain calm and use the commonly adopted Advanced Trauma Life Support (ATLS) principles.

- A—Airway
- B—Breathing
- C—Circulation
- D—Disability (Glasgow coma scale)/Drugs (which medications has the patient been taking or which drugs have been given)/Disability
- E—Environmental/exposure control

Establishing an airway almost always supersedes any other pressing issue. Patients with upper airway obstruction primarily present with stridor. Stridor (noisy breathing) is due to turbulent airflow caused by a narrowing in the upper respiratory tract at the level of the larynx. However, obstruction can also originate from the oral or nasal cavities, pharynx, or trachea. It is useful to understand and divide obstruction into three categories:

1. "*Functional obstruction*" due to inflammatory changes or edema. This usually responds to medical therapy, e.g., oxygen supplementation, epinephrine nebulization, intravenous steroids, and broad-spectrum antibiotics.
2. "*Structural obstruction,*" be it due to mass effect from a tumor, expanding hematoma, or a foreign body. Obstruction can be due to extra-luminal compression, intramural growth and narrowing, or endoluminal obstruction. This may require orotracheal or nasotracheal intubation or some surgical intervention to bypass the obstruction, like an emergency surgical airway (cricothyroidotomy or tracheostomy) or urgent bronchoscopic intubation under general anesthesia.
3. Combinations of "*Functional and Structural*" obstruction may occur, e.g., a deep neck space abscess causing distortion and inflammation of the larynx and upper airway. There is usually a partial response to medical therapy in such cases, but definitive structural (surgical) intervention or airway manipulation may be required.

Common Causes for Upper Airway Obstruction in Adults

- Neoplastic
  - Benign
  - Malignant
- Infective
  - Acute epiglottitis—H. Influenza
  - Deep neck space abscess
  - Respiratory papillomatosis
  - Tracheitis
  - Diphtheria
  - TB (Tuberculosis) of the larynx
  - Ludwig's angina
- Inflammatory
  - Angioneurotic oedema
  - Trauma—blunt or sharp

V. Pretorius (✉)
Department of ENT, University of Cape Town, Cape Town, South Africa
e-mail: vincent.pretorius@westerncape.gov.za

S. Atallah, J. Dragoljevic (eds.), *Fundamentals of Surgery for Physician Assistants*,
https://doi.org/10.1007/978-3-032-21069-2_47

  - Inhalational injury—chemical or thermal
  - Auto-immune—IgG4 disease, sarcoidosis
- Structural
  - Bilateral vocal cord palsy (Thyroid neoplasm/post thyroidectomy/trauma/neurological)
  - Subglottic/tracheal stenosis—often after intubation
- Foreign body

With airway emergencies, it is important to recruit the help of colleagues as soon as possible. Your ENT colleague should get involved for urgent upper airway flexible video nasopharyngolaryngoscopy or rigid endoscopy in the operating room.

With experience comes the ability to identify patients who will imminently decompensate and to act sooner rather than later to secure an airway. Should the patient require orotracheal intubation, it is important to identify which patients might be assessed as a potential difficult intubation risk.

Once the airway has been stabilized, further investigation will be determined by the patient history.

Questions to Ask:

1. A short onset history would indicate something acute, that is inflammatory or infective or traumatic or even toxin exposure in the form of ingestion or inhalational injury or even a possible foreign body.
2. A slowly progressive onset would indicate something neoplastic, be it benign or malignant.
3. Hoarseness of longer than 2–3 weeks with referred otalgia indicates a malignancy of the larynx and/or pharynx until proven otherwise. Such patients might also have dysphagia or odynophagia.

Management

- Call for help
- A, B, Cs
- Give humidified oxygen with atomized epinephrine: 1 ml of 1:1000 concentration diluted with 1 ml saline.
- Keep the patient nil by mouth and determine when their last meal was.
- Establish intravenous access and do arterial blood gas assessment.
- Give intravenous corticosteroid, Dexamethasone 8 mg, +/− a broad-spectrum antibiotic if sepsis is suspected and after doing a blood culture.
- Should the patient be stable enough for imaging, consider an A-P and lateral neck x-ray or a contrasted CT of the neck and chest.
- Assess and determine the need for intubation as listed below:
  - Hypoxia
  - Hypercapnea
  - Fatigue
  - Poor cardiopulmonary reserve
  - No access to an operating room
  - Change in level of consciousness

Predictors of Difficult Intubation That May Indicate the Need for a Surgical Airway

- Lemon score assess for features of a possible difficult intubation [1].

Evaluation criteria	Points
L = Look externally	
Facial trauma	1
Large incisors	1
Beard or moustache	1
Large tongue	1
E = Evaluate the 3-3-2 rule	
Incisor distance-3 finger breadths	1
Hyoid-mental distance-3 finger breadths	1
Thyroid-to-mouth distance-2 finger breadths	
M = Mallampati (Mallampati score > 3)	1
O = Obstruction (presence of any condition like epiglottitis, peritonsillar abscess, trauma)	1
N = Neck mobility (limited neck mobility)	1
Total	**10**

- Fibrotic neck due to previous radiation
- Trismus
- History of difficult intubation
- Poor cardiopulmonary reserve
- Tumor location and size
  - Base of tongue tumors
  - Supraglottic tumors
  - Large or bleeding tumors
  - Any tumor displacing or distorting the anatomy and position of the larynx

Intubation Options

- Orotracheal intubation with a standard laryngoscopy blade and a bougie
- Videolaryngoscopic intubation (C-MAC blades)—should preferably be used in any difficult-to-intubate scenario
- Flexible or rigid fiberoptic/video intubation
- "ENT" intubation—using an operating laryngoscope or rigid bronchoscope under general anesthetic

Surgical Airway Options

- Needle cricothyrotomy (to buy a few minutes of time only)
- Cricothyroidotomy
- Tracheostomy—awake vs intubated under general anesthesia

For further reading on technique see "Cricothyroidotomy and needle cricothyrotomy" and "Tracheostomy": https://health.uct.ac.za/entdev/guides/open-access-atlas-otolaryngology-head-neck-operative-surgery

Rhinology

Epistaxis

The term epistaxis is derived from the Greek word epistazein, which means to bleed/drip from the nose. It is key to have a basic understanding of the anatomy and blood supply of the nose. Epistaxis can be divided into anterior or posterior epistaxis according to the origin of the bleeding relative to the piriform aperture of the nose. It can further be classified into primary (idiopathic) epistaxis, which accounts for 70–80%, or secondary epistaxis, where a specific cause can be found, e.g., trauma, anticoagulants, hemophilia, etc.

Key Clinical Areas

Two areas of the nose have historically been considered clinically important. Little's area or Kiesselbach's plexus is a vascular plexus situated on the anterior nasal septum. Woodruff's plexus is situated inferior to the posterior end of the inferior turbinate, which may be responsible for most posterior bleeds. More recently, studies have shown a bleeding point on the septum, just medial to the head of the middle turbinate, from a septal branch of the anterior ethmoidal artery to be a common cause as well. This must be screened during endoscopic evaluation of the nasal cavity.

Causes of Epistaxis

Local

- Trauma (digital, blunt force, nasal fractures, etc.)
- Rhinitis or sinusitis
- Iatrogenic—complications of surgery
- Topical medication like nasal sprays
- Recreational drugs, e.g., cocaine
- Foreign body, especially in children or psychiatric patients

Systemic

- Anticoagulation
- Family history of bleeding diatheses
- Poorly controlled blood pressure
- Organ failure—hepatic or renal

Management

- Wear protective clothing—visor/goggles/apron/gloves.
- Good lighting.
- First aid measures: pinch the soft part of the nose at the level of the nasal alae while leaning forward for at least 5–10 min.
- Apply standard A, B, C (ATLS) principles.
- Prepare equipment for packing and/or cautery.
- If the bleeding has stopped with the above measures, place a length of ribbon gauze soaked in oxymetazoline or diluted epinephrine into both nasal cavities and wait at least another 15 min.
- Remove the packs and start with anterior nasal inspection using a Thudicum or Killian speculum and a good headlight.
- If an anterior septal bleeding point is identified, cauterize it with a silver nitrite (AgNO3) stick. Ensure that the solution does not run down the nasal cavity or onto the lips, as this will cause a chemical burn.
- If an anterior bleeding source is not seen, refer to an ENT for nasal endoscopy.
- Should the bleeding persist after nasal compression, proceed with placing a nasal BIPP pack (Bismuth Iodoform paraffin paste), or Rapid Rhino® or Merocel® pack.
- Keep the packs in situ for 24–48 h, depending on whether the patient has other risk factors for bleeding.
- If the patient is packed for more than 24 h, prophylactic broad-spectrum antibiotics should be initiated.
- Inspect the oropharynx for bleeding down the nasopharynx.
- Should the patient continue to bleed past the pack down the nasopharynx, proceed with a posterior pack.
- Examine the oral cavity for telangiectasia lesions, sclera for jaundice (liver failure), joints for hemarthrosis, stools for melena, and urine for hematuria.

It is important to note: In cases with recurrent nosebleeds in a teenage male with ipsilateral progressive nasal obstruction, juvenile angiofibroma needs to be high on your list of differential diagnoses and ENT referral is required to exclude this.

For further reading on posterior packing technique: *Leadon M, Hohman MH. Posterior Epistaxis Nasal Pack. [Updated 2023 Mar 1]. In: StatPearls [Internet]. Treasure Island (FL): StatPearls Publishing; 2024 Jan-. Available from:* https://www.ncbi.nlm.nih.gov/books/NBK576436/

Allergic Rhinitis

Allergic rhinitis (AR) is an inflammatory, IgE-mediated disease characterized by nasal congestion, rhinorrhea (nasal drainage), sneezing, and/or nasal itching. A concurrent diagnosis of asthma may be present in 15–38% of patients with AR compared to 3–5% in the general population [2].

Diagnosis

- The diagnosis is made based on the history and clinical findings as described above.
- Patients who do not respond to empiric therapy may be referred for IgE-specific skin prick testing or serum testing to confirm the diagnosis.
- Based on these results, advise patients to avoid possible environmental triggers.
- Routine imaging is not recommended.
- Exclude other comorbidities or conditions related to atopy, like eczema, asthma, conjunctivitis, otitis media, sinusitis, and sleep-disordered breathing.

Treatment

- Allergen avoidance.
- Topical intranasal or oral decongestant for no more than 10 days.
- A second-generation oral antihistamine is recommended if the main complaint is itching and sneezing.
- Intranasal topical corticosteroid is recommended in patients where symptoms negatively impact quality of life.
- Leukotriene receptor antagonists are only recommended for moderate to severe AR, not adequately controlled with the aforementioned medication.
- For anti-allergic Cromones and immunotherapy (sublingual or subcutaneous), refer the patient to an Allergologist for further treatment.

Rhinosinusitis

Rhinosinusitis in adults is defined as:

- Inflammation of the nose and paranasal sinuses characterized **by two or more symptoms**, one of which should be either nasal blockage/obstruction/congestion or nasal discharge (anterior/posterior nasal drip): ± facial pain/pressure ± reduction or loss of smell **and**
- Either endoscopic evidence of nasal polyps, and/or mucopurulent discharge primarily from the middle meatus and/or edema/mucosal obstruction primarily in the middle meatus **and/or**
- CT changes with evidence of mucosal changes within the ostiomeatal complex and/or sinuses [3, 4].

Acute rhinosinusitis (ARS): Abovementioned criteria with a duration of <12 weeks.

Recurrent acute rhinosinusitis (ABRS): Four or more episodes a year with symptom-free intervals.

Chronic rhinosinusitis (CRS): Abovementioned criteria with a duration of 12 weeks or longer.

Acute Viral rhinosinusitis (AVRS): Acute rhinosinusitis signs and symptoms present for <10 days and without worsening of symptoms after initial improvement.

Acute Bacterial Rhinosinusitis (ABRS): Acute rhinosinusitis signs and symptoms that fail to improve within 10 days or more from the time of onset or worsening of signs and symptoms within 10 days of onset after initial improvement ("double worsening").

Imaging

- Routine imaging in acute rhinosinusitis is not indicated.
- A pre- and post-contrasted CT is recommended in acute sinusitis with associated "red flags" (see below).
- A non-contrasted CT is generally recommended for elective preoperative planning.

Red Flags/Danger Signs

- **Periorbital edema**
- **Ophthalmoplegia**
- **Diplopia**
- **Chemosis**
- **Proptosis**
- **Any decrease in visual acuity**
- **Decreased level of consciousness**
- **Boggy swelling over the forehead**
- **Unilateral facial swelling**
- **Clinical signs of meningism**
- **Focal neurology**
- **Black areas of demarcation intranasally or intraorally in the immunosuppressed patient (Diabetes, HIV, Chemotherapy, and Cancer)**

Treatment

- In acute viral and bacterial rhinosinusitis, supportive care is advised:
  - Simple analgesics.
  - Nasal decongestants for <10 days.

- Saline nasal rinses.
- Routine prescription of antihistamines is not recommended.
- Use of nasal corticosteroids is only recommended in select cases of post-viral ARS if deemed necessary to improve symptoms.
- Routine antibiotics are not advised.
- Antibiotics may be given in cases of high fever, in cases where there is failure to improve after 7 days, with an elevated ESR, or if any "red flags" are present.
- In the setting of CRS, intranasal steroid spray is recommended for 6–12 weeks. Counsel patients on the correct technique for using a nasal spray and emphasize the importance of compliance with medical therapy.
- Immediate referral to an ENT specialist is advised if any "red flags" are present (see below).
- Referral to an ENT specialist is advised in recalcitrant cases or where surgery is indicated.

Surgical Management

This is recommended if, after 12 weeks, maximum medical therapy has failed. Functional endoscopic sinus surgery (FESS) is performed to improve drainage of the affected sinuses as well as to increase the access for the nasal spray to work in chronic rhinosinusitis with nasal polyps.

Postoperative Care

- Nasal stuffiness and crusting can be expected for 3–6 weeks.
- To control excessive bloody oozing, an ice pack may be applied over the nose and cheeks while leaning forward.
- Routine analgesia should be prescribed.
- Oxymetazoline 2 drops per nostril every 6 h for 5 days may be used for vasoconstriction.
- Saline rinses are recommended from day 1 after surgery, as advised by the ENT surgeon.
- Steroid nasal spray may be restarted after the first postoperative visit.
- The patient may return to work after 1 week, but full recovery takes approximately 6–8 weeks.

Otology

It is useful to divide the ear into the external ear, the middle ear, and the inner ear.

External ear: Pinna up to tympanic membrane
Middle ear: Tympanic membrane up to the oval window
Inner ear: Oval window up to the vestibulocochlear nerve

External Ear

Perichondritis

Inflammation of the perichondrium or cartilage of the auricle, which, if left untreated, may cause deformation of the auricle (cauliflower ear).

Pseudomonas is the most common causative organism causing infection following trauma, piercings, or insect bites. Autoimmune diseases like relapsing polychondritis may be responsible for noninfective cases.

Treatment

- With abscess formation (*see* Fig. 47.1)—admission for incision, drainage, and debridement of necrotic tissue with a compressive dressing and intravenous antibiotics.
- Without abscess formation: Oral antibiotics for at least two weeks and close follow up is required is usually safe in the setting where the patient is not immunocompromised, i.e., diabetic, HIV positive, or on immunosuppressive therapy.

Otitis Externa

Inflammation and infection of the external ear canal up to the tympanic membrane. Commonly seen in swimmers (swimmer's ear), due to cotton tip use, hot and humid environments, lack of cerumen, or with chronic inflammatory skin conditions like eczema or psoriasis.

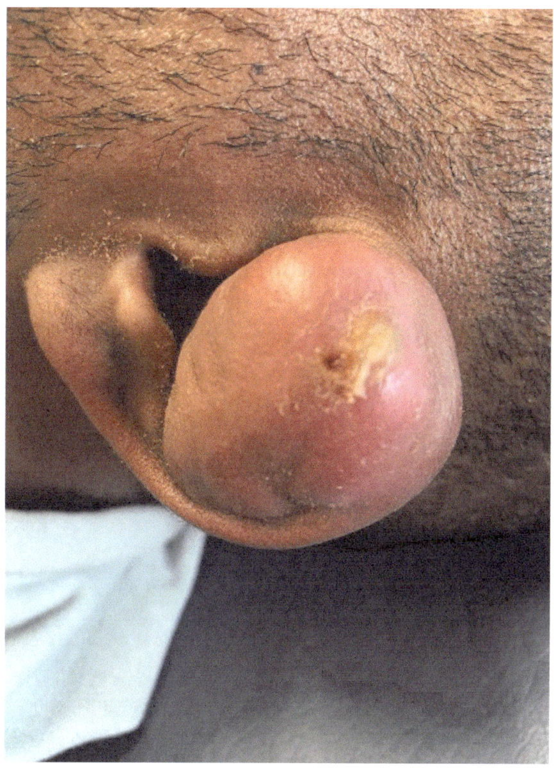

Fig. 47.1 A large abscess of the external ear is shown. The treatment for an abscess is incision and drainage

Focal inflammation: Infected hair follicle termed a "furuncle." Commonly caused by *Staphylococcus aureus*. Causes severe otalgia, especially at night. Often requires incision and drainage.

Diffuse inflammation: edema, swelling, and inflammation of the entire ear canal with or without discharge and hearing loss. Commonly caused by *Pseudomonas*. The tympanic membrane is normal.

Treatment

- Aural toilet in outpatients if the patient will allow (can be very painful).
- Adequate analgesia.
- Topical combination therapy consisting of a fluoroquinolone antibiotic and steroid drops. If the canal edema impairs instillation of drops, an otowick may be inserted soaked in the aforementioned medication. Treatment duration should be at least 10 days.
- Exclude diabetes mellitus. Ensure strict glucose control and compliance with diabetic medication.
- In immunocompromised patients with systemic symptoms and poorly controlled glucose, admission is required for observation and intravenous therapy.

Necrotizing Otitis Externa (Skull Base Osteomyelitis)

- Also called malignant otitis externa, which is a misnomer as it is not a neoplastic condition. It most often occurs in immunosuppressed (Diabetic, HIV, Oncology) patients.
- The infection of the ear canal spreads to the surrounding bone, causing a skull base osteomyelitis that may lead to multiple cranial nerve palsies.
- Causative organism: almost always due to *Pseudomonas* infection.
- **If not treated promptly, has a high mortality rate.**
- The attending ENT should be called immediately if this is suspected.

Management

- Urgent admission.
- Intravenous antipseudomonal antibiotics should promptly be initiated and discussed with infectious diseases colleagues.
- Aural toilet under microscopy and send pus for culture and sensitivities.
- Change antibiotics according to cultures and sensitivities.
- An otowick soaked with antipseudomonal (fluoroquinolone/steroid combination) topical drops should be placed in the ear canal and regularly changed.
- A non-contrasted CT of the temporal bones is a good first-line radiological investigation.
- Prolonged treatment is required.

Middle Ear

Acute Otitis Media

Inflammation of the middle ear cleft medial to the tympanic membrane. Infection of the middle ear may be viral, bacterial, or a coinfection.

The history is usually of short onset and associated with an upper respiratory tract infection. The most commonly implicated organisms are *Streptococcus pneumonia*, *Haemophilus influenzae*, and *Moraxella catarrhalis*.

Clinical Presentation

- Otalgia
- Fever
- Malaise
- Hearing loss
- An ear discharge may or may not be present

Otoscopy shows a bulging, red, and inflamed tympanic membrane **with or without** a perforation, and a normal external auditory canal (Fig. 47.2).

Management

- *Conservative:* In children older than 2 years with milder symptoms or children who are not classified as at-risk (Trisomy 21, craniofacial abnormalities, immunodeficiencies), simple analgesics and observation for 48–72 h will suffice.
- *Antibiotic therapy*: Antibiotics are indicated in children younger than 2 years of age, for bilateral acute otitis media and for acute otitis media with otorrhea.

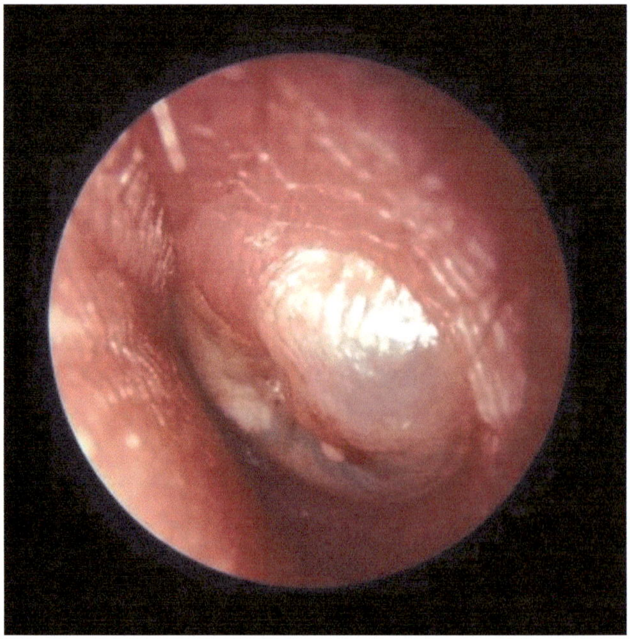

Fig. 47.2 Otoscopy shows a bulging, red, and inflamed tympanic membrane

- Amoxicillin at 90 mg/kg for 5 days or erythromycin or clarithromycin may be given in penicillin allergic cases. Topical antibiotics are as effective as oral antibiotics in the presence of a perforation. In unresponsive cases, high-dose amoxicillin-clavulanate is recommended.

Chronic Otitis Media (COM)

Inflammation of the middle ear cleft lasting more than 12 weeks in the presence of a perforation of the tympanic membrane.

Unlike acute otitis media, COM is not painful. It can be classified into "active" or "inactive" depending on the presence of a discharge. Active COM can be classified into mucosal discharge (mesotympanic disease), typically with a perforation of the pars tensa (*see* Fig. 47.3), or a squamosal discharge associated with a cholesteatoma (normally epitympanic space of the middle ear and the superior part of the tympanic membrane is involved (see Fig. 47.4), which requires ENT referral for surgical management.

Management

- Fluoroquinolone antibiotic drops topical therapy is indicated for active disease, with or without a combination of steroid drops, depending on the severity of the inflammation. It is recommended to perform oto-wick aural toilet prior to instilling any ear drops in any discharging ear.
- All patients with COM must be referred to an ENT for formal audiological assessment.

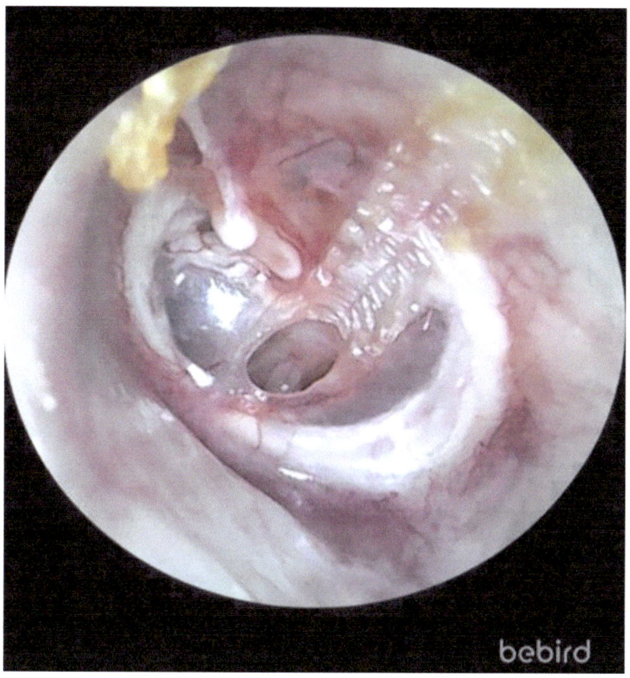

Fig. 47.3 Chronic otitis media (COM) showing perforation of the pars tensa

Cholesteatoma

Cholesteatoma is the accumulation of squamous debris in the middle ear cleft or other parts of the temporal bone outside of the ear canal. This causes a chronic inflammatory response with watery discharge unresponsive to medical therapy, where lytic and inflammatory enzymes cause destruction of the surrounding structures (ossicles, semicircular canals, nerves, etc.).

- It is a clinical diagnosis made on otoscopy/microscopy.
- A squamous, offensive discharge is seen on otoscopy coming from a retraction pocket or a perforation with surrounding granulation.
- The full extent of the retraction can often not be seen.
- The retraction is often found in the pars flaccida (attic or epitympanum).

Management

- The treatment in almost all cases is surgical, following a preoperative, non-contrasted CT scan of the temporal bone for surgical planning.
- The surgical options are broadly divided into mastoidectomy, where the canal wall is either preserved (normal anatomy and function preserved) or taken down, leaving the patient with a large, nonself-cleansing cavity.
- With the "canal wall up" approach, follow-up imaging with a diffusion weighted, non-epi MRI is required to exclude recurrence.
- With a "canal wall down" approach, the patient has a higher likelihood of having a discharging ear, but the disease is visible on microscopy and can be cleared in the outpatient setting. There is a lesser chance of complicated mastoiditis compared to a "canal wall up" approach, should there be a recurrence.

Cholesteatoma may eventually lead to acute mastoiditis and intracranial or extracranial complications. Acute mas-

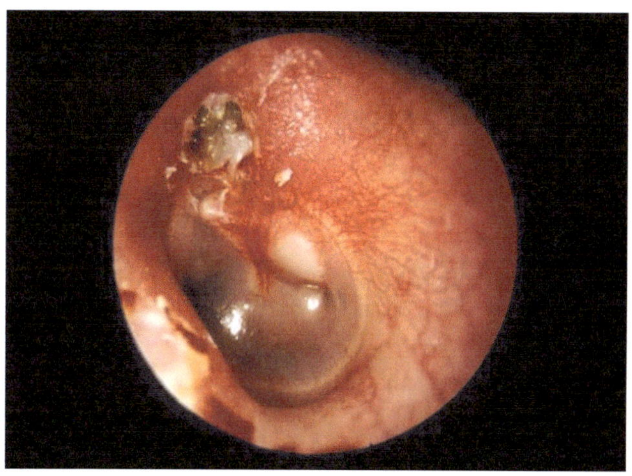

Fig. 47.4 Chronic otitis media (COM) demonstrating squamosal dischage

toiditis is an emergency and should be discussed with the attending ENT as soon as possible.

Acute Mastoiditis

Inflammation of the mastoid air cells that leads to suppuration.

Clinically

- Fever
- Peri-auricular oedema and erythema
- Mastoid tenderness
- Often otorrhoea
- Pinna may be pushed forward

Management

- Uncomplicated mastoiditis
  - Admit and resuscitate
  - Initiate intravenous broad-spectrum antibiotic: amoxicillin-clavulanate
  - Send a pus swab specimen for cultures and sensitivities
  - Pre- and post-contrasted CT imaging of the brain and neck.
  - Call the attending ENT immediately
- Complicated mastoiditis (meningism, focal neurology, or decreased level of consciousness)
  - Urgent admission and resuscitation
  - Pre- and post-contrasted CT imaging of the brain and neck
  - Initiate intravenous antibiotics that cross the blood-brain barrier—third generation cephalosporins
  - Call the attending ENT immediately
  - Keep nil by mouth—may need to go the operating room for surgical decompression

Inner Ear

Sudden Onset Hearing Loss

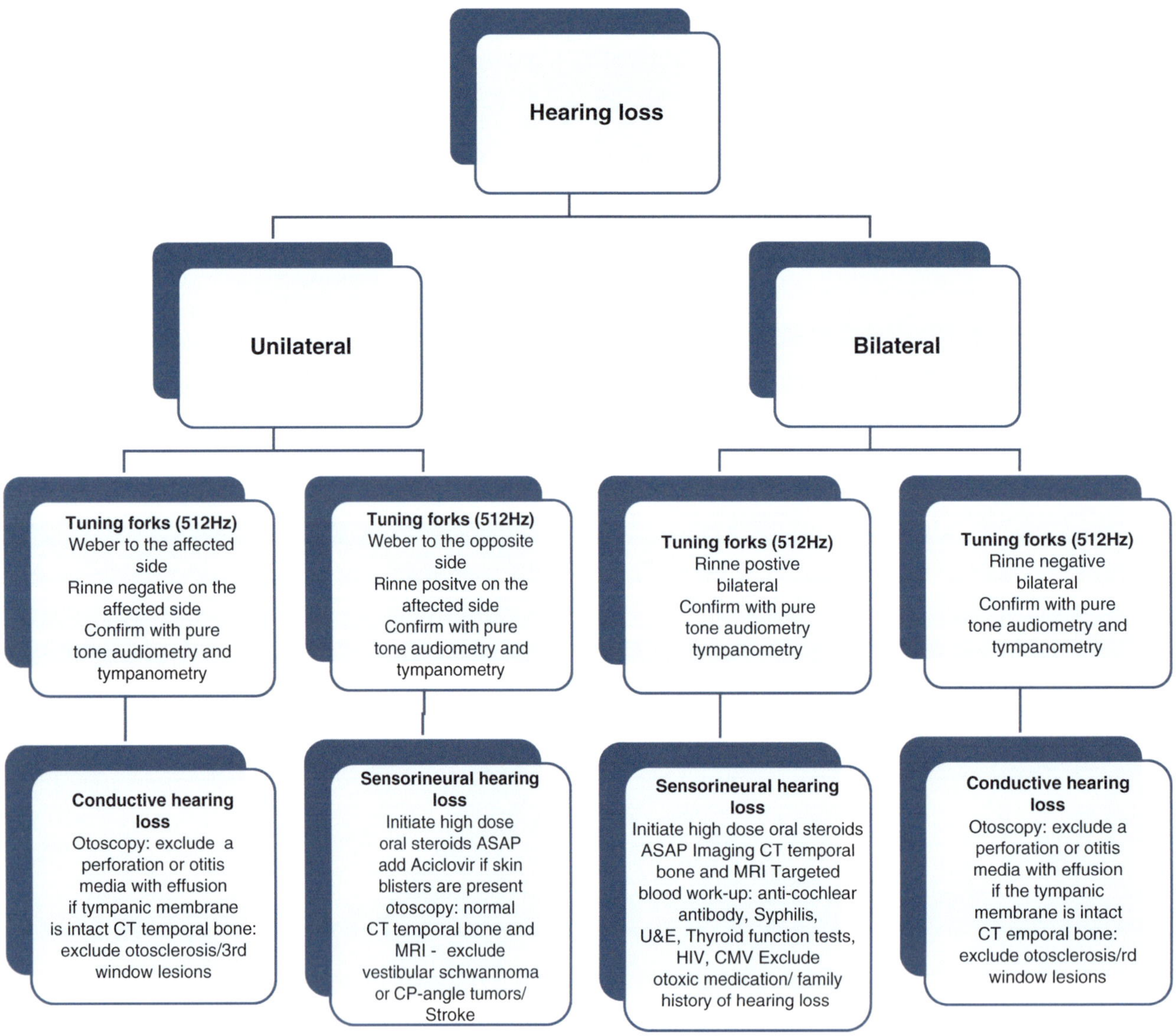

CP angle: cerebellopontine angle; HIV: Human Immunodeficiency Virus; CMV: Cytomegalovirus; U&E: urea, creatinine, and electrolytes; third window lesions: semicircular canal dehiscence/enlarged vestibular aqueduct.

Idiopathic (Bell's) Facial Palsy

Idiopathic facial palsy is a condition that a clinician commonly presents with as an emergency department consultation or as an urgent referral from a family practitioner.

It is important to note that it is a diagnosis of exclusion guided by the history and clinical examination.

Patients typically present with unilateral weakness of the facial muscles of sudden onset, commonly preceded by a prodromal phase of malaise and auricular or peri-auricular pain. The weakness is in the frontal, mid-face, as well as in the distribution of the marginal mandibular branch of the facial nerve. Thirteen percent may have a recurrent idiopathic palsy. This risk is doubled if there is a positive family history.

The etiology of Bell's palsy remains unclear, although a viral etiology has been proposed. Roughly two-thirds of patients will regain full function within 3 months, with most patients making a full recovery. No further improvement of function can be expected after 6 months.

Poor Prognostic Factors

- Complete paralysis at the onset of symptoms
- Old age
- Dry eye
- Absent stapedial reflex
- Postauricular pain
- Loss of taste

Red Flags

A red flag means the symptoms should raise suspicion of a possible neoplastic cause and a patient who requires further imaging (MRI) and investigation.

- **Progressive weakness over a 3-week period or more**
- **Incomplete palsy that fails to improve after 3–6 weeks**
- **Recurrent facial palsy**

Further Reading *Facial weakness grading system, see the House-Brackmann grading system.*

Differential Diagnosis

- Ramsey Hunt syndrome (Herpes Zoster Oticus)—Look for blisters or crusting in the external ear canal. Look for other cranial nerve involvement.
- Skull base fractures, lacerations, penetrating wounds, and birthing trauma
- Congenital/genetic: Moebius syndrome, Melkersson-Rosenthal syndrome, and congenital lower lip paralysis
- Middle ear infections or cholesteatoma involving the facial canal

Management

Treatment should preferably be initiated within the first 14 days of the onset of weakness.

- *Eye Care:* With incomplete eye closure, it is important to avoid the risk of corneal ulceration with frequent application of an artificial tear solution. A tear gel or ointment is recommended at night
- *Medical:* **Combination** therapy of a corticosteroid and antiviral.
  - Adequate analgesia
  - Prednisone 1 mg/kg/day for 10 days within 72 h of onset of the palsy
  - Oral Aciclovir 400 mg five times a day for ten days within 72 h of the onset of the palsy, always in combination with a steroid.
  - Routine laboratory tests are not recommended in new-onset Bell's palsy.
  - Routine diagnostic imaging is not recommended for new-onset Bell's palsy.
  - Routine electrodiagnostic testing is not recommended in a partial facial paresis but may be done in cases of complete facial paralysis [5].

Throat

Tonsillitis

Acute inflammation and infection of the palatine tonsils is another condition commonly seen and managed by family practitioners. Complications like peritonsillar abscess (quinsy) and deep neck space sepsis (parapharyngeal abscess) require urgent ENT referral for surgical drainage.

Etiology

- Group A beta-hemolytic streptococci, along with *Streptococcus pneumonia*, *Hemophilus influenza* and *Staphylococcus* are most commonly responsible for acute tonsillitis.
- However, it often has a viral etiology caused by the Adenovirus, Epstein-Barr virus, Coxsackie virus, or Rhinovirus.

Clinical Presentation

- Fever (>38.3 degree Celsius)
- Malaise
- Sore throat
- Exudate over tonsils
- Tender cervical adenopathy
- Anorexia
- Drooling and odynophagia
- Halitosis

Indications for Tonsillectomy

The Paradise outcome study, published in 1984, states that there is a benefit for tonsillectomy if the following criteria are met:

- 7 episodes in the previous year OR
- 5 episodes in the previous 2 years OR
- 3 episodes in the previous 3 years.

Peritonsillar Abscess

A peritonsillar abscess is an exudative purulent collection between the tonsillar capsule medially and the superior constrictor muscle laterally.

Clinical Features

- Asymmetrical swelling of the tonsils
- The uvula is displaced to the opposite side
- Unilateral otalgia
- Persistent fever in spite of antibiotic therapy
- Trismus
- Hot potato voice with drooling or inability to swallow

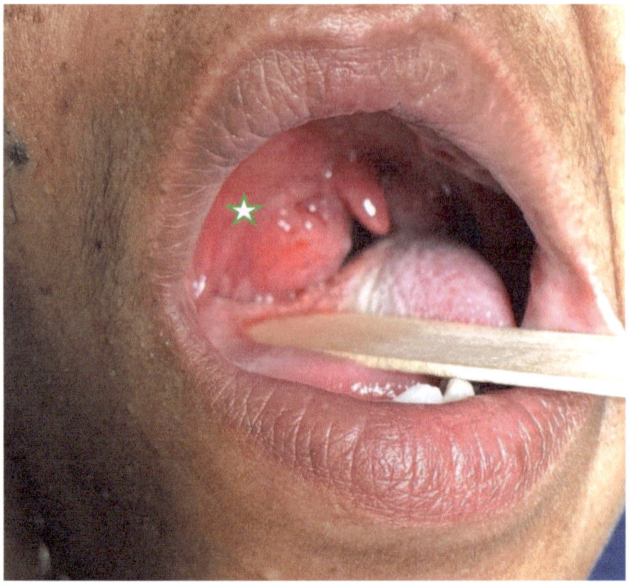

Landmark to aspirate: Draw a horizontal line through the base of the uvula intersecting with a vertical line taken inside the last upper molar tooth.

Management

- Transoral needle aspiration of the peritonsillar abscess—Useful in a cooperative patient without significant trismus.
- Incision and drainage—Following topical anesthesia, make a stab incision with an 11-blade taped to a tongue depressor with only a short bit of the tip protruding. Once the abscess cavity is entered, use mosquito forceps to open and drain the cavity further. Both the above methods have a chance of recurrence.
- "Hot tonsillectomy"—Tonsillectomy is done under general anesthesia in the acute setting. This has the benefit of optimal access in a controlled environment and eliminates the risk of recurrence.
- Elective tonsillectomy after second quinsy: Treat the initial episode with aspiration or open drainage and electively schedule a tonsillectomy without the presence of concurrent inflammation and infection.

Post-tonsillectomy Care

- Routine analgesia—acetaminophen and nonsteroidal anti-inflammatories.
- Do NOT routinely give opiates.
- A routine diet may be followed immediately after surgery if tolerated.
- Patients may be booked off work for 10 days to recover.
- Routine antibiotics are not recommended.

Neck Masses

When approaching patients with neck masses, it is helpful to look at the age of the patient. In younger patients, inflammatory and congenital lesions are more likely. *In older patients, especially those who smoke and abuse alcohol, a non-benign lesion should be assumed until proven otherwise*. It can be helpful to divide neck masses into midline neck masses versus lateral neck masses.

Age <20 Years

- Inflammatory/infective lymph node
- Abscess
- Thyroglossal duct cyst
- Branchial cleft cyst
- Midline dermoid cyst
- Haemangioma
- Cystic hygroma
- Lymphoma

Age 20–40 Years

- Reactive or pathological lymph node
- Abscess
- Salivary gland pathology—infective/inflammatory vs neoplastic
- Branchial cleft cyst
  - ***It is important to note that oropharyngeal squamous cell carcinomas that are associated with coinfection with the Human Papillomavirus (HPV) infection and skin cancers commonly have cystic metastases. It should therefore not be assumed that a cystic mass is congenital or benign.***
- Laryngocoele
- Thyroid mass
- Lymphoma

Age >40 Years

- **Metastases**
- **Primary malignancy**

Relevant History

- An asymptomatic mass present for more than 2 weeks in an adult should be suspicious of malignancy.
- Patients who smoke, consume alcohol, or chew tobacco/betelnut are at higher risk of a head-and-neck malignancy.
- Dysphonia for 3 weeks or more with referred unilateral otalgia is suspicious for laryngeal or hypopharyngeal cancer.
- Question about any skin lesions excised in the head-and-neck area.
- Ask about reflux symptoms and the presence of dysphagia or odynophagia.
- Head and neck cancers have a fairly predictable drainage pattern of metastatic nodal spread, so the location of a nodal neck mass may indicate the likely location of a primary cancer.

Management

- A physical exam of the neck, starting with inspection and palpation of every neck level.
- Try to identify a primary tumor.
- Examine the nose, nasopharynx, oral cavity, oropharynx, hypopharynx, larynx, skin, and thyroid gland.
- Palpate tonsils, base of tongue, and retract tonsillar pillars, and then examine for any contact bleeding.
- Get a detailed description of the characteristics of the mass:
  - Is it mobile?
  - Is it fixed?
  - Is it solid/cystic or mixed?
  - Is it well circumscribed?
  - Is it pulsatile?
  - Is it tender?
  - Is there more than one mass?
  - At which neck level is it situated?
  - Are there any overlying skin changes?
- A cytological or histological diagnosis is essential. A free-hand, fine needle aspiration cytology aspirate (FNAC) should be the first step. Should the first sample be nondiagnostic, it should be repeated. In facilities where

resources are available, the repeat FNAC may be done under ultrasound guidance.

*For further reading, see "**Head and neck lymph node and tumour biopsy techniques**":* https://health.uct.ac.za/entdev/guides/open-access-atlas-otolaryngology-head-neck-operative-surgery

- For standardized descriptive purposes, the neck is divided into six levels and three sublevels [6]:

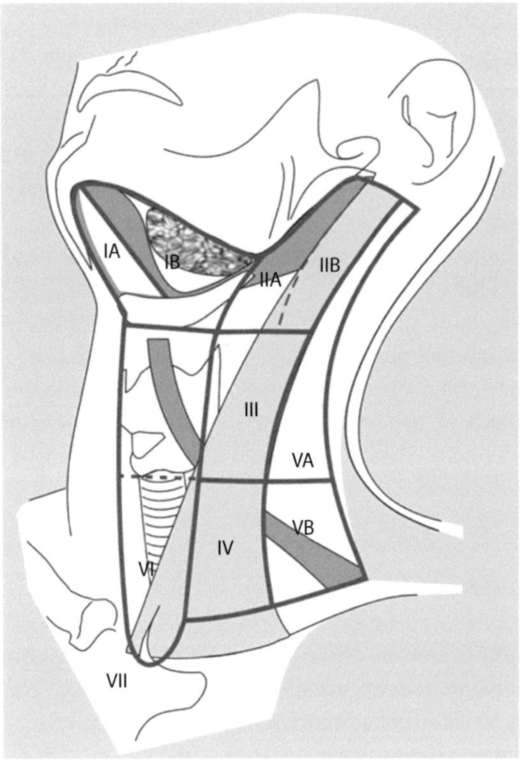

- Nodal location and laterality suggest location of primary [7].
  - Levels I A, B: Oral cavity, nose, sinuses.
  - Levels II, III: Oral cavity, oropharynx, hypopharynx, larynx, nose, sinuses.
  - Level IV: Larynx, hypopharynx, thyroid, oral tongue, floor of mouth.
  - Level V: Nasopharynx, posterior scalp, thyroid.
  - Level VI: Thyroid, subglottis, hypopharynx, oesophagus.
  - Nodes along external jugular vein: Facial skin.
  - Bilateral nodal involvement should be suspected in masses located in the midline, base of tongue, soft palate, supraglottis, hypopharynx, or nasopharynx (NPC).
- Exclude distant metastases as part of staging. A chest x-ray as an initial investigation should suffice. CT of the neck, head, neck, and chest area can evaluate the primary and exclude metastases to the chest.
- Head and neck cancers are staged according to the Tumor size, Nodal size and distribution and Metastases (TNM) system. This has some correlation to the prognosis of the patient, and if single modality (early disease) vs multimodality treatment (advanced disease) will be required.
- Head-and-neck cancers should ideally be referred to a multidisciplinary team to including a head-and-neck surgeon, reconstructive surgeon, oncologist, dietician, etc.
- Long-term follow-up will be required for all oncology patients with individualized departmental protocols.

References

1. Soyuncu S, Eken C, Cete Y, Bektas F. Determination of difficult intubation in the ED. Am J Emerg Med. 2009;27:905–10.
2. Brożek JL, et al. Allergic rhinitis and its impact on asthma (ARIA) guidelines—2016 revision. J Allergy Clin Immunol. 2017;140:950–8.
3. Fokkens WJ, et al. Executive summary of EPOS 2020 including integrated care pathways. Rhinol J. 2020;58:82–111.
4. Rosenfeld RM, et al. Clinical practice guideline (update): Adult sinusitis executive summary. Otolaryngol—Head Neck Surg (United States). 2015;152:598–609.
5. Schwartz R, Murray C, Deckard NA. Clinical practice guideline summary. Bell's Palsy; 2013. p. 34–5.
6. Robbins KT, et al. Consensus statement on the classification and terminology of neck dissection. Arch Otolaryngol Neck Surg. 2008;134:536–8.
7. AfHNS guidelines for evaluation and treatment of oral cancer_ Scenario 4—African Head & Neck Society (AfHNS) Clinical Practice Guidelines for Head & Neck Cancers in Developing Countries and Limited Resource Settings.pdf.

48 Neurosurgery

Elizabeth Dunham and W. Christopher Fox

Cranial

Epidural Hematoma (EDH)

Definition A collection of blood between the ***skull*** and the outermost covering of the brain called the ***dura mater.*** [44] They are often arterial in origin, commonly associated with injury to the ***middle meningeal artery*** [4].

Clinical Presentation

- Patients often report an ***initial loss of consciousness followed by a lucid interval***. Rapid neurologic deterioration can occur with the expansion of an EDH. [26].
- Presenting symptoms include headache, nausea, vomiting, hemiparesis, lethargy, and seizure [62], often in the setting of recent head injury.
- Evaluate for signs of *increased intracranial pressure (ICP)* or brain herniation requiring emergent management [2, 33].
  - Cushing reflex: hypertension, bradycardia, respiratory depression.
  - Decreased level of consciousness.
  - Unilaterally dilated or sluggish pupils.
  - Extensor posturing.

Work-Up and Examination

- A **full neurologic examination** should be performed, as well as a **Glasgow Coma Scale (GCS),** which can help assess the severity of a head injury.
- **Non-contrast CT scan**
  - When EDH is present, CT often reveals a **lens** or **biconvex-shaped hemorrhage** [10] see Fig. 48.1. This is most dangerous when focused on the temporal lobe

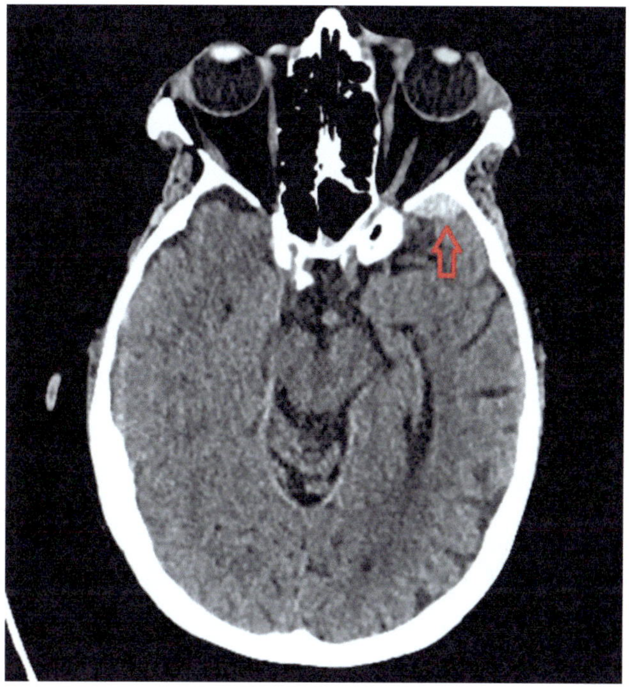

Fig. 48.1 A non-contrast CT of the head reveals a left temporal pole epidural hematoma as outlined by the red arrow

- *Always look for an underlying skull fracture, as these are often associated with epidural hematomas* [57]
- CBC, PTT, PT/INR, BMP

Treatment and Surgical Indications

- Nonsurgical management can be considered when hemorrhage size is <30 cm^3, thickness < 15 mL, midline shift <5 mm, GCS > 8, and without focal neurological deficit [11]
  - Neurologic and radiographic surveillance with frequent neuro checks and serial CT scans [6]
  - Reversal of anticoagulation
  - Blood pressure management

E. Dunham (✉) · W. C. Fox
Department of Neurosurgery, Mayo Clinic, Jacksonville, FL, USA
e-mail: Dunham.Elizabeth@mayo.edu

S. Atallah, J. Dragoljevic (eds.), *Fundamentals of Surgery for Physician Assistants*, https://doi.org/10.1007/978-3-032-21069-2_48

  - Avoiding hypertension, which can cause expansion of hematoma and hypotension, which can cause a decrease in cerebral perfusion pressure [2]
- Surgical evacuation via burr holes or craniotomy should be performed with the following: [11]
  - Hematoma volume > 30 cm^3, regardless of GCS
  - GCS < 9 and anisocoria
  - Surgery can also be considered with EDH associated with a depressed skull fracture

Subdural Hematoma (SDH)

Definition a collection of blood between the ***dura*** *mater* and the ***brain (arachnoid membranes).*** They can occur from cortical lacerations or rupture of ***bridging veins*** [2].

Clinical Presentation

- Traumatic subdural hematomas are often seen in the acute setting *following a fall or motor vehicle accident* [2] in which the patient has suffered a traumatic brain injury (TBI).
- Nontraumatic hematomas occur due to *cerebral atrophy* and are seen more frequently due to the increasing use of antiplatelet and anticoagulation in the elderly [2]. With brain atrophy, veins "bridging" the subdural space may stretch and tear, leading to SDH.
- Presenting symptoms can include headaches, nausea, vomiting, focal neurologic deficit, and seizures [46, 67].
- Evaluate for signs of increased intracranial pressure or brain herniation [67].

Work-Up and Examination

- A **GCS score** and full neurologic examination should be performed
- **Non-contrast CT head**
  - Often reveals a **crescent shape** blood pattern, as seen in Fig. 48.2a [41, 60]
- Acute blood will appear hyperdense, subacute products are isodense, and chronic blood product hypodense. In chronic SDH, it is common to see hemorrhage of varying ages
- CBC, BMP, PTT, PT/INR

Treatment and Surgical Indications

- Nonsurgical management is similar to EDH management, including blood pressure control, close neurologic and radiographic surveillance, reversal of anticoagulation, and use of antiepileptic medications if the patient presents with seizures.

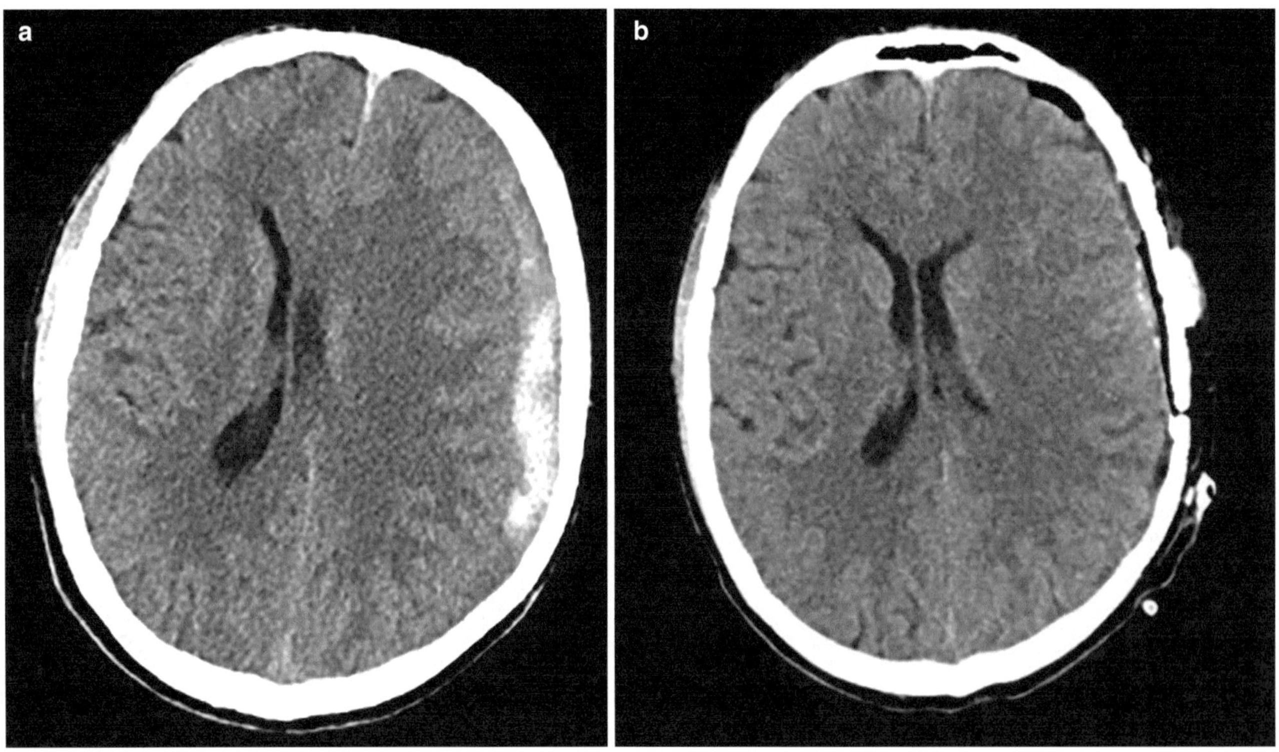

Fig. 48.2 (**a**) A non-contrast CT of the brain reveals a mixed-density, left-sided subdural hematoma with midline shift. (**b**) A non-contrast CT of the brain following craniotomy for subdural evacuation with significant improvement in midline shift and successful evacuation of subdural hematoma

- Surgical evacuation via burr holes or craniotomy should be performed with the following: [12]
  - Thickness > 10 mm or midline shift >5 mm
  - GCS < 9—consider ICP monitoring
  - GCS < 9, < 10 mm, shift <5 mm if GCS score decreased by more than 2 points since time of injury and hospital admission, or if asymmetric or fixed/dilated pupils
- Craniotomy is a more common treatment for acute SDH, while burr holes are typically limited to drainage of chronic SDH. See Fig. 48.2b.
- Middle meningeal artery embolization can be considered as a minimally invasive treatment option to prevent progression of chronic subdural hematomas [31].

Intraparenchymal Hemorrhage

Definition Bleeding into the brain parenchyma. This can be due to *hypertension, amyloid angiopathy, tumor, coagulopathy, infection, vasculitis, trauma, or an underlying vascular abnormality* [22] such as arteriovenous malformation or cavernous malformation.

Clinical Presentation

- Presenting symptoms can include headache, nausea, vomiting, seizure, focal neurological deficit, altered mental status, and coma
- Assess for clinical signs of elevated ICP
- May be hypertensive in nature
- Facial or other bodily signs of trauma

Work-Up and Examination

- **Glasgow Coma Scale** and **full neurologic examination** should be performed
- **Non-contrast head CT**
- Consider CT angiography (CTA) if concern for underlying vascular abnormality or MRI if tumor suspected
- CBC, PT/INR, PTT, BMP, serum glucose

Treatment and Surgical Indications

- Blood pressure management
- Reversal of antiplatelet or anticoagulant use
- Radiographic and neurologic surveillance
- Nonsurgical management of increased intracranial pressure includes elevating HOB, hypertonic/hyperosmolar agents, transient hyperventilation, sedation, and paralysis
- Consider emergent ventriculostomy placement if the patient presents with evidence of high intracranial pressure, obstructive hydrocephalus, or intraventricular extension of hemorrhage
- Decompressive craniectomy
  - Can reduce mortality, but does not typically reduce morbidity, in patients with significant midline shift or elevated ICP not responsive to medical management [23]
  - Role in improving long-term functional outcomes is inconclusive
  - Minimally invasive surgical evacuation of intracranial hemorrhage can be considered in patients who present with lobar hemorrhage. While traditionally the surgical treatment of intracranial hemorrhage has been controversial, a recent study [55] has shown functional benefit in select patients

Hydrocephalus

Definition an increase in size of the ventricular system due to an ***accumulation of cerebrospinal fluid.*** This can occur *with* or *without* an increase in intracranial pressure [27].

Types of hydrocephalus:

- Communicating, obstructive, normal pressure, hydrocephalus ex vacuo (due to brain atrophy and relative increase in ventricular size).

Monro-Kellie hypothesis: The skull is a rigid and fixed structure. Any change in either brain tissue, blood volume, or CSF volume should result in a compensatory reaction from one or both of the other two. *If there is no compensatory reaction, this can result in an increase in ICP, as often seen in acute hydrocephalus* [45].

Clinical Presentation [69]

- Presenting symptoms can include headaches, dizziness, visual changes, concentration problems, vomiting, papilledema, and altered mental status.
- **Normal pressure hydrocephalus**: **classic triad of *dementia, gait instability, and urinary incontinence*** ("whacky, wobbly, and wet").

Work-Up and Examination

- A full neurologic examination
- Non-contrast CT head (for patients presenting acutely) or MRI of the brain (for subacute to chronic complaints)
- **Lumbar puncture** may be required for the diagnosis of normal pressure hydrocephalus. This will reveal a normal opening pressure and improvement in symptoms after removal of CSF [64]
- Ophthalmology evaluation for papilledema in the chronic setting [19, 69]

Treatment and Surgical Consideration

- Nonsurgical management can include *acetazolamide* or *hyperosmolar therapy* in the acute setting [5, 30]
- *Continuous CSF drainage* either by external ventricular or lumbar drain in the acute setting, or placement of ventriculoperitoneal shunt, lumboperitoneal shunt, or endoscopic third ventriculostomy for more permanent treatment [27].

Seizures

Definition A transient episode of neurologic signs or symptoms due to abnormal, excessive, or synchronous neuronal activity in the brain [21].

Seizures are now classified as focal, generalized, or unknown onset [34].

As a neurosurgical PA, you will often encounter seizures in the postoperative setting or in patients with a new diagnosis of brain lesion.

Clinical Presentation

- Symptoms can include sustained rhythmical jerking, weak or limp muscles, tense or rigid muscles, muscle twitching, spasms, clapping or rubbing of hands, lip smacking or chewing, staring spells [34]
- Non-motor symptoms can be changes to sensation, emotions, thinking, or cognition

Todd's Paralysis a *transient neurologic deficit* that occurs after a seizure, which is characterized by temporary weakness or paralysis, *typically on one side of the body.* Aphasia, gaze palsy, confusion, and visual changes can also occur. This typically resolves within 36 h [58].

Work-Up and Examination

- Blood glucose, electrolyte panel, CBC [18]
- Non-contrast CT of the head
  - Used to rule out hemorrhage or cerebral edema in the postoperative setting; also used for efficient evaluation of patients presenting acutely
- MRI may be indicated to obtain more detailed information on the underlying brain/mechanism of seizure
- Continuous or spot EEG for suspected subclinical seizures
- Drug screen or lumbar puncture can be considered in the emergency setting to evaluate for drug-induced seizure or infection

Treatment and Surgical Indications

- Antiepileptic drugs are first-line treatment
  - ***Levetiracetam*** is frequently used in the neurosurgical setting. This medication has minimal drug interactions and side effects [18] compared to more traditional drugs like phenytoin
  - A second agent or increased dosage may be needed when a patient is already on antiepileptic drugs and has a breakthrough seizure
  - Treatment is tailored to the exact type of seizure and individual patient factors. Neurology should be consulted for guidance regarding treatment in the acute setting and long-term management
- ***For seizures that last more than 5 min (status epilepticus)****, a* ***benzodiazepine*** *(i.e., midazolam, diazepam) should be administered* [7], *in addition to an IV loading dose of* ***antiepileptic medication*** *and progressive escalation of treatment to stop the seizures.*
- Vagus nerve stimulation, laser interstitial thermal therapy, temporal lobe resection, resection of epileptic foci or underlying lesions, responsive neurostimulation, and deep brain stimulation are all neurosurgical procedures performed for the treatment of drug-resistant epilepsy [42].

Brain Tumor

Brain lesions can either be primary or metastatic and are a daunting diagnosis for patients. Metastatic brain lesions are far more common than primary lesions and most commonly metastasize from *lung, breast, melanoma, and colon cancer* [24]. Common primary lesions include **gliomas** and **meningiomas.**

Clinical Presentation [24]

- Common presenting symptoms include headaches, nausea, vomiting, weakness, sensory changes, cranial nerve dysfunction, speech disturbance, problems with coordination or balance, seizures, endocrine dysfunction, altered mental status, or changes in personal behavior. These will depend on the location, size, and grade of tumor.
- Symptoms tend to gradually worsen over time, either weeks to months, or even years.
- Increased intracranial pressure, hydrocephalus, or hemorrhage can cause an acute onset of symptoms.

Work-Up and Examination [24]

- A **full neurologic assessment** is required. Exam findings can help clue you in on the localization of the tumor prior to imaging being completed. A thorough history is important to identify patients at the highest risk of metastatic lesions.
- Imaging studies should include a **non-contrast CT of the brain** and an **MRI of the brain with and without contrast.** Sometimes a CT or MR angiogram or venogram is required if the tumor is located close to a major vein (typically one of the dural sinuses) or artery.

- Angiography can be considered if the tumor is highly vascularized, requiring embolization prior to surgical operation.
- A full oncologic work-up is important to help distinguish between a primary and metastatic brain lesion. This will include a CT chest, abdomen, and pelvis, basic lab work, and other diagnostic testing based on presenting symptoms.
- These patients should be evaluated by neurology, oncology, radiation oncology, and an internal medicine team in the hospital setting.

Treatment [24]

- *Treatment depends on the type, location, size, and grade of tumor.* Treatment options include the following:
  - Serial imaging observation
  - Radiation
  - Chemotherapy
  - Corticosteroids for surrounding cerebral edema
  - Antiepileptic drugs for seizure management
  - Surgical resection—required for pathological diagnosis or for larger lesions causing mass effect

Vascular

Subarachnoid Hemorrhage (SAH)

Definition bleeding into the subarachnoid spaces of the brain. This can be traumatic in nature or spontaneous. Nontraumatic cases are usually secondary to a ***ruptured aneurysm*** [43].

Risk factors for **nontraumatic aneurysmal subarachnoid hemorrhage** [16]

- *Smoking, hypertension, alcohol use, cocaine use, personal or family history of cerebral aneurysms, or prior subarachnoid hemorrhage*

Perimesencephalic subarachnoid hemorrhage is a subtype of nonaneurysmal subarachnoid hemorrhage. Blood is localized to the perimesencephalic cisterns and is thought to be venous in nature. These patients typically have a more favorable prognosis [29]. Diagnosis of perimesencephalic hemorrhage is often one of exclusion, after multiple vascular imaging studies, including CT Angiography (CTA), MR Angiography (MRA), and Digital Subtraction Angiography (DSA), have ruled out an underlying arterial vascular lesion such as aneurysm.

Clinical Presentation [16]

- **Patients will often present with a sudden, severe headache. This is often described as the *"worst headache of their life,"* also known as a *thunderclap headache.***
- A warning headache or "sentinel" headache can often occur days prior to the presenting event. This often represents a warning leak or initial bleed.
- Altered mental status or meningismus may be presenting symptoms.
- Nausea, vomiting, neck pain, focal neurologic deficit, photophobia, lightheadedness, or dizziness are also common.
- Some patients may present with coma.

Work-Up and Examination [16]

- A **full neurologic examination** should be performed, including a Glasgow Coma Score and Hunt Hess Scale
- **Non-contrast head CT**
  - This should be used to calculate the Fisher Scale, a marker of the severity of SAH
  - See Fig. 48.3
- **CT angiogram** to evaluate for aneurysm
- If CT is negative and suspicion for SAH remains high, **lumbar puncture** should be performed to evaluate for xanthochromia

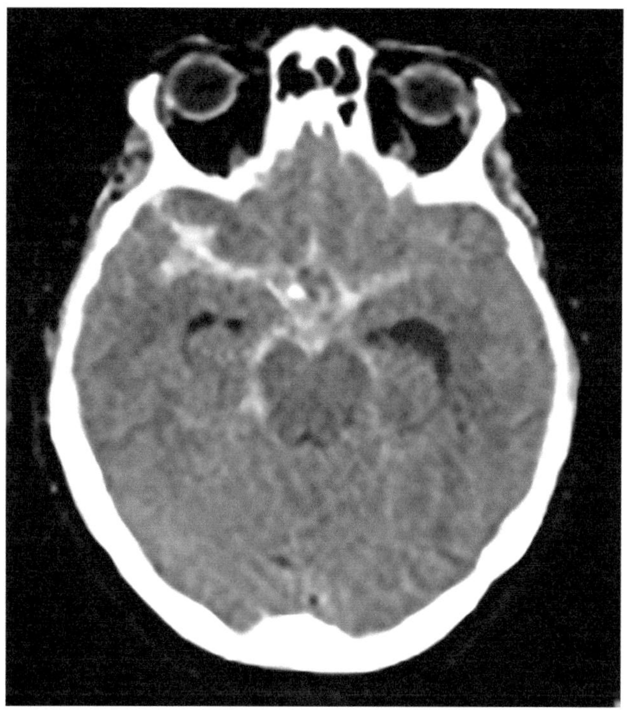

Fig. 48.3 A non-contrast CT of the brain showing subarachnoid blood in the basal cisterns, also known as the "star sign"

- If aneurysmal SAH is suspected and CTA is negative, a catheter angiogram (DSA) should be performed upon initial diagnosis and 7 days following, if the first study is negative, to ensure no underlying vascular abnormality
- Clinical grading tools include:
  - Hunt and Hess Severity Scale
  - World Federation of Neurologic Surgeons Scale
  - Fisher Scale and Modified Fisher Scale

Treatment and Surgical Considerations:

- Management includes *close observation in a neurocritical care unit.* Initial resuscitation with intubation may be required. Blood pressure management, coagulopathy correction, and analgesia are also important [43]
- In aneurysmal SAH, treatment of the aneurysm is required either by *microvascular neurosurgical clipping or endovascular embolization.* This helps decrease the risk of rebleed and should occur within 24–48 h of presentation [28]
- If there is evidence of increased intracranial pressure, hydrocephalus, or significant intraventricular hemorrhage, an emergent external ventricular device (EVD) should be considered
  - Occasionally, the patient does not tolerate weaning of the EVD and will require more permanent CSF diversion via a ventriculoperitoneal shunt
- Hyponatremia, hypovolemia, and hypervolemia should be avoided in these patients
- *Vasospasm and delayed cerebral ischemia can be a serious complication of subarachnoid hemorrhage.* Vasospasm most commonly occurs 4–14 days after the initial bleed
  - Nimodipine should be prescribed for 21 days to help reduce the risk of vasospasm
  - Daily transcranial dopplers should be performed to assess for intracranial vasospasm
  - Patients with a focal neurologic decline should get a CT angiogram with perfusion study or DSA to evaluate for vasospasm and tissue at risk for ischemia
  - Intrathecal nicardipine, intra-arterial injection of vasodilator therapy, or balloon angioplasty can be considered for treatment of vasospasm
- Traumatic subarachnoid hemorrhages will still require close observation, serial imaging to ensure stability of bleed, and similar medical management as aneurysmal bleeds.

Acute Ischemic Stroke (AIS)

Definition a disruption of blood flow to the brain due to a thrombus or embolus that results in infarcted tissue.

Approximately 85% of all strokes are ***ischemic***. They are the leading cause of serious long-term disability [66].

Risk factors include *hypertension, hyperlipidemia, atrial fibrillation, diabetes, smoking, and obesity* [40].

Clinical Presentation

- Patients will present with an ***acute neurologic deficit corresponding to the vascular territory.*** Symptoms include hemiparesis, facial droop, sudden visual loss, dysarthria, or aphasia.
- Remember the "**BE FAST**" mnemonic (**balance, eyes, face, arms, speech, time**) to help you quickly diagnose an acute stroke.
- Time is brain; the faster stroke is identified and treated, the more likely patients are to recover after a stroke.

Work-Up and Examination

- Blood pressure, oxygen saturation, glucose levels
- Comprehensive neurologic examination using the **National Institutes of Health Stroke Scale (NIHSS)**
- **Non-contrast CT scan** to rule out intracranial hemorrhage
- **CT angiogram and perfusion** will reveal the site of occlusion, assess the severity of infarction vs salvageable tissue, and help guide treatment, both medical and surgical (endovascular thrombectomy)
- MRI is the most sensitive and specific imaging study, but is not as readily available acutely and is time-consuming [53]

Treatment and Surgical Indications

- **IV thrombolytics**, such as tenecteplase or alteplase, should be considered **within 4.5 h** after symptom onset in patients who meet specific requirements [53]. ***There are many patient characteristics that prevent treatment with thrombolytics, and these must be considered in the patient presenting with AIS***
- If a large vessel occlusion is present, *mechanical thrombectomy* should be performed as soon as possible in patients presenting within 24 h of symptom onset [54]
  - Large vessel occlusion includes a blockage in the internal carotid artery (ICA), anterior cerebral artery, middle cerebral artery (MCA), or basilar artery.
  - Select patients presenting with more distal occlusions might also be candidates for thrombectomy
  - Hemorrhagic conversion, access site complications, and worsening stroke are all risks associated with mechanical thrombectomy [37]
- If a patient does not qualify for IV thrombolysis or mechanical thrombectomy, dual antiplatelet therapy with clopidogrel and aspirin should be considered to decrease the risk of recurrent stroke [54]
- Large infarcts within the MCA and ICA territories are at a higher risk of developing malignant cerebral edema, which

can lead to acute neurologic deterioration requiring surgical intervention. These patients should be closely monitored in an ICU setting with a focus on medical management to reduce brain swelling. They can be considered for surgical decompressive hemicraniectomy if neurologic decline occurs despite maximized medical management. It is important to note that in this setting, decompressive surgery is lifesaving and will likely not result in significant improvement in neurologic function [25].

Spine

Spinal Cord Injury (SCI)

Definition damage to the spinal cord that results in impaired motor and sensory function. This can either be traumatic or nontraumatic in nature. They are further classified as complete or incomplete [36].

Spinal shock is the temporary loss of all or most spinal reflexes below the level of injury [3].

Clinical Presentation

- Often occurring following motor vehicle accidents, falls, or sports injuries [70]
- Nontraumatic causes can include malignancy, infection, degenerative spine disease [47], leading to compression of neurologic tissue
- Presenting symptoms include paralysis or weakness in the extremities, numbness, tingling or loss of sensation, loss of bowel or bladder control, difficulty walking or breathing, and sexual dysfunction
- Incomplete Spinal Cord Syndromes [9, 35, 38]
  - Anterior Cord Syndrome
    - Deficit: ***sudden-onset paraplegia or quadriplegia, loss of pain, and temperature below the level of the lesion,*** and preserved posterior column function; typically caused by a vascular event affecting the anterior spinal artery
  - Central Cord syndrome
    - The most common spinal cord syndrome
    - Deficit: motor deficits affecting the ***upper extremities > lower, distal > proximal***, sensory findings may vary, patient often with a history, known or unknown, of degenerative cervical spine disease.
  - Posterior Cord Syndrome
    - Deficit: ***pain and paresthesia***
  - Brown-Sequard Syndrome
    - ***Ipsilateral* motor paralysis, loss of proprioception, vibration sense, with *contralateral* loss of pain and temperature**

Work-Up and Examination [17]

- ASIA (American Spinal Injury Association) score should be performed
- Other injury classification systems used include the thoracolumbar injury classification system (TLICS) or AO spine thoracolumbar or subaxial cervical spine injury classification system [50–52]
  - These can help determine whether the patient is likely to benefit from surgical intervention
- Non-contrast CT scan to evaluate bony injury and for surgical planning
- MRI without contrast to evaluate for the extent of ligamentous and spinal cord injury. The addition of contrast is typically used in patients presenting with spinal tumors
- Spinal precautions and utilization of bracing should be taken seriously until imaging is completed

Treatment and Surgical Considerations [17, 20]

- Initial airway, breathing, and circulation assessment should be performed
  - Low threshold for intubation, particularly with injury above C5
- Mean arterial pressure goals >85, and avoiding hypotension is recommended
- Steroid administration is still controversial. Consult your hospital policy regarding steroid administration in the setting of SCI, although in most patients, steroids will be contraindicated
- ***Early decompressive surgery is recommended, ideally within 24 h of injury***
  - Indications for surgery include cord compression with neurological deficit or unstable vertebral fractures.

Cauda Equina Syndrome [56]

Definition The cauda equina is a bundle of nerves located at the end of the spinal cord, typically just below the thoracolumbar junction, that innervates motor and sensory tracts throughout the lumbar, sacral, and coccygeal areas [56]. Cauda equina syndrome is a result of these nerves being compressed.

Clinical Presentation

- Presenting symptoms include ***back pain, sciatica, lower extremity weakness and sensory changes, saddle anesthesia, urinary retention, difficulty voiding, urinary incontinence, and bowel incontinence.*** Classically, patients with cauda equina syndrome present acutely.

Work-Up and Examination

- A thorough neurologic motor and sensory examination in the lower extremities should be performed
- Areflexia, hypotonia, or atrophy may be found in chronic cases
- Assess for rectal tone and the saddle area for loss of sensation
- A bladder scan with post-void residual can be helpful to confirm urinary retention
- MRI of the lumbar spine without contrast should be performed in an urgent manner if there is any clinical suspicion for cauda equina syndrome. Consider the addition of contrast if a tumor or infection is suspected. See Fig. 48.4a, b

Treatment and Surgical Considerations

- ***Urgent decompressive surgery*** should be performed when radiographic confirmation of cauda equina syndrome is present. The exact surgical operation should be tailored based on the etiology of compression. The most common cause is secondary to lumbar disc herniation, which is most commonly treated with lumbar laminectomy with discectomy. Other causes can include tumor, hematoma, or abscess.
- It is important to counsel patients presenting with cauda equina syndrome that the sooner pressure is removed from the nervous tissue, the more likely they are to improve, although this is not guaranteed. In addition, pain and motor deficits often improve faster than sensory or urinary symptoms, and some deficits may remain after surgery due to variable recovery of injured neurologic tissue.

Cervical or Lumbar Radiculopathy

Definition Radiculopathy refers to compression or irritation of a spinal nerve root as it exits the spinal column. This can occur throughout the entirety of the spine, but cervical and lumbar radiculopathy are most common [14].

Radiculopathy is most frequently caused by *disc herniations* or *degenerative changes in the spine* [15, 61].

Clinical Presentation

- Presenting symptoms include pain, weakness, numbness, or paresthesia often in a ***dermatomal distribution***, pain in the neck or back [14]
- Pain radiating into the posterior shoulder and periscapular region frequently occurs with cervical radiculopathy [14, 39]
- Pain is often described as sharp, dull, aching, burning, or throbbing [61]
- Pain related to a disc herniation can be exacerbated by straining, coughing, or bending forward [61]
- Pain in the back or legs related to lumbar stenosis often improves with bending forward, sitting, or lying down and worsens with walking [61]

Work-Up and Examination

- A thorough motor and sensory examination should be performed, focused on deficits in a radicular distribution that correlate with the suspected clinical level [61].
- Diminished reflexes are often present
- **Spurling test** involves passively moving the patient's neck into *lateral flexion and extension,* then *applying*

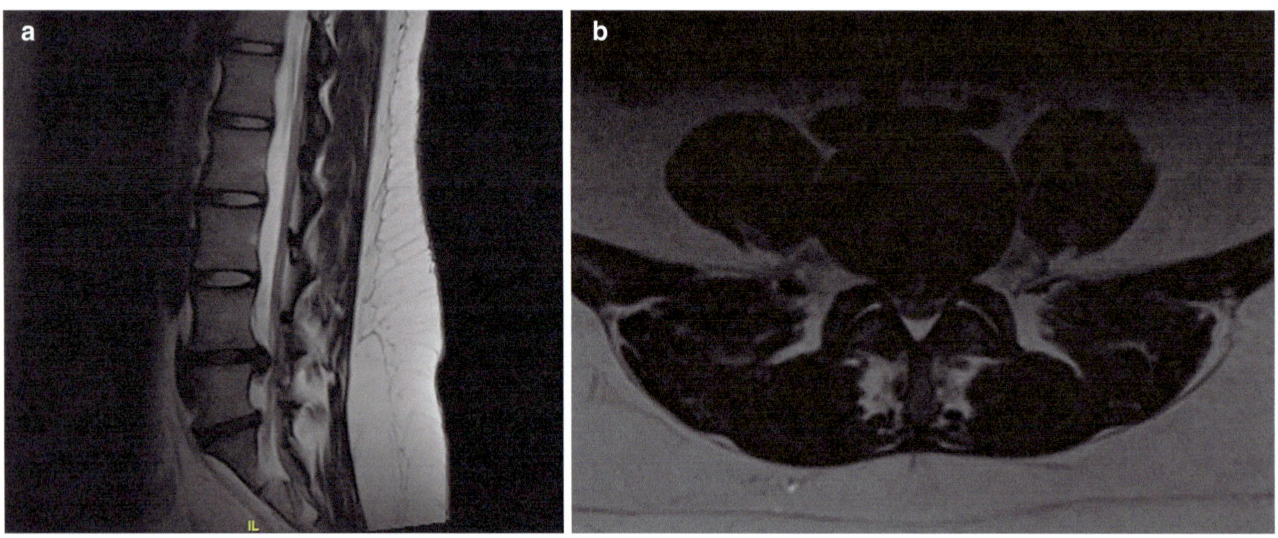

Fig. 48.4 (**a**) A sagittal T2 MRI of the lumbar spine reveals a large central disc herniation at L4–5. This patient required urgent surgical decompression after presenting with bladder incontinence, lower extremity weakness, and numbness. (**b**) Axial T2 imaging of the same patient reveals central compression of the thecal sac and cauda equina

downward axial pressure, positive result reproduces cervical radicular symptoms [14]. Patients will often provide a clinical history consistent with Spurling's sign, noting that certain neck movements exacerbate radicular symptoms
- **Straight leg raise** is a test in which you place one hand on the iliac crest of the affected side and have the patient lie supine. Slowly elevate the heel while keeping the knee straight. *This test is positive if radicular symptoms are reproduced with elevation above 30 degrees.* This test can be indicative of a disc herniation [13, 61]. Again, patients will often provide a history of difficulty raising the affected leg that makes it difficult to perform certain tasks such as putting on socks
- Initial imaging evaluation includes cervical or lumbar x-rays, which should be obtained while standing to evaluate for underlying instability. Flexion-extension films are useful for this as well
- MRI should be obtained when there is progressive neurologic deficit despite conservative treatment [14, 61].
- EMG can be useful when the diagnosis is unclear or to help differentiate a peripheral neuropathy [61, 68] from cervical or lumbar radiculopathy
- **Red flags in the evaluation of neck or back pain that require further work-up include *fever, history of cancer, pain at night, weight loss, IV-drug use, history of immunocompromise, and signs of myelopathy*** [14]

Treatment and Surgical Considerations

- *Conservative therapy is considered first line treatment.* This includes physical therapy, home exercises, nonsteroidal anti-inflammatory medications, muscle relaxants, and careful consideration of limited-use prescription pain medication [14]
- Interventional therapy with steroid injections can be considered if symptoms persist despite conservative management
- Surgery should be considered in patients who have failed conservative therapy, present with a progressive neurologic deficit, and when imaging reveals evidence of nerve root impingement that correlates with physical exam findings.

Myelopathy

Definition spinal cord dysfunction caused by compression of the spinal cord [1].

Myelopathy is most frequently caused by *degenerative disease*, and is more commonly seen in the *cervical spine*; however, it can occur anywhere throughout the spinal cord. Metastatic disease, primary neoplasms, infection, inflammatory, neurodegenerative, vascular, nutritional, and idiopathic disorders can all cause myelopathy [1, 63].

Clinical Presentation

- Presenting symptoms include neck or back pain/stiffness, extremity weakness, sensory loss, balance abnormalities, unstable gait, decline in hand dexterity, difficulty with fine motor tasks, bowel or bladder incontinence [32, 65].

Work-Up and Examination

- A thorough motor, sensory, and reflexive examination should be performed
- Evaluate for *upper motor neuron signs* such as a **Hoffman's reflex** or **Babinski sign** [8, 32]
- Other physical exam findings can include hyperreflexia, spasticity, or a wide-based ataxic gait [8, 32]
- **Lhermitte's sign:** *electric, shock-like sensation down the back and extremities with neck flexion* [8] *or axial loading*
- **MRI without contrast** is the preferred imaging modality [32, 59]. Contrast can be added in patients with a history of a tumor or other, less typical presentations such as syrinx.
- CT myelogram can be considered in patients who are unable to undergo MR [49]
- Consider radiographic flexion/extension views to evaluate for spine instability
- ***Vitamin B12 deficiency** is a common reversible cause of myelopathy;* this should be tested when myelopathy is suspected and no structural etiology is found on imaging [8]. Neurology evaluation should also be considered in patients in whom cord compression on imaging does not match the severity of clinical symptoms.

Treatment and Surgical Considerations

- *An incidental finding of cord compression in an asymptomatic patient should be treated conservatively.* [32, 48] Surgery might be considered in younger patients and those with low risk of perioperative complications with severe compression or cord edema (myelomalacia) to prevent the development or progression of symptoms over time.
- Management should be guided toward the underlying etiology of cord disease.
- *Surgical management is indicated in patients with myelopathic signs and symptoms and evidence of cord compression on imaging.*
- The goal of decompressive surgery is to prevent further decline in neurologic symptoms. It is important for patients to understand that reversal of symptoms is not guaranteed even after surgical decompression.

Although pediatric and functional neurosurgery are outside the scope of this chapter, similar principles apply to pathologies that are found in both pediatric and adult patients. Please refer to the suggested readings, which will have further information regarding these topics.

Suggested Readings

Fundamentals of Neurosurgery—Nitin Agarwal, MD

Tarascan Neurosurgery Pocketbook—Melaine G. Hayden Gephart, MD, MAS

Fast Facts about Neurocritical Care—Diane McLaughlin DNP, AGACNP-BC

Handbook of Neurosurgery—Mark S. Greenberg, MD, FAANS

References

1. Agarwal V, Shah LM, Parsons MS, et al. ACR appropriateness criteria® myelopathy: 2021 update. J Am Coll Radiol. 2021;18:S73–82. https://doi.org/10.1016/j.jacr.2021.01.020.
2. Al-Mufti F, Mayer SA. Neurocritical care of acute subdural hemorrhage. Neurosurg Clin N Am. 2017;28:267–78. https://doi.org/10.1016/j.nec.2016.11.009.
3. Atkinson PP, Atkinson JLD. Spinal shock. Mayo Clin Proc. 1996;71:384–9. https://doi.org/10.4065/71.4.384.
4. Babu JM, Patel SA, Palumbo MA, Daniels AH. Spinal emergencies in primary care practice. Am J Med. 2019;132:300–6. https://doi.org/10.1016/j.amjmed.2018.09.022.
5. Barbuskaite D, Oernbo EK, Wardman JH, et al. Acetazolamide modulates intracranial pressure directly by its action on the cerebrospinal fluid secretion apparatus. Fluids Barriers CNS. 2022;19 https://doi.org/10.1186/s12987-022-00348-6.
6. Basamh M, Robert A, Lamoureux J, et al. Epidural hematoma treated conservatively: when to expect the worst. Can J Neurol Sci. 2015;43:74–81. https://doi.org/10.1017/cjn.2015.232.
7. Bazil C, Bank A. Emergency Management of Epilepsy and Seizures. Semin Neurol. 2019;39:073–81. https://doi.org/10.1055/s-0038-1677008.
8. Bhattacharyya S. Spinal cord disorders: myelopathy. Am J Med. 2018;131:1293–7. https://doi.org/10.1016/j.amjmed.2018.03.009.
9. Blumenfeld H. Neuroanatomy through clinical cases. New York: Sinauer associates, an imprint of Oxford University Press; 2022.
10. Broder J, Preston R. Imaging the head and brain. Diagnostic Imaging for the Emergency Physician. 2011:1–45. https://doi.org/10.1016/B978-1-4160-6113-7.10001-8.
11. Bullock MR, Chesnut R, Ghajar J, et al.. (2006)Surgical management of acute epidural hematomas. Neurosurgery. 58:S2–7–S2–15. https://doi.org/10.1227/01.NEU.0000210363.91172.A8.
12. Celmer P (2023) Guidelines for the management of severe TBI, 4th edition. In: Brain trauma foundation. https://braintrauma.org/coma/guidelines/guidelines-for-the-management-of-severe-tbi-4th-ed. Accessed 20 Oct 2024.
13. Charnley J. Orthopædic signs in the diagnosis of disc protrusion. Lancet. 1951;257:186–92. https://doi.org/10.1016/s0140-6736(51)93353-3.
14. Childress M, Becker B. Nonoperative management of cervical radiculopathy. Am Fam Physician. 2016;93:746–54.
15. Clark R, Weber RP, Kahwati L. Surgical management of lumbar radiculopathy: a systematic review. J Gen Intern Med. 2019;35:855–64. https://doi.org/10.1007/s11606-019-05476-8.
16. Cohen-Gadol AA, Bohnstedt BN. Recognition and evaluation of nontraumatic subarachnoid hemorrhage and ruptured cerebral aneurysm. Am Fam Physician. 2013;88:451–6.
17. Eli I, Lerner DP, Ghogawala Z. Acute Traumatic Spinal Cord Injury. Neurol Clin. 2021;39:471–88. https://doi.org/10.1016/j.ncl.2021.02.004.
18. Englot DJ, Chang EF, Vecht CJ. Epilepsy and brain tumors. Handb Clin Neurol. 2016:267–85. https://doi.org/10.1016/B978-0-12-802997-8.00016-5.
19. Eymann R. Klinische Symptome des Hydrozephalus. Radiologe. 2012;52:807–12. https://doi.org/10.1007/s00117-012-2327-y.
20. Fehlings MG, Tetreault LA, Wilson JR, et al. A clinical practice guideline for the management of patients with acute spinal cord injury and central cord syndrome: recommendations on the timing (≤24 hours versus >24 hours) of decompressive surgery. Global Spine J. 2017;7:195S–202S. https://doi.org/10.1177/2192568217706367.
21. Fisher RS, Boas W v E, Blume W, et al. Epileptic seizures and epilepsy: definitions proposed by the International League Against Epilepsy (ILAE) and the International Bureau for Epilepsy (IBE). Epilepsia. 2005;46:470–2. https://doi.org/10.1111/j.0013-9580.2005.66104.x.
22. Freeman WD, Aguilar MI. Intracranial hemorrhage: diagnosis and management. Neurol Clin. 2012;30:211–40. https://doi.org/10.1016/j.ncl.2011.09.002.
23. Greenberg SM, Ziai WC, Cordonnier C, et al. 2022 guideline for the management of patients with spontaneous intracerebral hemorrhage: a guideline from the American Heart Association/American Stroke Association. Stroke. 2022;53 https://doi.org/10.1161/STR.0000000000000407.
24. Hayat MA. Introduction, vol. 3. Tumors of the central nervous system; 2011. p. 1–3. https://doi.org/10.1007/978-94-007-1399-4_1.
25. Hawkes MA, Rabinstein AA. Treatment of Malignant Cerebral Edema in Acute Ischemic Stroke. Curr Treat Options Neurol. 2024;26:243–59. https://doi.org/10.1007/s11940-024-00793-8
26. Heinzelmann M, Platz A, Imhof HG. Outcome after acute extradural haematoma, influence of additional injuries and neurological complications in the ICU. Injury. 1996;27:345–9. https://doi.org/10.1016/0020-1383(95)00223-5.
27. Hochstetler A, Raskin J, Blazer-Yost BL. Hydrocephalus: historical analysis and considerations for treatment. Eur J Med Res. 2022;27 https://doi.org/10.1186/s40001-022-00798-6.
28. Hoh BL, Ko NU, Amin-Hanjani S, et al. 2023 guideline for the management of patients with aneurysmal subarachnoid hemorrhage: a guideline from the American Heart Association/American Stroke Association. Stroke. 2023;54 https://doi.org/10.1161/STR.0000000000000436.
29. Hou K, Yu J. Current status of perimesencephalic non-aneurysmal subarachnoid hemorrhage. Front Neurol. 2022;13 https://doi.org/10.3389/fneur.2022.960702.
30. Jantzen J-PAH. Prevention and treatment of intracranial hypertension. Best Pract Res Clin Anaesthesiol. 2007;21:517–38. https://doi.org/10.1016/j.bpa.2007.09.001.
31. Joyce E, Bounajem MT, Scoville J, et al. Middle meningeal artery embolization treatment of nonacute subdural hematomas in the elderly: a multiinstitutional experience of 151 cases. Neurosurg Focus. 2020;49:E5. https://doi.org/10.3171/2020.7.FOCUS20518.
32. Kane S, Abadie K, Wilson A. Degenerative cervical myelopathy: recognition and management. Am Fam Physician. 2020;102:740.
33. Khairat A, Waseem M (2023) Epidural hematoma. In: StatPearls [Internet]. https://www.ncbi.nlm.nih.gov/book/NBK518982/. Accessed 3 Sept 2024.

34. Kiriakopoulos E (2022) Types of seizures. In: Epilepsy Foundation. https://www.epilepsy.com/what-is-epilepsy/seizure-types#How-Are-Seizures-Classified-Now. Accessed 20 Oct 2024.
35. Kirshblum SC, Burns SP, Biering-Sorensen F, et al. International standards for neurological classification of spinal cord injury (revised 2011). J Spinal Cord Med. 2011;34:535–46. https://doi.org/10.1179/204577211X13207446293695.
36. Kretzer RM. A clinical perspective and definition of spinal cord injury. Spine. 2016;41:S27. https://doi.org/10.1097/BRS.0000000000001432.
37. Krishnan R, Mays W, Elijovich L. Complications of mechanical thrombectomy in acute ischemic stroke. Neurology. 2021;97 https://doi.org/10.1212/WNL.0000000000012803.
38. Kunam VK, Velayudhan V, Chaudhry ZA, et al. Incomplete cord syndromes: clinical and imaging review. Radiographics. 2018;38:1201–22. https://doi.org/10.1148/rg.2018170178.
39. Levine MJ, Albert TJ, Smith MD. Cervical radiculopathy: diagnosis and nonoperative management. J Am Acad Orthop Surg. 1996;4:305–16. https://doi.org/10.5435/00124635-199611000-00003.
40. Libruder C, Ram A, Hershkovitz Y, et al. The contribution of potentially modifiable risk factors to acute ischemic stroke burden—comparing young and older adults. Prev Med. 2022;155:106933. https://doi.org/10.1016/j.ypmed.2021.106933.
41. Lim M, Kheok SW, Lim KC, et al. Subdural haematoma mimics. Clin Radiol. 2019;74:663–75. https://doi.org/10.1016/j.crad.2019.04.013.
42. Liu G, Slate N, Perkins A. Epilepsy: treatment options. Am Fam Physician. 2017;96:87–96.
43. Long B, Koyfman A, Runyon MS. Subarachnoid hemorrhage. Emerg Med Clin North Am. 2017;35:803–24. https://doi.org/10.1016/j.emc.2017.07.001.
44. Maas AIR, Adams H, et al. Traumatic brain injury: integrated approaches to improve prevention, clinical care, and research. Lancet Neurol. 2017;16(12):987–1048.
45. Mokri B. The Monro–Kellie hypothesis. Neurology. 2001;56:1746–8. https://doi.org/10.1212/WNL.56.12.1746.
46. Mulcahy MJ, Chaganti J, Dower A, Al-Khawaja D. Spontaneous acute arterial subdural hematoma. World Neurosurg. 2018;110:403–6. https://doi.org/10.1016/j.wneu.2017.
47. Müller-Jensen L, Ploner CJ, Kroneberg D, Schmidt WU. Clinical presentation and causes of non-traumatic spinal cord injury: an observational study in emergency patients. Front Neurol. 2021;12 https://doi.org/10.3389/fneur.2021.701927.
48. Naito K, Yamagata T, Ohata K, Takami T. Management of the patient with cervical cord compression but no evidence of myelopathy. Neurosurg Clin N Am. 2018;29:145–52. https://doi.org/10.1016/j.nec.2017.09.010.
49. Oyinkan Marquis B, Capone PM. Myelopathy. Handb Clin Neurol. 2016:1015–26. https://doi.org/10.1016/B978-0-444-53486-6.00052-1.
50. Park HJ, Lee SY, Park NH, et al. Modified thoracolumbar injury classification and severity score (TLICS) and its clinical usefulness. Acta Radiol. 2015;57:74–81. https://doi.org/10.1177/0284185115580487.
51. Pizones J, Álvarez-González P, Sánchez-Mariscal F, et al. Letters. Spine. 2014;39:783.
52. Vaccaro AR, Koerner JD, Radcliff KE, et. al. AOSpine subaxial cervical spine injury classification system. Eur Spine J. 2016;25:2173–84. https://doi.org/10.1097/BRS.0000000000000279.
53. Powers WJ. Acute ischemic stroke. N Engl J Med. 2020;383:252–60. https://doi.org/10.1056/NEJMcp1917030.
54. Powers WJ, Rabinstein AA, Ackerson T, et al. Guidelines for the early management of patients with acute ischemic stroke: 2019 update to the 2018 guidelines for the early management of acute ischemic stroke: a guideline for healthcare professionals from the American Heart Association/American Stroke Association. Stroke. 2019;50
55. Pradilla G, Ratcliff JJ, Hall AJ, et al. Trial of early minimally invasive removal of intracerebral hemorrhage. N Engl J Med. 2024;390:1277–89.
56. Quaile A. Cauda equina syndrome—the questions. International Orthopaedics (SICOT). 2018;43:957–61. https://doi.org/10.1007/s00264-018-4208-0.
57. Rahimi A, Corley JA, Ammar A, et al. The unmet global burden of cranial epidural hematomas: a systematic review and meta-analysis. Clin Neurol Neurosurg. 2022;219:107313. https://doi.org/10.1016/j.clineuro.2022.107313.
58. Rolak LA, Rutecki P, Ashizawa T, Harati Y. Clinical features of Todd's post-epileptic paralysis. J Neurol Neurosurg Psychiatr. 1992;55:63–4. https://doi.org/10.1136/jnnp.55.1.63.
59. Roth CJ, Angevine PD, Aulino JM, et al. ACR appropriateness criteria myelopathy. J Am Coll Radiol. 2016;13:38–44. https://doi.org/10.1016/j.jacr.2015.10.004.
60. Stoffey RD, Nadgir R, Yousem D. Head trauma. In: Neuroradiology: the requisites. Philadelphia, PA: Elsevier; 2017. p. 150–73.
61. Tarulli AW, Raynor EM. Lumbosacral radiculopathy. Neurol Clin. 2007;25:387–405. https://doi.org/10.1016/j.ncl.2007.01.008.
62. Tenny S (2024) Intracranial hemorrhage. In: StatPearls [Internet]. https://www.ncbi.nlm.nih.gov/books/NBK470242/. Accessed 19 Oct 2024.
63. Tettenborn B, Hägele-Link S. Spinal cord disorders. Eur Neurol. 2015;74:141–6. https://doi.org/10.1159/000437417.
64. Thakur SK, Serulle Y, Miskin NP, et al. Lumbar puncture test in normal pressure hydrocephalus: does the volume of CSF removed affect the response to tap? AJNR Am J Neuroradiol. 2017;38:1456–60. https://doi.org/10.3174/ajnr.A5187.
65. Toledano M, Bartleson JD. Cervical spondylotic myelopathy. Neurol Clin. 2013;31:287–305. https://doi.org/10.1016/j.ncl.2012.09.003.
66. Tsao CW, Aday AW, Almarzooq ZI, et al. Heart disease and stroke statistics—2023 update: a report from the American Heart Association. Circulation. 2023;147 https://doi.org/10.1161/CIR.0000000000001167.
67. Westermaier T, Eriskat J, Kunze E, et al. Clinical features, treatment, and prognosis of patients with acute subdural hematomas presenting in critical condition. Neurosurgery. 2007;61:482–8. https://doi.org/10.1227/01.NEU.0000290893.85072.F9.
68. Wilbourn AJ, Aminoff MJ. AAEE minimonograph #32: the electrophysiologic examination in patients with radiculopathies. Muscle Nerve. 1988;11:1099–114. https://doi.org/10.1002/mus.880111102.
69. Wolfsegger T, Assar H. Assessment of neurological symptoms in adult hydrocephalus occlusus. A pilot study. J Clin Neurosci. 2021;90:89–93. https://doi.org/10.1016/j.jocn.2021.05.054.
70. National Spinal Cord Injury Statistical Center, Recent Trends in Causes of Traumatic Spinal Cord Injury. (2023) Birmingham, AL: University of Alabama at Birmingham.

Endocrine Surgery

49

Shaghayegh Sabbaghan Kermani and Roy Phitayakorn

Thyroid Diseases

Thyroid Anatomy and Physiology

The thyroid gland is a butterfly-shaped organ located in the front of the neck and is pivotal in regulating numerous metabolic processes through the secretion of thyroid hormones. These hormones, thyroxine (T4) and triiodothyronine (T3), are fundamental to regulating the body's metabolic rate, heart and digestive function, muscle control, brain development, and bone maintenance. The thyroid gland originates embryologically from the primitive pharynx and the neural crest. It forms a bilobed structure that then descends in the midline of the neck, giving rise to the thyroid's eventual anatomical placement. The thyroid receives its blood supply from the superior and inferior thyroid arteries and is drained by corresponding veins, which ensures efficient uptake and distribution of thyroid hormone [1–16].

Goiter

A goiter is an enlarged thyroid gland. While not inherently dangerous, it can be a sign of thyroid dysfunction and may require medical attention.

Epidemiology

Goiter is a global health issue, affecting over 740 million people worldwide, primarily due to iodine deficiency, which remains the leading cause. This condition is particularly prevalent in areas where the soil and diet provide insufficient iodine. Goiters can be classified based on their causative mechanisms and include endemic versus sporadic goiters. Endemic Goiters occur in geographic regions with iodine deficiency affecting more than 10% of the local population. On the other hand, sporadic goiter arises independently of geographic or dietary influences and can be attributed to factors like genetic defects or certain drugs that interfere with thyroid hormone synthesis. Goiter occurs 2–10 times more frequently in women compared to men.

Clinical Presentation

The term goiter stems from the Latin word "guttur," meaning throat, reflecting its most evident physical symptom. The enlargement may vary, affecting one or both lobes of the thyroid. The underlying pathophysiology of goiter involves the thyroid gland's response to insufficient thyroid hormone production. To compensate, the gland enlarges to enhance its capability to trap available iodine, which can lead to the visible swelling known as a goiter. The main sign of a goiter is the visible enlargement of the thyroid gland. Symptoms may escalate to cause discomfort, including difficulty in swallowing or breathing, if the goiter significantly enlarges.

Diagnosis and Management

Diagnosis typically involves a physical examination, thyroid function tests, and imaging studies such as thyroid ultrasound to determine the extent of the gland enlargement and its impact on surrounding structures. If there is suspicion that

S. Sabbaghan Kermani (✉)
Department of Surgery, Massachusetts General Hospital, Harvard Medical School, Boston, MA, USA
e-mail: ssabbaghankermani@mgh.harvard.edu

R. Phitayakorn
UIC College of Medicine, Chicago, IL, USA

Division of Surgical Oncology, Department of Surgery, UI Health, Chicago, IL, USA

S. Atallah, J. Dragoljevic (eds.), *Fundamentals of Surgery for Physician Assistants*,
https://doi.org/10.1007/978-3-032-21069-2_49

the goiter extends below the sternal notch into the mediastinum/chest, a contrast CT scan should be used to better visualize the extent of the gland. Since intravenous contrast contains iodine analogues, it is very important to ensure that the patient is not hyperthyroid before giving the contrast to avoid thyroid storm, which is a life-threatening condition (see below).

The management for goiter varies based on the cause and severity. Mild cases may only require monitoring and dietary iodine supplementation. TSH suppression may also be helpful to reduce the goiter rate. More significant or symptomatic goiters might need pharmacological treatment with thyroid hormones or even surgical intervention. The decision for surgery is generally reserved for cases where the goiter causes obstructive symptoms or if there is a suspicion of malignancy within a thyroid nodule inside the goiter (see below).

Hyperthyroidism

Hyperthyroidism refers to the clinical condition resulting from the excessive production of thyroid hormones, termed thyrotoxicosis. Hyperthyroidism has several different presentations, the most prevalent being Graves' disease and toxic multinodular goiter (TMNG). Other forms include toxic adenoma and more transient conditions such as subacute thyroiditis or iodine-induced hyperthyroidism.

Epidemiology

Hyperthyroidism affects about 0.5% of the population, with another 0.8% exhibiting subclinical forms where thyroid-stimulating hormone (TSH) levels are suppressed, yet the circulating thyroid hormone levels remain within the normal range. The condition's prevalence varies by geographical region and dietary iodine intake, impacting the distribution of causes like Graves' disease and TMNG.

Clinical Presentation

The symptoms of hyperthyroidism vary widely, including weight loss, heat intolerance, increased heart rate, fatigue, anxiety, and insomnia. In more severe cases, patients may experience muscle weakness, dyspnea, or advanced ocular symptoms in Graves' disease, such as proptosis and periorbital edema.

Graves' Disease

Graves' or Basedow's Disease is the most common cause of hyperthyroidism and is an autoimmune disorder marked by the presence of IgG autoantibodies stimulating the thyroid. This stimulation results in the gland producing excess hormone. Clinical features specific to Graves' disease can include diffuse goiter, exophthalmos, and pretibial myxedema. Diagnosis is confirmed through the detection of autoantibodies called thyroid-stimulating immunoglobulins (TSI) and elevated thyroid hormone levels, with suppressed TSH.

Toxic Multinodular Goiter

This condition involves the development of autonomously functioning nodules within the thyroid, each producing thyroid hormones independently of TSH regulation. It is more common in older populations and can manifest without a significant goiter.

Toxic Solitary Adenoma

A single autonomously functioning thyroid nodule that produces an excessive amount of thyroid hormones. Unlike Graves' or Plummer's diseases, this is typically confined to a solitary nodule.

Diagnosis and Management

The diagnostic evaluation for hyperthyroidism begins with serum TSH, total T3, and free T4 levels. In hyperthyroidism, TSH is usually suppressed due to negative feedback mechanisms, while T4 and T3 are elevated. Thyroid scintigraphy with radioactive iodine can help differentiate types of hyperthyroidism based on the pattern of iodine uptake, identifying areas of autonomy in the gland, with diffuse uptake being pathognomonic for Graves' disease.

The treatment strategies for hyperthyroidism include antithyroid medications, radioactive iodine therapy, and thyroidectomy. The choice of treatment depends on the cause of hyperthyroidism, the severity of symptoms, and patient-specific factors such as age and potential pregnancy.

- **Antithyroid Medications:** These drugs, such as methimazole and propylthiouracil, are used to reduce thyroid hormone synthesis and are particularly useful in young adults, pregnant women, or individuals preparing for radioactive iodine therapy or surgery.
- **Radioactive Iodine Therapy:** Often selected for its ability to ablate hyperactive thyroid tissue effectively, this treatment is suitable for nonpregnant adults and may be associated with an increased risk of secondary malignancy at high dosages.
- **Surgery:** Recommended in patients with large goiters, suspicious nodules, or those who cannot undergo or wish

to avoid radioactive treatments. Surgery may involve removing all or part of the thyroid gland, depending on the extent of the disease and the presence of nodules.

In general, the treatment of hyperthyroidism should include a detailed conversation between the patient and their endocrinologist or endocrine surgeon to address the underlying cause while minimizing the risk of recurrence and adverse effects.

Hypothyroidism

Hypothyroidism reflects an underproduction of thyroid hormones, resulting in a slowing of the metabolic processes.

Epidemiology

In areas where iodine levels are sufficient, spontaneous hypothyroidism affects approximately 1–2% of the population. It is more prevalent in older women and occurs about ten times more frequently in women compared to men.

Clinical Presentation

Symptoms are often nonspecific and can include fatigue, weight gain, cold intolerance, depression, and constipation. Physical signs might include bradycardia, dry skin, and puffiness around the eyes. Subclinical hypothyroidism, where symptomatic manifestations are minimal despite abnormal lab values, is also common.

Diagnosis and Management

Diagnosis is primarily based on elevated TSH and low free T4 levels. Treatment generally involves lifelong thyroid hormone replacement therapy with artificial T4 supplementation (levothyroxine) or animal-based mixed T3 and T4 supplementation (Armor).

Thyroiditis

Thyroiditis refers to a variety of conditions characterized by inflammation of the thyroid gland, which can present with varying clinical pictures depending on the etiology and progression of the disease. There are several common types of thyroiditis that each require different management strategies.

Epidemiology

Thyroiditis accounts for around 20% of all thyroid conditions and can arise from multiple causes. Autoimmune disorders are the most prevalent underlying factors. Approximately 1 in 100 people will experience overt autoimmune thyroiditis, and thyroid autoantibodies can be detected in up to 10% of the general population.

Clinical Presentation

Hashimoto's Thyroiditis This disease is the most common form of autoimmune thyroiditis, often associated with alternating hyper- and hypothyroidism and eventual permanent hypothyroidism. Hashimoto's features a diffuse infiltration of the thyroid gland by lymphocytes and plasma cells, which can lead to glandular atrophy and fibrosis over time. Patients might experience gradual thyroid failure with symptoms such as fatigue, weight gain, and cold intolerance.

Subacute Thyroiditis (De Quervain's) This condition is usually preceded by an upper respiratory infection and presents with painful, tender thyroid enlargement. It may cause transient hyperthyroidism due to the destruction of thyroid cells, releasing thyroid hormone into the bloodstream.

Riedel's Thyroiditis Characterized by a dense fibrous replacement of the thyroid tissue, this rare form of thyroiditis presents similarly to a thyroid malignancy because of its firm and invasive nature. It may cause compressive symptoms and requires a biopsy for definitive diagnosis.

Postpartum Thyroiditis Typically occurring in women after childbirth, this condition can present in phases: an initial thyrotoxic phase followed by a hypothyroid phase. Most women recover normal thyroid function, although some may develop permanent hypothyroidism.

Diagnosis and Management

Hashimoto's Thyroiditis Diagnostically, high levels of *thyroid peroxidase* and *antithyroglobulin antibodies* are typically present in the serum. Thyroid hormone replacement therapy is required if hypothyroidism develops on lab work. Nonsteroidal anti-inflammatory medications may help with acute flares and selenium may help with overall immune modulation.

Subacute Thyroiditis The condition is self-limiting, and treatment usually involves pain relief and beta-blockers to manage symptoms.

Riedel's Thyroiditis Riedel's Thyroiditis requires a biopsy for definitive diagnosis, and management often involves surgical intervention to relieve compressive symptoms. Corticosteroids may also be used to control inflammation.

Postpartum Thyroiditis Postpartum Thyroiditis is treated supportively, focusing on managing symptoms during both the thyrotoxic and hypothyroid phases. Most women recover normal thyroid function, although some may develop permanent hypothyroidism.

Thyroid Nodules

Epidemiology

Thyroid nodules are commonly detected during physical examinations or incidentally through imaging, with prevalence increasing with age. While most nodules are benign, a small but significant percentage may harbor malignancy, necessitating thorough evaluation.

Clinical Presentation

Patients may present asymptomatically or with symptoms ranging from a palpable lump in the neck to changes in voice, swallowing difficulties, or signs of thyroid dysfunction. The presentation can vary widely based on the size and location of the nodule within the thyroid gland.

Diagnostic Evaluation

The initial evaluation of a thyroid nodule involves biochemical tests to assess thyroid function, primarily focusing on TSH and thyroid hormone levels. Imaging studies, particularly ultrasonography, play a crucial role in characterizing nodules, assessing their size, composition, and potential for malignancy.

The Thyroid Imaging Reporting and Data System (TIRADS) is a classification system developed to standardize the reporting of thyroid ultrasound findings and to assess the risk of malignancy in thyroid nodules. It is designed to help guide management decisions, such as whether a thyroid nodule needs a biopsy or can be safely monitored. This classification system is based on five risk stratification criteria: composition, echogenicity, shape, margins, and echogenic foci or presence of microcalcification. Based on these parameters, thyroid nodules are scored 1–5 in the TIRADS system (see Table 49.1). The higher the score, the higher the risk of malignancy and the indication for fine needle aspiration (FNA) biopsy (see Table 49.2). Ultrasound-guided FNA is typically utilized for cytological evaluation, providing essential insights into the nodule's nature, whether benign or malignant.

Table 49.1 Sonographic features in Thyroid Imaging Reporting and Data System (TIRADS)

Category	Options	Points	Category	Options	Points
Composition			**Margin**		
	Cystic or almost completely cystic	0 points		Smooth	0 points
	Spongiform	0 points		Ill-defined	0 points
	Mixed cystic and solid	1 point		Lobulated/irregular	2 points
	Solid or almost completely solid	2 points		Extra-thyroidal extension	3 points
Echogenicity			**Echogenic foci**		
	Anechoic	0 points		None or large comet-tail artifact	0 points
	Hyper- or isoechoic	1 point		Macrocalcifications	1 point
	Hypoechoic	2 points		Peripheral/rim calcifications	2 points
	Very hypoechoic	3 points		Punctate echogenic foci	3 points
Shape					
	Wider than tall	0 points			
	Taller than wide	3 points			

Table 49.2 Thyroid Imaging Reporting and Data System (TIRADS) and clinical management

0 points	TR1	Benign	No FNA
2 points	TR2	Not suspicious	No FNA
3 points	TR3	Mildly suspicious	FNA if >2.5 cm Follow-up if >1.5 cm
4–6 points	TR4	Moderately suspicious	FNA if >1.5 cm Follow-up if >1 cm
7 points or more	TR5	Highly suspicious	FNA if >1 cm Follow-up if >0.5 cm

Table 49.3 Staging Criteria for Follicular Thyroid Cancer (FTC) and Papillary Thyroid Cancer (PTC)

Category	Description
Overview of the TNM system	The American joint committee on cancer (AJCC) TNM system outlines cancer stages using three main elements: T (tumor), N (nodes), and M (metastasis).
T categories for thyroid cancer	**TX**: Unable to evaluate the primary tumor. **T0**: No evidence of a primary tumor. **T1**: Tumor is ≤2 cm; **T1a** ≤1 cm, **T1b** >1 cm but ≤2 cm. **T2**: Tumor size >2 cm and ≤ 4 cm. **T3**: Tumor size >4 cm; confined to the thyroid (**T3a**) or of any size with gross extrathyroidal extension involving strap muscles (**T3b**). **T4a**: Tumor of any size extending beyond the thyroid into soft neck tissues, trachea, larynx, esophagus, or recurrent laryngeal nerve. **T4b**: Tumor extends to the prevertebral fascia or nearby major blood vessels.
N categories for thyroid cancer	**NX**: Regional lymph nodes cannot be evaluated. **N0**: No spread to lymph nodes, either histologically (**N0a**) or clinically/radiologically (**N0b**). **N1a**: Spread to level VI or VII lymph nodes in the neck. **N1b**: Involvement of unilateral, bilateral, or contralateral level I–V lymph nodes or retropharyngeal nodes.
M categories for thyroid cancer	**MX**: Distant metastasis cannot be assessed. **M0**: No distant metastasis. **M1**: Distant metastasis present, involving remote lymph nodes, organs, bones, etc.
Staging for patients younger than 55	**Stage I**: Any T, any N, M0—Tumor can be of any size, may involve lymph nodes, but no distant metastasis. **Stage II**: Any T, any N, M1—Tumor may be of any size and may involve lymph nodes, with distant metastasis present.
Staging for patients aged 55 and older	**Stage I**: T1 or T2, N0, M0—Tumor ≤4 cm, no regional lymph node or distant metastasis. **Stage II**: T1 to T3, N1, M0 or T3, N0, M0—Tumor may be any size with lymph node spread but no distant metastasis; tumor >4 cm confined to the thyroid without lymph node or distant spread; or any tumor with gross extension to strap muscles but no regional lymph node or distant spread. **Stage III**: T4a, N0/N1, M0—Tumor of any size with extensive local spread, may or may not involve lymph nodes, without distant metastasis. **Stage IVA**: T4b, N0/N1, M0—Tumor extends to prevertebral fascia or major vessels, with or without lymph node spread, no distant metastasis. **Stage IVB**: T1 to T4, N0/N1, M1—Tumor of any size, potentially with local or lymph node involvement, with distant metastasis.

Management Strategies

The management of thyroid nodules is tailored to the risk profile indicated by initial assessments. A commonly used criteria are the Bethesda criteria (see Table 49.3) which includes six diagnostic categories: (I) nondiagnostic, (II) benign, (III) atypia of undetermined significance, (IV) follicular neoplasm, (V) suspicious for malignancy, and (VI) malignant.

Low-Risk Nodules (Bethesda Categories II and III) Observation and routine monitoring may suffice, with periodic ultrasound examinations to assess for growth or changes in the nodule's characteristics. These nodules have a low risk of malignancy, and active surveillance is generally recommended unless significant changes are observed over time.

High-Risk Nodules (Bethesda Categories IV, V, and VI) Surgical removal is often recommended, particularly if the nodule is large, exhibits rapid growth, or has suspicious features on ultrasound or fine needle aspiration (FNA) results. The approach to surgery will depend on factors like the size and location of the nodule, the patient's overall health, and the presence of any potential complications such as thyroiditis or concurrent thyroid disorders. Depending on the extent and nature of the nodule, a partial or total thyroidectomy may be necessary to ensure complete removal of the high-risk tissue and to prevent the progression of malignancy (see below).

Thyroid Cancer

Epidemiology

Thyroid cancer is relatively uncommon, representing less than 1% of all cancers and contributing marginally to overall cancer deaths. However, the incidence rates vary, affecting approximately 3.7–4.7 individuals per 100,000 of the population.

The prognosis for thyroid cancer is generally favorable, especially when detected early and managed appropriately, although long-term management strategies and optimal treatment approaches remain areas of ongoing research and debate due to the lack of large, randomized studies.

Thyroid cancer arises from complex genetic changes within the thyroid cells, which may include mutations in oncogenes such as those from the RAS family, and growth factors like epidermal growth factor (EGFR) and insulin-like growth factor (IGF-1). RET proto-oncogene mutations are particularly noted in medullary thyroid cancers. These genetic alterations can lead to the uncontrolled growth and division of thyroid cells, forming tumors [17–19].

Clinical Presentation

Papillary Thyroid Carcinoma *This is the most common form of thyroid cancer*, accounting for 70–80% of all cases. It is particularly prevalent among children and young adults and is linked to a history of radiation exposure. Patients with PTC are often asymptomatic, typically presenting with either a single thyroid nodule or multiple nodules within the thyroid gland. In some cases, a palpable cervical lymph node may also be detected.

Follicular Thyroid Carcinoma Comprising 15–20% of thyroid cancers, follicular carcinoma has a higher prevalence in regions with iodine deficiency and is more likely to invade blood vessels and metastasize distantly compared to papillary carcinoma. In most cases, a single thyroid nodule is detected either during a physical exam by the patient or physician, or incidentally through imaging. Most patients are asymptomatic.

Medullary Thyroid Cancer Arising from parafollicular C-cells which secrete calcitonin, Medullary Thyroid Cancer (MTC) makes up about 5–8% of thyroid cancers. *This type is notable for its association with genetic conditions like Multiple Endocrine Neoplasia (MEN) syndromes*, demanding early and precise diagnostic and treatment approaches due to its aggressive nature. Around 15% of patients with MTC present with symptoms of locally advanced disease, such as hoarseness, difficulty breathing (dyspnea), or difficulty swallowing (dysphagia).

Anaplastic Thyroid Carcinoma Highly aggressive and typically occurring in older patients, this rare form of thyroid cancer rapidly progresses and is often fatal. Anaplastic Thyroid Carcinoma (ATC) is resistant to most conventional therapies and frequently presents with significant complications due to its rapid growth and invasion into surrounding structures. Most patients with ATC present with a rapidly growing neck mass. Some may also exhibit symptoms of hyperthyroidism, resulting from pseudo-thyroiditis caused by the rapid destruction of normal thyroid follicles due to ATC invasion.

Diagnosis and Management

The primary treatment for well-differentiated thyroid cancer, which includes papillary and follicular types, is surgical removal of the thyroid gland (thyroidectomy). Depending on the extent of the disease, this may range from lobectomy to total thyroidectomy, possibly accompanied by removal of affected lymph nodes. Radioactive iodine therapy may be employed postsurgery to eliminate residual thyroid tissue or metastatic disease. For medullary and anaplastic carcinomas, treatment strategies also include targeted therapies and chemotherapy, acknowledging their unique biological behaviors and poorer prognosis.

Prognostic Factors

The prognosis for thyroid cancer patients depends significantly on the cancer type, stage at diagnosis, patient's age, and the tumor's genetic makeup. Papillary and follicular thyroid cancers often have an excellent prognosis, with high survival rates when treated appropriately, whereas medullary and especially anaplastic carcinomas have a less favorable outlook due to their propensity for early metastasis and resistance to standard treatments.

Complications of Thyroidectomy

Thyroidectomy, while generally safe, carries potential risks and complications that vary depending on the extent of surgery and the patient's preexisting conditions. Here are some of the key complications:

Recurrent Laryngeal Nerve Injury *Injury to the recurrent laryngeal nerve (RLN) is one of the most significant complications, which can result in vocal cord paralysis, leading to hoarseness, voice changes, or, in severe cases, airway obstruction.* This complication is rare but can be minimized through the careful identification and preservation of the nerve during surgery. An RLN monitor may increase the speed of positive identification of the nerve and ensure that it is functional during surgery.

Hypoparathyroidism Inadvertent removal or damage to the parathyroid glands during thyroidectomy can lead to hypoparathyroidism, resulting in low calcium levels, which may cause muscle cramps, tingling, or cardiac issues. This complication necessitates prompt treatment with calcium and vitamin D supplementation.

Hemorrhage Bleeding can occur after the operation, which might require reoperation. Significant bleeding can lead to decreased venous return, which in turn causes vocal cord swelling and eventual closure of the airway, necessitating urgent medical intervention.

Infection Although uncommon, there is a risk of infection at the incision site or within the neck, which can generally be managed with antibiotics and proper wound care.

Thyroid Storm A rare but life-threatening complication of thyroidectomy, especially in patients with hyperthyroidism who are not adequately prepared preoperatively with antithyroid medications. It is characterized by a sudden and severe exacerbation of hyperthyroid symptoms, typically during the thyroidectomy, which requires immediate emergency treatment. Intraoperative management primarily focuses on supportive care, which may involve the use of beta blockers and vasodilators to stabilize hemodynamics, along with cooling blankets to address hyperthermia. A recommended approach includes a combination of thionamide, beta blocker, glucocorticoid, and iodine.

External Branch of the Superior Laryngeal Nerve Injury Damage to this nerve can affect vocal pitch and projection, particularly impacting professional singers and speakers.

Each of these complications necessitates specific preventive measures, such as careful surgical technique and preoperative preparation, to minimize risks and ensure patient safety. Additionally, a thorough understanding of the anatomy and careful monitoring during the postoperative period are critical to preventing and managing these complications effectively.

Parathyroid

This section reviews the anatomy and physiology of the parathyroid glands, the most common forms of hyperparathyroidism, parathyroid carcinoma, and managing postoperative complications after parathyroid surgery [20–44].

Anatomy and Physiology

Parathyroid glands (PTG) are nodular structures that are usually located along the posterior wall of the thyroid. Typically, there are four parathyroid glands—two superior and two inferior. However, anatomical variations, such as supernumerary parathyroid glands, have been documented. Additionally, ectopic positioning of these glands is possible, including the mediastinum, retro-esophageal region, or in the lateral neck.

The regulation of calcium is vital for numerous bodily functions, including enzymatic activities, muscle contraction, and neurotransmission. Most body calcium is stored in the skeleton, making up about 2% of body weight. Serum calcium levels are maintained through a regulatory axis involving parathyroid hormone (PTH), calcium receptors, kidneys, intestines, and bones. PTH secretion responds to minute decreases in serum calcium, mobilizing calcium from bone, reducing renal calcium excretion, and increasing intestinal calcium absorption. High serum calcium inhibits PTH secretion and vice versa. Diseases of the parathyroid often manifest as calcium metabolism disorders, with hypercalcemia as the most common presentation.

Primary Hyperparathyroidism

Epidemiology

Primary hyperparathyroidism (PHPT) results from the overproduction of parathyroid hormone (PTH) by one or more autonomously hyperfunctioning parathyroid glands, leading to hypercalcemia. It is predominantly caused by a single parathyroid adenoma (85%), while up to 15% of cases involve multi-gland disease (MGD) in which more than one parathyroid gland is secreting excess PTH. Parathyroid carcinoma is extremely rare and is discussed in a separate section below.

PHPT is the leading cause of hypercalcemia in outpatient settings, with around 100,000 new cases annually in the United States. Its prevalence has increased with routine laboratory testing, increasing from 0.1% to 0.4%. PHPT can present at any age, but it is most common in patients over 45 years, with a higher incidence in women, possibly due to estrogen deficiency unmasking underlying hyperparathyroidism.

Clear risk factors for PHPT are identifiable in only a limited number of patients. Genetic abnormalities such as multiple endocrine neoplasia (MEN) syndromes and familial isolated hyperparathyroidism (FIHPT) are significant. Radiation exposure, even at low doses during teenage years, also increases the risk.

Clinical Presentation

The clinical presentation of PHPT has changed over time. Classical symptoms included osteitis fibrosa cystica, nephrocalcinosis, peptic ulcer disease, and severe proximal myopathy. Today, common signs and symptoms include bone pain, nephrolithiasis, fatigue, weakness, mood swings, irritability, anxiety, depression, poor concentration, and memory loss. However, up to 80% of patients may have nonspecific or no noticeable symptoms.

Diagnostic Evaluation

Diagnosis of PHPT begins with biochemical confirmation of hypercalcemia. Elevated total serum calcium or ionized calcium levels indicate hypercalcemia, and PTH levels are measured to confirm PHPT. Other conditions causing hypercalcemia, such as medications (thiazides, lithium), malignancies, and granulomatous diseases, must be excluded.

Imaging studies like ultrasonography, technetium pertechnetate (^{99m}Tc) sestamibi scans, CT, and MRI help localize the hyperfunctioning gland(s) if surgery is planned. Less commonly, patients may present with normocalcemic HPT, which is when serum calcium levels may be high normal with an inappropriately high normal PTH level. Management of this entity is controversial, and these patients should be referred to an endocrinologist and endocrine surgeon for a discussion of next steps.

Management

Management of PHPT involves surgical intervention in symptomatic patients and in certain asymptomatic patients with specific criteria, such as significant hypercalcemia, reduced renal function, osteoporosis, age under 50 years, poor patient compliance, and patient desire for surgical treatment. Surgery involves parathyroidectomy, with options like bilateral neck exploration, unilateral neck exploration, and minimally invasive radio-guided parathyroidectomy. Postoperative monitoring of serum calcium levels is essential to ensure cure and monitor for recurrence.

Secondary and Tertiary Hyperparathyroidism

Secondary hyperparathyroidism (SHPT) occurs due to a non-parathyroid cause, such as vitamin D deficiency, chronic kidney disease, or end-stage renal disease (ESRD), leading to increased PTH secretion. **Chronic kidney disease** (CKD) is associated with hypocalcemia due to decreased renal conversion of 25-hydroxyvitamin D to 1,25-dihydroxyvitamin D (the more active form). Concurrently, decreased glomerular filtration leads to inadequate clearance of plasma phosphate. The resulting hypocalcemia and hyperphosphatemia lead to parathyroid hyperplasia and stimulate secretion of PTH, leading to high circulating PTH levels (i.e., secondary hyperparathyroidism).

Tertiary hyperparathyroidism (THPT) results from prolonged secondary stimulation, where the parathyroid glands become unresponsive to serum calcium, becoming autonomously hypersecretory. In patients with long-standing CKD, especially those who received a kidney transplant, chronic parathyroid stimulation can lead to parathyroid disease. This is associated with autonomous PTH secretion (i.e., not suppressed by rising calcium levels) due to downregulation of calcium-sensing receptor and vitamin D receptor in the parathyroid glands.

Epidemiology

SHPT is commonly linked to end-stage renal disease (ESRD), with 65–75% of these patients affected, and about 5% requiring surgery. THPT can develop following prolonged SHPT. In patients with ESRD and SHPT who undergo kidney transplants, around 5–7% develop tertiary disease.

Risk factors for SHPT and THPT relate to the underlying metabolic disturbances. Chronic renal failure, malnutrition, malabsorption, cholestatic liver disease, certain drugs, and advanced age increase SHPT risk. THPT risk is primarily the duration of SHPT.

Clinical Presentation

Patients with SHPT related to chronic renal failure often exhibit bone pain, GI dysfunction, arthritis, myopathy, tendon rupture, pruritis, and extra-skeletal calcifications. Advances in medical management can render these symptoms less pronounced. Skeletal abnormalities due to PTH-induced bone resorption are common, including osteitis fibrosa cystica and mixed osteomalacia. Cardiovascular complications like calciphylaxis, affecting large and small vessels, are significant morbidity and mortality contributors in ESRD patients.

Diagnostic Evaluation

Diagnosis of SHPT involves persistently elevated intact PTH levels despite low or normal calcium levels. THPT is characterized by:

- **Very high serum PTH levels** (2–9 times above the upper limit of normal).
- **Hypercalcemia** due to mobilization from bone.
- **Hyperphosphatemia** due to renal phosphate retention.

In ESRD patients, elevated serum phosphorus and alkaline phosphatase levels confirm the diagnosis. Radiographs may also reveal bone changes typical of SHPT.

Management

Medical Management Medical treatment focuses on preventing glandular hyperplasia by maintaining serum calcium and phosphate levels within normal limits. This includes dietary manipulation, vitamin D supplementation, and oral phosphate binders. New therapies targeting calcium-sensing receptors offer tighter PTH level control.

Indications for Surgery Surgical intervention is considered for patients with symptoms unresponsive to medical therapy, severe bone disease, calciphylaxis, or failed renal transplant. Preoperative imaging localizes parathyroid tissue and ensures that there are no ectopic parathyroid glands.

Surgical Approaches Surgical options include subtotal parathyroidectomy (more common) and total parathyroidectomy with auto-transplantation (less common). Preoperative imaging identifies ectopic glands or supernumerary glands to improve surgical outcomes.

Parathyroid Carcinoma

Epidemiology

Parathyroid carcinoma (PC) is an uncommon endocrine cancer, representing less than 1% of all instances of sporadic primary hyperparathyroidism (PHPT). Parathyroid carcinoma generally affects men and women equally, typically occurring between the ages of 45 and 59. This differs somewhat from benign hyperparathyroidism, which tends to present at an older age and shows a marked female predominance.

Clinical Presentation

Parathyroid carcinoma is biochemically functional in 96% of cases, presenting with signs of PHPT and hypercalcemia, such as bone pain, renal insufficiency, and gastrointestinal disturbances. Renal calculi occur in 30–64% of cases, and abdominal complications like peptic ulcer disease occur in 10–18% of cases. Hypercalcemic crises, with severe dehydration, renal failure, and reduced consciousness, are seen in 8–17% of cases. Radiographic features often include osteitis fibrosa cystica.

Diagnostic Evaluation

Evaluation involves biochemical and imaging investigations. Parathyroid cancer is associated with significant elevation of serum calcium and PTH and may be differentiated from benign causes of hyperparathyroidism on biochemical criteria alone. Ultrasound, sestamibi scanning, CT, or MRI can localize the tumor and exclude ectopic glands.

Management

Medical Management Fluid hydration, diuresis, bisphosphonate, etc.

Surgical Management Preoperative vocal cord function assessment and management of hypercalcemia are critical. Curative surgery involves en bloc resection of the tumor with adjacent structures to ensure complete removal. This may include thyroid lobectomy and resection of the involved recurrent laryngeal nerve, strap muscles, esophagus, or trachea with subsequent reconstruction.

Postoperative Management Monitoring serum calcium and PTH levels postsurgery is essential due to risks such as hungry bone syndrome. Lifelong surveillance is necessary to detect recurrence, as recurrent disease occurs in 40–67% of cases. External-beam radiation therapy (EBRT) may reduce recurrence risk.

Management of Recurrent Disease Recurrent disease requires imaging to localize and manage new growths. Surgical resection is the primary treatment, with EBRT or chemotherapy for inoperable cases. Bisphosphonates and cinacalcet can manage hypercalcemia.

Complications After Parathyroid Surgery

Postoperative Bleeding and Hematoma

Postoperative bleeding and hematoma, though rare, can be life-threatening, with an incidence rate reported at 0.6% [30]. Hematomas can exert pressure on the trachea, leading to venous congestion of the airway structures and resulting in potential airway obstruction. Immediate action, including wound reopening and surgical evacuation or reexploration, is necessary to relieve the airway compression. Prompt intubation should not be postponed.

Hypoparathyroidism and Hypocalcemia

Postoperative hypocalcemia can present with symptoms such as numbness around the mouth, tingling in the fingertips, Chvostek's and Trousseau's signs, and in severe cases, tetany, irregular heart rhythms, and seizures. While most cases are temporary, permanent hypocalcemia occurs in only 0.5–3.8% of cases. A common reason for postsurgical hypoparathyroidism and hypocalcemia is the accidental removal, injury, or loss of blood supply to the parathyroid glands. Additionally, hypocalcemia postsurgery may result from "hungry bone syndrome," characterized by low serum calcium as bone remineralizes due to the reduced stimulus for high bone turnover after parathyroid surgery. According to the American Association of Endocrine Surgeons Guidelines, individuals with temporary postoperative hypoparathyroidism should receive calcium and potentially calcitriol supplementation, which can be reduced as the condition improves. For those with lasting hypoparathyroidism, recombinant PTH therapy may be an option.

Persistent or Recurrent Hyperparathyroidism

Persistent or recurrent hyperparathyroidism is reported in 2–5% of individuals with sporadic primary hyperparathyroidism. Persistent hyperparathyroidism is defined as the inability to reach normal calcium levels within 6 months following parathyroidectomy, while recurrent hyperparathyroidism refers to the return of elevated calcium levels after an initial period of normal calcium, occurring more than 6 months postsurgery. Common factors contributing to persistent or recurrent hyperparathyroidism include unrecognized four-gland hyperplasia or ectopic parathyroid glands. A repeat surgery is often suggested to attain biochemical normalization.

Adrenal Disorders

Anatomy

The adrenal glands are two retroperitoneal organs located above the kidneys, each with a distinct shape and slightly different positions. The right adrenal gland is pyramid-shaped and situated at the upper pole of the right kidney. The left adrenal gland, on the other hand, has a crescent shape and lies on the upper medial part of the left kidney, with the tail of the pancreas sometimes covering its lower portion. Both glands are composed of two main regions: an outer cortex, which is involved in the production of steroid hormones, and an inner medulla, which produces catecholamines. These glands have a golden appearance due to the cholesterol content in their cortex and typically weigh between 5 and 7 grams in an adult male.

Hypercortisolism (Cushing's Syndrome)

Definition

Hypercortisolism, commonly known as Cushing's syndrome, is a condition characterized by prolonged exposure to elevated levels of cortisol. Cortisol is a glucocorticoid hormone produced by the adrenal cortex, which plays a critical role in regulating metabolism, immune response, and stress. Cushing's syndrome can result from exogenous sources (iatrogenic), such as prolonged corticosteroid therapy, or endogenous sources due to adrenocorticotropic hormone (ACTH)-dependent or ACTH-independent mechanisms [45–47].

Epidemiology

Cushing's syndrome is a relatively rare disorder with an estimated annual incidence of 1–2 cases per million people. It predominantly affects adults aged 20–50 years, with a higher prevalence in women compared to men. The endogenous form of Cushing's syndrome is often categorized into ACTH-dependent, primarily caused by Cushing's disease (pituitary adenomas), and ACTH-independent, resulting from adrenal tumors or hyperplasia.

Clinical Presentation

The clinical manifestations of Cushing's syndrome are diverse and often develop insidiously. Common signs and symptoms include:

- **Central Obesity**: Patients typically present with weight gain, particularly around the abdomen, face (moon face), and upper back (buffalo hump).
- **Skin Changes**: Thinning of the skin, easy bruising, purple striae (stretch marks), and slow wound healing are common dermatologic features.
- **Muscle Weakness**: Proximal muscle weakness and wasting are frequently observed.
- **Metabolic Disturbances**: Hyperglycemia, hypertension, and dyslipidemia are common due to cortisol's metabolic effects.
- **Neuropsychiatric Symptoms**: Patients may experience mood swings, depression, anxiety, and cognitive dysfunction.
- **Reproductive Issues**: Women may present with menstrual irregularities, hirsutism, and infertility, while men may experience decreased libido and erectile dysfunction.

Diagnostic Evaluation

The diagnostic evaluation of suspected Cushing's syndrome involves a combination of clinical assessment, biochemical testing, and imaging studies.

- **Biochemical Testing**:
  - **Initial Screening Tests**: These include the 24-h urinary free cortisol measurement, late-night salivary cor-

tisol test, and the low-dose dexamethasone suppression test. Elevated cortisol levels in these tests suggest hypercortisolism.
  - **Confirmatory Tests**: If initial tests are positive, further evaluation includes the high-dose dexamethasone suppression test and plasma ACTH levels to differentiate between ACTH-dependent and ACTH-independent causes.
- **Imaging Studies**:
  - **Pituitary Imaging**: MRI of the pituitary gland may be performed if Cushing's disease is suspected.
  - **Adrenal Imaging**: CT or MRI of the adrenal glands is indicated to identify adrenal adenomas, carcinomas, or hyperplasia.
- **Inferior Petrosal Sinus Sampling**: In cases where the source of ACTH is unclear, IPSS can help distinguish between pituitary and ectopic ACTH secretion.

Management

The management of Cushing's syndrome aims to normalize cortisol levels, alleviate symptoms, and address the underlying cause.

- **Surgical Treatment**: Surgery is the treatment of choice for most cases of Cushing's syndrome.
  - **Transsphenoidal Surgery**: *This is the preferred approach for removing ACTH-secreting pituitary adenomas.*
  - **Adrenalectomy**: Surgical removal of adrenal tumors is indicated for ACTH-independent Cushing's syndrome.
  - **Ectopic ACTH Syndrome**: Surgical resection of the ACTH-producing tumor, if identified, is necessary.
- **Medical Therapy**: In cases where surgery is not feasible or as an adjunct to surgery, medical therapy can be employed to control hypercortisolism.
  - **Steroidogenesis Inhibitors**: Drugs such as ketoconazole, metyrapone, and mitotane reduce cortisol production.
  - **Pituitary-Directed Therapies**: Medications like pasireotide and cabergoline target ACTH-secreting pituitary tumors.
  - **Glucocorticoid Receptor Antagonists**: Mifepristone can be used to counteract the effects of excess cortisol.
- **Radiation Therapy**: For patients with residual or recurrent pituitary adenomas postsurgery, radiotherapy may be considered.
- **Long-term Follow-up**: Lifelong monitoring is essential to detect recurrence, manage adrenal insufficiency, and address complications associated with prolonged hypercortisolism.

Hyperaldosteronism (Conn's Syndrome)

Definition

Hyperaldosteronism, also known as Conn's syndrome, is a condition characterized by excessive production of aldosterone by the adrenal glands. Aldosterone is a mineralocorticoid hormone that plays a critical role in regulating sodium and potassium balance, as well as blood pressure. The overproduction of aldosterone leads to hypertension and hypokalemia [48–50].

Epidemiology

Hyperaldosteronism is considered one of the most common causes of secondary hypertension, accounting for approximately 5–10% of hypertensive patients. It is more frequently diagnosed in individuals with resistant hypertension and those with a family history of early-onset hypertension or cerebrovascular accidents. The prevalence of primary aldosteronism increases with age and is slightly higher in women compared to men.

Clinical Presentation

The clinical presentation of hyperaldosteronism varies depending on the severity and duration of the condition. Common signs and symptoms include:

- **Hypertension**: Persistent high blood pressure that is often resistant to standard antihypertensive therapy is a hallmark of hyperaldosteronism.
- **Hypokalemia**: Low potassium levels can lead to muscle weakness, cramps, fatigue, and in severe cases, cardiac arrhythmias.
- **Metabolic Alkalosis**: Excess aldosterone can cause an increase in bicarbonate levels, leading to metabolic alkalosis.
- **Polydipsia and Polyuria**: Patients may experience increased thirst and frequent urination due to the renal effects of hypokalemia.

Diagnostic Evaluation

The diagnostic evaluation of hyperaldosteronism involves a combination of biochemical testing and imaging studies.

- **Biochemical Testing**:
  - **Screening Tests**: The plasma aldosterone concentration to plasma renin activity ratio is the initial screening test for hyperaldosteronism. An elevated

aldosterone-to-renin ratio (ARR) suggests primary aldosteronism.
  - **Confirmatory Tests**: If the ARR is elevated, confirmatory tests such as the saline infusion test, oral sodium loading test, or captopril challenge test are performed to confirm the diagnosis.
- **Imaging Studies**:
  - **Adrenal CT or MRI**: Imaging studies are used to identify the presence of an adrenal adenoma or hyperplasia. Adrenal CT is the preferred imaging modality to differentiate between unilateral and bilateral adrenal disease.
  - **Adrenal Venous Sampling (AVS)**: AVS is the gold standard for distinguishing between unilateral and bilateral hyperaldosteronism, particularly in patients being considered for surgical treatment.

Differential Diagnosis

The differential diagnosis of hyperaldosteronism includes other conditions that can cause hypertension and hypokalemia:

- **Essential Hypertension**: Primary hypertension without a secondary cause.
- **Renal Artery Stenosis**: Narrowing of the renal arteries leading to secondary hyperaldosteronism.
- **Cushing's Syndrome**: Excess cortisol production can mimic features of hyperaldosteronism.
- **Liddle Syndrome**: A rare genetic disorder causing hypertension and hypokalemia due to increased sodium reabsorption in the kidneys.

Management

The management of hyperaldosteronism aims to normalize aldosterone levels, control blood pressure, and correct hypokalemia. Treatment options include medical therapy and surgical intervention.

- **Medical Therapy**:
  - **Mineralocorticoid Receptor Antagonists**: Spironolactone and eplerenone are the mainstay of medical treatment for hyperaldosteronism. These drugs block the effects of aldosterone, helping to control blood pressure and correct hypokalemia.
  - **Antihypertensive Medications**: Additional antihypertensive agents may be required to achieve optimal blood pressure control.
- **Surgical Treatment**:
  - **Adrenalectomy**: Surgical removal of the affected adrenal gland is indicated for patients with unilateral aldosterone-producing adenomas. Laparoscopic adrenalectomy is the preferred approach due to its minimally invasive nature and faster recovery times.
  - **Postoperative Management**: Patients require close monitoring of electrolytes and blood pressure following adrenalectomy. Some patients may develop transient or permanent adrenal insufficiency, necessitating corticosteroid replacement therapy.
- **Lifestyle Modifications**: Dietary modifications, including sodium restriction and potassium supplementation, may be beneficial in managing hyperaldosteronism.

Pheochromocytoma and Paraganglioma

Definition

Pheochromocytomas and paragangliomas are rare neuroendocrine tumors originating from chromaffin cells. Pheochromocytomas arise from the adrenal medulla, while paragangliomas can develop in various locations outside the adrenal glands along the sympathetic and parasympathetic chains. These tumors often secrete catecholamines, leading to significant clinical symptoms and complications [51–53].

Epidemiology

The incidence of pheochromocytomas and paragangliomas is estimated at 2–8 cases per million people annually. These tumors can occur at any age but are most commonly diagnosed in adults between 30 and 50 years. There is no significant gender predilection. Approximately 30–40% of cases are hereditary, associated with genetic syndromes such as Multiple Endocrine Neoplasia type 2 (MEN2), von Hippel-Lindau (VHL) disease, and neurofibromatosis type 1 (NF1).

Clinical Presentation

The clinical presentation of pheochromocytomas and paragangliomas is highly variable and depends on the tumor's location and catecholamine secretion levels. Common symptoms include:

- **Hypertension**: Often paroxysmal, leading to episodic severe headaches, sweating, palpitations, and anxiety.

- **Cardiovascular Symptoms**: Tachycardia, arrhythmias, and orthostatic hypotension are common due to excessive catecholamine release.
- **Metabolic Effects**: Hyperglycemia and weight loss may occur.
- **Other Symptoms**: Abdominal pain, nausea, and constipation can be present, especially with larger tumors or those located in the abdomen.

Diagnosis

The diagnosis of pheochromocytomas and paragangliomas involves biochemical testing and imaging studies.

- **Biochemical Testing**:
  - **Plasma-Free Metanephrines and Normetanephrines**: These are sensitive markers for detecting catecholamine-secreting tumors.
  - **24-h Urinary Catecholamines and Metanephrines**: Used to confirm excessive catecholamine production.
- **Imaging Studies**:
  - **Computed Tomography (CT) and Magnetic Resonance Imaging (MRI)**: These imaging modalities are used to localize the tumor. CT is often the first-line imaging study, while MRI is useful for detecting extra-adrenal and metastatic lesions.
  - **Iodine-metaiodobenzylguanidine (MIBG) Scintigraphy and PET Scans**: These nuclear medicine studies can help identify metastatic disease and determine the extent of the tumor.

Management

The management of pheochromocytomas and paragangliomas involves preoperative medical preparation, surgical resection, and long-term follow-up.

- **Preoperative Medical Preparation**:
  - **Alpha-adrenergic Blockade**: Phenoxybenzamine or selective alpha-blockers are used to control hypertension and prevent intraoperative hypertensive crises.
  - **Beta-blockers**: Added after adequate alpha-blockade to control tachycardia and arrhythmias.
- **Surgical Resection**:
  - **Adrenalectomy**: Laparoscopic adrenalectomy is the preferred approach for pheochromocytomas. Open surgery may be required for large or invasive tumors.
  - **Paraganglioma Resection**: The surgical approach depends on the tumor's location and size.
- **Medical Therapy for Inoperable or Metastatic Disease**:
  - **Metyrosine**: Used to reduce catecholamine synthesis.
  - **Chemotherapy and Radiotherapy**: Considered for metastatic or unresectable tumors.

Prognosis and Surveillance

The prognosis for patients with pheochromocytomas and paragangliomas depends on the completeness of tumor resection and the presence of metastases. Early detection and surgical intervention can lead to favorable outcomes.

- **Surveillance**: Lifelong follow-up is necessary due to the risk of recurrence or metastasis. Regular biochemical testing and imaging studies are recommended to monitor for disease recurrence.
- **Genetic Counseling and Testing**: Recommended for patients with hereditary forms of the disease to identify at-risk family members and guide long-term surveillance strategies.

Adrenocortical Carcinoma

Definition and Epidemiology

Adrenocortical carcinoma (ACC) is a rare and aggressive malignancy originating from the adrenal cortex. It accounts for about 0.02–0.2% of all cancers and has an annual incidence of 1–2 cases per million people. ACC can occur at any age but has a bimodal age distribution, with peaks in early childhood and middle adulthood. There is a slight female predominance [54–59].

Clinical Presentation

The clinical presentation of ACC varies and can be due to hormone excess or the mass effect of the tumor.

- **Hormonal Excess**: Approximately 60% of ACCs are hormonally active, producing excess cortisol, androgens, estrogens, or aldosterone. Symptoms include Cushing's syndrome (weight gain, hypertension, diabetes, and osteoporosis), virilization in women (hirsutism, acne, deepening voice), feminization in men (gynecomastia, impotence), and hyperaldosteronism (hypertension, hypokalemia).
- **Mass Effect**: Large tumors can cause abdominal pain, fullness, and palpable masses. Symptoms related to metastases may also be present, such as bone pain or neurological deficits.

Diagnostic Evaluation

Imaging

- **Computed Tomography (CT) and Magnetic Resonance Imaging (MRI)**: These are the primary imaging modalities used to evaluate ACC. CT scans provide detailed information about the tumor's size, shape, and involvement of surrounding structures. MRI is useful for assessing vascular invasion and distinguishing ACC from benign adrenal lesions.

Size

1. Tumors larger than 4 cm are more likely to be malignant. Size, along with imaging characteristics such as irregular borders, heterogeneity, and local invasion, helps in differentiating ACC from benign adenomas.

Histopathology

- Histopathological examination is essential for the definitive diagnosis of ACC. The Weiss criteria, which include features such as high mitotic rate, atypical mitoses, and necrosis, are used to differentiate ACC from benign adrenal tumors. Immunohistochemical staining for markers like Ki-67, inhibin, and Melan-A can also aid in diagnosis.

Staging and Prognosis

Staging of ACC is based on the Tumor, Node, Metastasis (TNM) system (see Table 49.4), which considers the size of the tumor, involvement of lymph nodes, and presence of distant metastases. The prognosis for ACC is generally poor, with a 5-year survival rate of approximately 35–55%. Factors affecting prognosis include tumor stage, completeness of surgical resection, and hormonal activity.

Table 49.4 TNM Classification of Adrenocortical Carcinoma

Tumor	
Tx	Cannot be assessed
T0	No primary tumor present
T1	Tumor 5 cm or less, localized within adrenal gland
T2	Tumor greater than 5 cm, localized within adrenal gland
T3	Tumor of any size with invasion but not involving adjacent organs
T4	Tumor of any size with invasion into kidney, diaphragm, great vessels, pancreas, and spleen
Lymph node	
Nx	Local lymph nodes cannot be assessed
N0	No local lymph node involvement
N1	Local lymph nodes are involved
Metastasis	
M0	No distant metastasis
M1	Confirmed distant metastasis

Treatment

Perioperative Management

Preoperative management includes optimizing hormonal imbalances, particularly in patients with Cushing's syndrome, to reduce perioperative complications. This may involve the use of medications like ketoconazole or metyrapone.

Surgery

Surgical resection is the mainstay of treatment for localized ACC. Complete en bloc resection with negative margins (R0 resection) offers the best chance for cure. Laparoscopic adrenalectomy is generally not recommended due to the risk of tumor spillage and incomplete resection.

Postoperative Management

Adjuvant therapies are often considered for high-risk patients or those with incomplete resections. These may include mitotane, a chemotherapeutic agent specific for adrenocortical tissue, as well as conventional chemotherapy and radiation therapy. Mitotane therapy requires close monitoring of drug levels and management of side effects, including adrenal insufficiency.

Surveillance and Follow-Up

Lifelong surveillance is necessary for patients with ACC due to the high risk of recurrence. Follow-up protocols typically include periodic clinical evaluations, hormonal assessments, and imaging studies (CT or MRI) every 3–6 months for the first 2 years, then annually. Surveillance aims to detect recurrences early when they are potentially resectable.

Familial Endocrine Syndrome

Multiple Endocrine Neoplasia Type 1 (MEN 1)

Definition and Epidemiology

Multiple Endocrine Neoplasia Type 1 (MEN 1) is an inherited disorder characterized by the development of tumors in multiple endocrine glands. MEN 1 is caused by mutations in the MEN1 gene, which encodes the protein menin. The condition follows an autosomal dominant inheritance pattern, meaning a single copy of the mutated gene can cause the disorder. MEN1 is estimated to occur in approximately 1 in 30,000 individuals, with no specific association with race or geographic region. However, incomplete recognition of the syndrome can result in underreporting and an underestimation of its true prevalence [60–62].

Clinical Presentation

Patients with MEN 1 commonly present with tumors in the parathyroid glands, pancreatic islet cells, and the anterior pituitary. The primary clinical manifestations include:

- **Hyperparathyroidism**: Caused by parathyroid adenomas, leading to hypercalcemia, kidney stones, and osteoporosis.
- **Pancreatic Neuroendocrine Tumors (NETs)**: These can secrete various hormones, leading to conditions such as gastrinoma (Zollinger-Ellison syndrome), insulinoma, and glucagonoma.
- **Pituitary Adenomas**: These can produce excess prolactin, growth hormone, or ACTH, resulting in conditions like prolactinoma, acromegaly, or Cushing's disease.

Diagnostic Evaluation

Diagnosis of MEN 1 involves genetic testing for MEN1 gene mutations, along with clinical and biochemical assessments to identify the presence of endocrine tumors. Imaging studies such as MRI, CT scans, and functional imaging are also utilized to localize and characterize the tumors.

Management

Management of MEN 1 focuses on addressing the specific endocrine tumors and associated hormonal imbalances. Surgical resection is often required for symptomatic or growing tumors. Medical therapies may include hormone suppression or replacement, depending on the type of tumor and its hormonal activity. Regular surveillance and monitoring are essential for early detection and management of new or recurrent tumors.

Multiple Endocrine Neoplasia Type 2 (MEN 2)

Definition and Epidemiology

Multiple Endocrine Neoplasia Type 2 (MEN 2) is an inherited disorder associated with mutations in the RET proto-oncogene. Like MEN 1, MEN 2 follows an autosomal dominant inheritance pattern. MEN 2 is divided into three subtypes: MEN 2A, MEN 2B, and Familial Medullary Thyroid Carcinoma (FMTC).

Clinical Presentation

MEN 2 is primarily characterized by:

- **Medullary Thyroid Carcinoma (MTC)**: A common feature in all subtypes, often presenting as an early sign of the disease.
- **Pheochromocytoma**: Tumors of the adrenal medulla, causing episodic hypertension, palpitations, and headaches.
- **Hyperparathyroidism**: Primarily seen in MEN 2A, leading to hypercalcemia and its associated complications.

Diagnostic Evaluation

Diagnosis of MEN 2 involves genetic testing for RET mutations. Biochemical testing for elevated calcitonin levels (indicative of MTC) and catecholamines/metanephrines (for pheochromocytoma) is critical. Imaging studies, including neck ultrasound, MRI, and CT, are used to evaluate tumor extent and involvement.

Management

Management strategies for MEN 2 include:

- **Prophylactic Thyroidectomy**: Recommended for individuals with identified RET mutations to prevent the development of MTC.
- **Surgical Resection**: Removal of pheochromocytomas and parathyroid adenomas is necessary to manage symptoms and prevent complications.
- **Medical Therapy**: Includes hormone replacement or suppression therapies, as needed.

Surveillance and Follow-Up

Regular and lifelong surveillance is essential for individuals with MEN 1 and MEN 2 to monitor for new tumor development and manage existing conditions. This includes periodic biochemical testing, imaging studies, and clinical evaluations.

References

1. Khan YS, Farhana A. Histology, thyroid gland. [Updated 2022 Dec 5]. In: StatPearls [Internet]. Treasure Island (FL): StatPearls Publishing; 2024.
2. Morita SY, Dackiw APB, Zeiger MA, et al. McGraw-Hill manual of endocrine surgery. 1st ed. McGraw-Hill; 2010.
3. Benoist BD, Andersson M, Egli I, et al. *Iodine status worldwide*. Geneva: World Health Organization; 2004.
4. Knudsen N, Laurberg P, Perrild H, et al. Risk factors for goiter and thyroid nodules. Thyroid. 2002;12(10):879–88.
5. Knobel M. Etiopathology, clinical features, and treatment of diffuse and multinodular nontoxic goiters. J Endocrinol Investig. 2016;39(4):357–73. https://doi.org/10.1007/s40618-015-0391-7. Epub 2015 Sep 21
6. Aghini-Lombardi F, Antonangeli L, Martino E, et al. The spectrum of thyroid disorders in an iodine-deficient community: the Pescopagano survey. J Clin Endocrinol Metab. 1999;84(2):561–6.

7. Bonnema SJ, Bennedbaek FN, Ladenson PW, Hegedus L. Management of the nontoxic multinodular goiter: a North American survey. J Clin Endocrinol Metab. 2002;87(1):112–7.
8. Hollowell JG, Staehling NW, Flanders WD, et al. Serum TSH, T(4), and thyroid antibodies in the United States population (1988 to 1994): National Health and nutrition examination survey (NHANES III). J Clin Endocrinol Metab. 2002;87(2):489–99.
9. Laurberg P, Bulow Pedersen I, Knudsen N, et al. Environmental iodine intake affects the type of nonmalignant thyroid disease. Thyroid. 2001;11(5):457–69.
10. Vanderpump MP. The epidemiology of thyroid disease. Br Med Bull. 2011;99:39–51.
11. Sheu SY, Schmid KW. Entzündliche Schilddrüs- enerkrankungen. Pathologe. 2003;24:339–47.
12. Khan A, Nosé V. Pathology of the thyroid gland. In: Lloyd RV, editor. Endocrine pathology. Totowa: Humana; 2004. p. 153–89.
13. Tunbridge WM, Evered DC, Hall R, et al. The spectrum of thyroid diseases in a community: the Whickham survey. Clin Endocrinol. 1977;7:481–93.
14. Weetman AP. Determinants of autoimmune thyroid disease. Nat Immunol. 2001;2:769–70.
15. Hegedu L. Clinical practice. The thyroid nodule. N Engl J Med. 2004;351(17):1764–71.
16. Tessler FN, Middleton WD, Grant EG, Hoang JK, Berland LL, Teefey SA, Cronan JJ, Beland MD, Desser TS, Frates MC, Hammers LW, Hamper UM, Langer JE, Reading CC, Scoutt LM, Stavros AT. ACR thyroid imaging, reporting and data system (TI-RADS): white paper of the ACR TI-RADS Committee. J Am Coll Radiol. 2017;14(5):587–95. https://doi.org/10.1016/j.jacr.2017.01.046. Epub 2017 Apr 2
17. Cibas ES, Ali SZ. The 2017 Bethesda system for reporting thyroid cytopathology. Thyroid. 2017;27(11):1341–6. https://doi.org/10.1089/thy.2017.0500.
18. Thompson NW, Nishiyama RH, Harness JK. Thyroid carcinoma: current controversies. Curr Probl Surg. 1978;15(11):1–67. https://doi.org/10.1016/s0011-3840(78)80004-5.
19. Hundahl SA, Fleming ID, Fremgen AM, Menck HR. A National Cancer Data Base report on 53,856 cases of thyroid carcinoma treated in the U.S., 1985–1995 [see comments]. Cancer. 1998;83(12):2638–48.
20. Christou N, Mathonnet M. Complications after total thyroidectomy. J Visc Surg. 2013;150(4):249–56. https://doi.org/10.1016/j.jviscsurg.2013.04.003. Epub 2013 Jun 6
21. Schaefer AW, Solorzano PJ, Mavarez AC, Muñoz-Monaco GM. Diagnosis and management of intraoperative thyroid storm in a child with undiagnosed Graves' disease: a case report. JA Clin Rep. 2022;8(1):52. https://doi.org/10.1186/s40981-022-00543-2.
22. Bland KI, Sarr MG, Büchler MW, Csendes A, Garden OJ, Wong J. Endocrine surgery: handbooks in general surgery. Springer; 2011.
23. Clark OH, Duh QY, Kebebew E, Gosnell JE, Shen WT. Textbook of endocrine surgery. 3rd ed. Jaypee Brothers Medical Pub; 2016.
24. Haugen BR, Alexander EK, Bible KC, Doherty GM, Mandel SJ, Nikiforov YE, et al. 2015 American Thyroid Association management guidelines for adult patients with thyroid nodules and differentiated thyroid cancer: the American Thyroid Association guidelines task force on thyroid nodules and differentiated thyroid cancer. Thyroid. 2016;26(1):1–133. https://doi.org/10.1089/thy.2015.0020.
25. Jonklaas J, Bianco AC, Bauer AJ, Burman KD, Cappola AR, Celi FS, American Thyroid Association Task Force on Thyroid Hormone Replacement, et al. Guidelines for the treatment of hypothyroidism: prepared by the American Thyroid Association task force on thyroid hormone replacement. Thyroid. 2014;24(12):1670–751. https://doi.org/10.1089/thy.2014.0028.
26. Lennard TWJ. Endocrine surgery: a companion to specialist surgical practice. 3rd ed. Saunders Ltd; 2006.
27. Oertli D, Udelsman R. Surgery of the thyroid and parathyroid glands. 1st ed. Springer Verlag; 2007.
28. Ross DS, Burch HB, Cooper DS, Greenlee MC, Laurberg P, Maia AL, et al. 2016 American Thyroid Association guidelines for diagnosis and management of hyperthyroidism and other causes of thyrotoxicosis. Thyroid. 2016;26(10):1343–421. https://doi.org/10.1089/thy.2016.0229.
29. Wermers RA, Khosla S, Atkinson EJ, et al. Incidence of primary hyperparathyroidism in Rochester, Minnesota, 1993–2001: an update on the changing epidemiology of the disease. J Bone Miner Res. 2006;21:171.
30. Belezikian JP, Potts JP. Asymptomatic primary hyperparathyroidism: new issues and questions. J Bone Miner Res. 2002;17(suppl 2):N57–67.
31. Taterra D, Wong LM, Vikse J, Sanna B, Pękala P, Walocha J, et al. The prevalence and anatomy of parathyroid glands: a meta-analysis with implications for parathyroid surgery. Langenbeck's Arch Surg. 2019;404(1):63–70. https://doi.org/10.1007/s00423-019-01751-8.
32. Palumbo VD, Palumbo VD, Damiano G, Messina M, Fazzotta S, Lo Monte G, et al. Tertiary hyperparathyroidism: a review. Clin Ter. 2021;172(3):241–6. https://doi.org/10.7417/CT.2021.2322.
33. Cetani F, Pardi E, Marcocci C. Parathyroid carcinoma. Front Horm Res. 2019;51:63–76. https://doi.org/10.1159/000491039. Epub 2018 Nov 19
34. Goswamy J, Lei M, Simo R. Parathyroid carcinoma. Curr Opin Otolaryngol Head Neck Surg. 2016;24(2):155–62. https://doi.org/10.1097/MOO.0000000000000234.
35. Lee PK, Jarosek SL, Virnig BA, Evasovich M, Tuttle TM. Trends in the incidence and treatment of parathyroid cancer in the United States. Cancer. 2007;109(9):1736–41. https://doi.org/10.1002/cncr.22599.
36. Wynne AG, van Heerden J, Carney JA, Fitzpatrick LA. Parathyroid carcinoma: clinical and pathologic features in 43 patients. Medicine (Baltimore). 1992;71(4):197–205.
37. Iihara M, Okamoto T, Suzuki R, et al. Functional parathyroid carcinoma: long-term treatment outcome and risk factor analysis. Surgery. 2007;142(6):936–43; discussion 943 e931.
38. Munson ND, Foote RL, Northcutt RC, et al. Parathyroid carcinoma: is there a role for adjuvant radiation therapy? Cancer. 2003;98(11):2378–84.
39. Busaidy NL, Jimenez C, Habra MA, et al. Parathyroid carcinoma: a 22-year experience. Head Neck. 2004;26(8):716–26.
40. Wang Y, Ladie DE. Parathyroidectomy. [Updated 2024 Sep 10]. In: StatPearls [Internet]. Treasure Island (FL): StatPearls Publishing; 2024.
41. Rosenbaum MA, Haridas M, McHenry CR. Life-threatening neck hematoma complicating thyroid and parathyroid surgery. Am J Surg. 2008;195(3):339–43; discussion 343.
42. Steen S, Rabeler B, Fisher T, Arnold D. Predictive factors for early postoperative hypocalcemia after surgery for primary hyperparathyroidism. Proc (Bayl Univ Med Cent). 2009;22(2):124–7.
43. Witteveen JE, van Thiel S, Romijn JA, Hamdy NA. Hungry bone syndrome: still a challenge in the post-operative management of primary hyperparathyroidism: a systematic review of the literature. Eur J Endocrinol. 2013;168(3):R45–53.
44. Wilhelm SM, Wang TS, Ruan DT, Lee JA, Asa SL, Duh QY, Doherty GM, Herrera MF, Pasieka JL, Perrier ND, Silverberg SJ, Solórzano CC, Sturgeon C, Tublin ME, Udelsman R, Carty SE. The American Association of Endocrine Surgeons Guidelines for definitive Management of Primary Hyperparathyroidism. JAMA Surg. 2016;151(10):959–68.
45. Mazotas IG, Yen TWF, Doffek K, Shaker JL, Carr AA, Evans DB, Wang TS. Persistent/recurrent primary hyperparathyroidism: does the number of abnormal glands play a role? J Surg Res. 2020;246:335–41.

46. Porterfield JR, Thompson GB, Young WF, et al. Surgery for Cushing's syndrome: a historical review and recent ten-year experience. World J Surg. 2008;32(5):659–77.
47. Stewart PM. The adrenal cortex. In: Larsen PR, Knonenberg HM, Melmed S, Polansky KS, editors. Williams textbook of endocrinology. 10th ed. Philadelphia: Saunders; 2003. p. 491–548.
48. Funder JW, Carey RM, Mantero F, Murad MH, Reincke M, Shibata H, et al. The management of primary aldosteronism: case detection, diagnosis, and treatment: an Endocrine Society clinical practice guideline. J Clin Endocrinol Metab. 2016;101:1889–916.
49. Yang J, Fuller PJ, Stowasser M. Is it time to screen all patients with hypertension for primary aldosteronism? Med J Aust. 2018;209:57–9.
50. Yoon M, Hong N, Ha J, Lee CJ, Ku CR, Rhee Y, et al. Prevalence and clinical characteristics of primary aldosteronism in a tertiary-care center in Korea. Hypertens Res. 2022;45:1418–29.
51. Kiernan CM, Solórzano CC. Pheochromocytoma and Paraganglioma: diagnosis, genetics, and treatment. Surg Oncol Clin N Am. 2016;25:119–38. https://doi.org/10.1016/j.soc.2015.08.006.
52. Chen H, Sippel RS, O'Dorisio MS, Vinik AI, Lloyd RV, Pacak K. North American neuroendocrine tumor society (NANETS) the north American neuroendocrine tumor society consensus guideline for the diagnosis and management of neuroendocrine tumors: pheochromocytoma, paraganglioma, and medullary thyroid cancer. Pancreas. 2010;39:775–83. https://doi.org/10.1097/MPA.0b013e3181ebb4f0.
53. Favier J, Amar L, Gimenez-Roqueplo AP. Paraganglioma and phaeochromocytoma:from genetics to personalized medicine. Nat Rev Endocrinol. 2015;11:101–11. https://doi.org/10.1038/nrendo.2014.188.
54. Allolio B, Fassnacht M. Clinical review: adrenocortical carcinoma: clinical update. J Clin Endocrinol Metab. 2006;91:2027–37.
55. Wajchenberg BL, Albergaria Pereira MA, et al. Adrenocortical carcinoma: clinical and laboratory observations. Cancer. 2000;88:711–36.
56. Schteingart DE, Doherty GM, Gauger PG, et al. Management of patients with adrenal cancer: recommendations of an international consensus conference. Endocr Relat Cancer. 2005;12:667–80.
57. Else T, Kim AC, Sabolch A, Raymond VM, Kandathil A, Caoili EM, Jolly S, Miller BS, Giordano TJ, Hammer GD. Adrenocortical carcinoma. Endocr Rev. 2014;35(2):282–326. https://doi.org/10.1210/er.2013-1029. Epub 2013 Dec 20. PMID: 24423978; PMCID: PMC3963263.
58. Crucitti F, Bellantone R, Ferrante A, et al. The Italian registry for adrenal cortical carcinoma: analysis of a multiinstitutional series of 129 patients. The ACC Italian Registry Study Group. Surgery. 1996;119(2):161–70.
59. Icard P, Goudet P, Charpenay C, et al. Adrenocortical carcinomas: surgical trends and results of a 253-patient series from the French Association of Endocrine Surgeons study group. World J Surg. 2001;25(7):891–7.
60. Phay JE, Moley JF, Lairmore TC. Multiple endocrine neoplasias. Semin Surg Oncol. 2000;18:324–32.
61. Glascock J, Carty S. Multiple endocrine neoplasia type 1: fresh perspective on clinical features and penetrance. Surg Oncol. 2002;11:143–50.
62. White ML, Doherty GM. Multiple endocrine neoplasia. Surg Oncol Clin North Am. 2008;17(2):439–59.

Facial Aesthetics and Cosmetic Procedures

50

Melina Norberto

Introduction

Cosmetic injectables encompass a wide range of treatments aimed at enhancing the appearance of the face by addressing concerns such as wrinkles, volume loss, sagging, and asymmetry. This chapter will provide you with the scenarios frequently encountered in the field of facial aesthetics. A substantial number of patients are nowadays treated with *botulinum toxin* and *hyaluronic acid fillers* (or their various analogs). The following is a basic summary of the most common facial injectables used.

Cosmetic Injection Therapy: Getting Started

Several things need to be considered when performing cosmetic injection-based procedures. It is important for medical professionals to have a thorough understanding of the different layers of facial anatomy, the action of each muscle group, and the associated antagonist muscle group. It is also important to be knowledgeable about the pharmacologic properties and potential side effects of the products being injected. Proper training and certification of the medical professional, as well as patient selection and posttreatment care, are essential to ensure safe and effective treatment outcomes for patients. Additionally, medical professionals should carefully assess each patient's individual concerns and goals to develop a customized treatment plan that addresses their specific needs, while at the same time setting realistic expectations.

Neurotoxin Injection

Botulinum toxin is a neurotoxin produced by *Clostridium botulinum.* It blocks nerve signals to muscles, causing muscle paralysis. Today, it is one of the most common facial aesthetic injectables used worldwide. **Botulinum Toxin Type A (BTX-A)** is considered a **neuromodulator** and includes a variety of formulations, such as **onabotulinumtoxinA** *(Botox®),* ***abotulinumtoxinA*** *(Dysport®),* **incobotulinum-toxinA** *(Xeomin®), and* ***prabotulinumtoxinA*** *Jeauveau®.* BTX-A *is primarily used for cosmetic, while botulinum toxin type B (**rimabotulinumtoxinB,** Myobloc®) is mainly used for medical conditions like* **cervical dystonia.** BTX-A injections are used to temporarily relax muscles that cause *dynamic wrinkles* (wrinkles created by contracting facial muscles), such as the horizontal forehead lines formed by raising the eyebrows, the vertical lines between the eyebrows created by furrowing the brows, and the lines that radiate outward from the eyes from squinting or smiling (crow's feet). Static wrinkles are lines that are constant and do not change due to muscle contractions (such as nasolabial folds and marionette lines, which will be addressed next under *hyaluronic acid fillers*).

Botulinum toxin inhibits muscle contraction by **blocking acetylcholine release from nerve terminals**. It is important to know that botulinum toxin is *not* safe to administer to *all* patients. **For example,** it is contraindicated in patients with **myasthenia gravis**, as botulinum toxin Type A can worsen symptoms and even activate latent disease. It is important to take a medical history on all patients prior to administering this neurotoxin.

By preventing muscle contractions, botulinum toxin can help smooth out and soften existing dynamic wrinkles and prevent the formation of new ones as long as treatments are done regularly (usually every 3–4 months). The various facial muscle groups and targets for cosmetic neurotoxin injection are shown in Fig. 50.1. Botulinum toxin is not only used for cosmetic purposes, but can also be used therapeutically to temporarily treat conditions caused by strong or hypertrophic muscles, such as the masseter muscles in a patient with **temporomandibular joint pain (TMJ)** and **bruxism**. In addition, it can be used to treat frequent headaches caused by excessive strength and tension in the trape-

M. Norberto (✉)
Lakeland, FL, USA

S. Atallah, J. Dragoljevic (eds.), *Fundamentals of Surgery for Physician Assistants*,
https://doi.org/10.1007/978-3-032-21069-2_50

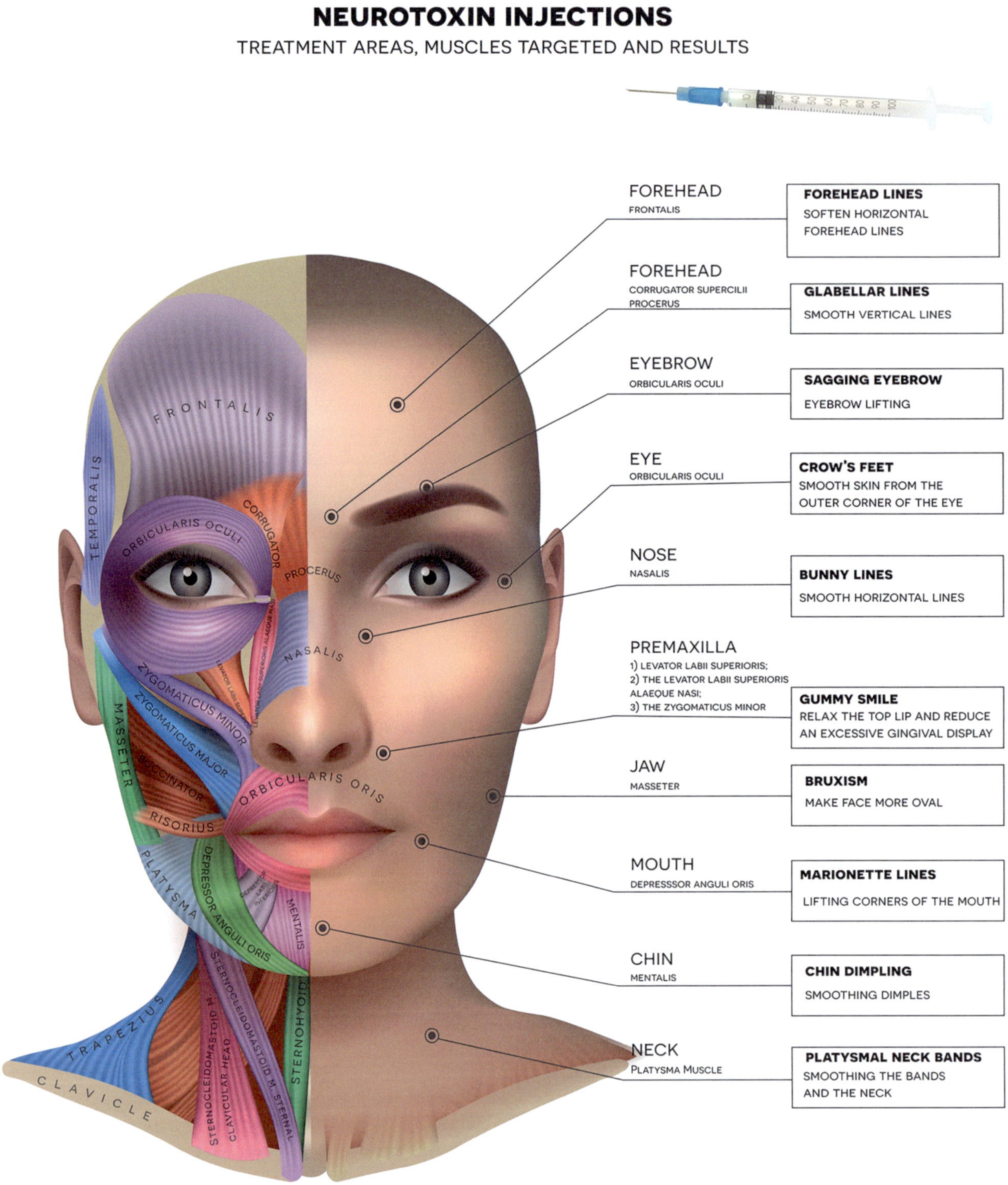

Fig. 50.1 Target muscle groups for cosmetic neurotoxin injection are illustrated

Table 50.1 Different applications of neurotoxins in clinical medicine

Neurotoxin	Medical application	Condition treated	Expected outcome
Botulinum Toxin Type A	**Cosmetic and Medical Uses**	Wrinkle reduction (e.g., forehead lines, crow's feet, frown lines)	Smoother skin, reduction in fine lines and wrinkles
Botulinum Toxin Type A	**Chronic Migraine**	Chronic migraine (headaches occurring 15+ days/month)	Reduction in headache frequency and severity
Botulinum Toxin Type A	**Hyperhidrosis**	Excessive sweating (underarms, hands, feet, face)	Reduction in sweat production
Botulinum Toxin Type A	**Cervical Dystonia**	Abnormal neck muscle contractions, causing pain or stiffness	Reduction in muscle spasms and neck pain
Botulinum Toxin Type A	**Strabismus**	Misalignment of the eyes (crossed eyes or lazy eye)	Improvement in eye alignment
Botulinum Toxin Type A	**Blepharospasm**	Involuntary eyelid twitching	Relief from eye twitching and eyelid spasms
Botulinum Toxin Type A	**Overactive Bladder**	Frequent and urgent need to urinate, incontinence	Improved bladder control and reduced urinary urgency
Botulinum Toxin Type A	**TMJ Disorders (Temporomandibular Joint)**	Jaw muscle tension, teeth grinding, jaw pain	Reduction in jaw pain and teeth grinding
Botulinum Toxin Type B	**Cervical Dystonia**	Abnormal neck muscle contractions, causing pain or stiffness	Similar to Type A toxins, but may be used for patients who do not respond to Type A
Botulinum Toxin Type B	**Chronic Migraine**	Chronic migraines (alternative to Type A if ineffective)	Similar outcomes as Type A

zius muscles, as well as **hyperhidrosis** (excessive sweating). Table 50.1 summarizes some of the common medical applications of botulinum toxin types A and B.

Technical Tips and Patient Considerations for Neurotoxin Injection

A quick explanation of facial anatomy to patients who have not previously undergone cosmetic injections can provide them with important background. They may initially express concern over just one area of their face to be treated with botulinum toxin, for example, horizontal forehead lines. It is important to explain that those specific lines on the *frontalis muscle* (which is an elevator muscle) cannot be treated without also treating the **antagonizing depressor muscle group,** the *glabellar complex* (mainly the procerus muscle and corrugator muscles, which form a V-shaped muscle bulge and vertical lines between the eyebrows when contracted) (Fig. 50.2). This is one of the most common scenarios a cosmetic injector faces daily and a prime example of the importance of knowing the action of muscles along with their antagonizing muscle group.

The action of the frontalis muscle is to elevate the eyebrows, which creates the horizontal forehead lines when contracted. Therefore, if botulinum toxin was to be injected *only* into the frontalis muscle, the weakened or paralyzed muscle will no longer elevate the eyebrows, and the result will be *flattening and lowering of the eyebrows*. This is why it is important to also inject the frontalis' antagonizing depressor muscle group, the *glabellar complex* (focusing on the procerus and corrugator muscles) (Figs. 50.3 and 50.4). The contraction of the corrugator muscles lowers the eyebrows inferiorly and medially, creating the vertical glabellar lines often called "the 11's," while contraction of the procerus muscle moves inferiorly and creates the horizontal line where the nose meets the forehead. Consequently, when botulinum toxin is injected into the glabellar complex, it raises the eyebrows and beautifully balances out the frontalis muscle injections, which can be done with a gentle tapping maneuver for patient comfort (Figs. 50.5 and 50.6).

If botulinum toxin was to be injected only into the glabellar complex without targeting the frontalis muscle, the eyebrows will elevate to the point at which the brow arch becomes exaggeratedly pointed laterally and angular when the forehead is raised, which is sometimes referred to as "Spock brow" or "Spocking." Therefore, the frontalis also needs to be injected in order to prevent "Spocking." *Injecting the* ***muscle agonist and antagonist together*** *is key to achieving good results and leaving your patients happy.*

Therapeutic uses for botulinum toxin (Table 50.1) include injections to temporarily relieve hyperhidrosis, as well as masseter muscle and trapezius muscle injections. Superficial injections into the dermis can temporarily paralyze the targeted sweat glands and reduce excessive sweating in patients with symptomatic hyperhidrosis. ***Masseter muscle*** *injections* help reduce (a) **bruxism** (which is the involuntary and habitual teeth grinding, *esp.* during sleep) and (b) **temporomandibular joint (TMJ) pain.**

Strong masseter muscles contribute to bulk in the lower face and can cause the face to look square-shaped. As those muscles weaken and atrophy posttreatment, the associated cosmetic result is slimming of the lower face (Fig. 50.7).

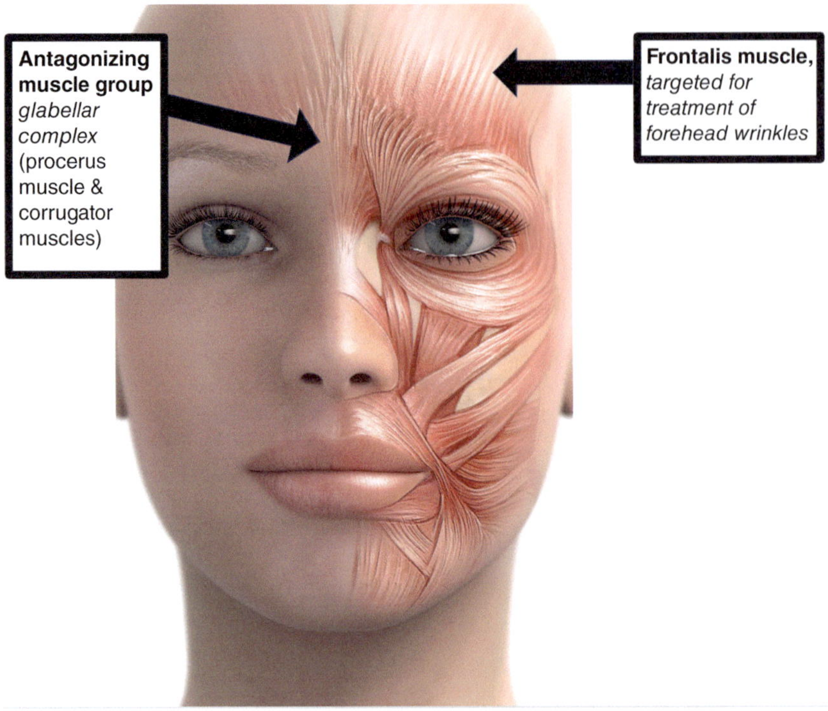

Fig. 50.2 Proper neurotoxin injection to treat forehead wrinkles must also address and treat the antagonizing muscle group. Thus, the frontalis muscle treatment also requires treatment of the glabellar muscle complex (shown)

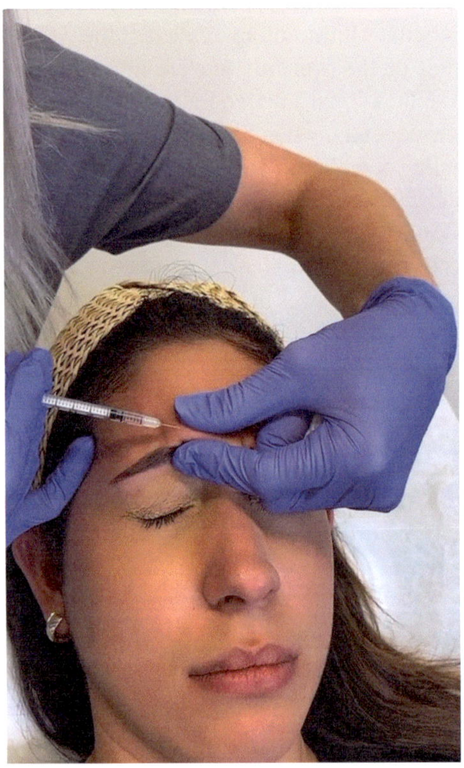

Fig. 50.3 Grasping the corrugator muscle as it is being contracted and injecting the corrugator tail superficially (compared to the corrugator head, which is a deeper injection)

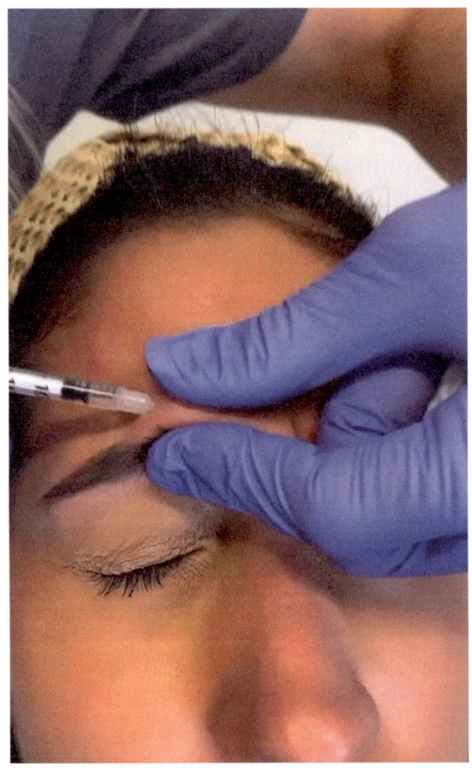

Fig. 50.4 Corrugator muscle tail being injected with BTX-A at an oblique angle. The average treatment of the glabella complex is 15–25 Units BTX-A

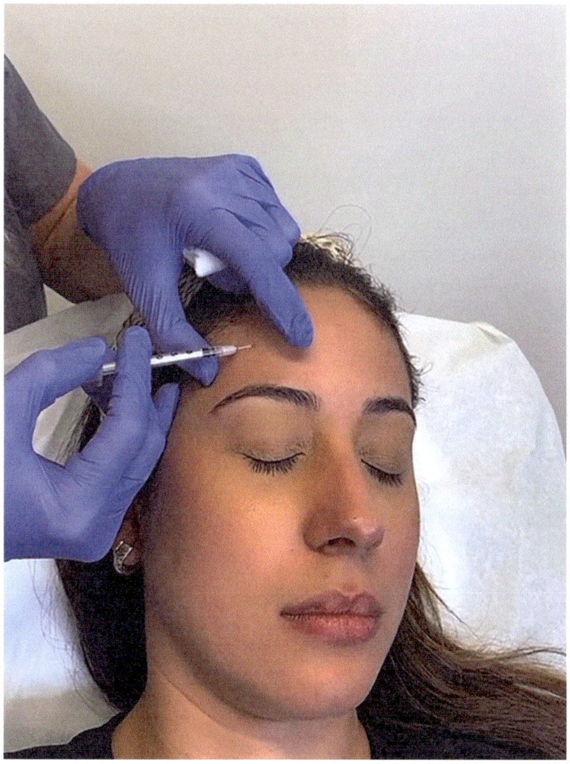

Fig. 50.5 Injecting the frontalis muscle while using a tapping technique as a distractor, for the patient's comfort

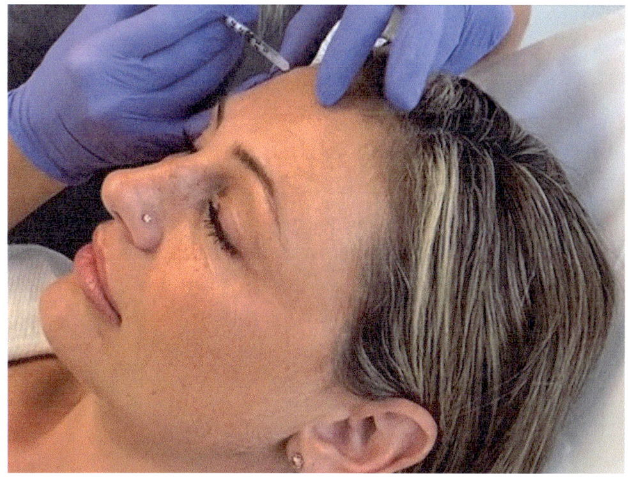

Fig. 50.6 Frontalis muscle neurotoxin injection using a 31-gauge needle and TB syringe. Typical treatment for this muscle group ranges between 10 and 20 Units BTX-A

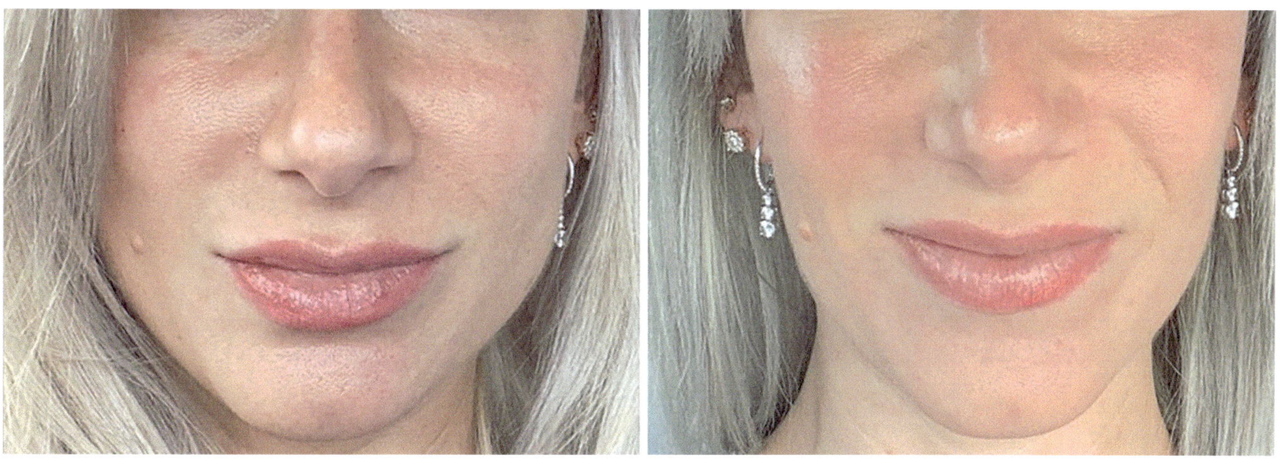

Fig. 50.7 Before (L) and after (R) masseter (and chin) botulinum toxin injections. Note the effect of slimming the face, which has a visibly less square appearance postinjection

Some tension headaches may be caused by strong trapezius muscles, so injecting botulinum toxin into those muscles can help reduce the severity of the headaches. As the trapezius muscles weaken, the aesthetic results are slimming of the trapezius muscles, which gives an often aesthetically desirable appearance of a longer neckline.

Botulinum toxin injection results peak around 14 days postinjection, and the body gradually metabolizes it until the effects completely wear off, which is about 3 months for the majority of patients, depending on their metabolism and activity level. As a general rule, patients with a high metabolism who are very active physically see the effect of BTX-A wear off quicker than those who live a more sedentary lifestyle.

Neurotoxin After Care and Considerations

Explaining botulinum toxin aftercare to the patient is crucial for optimal results. This includes maintaining the head upright for 4 h postinjection, avoiding saunas, excessive sweating, and exercise for 24–72 h postinjection, and avoiding pressure on the areas injected for 2 weeks postinjection.

The most important aftercare rule is *maintaining the head upright for 4 h.* The liquid toxin needs to be fully absorbed by the targeted muscle, so if the head is tilted up or down within the first 4 h, the liquid toxin can potentially migrate to a different muscle and cause unwanted results, including facial asymmetry.

When injecting the glabellar complex, the head of the corrugator muscle (medially) lies deeper to the frontalis muscle (which requires a deep injection to target that muscle), and the tail of the corrugator muscle (laterally) is superficial to the frontalis muscle (which requires a superficial and angled injection to target that portion of the muscle). Thus, if the botulinum toxin has not yet been fully absorbed by the corrugator muscles, tilting the head up or down within the first 4 h postinjection can result in unwanted migration to the frontalis muscle either superficially at the corrugator head or deep at the corrugator tail, causing **brow ptosis.**

With masseter injections, as the **risorius muscle** lies medially to the masseter, tilting the head down can cause the botulinum toxin to migrate to the risorius muscle and prevent the patient from being able to fully smile on the affected side. These examples effectively convey the importance of proper head positioning posttreatment. Explaining the rationale behind the 4-h rule to patients helps them to not only remember this, but also seems to make aftercare easier to follow, as it has the effect of improving patient compliance.

Dermal Fillers: Dermal fillers have evolved over time (Table 50.2), with hyaluronic acid fillers being the ones most commonly used in modern clinical practice.

Hyaluronic Acid Fillers: Hyaluronic acid (HA) is a linear glycosaminoglycan (GAG), anionic, gel-like polysaccharide, found in the extracellular matrix of epithelial and connective tissues of vertebrates (Fig. 50.8). HA fillers, such as Juvederm® and Restylane®, have hydrophilic properties that attract water molecules to restore volume, enhance facial contours, and soften some lines such as nasolabial folds, marionette lines, and perioral lines (Fig. 50.9). They can be used to augment the lips, lift the cheeks, contour the chin and jawline, and fill hollow tear troughs.

Other Dermal Fillers: Not all fillers are HA-based. For example, Radiesse® is a somewhat complex implant composed of smooth calcium hydroxylapatite (CaHA) microspheres (diameter of 25–45 μm) suspended in a sodium carboxymethylcellulose gel carrier (30% CaHA and 70% gel carrier by vol). Over time, the gel is absorbed, and fibroblasts arrive. Radiesse®w stimulates collagen III. Sculptra® is a poly-L-lactic acid (PLLA-SCA) facial injectable. Table 50.3 summarizes common dermal fillers used in clinical practice today.

Table 50.2 The historical development and evolution of dermal fillers, with a brief description

Year	Dermal filler	Description
1893	**Paraffin Wax**	The first injectable filler, used to treat scars and wrinkles.
1940s	**Liquid Silicone**	Used for facial wrinkles and contouring, but later deemed unsafe due to complications.
1970s	**Collagen (Bovine)**	Derived from cows, it became the first FDA-approved filler in 1981.
1980s	**Hyaluronic Acid (HA)**	First introduced as a filler and later became widely popular for its natural look and resorbable nature.
1990s	**Calcium Hydroxylapatite**	Developed for more permanent facial volume restoration.
2003	**Restylane® (Hyaluronic Acid)**	First hyaluronic acid-based filler approved by the FDA for wrinkle treatment.
2006	**Juvederm® (Hyaluronic Acid)**	Another hyaluronic acid filler, introduced as a smoother version of Restylane.
2009	**Radiesse® (Calcium Hydroxylapatite)**	A volumizing filler for deeper wrinkles and folds now commonly used for facial volume loss.
2010s	**Scuptra® (Poly-L-lactic Acid)**	Introduced as a filler for facial volume loss and to stimulate collagen production.
2012	**Voluma® (Hyaluronic Acid)**	A thicker version of hyaluronic acid designed for deeper injections

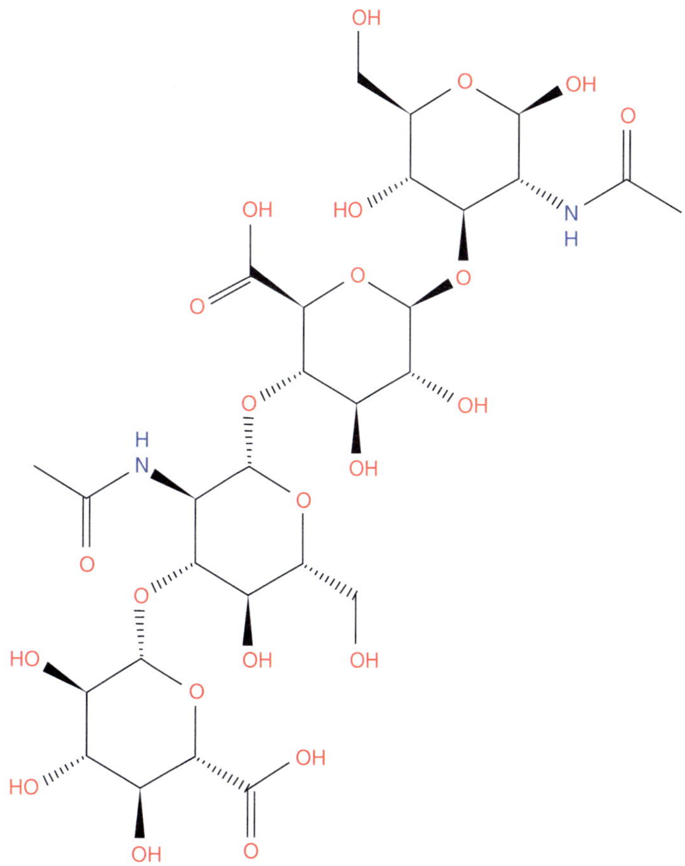

Fig. 50.8 The chemical structure of hyaluronic acid (HA) is shown. HA is a linear glycosaminoglycan (GAG) polymer and an anionic polysaccharide. It is found in the extracellular matrix of epithelial and connective tissues of vertebrates. Cosmetically, it is one of the most common dermal fillers used in clinical practice today

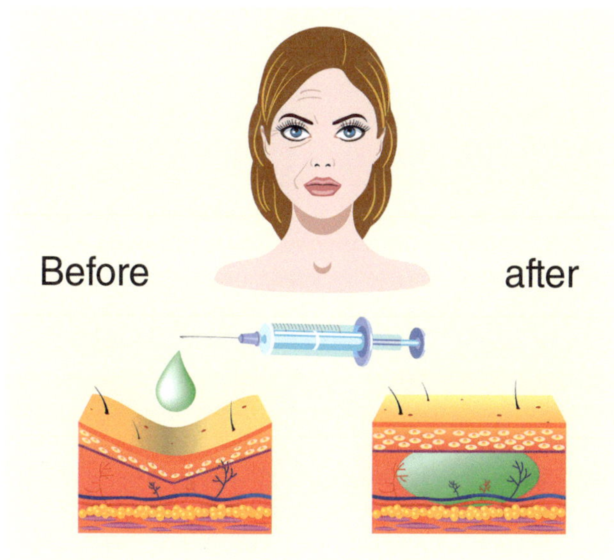

Fig. 50.9 Dermal fillers do not act the same way as neurotoxins do. When applied correctly, fillers restore lost volume. Some fillers can also promote new collagen deposition. Restoring lost volume in this manner, and as illustrated here, can restore a more youthful appearance

Table 50.3 Summary of the most commonly used dermal fillers, their composition, primary uses, and the typical duration of their effects

Filler type	Composition	Primary uses	Duration of effect
Hyaluronic Acid (HA)	Hyaluronic acid (natural substance found in the skin)	Wrinkle reduction, lip enhancement, cheek volume restoration, nasolabial folds	6–18 months
Calcium Hydroxylapatite	Calcium hydroxylapatite (a substance naturally found in bones)	Deep wrinkles, volume loss in cheeks, chin, and jawline	12–18 months
Poly-L-lactic Acid (PLLA)	Synthetic biodegradable polymer	Stimulates collagen production; used for facial volume restoration, deep wrinkles	2+ years
Polymethyl Methacrylate (PMMA)	PMMA microspheres suspended in a collagen gel	Deep wrinkles, acne scars, and facial contouring	Permanent
Autologous Fat Injections	Fat harvested from the patient's own body	Lip augmentation, wrinkle reduction, and restoration	1–3 years (variable)
Belotero®	Hyaluronic acid	Fine lines, especially around the eyes and lips	6–12 months
Radiesse®	Calcium hydroxylapatite + gel	Wrinkle reduction, volume restoration in cheeks and jawline	12–18 months
Sculptra®	Poly-L-lactic acid (PLLA)	Volume loss, deep wrinkles, and overall facial rejuvenation	2+ years

Technical Tips and Considerations for Dermal Filler Injections

HA fillers vary in density and hyaluronic acid concentration, and each is intended for a specific area of the face. They can be used to (a) *shape and enhance lip volume,* (b) *fill and brighten hollowing under the eyes,* and (c) *enhance facial contours.* Aestheticians often assess patients for facial *balancing and contouring,* and may often first focus on the **midface**, as this is typically the first area to be addressed.

With aging, **volume loss occurs,** which causes the skin to sag, giving the appearance of facial drooping, which results in more pronounced **nasolabial folds** (the fold that starts lateral to the nostrils down to the mouth corners) and **marionette lines** (the lines that start from the mouth corners down to the jawline). *Directly* targeting those lines and folds with HA filler results in adding volume to those areas, and may not look as natural and aesthetically pleasing compared to lifting the midface *first*.

Lifting the cheeks and adding lateral cheek contour with filler will lift the sagging skin around the nasolabial folds and marionette lines without adding volume to those lines and folds. It might not completely remove the nasolabial folds and marionette lines, but that result is preferred compared to directly filling those lines and adding volume in those midface areas. As a useful analogy, one can compare this to fabric. Imagine if you had creases in the center of a piece of fabric. The best way to diminish the creases would not be to add more fabric in the creases, ***but instead to lift and pull the fabric on its edges to flatten the creases out.*** Thus, addressing midface concerns often means focusing *lateral to the midface!*

Cheek filler injections are placed in the **supra-periosteal plane,** in order to get the product *under* the muscles and ligaments to provide a more natural lift. If the product is injected superficially into the ligaments, it will simply add bulk *without lifting,* so the *depth* of the product (filler) placement as well as *injecting with precision* is vital for an injector to achieve good results. Always locate my exact injection points and physically lift the skin superiorly and laterally in order to get as much lift as possible prior to inserting the needle. Next, you should aspirate and inject 0.01 mL at a time.

When using filler for *undereye hollows*, it is preferred to use less viscous products (e.g., Juvederm® Volbella®) with the smallest hyaluronic acid concentration. The reason is that it is not an area where a lot of "plumping" is desirable. Injections in this area can be done by backfilling a very small amount (0.05 mL) into multiple (insulin) syringes (a 1 mL syringe of Juvederm Volbella fills 20 syringes), and then injecting only once per syringe.

The filler is injected directly onto the orbital rim. Immediately after injection, a brief massage is done at each injection point to smooth out the area. This approach keeps the *patient as comfortable as possible* since it *prevents the needle from becoming dull* from multiple injections (a new needle for every injection). Importantly, this technique also allows the injector to maintain control of the *precise amount of product being injected,* so the area can be evaluated after each injection and ensures the area will not become overfilled (Fig. 50.10a and b).

Another option an injector has when injecting filler is to *replace the needle of the filler syringe with a* ***cannula.*** *A cannula can be used to evenly distribute filler in small amounts over an area and reduce the number of injection points when injecting an area such as the temples, chin, and jawline* (Figs. 50.11 and 50.12a and b). Using a cannula can also help reduce the risk of puncturing a blood vessel due to its blunt tip. Filler is deposited evenly in the targeted plane as the can-

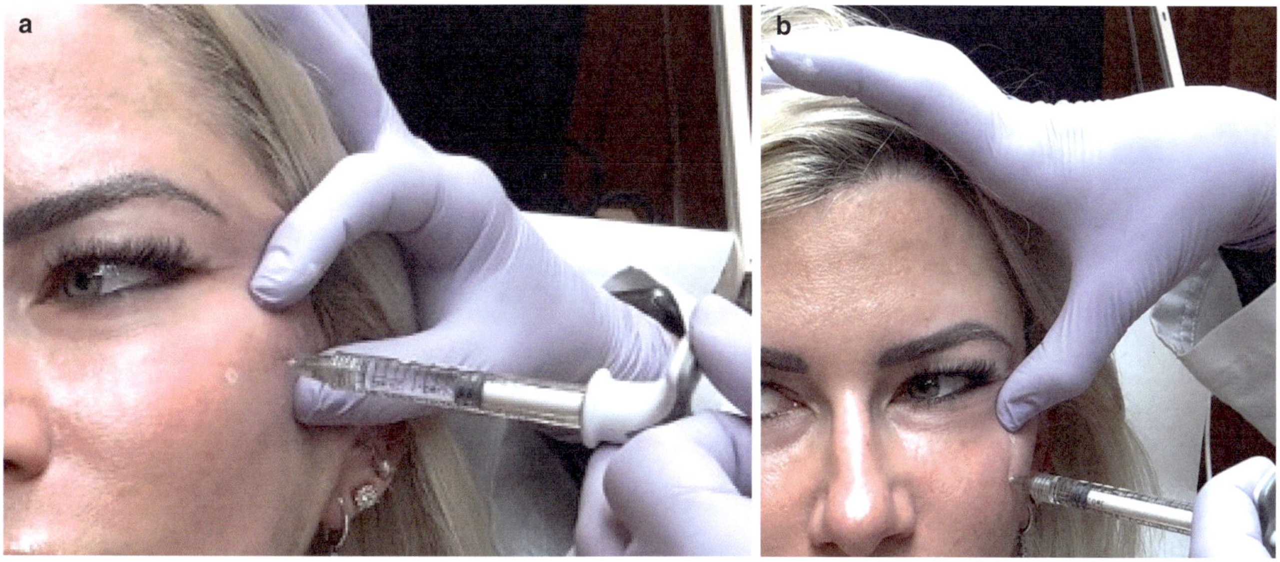

Fig. 50.10 (**a** and **b**) Lateral cheek dermal filler injection. (**a**) The lifting technique in which the skin is pulled superiorly and posteriorly prior to inserting the needle, and held in that position for the duration of each injection. (**b**) The lifting technique, close-up

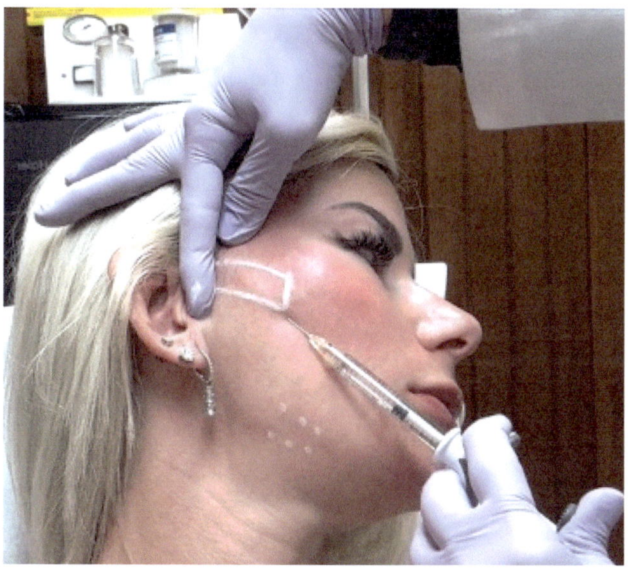

Fig. 50.11 Using a cannula technique to inject the area just inferior and lateral to the cheekbone, to further lift and define the cheekbone region

nula moves back and forth, with the bevel pointed up. An example with one half of the face treated is shown (Fig. 50.13).

Lip filler can be injected using different techniques to achieve different results. ***A linear technique*** (also known as the *fanning technique*) is the simplest and is used to achieve a subtle plump (Fig. 50.14). Whereas the ***Russian lip technique*** involves significantly more injection points with the needle being placed vertically to maximize the height of the lip (Fig. 50.15a–c). A cannula can also be used to inject a small bolus into each quadrant of the lip, and the product is massaged throughout that quadrant (Fig. 50.16). As the majority of lip volume is in the *center area* of the lip, the cannula injection points are placed *on the vermillion border* of each "cupid's bow" for the upper lip, and on the vermillion border inferior to the lip tubercles of the lower lip.

Overall, dermal fillers result in a quite noticeable change in overall aesthetic appearance. It provides a more youthful look and is a relatively newer alternative to surgical procedures, which were the mainstay of facial cosmetics prior to the advent of dermal fillers. Examples of before and after treatment are shown (Fig. 50.17a and b). Patient satisfaction is often derived from improving self-image and confidence, which has an overall positive impact on their well-being.

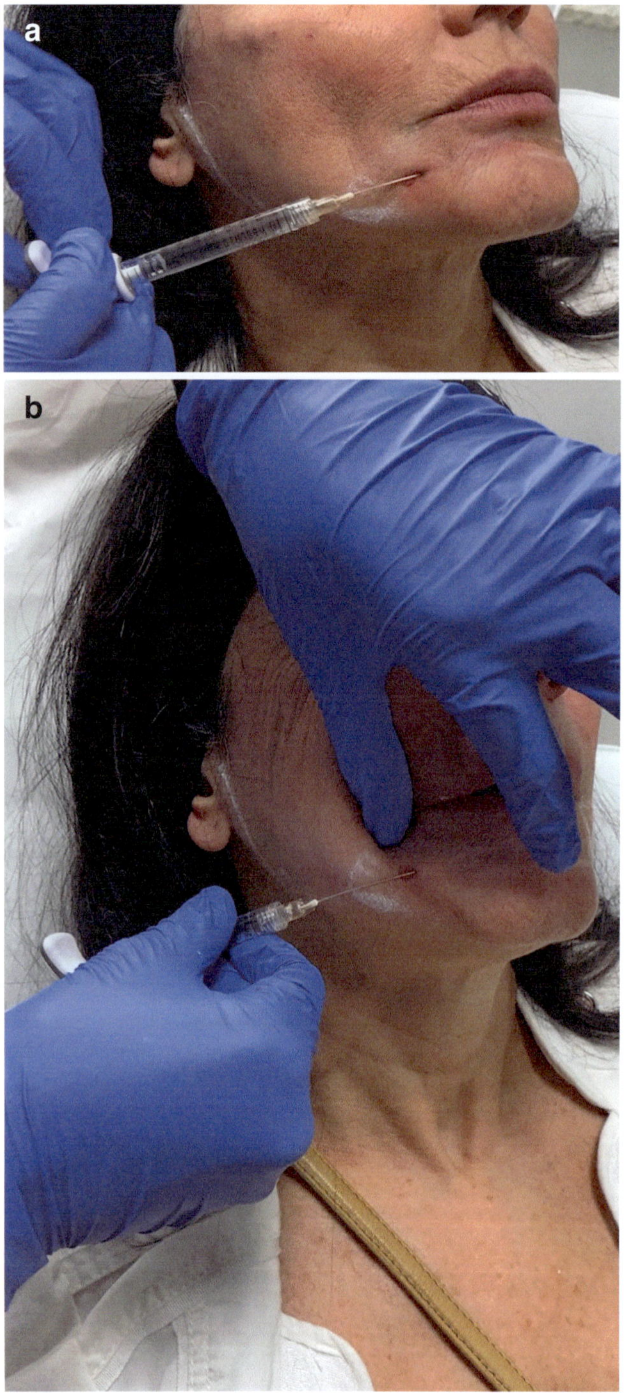

Fig. 50.12 (**a**) Cannula being used to deposit filler in the chin and mental crease areas. (**b**) Skin being pulled taut in order to ease the cannula through the tissue and evenly distribute the filler

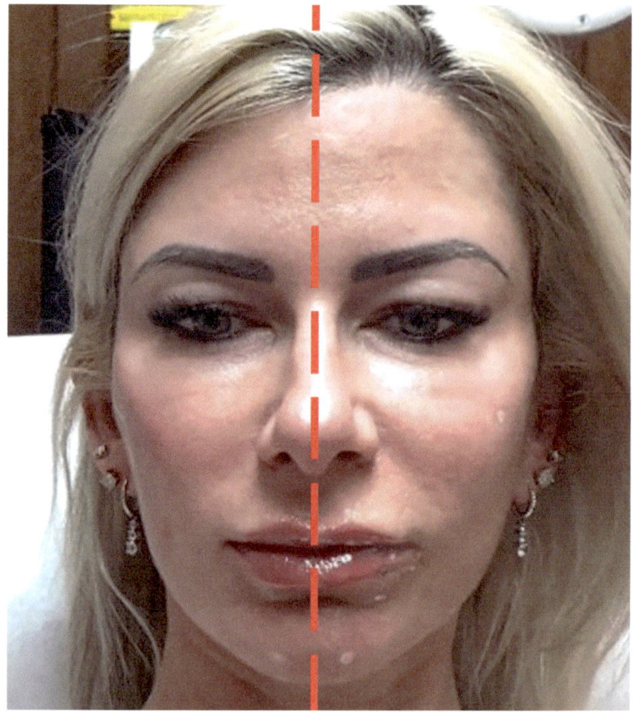

Fig. 50.13 A half-and-half before and after photograph. Cheek contouring filler completed on the patient's *right side* using a needle technique on the cheekbone and a cannula technique inferior to the cheekbone. Notice the definition of the *right cheek and how it lifted the lower face* compared to the left side, which is softer and wider, and has not yet been injected

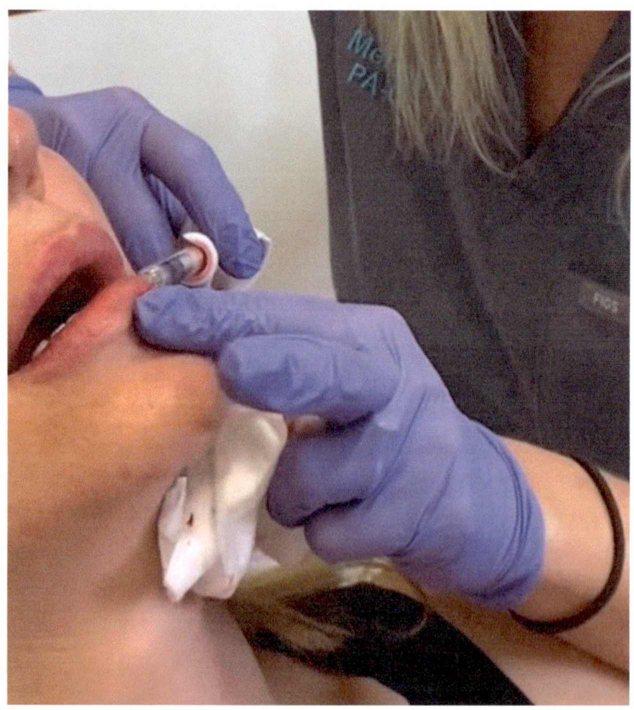

Fig. 50.14 Lip dermal filler injection using a linear technique

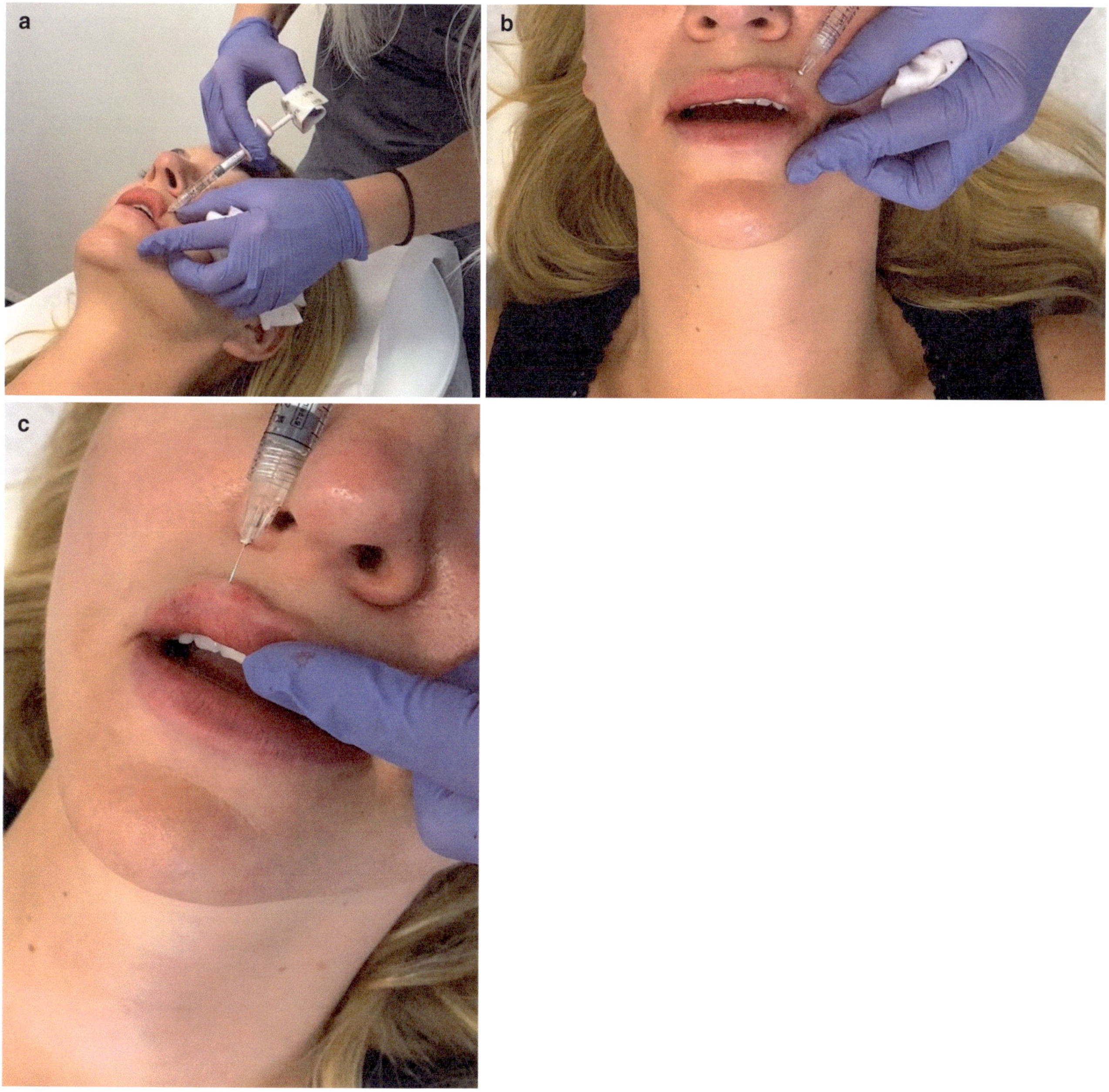

Fig. 50.15 (**a**) Using the Russian lip filler technique. (**b** and **c**) Close-up photographs demonstrating the Russian lip filler injection technique

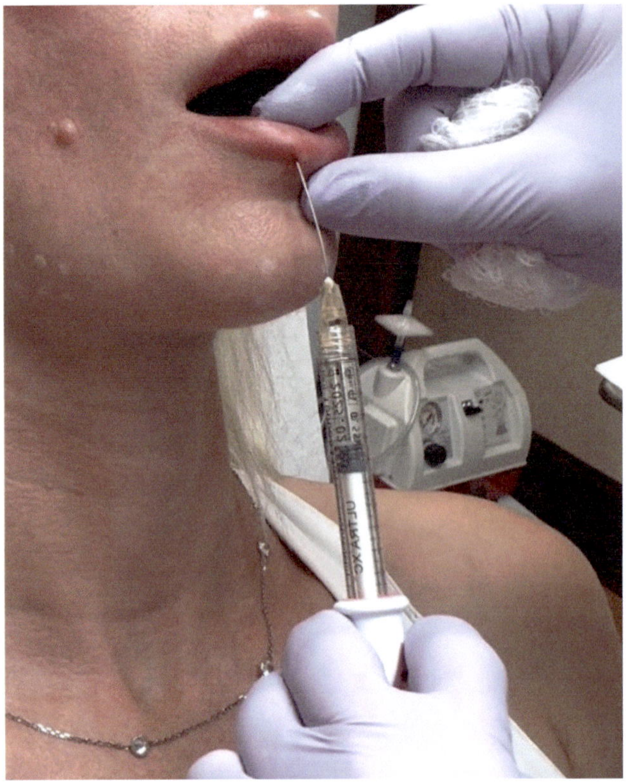

Fig. 50.16 Lip filler using a cannula technique, in which the lip was divided into quadrants prior to injecting a bolus, followed by massaging the product throughout each quadrant of the lip while depositing the majority of the volume nearest to midline

Fig. 50.17 (a and b) *Before and after* photographs immediately postinjection **with** (**a**) frontal and (**b**) lateral views shown. Dermal filler has been applied to the cheek and jawline for contouring, as well as the under eyes and lips. Notice how the cheeks are lifted and the nasolabial folds softened. Lifting with filler has almost eliminated the marionette lines and softened and brightened the undereye hollows. The lips are visibly more plump and youthful appearing

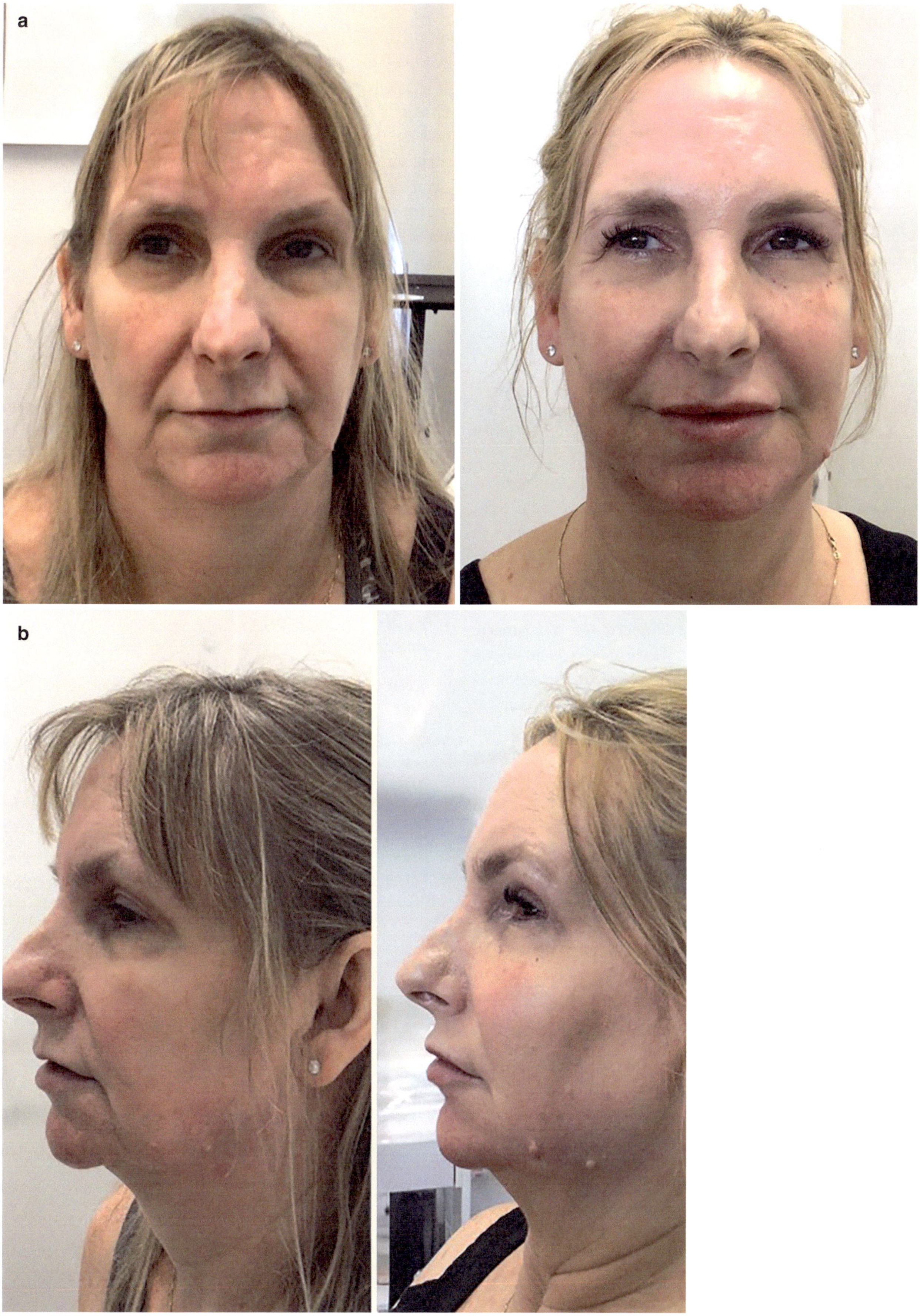
a
b

Dermal Filler After Care

As with botulinum toxin, dermal fillers are also metabolized by the body, and depending on the product used and the location, *the results can last 1–2 years.* Aftercare for filler injections is less stringent compared to botulinum toxin, as all fillers are more viscous and thus less likely to migrate. Makeup and other products should be avoided for 12 h postinjection to avoid infection, and pressure on the face should be avoided for 2 weeks to prevent the product from migrating as the product settles.

Swelling and tenderness are normal for the next few days due to the inflammatory response, secondary to the injections. For patients with thinner faces, the initial appearance of cheek injections appears as a sharp contour due to the density of the product. The final results can take about 2 weeks as the dense hyaluronic acid gel attracts water molecules, and it softens and spreads out, and the sharp contour looks more natural and blended with time.

Posttreatment bruising, swelling, tenderness, and redness posttreatment from dermal fillers are common and self-limited. To limit the risk of infection, it is best practice to cleanse the face prior to an injection session. Different cleansing agents can be used, for example, a mixture of chlorhexidine and alcohol.

The most important safety concern for a cosmetic injector is vascular occlusion, *which can lead to tissue necrosis and is considered an emergency.* After the needle is in place, it is absolutely crucial for the injector to aspirate for a few seconds prior to pushing down on the plunger and injecting the product, to ensure the product is not entering a blood vessel. **Ultrasonography** can be a useful aid to help identify and avoid blood vessels that may course near a planned injection site. Rarely, vascular occlusion can occur without a positive aspiration, which can be noticed either immediately or even within the next few hours. Patients should be counseled on the possible signs and symptoms of necrosis, which can include skin blanching or significant *swelling with pain out of proportion and increasing in intensity*—which requires emergent reevaluation. It is possible to break down the occlusion by massaging the area with moderate direct pressure and applying a warm compress for vasodilation. If these measures are unsuccessful, **hyaluronidase** (an enzyme that rapidly breaks down hyaluronic acid) needs to be immediately injected until there is no more evidence of vascular compromise and capillary refill is restored. It is worth mentioning two things. First, vascular occlusion, although uncommon, does occur in clinical practice and all aesthetic injectors should be very familiar with the management of a patient who presents with vascular occlusion. Second, not all fillers are HA-based, and thus hyaluronidase will not dissolve those products. It is for this reason that some cosmetic injectors avoid using ***non**-HA-based products*—such as Sculptra® and Radiesse®.

Closing Comments

Ongoing education and training are essential to stay updated on the latest advancements and best practices in aesthetic medicine. By understanding the principles of cosmetic injectables, medical professionals can provide comprehensive care and guidance to patients seeking nonsurgical facial rejuvenation and enhancement.

Suggested Reading

1. Kontis TC, Lacombe VG. Cosmetic injection techniques: a text and video guide to neurotoxins and fillers. Thieme; 2013.
2. Kontis TC, Rivkin A. The history of injectable facial fillers. Facial Plast Surg. 2009;25(2):67–72. https://doi.org/10.1055/s--0029-1220645. Epub 2009 May 4
3. Glenn G. Cosmetic injection: understanding all about cosmetic injection therapy and easy procedural guide to everything you need to know from basic to pro. Amazon Digital Services LLC - Kdp; 2024.
4. Stefan DK. Cosmetics injection techniques for beginners: mastering Botox, fillers, and aesthetic injections: essential techniques, safety tips, and step-by-step guidance for novice. Amazon Digital Services LLC - Kdp; 2024.
5. Luka DJ. Complete guide to cosmetic injection: empowering practitioners with knowledge, skills, best practices, techniques, safety protocols, and patient care for optimal results. Amazon Digital Services LLC - Kdp; 2024.
6. Lipham WJ, Mellicher J. Cosmetic and clinical applications of Botox and dermal fillers. CRC Press; 2024.
7. Stefan DK. Dermal fillers and Botox techniques for beginners: mastering cosmetic injections: essential methods, safety tips, and expert guidance for flawless results. Amazon Digital Services LLC - Kdp; 2024.

Avoiding Burnout and Promoting Well-Being

51

Carlina A. Maria

Introduction

Since the COVID-19 pandemic, growing concerns about exhaustion, staff shortages, and mental health crises have kept the topic of burnout at the forefront of many conversations within the healthcare industry. In 1974, Dr. Herbert J. Freudenberger first discussed **burnout** as a preventable psychological condition caused by long-term work-related stress [6]. With the help of his theory, physician and nurse burnout has already been on the radar of hospital administrators for several decades. In today's ever-changing healthcare landscape, administrators recognize that burnout can impact all healthcare team members, including physician assistants and physician assistant students.

Christina Maslach and Michael Leiter [13] expanded Dr. Freudenberger's basic burnout description into a three-dimensional definition. Figure 51.1 shows a summary of the three dimensions. The first dimension of burnout is **exhaustion**, which includes complete mental or physical exhaustion. This type of exhaustion does not get better with rest or a vacation. Fatigue and mental exhaustion are conditions that may require years of medical treatment. **Depersonalization** is the second dimension, which deals with feelings of negativity and cynicism. A person going through depersonalization will likely withdraw from professional and social situations and distance themselves from coworkers and personal relationships. Lastly, the third dimension turns inward on a more personal feelings level: **inefficacy and ineffectiveness**. While

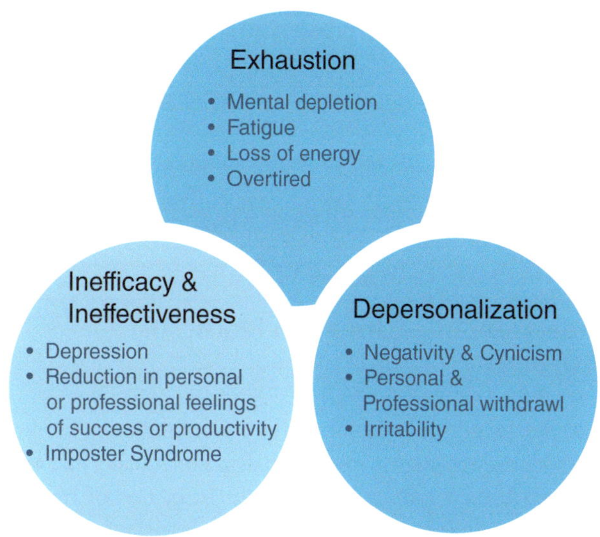

Fig. 51.1 The three dimensions of burnout: exhaustion, depersonalization, and inefficacy and ineffectiveness

C. A. Maria (✉)
MassGeneral Brigham, Boston, MA, USA
e-mail: cmaria@mghihp.edu

S. Atallah, J. Dragoljevic (eds.), *Fundamentals of Surgery for Physician Assistants*,
https://doi.org/10.1007/978-3-032-21069-2_51

depersonalization is negative opinions about work and life, inefficacy and ineffectiveness are about a negative opinion toward oneself. This dimension can increase feelings of depression or anxiety and reduce feelings of accomplishment, success, or productivity. It can even lead to Imposter Syndrome, a psychological condition where intellectual and successful individuals doubt their skills and abilities [9].

Feelings of burnout may be unavoidable when working in the healthcare industry. High stress, administrative burden, and heavy patient loads are the new norm, regardless of the specialty one joins. Adapting and recovering from stress is crucial in an industry where high-stakes situations frequently change and stress levels constantly rise. With back-to-back and 24-hour shifts, it is easy for burnout symptoms to set in quickly. Fortunately, there are many ways to mitigate the symptoms of burnout, including maintaining healthy well-being, practicing self-care, and focusing on mental health.

Chapter Objectives

- Review the prevalence of burnout among physician assistants and how the impacts of burnout vary depending on different factors such as race and gender.
- Compare contributing factors of burnout from within the workplace.
- Understand the impact burnout can have on the individual, the team, and the organization.
- Understand the signs and symptoms of burnout on a physical, emotional, and behavioral level.
- Summarize personal preventative strategies for implementation at work.
- Identify well-being and self-care practices for personal use.
- Understand well-being strategies to promote a supportive work environment.
- Understand when to seek help and what resources to use.

Understanding Burnout in Physician Assistants

To understand how to make strides toward reducing burnout in physician assistants, one must first understand just how widespread the problem is and what the causes of burnout are. Addressing burnout in physician assistants requires understanding these varied influences and developing strategies tailored to support their mental and emotional well-being across the different stages of their careers. Implementing different burnout interventions can help diminish the impact burnout has on the individual, the team, and the organization.

The Prevalence of Burnout Among Physician Assistants

Burnout is becoming more prevalent in many industries worldwide. In 2019, although one may not believe it to be true, the healthcare industry was not even the top industry experiencing burnout—it was the hotel, food services, and hospitality industry [18]. The healthcare industry was third on that list. According to the American Academy of Physician Associates [2], about 41% and 56% of physician assistants and physician assistant students, respectively, report at least one or more symptoms of burnout or are completely burnt out. Think about that: almost half of the physician assistant workforce and more than half of our physician assistant students, who are training to help relieve the stress of that 41%, are either working toward becoming or are already entirely burnt out. Practicing physician assistants are pushing through with the hope that relief is coming, but that relief is coming in already experiencing burnout.

Like other healthcare team members, physician assistants experience different burnout levels based on their specialty of medicine. The list below reflects the percentage of physician assistants who reported at least one symptom of burnout by specialty. The top physician assistant specialty experiencing burnout is emergency medicine, with 42.2% reporting at least one symptom of burnout. While not stated below, the specialty with the lowest reported burnout was dermatology, with 26.1% experiencing at least one symptom of burnout [8].

Top 10 Physician Assistant Specialties Experiencing Burnout

1. Emergency Medicine (42.2%)
2. Gastroenterology (38.5%)
3. Critical Care Medicine (38.5%)
4. Family Medicine/General Medicine (37.2%)
5. Hospital Medicine (37%)
6. Oncology (36.7%
7. Primary care (36.6%)
8. Internal Medicine/General Practice (36.3%)
9. Psychiatry (35.2%)
10. Neurosurgery (34.6%)

Other causes can play a role in the prevalence of burnout. An individual's **age** can have different impacts on burnout. The Boomer generation (60–80-year olds) report burnout at a rate of 38% [1]. They are the least burnt-out generation, and this may be because they have lighter workloads and a higher sense of professional achievement. Overall, they have greater job satisfaction. Next are Generation X (40–60-year olds) with 57% and Millennials (30–40-year olds) with 65% [1]. These generations make up the bulk of the workforce today. Causes of higher burnout could include increased workloads from retiring Boomers and training younger generations, less time for scholarly work leading to less professional achievement, and greater levels of depersonalization, pushing toward higher job dissatisfaction. The youngest generation, Generation Z (18–29-year olds), who are just starting to enter the workforce, report that 71% are experiencing symptoms of burnout [1]. This younger generation seems plagued by newer concerns that older generations did not have to worry about, such as rising cost of living, increasing isolation, reduced social skills, and an inability to disconnect from the Internet [15].

Burnout is experienced differently between **genders**. Not only does gender inequality still exist in the workplace, but now, because of it, women are experiencing burnout at significantly higher rates than men [10]. Women feel obligated to take on greater workloads, spend more time with patients, and spend more time charting in electronic medical record systems. Additionally, inequality in pay, whether actual or perceived, can be a significant stressor. Unlike gender and age, **race** has not been statistically significant in those experiencing higher levels of burnout. However, it *has* shown that members of the healthcare team of minority descent are less likely to report their symptoms of burnout compared to their white counterparts [7]. The reasons they do not report their symptoms can lead down the path of social determinants of health. Why are they not reporting—lack of insurance? Lack of quality healthcare? Lack of transportation? Lack of financial support? Lack of education? Mental health stigma? Cannot get time off from work? It can be any number of factors.

Contributing Factors of Burnout

Various factors can contribute to the development of burnout symptoms, and they can be sorted into three categories: organizational, leadership, and individual. When someone asks, “Who is to blame for burnout?” organizations, leadership, and individuals all point the finger at each other. No one wants to accept the blame themselves, but the truth is, they are all to blame. It is never just one factor that is the sole cause of burnout. At the **organizational level** are the situations that happen in the workplace that affect an employee’s job that are beyond their control. These are the higher level, institutional problems dictated to the employees. For example, staffing shortages are a significant factor contributing to burnout. They lead to longer hours, busier schedules, and heavier and excessive workloads. No one wants to work under these conditions, but sometimes they are asked to when faced with a shortage. Another problem at the organizational level is institutional support. A lack of support can make an employee feel unheard, unrecognized, and underappreciated. Institutional support is more than having appropriate facilities and equipment to do the job. It also means having the funding to pursue continuing education opportunities, research projects, and professional development. When an organization invests in an employee, the employee will feel more invested in themselves.

It is expected that hospital administrators at the organizational level have a bird’s-eye view of the hospital’s employees. It would not be typical for them to know each of their employees personally. However, management and leaders at the **leadership level** generally have a closer relationship with their employees and should take keener notice of attitudes, behaviors, work performance, and the work environment. Often, leaders are promoted to management positions without training; they do not know how to recognize burnout in their employees, do not know how to prevent it, and do not know that some of their behaviors contribute to it. For instance, some leaders set unrealistic expectations or do not respect boundaries. They expect their employees to work through their lunch break, put in extra time off the clock, and check emails through the night or while on vacation. These expectations include extra work time the employee puts in instead of disconnecting and resetting that burnout clock. Another example of a new, untrained manager is someone who delegates every task or does not delegate anything. This behavior can be stressful to an employee who may feel overwhelmed by all their new tasks or feel useless and untrustworthy due to the lack of tasks. New or untrained managers unknowingly contribute to toxic work environments by creating unnecessary stress and heavier workloads. They have another responsibility to pay attention to their employees’ physical and mental health. This concept does not mean they must bring a box of tissues to an employee every time they sneeze. However, if an employee starts exhibiting symptoms of depression and becomes withdrawn, a leader should reach out to that employee to offer help. If they notice an employee becoming anxious or struggling to meet deadlines, they should intervene before the problem becomes something like burnout.

As much as blaming others is simpler, sometimes the finger has to be pointed at ourselves. As previously mentioned, race, age, and gender can make a person more or less susceptible to burnout. Other factors on the **individual level** can contribute to burnout just as much. A resilient and tough support system can be integral to overcoming burnout. They provide a shoulder to cry on, an ear to talk to, advice to offer, hugs to give, and much more to someone who needs them. Not having a support system can contribute to burnout, making a person unable to vent or cry, forcing them to suppress emotions. Countless factors could happen in a person’s life that a professional administrator or colleague may not know about (or even a personal friend). A short list of events includes divorce, pregnancy complications, domestic violence, the death of a family member or friend, financial stress, parenting difficulties, or struggling with addiction. In addition to these events, a poor work–life balance can further contribute to burnout and have a profound impact on mental health and personal relationships. Lastly, sometimes, a person lacks the skills needed to cope with stress, such as interpersonal and communication skills, resiliency, and stress management skills.

The Impact of Burnout on the Organization, the Team, and the Individual

Burnout can significantly impact the organization, the team, and the individual in ways that are not often considered. Managers frequently consider the organization in the present; however, they should consider the big picture with the organization's bottom line in mind. One of the most substantial impacts of burnout is on patient care. Burnt-out healthcare professionals typically spend less time with patients and have increased reports of medical errors [17]. This fact seems simple enough, but when considered further, these actions can decrease patient satisfaction, increase malpractice lawsuits, and even decrease the institutional reputation. Now, take it even further and think about the organization's bottom line. Burnout not only means unhappy patients but also unhappy employees—job dissatisfaction. Job dissatisfaction inevitably leads to job turnover. Employees leave for better work–life balance, higher pay, more manageable workloads, or better benefits, leaving organizations with open positions and the unpleasant tasks of trying to fill them. In today's economy, recruiting and training a new physician can cost an organization between $50,000 and $1,000,000 [17]. Multiply those figures by several open positions, and the organization's bottom line will undoubtedly take a hit.

Burnout on the team level can impact the individual, their teammates, and their team leader. The individual experiencing burnout may not be communicating efficiently with their team. They may be working at a reduced productivity rate or may not be doing the work at all. These behaviors can lead to missed deadlines and problems in team dynamics, including feelings of distrust and resentment. Team leaders must also be aware of employee production and performance, which could cost the department more money than necessary. For example, absenteeism and presenteeism are two ways an employee can cost a department money while not accomplishing anything. **Absenteeism** is when an employee calls into work and uses paid vacation or sick leave. They will still be paid for the day but will not produce any work. **Presenteeism** is when an employee physically shows up for work but cannot accomplish or produce anything. While job turnover does impact organizations, the departments and teams will feel the impact a lot more. The individuals on those teams will have to step in to cover the open positions. The same will need to happen when a team member is experiencing burnout. The work left by an open position or a colleague experiencing burnout still needs to be completed. It becomes a cyclical burnout epidemic. The work gets passed to another employee who becomes overwhelmed and burnt out from the excessive workload; they take time off to recover; their work and the original work get passed to another employee, who becomes overwhelmed and burned out; and so forth and so on.

Finally, the individual impacts of burnout can be some of the most devastating and unexpected. While it does happen sometimes, most individuals who suffer from burnout do not recover with a short respite of relaxation. Individuals who suffer from burnout can be affected by it for months or even years. Burnout symptoms have been linked to long-term psychological and physical health effects, such as posttraumatic stress disorder (PTSD) and heart disease. Burnout can also have a significant impact on personal and professional relationships. Unfortunately, people often do not realize the irreparable damage they do to their relationships when going through burnout. Many families, friendships, and professional relationships have been devastated due to burnout behaviors, unable to recover from burnout's lasting impacts.

Burnout can force people to believe they have no alternative but to give up their careers. They do not see a way to improve their job or workplace, so they leave searching for happiness, often starting over in a new career. In 2023, Deloitte reported that about 70% of executives were unhappy and wanted to give up their careers in search of a better work–life balance [5]. As previously mentioned, various events in an individual's life contribute to burnout and the ability to effectively manage it. For example, an individual goes through a divorce and ends up homeless, or an individual develops a dependency on alcohol and now needs a liver transplant.

Recognizing the Signs of Burnout

Being able to recognize the signs and symptoms of burnout is a valuable skill to possess. Individuals with this skill are better positioned to identify if they or someone close to them (a colleague, family member, or friend) is experiencing burnout symptoms and can seek help sooner. Implementing a burnout intervention earlier allows for a greater chance of success and more time to make adjustments if needed. This section will explore the physical, emotional, and behavioral signs and symptoms of burnout and how to recognize them when they might not be easy to notice.

Physical Signs and Symptoms of Burnout

The **physical** signs and symptoms of burnout are not a simple list of standard and easy-to-recognize symptoms, but rather a long list of contradictory, everyday, and complex symptoms that can range from the common cold to hives. The physical symptoms that are most frequently reported are being fatigued or having insomnia, constantly sick with a cold or the flu, stomach aches, nausea, indigestion, diarrhea, constipation, recurrent headaches, musculoskeletal pain (back pain, joint pain, muscle tension), increased blood pressure, chest pain, heart palpitations, atrial fibrillation, increased risk of heart attack or stroke, excessive sweating, hair loss, increased itching, and hives. These symptoms are just the beginning of the list; burnout can manifest in just about any physical form and depends on how a person's body manages stress. When experiencing burnout symptoms, staying open and honest with the general practitioner is incredibly important. A combination of these symptoms can lead to more extensive health issues requiring monitoring and treatment.

Emotional Signs and Symptoms of Burnout

Emotional signs and symptoms of burnout can be more challenging to diagnose and even more complicated to offer help to an individual experiencing these symptoms. Individuals going through emotional symptoms might be feeling embarrassed or unwilling to share what they are going through and may try to hide their emotions, making openly talking about them problematic. An individual experiencing emotional symptoms of burnout may be feeling depressed, anxious, or paranoid. Visual cues may not always be present, so paying attention to verbal messages is also important. They may also be feeling angry or irritable—visual cues are sometimes more noticeable with these feelings. Experiencing burnout may cause someone difficulty processing their emotions—they may switch between emotions frequently, including laughing at inappropriate moments or spontaneously crying. Burnout can leave an individual feeling overwhelmed or constantly frazzled. The individual does not seem like they can get organized or figure out the task they are trying to do. On the other hand, they may also seem completely detached, as if they do not care about the task or the organization. There is a complete lack of motivation, urgency, and concentration.

In extreme cases of burnout, individuals have even turned to suicide and suicidal ideation. While there is limited research on the number of physician assistant suicides relating to burnout, there is no lack of research on physician and nurse burnout and suicide. A harrowing statistic to take in is that in the United States, 300–400 physicians die by suicide each year, and nurses commit suicide at a rate of two times that of the general population [14, 16]. Part of the blame for burnout-related physician and nurse suicide is put on the mental health stigma that healthcare professionals face. This barrier to treatment places stigmatization on mental illnesses and suggests negative attitudes, ostracization, and discriminatory judgment toward healthcare professionals who seek help or treatment for mental health illnesses. As a result, many healthcare professionals with mental health illnesses go untreated.

Behavioral Signs and Symptoms of Burnout

The final category of signs and symptoms of burnout is **behavioral,** which is usually the most straightforward and apparent category of symptoms to spot. Someone who is experiencing behavioral symptoms is simply not acting like themselves. They could act out of character like a pre-teen by rolling their eyes, walking away from conversations, and saying things like "whatever." Conversely, their behavior could become aggressive and combative toward others. The individual may start yelling at others, criticizing them, or potentially physically attacking them. Other changes in behaviors that administrators and leaders should address could include self-harm, self-medicating with drugs or alcohol, or other forms of addictive behaviors like gambling or overeating, purposeful isolation, procrastination, or forgetfulness. Administrators and leaders should immediately address any behavior that seems out of the norm, recurrent, and disruptive for an individual.

Professional Burnout Interventions for the Individual

As Freudenberger theorized, burnout is caused by stress in the workplace [6]. Developing and implementing interventions can help individuals create barriers to protect themselves from burnout in the place where it is most likely to start. The following interventions may, to the mind, make sense as practical interventions to develop, but may prove to be strenuous in the implementation phase. The most valuable techniques in a professional setting for mitigating burnout symptoms are setting realistic goals and expectations, improving time management and prioritization techniques, setting boundaries, learning to say "no," and delegating.

Setting Realistic Goals and Expectations

Having goals and expectations that are realistic, clear, and attainable is an effective strategy for managing stressful workloads, giving individuals a sense of purpose in their work, and staying motivated [12]. Individuals who are burnt out often feel detached from their work, as if it does not make a difference in the lives of others, leading to greater job dissatisfaction. Setting realistic goals and expectations can provide more clarity and a stronger sense of direction to individuals feeling lost or overwhelmed. Some individuals who like to feel a sense of accomplishment take the time to break down their goals into smaller, more achievable tasks. This approach can help the individual and leaders track progress, manage time better, and allow for a better work–life balance.

Many organizations that utilize goal setting for annual review monitoring also require individuals to use the SMART goals concept to develop their goals. Five key elements comprise a **SMART goal**: Specific, Measurable, Achievable, Relevant, and Time-Bound.

Specific: Specific goals are clearly defined, including what is to be accomplished, who is involved, and the actions needed to accomplish the goal.

Measurable: Measurable goals have a quantifiable means to track the goal's progress. Explain how the goal's success will be determined.

Achievable: Achievable Goals should motivate individuals to achieve them. Breaking down goals into smaller goals can help accomplish more heavy goals.

Relevant: Relevant goals should align with the individual's job description, the department's goals, and/or the organization's mission and vision. Developing a goal that does not benefit the organization may be rejected.

Time-Bound: Time-Bound goals should have a deadline for evaluating the success of the goals and setting new goals. For most organizations that tie goals to annual reviews, the deadline is annually.

When setting goals and expectations, asking for feedback from direct management and leadership is a necessary part of the process and is often done before the process even begins. Management and leadership likely have ideas about what they want to see for goals in the upcoming year. Perhaps they have a particular skill set they would like to see an individual work on or a specific project they would like to assign. By considering their ideas when developing goals, an individual can ensure that an organization's and department's needs are met.

Time Management and Prioritization Techniques

Poor **time management skills** can undoubtedly lead to increased symptoms of burnout like increased stress, feeling overwhelmed, anxiety, and lack of focus. Constantly feeling under pressure to perform, that everything is urgent, and that tasks came out of nowhere are common feelings with poor time management skills. Improving these skills can reduce symptoms of burnout by reducing anxiety, creating a greater sense of accomplishment, and increasing job satisfaction. However, time management is a learned behavior, meaning that it is a skill learned through habituation, rewards or punishment, watching others, and even physiological responses [20]. Changing a learned behavior takes positivity, hard work, dedication, commitment, and a strong desire to change. Understanding that failure is always possible, being willing to start repeatedly is essential to changing a learned behavior.

How does an individual know that they are managing their time effectively? Individuals with successful time management skills have complete control over their schedule; they do not get overwhelmed when asked to do last-minute projects or take on new projects. Successful time management skills can increase productivity and a better work–life balance. One can improve their time management skills using numerous approaches, including task prioritization, calendar time blocking, delegating tasks, and time management techniques like the Pomodoro Method and the Eisenhower Matrix.

Task prioritization is a practical time management tool that allows individuals to sort tasks based on how urgently they need to be completed and how important they are. Using the **Eisenhower Matrix**, individuals can accomplish this prioritization easily. Figure 51.2 is an example of the Eisenhower Matrix template. Sort tasks that are urgent and important into the "Do" quadrant (top left). These tasks have approaching deadlines, clear-cut consequences if not completed, and have a direct correlation to long-term goals. The

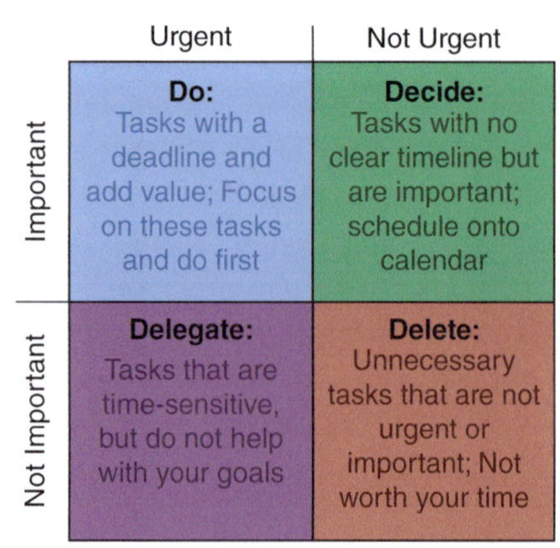

Fig. 51.2 The Eisenhower Matrix

tasks in the "Do" quadrant should be the primary focus of an individual's time. The second quadrant is "Decide" (top right). The tasks sorted into the "Decide" category are not urgent but are still essential to the organization and long-term goals. Schedule these tasks for later completion; allow an appropriate amount of time for the task and set reminders to stay on top of completing the task.

The "Delegate" quadrant (Lower Left) is reserved for urgent tasks that are not important. These tasks require follow-up immediately but do not necessarily need a specific individual to complete or tie to specific goals. Delegating tasks under this category aids in efficiently managing workloads and allows other team members to utilize their skill sets. The last quadrant, "Delete" (Lower Right), consists of tasks that are neither urgent nor important. These are distractor tasks disguised to seem like they need to be completed, but in reality, they are not relevant to the organization's needs or an individual's long-term goals. They are not worth considering further.

Calendar time blocking and the **Pomodoro Method** are effective techniques for successfully keeping up with scheduled tasks. Time blocking allows individuals to build time into their calendars to balance their workloads, ensure break times, and keep their goals and expectations realistic. The Pomodoro Method is a structured method of timing periods of focus and allowing break times. Individuals select the task they want to complete, set a timer, and work straight for 25 min. When the 25 min are up, they take a 5-minute break and then repeat from the beginning four more times. Once completed, they take an extended 30-minute break and then repeat. This method is a successful time management technique for individuals who struggle with Attention-Deficit Hyperactivity Disorder (ADHD) [4].

Setting Boundaries and Learning to Say No

Perhaps the toughest intervention to implement in the workplace to mitigate burnout symptoms is setting boundaries and learning to say no. Many employees believe they should do as told and are not allowed to say no. This belief is a common misconception passed down from generations when this behavior was the norm. Today, employees have the right to set workplace and personal boundaries and can say no in order to prioritize their self-care. Setting boundaries empowers individuals to decide what they will and will not accept into their lives. It puts the individual back in control of their life and reduces stressful situations. The power of saying no allows individuals to reflect on boundaries and manage a better work–life balance by releasing unnecessary commitments. It can increase their confidence and lead to a healthier lifestyle, reducing burnout symptoms.

Similarly to changing time management learned behaviors, **boundary setting** requires dedication and a solid motivation to change. For some individuals, their fears and desires can act as barriers that prevent them from standing strong for their newly set boundaries. A fear of disappointing others or a desire to make others happy can cause individuals to betray their boundaries. Additionally, a need to have the approval or validation of others or being a perfectionist can make an individual vulnerable to going against their boundaries. However, if an individual can overcome these barriers, setting boundaries is one of the most effective ways to mitigate burnout in the workplace.

The first step to setting boundaries is to clearly define what needs of the individual the boundary addresses and what the expectations of others will be. It is important to remember that setting boundaries for reducing burnout and improving mental health is essential as long as the boundaries do not interfere with an organization's goals, a department's expectations, or an individual's job role. For example, if an individual is expected to work until 4:00 pm, they cannot simply set a boundary that their workday will end at 2:00 pm in order to increase family time. The personal boundary does not supersede the department's expectations. The next step is communicating new boundaries openly and politely with those impacted professionally. The last step is to be consistent and uphold the boundary. Do not allow others' behaviors to break the boundary; politely correct the action and issue a reminder of the boundary. Make sure to document all incidents. If the behavior continues, bring it to the attention of management. Remaining consistent with the boundary will encourage colleagues to take it seriously.

The power of **saying no** is another helpful tool to diminish burnout symptoms. People often feel guilty about saying no or do not want to disappoint others. However, saying no is not about the needs of others but about the needs of oneself. Saying no can be utilized in social settings and the workplace, and both can alleviate burnout symptoms. Still, one must consider saying no at appropriate times. They should consider proposals fully before saying no; if a proposal may benefit long-term goals, it may be worth taking on. Remember that the decision to say no was made for a reason and should be maintained unless circumstances change.

Professional Health: Continuing Education, Professional Associations, Mentorship, and Professional Development

The final individual intervention that effectively mitigates burnout symptoms in the workplace is improving professional health. Professional health includes opportunities that contribute to education, research, and development, anything that makes an individual more valuable to an organization. **Continuing education** is when an individual returns to formal education or training to develop a skill, receive training for a job, or earn a higher degree. Sometimes, an organization may ask an individual to specifically attend a skills training workshop at the organization's expense. These opportunities are a confidence booster, showing the individual that the organization is investing in their future. Additionally, continuing education is vital to healthcare professionals who need it for recertification. Physician assistants in the United States must earn at least 100 continuing medical education (CME) credits every two years to keep their certification current with the National Commission on Certification of Physician Assistants (NCCPA).

Joining **professional associations** is an informal way to grow support systems, which, as previously mentioned, can reduce burnout-related stress. With the rapid progression of the Internet came easier accessibility to any professional association an individual may want to join. Linking up with fellow physician assistants, healthcare professionals, surgical physician assistants, students, or soccer fans from the United States or worldwide is now just at the click of a button. Students can join groups studying for the Physician Assistant National Certifying Examination (PANCE) and share study questions, test-taking tips, and tricks. There are even support groups for physician assistants new to clinical work, academia, and changing careers. Some of the universal professional associations that physician assistants join are the American Academy of Physician Associates (AAPA) (https://www.aapa.org), the Student Academy of the AAPA (https://www.aapa.org/governance/student-academy/), and the Physician Assistant Education Association (PAEA) (https://www.paeaonline.org).

Research shows that individuals who participated in a **mentoring** relationship were less likely to experience symptoms of burnout than those who did not participate in the relationships [3]. This intervention reduces burnout symptoms by allowing an individual to work on their professional development with someone who knows the industry and the career, and it also provides psychosocial support for the individual and the mentor. An individual does not have to find a mentorship program to acquire a mentor, although it is the easiest route. A mentor can be anyone that the individual is motivated by, respects, feels that they can learn from, and that the mentor will challenge them. Networking and asking others for recommendations can draw an individual closer to an appropriate mentor. When searching for a mentor, an individual should remember their long-term and short-term goals and practice an elevator pitch on why the mentor should take them on as a mentee and what they hope to gain from the relationship.

A relationship does not always work out perfectly; sometimes, an individual needs to end their relationship with a mentor and begin the search again. Fostering the relationship is fundamental to survival when a suitable mentor relationship forms. This action requires an individual to maintain contact and update their mentor on progress. Scheduling meetings consistently based on the mentor's and mentee's schedules can ensure this responsibility is not forgotten. Just as an individual has boundaries they expect their mentor to respect, they must also respect their mentor's boundaries. Another benefit to scheduling meetings is that it guarantees that an individual does not disrespect a mentor's boundaries. Mentoring relationships are not solely about the mentor helping the mentee. They dedicate their time, energy, and resources to helping individuals achieve their goals. Do not be afraid to give back to the mentor. Offer skills and time to help with any projects they might have going on.

Lastly, one of the most effective ways to reduce burnout symptoms and improve job satisfaction is to dedicate time to **professional development**. Most people recognize professional development as any activity that advances skills in one's career. Continuing education and professional development seem to accomplish the same things, but are very different. Continuing education often comes with a price attached to it. Sitting through a CME course, attending a conference, and earning a new degree all cost money, while professional development does not necessarily cost money. It can be free, such as watching a Microsoft Excel video on YouTube or taking a workshop at the office on having difficult conversations with patients.

Continuing education often requires the approval of management and leaders, especially if time off is needed to attend classes or a conference. Professional development courses and webinars are usually short and can be completed during the workday. Each year, individuals should identify skills they want to develop that directly correlate to their annual goals. Spending time devoted to advancing these skills will allow them to add value to their portfolio, gain a skill that will help them achieve their goal more effectively, and allow management and leadership to see their dedication to the job role while overarchingly improving their job satisfaction.

Organizational Strategies to Promote Well-Being and Mitigate Burnout

Since organizations play a role in generating stress that leads to employee burnout, there are strategies management and leaders can utilize to counteract the stress they create. While higher pay and more time off are ideal, they are not always feasible. Making a more supportive work environment can improve employee job satisfaction and reduce burnout symptoms. Management can also intervene in employees' work roles to protect their well-being. They can also encourage open communication and feedback in the workplace to allow for a greater flow of ideas and collaboration.

Creating a Supportive Work Environment

A toxic work environment can substantially impact an individual's burnout levels. Several characteristics classify a work environment as "toxic," such as poor work–life balance, leadership that does not protect employees' rights, bad leadership, poor communication, and high job turnover rates. These can all lead to high reports of job dissatisfaction, more turnover, and decreased job productivity. There is a lot that management and leadership can do to make a work environment more supportive of promoting their departments' well-being and mitigating burnout symptoms in their employees.

1. Engage in **Active Listening**. This technique is when an individual gives a speaker their full attention and then responds by paraphrasing and reflecting on what was said rather than reacting.
2. Offer **Recognition** and **Praise**. More often, management and leadership offer criticism and feedback to employees than praise them, which can reduce confidence and cause feelings of inefficacy. It is just as important for employees to hear the recognition and praise as it is to hear the criticism and feedback. Recognizing and praising employees (in public, not just behind closed doors) can boost their confidence and help them see the purpose of their job roles, leading to fewer burnout symptoms and greater job satisfaction.
3. **Reduce the Stigma** surrounding mental health and burnout. Employees should understand that they are not being judged or penalized for seeking mental health treatment. Ensure employees are given the appropriate time off when needed and are not a burden, a widespread feeling among those stigmatized. Additionally, their medical records should be kept confidential and not discussed with people who are not on a need-to-know basis.
4. Comprehend state and federal laws and uphold **Employee Rights**. State and federal laws and regulations protect employees and organizations from any wrongdoing in the workplace. For example, some laws mandate how often and how long employees should take a break. Furthermore, accrediting bodies set standards for academic institutions that protect students and faculty. Knowing and understanding these laws and regulations will help to avoid breaking them, contributing to employee burnout and being sued by employees.
5. Ensure employees **Know the Resources** available to them regarding well-being and mental health support. Too many times, employees do not seek help and mental health treatment because they do not know where to start. Managers should be responsible for knowing what resources are available inside and outside the organization. Should the need arise, managers can effortlessly provide an employee with the information.

Interventions to Prevent Overwork and Reduce Stress

Management and leadership can intervene to prevent overworking employees, manage workloads, and reduce employee stress. Monitoring workloads is an easy way to keep track of what employees are working on, track progress, and intervene when employees feel overwhelmed or struggle with a project. At this point, management can reassign a task to another employee with a lighter workload or more skills to handle the task, or they could break down the task into something more manageable for the employee. Management can also use this opportunity to offer professional development to the employee to work on skills that may make the goal of the task more attainable. Delegation, making tasks more manageable, and professional development are all approaches management can take to help reduce employee stress levels and mitigate burnout symptoms.

As mentioned, some managers are not adequately trained for the role and can become poor leaders. To avoid being labeled a "bad leader," managers should avoid unhealthy leader behaviors that cause employees stress, such as micromanaging, last-minute work assignments, not respecting boundaries, abusive language, and being disrespectful toward an employee's ideas. To promote healthy work–life balance, managers should encourage and respect boundaries, avoid showing signs of favoritism, and lead by example. Employees are more likely to follow a manager's advice if they demonstrate the behavior themselves.

Encouraging Open Communication and Feedback

Open communication and having a safe space to speak in can significantly reduce an employee's anxiety and burnout. When employees do not feel their work environment is safe to offer ideas, speak up against something, or even ask a question, they will hold back their thoughts, which can build up emotions and anxieties. Creating a safe work environment where employees are encouraged to communicate openly and offer (and receive) feedback will drastically reduce these anxieties and increase collaboration among colleagues. Managers should keep an open-door policy where employees can speak to their manager anytime. Moreover, managers should try to remain transparent about situations involving their employees from upper management. Employees can become distrustful when they know something is happening, but no one will update them. If a manager practices transparency and an open-door policy, their employees will likely respond with the same.

Management should foster intradepartmental and interdisciplinary collaboration. Collaboration is an exciting way to encourage employees to network, engage in research and scholarly work, build a positive work environment, and increase productivity. Employees may see a boost in their confidence from collaboration; they may learn a new skill and even increase their job satisfaction. Reducing burnout is a benefit of collaboration and is a cost-effective method (talking to people is free).

Personal Well-Being and Self-Care Practices

Individuals are just as responsible for their well-being and alleviating symptoms of burnout as their workplace. Practicing self-care and maintaining healthy well-being can be difficult with a busy schedule, but activities do not have to be grandiose to make a difference. Even minimalistic activities can improve an individual's physical, mental, and emotional health.

Physical Health

Improving physical health can be a difficult feat for some people. They spend all their time dieting but do not see any improvements. Self-care practices to improve physical health do not have to include dieting or weight loss at all. Improving physical health includes any activity that makes the body feel good and makes an individual feel good about their body.

- **Exercise**—Keeping a regular exercise routine can positively impact heart health and release endorphins. It is also a great way to reduce stress and manage symptoms of depression. Plan walk breaks into the daily schedule to guarantee exercise time.
- **Nutrition**—Starving oneself is not on the dinner menu tonight. Eating balanced meals and healthy snacks can ensure one gets the nutrients and vitamins needed for energy throughout the day. If this is a struggle, consider seeking the help of a licensed nutritionist.
- **Sleep**—Sleep may only seem like a fantasy for a practicing physician assistant or a student studying to be a physician assistant. However, getting restful sleep every night is essential to allow the body to recharge. Try sleeping with a sunrise alarm that will allow one to wake naturally with the sunrise.
- Other activities that can make the body feel good and reduce stress: going to the hair salon for a blowout, having a dance party, getting a massage, practicing safe sex with a consensual partner, taking a walk in the sunshine, munching on a favorite snack, and having a quick nap under a cozy blanket.

Mental Health

Mental health focuses on the cognitive functioning of an individual's psychological well-being. It helps individuals build relationships, make decisions, and deal with stress while being influenced by physical and emotional health, genetics, lifestyle, and social environment [11]. Taking care of mental health can be challenging, especially if an individual does not recognize the problem.

- **Mindfulness Practice**—One of the successful techniques to reduce burnout symptoms is practicing mindfulness. This technique involves an individual being aware and reflective about what they are experiencing without passing any judgment. Research on mindfulness practice shows that it reduces anxiety and stress levels [19]. Quiet meditation is the most frequent form of mindfulness practice.
- **Seek Professional Help**—Sometimes, individuals cannot beat burnout alone and require the help of a professional. Reaching out to a therapist or a mental health counselor can provide individuals with the support they need to develop a plan of action. Whether that plan includes medications or treatment facilities, it is critical that the individual agrees to a plan that they are comfortable with and that they feel is achievable.
- Other activities that can improve mental well-being and decrease high levels of stress: reading a book, taking a bath, listening to music, spending time with friends and family, and spending time outdoors.

Emotional Health

Finally, emotional health is an individual's ability to identify and manage their emotions and the emotions of others. Not coping with one's emotions makes them more susceptible to feeling overwhelmed and stressed in chaotic situations, and they often cannot bounce back afterward. Emotional health plays a significant role in burnout and is a fundamental contributor to mental health. Unstable emotional health can be the rocky foundation on which burnout can be built.

- **Resiliency Training**—Much of the research on burnout focuses on resiliency training as the premier intervention for reducing symptoms and preventing burnout. Resiliency is the ability to recover and adapt to stress quickly. One of the reasons resiliency training has been the most effective at reducing burnout symptoms is that individuals possess the skills that allow them to recognize their emotions and adapt to stressful situations in real time. Despite adversity, they maintain their composure and well-being, increasing their problem-solving ability and handling crises. Resiliency training can improve confidence and make individuals more emotionally aware, allowing them to control their emotions and focus on the problem.

- **Developing and Maintaining a Support System**—As mentioned, not having a support system can be detrimental to recovering from burnout or suppressing symptoms. Individuals should develop a strong support system that they can depend on, and that can depend on them as well. Besides friends and family and the previously mentioned professional associations, individuals can find support groups at local hospitals, on the Internet, and in their local community. A group does not have to be related to a career. It can focus on a hobby or a musical group, families and caregivers, and religious beliefs. Individuals can even find others who suffer from burnout and are going through the same experiences as them. The hardest part of creating a connection is saying hello.
- Other activities that can improve emotional health and reduce burnout: practicing gratitude by creating a daily list, reducing screentime, practicing self-compassion, building a social support network, challenging any negative thoughts, and practicing forgiveness.

Conclusion

In conclusion, burnout among healthcare professionals, especially physician assistants, is a critical issue with far-reaching implications for individuals, teams, and healthcare organizations. Recognizing the signs, understanding the contributing factors, and addressing the impact of burnout are essential for creating a supportive, resilient healthcare environment. Implementing both personal strategies, like self-care and time management, and organizational strategies, such as fostering open communication and supporting well-being, can mitigate burnout. By actively promoting a culture of mental health awareness and prioritizing well-being, the healthcare industry can improve job satisfaction, enhance patient care, and build a more sustainable workforce for the future.

References

1. Aflac. Workplace benefits trends: employee well-being and mental health. Aflac WorkForces Report; 2023. https://www.aflac.com/business/resources/aflac-workforces-report/default.aspx
2. American Academy of Physician Associates. PA Wellness. AAPA. 2024 August 6. https://www.aapa.org/career-central/pa-wellness/.
3. Cavanaugh K, Cline D, Belfer B, Chang S, Thoman E, Pickard T, Holladay CL. The positive impact of mentoring on burnout: organizational research and best practices. J Interprof Educ Pract. 2022;28:100521. https://doi.org/10.1016/j.xjep.2022.100521.
4. Cirillo F. The Pomodoro Tehcnique. About The Pomodoro® Technique; 2024. https://www.pomodorotechnique.com/
5. Fisher J, Silverglate PH. The C-suite's role in well-being. Deloitte Insights. 2022 June 22. https://www2.deloitte.com/us/en/insights/topics/leadership/employee-wellness-in-the-corporate-workplace.html.
6. Freudenberger HJ. Staff burnout. J Soc Issues. 1974;30(1):159–65. https://doi.org/10.1111/j.1540-4560.1974.tb00706.x.
7. Garcia LC, Shanafelt TD, West CP, Sinsky CA, Trockel MT, Nedelec L, Maldonado YA, Tutty M, Dyrbye LN, Fassiotto M. Burnout, depression, career satisfaction, and work-life integration by physician race/ethnicity. JAMA Netw Open. 2020;3(8). https://doi.org/10.1001/jamanetworkopen.2020.12762.
8. Gooch K. PA burnout, by specialty. Becker's Hospital Review. 2024 July 30. https://www.beckershospitalreview.com/workforce/pa-burnout-by-specialty.html.
9. Huecker MR. Imposter phenomenon. StatPearls [Internet]. 2023 July 31. https://www.ncbi.nlm.nih.gov/books/NBK585058/.
10. Karakcheyeva V, Willis-Johnson H, Corr PG, Frame LA. The well-being of women in healthcare professions: a comprehensive review. Glob Adv Integr Med Health. 2024;13. https://doi.org/10.1177/27536130241232929.
11. Kunasegaran K, Ismail AM, Ramasamy S, Gnanou JV, Caszo BA, Chen PL. Understanding mental fatigue and its detection: a comparative analysis of assessments and tools. PeerJ. 2023;11. https://doi.org/10.7717/peerj.15744.
12. Lee-Hawkins Y. Setting clear goals to escape and prevent burnout. Medium. 2024 August 21. https://medium.com/@yvonneleehawkins/setting-clear-goals-to-escape-and-prevent-burnout-855626e77ef8.
13. Maslach C, Leiter MP. Understanding the burnout experience: recent research and its implications for psychiatry. World Psychiatry. 2016;15(2):103–11. https://doi.org/10.1002/wps.20311.
14. McFarland DC, Hlubocky F, Susaimanickam B, O'Hanlon R, Riba M. Addressing depression, burnout, and suicide in oncology physicians. Am Soc Clin Oncol Educ Book. 2019;39:590–8. https://doi.org/10.1200/edbk_239087.
15. Medaris A. Gen Z adults and younger millennials are "completely overwhelmed" by stress. American Psychological Association. 2023 November 1. https://www.apa.org/topics/stress/generation-z-millennials-young-adults-worries.
16. Menon NK, Shanafelt TD, Sinsky CA, Linzer M, Carlasare L, Brady KJ, Stillman MJ, Trockel MT. Association of Physician Burnout with suicidal ideation and medical errors. JAMA Netw Open. 2020;3(12). https://doi.org/10.1001/jamanetworkopen.2020.28780.
17. Patel RS, Bachu R, Adikey A, Malik M, Shah M. Factors related to physician burnout and its consequences: a review. Behav Sci. 2018;8(11):98. https://doi.org/10.3390/bs8110098.
18. Paychex, Inc. Feeling the burn(out): exploring how employees overcome burnout. Paychex. 2019 February 25. https://www.paychex.com/articles/human-resources/impact-of-employee-burnout.
19. Sadowski C, Taylor L, Sharaf E. Mindfulness training and practice in physician assistant education. Internet J Allied Health Sci Pract. 2021; https://doi.org/10.46743/1540-580x/2021.2015.
20. Tierney AJ. The evolution of learned and innate behavior: contributions from genetics and neurobiology to a theory of behavioral evolution. Anim Learn Behav. 1986;14(4):339–48. https://doi.org/10.3758/bf03200077.

Index

S. Atallah, J. Dragoljevic (eds.), *Fundamentals of Surgery for Physician Assistants*,
https://doi.org/10.1007/978-3-032-21069-2

J

K

L